Mosby's
PEDIATRIC CLINICAL ADVISOR
Instant Diagnosis and Treatment

Visit our website at www.mosby.com

Mosby's
PEDIATRIC CLINICAL ADVISOR

Instant Diagnosis and Treatment

Editors

LYNN C. GARFUNKEL, M.D.
Associate Professor of Pediatrics
University of Rochester School of Medicine and Dentistry
Department of Pediatrics
Rochester General Hospital
Rochester, New York

JEFFREY KACZOROWSKI, M.D.
Assistant Professor of Pediatrics
University of Rochester School of Medicine and Dentistry
Strong Children's Hospital
Department of Pediatrics
Rochester, New York

CYNTHIA CHRISTY, M.D.
Associate Professor of Pediatrics
University of Rochester School of Medicine and Dentistry
Department of Pediatrics
Rochester General Hospital
Rochester, New York

with 166 contributors

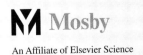

An Affiliate of Elsevier Science

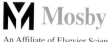

Acquisitions Editor: Liz Fathman
Senior Managing Editor: Kathryn Falk
Project Manager: Patricia Tannian
Project Specialist: Suzanne C. Fannin
Book Design Manager: Gail Morey Hudson
Cover Designer: Teresa Breckwoldt

Mosby, Inc.
An Affiliate of Elsevier Science
11830 Westline Industrial Drive
St. Louis, Missouri 63146

Printed in the United States of America

ISBN: 0-323-01049-0

02 03 04 05 GW/RDW 9 8 7 6 5 4 3 2

CONTRIBUTORS

CHLOE G. ALEXSON, M.D.
Professor Emeritus
Department of Pediatrics
Strong Children's Hospital
Rochester, New York

C. ANDREW ALIGNE, M.D.
Rochester, New York

PAULA ANNUNZIATO, M.D.
Associate Professor of Clinical Pediatrics
Columbia University
College of Physicians & Surgeons
Attending Physician, Department of Pediatrics
Presbyterian Hospital
New York, New York

MARC S. ARKOVITZ, M.D.
Assistant Professor
Department of Pediatric Surgery
University of Cincinnati College of Medicine
Pediatric Surgeon
Department of Pediatric Surgery
Children's Hospital Medical Center
Cincinnati, Ohio

GEORGIANNE L. ARNOLD, M.D.
Associate Professor of Pediatrics and Genetics
Department of Pediatrics
University of Rochester School of Medicine and Dentistry
Attending Physician
Strong Children's Hospital
Rochester, New York

BARBARA L. ASSELIN, M.D.
Associate Professor of Pediatrics and Oncology
University of Rochester School of Medicine and Dentistry
Department of Pediatrics
Strong Children's Hospital
Rochester, New York

SUSAN A. BIRNDORF, D.O.
Division of Adolescent Medicine
Department of Pediatrics
University of Rochester School of Medicine and Dentistry
Rochester, New York

CHRISTOPHER F. BOLLING, M.D.
Voluntary Associate Professor
Department of General and Community Pediatrics
University of Cincinnati
Cincinnati, Ohio
Attending Physician
Department of Pediatrics
St. Elizabeth Medical Center
Edgewood, Kentucky
Pediatric Associates, PSC
Crestview Hills, Kentucky

PETER N. BOWERS, M.D.
Assistant Professor, Department of Pediatric Cardiology
Yale University School of Medicine
Attending Physician
Department of Pediatric Cardiology
Yale–New Haven Hospital
New Haven, Connecticut

PAULA K. BRAVERMAN, M.D.
Associate Professor of Pediatrics
MCP Hahnemann University School of Medicine
Chief, Section of Adolescent Medicine
St. Christopher's Hospital for Children
Philadelphia, Pennsylvania

CARMELITA BRITTON, M.D.
Clinical Associate Professor of Pediatrics
University of Rochester School of Medicine and Dentistry
Associate Chief of Pediatrics
Rochester General Hospital
Rochester, New York

ANN MARIE BROOKS, M.D.
Department of Pediatric Pulmonology
Nemours Children's Clinic
Orlando, Florida

ROBERT A. BROUGHTON, M.D.
Chief, Division of Pediatric Infectious Diseases
Professor of Pediatrics
Division of Pediatric Critical Care
University of Kentucky Medical Center
Lexington, Kentucky

RACHEL BUDIANSKY, M.D.
Associate Clinical Instructor in Pediatrics
Strong Children's Hospital
Pittsford Pediatrics
Pittsford, New York

GALE R. BURSTEIN, M.D., M.P.H.
Medical Officer
Division of HIV/AIDS Prevention
Centers for Disease Control and Prevention
Atlanta, Georgia

JAMES R. CAMPBELL, M.D., M.P.H.
Associate Professor of Pediatrics
University of Rochester School of Medicine and Dentistry
Staff Physician, Department of Pediatrics
Rochester General Hospital
Rochester, New York

LYNN R. CAMPBELL, M.D.
Associate Professor of Pediatrics
Director, Pediatric Residency Program
University of Kentucky Medical Center
Lexington, Kentucky

PATRICK L. CAROLAN, M.D.
Clinical Associate Professor of Pediatrics, Family Practice, and Community Health
University of Minnesota Medical School
Medical Director, Minnesota Sudden Infant Death Center
Children's Hospitals and Clinics
Minneapolis, Minnesota

MARY T. CASERTA, M.D.
Associate Professor of Pediatrics
University of Rochester School of Medicine and Dentistry
Attending Physician, Department of Pediatrics
Strong Children's Hospital
Rochester, New York

KATHRYN A. CASTLE, Ph.D.
Senior Instructor of Psychiatry and Pediatrics
Department of Psychiatry
University of Rochester Medial Center
Rochester, New York

HEATHER A. CHAPMAN, M.D.
Staff Pediatrician
St. Joseph Health Services of Rhode Island
Medical Director
St. Joseph Lead Clinic
Providence, Rhode Island

SHARON F. CHEN, M.D.
Fellow
Pediatric Infectious Disease
Stanford University School of Medicine
Stanford, California

EULALIA R.Y. CHENG, M.D.
Assistant Clinical Professor of Pediatrics
Division of Pediatric Pulmonology
University Rochester School of Medicine and Dentistry
Department of Pediatrics
University of Rochester Medical Center
Strong Children's Hospital
Rochester, New York

ELIZABETH CHEROT, M.D.
Strong Children's Hospital
Rochester, New York

PATRICIA R. CHESS, M.D.
Assistant Professor of Pediatrics
Division of Neonatology
University of Rochester School of Medicine and Dentistry
Strong Children's Hospital
Rochester, New York

BARBARA A. CHINI, M.D.
Assistant Professor of Pediatrics
Division of Pulmonary Medicine
Children's Hospital Medical Center
Cincinnati, Ohio

CYNTHIA CHRISTY, M.D.
Associate Professor of Pediatrics
University of Rochester School of Medicine and Dentistry
Department of Pediatrics
Rochester General Hospital
Rochester, New York

CAROLYN T. CLEARY, M.D.
Clinical Instructor, Department of Pediatrics
University of Rochester School of Medicine and Dentistry
Practicing Pediatrician
Elmwood Pediatrics Group
Rochester, New York

LISA LOEB COLTON, M.D.
Clinical Instructor, Department of Pediatrics
University of Rochester School of Medicine and Dentistry
Practicing Pediatrician
Panorama Pediatric Group
Rochester, New York

GREGORY P. CONNERS, M.D., M.P.H.
Associate Chair of Emergency Medicine for Academic Affairs
Assistant Professor, Departments of Emergency Medicine and Pediatrics
University of Rochester School of Medicine and Dentistry
Rochester, New York

CHRISTOPHER C. COPENHAVER, M.D.
Department of Pediatrics
University of Rochester School of Medicine and Dentistry
Strong Children's Hospital
Rochester, New York

THERESE CVETKOVICH, M.D.
Medical Officer, Division of Antiviral Drug Products
Center for Drug Evaluation and Review
U.S. Food and Drug Administration
Rockville, Maryland

KRISTEN SMITH DANIELSON, M.D.
Fellow, Department of Pediatrics
University of Rochester School of Medicine and Dentistry
Rochester, New York

ROSEMARY AMOFAH DAYIE, M.D.
Children's Hospital of Pittsburgh
Pittsburgh, Pennsylvania

CYNTHIA A. DeLAAT, M.D.
Associate Professor of Pediatrics
Department of Pediatric Hematology/Oncology
University of Cincinnati
Children's Hospital Medical Center
Cincinnati, Ohio

DOROTHY M. DELISLE, M.D.
Staff Pediatrician, Department of Pediatrics
Children's Hospital of Wisconsin
Milwaukee, Wisconsin

LARRY DENK, M.D.
Clinical Assistant Professor of Pediatrics
University of Rochester School of Medicine and Dentistry
Department of Pediatrics
Rochester General Hospital
Rochester, New York

LEE A. DENSON, M.D.
Associate Research Scientist
Department of Pediatrics
Yale School of Medicine
Attending, Department of Pediatrics
Yale–New Haven Hospital
New Haven, Connecticut

CAROLYN PIVER DUKARM, M.D.
Director, Eating Disorder Program
Department of Pediatrics
Sisters' Hospital
Buffalo, New York

GUS G. EMMICK, M.D.
Departments of Internal Medicine and Pediatrics
University of Rochester School of Medicine
Rochester, New York

JASON GIBBONS EMMICK, M.D.
Chief Resident in Pediatrics
Resident in Medicine and Pediatrics
University of Rochester Medical Center
Strong Children's Hospital
Rochester, New York

ROBERT ENGLANDER, M.D., M.P.H.
Assistant Professor of Pediatrics
University of Maryland School of Medicine
Associate Director, Pediatric Education
Department of Pediatrics
University of Maryland
Baltimore, Maryland

ANNA F. FAKADEJ, M.D.
Chairman, Division of Ophthalmology
Carolina Eye Associates
Southern Pines, North Carolina

THOMAS J. FISCHER, M.D.
Professor of Clinical Pediatrics
University of Cincinnati College of Medicine
Division of Pulmonary Medicine and Allergy
Children's Hospital Medical Center
Cincinnati, Ohio

DONNA J. FISHER, M.D.
Assistant Professor of Pediatrics
Department of Pediatric Infectious Diseases
Tufts University School of Medicine
Boston, Massachusetts
Department of Pediatric/Pediatric Infectious Disease
Baystate Medical Center Children's Hospital
Springfield, Massachusetts

CHIN-TO FONG, M.D.
Clinical Associate Professor
Departments of Pediatrics, Genetics, and Dentistry
University of Rochester School of Medicine and Dentistry
Strong Children's Hospital
Rochester, New York

CHARLES B. FOSTER, M.D.
Senior Clinical Fellow
Pediatric Oncology Branch
National Cancer Institute
National Institutes of Health
Bethesda, Maryland

D. STEVEN FOX, M.D., M.SC.
Senior Resident
Departments of Internal Medicine and Pediatrics
University of Rochester School of Medicine and Dentistry
Rochester, New York

ROBERT J. FREISHTAT, M.D.
Associate Instructor
Departments of Pediatrics and Emergency Medicine
The George Washington University School of Medicine
   and Health Sciences
Fellow, Pediatric Emergency Medicine
Children's National Medical Center
Washington, DC

LYNN C. GARFUNKEL, M.D.
Associate Professor of Pediatrics
University of Rochester School of Medicine and Dentistry
Department of Pediatrics
Rochester General Hospital
Rochester, New York

M. ELLEN GELLERSTEDT, M.D.
Clinical Associate Professor, Department of Pediatrics
University of Rochester School of Medicine and Dentistry
Director, Behavioral Pediatrics Program
Department of Pediatrics
Rochester General Hospital
Rochester, New York

ALKA GOYAL, M.D.
Assistant Professor of Pediatrics
University of Pittsburgh School of Medicine
Assistant Professor of Pediatrics
Division of Pediatric Gastroenterology
Children's Hospital of Pittsburgh
Pittsburgh, Pennsylvania

MELISSA J. GREGORY, M.D.
Clinical Assistant Professor
Department of Pediatric Nephrology
University of Michigan School of Medicine
Clinical Chief of Pediatric Nephrology
C.S. Mott Children's Hospital
Ann Arbor, Michigan

MICHELLE ANN GRENIER, M.D.
Pediatric Cardiologist
South Texas Pediatric Cardiology Associates
Corpus Christi, Texas

MARK GUSTAFSON, M.D.
Carrollton Ear, Nose and Throat
Carrollton, Georgia

JILL S. HALTERMAN, M.D., M.P.H.
Assistant Professor of Pediatrics
University of Rochester School of Medicine and Dentistry
Children's Hospital at Strong
Rochester, New York

DAVID W. HANNON, M.D.
Associate Professor of Pediatrics
East Carolina University
Brody School of Medicine
Section Head, Pediatric Cardiology
University Health Systems
Greenville, North Carolina

WILLIAM G. HARMON, M.D.
Senior Instructor, Division of Pediatric Critical Care
Fellow, Division of Pediatric Cardiology
University of Rochester School of Medicine and Dentistry
Strong Children's Hospital
University of Rochester Medical Center
Rochester, New York

J. PETER HARRIS, M.D.
Professor of Pediatrics
Pediatric Cardiology
University of Rochester School of Medicine and Dentistry
Director, Pediatric Residency Training Program
Strong Children's Hospital
Rochester, New York

NEIL E. HERENDEEN, M.D.
Clinical Assistant Professor of Pediatrics
University of Rochester School of Medicine and Dentistry
Director, Pediatric Practice at Strong
Strong Children's Hospital
Rochester, New York

JOELI HETTLER, M.D.
Instructor
Department of Pediatrics
Harvard Medical School
Assistant
Department of Medicine
Children's Hospital
Boston, Massachusetts

JOHN L. HICK, M.D.
Assistant Professor of Clinical Emergency Medicine
Emergency Medicine Program
University of Minnesota School of Medicine
Faculty, Emergency Medicine
Hennepin County Medical Center
Minneapolis, Minnesota

ANDREA S. HINKLE, M.D.
Assistant Professor, Department of Pediatrics
Division of Pediatric Hematology/Oncology
University of Rochester School of Medicine and Dentistry
Strong Children's Hospital
Rochester, New York

ALEJANDRO HOBERMAN , M.D.
Associate Professor of Pediatrics
University of Pittsburgh School of Medicine
Children's Hospital of Pittsburgh
Pittsburgh, Pennsylvania

CHRISTOPHER H. HODGMAN, M.D.
Professor of Psychiatry and Pediatrics
University of Rochester School of Medicine and Dentistry
Psychiatrist, Strong Children's Hospital
Rochester, New York

ALLISON L. HOLM, M.D.
Assistant Professor of Dermatology and Pediatrics
University of Rochester School of Medicine and Dentistry
Strong Children's Hospital
Rochester, New York

MARK A. HOSTETLER, M.D., M.P.H.
Instructor, Department of Pediatrics
Division of Emergency Medicine
Washington University School of Medicine
Attending Pediatrician
Division of Emergency Medicine
St. Louis Children's Hospital
St. Louis, Missouri

CYNTHIA R. HOWARD, M.D., M.P.H.
Associate Professor of Pediatrics
University of Rochester School of Medicine and Dentistry
Pediatric Director, Mother Baby Unit
Rochester General Hospital
Rochester, New York

EMMA HUGHES, M.D.
Worcester, Massachusetts

WILLIAM C. HULBERT, M.D.
Associate Professor
Department of Urology
Division of Pediatric Urology
University of Rochester School of Medicine and Dentistry
Strong Children's Hospital
Rochester, New York

SUSAN L. HYMAN, M.D.
Assistant Professor of Pediatrics
University of Rochester School of Medicine and Dentistry
Strong Center for Developmental Disabilities
Strong Children's Hospital
Rochester, New York

ERIC F. INGEROWSKI, M.D.
Clinical Instructor of Pediatrics
University of Rochester School of Medicine and Dentistry
Strong Children's Hospital
Rochester, New York

MARY ANNE JACKSON, M.D.
Professor or Pediatrics
University of Missouri–Kansas City
School of Medicine
Children's Mercy Hospital
Kansas City, Missouri

ANDREE A. JACOBS-PERKINS, M.D.
Clinical Instructor
Department of Pediatrics
University of Rochester School of Medicine and Dentistry
Attending Physician
Strong Children's Hospital
Rochester General Hospital
Highland Hospital
Rochester, New York

JULIE A. JASKIEWICZ, M.D.
Pediatrician
Eastgate Pediatric Center
Cincinnati, Ohio

STANLEY D. JOHNSEN, M.D.
Associate Professor of Pediatrics and Neurology
Department of Child Neurology
Texas Children's Hospital
Director, Blue Bird Clinic for Child Neurology
Houston, Texas

NICHOLAS JOSPE, M.D.
Associate Professor of Pediatrics
University of Rochester School of Medicine and Dentistry
Strong Children's Hospital
Rochester, New York

STEVEN PAUL JOYCE, M.D.
Assistant Professor of Internal Medicine and Pediatrics
University of Iowa School of Medicine
Iowa City, Iowa
Associate Program Director
Siouxland Medical Education Foundation
Sioux City, Iowa

JEFFREY KACZOROWSKI, M.D.
Assistant Professor of Pediatrics
University of Rochester School of Medicine and Dentistry
Strong Children's Hospital
Department of Pediatrics
Rochester, New York

INDRA A. KANCITIS, M.D.
Assistant Professor of Pediatrics
Virginia Commonwealth University
Medical College of Virginia Hospitals
Richmond, Virginia

MAUREEN A. KAYS, M.D.
Clinical Assistant Professor
Department of Pediatrics
University of Florida College of Medicine
Shands at the University of Florida
Gainesville, Florida

JAMES W. KENDIG, M.D.
Professor of Pediatrics
Penn State College of Medicine
Attending Neonatologist, Department of Pediatrics
Division of Newborn Medicine
Penn State Children's Hospital
Hershey, Pennsylvania

JOHN R. KNIGHT, M.D.
Assistant Professor of Pediatrics
Harvard Medical School
Director, Center for Adolescent Substance Abuse Research
Children's Hospital
Boston, Massachusetts

CHERYL KODJO, M.D., M.P.H.
Senior Instructor in Adolescent Medicine
Department of Pediatrics
University of Rochester School of Medicine and Dentistry
Rochester, New York

DAVID N. KORONES, M.D.
Associate Professor of Pediatrics and Oncology
University of Rochester School of Medicine and Dentistry
Strong Children's Hospital
Rochester, New York

PETER A. KOUIDES, M.D.
Associate Professor of Medicine
University of Rochester School of Medicine and Dentistry
Associate Medical Director
Mary M. Gooley Hemophilia Treatment Center
Rochester, New York

RICHARD E. KREIPE, M.D.
Division of Adolescent Medicine
Department of Pediatrics
Strong Children's Hospital
University of Rochester School of Medicine and Dentistry
Rochester, New York

MARC S. LAMPELL, M.D.
Clinical Assistant Professor of Emergency Medicine
    and Pediatrics
University of Rochester School of Medicine and Dentistry
Clinical Director, Pediatric Emergency Services
Department of Pediatrics
Rochester General Hospital
Rochester, New York

NANCY LANPHEAR, M.D.
Assistant Professor of Pediatrics
University of Cincinnati School of Medicine
Cincinnati Center for Developmental Disorders
Children's Hospital Medical Center
Cincinnati, Ohio

JEFFREY H. LEE, M.D.
Instructor of Medicine and Pediatrics
University of Massachusetts Medical School
Community Medical Group
Departments of Internal Medicine and Pediatrics
UMass Medical Center
Worcester, Massachusetts

LUCIA LEE, M.D.
Food and Drug Administration
Rockville, Maryland

THOMAS J. A. LEHMAN, M.D.
Professor of Pediatrics
Sanford Weil Medical Center
Cornell University
Chief, Pediatric Rheumatology
Hospital of Special Surgery
New York, New York

PAUL F. LEHOULLIER, M.D., Ph.D.
Clinical Instructor
Department of Pediatrics
Rochester General Hospital
Rochester, New York

ANN M. LENANE, M.D.
Assistant Professor of Emergency Medicine and Pediatrics
University of Rochester School of Medicine and Dentistry
Rochester, New York

NORMA B. LERNER, M.D
Clinical Associate Professor of Pediatrics
Department of Hematology/Oncology
University of Rochester School of Medicine and Dentistry
Strong Children's Hospital
Rochester, New York

GREGORY S. LIPTAK, M.D., M.P.H.
Associate Professor of Pediatrics
University of Rochester School of Medicine and Dentistry
Attending Pediatrician
Strong Children's Hospital
Rochester, New York

STUART T. LOEB, M.D.
Clinical Instructor
Department of Psychiatry
University of Rochester School of Medicine and Dentistry
Medical Director
Hillside Children's CenterRochester, New York

JOSEPH E. LOSEE, M.D.
Pediatric Plastic and Craniofacial Surgery
University of Rochester School of Medicine and Dentistry
Strong Children's Hospital
Rochester, New York

KRISTINA LYNCH-GUYETTE, M.D.
Ophthalmologist
Albany Eye Associates at
Albany Memorial Hospital
Albany, New York

FRANK B. MAGILL, Jr., M.D.
Departments of Internal Medicine and Pediatrics
Jefferson General Hospital
Port Townsend, Washington

ELIZABETH MANNICK, M.D.
Assistant Professor
Departments of Pediatrics and Pathology
Louisiana State University Health Sciences Center
New Orleans, Louisiana

H. REID MATTISON, M.D.
Infectious Disease of Indiana
Methodist Hospital of Indiana
Indianapolis, Indiana

CHRISTINA M. McCANN, Ph.D.
Clinical Instructor of Pediatrics
University of Rochester School of Medicine and Dentistry
Rochester, New York

CAROL A. McCARTHY, M.D.
Associate Professor of Pediatrics
University of Vermont
Director, Pediatric Infectious Disease
Maine Medical Center
Portland, Maine

MICHAEL McCONNELL, M.D.
Department of Cardiology
East Carolina University School of Medicine
Greenville, North Carolina

COLSTON F. McEVOY, M.D.
Assistant Clinical Professor
Department of Pediatrics
Yale University School of Medicine
New Haven, Connecticut

ALAN M. MENDELSOHN, M.D.
Associate Professor
Department of Pediatrics
University of Rochester School of Medicine and Dentistry
Department of Pediatric Cardiology
University of Rochester Medical Center
Rochester, New York

RAM K. MENON, M.D.
Associate Professor of Pediatrics
University of Pittsburgh School of Medicine
Associate Professor of Endocrinology
Children's Hospital of Pittsburgh
Pittsburgh, Pennsylvania

ROBERT ALAN MEVORACH, M.D.
Assistant Professor
Department of Urology and Pediatrics
University of Rochester
Strong Children's Hospital
Rochester General Hospital
Rochester, New York

AYESA N. MIAN, M.D.
Assistant Professor of Pediatrics
Department of Pediatric Nephrology
Medical College of Georgia
Assistant Professor
Department of Pediatrics
Children's Medical Center
Augusta, Georgia

M. SUSAN MOYER, M.D.
Chief, Section of Gastroenterology/Hepatology
Department of Pediatrics
Yale School of Medicine
Attending Physician, Department of Pediatrics
Yale–New Haven Children's Hospital
New Haven, Connecticut

CHARLES M. MYER III, M.D.
Professor, Department of Otolaryngology–Head
    and Neck Surgery
University of Cincinnati College of Medicine
Professor, Department of Pediatric Otolaryngology
Children's Hospital Medical Center
Cincinnati, Ohio

RAN NAMGUNG, M.D., Ph.D.
Professor of Pediatrics
Yonsei University College of Medicine
Seoul, Korea

JONATHAN F. NASSER, M.D.
Chief Resident
Department of Internal Medicine–Pediatrics
Strong Memorial Hospital
Rochester, New York

ROBERT NEEDLMAN, M.D.
Associate Professor, Adjunct
Department of Pediatrics
Case Western Reserve University School of Medicine
Cleveland, Ohio
Vice President for Developmental-Behavioral Pediatrics
The Dr. Spock Company
Menlo Park, California

CHRISTOPHER T. NELSON, M.D.
Pediatric Infectious Disease Specialist
Department of Pediatrics
University of Kentucky
Lexington, Kentucky

JOSEPH A. NICHOLAS, M.D.
Resident
Department of Internal Medicine and Pediatrics
University of Rochester School of Medicine and Dentistry
Strong Children's Hospital
Department of Pediatrics
Rochester, New York

SAMUEL NURKO, M.D., M.P.H.
Assistant Professor of Pediatrics
Harvard Medical School
Director, Gastrointestinal Motility Program
Department of Medicine
Children's Hospital
Boston, Massachusetts

MARIA S. OGDEN, Ph.D.
Department of Psychiatry
University of Rochester Medical Center
Rochester, New York

CRAIG C. ORLOWSKI, M.D.
Clinical Associate Professor of Pediatrics
University of Rochester School of Medicine and Dentistry
Attending Pediatrician
Strong Children's Hospital
Rochester, New York

LORA L. PAK, M.D.
Department of Pediatrics
Cox Health Systems
Springfield, Missouri

JAMES PALIS, M.D.
Associate Professor of Pediatrics, Cancer Center,
    Human Genetics and Molecular Pediatric Disease
University of Rochester School of Medicine and Dentistry
Attending Physician, Department of Pediatrics
Strong Children's Hospital
Rochester, New York

MURRAY H. PASSO, M.D.
Professor of Clinical Pediatrics
University of Cincinnati College of Medicine
Clinical Director, Division of Rheumatology
Children's Hospital Medical Center
Cincinnati, Ohio

WALTER PEGOLI, Jr., M.D.
Associate Professor, Department of Surgery
University of Rochester School of Medicine and Dentistry
Section Chief, Pediatric Surgery
Strong Children's Hospital
Rochester, New York

KAREN S. POWERS, M.D.
Associate Professor of Pediatrics
Pediatric Critical Care
University of Rochester School of Medicine and Dentistry
Associate Director, Strong Critical Care Center
Strong Children's Hospital
Rochester, New York

SUSAN HALLER PSAILA, M.D.
Clinical Instructor
Departments of Pediatrics and Dermatology
University of Rochester School of Medicine and Dentistry
Strong Children's Hospital
Rochester General Hospital
Rochester, New York

RONALD RABINOWITZ, M.D.
Professor of Urology and Pediatrics
Associate Chair, Department of Urology
University of Rochester School of Medicine and Dentistry
Chief, Pediatric Urology
Strong Children's Hospital
Rochester General Hospital
Rochester, New York

MARC A. RASLICH, M.D.
Assistant Professor of Internal Medicine and Pediatrics
Wright State University School of Medicine
Dayton, Ohio

KAREN L. RESCH, M.D.
Clinical Instructor, Department of Pediatrics
University of Minnesota School of Medicine
Faculty Physician
Department of Pediatric Emergency Medicine
Children's Hospital
Minneapolis, Minneapolis

MATTHEW W. RICHARDSON, M.D.
Fellow, Department of Pediatrics
Division of Pediatric Hematology/Oncology
University of North Carolina School of Medicine at Chapel Hill
University of North Carolina Hospital at Chapel Hill
Chapel Hill, North Carolina

BRETT ROBBINS, M.D.
Assistant Professor of Medicine and Pediatrics
Department of Medicine and Pediatrics
University of Rochester School of Medicine and Dentistry
Rochester, New York

DENNIS R. ROY, M.D.
Professor of Orthopaedics Surgery
University of Cincinnati
Director, Hip Surgery
Associate Director, Department of Pediatric Orthopaedics
Children's Hospital Medical Center
Cincinnati, Ohio

SHERYL A. RYAN, M.D.
Assistant Professor of Pediatrics
University of Rochester School of Medicine and Dentistry
Director of Adolescent Services
Department of Pediatrics
Rochester General Hospital
Rochester, New York

FREDERICK C. RYCKMAN, M.D.
Professor of Surgery and Pediatric Surgery
University of Cincinnati School of Medicine
Professor of Surgery and Pediatric Surgery
Children's Hospital Medical Center
Cincinnati, Ohio

STEPHANIE SANSONI, M.D.
Group Pediatric Practice
Towson, Maryland

CHARLES J. SCHUBERT, M.D.
Associate Professor of Clinical Pediatrics
Department of Pediatrics
University of Cincinnati
Associate Professor
Department of Pediatric Emergency Medicine
Children's Hospital Medical Center
Cincinnati, Ohio

GEORGE J. SCHWARTZ, M.D.
Professor and Chief of Pediatric Nephrology
Departments of Pediatrics and Medicine
University of Rochester School of Medicine and Dentistry
Attending Physician, Department of Pediatrics
Strong Children's Hospital
Rochester, New York

STEVEN SCOFIELD, M.D.
Assistant Professor
Departments of Internal Medicine and Pediatrics
University of Rochester School of Medicine and Dentistry
Department of Medicine
Highland Hospital
Strong Children's Hospital
Department of Pediatrics
Rochester, New York

GEORGE B. SEGEL, M.D.
Professor of Pediatrics, Medicine, Genetics, and Oncology
Department of Pediatric Hematology/Oncology
University of Rochester School of Medicine and Dentistry
Strong Children's Hospital
Rochester, New York

EDGARD A. SEGURA, M.D.
Attending Physician, Department of Pediatrics
Loudoun Hospital Center
Lansdowne, Virginia

RONALD L. SHAM, M.D.
Associate Professor of Medicine
Department of Medicine
University of Rochester School of Medicine and Dentistry
Faculty, Department of Hematology
Rochester General Hospital
Rochester, New York

SAM REED SHIMAMOTO, M.D.
Chief Resident
Department of Pediatrics
St. Joseph's Hospital and Medical Center
Phoenix, Arizona

LAURA JEAN SHIPLEY, M.D.
Clinical Assistant Professor
Department of Pediatrics
University of Rochester School of Medicine and Dentistry
Rochester, New York

BENJAMIN L. SHNEIDER, M.D.
Associate Professor of Pediatrics
Mount Sinai School of Medicine
Director, Pediatric Liver Program
Department of Pediatrics
Mount Sinai Medical Center
New York, New York

DAVID M. SIEGEL, M.D., M.P.H.
Associate Professor of Pediatrics and Internal Medicine
Co-Director, Pediatric Rheumatology
University of Rochester School of Medicine and Dentistry
Chief of Pediatrics
Rochester General Hospital
Rochester, New York

MARK SCOTT SMITH, M.D.
Associate Professor of Pediatrics
Chief, Adolescent Medicine Section
Division of General Pediatrics
University of Washington
Chief, Adolescent Services
Children's Hospital & Regional Medical Center
Seattle, Washington

R. DENNIS STEED, M.D.
Associate Professor, Department of Pediatrics
Division of Cardiology
East Carolina University School of Medicine
Greenville, North Carolina

KATHLEEN A. TIGUE, M.D.
Private Practice
Scranton, Pennsylvania

DEBBIE S. TODER, M.D.
Assistant Professor of Pediatrics
Wayne State University School of Medicine
Director, Cystic Fibrosis Center
Pulmonary Medicine Division
Children's Hospital of Michigan
Detroit, Michigan

MARLAH TOMBOC, M.D.
Post-Doctoral Fellow
Department of Pediatrics
University of Pittsburgh School of Medicine
Associate Professor of Endocrinology
Children's Hospital of Pittsburgh
Pittsburgh, Pennsylvania

CARLOS F. TORRES, M.D.
Associate Professor of Neurology and Pediatrics
Department of Neurology
University of Rochester School of Medicine and Dentistry
Strong Children's Hospital
Rochester, New York

JOHN J. TREANOR, M.D.
Associate Professor of Medicine
Infectious Diseases Unit
University of Rochester School of Medicine and Dentistry
Attending Physician, Department of Medicine
Strong Children's Hospital
Rochester, New York

C. ELIZABETH TREFTS, M.D.
Penobscot Pediatrics, PA
Bangor, Maine
Assistant Clinical Professor of Pediatrics
Tufts University School of Medicine
Boston, Massachusetts

REGINALD TSANG, M.B.B.S.
Professor Emeritus of Pediatrics
Cincinnati Children's Hospital
Cincinnati, Ohio

HEATHER VAHLE, M.D.
Assistant Professor
Department of Pediatrics
Truman Medical Center
Assistant Professor
Department of Pediatrics
Children's Mercy Hospital
Kansas City, Missouri

JON A. VANDERHOOF, M.D.
Professor of Pediatrics
Director, Joint Section of Pediatric Gastroenterology
   and Nutrition
University of Nebraska Medical Center
Creighton University
Omaha, Nebraska

ÉLISE W. van der JAGT, M.D., M.P.H.
Associate Professor of Pediatrics and Critical Care
University of Rochester School of Medicine and Dentistry
Director, Pediatric General Inpatient Units
Department of Pediatrics
Strong Children's Hospital
Rochester, New York

WILLIAM S. VARADE, M.D.
Associate Professor of Pediatrics
University of Rochester School of Medicine and Dentistry
Attending Pediatrician
Strong Children's Hospital
Rochester, New York

KATHLEEN M. VENTRE, M.D.
Fellow, Department of Anaesthesia/Critical Care Medicine
Harvard Medical School
Children's Hospital, Boston
Boston, Massachusetts

MICHAEL K. VISICK, M.D.
Department of Internal Medicine-Pediatrics
IHC Budge Clinic
Logan, Utah

BRAD W. WARNER, M.D.
Professor of Surgery
University of Cincinnati College of Medicine
Attending Surgeon
Division of Pediatric Surgery
Children's Hospital Medical Center
Cincinnati, Ohio

GEOFFREY A. WEINBERG, M.D.
Associate Professor of Pediatrics
University of Rochester School of Medicine and Dentistry
Director, Pediatric HIV Program
Strong Children's Hospital
Rochester, New York

SUSAN E. WILEY, M.D.
Adjunct Assistant Professor
Division of Developmental Disorders
University of Cincinnati
Children's Hospital Medical Center
Cincinnati, Ohio

ROBERT R. WITTLER, M.D.
Associate Professor of Pediatrics
University of Kansas School of Medicine-Wichita
Wichita, Kansas

JONATHAN P. WOOD, M.D.
Assistant Professor, Pediatric Critical Care
Department of Pediatrics
University of Massachusetts Medical School
Worcester, Massachusetts

ROGER A. YEAGER, Ph.D.
Clinical Psychologist
Behavioral Pediatric Program
Department of Pediatrics
Rochester General Hospital
Rochester, New York

To our spouses
Craig Orlowski,
Laura Jean Shipley, and
Ralph Manchester

To our children
Zachary and **Rachel Orlowski,**
Daniel Shipley, and
Eric, Alison, and **Ian Manchester**

and to
our parents, mentors, colleagues, students, and **friends**
who have encouraged and inspired us

Thank you all,
LCG, JK, CC

PREFACE

You are between patients, the waiting room is full, and you are falling further behind. You need to review a clinical topic, broaden your differential diagnosis, initiate a diagnostic workup, or remember the latest treatment of a less common disease—this is what we had in mind when we created *Mosby's Pediatric Clinical Advisor.*

This textbook is meant to be a user-friendly, ready reference for the primary care physician, nurse practitioner, physician assistant, resident, or student. It is organized to lead you from signs and symptoms to comprehensive information about specific diseases and clinical problems, with supporting diagrams, tables, and formulas.

Part I presents differential diagnoses of more than 40 common signs and symptoms paired with diagnostic algorithms. **Part II** covers more than 350 clinical topics in a bulleted format including ICD-9CM codes, etiology, epidemiology and demographics, differential diagnosis, diagnostic workup, and therapeutic plans; it also contains pertinent websites and references. **Part III** includes those frequently sought graphs, equations, and charts that you can never seem to get your hands on, such as endocarditis prophylaxis, developmental screening tools, and the body mass index calculation with normative tables.

We wish to express our deepest appreciation to Jean Brockmann, our coordinator, who has worked kindly and tirelessly to facilitate and organize the production of this book. Thanks, Jean.

LCG, JK, CC

CONTENTS

PART I

Differential Diagnosis and Clinical Algorithms

ABDOMINAL MASS

The clinical classification of abdominal masses in children can be divided into neonatal and postneonatal causes. Approximately half of abdominal masses in newborns involve the urinary tract. Constipation is the most common cause of an abdominal mass in the older child.

■ **DIFFERENTIAL DIAGNOSIS**

Neonate

I. Urinary tract
   A. Hydronephrosis (obstructive uropathy)
      1. Posterior urethral valves
      2. Ureterocele
      3. Prune-belly syndrome
   B. Renal cystic dysplasia
   C. Polycystic kidney disease
   D. Glomerulocystic kidney disease
   E. Medullary cystic disease/juvenile nephronophthisis
   F. Simple renal cysts
   G. Wilms' tumor
   H. Renal vein thrombosis
   I. Renal hamartoma (mesoblastic nephroma)
   J. Ectopic kidney
   K. Other congenital abnormalities of the kidneys
   L. Renal or perinephric abscess
   M. Distended bladder

II. Gastrointestinal
   A. Pyloric stenosis
   B. Ileus
      1. Meconium
   C. Bowel duplication
   D. Choledochal cyst
   E. Hydrops of the gallbladder

III. Hepatomegaly
   A. Congestive heart failure
   B. Sepsis
   C. Congenital infections
      1. Cytomegalovirus
      2. Toxoplasmosis
      3. Enterovirus
      4. Herpes simplex
      5. Syphilis
      6. Rubella
   D. Biliary atresia
   E. Hemolytic anemia
   F. Neonatal hepatitis
   G. Peripheral hyperalimentation
   H. Hepatic cysts
   I. Hemangioma

IV. Splenomegaly
   A. Sepsis
   B. Congenital infections (as earlier under "Hepatomegaly")
   C. Hemolytic anemia
   D. Portal vein thrombosis
      1. Omphalitis
      2. Umbilical vein catheterization

V. Neoplasms
   A. Neuroblastoma
   B. Teratoma
   C. Renal tumors (as listed previously)

Postneonatal

I. Urinary tract causes (as noted in previous section)

II. Gastrointestinal
   A. Constipation
      1. Diet related
      2. Hirschsprung's disease (congenital aganglionic megacolon)
      3. Neurologic disorders
      4. Hypothyroidism
      5. Drugs
      6. Behavioral/psychologic
   B. Intussusception
   C. Pancreatic pseudocyst
   D. Intestinal or appendiceal abscess
   E. Ileus
   F. Choledochal cyst
   G. Hydrops of the gallbladder
   H. Mesenteric cyst

III. Hepatomegaly (see causes in "Hepatomegaly/Hepatosplenomegaly")

IV. Splenomegaly (see causes in "Splenomegaly," p. 94)

V. Genital tract
   A. Pregnancy
   B. Ovarian cyst
   C. Ovarian torsion
   D. Ovarian tumor
   E. Pelvic abscess
   F. Hematocolpos (imperforate hymen or vaginal atresia)

VI. Neoplasm
   A. Neuroblastoma
   B. Teratoma
   C. Lymphoma
   D. Sarcoma
   E. Adrenal tumor
   F. Renal and ovarian tumors (as noted earlier)

Author: **Jeffrey Kaczorowski, M.D.**

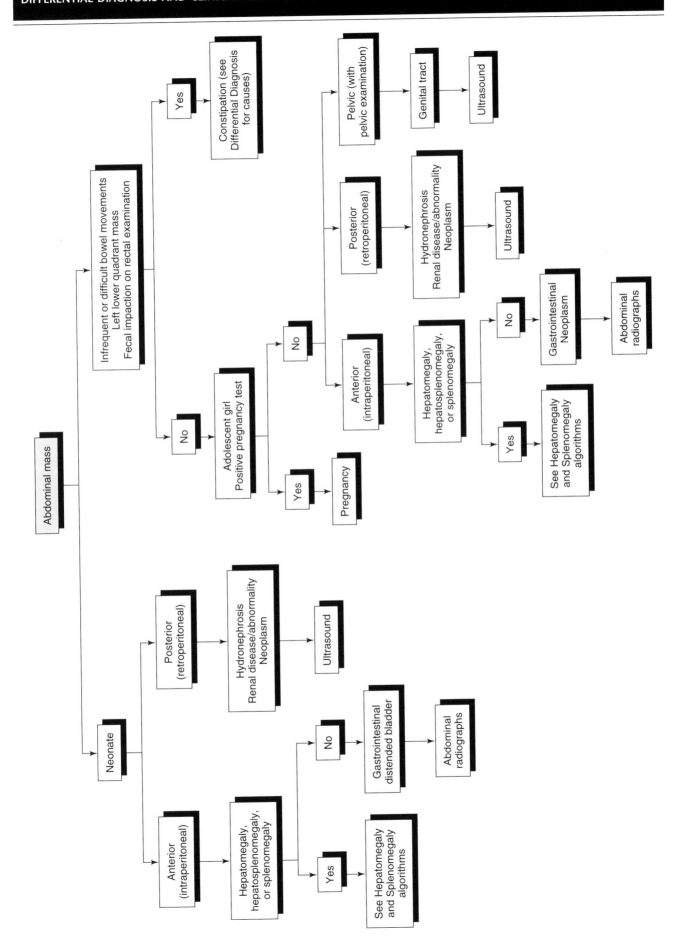

ABDOMINAL PAIN

■ **DEFINITION**

Any abdominal discomfort that may be acute or chronic, constant or intermittent, or sudden or insidious. It may or may not be associated with other gastrointestinal (diarrhea, vomiting), genitourinary (dysuria, discharge, menorrhagia), infectious (fever, sore throat, headache, malaise), or systemic (lethargy, irritability, rash) findings.

Chronic

I. **Common, general**
   A. Chronic recurrent abdominal pain, also known as *chronic nonspecific abdominal pain of childhood* and *functional abdominal pain*
   B. Lactose intolerance
   C. Psychogenic, anxiety related
   D. Irritable colon
   E. Constipation
   F. Dysmenorrhea
   G. Medications
      1. Nonsteroidal antiinflammatory agents
      2. Antibiotics
      3. Bronchodilators
      4. Methylphenidate (Ritalin)

II. **Less common, but worth considering**
   A. Reflux esophagitis
   B. Gastritis
   C. Peptic ulcer disease
      1. *Helicobacter pylori* infection
   D. Inflammatory bowel disease
   E. Endometriosis
   F. Chronic pyelonephritis
   G. Abdominal tumors/masses

III. **Uncommon**
   A. Heavy metal poisoning (lead, arsenic, mercury)
   B. Abdominal migraine
   C. Abdominal epilepsy
   D. Porphyria
   E. Collagen vascular disease
   F. Discitis
   G. Other spinal cord or spine diseases
      1. With or without constipation
      2. With or without urinary findings
      3. With or without gait difficulties
   H. Addison's disease
   I. Cystic fibrosis
      1. With or without meconium plug or obstruction
      2. Resulting from hypoxia
      3. Pneumonia
      4. Medications

   J. Arrhythmias—palpitations and nausea
   K. Hematocolpos
   L. Superior mesenteric artery syndrome, especially with recent significant weight loss, usually with vomiting
   M. Duplications anywhere along gastrointestinal tract; usual presentation is obstruction
   N. Mesenteric cysts

Acute

Many of the chronic causes of abdominal pain can present acutely. Other acute presentations are listed here.

I. **Infectious**
   A. Infectious gastroenteritis, gastroenterocolitis
   B. Pharyngitis/tonsillitis
   C. Appendicitis
   D. Pneumonia
   E. Pyelonephritis
   F. Food poisoning
   G. Pelvic inflammatory disease, Fitz-Hugh-Curtis (perihepatitis)
   H. Hepatitis
   I. Peritonitis
   J. Cholecystitis
   K. Pancreatitis (may be recurrent) or pancreatic cyst or pseudocyst
   L. Abdominal, pelvic or abdominal wall abscess
   M. Acute rheumatic fever
   N. Zoster
   O. Pericarditis

II. **Obstruction**
   A. Meckel's diverticulum
   B. Volvulus
   C. Intussusception
   D. Inguinal or femoral hernia with bowel strangulation or torsion
   E. Adhesions
   F. Ovary or ovarian cyst, torsion
   G. Choledochal or choledochal duct cyst
   H. Cholelithiasis (may be recurrent)
   I. Acute hydrops
   J. Testicular torsion
   K. Renal stones (may be recurrent)
   L. Ectopic pregnancy

III. **Other, not specifically categorized**
   A. Acute abdomen resulting from vasoocclusive crisis in sickle cell disease
   B. Diabetic ketoacidosis
   C. Hemolytic uremic syndrome

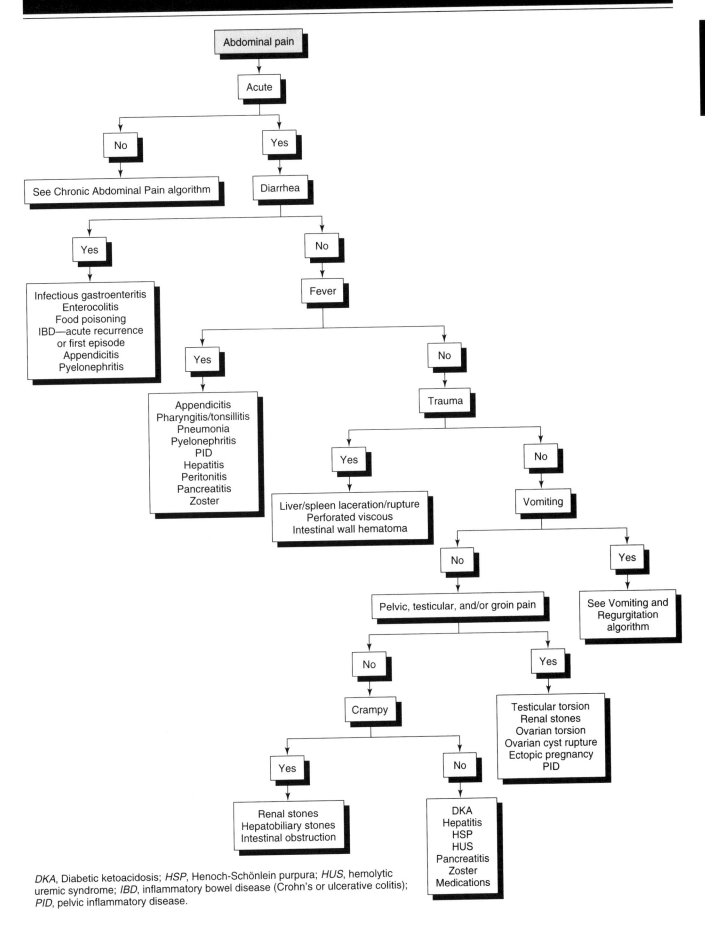

DKA, Diabetic ketoacidosis; *HSP*, Henoch-Schönlein purpura; *HUS*, hemolytic uremic syndrome; *IBD*, inflammatory bowel disease (Crohn's or ulcerative colitis); *PID*, pelvic inflammatory disease.

D. Peritonitis, caused by bleeding
E. Ovarian cyst rupture
F. Mittelschmerz (recurrent)
G. Abdominal muscle wall injury
H. Splenic rupture
I. Liver laceration or hematoma
J. Perforated viscus or abdominal blood vessel
K. Electrolyte abnormalities (ileus with hypo-kalemia, cramping with hypocalcemia, acute abdomen with acidosis)
L. Mesenteric artery occlusion

M. Familial dysautonomia
N. Hyperlipoproteinemia
O. Hemolytic crises
P. Spider bite (especially Black Widow)

IV. Inflammatory
A. Peritoneal inflammation (rheumatologic, vascular, familial Mediterranean fever)
B. Hereditary angioneurotic edema (recurrent)
C. Vasculitis

Author: **Lynn C. Garfunkel, M.D.**

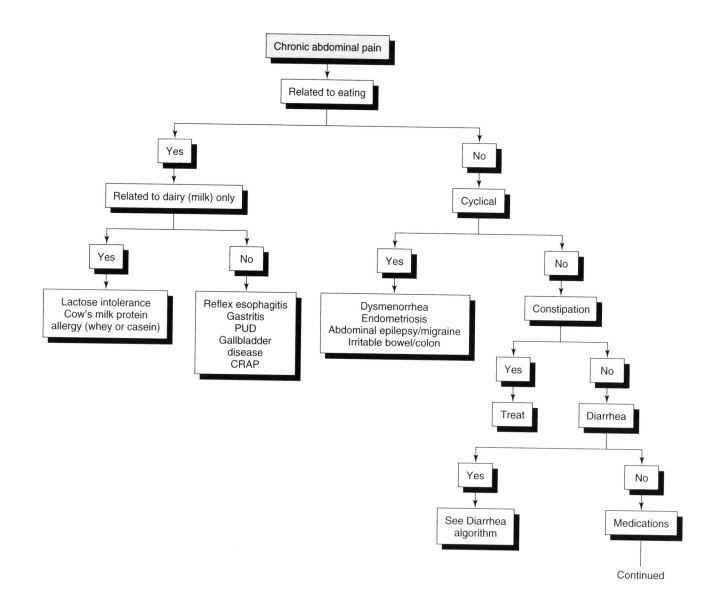

Continued

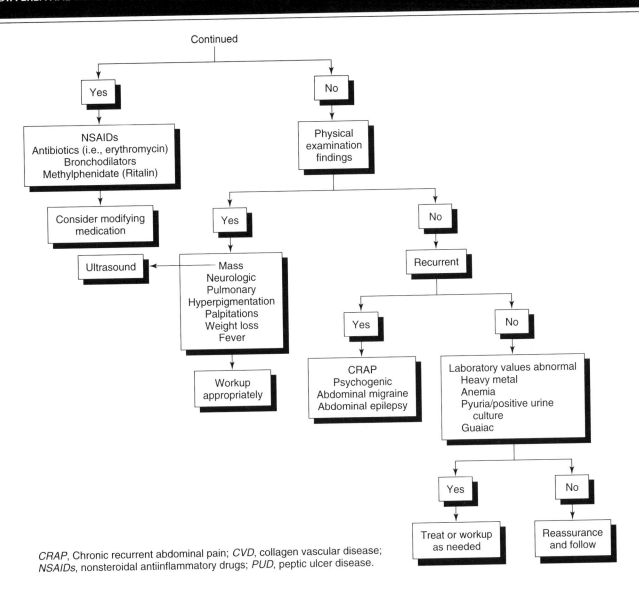

CRAP, Chronic recurrent abdominal pain; CVD, collagen vascular disease; NSAIDs, nonsteroidal antiinflammatory drugs; PUD, peptic ulcer disease.

ALOPECIA/HAIR LOSS

■ DEFINITION

Hair loss from the scalp. This section deals with *acute* causes of alopecia.

■ DIFFERENTIAL DIAGNOSIS

I. **Tinea capitis (fungal infection)**

II. **Trauma**
   A. Traction alopecia
   B. Trichotillomania (pulling out of hair)
   C. Chemical burn
   D. Thermal burn
   E. Radiation
   F. Chemotherapy (anagen effluvium)

III. **Alopecia areata (autoimmune)**
   A. Alopecia totalis (loss of all hair on the scalp)
   B. Alopecia universalis (loss of all hair on the body)

IV. **Telogen effluvium**
   A. Significant stress (hospitalization, childbirth, surgery, malnutrition, psychosocial)
   B. Drugs
      1. Valproic acid
      2. Warfarin
      3. Heparin
      4. Propanolol

V. **Male-pattern baldness**

VI. **Systemic diseases**
   A. Systemic lupus erythematosus
   B. Scleroderma (morphea)
   C. Acrodermatitis enteropathica
   D. Hypoparathyroidism

Author: **Jeffrey Kaczorowski, M.D.**

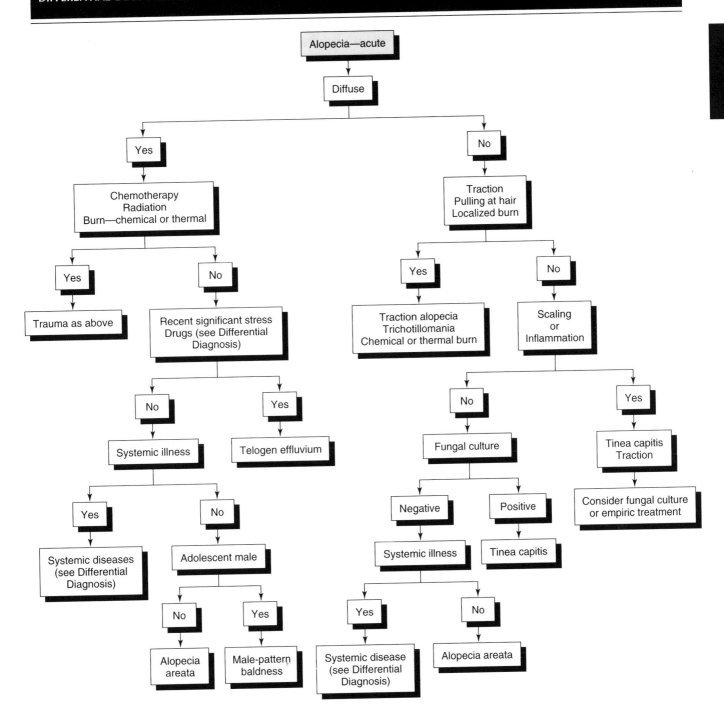

ALTERED MENTAL STATUS

■ **DEFINITION**

Includes several different states of consciousness. *Delirium* is confusion and irrational behavior sometimes accompanied by excitability. *Lethargy* refers to sleepiness and disinterest in the environment. *Stupor* or *obtundation* refers to a state of unconsciousness from which a child can momentarily be aroused. *Coma* is a prolonged state of unconsciousness.

■ **DIFFERENTIAL DIAGNOSIS**

I. Head trauma
   A. Subdural hematoma
   B. Epidural hematoma
   C. Intracerebral hemorrhage
   D. Intraventricular hemorrhage
   E. Subarachnoid hemorrhage
   F. Concussion
   G. Contusion
   H. Cerebral edema

II. Infectious
   A. Sepsis
   B. Meningitis
   C. Encephalitis
   D. Postinfectious encephalomyelitis
   E. Brain abscess
   F. Subdural empyema
   G. Shigella infections

III. Drug intoxication/overdose/reaction
   A. Alcohol
   B. Carbon monoxide
   C. Sedatives
   D. Benzodiazepines
   E. Narcotics
   F. Anticonvulsants
   G. Anticholinergics
   H. Neuroleptics
   I. Psychedelics
   J. Lead
   K. Aspirin
   L. Iron
   M. Cocaine
   N. Amphetamines
   O. Organophosphates
   P. Many others

IV. Seizures
   A. Status epilepticus
   B. Postictal

V. Neoplasms/brain tumors

VI. Hydrocephalus/shunt malfunction

VII. Hypertensive encephalopathy

VIII. Cerebrovascular disorders
   A. Arteriovenous malformation
   B. Venous thrombosis
   C. Aneurysm
   D. Stroke

IX. Metabolic
   A. Hypoglycemia
   B. Uremia
   C. Diabetic ketoacidosis
   D. Hepatic encephalopathy
   E. Reye's syndrome
   F. Adrenal insufficiency
   G. Hyponatremia and hypernatremia
   H. Hypocalcemia and hypercalcemia
   I. Hypomagnesemia
   J. Inborn errors of metabolism
      1. Amino acid disorders
         a. Urea cycle defects
         b. Tyrosinemia
         c. Nonketotic hyperglycinemia
      2. Organic acid disorders
         a. Methylmalonic acidemia
         b. Propionic acidemia
         c. Maple syrup urine disease
         d. Others
      3. Carbohydrate disorders
         a. Galactosemia
         b. Pyruvate dehydrogenase deficiency
         c. Ketotic hypoglycemia
         d. Others
      4. Fatty acid disorders
         a. Carnitine deficiencies
         b. Acyl-CoA dehydrogenase deficiency

X. Hypoxia/shock

XI. Hypothermia/hyperthermia

XII. Psychologic
   A. Psychosis
   B. Conversion reaction

XIII. Other
   A. Intussusception
   B. Hemolytic uremic syndrome
   C. Narcolepsy

Author: Jeffrey Kaczorowski, M.D.

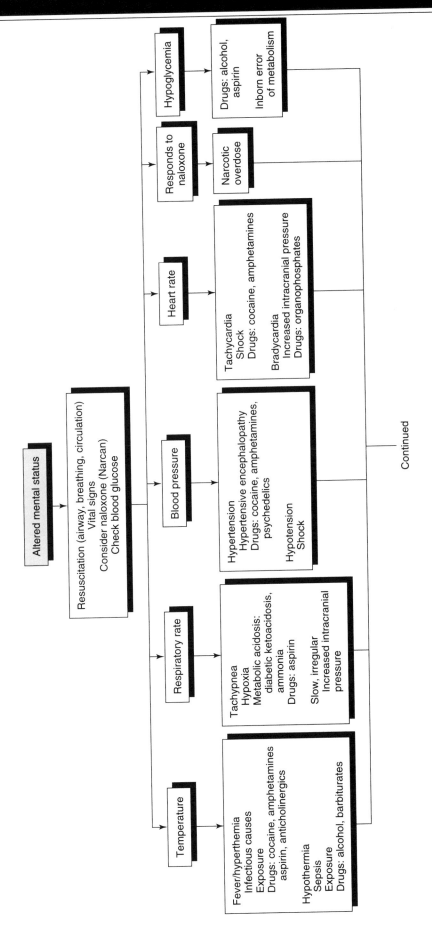

Altered mental status

Resuscitation (airway, breathing, circulation)
Vital signs
Consider naloxone (Narcan)
Check blood glucose

Temperature

Fever/hyperthermia
Infectious causes
Exposure
Drugs: cocaine, amphetamines
aspirin, anticholinergics

Hypothermia
Sepsis
Exposure
Drugs: alcohol, barbiturates

Respiratory rate

Tachypnea
Hypoxia
Metabolic acidosis:
diabetic ketoacidosis,
ammonia
Drugs: aspirin

Slow, irregular
Increased intracranial
pressure

Blood pressure

Hypertension
Hypertensive encephalopathy
Drugs: cocaine, amphetamines,
psychedelics

Hypotension
Shock

Heart rate

Tachycardia
Shock
Drugs: cocaine, amphetamines

Bradycardia
Increased intracranial pressure
Drugs: organophosphates

Responds to
naloxone

Narcotic
overdose

Hypoglycemia

Drugs: alcohol,
aspirin

Inborn error
of metabolism

Continued

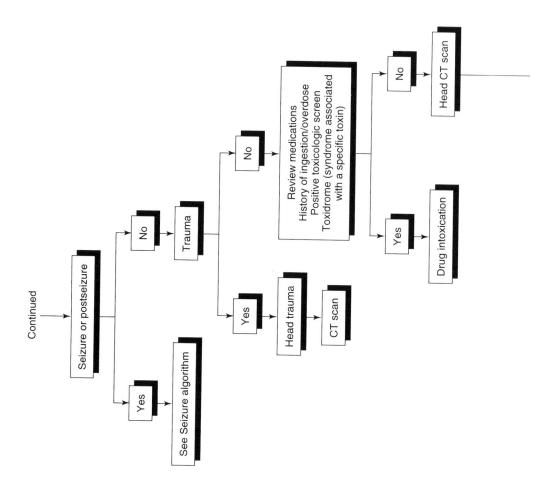

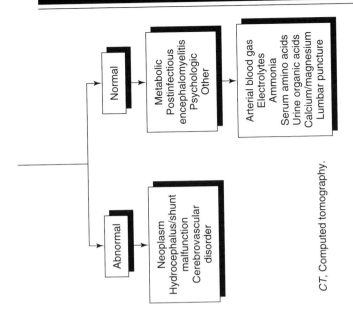

CT, Computed tomography.

AMENORRHEA

■ **DEFINITION**

Absence of menses. *Primary amenorrhea* is the absence of menarche by age 16 years in the presence of normal pubertal development *or* the absence of menarche by age 14 years in the absence of normal pubertal development *or* the absence of menarche 2 years after completion of sexual maturation. *Secondary amenorrhea* is the absence of menstruation for at least three cycles or at least 6 months in females who have already established menstruation. It is helpful to divide the evaluation of amenorrhea into three categories: amenorrhea with normal pubertal development, amenorrhea with delayed pubertal development, and amenorrhea with an abnormal genital examination.

■ **DIFFERENTIAL DIAGNOSIS**

I. **Pregnancy**

II. **Hormonal contraception**

III. **Hypothalamic**
   A. Chronic or systemic illness
   B. Eating disorder
   C. Hypothalamic-pituitary axis immaturity
   D. Infiltration
      1. Hemochromatosis
   E. Isolated gonadotropin-releasing hormone deficiency
   F. Kallmann's syndrome (defect in olfaction)
   G. Obesity
   H. Strenuous exercise
   I. Stress
   J. Substance abuse
   K. Tumor
      1. Craniopharyngioma

IV. **Pituitary**
   A. Hypopituitarism

   B. Infiltration
      1. Hemochromatosis
   C. Infarction
      1. Sheehan's syndrome
      2. Sickle cell disease
   D. Tumor
      1. Prolactinoma

V. **Adrenal**
   A. Congenital adrenal hyperplasia
      1. Classic
      2. Nonclassic

VI. **Ovarian**
   A. Agenesis (46,XX)
   B. Dysgenesis (Turner syndrome [45,XO] or variant)
   C. Hyperandrogenic chronic anovulation (polycystic ovary syndrome)
   D. Premature ovarian failure
      1. Autoimmune
      2. Chemotherapy
      3. Radiation
   E. Tumor

VII. **Uterus/cervix/vaginal abnormalities**
   A. Agenesis (Mayer-Rokitansky-Kuster-Hauser syndrome)
   B. Androgen insensitivity syndrome (testicular feminization)
   C. Imperforate hymen
   D. Synechiae (Asherman's syndrome)
   E. Transverse vaginal septum

VIII. **Other**
   A. Endocrinopathies
      1. Thyroid disease
      2. Cushing's syndrome
   B. Prader-Willi syndrome
   C. Laurence-Moon-Biedl syndrome

Author: **Stephanie Sansoni, M.D.**

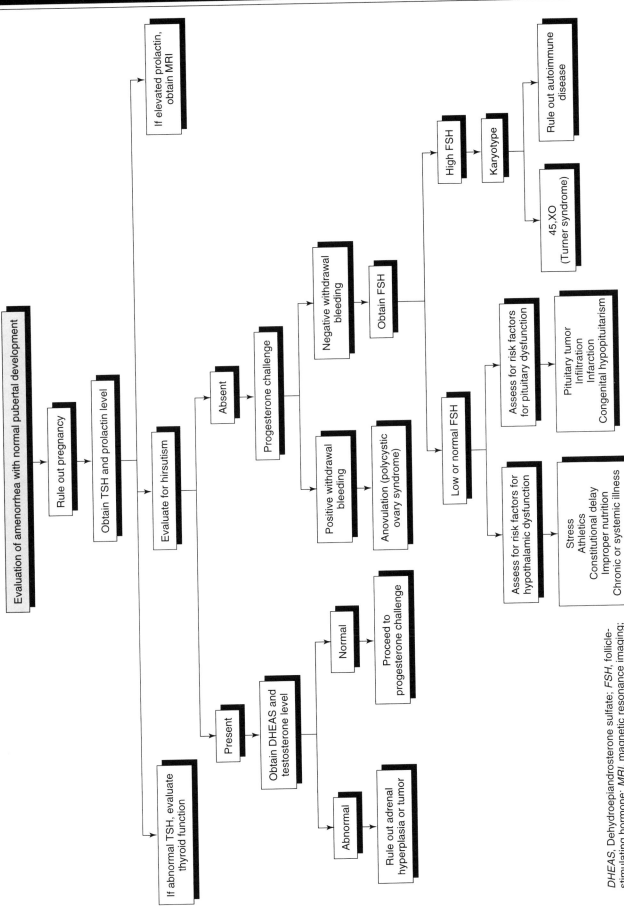

DHEAS, Dehydroepiandrosterone sulfate; FSH, follicle-stimulating hormone; MRI, magnetic resonance imaging; TSH, thyroid-stimulating hormone.

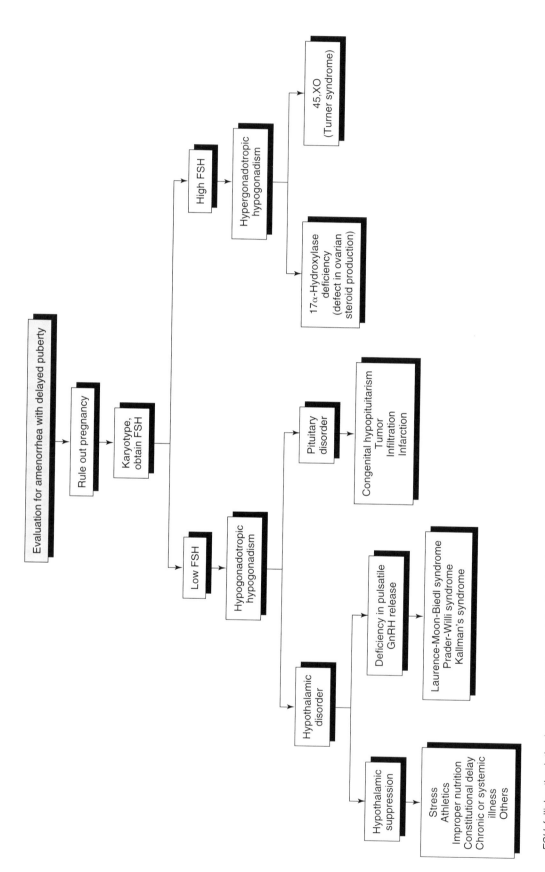

FSH, follicle-stimulating hormone; *GnRH*, gonadotropin-releasing hormone.

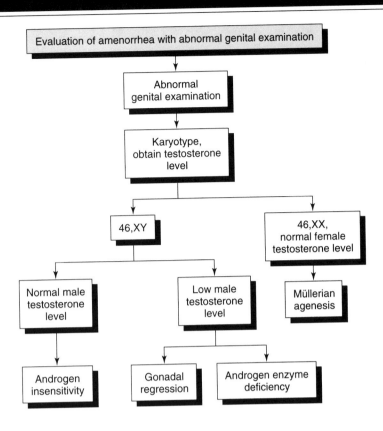

ARTHRITIS/JOINT SWELLING

■ DEFINITION

Swelling of a joint that is accompanied by limitation of motion, heat, pain, or tenderness. *Arthralgia* refers to pain or tenderness of a joint alone.

■ DIFFERENTIAL DIAGNOSIS

I. Trauma/mechanical
A. Hematoma/contusion
B. Fracture
  1. Stress fracture
  2. Osteochondritis dissecans
C. Dislocation
D. Ligament injuries (sprains)
E. Cartilage injuries
  1. Chondromalacia patella
F. Muscle injuries (strains)
G. Tendon injuries
H. Hemarthrosis
I. Bursitis
J. Foreign body
K. Overuse syndromes
  1. Osgood-Schlatter disease
  2. Little League elbow

II. Infectious/postinfectious
A. Septic arthritis (bacterial)
  1. *Staphylococcus aureus*
  2. Group A streptococcus
  3. *Streptococcus pneumoniae*
  4. Group B streptococcus
  5. *Haemophilus influenzae* type B
  6. *Neisseria gonorrhea*
  7. *Neisseria meningitidis*
  8. *Pseudomonas aeruginosa* (puncture wounds)
  9. *Salmonella* species (sickle cell disease)
  10. *Mycobacterium tuberculosis*
B. Postinfectious (bacterial)
  1. Group A streptococcus (acute rheumatic fever)
  2. *Neisseria gonorrhea*
  3. *Neisseria meningitidis*
  4. *Chlamydia*
  5. *Shigella*
  6. *Salmonella*
  7. *Yersinia*
  8. *Campylobacter*
C. Lyme disease
D. Rate-bite fever
E. *Mycoplasma*
F. Viral/postviral
  1. Rubella
  2. Hepatitis B virus
  3. Epstein-Barr virus
  4. Cytomegalovirus
  5. Parvovirus
  6. Herpesvirus-6
  7. Mumps
  8. Enterovirus
  9. Adenovirus
  10. Varicella-zoster virus
  11. Influenza viruses
G. Fungal
H. Bacterial endocarditis
I. Hemarthrosis or hematoma with infection

III. Rheumatic/collagen vascular disease
A. Juvenile rheumatoid arthritis
B. Systemic lupus erythematosus
C. Inflammatory bowel disease–associated arthritis
D. Behçet's syndrome
E. Henoch-Schönlein purpura
F. Kawasaki syndrome
G. Erythema nodosum–associated arthritis
H. Erythema multiforme (Stevens-Johnson syndrome)
I. Reiter's syndrome
J. Sclerodema
K. Dermatomyositis
L. Mixed connective tissue disorder
M. Ankylosing spondylitis
N. Polyarteritis nodosa
O. Sjögren's syndrome
P. Psoriatic arthritis
Q. Pigmented villonodular synovitis
R. Hypermobility syndrome

IV. Drugs
A. Serum sickness

V. Neoplasms
A. Leukemia
B. Neuroblastoma
C. Ewing's sarcoma
D. Osteogenic sarcoma

VI. Other
A. Hemophilia (hemarthrosis)
B. Sickle cell disease
C. Ehlers-Danlos syndrome (dislocations)
D. Sarcoidosis
E. Familial Mediterranean fever

Author: **Jeffrey Kaczorowski, M.D.**

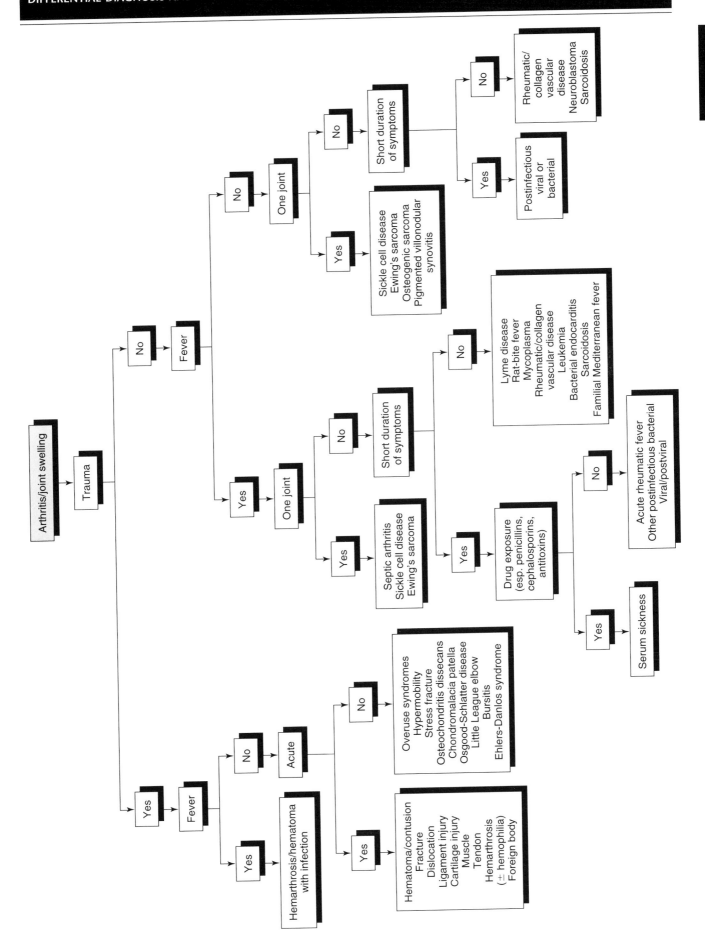

Arthritis/joint swelling

Trauma

No → Fever

No → One joint

No → Short duration of symptoms

No → Rheumatic/collagen vascular disease
Neuroblastoma
Sarcoidosis

Yes → Postinfectious viral or bacterial

Yes → Sickle cell disease
Ewing's sarcoma
Osteogenic sarcoma
Pigmented villonodular synovitis

Yes → One joint

No → Short duration of symptoms

No → Lyme disease
Rat-bite fever
Mycoplasma
Rheumatic/collagen vascular disease
Leukemia
Bacterial endocarditis
Sarcoidosis
Familial Mediterranean fever

Yes → Septic arthritis
Sickle cell disease
Ewing's sarcoma

Yes → Drug exposure (esp. penicillins, cephalosporins, antitoxins)

No → Acute rheumatic fever
Other postinfectious bacterial
Viral/postviral

Yes → Serum sickness

Yes → Fever

No → Acute

No → Overuse syndromes
Hypermobility
Stress fracture
Osteochondritis dissecans
Chondromalacia patella
Osgood-Schlatter disease
Little League elbow
Bursitis
Ehlers-Danlos syndrome

Yes → Hematoma/contusion
Fracture
Dislocation
Ligament injury
Cartilage injury
Muscle
Tendon
Hemarthrosis (± hemophilia)
Foreign body

Yes → Hemarthrosis/hematoma with infection

ATAXIA

■ **DEFINITION**

Impairment in coordination of movement without loss of muscle strength.

■ **DIFFERENTIAL DIAGNOSIS**

I. **Drugs/toxins**
   A. Anticonvulsants
      1. Barbiturates
      2. Phenytoin
      3. Carbamazepine
      4. Valproate
      5. Benzodiazepines
   B. Heavy metal poisoning
      1. Lead
      2. Mercury
      3. Arsenic
   C. Substance abuse
      1. Alcohol
      2. Glue sniffing
      3. Gasoline sniffing
   D. Sedatives
   E. Hypnotics
   F. Drug withdrawal
   G. Other agents

II. **Infectious**
   A. Meningitis
   B. Encephalitis
      1. Herpes
      2. Enterovirus
      3. Other infections
   C. Postinfectious encephalomyelitis
   D. Labyrinthitis
   E. Cerebellar abscess

III. **Acute cerebellar ataxia**

IV. **Central nervous system**
   A. Head trauma
      1. Cerebellar hemorrhage
      2. Posterior fossa subdural hematoma
      3. Concussion
   B. Tumor
      1. Posterior fossa
      2. Von Hippel-Lindau syndrome (cerebellar hemangioblastoma)
   C. Hydrocephalus
   D. Congenital anomalies of the cerebellum
      1. Cerebellar dysgenesis
      2. Dandy-Walker malformation
      3. Chiari malformation
      4. Vascular malformation of cerebellum/cerebellar hemorrhage
   E. Basilar artery migraine
   F. Cerebral palsy

V. **Peripheral nervous system**
   A. Guillain-Barré syndrome
   B. Tick bite paralysis

VI. **Metabolic disorders**
   A. Hypoglycemia
   B. Vitamin B_{12} deficiency
   C. Vitamin D deficiency
   D. Amino acid disorders
      1. Urea cycle defects
      2. Hartnup disease
   E. Organic acid disorders
      1. Maple syrup urine disease
      2. Isovaleric acidemia
      3. Multiple carboxylase deficiency
   F. Pyruvate metabolism disorders
      1. Leigh's disease (subacute necrotizing encephalomyelopathy)
      2. Pyruvate dehydrogenase complex deficiency
      3. Pyruvate decarboxylase deficiency

VII. **Systemic disorders**
   A. Friedreich's ataxia
   B. Ataxia telangiectasia
   C. Refsum's disease
   D. Multiple sclerosis
   E. Cockayne's syndrome
   F. Angelman's syndrome
   G. Abetalipoproteinemia
   H. Lipidoses (e.g., Tay-Sachs disease)
   I. Leukodystrophies

VIII. **Conversion disorder/psychogenic**

Author: Jeffrey Kaczorowski, M.D.

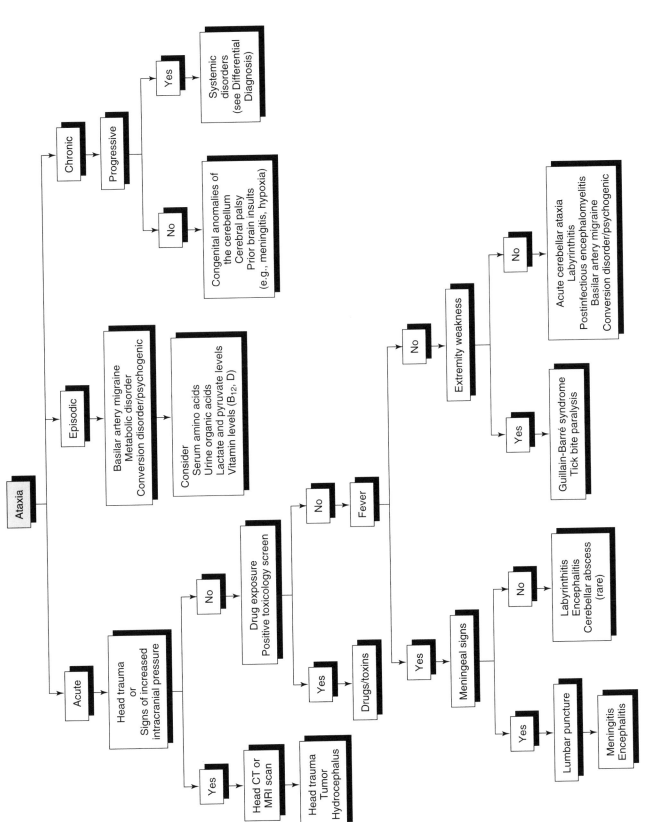

CT, Computed tomography; MRI, magnetic resonance imaging.

BACK PAIN

Back pain is less common in children than in adults. In general, the younger the child, the more likely back pain signifies serious disease.

■ DIFFERENTIAL DIAGNOSIS

I. Trauma/posttraumatic/recurrent stress
   A. Musculoskeletal strain
   B. Contusion
   C. Compression fracture
   D. Spondylolysis
   E. Spondylolisthesis
   F. Herniated disc
   G. Epidural hematoma

II. Infectious
   A. Spinal
      1. Discitis
      2. Vertebral osteomyelitis
      3. Epidural abscess
      4. Tuberculosis
   B. Extraspinal
      1. Pyelonephritis
      2. Pneumonia
      3. Meningitis
      4. Iliac osteomyelitis
      5. Sacroiliac pyoarthritis
      6. Paraspinal abscess
   C. Postinfectious: transverse myelitis

III. Collagen vascular disease
   A. Juvenile rheumatoid arthritis
   B. Ankylosing spondylitis
   C. Other spondylitis (inflammatory bowel disease, Reiter's syndrome, psoriasis)

IV. Tumors
   A. Vertebral tumors
      1. Ewing's sarcoma
      2. Osteogenic sarcoma
      3. Eosinophilic granuloma
      4. Osteoid osteoma
      5. Osteoblastoma
      6. Bone cysts
   B. Spinal cord tumors
      1. Neurofibromas
      2. Gliomas
      3. Lipomas
      4. Teratomas
   C. Extraspinal tumors
      1. Neuroblastoma
      2. Wilms' tumor
      3. Leukemia
      4. Lymphoma

V. Congenital/developmental spine disorders
   A. Congenital anomalies of the spine
   B. Scheuermann's disease (juvenile kyphosis)
   C. Disc space calcification
   D. Arteriovenous malformations

VI. Systemic disorders
   A. Sickle cell disease
   B. Muscular dystrophies
   C. Aortic aneurysm/dissection (hypertension, Marfan's syndrome)

VII. Referred pain
   A. Gallbladder disease
   B. Pancreatitis
   C. Appendicitis
   D. Renal colic
   E. Gastrointestinal cramping

VIII. Psychogenic

Author: Jeffrey Kaczorowski, M.D.

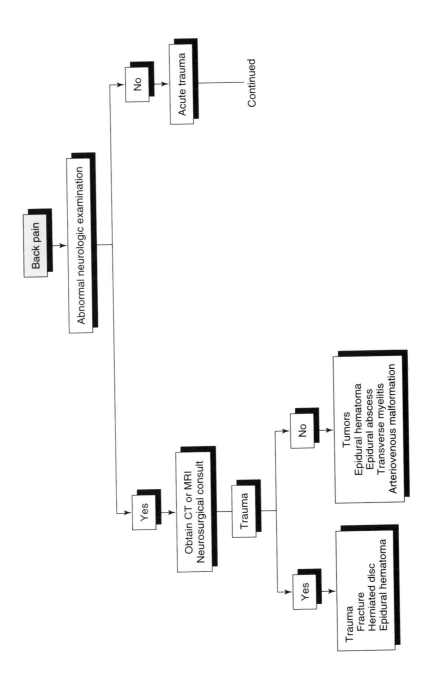

Back pain

Abnormal neurologic examination

No → Acute trauma → Continued

Yes → Obtain CT or MRI
Neurosurgical consult → Trauma

Yes →
Trauma
Fracture
Herniated disc
Epidural hematoma

No →
Tumors
Epidural hematoma
Epidural abscess
Transverse myelitis
Arteriovenous malformation

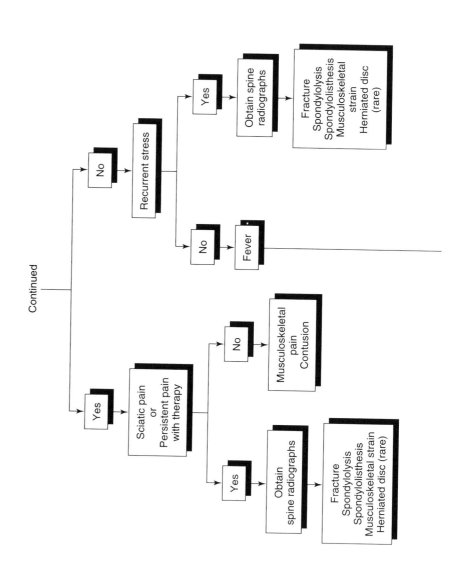

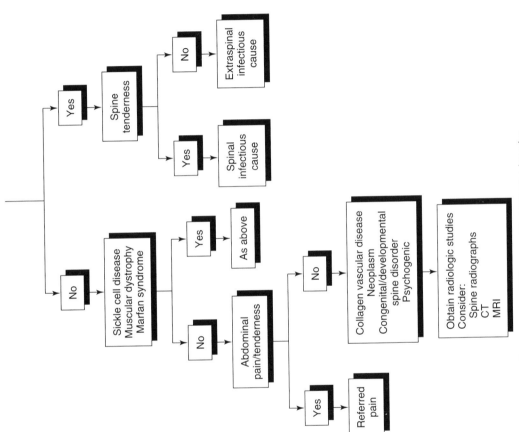

CT, Computed tomography; MRI, magnetic resonance imaging.

BREAST MASS/ENLARGEMENT

The differential diagnosis of a breast mass or enlargement is based on the age and sex of the child. Most breast masses in children and adolescents are benign. Obese children may sometimes appear to have breast enlargement without any actual breast tissue being present.

■ DIFFERENTIAL DIAGNOSIS

Any Age

I. **Infection**
   A. Cellulitis
   B. Abscess

II. **Drugs**
   A. Estrogen-containing medicines
   B. Spironolactone
   C. Cimetidine
   D. Imipramine
   E. Phenothiazines
   F. Isoniazid

III. **Trauma**
   A. Hematoma
   B. Fat necrosis
   C. Contusion

IV. **Chronic liver disease**

V. **Tumors (rare; see following)**

Infant

I. **Physiologic hypertrophy**

II. **Primary tumor**
   A. Hemangioma
   B. Others

Prepuberty
Male

I. **Precocious puberty (prepubertal gynecomastia) (see "Precocious Puberty" in Part II for causes)**

II. **Primary tumor**
   A. Lipoma
   B. Neurofibroma
   C. Others

Female

I. **Premature thelarche**

II. **Precocious puberty (see "Precocious Puberty" in Part II for causes)**

III. **Primary tumor**
   A. Lipoma
   B. Neurofibroma
   C. Others

Puberty
Male

I. **Physiologic gynecomastia (can be asymmetric)**

II. **Klinefelter syndrome (47,XXY karyotype)**

III. **Tumor**
   A. Primary
      1. Lipoma
      2. Neurofibroma
      3. Others
   B. Secondary: hormone producing
      1. Adrenal
      2. Testicular

Female

I. **Physiologic (can be asymmetric)**

II. **Pregnancy**

III. **Lactational changes**

IV. **Fibrocystic changes**

V. **Tumor**
   A. Fibroadenoma
   B. Giant fibroadenoma
   C. Cystosarcoma phylloides
   D. Intraductal papilloma
   E. Lipoma
   F. Breast carcinoma (rare)
   G. Breast sarcoma (rare)

VI. **Intramammary lymph node**

Author: Jeffrey Kaczorowski, M.D.

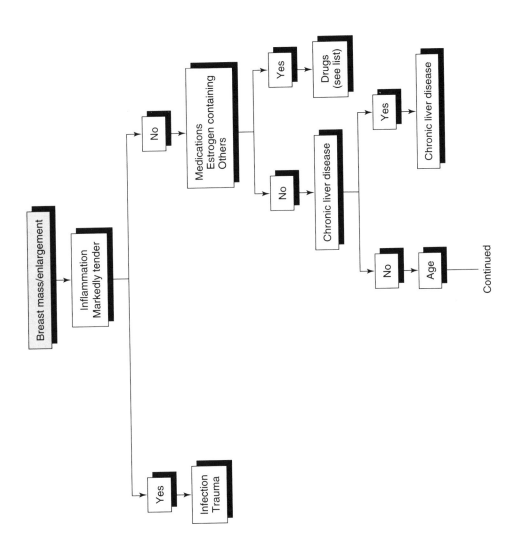

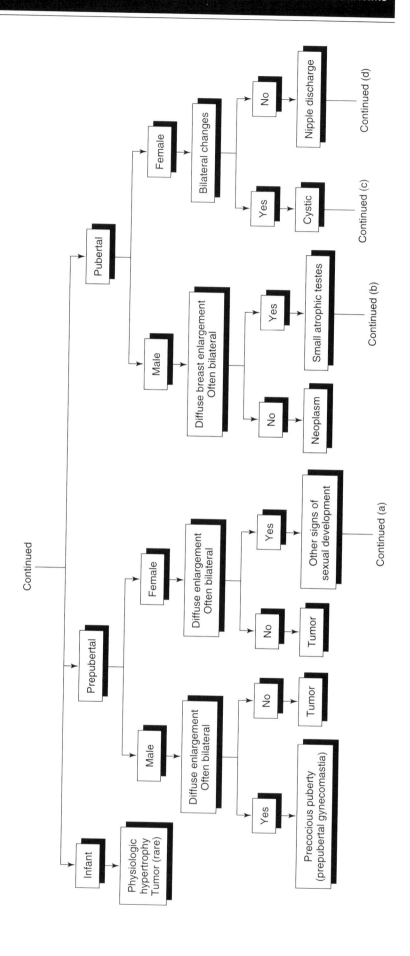

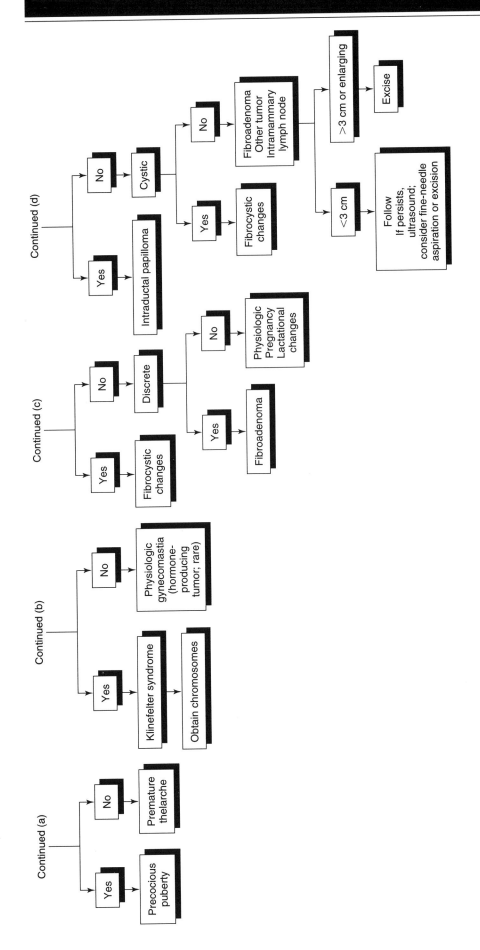

CHEST PAIN

Chest pain originates from inside or outside the chest. It may be referred from the abdomen. The most common causes include the following:

- Musculoskeletal: trauma, strain
- Psychogenic
- Costochondritis
- Esophagitis
- Asthma
- Cough
- Pneumonia
- Sickle cell disease

- **DIFFERENTIAL DIAGNOSIS**

  I. **Trauma/mechanical**
  - A. Chest wall strain
  - B. Costochondritis
  - C. Direct trauma
  - D. Slipping rib syndrome
  - E. Precordial catch: Texidor's twinge, benign pleuralgia

  II. **Infectious**
  - A. Devil's grip: epidemic pleurodynia, Bornholm disease
  - B. Varicella-zoster
  - C. Pleural effusion
  - D. Pneumonia
  - E. Pericarditis, myocarditis

  III. **Cardiac disease**
  - A. Arrhythmias (supraventricular tachycardia, premature ventricular contractions)
  - B. Structural abnormalities (hypertrophic congestive cardiomyopathy, aortic stenosis, pulmonary stenosis, mitral valve prolapse)
  - C. Coronary artery abnormalities
  - D. Coronary arteritis (Kawasaki syndrome)
  - E. Myocardial infarction, ischemia
  - F. Empyema, abscess
  - G. Myocarditis/pericarditis
  - H. Pneumopericardium
  - I. Rheumatic fever
  - J. Pulmonary hypertension
  - K. Dissecting aortic aneurysm
  - L. Marfan syndrome
  - M. Ehlers-Danlos syndrome
  - N. Takayasu arteritis
  - O. Pheochromocytoma

  IV. **Respiratory problems**
  - A. Cough
  - B. Pneumonia
  - C. Asthma
  - D. Pleural effusion
  - E. Pneumothorax
  - F. Pneumomediastinum
  - G. Cystic fibrosis

  V. **Gastrointestinal disorders**
  - A. Esophagitis
  - B. Esophageal foreign bodies
  - C. Caustic ingestions
  - D. Esophageal ulceration, stricture
  - E. Achalasia
  - F. Peptic ulcer disease
  - G. Pancreatitis, pancreatic pseudocyst
  - H. Hiatal hernia
  - I. Pylorospasm

  VI. **Idiopathic**

  VII. **Miscellaneous disorders**
  - A. Thoracic tumor
  - B. Breast mass
  - C. Sickle cell crisis
  - D. Cigarette smoking
  - E. Anxiety/psychologic
  - F. Hyperventilation

Author: **Cynthia Christy, M.D.**

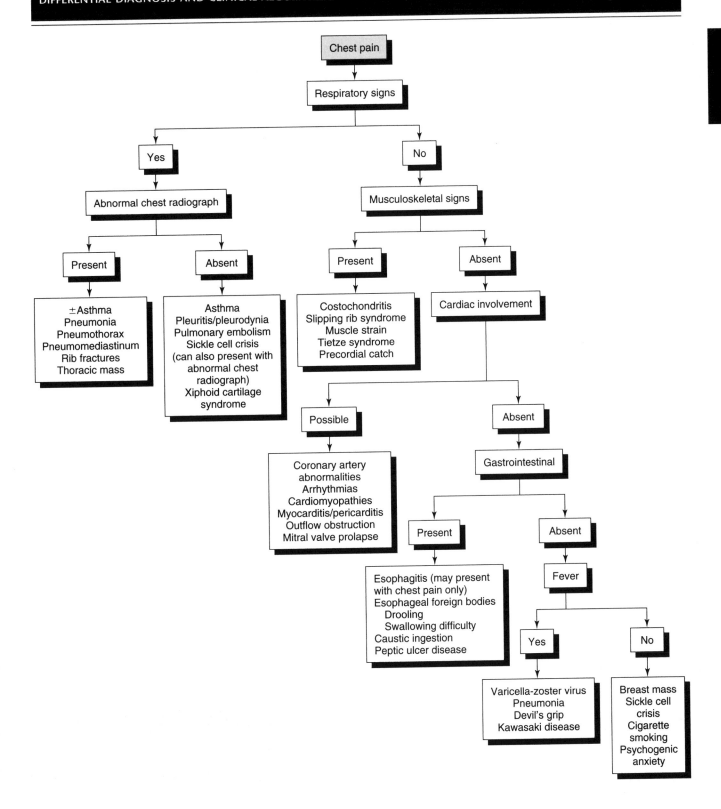

COUGH

■ **DEFINITION**

A reflexive action of deep inspiration followed by forced, rapid expiration, usually to protect and clear the airway of secretions, foreign material, or irritants.

I. **Congenital anomalies: compression or abnormality of airway**
   A. Connection of airway to esophagus (tracheoesophageal fistula [TEF])
   B. Tracheobronchomalacia
   C. Interstitial lung disease
   D. Aberrant mediastinal vessels
   E. Pulmonary sequestration
   F. Bronchopulmonary-foregut malformations
   G. Bronchogenic cysts
   H. Adductor vocal cord paralysis
   I. Congenital mediastinal tumors

II. **Other congenital**
   A. Cardiac malformations that lead to congestive heart failure
   B. Aspiration resulting from neurogenic abnormality

III. **Allergic**
   A. Rhinitis: allergic or vasomotor with postnasal drip
   B. Asthma/reactive airway: may begin with infectious upper airway disease
   C. Cough variant asthma: up to 40% of cases of chronic cough
   D. Allergic sinusitis

IV. **Infectious**
   A. Viral upper airway illnesses: upper respiratory infection
      1. Respiratory syncytial virus
      2. Adenovirus
      3. Parainfluenza virus
      4. Influenza virus
      5. Rhinovirus
      6. Corona virus
   B. Sinusitis
      1. *Streptococci*
      2. *Moraxella*
      3. Nontypable *Haemophilus influenzae*
   C. Pneumonia and lower respiratory tract infections
      1. *Chlamydia* in young infant
      2. *Mycoplasma pneumoniae*
      3. Viral pneumonia, bronchiolitis
      4. Bacterial pneumonias
         a. *Streptococcus pneumoniae*
         b. *Haemophilus influenzae*
         c. Gram-negative bacilli
         d. Anaerobes
      5. Fungal
   D. Whooping cough syndrome
      1. Pertussis
      2. Parapertussis
      3. Respiratory syncytial virus
      4. Adenovirus
      5. Influenza
      6. *Chlamydia*
      7. *Mycoplasma*
      8. Cystic fibrosis
   E. Suppurative lung disease with bronchiectasis or abscess
      1. Cystic fibrosis
      2. Dyskinetic cilia (immotile cilia, Kartagener syndrome)
      3. Foreign body
   F. Granulomatous lung disease
      1. Tuberculosis
      2. Fungi (histoplasma, coccidioidomycosis)
   G. Paranasal sinus infection

V. **Other, usually associated with infections**
   A. Immunodeficiency syndromes, including acquired immunodeficiency syndrome
   B. Abnormal mechanical clearance (cystic fibrosis, immotile cilia, bronchiectasis)

VI. **Foreign body aspiration or ingestion**
   A. Esophagus or tracheobronchial tree, most common in toddler years
   B. Tracheoesophageal (H-type) fistula

VII. **Tumors**

VIII. **Irritants**
   A. Chemical or physical
      1. Tobacco
      2. Firewood
      3. Dry and/or dusty air
      4. Volatile chemicals
   B. Aspiration associated with gastroesophageal reflux
   C. Aspiration from swallowing abnormality or TEF

IX. **Psychogenic/habitual: usually disappears during sleep; brassy tone, remarkable**

Author: Lynn C. Garfunkel, M.D.

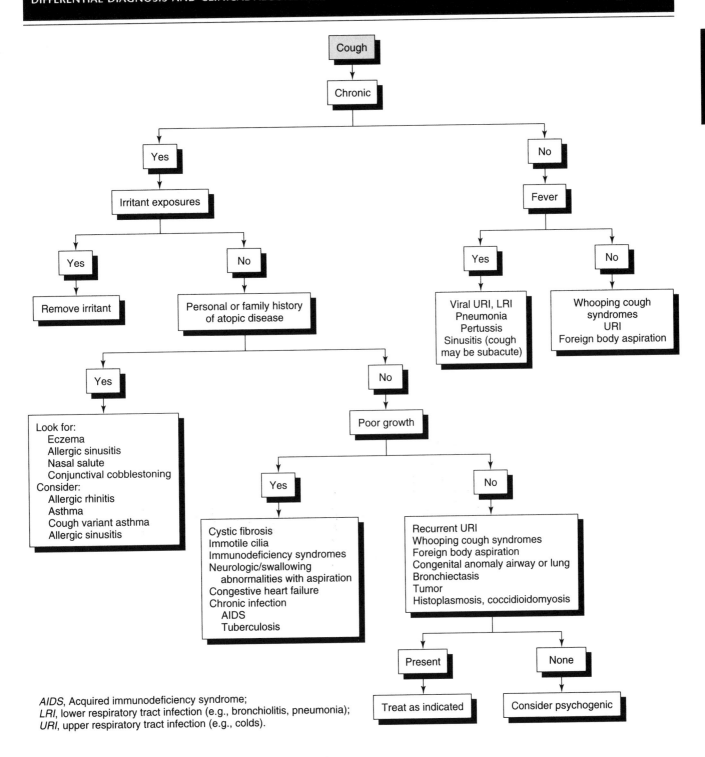

AIDS, Acquired immunodeficiency syndrome;
LRI, lower respiratory tract infection (e.g., bronchiolitis, pneumonia);
URI, upper respiratory tract infection (e.g., colds).

DIARRHEA

■ DEFINITION

An abnormally high stool volume and water content, usually associated with increased frequency of stool, although normal amounts vary dramatically among children. Typical stool volumes for infants are 5 to 10 g/kg body weight per 24 hours and 100 to 200 g/day for adults. Therefore an amount that is greater than 10 g/kg/day for an infant or greater than 200 g/day in an older child usually means diarrhea. The most common causes of altered motility and absorption are (1) colonization or invasion by bacteria, parasites, or viruses; (2) inflammatory processes; or (3) drugs.

I. **History: specific causes may be more likely with specific history**
   A. Fever, crampy pain, tenesmus: inflammatory bowel diseases (e.g., Crohn's, ulcerative colitis)
   B. Bloody stool: *Shigella, Escherichia coli,* amebiasis, *Salmonella, Yersinia, Campylobacter*
   C. Pain and fever (appendicitis-like): *Yersinia*
   D. Multiple cases/outbreak: less than 6 hours—staphylococci, *Bacillus;* more than 6 hours—*Clostridium perfringens*
   E. Seafood: *Vibrio cholera* (or similar)
   F. Immunosuppression (e.g., malnutrition, acquired immunodeficiency syndrome [AIDS]): *Salmonella,* rotavirus, isoporosis, cryptosporidium
   G. Persistent diarrhea may occur with the following:
      1. Malnutrition
      2. Diet changes
      3. Diarrhea after milk ingestion
      4. Antibiotic treatment
      5. Poor appetite
      6. Poor diet management

II. **Acute**
   A. Viral: acute gastroenteritis
      1. Rotavirus
      2. Norwalk-like virus
   B. Bacterial
      1. *Salmonella* species (antibiotics prolong carriage; treat if dysentery, age younger than 6 months, immunosuppressed)
      2. *Shigella* species (trimethoprim-sulfamethoxazole [TMP-SMX] or cephalosporin)
      3. *Yersinia* (consider TMP-SMX or intravenous [IV] gentamicin or chloramphenicol)
      4. *Campylobacter* (consider erythromycin, chloramphenicol, or IV gentamicin)
      5. *Clostridium difficile* (50% newborns colonized, if infant is positive, may be incidental): major treatment—discontinue antibiotic, consider vancomycin or metronidazole
      6. *E. coli* O157:H70 (antibiotics may increase risk of hemolytic uremic syndrome; treat only if toxic/septic; neonate: IV gentamicin or TMP-SMX)
      7. *Aeromonas hydrophilus* (consider TMP-SMX)
   C. Food poisoning, toxin mediated
      1. *Staphylococcus aureus*
      2. *Bacillus cereus*
      3. *C. perfringens*
   D. Other
      1. *V. cholera*
      2. *Giardia lamblia* (furazolidone or metronidazole, or quinacrine)
      3. *Cryptosporidium entamoeba*
      4. *Histolytica* (metronidazole)

E. Inflammatory bowel disease
  1. White blood cell (WBC) count and/or blood in stool with negative cultures
  2. Consider inflammatory bowel disease, endoscopy and biopsy looking for typical ulcerative colitis or Crohn's lesions
F. Drug induced

III. **Chronic: assess growth and development; onset in infancy, after infancy, school-age, or adolescent**
  A. Infancy
    1. Congenital monosaccharidase or disaccharidase deficiencies
    2. Pancreatic insufficiency (cystic fibrosis)
    3. Na-H transport deficiencies
    4. Chloride deficiency
    5. Short gut
    6. Microvillus abnormality
    7. Chronic intractable diarrhea of the newborn
    8. Malrotation/intermittent volvulus
  B. After infancy
    1. Overfeeding
    2. Excessive juice intake
    3. Specific food intolerance
    4. Laxative abuse, Munchausen syndrome by proxy
    5. Starvation stool
    6. Constipation with overflow encopresis
    7. Irritable bowel syndrome
  C. With growth insufficiency workup might also include the following (also see differential following workup):
    1. Workup
      a. Urine culture, blood urea nitrogen, creatinine (chronic renal insufficiency)
      b. Calcium, phosphorus, alkaline phosphatase (rickets)
      c. Electrolytes (acidosis, electrolyte abnormality)
      d. Magnesium, zinc (fat malabsorption)
      e. Carotene, cholesterol, human immunodeficiency virus (HIV) antibody or culture, immunoglobulins, trypsinogen, sweat chloride, *C. difficile* toxin, small bowel aspirate/culture, IgA and IgG antigliadin and antimesial antibodies, urine catecholamines, D-xylose
      f. Stool for ova and parasite (*Giardia* can present as chronic, nonspecific diarrhea)
      g. May also consider endoscopy or radiographic testing
    2. Cystic fibrosis
    3. Immunodeficiency
    4. AIDS/HIV
    5. Celiac disease
    6. Starvation stool

D. Fat malabsorption
1. Celiac disease
2. Cystic fibrosis
3. Shwachman syndrome
4. Intestinal lymphangiectasia
5. Abetalipoproteinemia
6. Trypsinogen deficiency
7. Enterokinase deficiency
8. Acrodermatitis enteropathica (zinc deficiency)
E. Colitis/obstruction
1. Hirschsprung's disease
2. Inflammatory bowel disease
3. Milk protein intolerance
4. Pseudoobstruction
F. Secretory (vasoactive polypeptide, prostaglandin, thyroid function testing, abdominal computed tomography scan)
1. Adrenal insufficiency
2. Thyroid disease
3. Tumor
   a. Ganglioneuroma
   b. Neuroblastoma
   c. Carcinoid
G. Later childhood, adolescence
1. Laxative abuse (anorexia nervosa)
2. Irritable bowel (colon) syndrome
3. Inflammatory bowel disease
4. Other systemic disease
5. *Giardia*
6. Carbohydrate intolerance
7. Celiac disease
8. Eosinophilic gastroenteritis
9. Bacterial overgrowth

Author: **Lynn C. Garfunkel, M.D.**

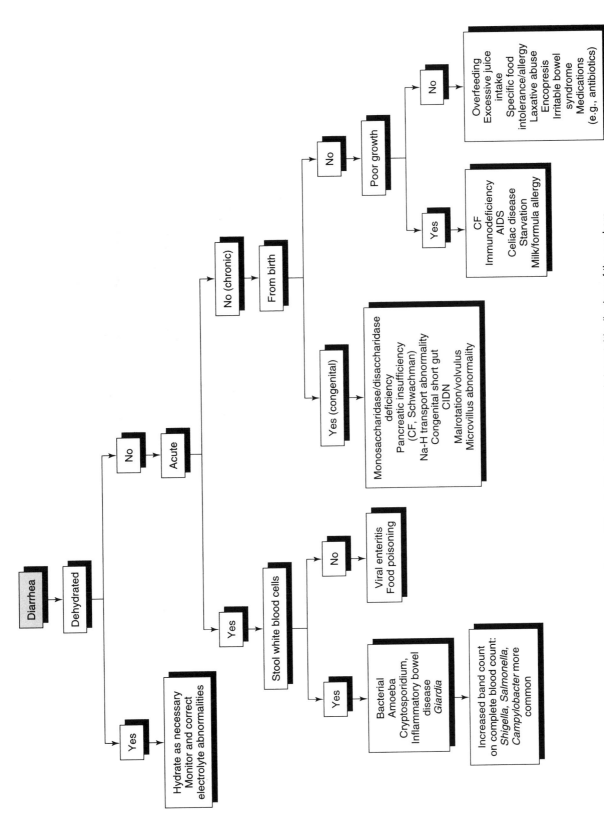

AIDS, Acquired immunodeficiency syndrome; *CF,* cystic fibrosis; *CIDN,* chronic intractable diarrhea of the newborn.

FEVER AND PETECHIAE
■ DEFINITION
Petechiae are less than 0.5 cm of circumscribed deposits of blood.

I. Noninfectious
   A. Leukocytoclastic vasculitis
   B. Platelet abnormalities
   C. Progressive pigmentary purpura
   D. Scurvy
   E. Senile (as a result of trauma)
   F. Leukemia

II. Infections with petechiae
   A. Bacteria
      1. *Neisseria meningitidis*
      2. *Neisseria gonorrhoeae*
      3. *Streptococcus pneumoniae*
      4. Group A streptococcus (*Streptococcus pyogenes*)
      5. *Borrelia* species (relapsing fever)
      6. *Staphylococcus aureus*
      7. *Capnocytophaga canimorsus*
      8. *Streptobacillus moniliformis*

   B. Viral illnesses
      1. Enterovirus
         a. Coxsackie A9
         b. Echovirus 9
      2. Epstein-Barr virus
      3. Cytomegalovirus
      4. Atypical measles
      5. Viral hemorrhagic fever
      6. Adenovirus
      7. Influenza
      8. Dengue virus
      9. Rubella
     10. Yellow fever
   C. Rickettsial disease
      1. Rocky Mountain spotted fever (*Rickettsia rickettsii*)
      2. Endemic *Rickettsia typhi/typhus* epidemic (*Rickettsia prowazekii*)
      3. Rickettsialpox (*Rickettsia akari*)
      4. Rat-bite fever (*Streptobacillus moniliformis*)
      5. Scrub or chigger typhus (*Rickettsia tsutsugamushi*)
   D. Malaria (*Plasmodium falciparum*)

Author: **Cynthia Christy, M.D.**

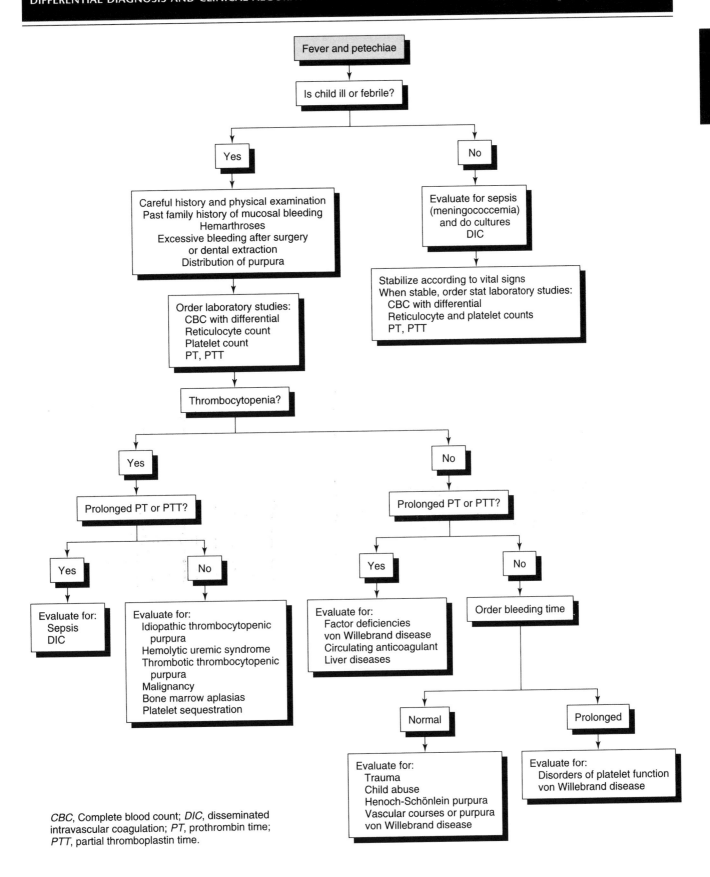

CBC, Complete blood count; DIC, disseminated intravascular coagulation; PT, prothrombin time; PTT, partial thromboplastin time.

GASTROINTESTINAL BLEEDING

■ DEFINITION

Upper gastrointestinal bleeding occurs proximal to the ligament of Treitz (between the third and fourth segments of the duodenum); lower gastrointestinal bleeding occurs distal to this ligament. *Hematemesis* refers to bright red or brown blood in the vomit; it is usually seen with upper gastrointestinal bleeding. *Hematochezia* is bright red, brown, or dark red blood from the rectum; it is usually caused by lower gastrointestinal bleeding but can be seen with brisk upper gastrointestinal bleeding. *Melena* is the passage of black tarry material (the product of degradation of blood in the small intestine) from the rectum; it is generally seen in upper gastrointestinal bleeding. Many food substances may mimic blood (e.g., red dyes, fruit juices, beets); confirmation of the presence of blood by Gastroccult (vomit) or guaiac (stool) tests is essential.

■ DIFFERENTIAL DIAGNOSIS

I. **Upper gastrointestinal bleeding**
   A. Oral or pharyngeal
      1. Swallowed blood from nose or oropharynx
   B. Esophagus
      1. Esophagitis
      2. Esophageal varices
   C. Stomach and duodenum
      1. Gastritis
      2. Ulcer
   D. Mallory-Weiss tears (junction of esophagus and stomach)
   E. Hemobilia (bleeding into the biliary tract)

II. **Lower gastrointestinal bleeding**
   A. Small intestine
      1. Cow's milk protein allergy
      2. Necrotizing enterocolitis
      3. Volvulus with malrotation
      4. Meckel's diverticulum
      5. Intussusception
      6. Crohn's disease
      7. Henoch-Schönlein purpura
      8. Mesenteric thrombosis/embolism
   B. Large intestine and rectum
      1. Infectious colitis
         a. *Escherichia coli* species
         b. *Salmonella* species
         c. *Shigella* species
         d. *Campylobacter jejuni*
         e. *Clostridium difficile*
         f. Entamoeba
         g. Parasites
      2. Intussusception
      3. Inflammatory bowel disease
      4. Intestinal polyps
         a. Juvenile polyps
         b. Familial multiple adenomatous polyposis
         c. Gardner's syndrome
         d. Peutz-Jeghers syndrome
         e. Benign lymphoid polyposis
      5. Henoch-Schönlein purpura
      6. Diverticulosis
      7. Hemolytic uremic syndrome
   C. Anus
      1. Hemorrhoids
      2. Fissure
      3. Trauma/abuse

III. **Either upper or lower gastrointestinal bleeding**
   A. Swallowed maternal blood
   B. Vascular malformation
      1. Arteriovenous malformations
      2. Hemangiomas
      3. Angiodysplasia
      4. Rendu-Osler-Weber syndrome (hereditary hemorrhagic telangiectasia)
   C. Duplication
   D. Toxic ingestion/drugs
      1. Aspirin/salicylates
      2. Anticoagulants
      3. Rat poison ("superwarfarins")
   E. Foreign body
   F. Bleeding disorders
      1. Hemorrhagic disease of the newborn
      2. Disseminated intravascular coagulation
      3. Hemophilia
   G. Neoplasms

Author: **Jeffrey Kaczorowski, M.D.**

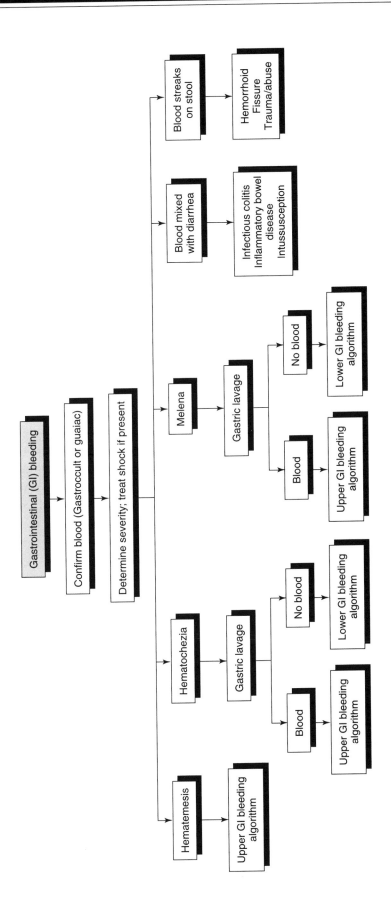

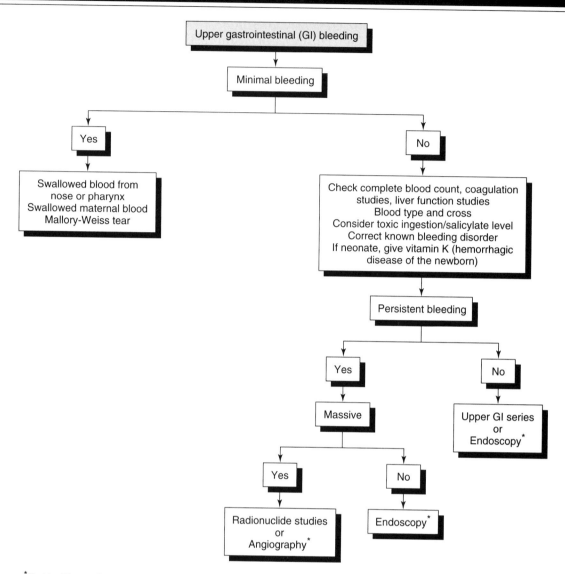

*To identify precise cause of bleeding: esophagitis, esophageal varices, gastritis, ulcer, hemobilia, vascular malformation, duplication, foreign body, neoplasm.

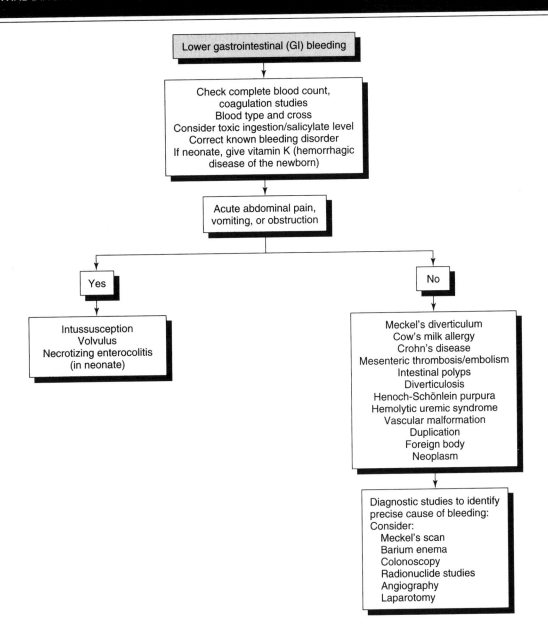

HEADACHE

Most headaches in children are not caused by serious disease. The differential diagnosis should initially focus on distinguishing serious causes from the more common causes.

■ DIFFERENTIAL DIAGNOSIS

I. **Vascular headache**
   A. Migraine
      1. Common
      2. Classic
      3. Complicated
   B. Hypertension
   C. Vasculitis
   D. Embolus/infarction
   E. Cluster headache

II. **Intracranial infections**
   A. Meningitis
   B. Encephalitis

III. **Altered intracranial pressure**
   A. Increased
      1. Tumor
      2. Intracranial hemorrhage or hematoma
      3. Abscess
      4. Cerebral edema
      5. Hydrocephalus
      6. Pseudotumor cerebri
      7. Venous sinus thrombosis
   B. Decreased
      1. Post–lumbar puncture

IV. **Disorders of the head and neck**
   A. Eyestrain
   B. Glaucoma
   C. Sinus infections
   D. Streptococcal sore throat
   E. Dental caries
   F. Malocclusion
   G. Temporomandibular joint dysfunction
   H. Cranial neuralgias

V. **Muscular headache**
   A. Tension
   B. Muscle strain
      1. Activity
      2. Posture
      3. Prolonged position

VI. **Trauma**
   A. Intracranial hemorrhage or hematoma
   B. Posttraumatic
   C. Muscle strain ("whiplash")

VII. **Psychogenic**

VIII. **Other**
   A. Systemic illness
   B. Drugs/poisoning
   C. Hyperventilation
   D. Hypoxia
   E. Seizure/postseizure

Table 1-1 reviews some characteristics that may be helpful in distinguishing between common causes of headache.

Author: Jeffrey Kaczorowski, M.D.

TABLE 1-1   Characteristics of Migraine, Tension, and Psychogenic Headaches

	MIGRAINE	TENSION	PSYCHOGENIC
Location	Typically unilateral	Bilateral—often occipital	Bilateral—anywhere
Character	Throbbing	Pressure	Pressure or no particular character
Severity	Moderate to severe	Mild to moderate	Usually mild
Aura	Sometimes	No	No
Associated symptoms	Vomiting, photophobia	Stress, muscle strain	Other somatic complaints, depression, anxiety

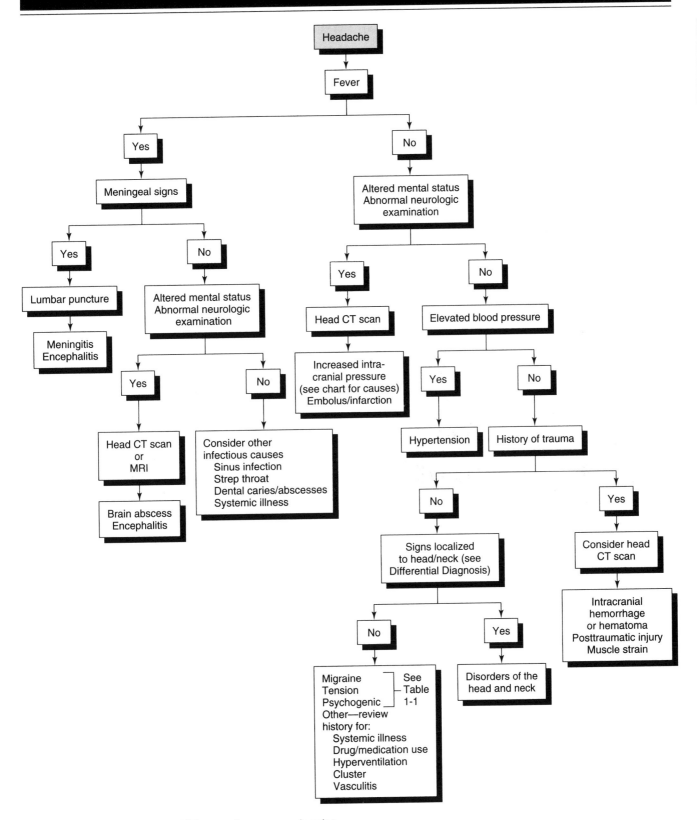

CT, Computed tomography; MRI, magnetic resonance imaging.

HEMATURIA

■ DEFINITION

The presence of red blood cells (RBCs) in the urine. Urine dipstick detects RBCs, hemoglobin, and myoglobin; microscopy can reveal only RBCs. The presence of more than 2 to 5 RBCs per high-power field (hpf) on a centrifuged urine specimen is generally considered abnormal. Hematuria on a single urinalysis occurs at some point in approximately 5% of children, but only 0.5% to 1% have persistent hematuria. *Clinically significant persistent hematuria* is the presence of more than 2 to 5 RBCs/hpf on at least two of three consecutive spun urine specimens obtained over a 2-month period. Bleeding from the glomeruli of the kidney often results in smoky (tea- or cola-colored) reddish-brown urine. The presence of RBC casts indicates bleeding from the glomeruli.

Hematuria can exist with or without proteinuria. Gross hematuria usually results in detection of urinary protein. This protein originates from RBCs. Microscopic hematuria combined with proteinuria strongly suggests glomerulonephritis, although it may be seen with acute tubular necrosis and systemic diseases (see the following differential diagnosis) as well.

Hemoglobinuria may result from any disorder causing hemolysis (e.g., RBC membrane defects, hemoglobinopathies, immune hemolytic disorders, mismatched blood transfusions, disseminated intravascular coagulation, sepsis, malaria, mechanical erythrocyte damage). *Myoglobinuria* is caused by damage to muscles (e.g., crush injury, electrical burns, prolonged seizures, malignant hyperthermia, myositis, rhabdomyolysis, extreme exercise). Hemoglobinuria can be differentiated from myoglobinuria by a variety of methods that directly test the urine. Other laboratory data may also be used to identify the source of urinary pigment indirectly. A low blood urea nitrogen:creatinine ratio and high creatine phosphokinase suggest myoglobinuria (creatinine is released from damaged muscles). Pink serum suggests hemoglobinuria; normal-colored serum suggests myoglobinuria.

■ DIFFERENTIAL DIAGNOSIS

I. Infection
A. Cystitis
B. Pyelonephritis
C. Urethritis
D. Balanitis
E. Tuberculosis

II. Trauma
A. Kidney
B. Bladder
C. Urethra

III. Drugs/toxins
A. Nonsteroidal antiinflammatory agents
B. Cyclophosphamide
C. Penicillins
D. Cephalosporins
E. Sulfa drugs
F. Furosemide
G. Aminoglycosides
H. Cyclosporine
I. Heavy metals

IV. **Exercise (vigorous)**

V. **Hypercalciuria**

VI. **Calculi**
   A. Congenital
   B. Infectious
   C. Metabolic disorder
      1. Hypercalcuria
      2. Hyperuricosuria
      3. Cystinuria
      4. Hyperoxaluria
   D. Idiopathic

VII. **Foreign body/instrumentation in urethra or bladder**
   A. Urinary catheterization
   B. Suprapubic aspiration

VIII. **Tumor**
   A. Wilms' tumor
   B. Leukemia
   C. Hemangioma
   D. Bladder cancer

IX. **Structural abnormality**
   A. Polycystic kidney disease
   B. Cystic kidneys
   C. Hydronephrosis
   D. Ureteropelvic junction obstruction
   E. Posterior urethral valves

X. **Hemoglobinopathies**
   A. Sickle cell hemoglobinopathies
   B. Others

XI. **Bleeding disorders**
   A. Hemophilias
   B. Thrombocytopenias

XII. **Renal vessel thrombosis/infarction**

XIII. **Acute tubular necrosis**
   A. Drugs/toxins (see earlier)
   B. Hypoxia
   C. Hypoperfusion

XIV. **Glomerulonephritis**
   A. Acute poststreptococcal
   B. IgA nephropathy
   C. Membranoproliferative
   D. Henoch-Schönlein purpura
   E. Alport's hereditary nephritis

XV. **Systemic diseases**
   A. Hemolytic uremic syndrome
   B. Systemic lupus erythematosus
   C. Polyarteritis nodosa
   D. Wegener's granulomatosis
   E. Goodpasture's syndrome

XVI. **Benign familial hematuria**

XVII. **Benign nonfamilial hematuria**
Author: **Jeffrey Kaczorowski, M.D.**

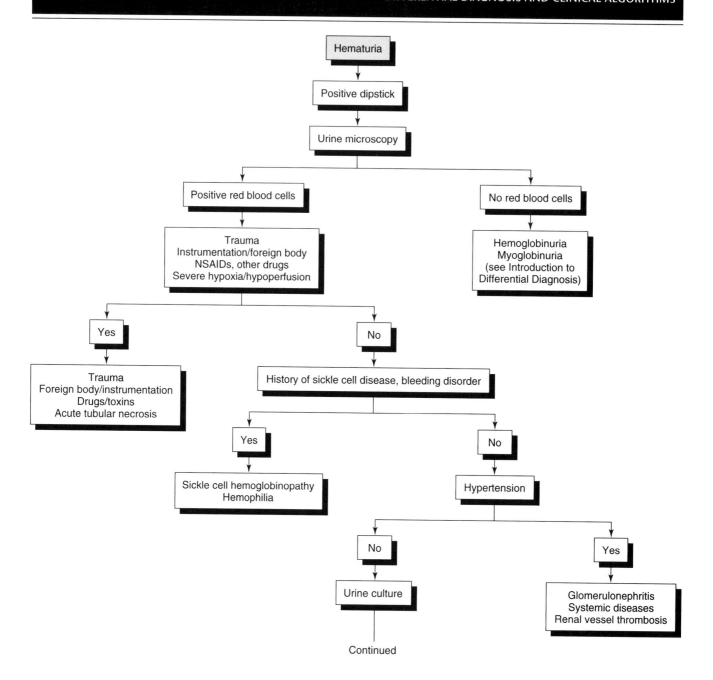

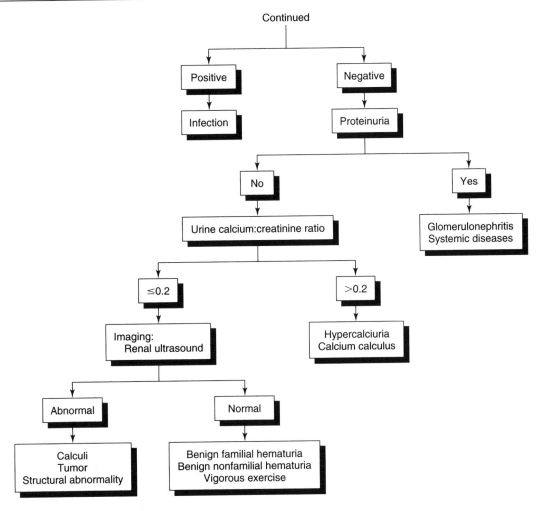

NSAIDs, Nonsteroidal antiinflammatory drugs.

HEPATOMEGALY AND HEPATOSPLENOMEGALY

■ DEFINITION

This section considers causes for hepatomegaly (enlargement of the liver) and hepatosplenomegaly (enlargement of the liver and spleen). Those causes that generally result in hepatomegaly (without splenomegaly) are noted with an *H*. For isolated splenomegaly, see the section "Splenomegaly."

■ DIFFERENTIAL DIAGNOSIS

I. Infection
  A. Viral
    1. Epstein-Barr virus
    2. Cytomegalovirus
    3. Herpes simplex virus
    4. Enterovirus
    5. Varicella-zoster virus
    6. Human immunodeficiency virus
    7. Congenital rubella
    8. Hepatitis (H)
  B. Bacterial
    1. Sepsis
    2. Endocarditis
    3. Tuberculosis
    4. Brucellosis
    5. Congenital syphilis
    6. Leptospirosis
    7. Liver abscess (H)
  C. Parasites
    1. Toxoplasmosis
    2. Visceral larva migrans
    3. Chagas' disease
    4. Amebiasis (H)
    5. Malaria
    6. Ascariasis (H)
    7. Others
  D. Fungal
    1. Histoplasmosis
  E. Rickettsial
    1. Rocky Mountain spotted fever

II. Trauma/liver injury (H)

III. Hemolytic anemia

IV. Neoplasms
  A. Leukemia
  B. Lymphoma
  C. Neuroblastoma
  D. Hemangioma (H)
  E. Hepatic tumor (H)

V. Collagen vascular disease
  A. Systemic lupus erythematosus
  B. Juvenile rheumatoid arthritis

VI. Cardiac
  A. Congestive heart failure (H)
  B. Pericardial tamponade (H)

VII. Idiopathic neonatal hepatitis (H)

VIII. Chronic hepatitis (H)
  A. Chronic active hepatitis
  B. Chronic persistent hepatitis

IX. Cirrhosis

X. Congenital hepatic fibrosis (H)

XI. Hepatic cysts (H)

XII. **Drugs/toxins (H)**
A. Acetaminophen
B. Ethanol
C. Carbon tetrachloride
D. Phenytoin
E. Valproate
F. Tetracycline
G. Isoniazid
H. Androgenic steroids
I. Antineoplastic/chemotherapeutic agents
J. Mushroom poisoning

XIII. **Biliary tract obstruction**
A. Extrahepatic
1. Biliary atresia (H)
2. Biliary hypoplasia (H)
3. Gallstone (H)
B. Intrahepatic
1. Intrahepatic biliary atresia (H)
2. Alagille syndrome (H)
3. Byler syndrome (H)

XIV. **Metabolic disorders**
A. Amino acid disorders
1. Tyrosinemia
B. Carbohydrate disorders
C. Galactosemia (H)
D. Hereditary fructose intolerance (H)
E. Fructose-1,6-diphosphatase deficiency (H)
F. Glycogen storage diseases (H)

G. Others
H. Lipidoses
1. Niemann-Pick disease
2. Gaucher's disease
3. Farber's disease
I. Mucopolysaccharidoses
J. Mucolipidoses
K. Glycoproteinoses
1. Fucosidosis
2. Mannosidosis
3. Sialidosis
L. Acid lipase deficiency
1. Wolman's disease
2. Cholesterol ester storage disease (H)
M. Peroxisomal disorders
1. Zellweger syndrome (H)
N. Lipoprotein disorders
1. Type I hyperlipoproteinemia

XV. **Other**
A. Peripheral hyperalimentation (H)
B. Malnutrition (H)
C. Cystic fibrosis (H)
D. Histiocytosis
E. Hemochromatosis (H)
F. Wilson disease (H)
G. α_1-Antitrypsin deficiency (H)
H. Reye's syndrome (H)
I. Sarcoidosis (H)

Author: **Jeffrey Kaczorowski, M.D.**

Hepatomegaly

Without splenomegaly

Trauma

Yes → Liver injury

No → Signs of congestive heart failure (tachypnea, tachycardia, cardiomegaly, abnormal cardiac examination)

No → Drugs/toxic exposures (see Differential Diagnosis)

Yes → Cardiac

Yes → Drug-induced hepatitis

No → Fever

Continued

With splenomegaly

Jaundice and hemolysis on blood smear

Yes → Hemolytic anemia Sepsis

No → Fever

No → Neoplasm Collagen vascular disease Metabolic disorder Histiocytosis

CBC, differential
Reticulocyte count
Liver function tests
Sedimentation rate
Serum amino acids
Serum lipids
Ultrasound
Referral to genetics/GI
if metabolic disorder suspected

Yes → Infectious Collagen vascular disease Neoplasm

CBC, differential
Reticulocyte count
Liver function tests
Sedimentation rate
Viral titers
Ultrasound

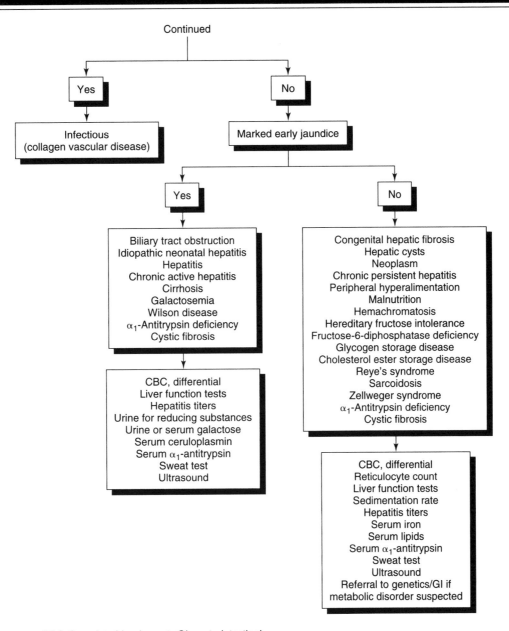

CBC, Complete blood count; GI, gastrointestinal.

HYPOGLYCEMIA

- **DEFINITION**

Hypoglycemia is a serum or plasma glucose level less than 40 mg/dl or a whole blood glucose level less than 35 mg/dl.

- **DIFFERENTIAL DIAGNOSIS**
  I. **Hyperinsulinemia**
     A. Infant of a diabetic mother
     B. Pancreatic or islet cell dysplasia/hyperplasia (formerly called *nesidioblastosis*)
     C. Islet cell adenoma or adenomatosis
     D. Beckwith-Wiedemann syndrome
     E. Exogenous administration of insulin (unintentional overdose, suicide attempt, Munchausen syndrome by proxy)

  II. **Poor intake or diminished glycogen stores**
     A. Low birth weight/small for gestational age
     B. Hepatitis
     C. Hepatic failure (congenital, infectious, inborn error of metabolism), cirrhosis
        1. Reye's syndrome
        2. α_1-Antitrypsin deficiency
     D. Malnutrition
     E. Malabsorption, chronic diarrhea
     F. Insufficient glucose administration postoperatively

  III. **Ketotic hypoglycemia**

  IV. **Counterregulatory hormone abnormalities**
     A. Hypothalamic defect or hypopituitarism
     B. Growth hormone deficiency or growth hormone receptor unresponsiveness (Laron dwarfism)
     C. Cortisol deficiency
        1. Addison's disease
        2. Adrenal failure
        3. Congenital adrenal insufficiency
     D. Adrenocorticotropic hormone deficiency or unresponsiveness
     E. Thyroid hormone deficiency
     F. Glucagon or catecholamine deficiency—both rare

  V. **Inborn errors of metabolism**
     A. Glycogen storage diseases (GSD)
        1. GSD type Ia, Ib (glucose-6-phosphatase deficiency)
        2. GSD type 0 (glycogen synthetase deficiency)
        3. Liver phosphorylase enzyme defects
     B. Gluconeogenesis enzyme abnormalities
        1. Fructose-1,6-diphosphatase
        2. Phosphoenolpyruvate carboxykinase
        3. Pyruvate carboxylase
     C. Galactosemia (galactose-1-phosphate uridyltransferase defect)
     D. Hereditary fructose intolerance (fructose-1-phosphate aldolase defect)
     E. Amino acid and organic acid abnormalities
        1. Maple syrup urine disease
        2. Propionic acidemia
        3. Methylmalonic aciduria
        4. Tyrosinosis
        5. 3-Hydroxy-3-methylglutaric aciduria
        6. Glutaric aciduria
     F. Enzymatic defects in fat metabolism
        1. Carnitine deficiency, transferase deficiency
        2. Long-chain and medium-chain acyl-CoA dehydrogenase deficiencies

  VI. **Drugs or poisons**
     A. Salicylates
     B. Alcohol
     C. Propranolol
     D. Hypoglycemic agents (e.g., sulfonylureas)
     E. Pentamidine
     F. Hypoglycin (from unripe ackees; Jamaican vomiting sickness)

  VII. **Other**
     A. Tumors
        1. Hepatoma
        2. Adrenocortical carcinoma
        3. Wilms' tumor
        4. Neuroblastoma
        5. Others
     B. Cyanotic congenital heart disease

Author: **Craig C. Orlowski, M.D.**

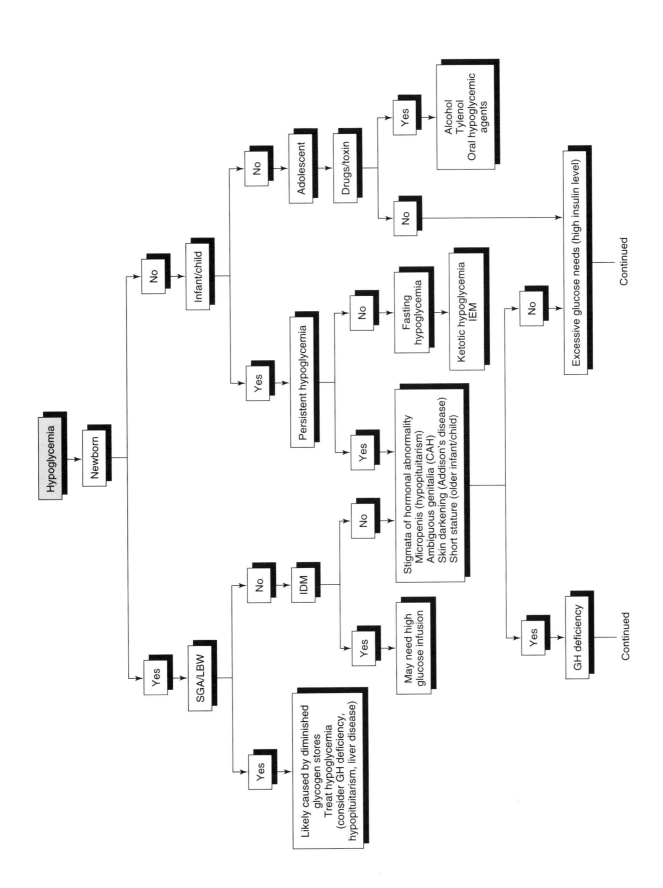

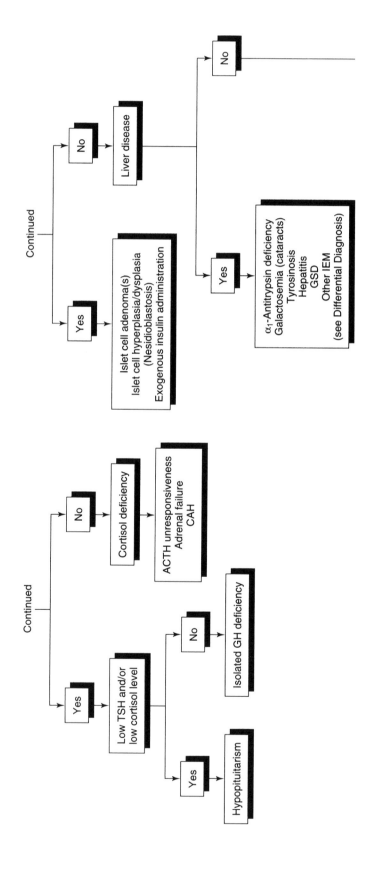

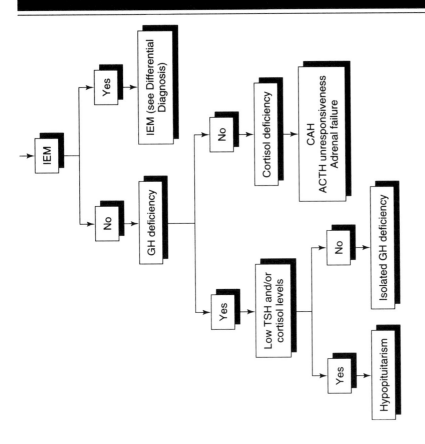

ACTH, Adrenocorticotropic hormone; *CAH*, congenital adrenal hyperplasia; *GH*, growth hormone; *GSD*, glycogen storage disease; *IDM*, infant of diabetic mother; *IEM*, inborn error of metabolism; *LBW*, low birth weight; *SGA*, small for gestational age; *TSH*, thyroid-stimulating hormone.

HYPOTONIA

■ **DEFINITION**

Decreased resistance to passive movement. It is usually associated with joint hypermobility and decreased reflexes. It may or may not be associated with weakness (diminished muscle power).

■ **DIFFERENTIAL DIAGNOSIS**

  I. **Generalized brain insults**
    A. Hypoxic-ischemic encephalopathy
    B. Postseizure
    C. Sepsis
    D. Meningitis
    E. Hypotonic cerebral palsy

  II. **Spinal cord disorders**
    A. Trauma
    B. Spinal dysraphism
      1. Meningomyelocele
    C. Abscess
    D. Neoplasm
    E. Transverse myelitis
    F. Anterior horn cell disorders
      1. Spinal muscular atrophy (Werdnig-Hoffman disease)
      2. Polio/other enteroviral infections

  III. **Peripheral nervous system disorders**
    A. Acute
      1. Guillain-Barré syndrome
    B. Chronic
      1. Hereditary motor sensory neuropathy
        a. Charcot-Marie-Tooth disease
        b. Refsum's disease
      2. Leukodystrophies

  IV. **Neuromuscular junction disorders**
    A. Botulism
    B. Myasthenia gravis
    C. Tick paralysis

  V. **Muscle disorders**
    A. Myopathies
      1. Congenital
      2. Mitochondrial
      3. Metabolic
        a. Glycogen storage diseases
        b. Carnitine deficiency
    B. Periodic paralysis
      1. Hypokalemic
      2. Hyperkalemic
      3. Normokalemic
    C. Muscular dystrophies
      1. Congenital
      2. Duchenne's muscular dystrophy
      3. Becker muscular dystrophy
      4. Limb-Girdle muscular dystrophy
      5. Fascioscapulohumeral muscular dystrophy
    D. Myotonic dystrophy
      1. Congenital
      2. Later onset
    E. Dermatomyositis
    F. Polymyositis

  VI. **Metabolic disorders**
    A. Amino acid disorders
    B. Organic acid disorders
      1. Methylmalonic acidemia
      2. Propionic acidemia
    C. Lipidoses (e.g., Tay-Sachs disease, Niemann-Pick disease)
    D. Leukodystrophies (e.g., Krabbe's disease)
    E. Mucopolysaccharidoses
    F. Mucolipidoses
    G. Peroxisomal disorders

  VII. **Endocrine disorders**
    A. Hypothyroidism
    B. Hypopituitarism

  VIII. **Chromosomal disorders and syndromes**
    A. Down syndrome
    B. Achondroplasia
    C. Ehlers-Danlos syndrome
    D. Marfan's syndrome
    E. Opitz syndrome
    F. Prader-Willi syndrome
    G. Velocardiofacial (Shprintzen's) syndrome
    H. Sotos' syndrome
    I. Others

  IX. **Benign essential hypotonia**

Author: **Jeffrey Kaczorowski, M.D.**

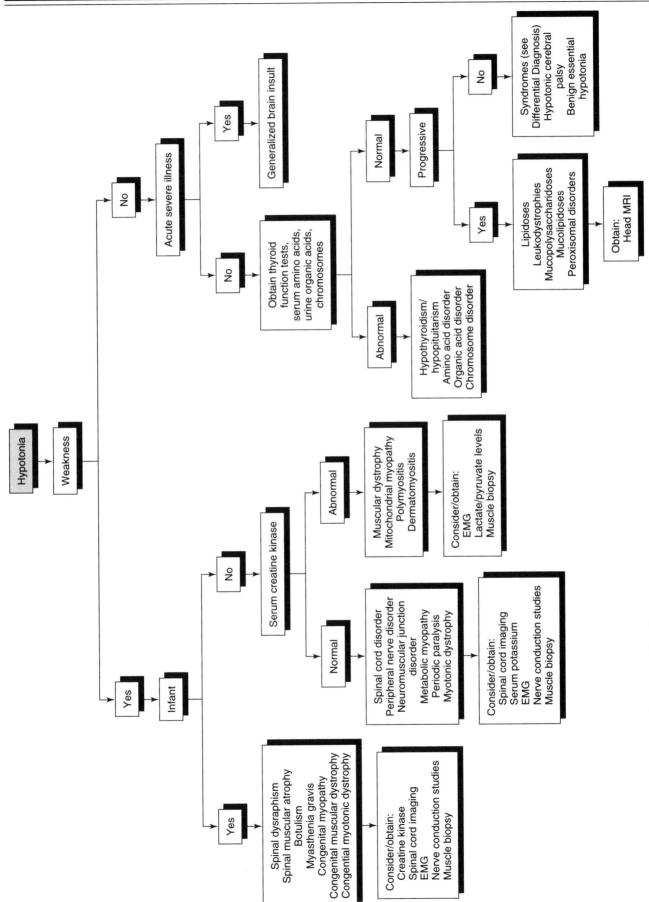

EMG, Electromyograph; *MRI*, magnetic resonance imaging.

JAUNDICE/HYPERBILIRUBINEMIA

■ DEFINITION

Jaundice refers to the yellow color of the skin and sclera caused by hyperbilirubinemia. Bilirubin is a breakdown product of heme, derived from red blood cells. Bilirubin is carried to the liver by albumin, where it is conjugated by glucuronyl transferase to a water-soluble form. Bilirubin is then excreted into the small intestine as bile and eliminated in the stool. *Hyperbilirubinemia* is classified as either unconjugated (indirect) hyperbilirubinemia or conjugated (direct—because it is directly measured) hyperbilirubinemia.

■ DIFFERENTIAL DIAGNOSIS: UNCONJUGATED HYPERBILIRUBINEMIA

Neonatal

I. Physiologic jaundice

II. Increased bilirubin production
   A. Cephalohematoma or other bleeding with resorption of heme
   B. Polycythemia
      1. Delayed umbilical cord clamping
      2. Twin-to-twin transfusion
      3. Maternal-fetal transfusion
      4. Maternal diabetes
   C. Isoimmunization
      1. Rh
      2. ABO
      3. Other
   D. Red blood cell enzyme defects
      1. Glucose-6-phosphate dehydrogenase deficiency
      2. Pyruvate kinase deficiency
      3. Other
   E. Red blood cell membrane defects
      1. Hereditary spherocytosis
      2. Hereditary elliptocytosis
      3. Other

III. Decreased bilirubin conjugation
   A. Glucuronyl transferase deficiency (Crigler-Najjar syndrome)
      1. Type I
      2. Type II
   B. Transient familial hyperbilirubinemia (Lucey-Driscoll syndrome)

IV. Decreased intestinal elimination
   A. Intestinal obstruction
      1. Pyloric stenosis
      2. Duodenal atresia
      3. Ileal atresia
      4. Other
   B. Lack of feeding
   C. Delayed passage of meconium
      1. Hirschsprung's disease
      2. Meconium ileus

V. Other
   A. Breastmilk-associated jaundice
   B. Hypothyroidism
   C. Hypoalbuminemia
   D. Drugs
      1. Sulfa drugs
      2. Cephalosporins
   E. Sepsis
   F. Hypoxia/acidosis

Postneonatal

I. Increased bilirubin production
   A. Hemolytic anemia
   B. Sepsis

II. Decreased bilirubin conjugation
   A. Gilbert's disease
   B. Glucuronyl transferase deficiency (Crigler-Najjar syndrome)

■ DIFFERENTIAL DIAGNOSIS: CONJUGATED HYPERBILIRUBINEMIA

Neonatal/Infancy

I. Infectious
   A. Toxoplasmosis
   B. Rubella
   C. Cytomegalovirus
   D. Herpes
   E. Syphilis
   F. Varicella-zoster virus
   G. Enterovirus
   H. Hepatitis B virus
   I. Sepsis/bacterial agents
   J. Urinary tract infection

II. **Biliary obstruction**
  A. Intrahepatic
    1. Congenital biliary atresia (hypoplasia of intrahepatic biliary ducts)
    2. Alagille syndrome
    3. Byler syndrome
  B. Extrahepatic
    1. Biliary atresia
    2. Congenital malformations of the biliary tree

III. **Total parenteral nutrition**

IV. **Metabolic disorders**
  A. α_1-Antitrypsin deficiency
  B. Cystic fibrosis
  C. Zellweger syndrome
  D. Galactosemia
  E. Glycogen storage disease
  F. Hereditary fructose intolerance
  G. Tyrosinemia
  H. Lipidoses: Niemann-Pick disease, Gaucher's disease, others
  I. Neonatal hemosiderosis

V. **Others**
  A. Idiopathic neonatal hepatitis
  B. Inspissated bile syndrome (persistent direct hyperbilirubinemia associated with isoimmune hemolytic disease)
  C. Postasphyxia

Postinfancy
  I. **Infectious**
    A. Hepatitis A, B, C, D, and E
    B. Epstein-Barr virus
    C. Cytomegalovirus
    D. Varicella-zoster virus
    E. Peritonitis
    F. Parasitic infections
    G. Liver abscess

II. **Chronic hepatitis**
  A. Chronic persistent hepatitis
  B. Chronic active hepatitis

III. **Drugs/chemicals**
  A. Acetaminophen
  B. Phenytoin
  C. Isoniazid
  D. Carbon tetrachloride
  E. Mushroom poisoning
  F. Chemotherapy agents
  G. Alcohol
  H. Others

IV. **Biliary tract disease**
  A. Cholelithiasis
  B. Cholecystitis
  C. Choledochal cyst
  D. Cholangitis
  E. Pancreatic malformations or disease

V. **Familial hepatic disorders**
  A. Dubin-Johnson syndrome
  B. Rotor's syndrome

VI. **Total parenteral nutrition**

VII. **Cirrhosis**

VIII. **Neoplasms**
  A. Primary hepatic
  B. Metastatic

IX. **Metabolic disorders**
  A. Wilson's disease
  B. Hemochromatosis
  C. Neonatal causes listed in preceding section

X. **Other**
  A. Reye's syndrome
  B. Ischemic liver injury
  C. Porphyria

Author: **Jeffrey Kaczorowski, M.D.**

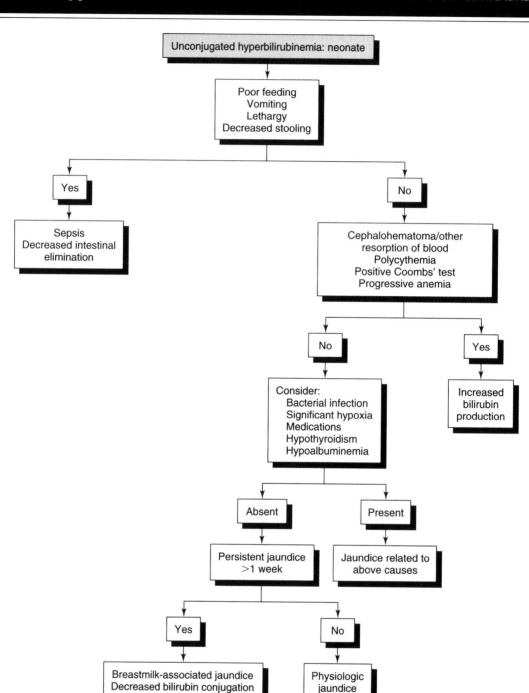

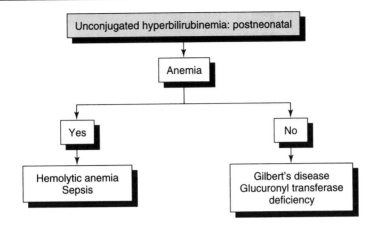

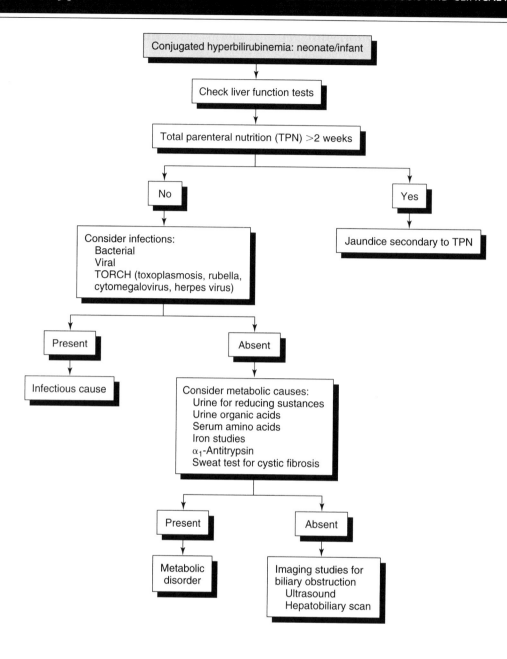

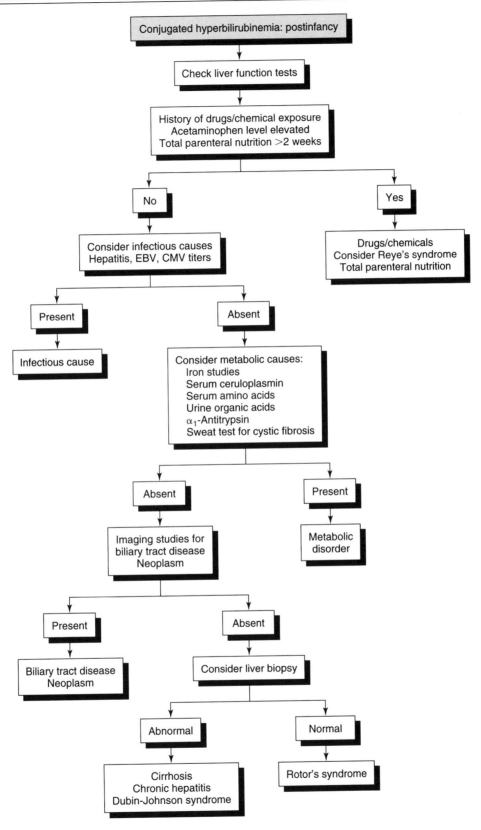

CMV, Cytomegalovirus; EBV, Epstein-Barr virus.

LIMP

■ **DEFINITION**

A limp is an abnormal gait with jerky movements. The differential diagnosis is extensive, with causes ranging from the spine to the foot to the central nervous system to soft tissue abnormalities.

I. **Leg length inequality**
   A. Congenital abnormality
   B. Hip dislocation, developmental dysplasia of the hip
   C. Bony malformation

II. **Neuromuscular disorders**
   A. Myalgia
   B. Trauma
   C. Recent intramuscular immunization
   D. Spinal cord neuropathy
   E. Patellofemoral syndrome
   F. Osgood-Schlatter disease
   G. Cerebral palsy

III. **Bone disorders**
   A. Legg-Calvé-Perthes (avascular necrosis of the femoral head)
   B. Slipped capital femoral epiphysis
   C. Osteochondritis dissecans

IV. **Infection**
   A. Arthritis (knee, hip, ankle)
   B. Bursitis
   C. Toxic synovitis
   D. Discitis
   E. Toxoplasmosis
   F. Trichinosis
   G. Osteomyelitis
   H. Plantar wart

V. **Systemic disorders**
   A. Systemic lupus erythematosus
   B. Acute rheumatic fever
   C. Polyarteritis nodosa
   D. Rheumatoid arthritis
   E. Polymyositis
   F. Dermatomyositis
   G. Thrombophlebitis
   H. Sickle cell disease

VI. **Neoplasm**
   A. Leukemia
   B. Neuroblastoma
   C. Osteogenic sarcoma
   D. Ewing's sarcoma

VII. **Trauma**
   A. Fracture (spine, pelvis, femur, tibia, fibula, any foot or toe bones)
   B. Stress fracture
   C. Sprain
   D. Injury to cartilage or ligaments
   E. Tendinitis
   F. Muscle strain
   G. Foreign body

Author: **Cynthia Christy, M.D.**

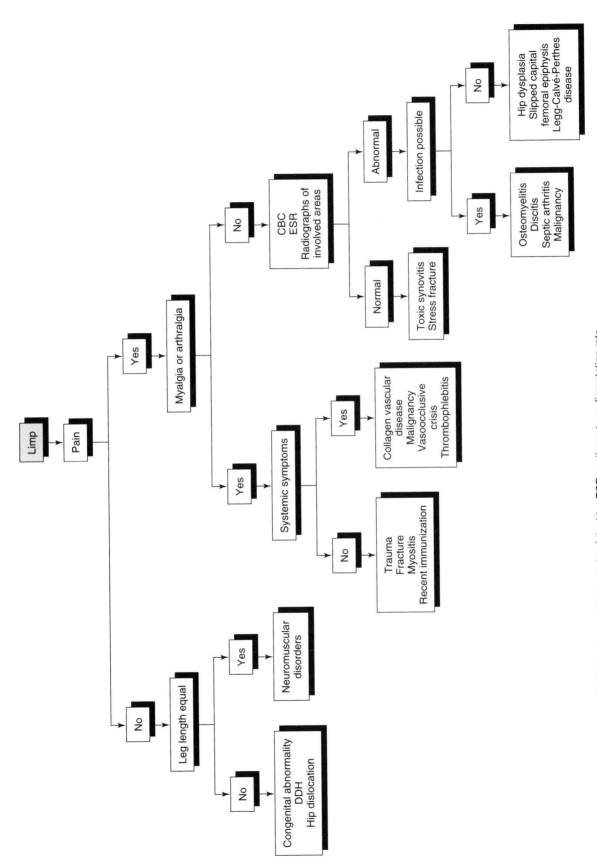

CBC, Complete blood count; *DDH*, developmental dysplasia of the hip; *ESR*, erythrocyte sedimentation rate.

MACROCEPHALY

■ DEFINITION

Large head size, generally defined as greater than the 99th percentile for age and sex on charts of head circumference. *Megalencephaly* refers to large brain size and is usually determined by radiologic studies.

■ DIFFERENTIAL DIAGNOSIS

I. Normal variation (familial)

II. Hydrocephalus
A. Noncommunicating hydrocephalus (obstruction within the ventricular system)
 1. Aqueductal stenosis
 2. Dandy-Walker malformation
 3. Masses (tumors, vascular malformations, arachnoid cysts)
B. Communicating hydrocephalus (block in resorption of cerebrospinal fluid)
 1. Arnold-Chiari malformations
 2. Sequelae of meningitis or intracranial hemorrhage
C. Excessive secretion of cerebrospinal fluid (CSF)
 1. Choroid plexus papilloma

III. Hydranencephaly (congenital malformation with absence of the cerebral hemispheres, replaced by CSF) and porencephaly (congenital malformation with cavities in the brain filled with CSF)

IV. Subdural hematoma

V. Tumor

VI. Pseudotumor cerebri (benign intracranial hypertension)

VII. Vascular malformation
A. Vein of Galen malformation
B. Arteriovenous malformation

VIII. Neurocutaneous syndromes
A. Neurofibromatosis
B. Tuberous sclerosis
C. Sturge-Weber syndrome

IX. Megalencephaly
A. Genetic/syndromic causes
 1. Achondroplasia
 2. Hypochondroplasia
 3. Sotos' syndrome
 4. Fragile X syndrome
 5. Weaver syndrome
B. Metabolic disorders
 1. Gangliosidoses (e.g., Tay-Sachs disease)
 2. Mucopolysaccharidoses
 3. Alexander disease
 4. Canavan's disease

X. Abnormal skull
A. Chronic, severe anemia
B. Genetic/syndromic causes
 1. Osteopetrosis syndromes

Author: **Jeffrey Kaczorowski, M.D.**

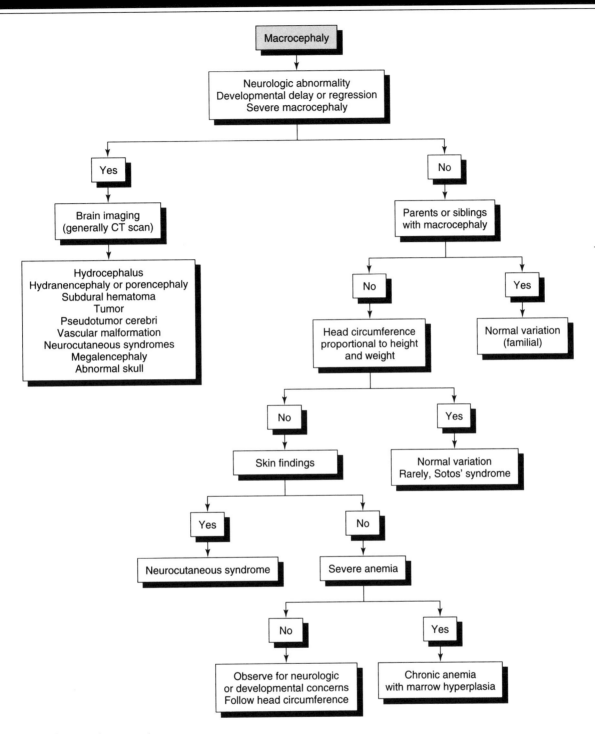

CT, Computed tomography.

MICROCEPHALY

■ **DEFINITION**

Head size less than the 1st percentile for age and sex on charts of head circumference.

■ **DIFFERENTIAL DIAGNOSIS**

I. **Normal variation**

II. **Genetic/syndromic causes**
   A. Autosomal dominant microcephaly
   B. Autosomal recessive microcephaly
   C. Chromosomal abnormalities
      1. Trisomy 21
      2. Trisomy 13
      3. Trisomy 18
      4. 5p-
   D. Dysmorphic syndromes
      1. Williams syndrome
      2. Velocardiofacial syndrome (Shprintzen's syndrome)
      3. Smith-Lemli-Opitz syndrome
      4. Angelman's syndrome
      5. Bloom syndrome
      6. Others

III. **Structural defects of the brain**
   A. Cerebral dysgenesis or hypoplasia

IV. **Infections**
   A. Congenital
      1. Rubella
      2. Cytomegalovirus
      3. Toxoplasmosis
      4. Herpes simplex virus
      5. Syphilis
   B. Meningitis (sequela)

V. **Trauma**

VI. **Radiation**

VII. **Hypoxic/ischemic insult**

VIII. **Malnutrition**

IX. **Maternal causes**
   A. Drugs
      1. Fetal alcohol syndrome
      2. Fetal hydantoin syndrome
      3. Fetal aminopterin syndrome
   B. Maternal phenylketonuria
   C. Severe maternal malnutrition

X. **Craniosynostosis**

Author: **Jeffrey Kaczorowski, M.D.**

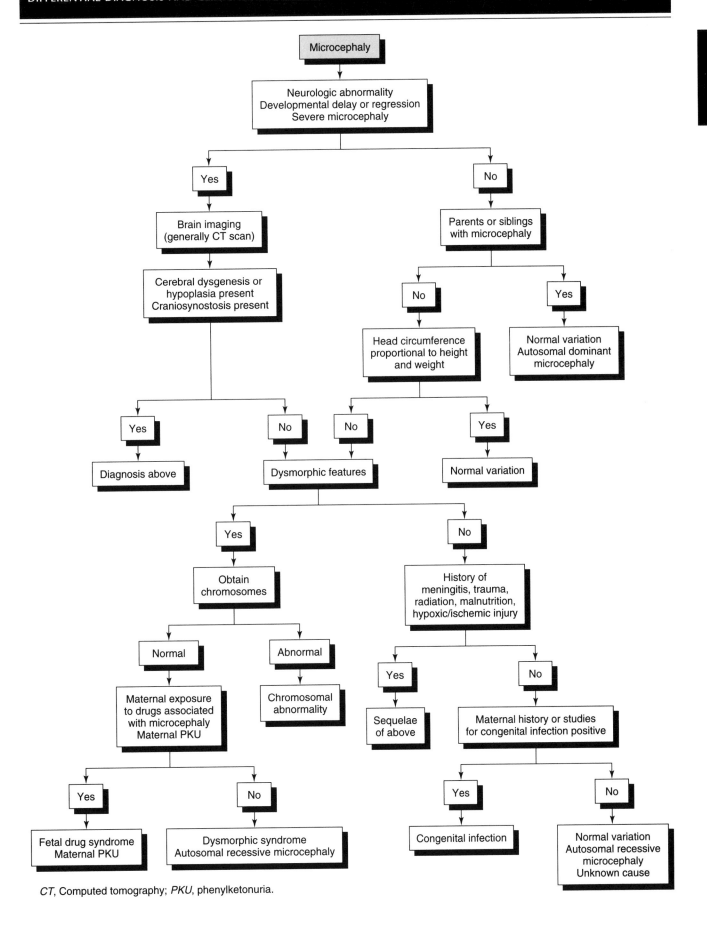

CT, Computed tomography; *PKU*, phenylketonuria.

NASAL DISCHARGE/RHINORRHEA

■ **DEFINITION**

Rhinorrhea refers to discharge from the nose. *Rhinitis* refers specifically to inflammation of the mucous membranes of the nose and may be caused by infectious and noninfectious processes.

■ **DIFFERENTIAL DIAGNOSIS**

I. **Infectious**
   A. Viral
   B. Bacterial/sinusitis

II. **Allergic**

III. **Irritant**
   A. Smoke, especially from cigarettes
   B. Cocaine
   C. Topical sympathomimetic nose drops
   D. Other

IV. **Foreign body**

V. **Cerebrospinal fluid**
   A. Trauma
   B. Skull defect

Author: **Jeffrey Kaczorowski, M.D.**

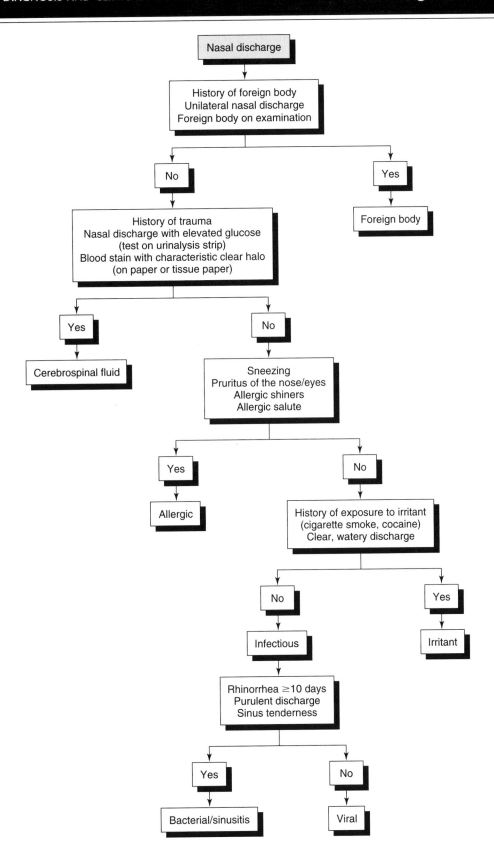

NECK MASS

■ DEFINITION

Most neck masses in children are enlarged lymph nodes caused by infection. *Lymphadenitis* is inflammation of a lymph node or nodes associated with enlargement, warmth, redness, tenderness, and sometimes fluctuance. *Lymphadenopathy* is enlarged, noninflamed lymph nodes.

■ DIFFERENTIAL DIAGNOSIS

I. Infection
A. Lymphadenitis
 1. Bacterial
  a. *Staphylococcus aureus*
  b. Group A streptococcus
  c. Cat-scratch disease *(Bartonella henselae)*
  d. Group B streptococcus
  e. Anaerobes
 2. Viral
 3. Fungal
 4. Mycobacterial
B. Local lymphadenopathy (head or neck infection)
C. Systemic lymphadenopathy
  a. Mononucleosis
  b. Cytomegalovirus
  c. Toxoplasmosis
  d. Human immunodeficiency virus
  e. Other
D. Salivary gland infection
 1. Parotitis
E. Infection of congenital anomaly/tract (see the following)

II. Congenital anomalies
A. Branchial cleft
B. Thyroglossal duct cyst
C. Dermoid cyst
D. Laryngocele
E. Cystic hygroma/lymphangioma
F. Fibrous dysplasia of the sternocleidomastoid (torticollis)

G. Squamous epithelial cyst

III. Thyroid
A. Thyroiditis
 1. Autoimmune (Hashimoto's disease)
 2. Bacterial
 3. Viral
B. Graves disease (hyperthyroidism)
C. Neoplasm
D. Idiopathic enlargement
E. Congenital
 1. Defective thyroid hormone synthesis
 2. Maternal Graves disease
 3. Maternal antithyroid drugs

IV. Tumor
A. Hemangioma
B. Neurofibroma
C. Keloid
D. Lipoma
E. Leukemia
F. Lymphoma
G. Neuroblastoma
H. Rhabdomyosarcoma
I. Histiocytosis X
J. Salivary gland tumor
K. Thyroid (as in preceding section)

V. Trauma
A. Hematoma
B. Subcutaneous emphysema
C. Foreign body

VI. Allergic reaction
A. Local bite or sting

VII. Other causes of lymphadenopathy
A. Kawasaki syndrome
B. Serum sickness
C. Collagen vascular disease

Author: **Jeffrey Kaczorowski, M.D.**

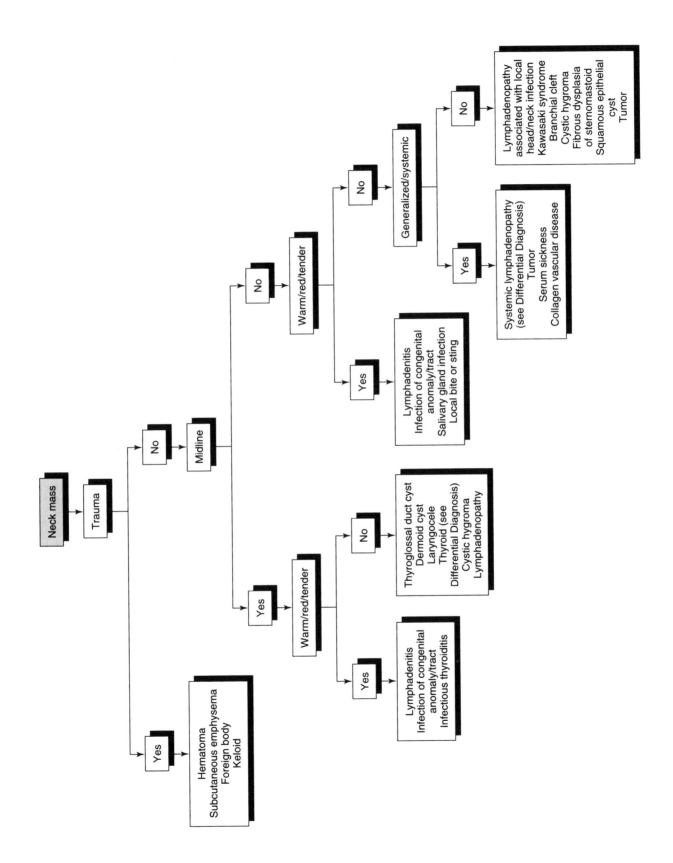

PINK EYE/RED EYE

■ DEFINITION

Erythema of the bulbar conjunctivae (conjunctivitis), often involving the cornea (keratitis).

■ DIFFERENTIAL DIAGNOSIS

I. Trauma
   A. Blunt
      1. Traumatic iritis—photophobia, decreased vision, small pupil
      2. Traumatic hyphema—blood in anterior chamber, which may make the cornea appear dark red
   B. Perforating trauma—obvious deformity to globe
   C. Corneal abrasion—use fluorescein and examine with Wood's lamp to assess for abrasions
   D. Burn
      1. Chemical
         a. Alkali and acid—alkali severe because of ongoing protein discoagulation
         b. Silver nitrate
         c. Petroleum
         d. Super glue/Crazy glue—no long-term damage but may take some time to resolve
      2. Thermal
   E. Foreign body

II. Congenital abnormality
   A. Nasolacrimal duct obstruction—usually epiphora (tear overflow onto cheek) and accumulation of mucoid discharge, with mild or no redness
   B. Congenital glaucoma—conjunctival injection late, with large eye, light sensitivity, excessive tear production, change in clarity of cornea

III. Infectious causes
   A. Conjunctivitis
      1. Viral
         a. Adenovirus
         b. Herpes virus
         c. Influenza virus
         d. Measles virus
      2. Bacterial
         a. *Haemophilus influenzae* (usually nontypable *H. influenzae*)
         b. *Streptococcus pneumoniae*
         c. *Staphylococcus aureus*
         d. Gonococcal
         e. Chlamydial

      3. Other
         a. Molluscum on lid may lead to inflammation of cornea and conjunctivae.
         b. Phthirus pubis (pubic lice) of eyelashes may present as conjunctivitis from feces of louse irritation on eye.
   B. Keratitis
      1. Dendritic
      2. Epidemic keratoconjunctivitis (adenovirus)

IV. Inflammatory
   A. Keratoconjunctivitis sicca—associated with collagen vascular diseases
   B. Uveitis—photophobia, tearing, deep aching, and prominent perilimbal blood vessels
   C. Episcleritis—mild patchy inflammation of tissue beneath conjunctiva
   D. Scleritis—patchy inflammation of sclera, severe pain

V. Allergic causes
   A. Immediate—itching is the hallmark
      1. Hayfever—rapid injection, chemosis, tearing, itching
   B. Delayed
      1. Contact dermatitis—eye cosmetics; usually lid erythema and edema without conjunctival infection
   C. Vernal conjunctivitis—recurring inflammation, presumed allergic, typically occurs in warm weather

VI. Orbital cellulitis—signs of orbital involvement, including proptosis, chemosis, diplopia (or inability to move eye), and pain with eye movement are all as, or more prominent than, injection

VII. Systemic diseases
   A. Ataxia telangiectasia—large tortuous vessels on bulbar conjunctiva
   B. Lyme disease—nonspecific conjunctivitis may be present before onset of erythema chronicum migrans
   C. Juvenile arthritis—anterior uveitis or iritis: perilimbal conjunctival injection
   D. Kawasaki syndrome—associated with conjunctivitis that spares the perilimbal area
   E. Leukemia
   F. Inflammatory bowel disease
   G. Stevens-Johnson syndrome

Author: **Lynn C. Garfunkel, M.D.**

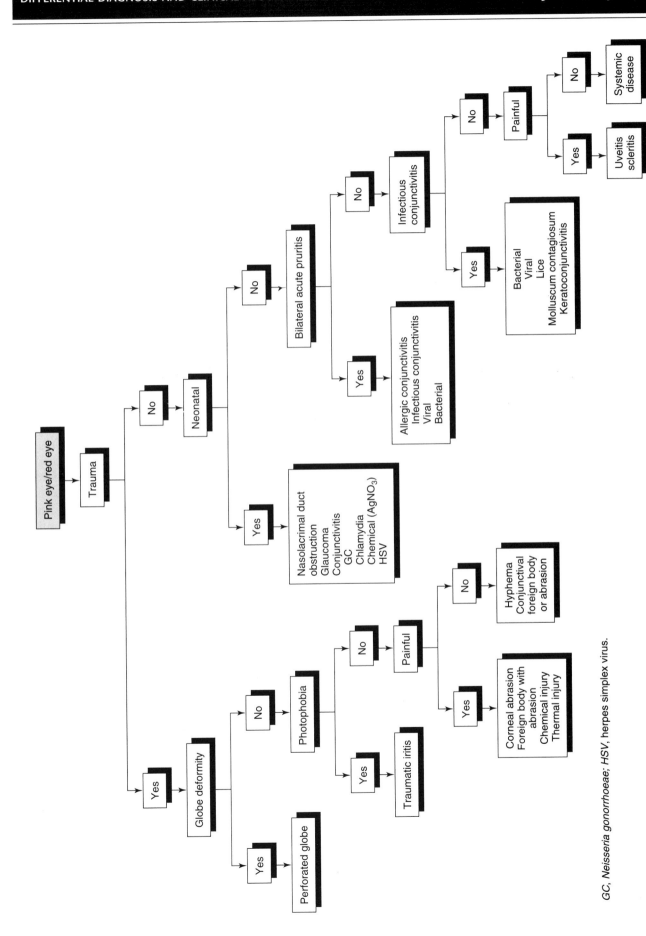

GC, Neisseria gonorrhoeae; HSV, herpes simplex virus.

PROTEINURIA—ISOLATED

■ DEFINITION

Transient proteinuria is seen in up to 12% of children; only 0.5% to 5% have persistent proteinuria. Urinary protein excretion is considered abnormal if it exceeds 4 mg/m^2/hr. This corresponds approximately to 2+ or greater protein on urine dipstick. Sulfosalicylic acid testing (combining sulfosalicylic acid with urine) is more reliable: increasing turbidity indicates protein and is graded from 1 to 4. A urine protein:creatinine ratio of greater than 0.2 on a random urine sample suggests significant proteinuria. A 24-hour urine collection is the most accurate method of protein detection. *Nephrotic range proteinuria* is urinary protein excretion of 40 mg/m^2/hr or greater.

Proteinuria may be seen with or without hematuria. Disorders involving both hematuria and proteinuria are discussed in the section "Hematuria." The differential diagnosis and algorithm presented here are strictly for isolated proteinuria.

■ DIFFERENTIAL DIAGNOSIS

   I. Persistent benign proteinuria

   II. Orthostatic (postural) proteinuria

   III. Fever

   IV. Dehydration

   V. Vigorous exercise

   VI. Extreme cold

   VII. Congestive heart failure

   VIII. Drugs/toxins
   A. Aminoglycosides
   B. Heavy metals
   C. Nonsteroidal antiinflammatory agents
   D. Captopril
   E. Lithium
   F. Outdated tetracycline

   IX. Nephrotic syndrome
   A. Minimal change disease
   B. Focal segmental glomerulosclerosis
   C. Membranous nephropathy
   D. Congenital nephrotic syndrome

   X. Congenital or structural anomalies
   A. Renal dysplasia
   B. Polycystic kidney disease
   C. Cystic kidneys
   D. Vesicoureteral reflux
   E. Obstructive uropathy

   XI. Pregnancy (preeclampsia, eclampsia)

   XII. Excessive serum protein
   A. Leukemias
   B. Myeloma
   C. Myoglobinuria
   D. Hemoglobinuria

Author: **Jeffrey Kaczorowski, M.D.**

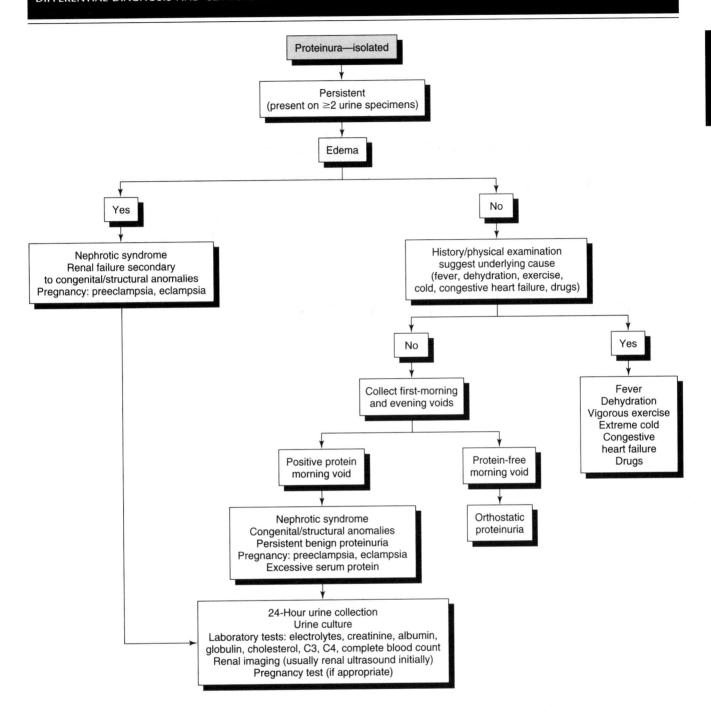

PURPURA

■ **DEFINITION**

Nonblanching skin lesions caused by hemorrhage into the skin. Purpura can be divided into petechiae and ecchymoses. *Petechiae* are less than 3 mm in size and macular. *Ecchymoses* are greater than 3 mm and may be macular or raised. Ecchymoses may also be tender. Purpura can be caused by disruption of vascular integrity, platelet deficiency or dysfunction, or coagulation defects. (See also Fever and Petechia differential diagnosis.)

■ **DIFFERENTIAL DIAGNOSIS**

I. Disruption of vascular integrity
  A. Trauma
    1. Accidental
    2. Abuse
    3. Violent coughing or vomiting
    4. Coining or cupping
    5. Iatrogenic (blood draws or intravenous line placement)
    6. Self-inflicted
  B. Infections
    1. Viral
    2. Group A streptococcus
    3. Sepsis
      a. *Neisseria meningitidis*
      b. *Neisseria gonorrhoeae*
      c. *Haemophilus influenzae* type B
      d. *Staphylococcus aureus*
      e. Others
    4. Bacterial endocarditis
    5. Rocky Mountain spotted fever (and other rickettsial diseases)
    6. Hemorrhagic fevers caused by arenaviruses and bunyaviruses (hantaviruses)
  C. Drugs
    1. Corticosteroids
  D. Vasculitis
    1. Henoch-Schönlein purpura
    2. Collagen vascular disorders
    3. Osler-Rendu-Weber disease (hereditary hemorrhagic telangiectasia)
  E. Connective tissue diseases
    1. Ehlers-Danlos syndrome
    2. Marfan's syndrome
    3. Osteogenesis imperfecta
  F. Other systemic diseases
    1. Vitamin C deficiency (scurvy)
    2. Histiocytosis X
    3. Erythema nodosum
    4. Cushing's syndrome
    5. Ataxia telangiectasia

II. Platelet deficiency (thrombocytopenia)
  A. Increased destruction of platelets
    1. Maternal-fetal
      a. Isoimmune thrombocytopenia (PlA 1 antigen)
      b. Maternal idiopathic thrombocytopenic purpura
      c. Maternal systemic lupus erythematosus
    2. Immune mediated
      a. Idiopathic thrombocytopenic purpura
      b. Drug induced
        (1) Sulfa drugs
        (2) Phenytoin
        (3) Carbamazepine
        (4) Acetazolamide
        (5) Quinidine
      c. Collagen vascular diseases (especially systemic lupus erythematosus)

3. Microangiopathic disorders
   a. Hemolytic uremic syndrome
   b. Thrombotic thrombocytopenic purpura
   c. Disseminated intravascular coagulation
4. Wiskott-Aldrich syndrome
5. Giant platelet disorders
   a. May-Hegglin anomaly
   b. Bernard-Soulier syndrome
B. Decreased production of platelets
1. Bone marrow infiltration
   a. Leukemia
   b. Neuroblastoma
   c. Other malignancies
   d. Osteopetrosis
2. Bone marrow suppression
   a. Sepsis
   b. Viral
   c. Congenital infections (syphilis, toxoplasmosis)
   d. Drugs
   e. Radiation
   f. Acquired aplastic anemia
   g. Congenital aplastic anemia (Fanconi's anemia)
3. Thrombocytopenia absent radius syndrome

C. Sequestration of platelets
1. Hypersplenism
2. Kasabach-Merritt syndrome (large hemangioma)

III. **Platelet dysfunction**
A. Congenital
   1. Bernard-Soulier syndrome
   2. Glanzmann's thrombasthenia
   3. Gray platelet syndrome
   4. Storage pool disorders
B. Acquired/drug induced
   1. Aspirin

IV. **Coagulation defect**
A. Vitamin K deficiency
B. Coagulation factor abnormalities
   1. Factor VIII deficiency (hemophilia A)
   2. Factor IX deficiency (hemophilia B, Christmas disease)
   3. von Willebrand disease
   4. Dysfibrinogenemias (factor I)
   5. Others
C. Liver disease
D. Disseminated intravascular coagulation
E. Drugs
   1. Warfarin
   2. Heparin
F. Anticoagulants associated with collagen vascular disease or malignancy

Author: **Jeffrey Kaczorowski, M.D.**

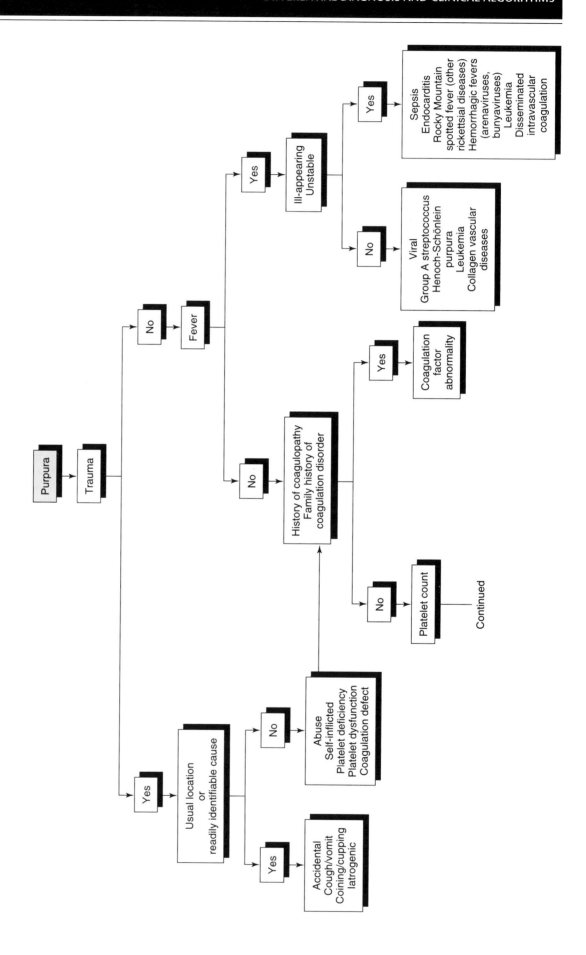

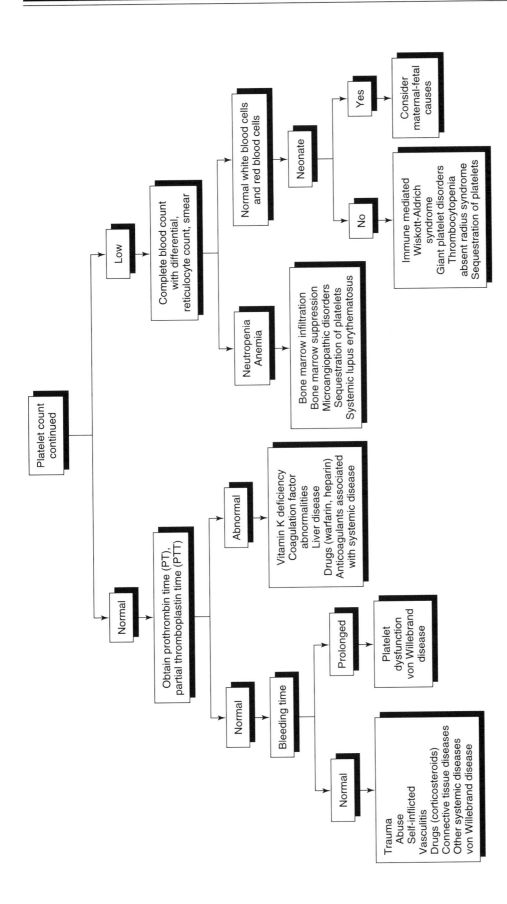

Platelet count continued

- Low
  - Complete blood count with differential, reticulocyte count, smear
    - Normal white blood cells and red blood cells
      - Neonate
        - Yes
          - Consider maternal-fetal causes
        - No
          - Immune mediated
            Wiskott-Aldrich syndrome
            Giant platelet disorders
            Thrombocytopenia
            absent radius syndrome
            Sequestration of platelets
    - Neutropenia Anemia
      - Bone marrow infiltration
        Bone marrow suppression
        Microangiopathic disorders
        Sequestration of platelets
        Systemic lupus erythematosus
- Normal
  - Obtain prothrombin time (PT), partial thromboplastin time (PTT)
    - Abnormal
      - Vitamin K deficiency
        Coagulation factor abnormalities
        Liver disease
        Drugs (warfarin, heparin)
        Anticoagulants associated with systemic disease
    - Normal
      - Bleeding time
        - Prolonged
          - Platelet dysfunction
            von Willebrand disease
        - Normal
          - Trauma
            Abuse
            Self-inflicted
            Vasculitis
            Drugs (corticosteroids)
            Connective tissue diseases
            Other systemic diseases
            von Willebrand disease

SCROTAL SWELLING

■ DEFINITION

Swelling in the scrotum may be caused by scrotal skin edema, fluid within the scrotal sac, or enlargement of the testis itself. The presence or absence of pain is the most useful characteristic in determining the cause of scrotal swelling/enlargement.

■ DIFFERENTIAL DIAGNOSIS

I. **Painful**
   A. Torsion of the testis
   B. Torsion of the appendix testis
   C. Trauma
      1. Hematoma
      2. Ruptured testis
      3. Minor trauma
   D. Epididymitis
   E. Orchitis
   F. Incarcerated inguinal hernia
   G. Scrotal cellulitis
   H. Contact dermatitis

II. **Painless**
   A. Hydrocele
   B. Inguinal hernia
   C. Varicocele
   D. Edema
      1. Henoch-Schönlein purpura
      2. Generalized edema
      3. Idiopathic scrotal edema
   E. Tumor
      1. Younger than 2 years of age: yolk sac carcinoma
      2. After puberty: germinal cell tumor
   F. Antenatal torsion of the testis (newborn)

Author: **Jeffrey Kaczorowski, M.D.**

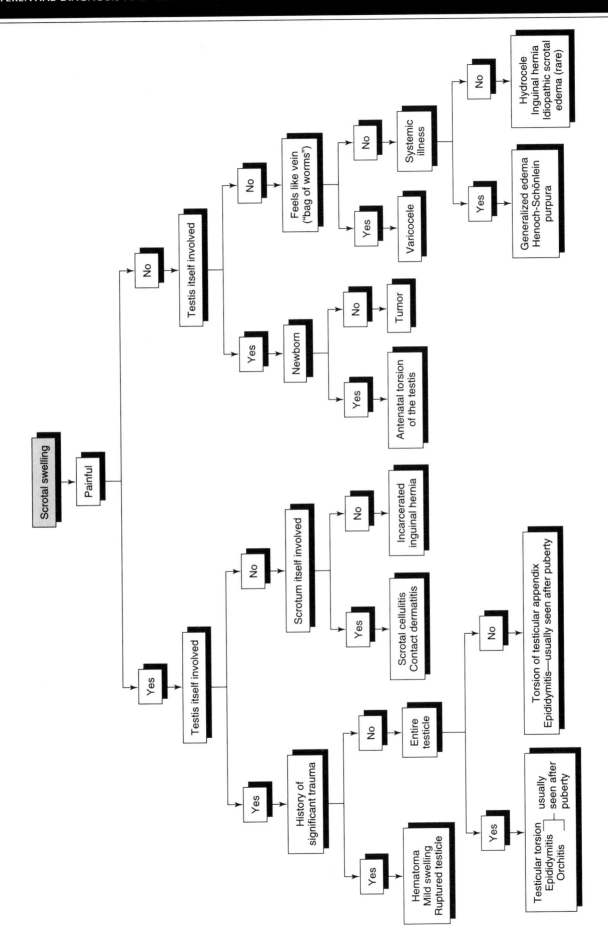

SEIZURES

■ **DEFINITION**

A *seizure* is an abnormal discharge of neurons in the cerebral cortex, generally manifested by motor, sensory, or autonomic dysfunction, with or without loss of consciousness. Seizures can sometimes be difficult to distinguish from syncope (see Table 1-2 in the section "Syncope") and other nonseizure movements (see the section "Seizures" in Part II). Seizures during childhood are most often febrile or idiopathic; an underlying cause is often not present. In the newborn period, most seizures have an underlying cause—and every effort should be made to determine the cause.

■ **DIFFERENTIAL DIAGNOSIS**

Neonatal

   I. **Infectious**
      A. Meningitis
      B. Encephalitis
         1. Herpes viruses
         2. Enteroviruses
         3. Other congenital infections
      C. Sepsis

   II. **Central nervous system/neurologic**
      A. Congenital anomalies, including chromosomal abnormalities
      B. Intracranial hemorrhage
      C. Vascular anomalies
      D. Embolus/infarction
      E. Venous thrombosis
      F. Hypoxic ischemic encephalopathy
      G. Bilirubin encephalopathy

   III. **Metabolic**
      A. Hypoglycemia
      B. Hypocalcemia
      C. Hypomagnesemia
      D. Hyponatremia
      E. Hypernatremia
      F. Uremia
      G. Inborn errors of metabolism

   IV. **Drug withdrawal**

   V. **Hypertension**

   VI. **Idiopathic (uncommon)**

Postneonatal

   I. **Infectious**
      A. Meningitis
      B. Encephalitis
      C. Brain abscess
      D. Parasites

   II. **Central nervous system/neurologic**
      A. Intracranial hemorrhage
      B. Tumor
      C. Cerebral contusion
      D. Congenital malformation
      E. Hypoxia/ischemia
      F. Vascular anomalies
      G. Embolus/infarction
      H. Vasculitis
      I. Venous thrombosis

III. **Metabolic**
   A. Hypoglycemia
   B. Hypocalcemia
   C. Hypomagnesemia
   D. Hyponatremia
   E. Hypernatremia
   F. Uremia
   G. Inborn errors of metabolism

IV. **Drugs/toxins**
   A. Intoxication
   B. Withdrawal

V. **Hypertension**

VI. **Neurocutaneous syndromes**
   A. Neurofibromatosis
   B. Tuberous sclerosis
   C. Sturge-Weber syndrome
   D. Epidermal nevus syndrome
   E. Others

VII. **Degenerative cerebral disorders**
   A. Lipidoses (e.g., Tay-Sachs disease, Niemann-Pick disease)
   B. Leukodystrophies (e.g., Krabbe's disease)
   C. Mucopolysaccharidoses
   D. Mucolipidoses

   E. Glycoprotein disorders
   F. Peroxisomal disorders
   G. Mitochondrial disorders
   H. Others

VIII. **Idiopathic (common)**

IX. **Febrile**

X. **Eclampsia**

XI. **Movements that may be confused with seizures**
   A. Pseudoseizures
   B. Hysteria
   C. Tics and tic disorders
   D. Movement disorders, such as chorea
   E. Syncope
   F. Breath-holding spells
   G. Night terrors
   H. Rage attacks
   I. Sandifer syndrome and gastroesophageal reflux
   J. Infantile masturbation, self-stimulation
   K. Head banging
   L. Benign sleep myoclonus
   M. Startle response
   N. Migraine

Author: **Jeffrey Kaczorowski, M.D.**

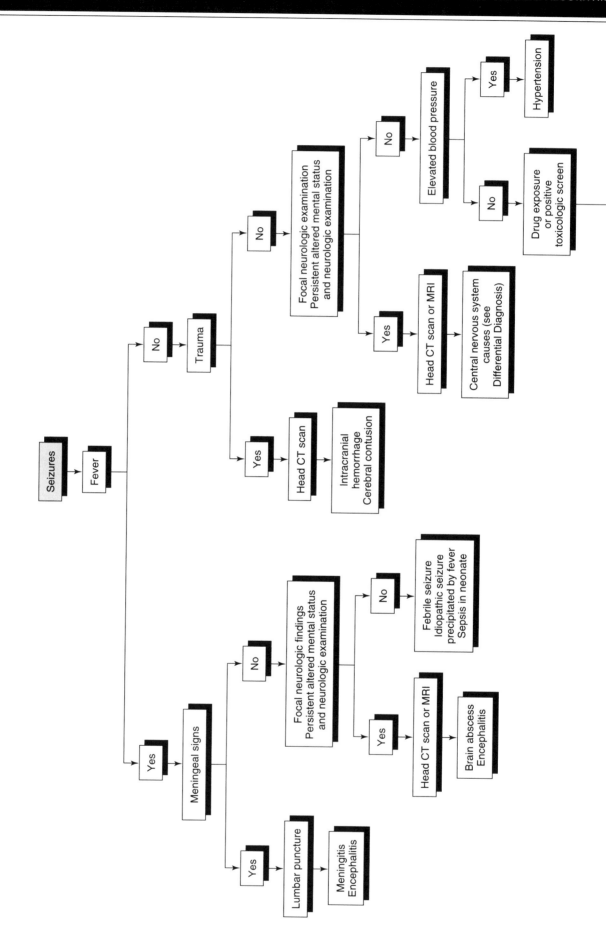

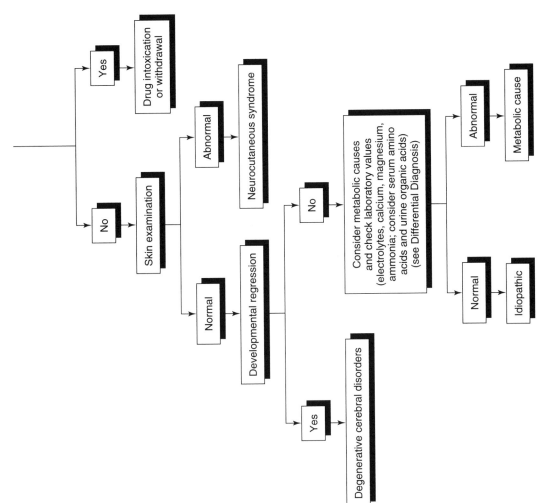

CT, Computed tomography; *MRI,* magnetic resonance imaging.

SKIN LESIONS—COMMON

Typical skin lesions can be divided into clear fluid–filled (vesicles, bullae), yellow or white fluid–filled (pustules), papular, scaling (papulosquamous), raised (papular), or nonscaling flat (macular) lesions. The differential of each category follows.

I. **Skin lesions associated with vesicles and bullae:** A *vesicle* is a raised skin or mucous membrane lesion filled with clear fluid; a *bulla* is a lesion larger than 1 cm filled with clear fluid.
   A. Miliaria crystallina
   B. Incontinentia pigmenti
      1. Linear rows of blisters on extremities in first few months of life
   C. Bullous impetigo
   D. Pemphigus
      1. Vulgaris
      2. Foliaceus
      3. Benign familial
   E. Epidermolysis bullosa
      1. Generalized
      2. Localized
      3. Simplex
      4. Dystrophic
   F. Recurrent bullous eruption (Weber-Cockayne disease)
   G. Dermatitis herpetiformis
   H. Immunoglobulin A dermatosis
   I. Chronic bullous dermatosis of childhood
   J. Staphylococcus scalded skin syndrome
   K. Stevens-Johnson syndrome/toxic epidermal necrolysis (have mucous membrane involvement as well)
   L. Sucking blisters
   M. Friction blisters
   N. Burns
   O. Herpes simplex
   P. Varicella/herpes zoster
      1. Chickenpox
      2. Shingles
   Q. Coxsackie: hand-foot-mouth and many other coxsackie infections
   R. Papular urticaria: may look vesicular
   S. Tinea pedis: may present with pustules or vesicles on dorsum, not interdigital
   T. Carpet beetle bites: flaccid bullae
   U. Bullous pemphigoid
   V. Polymorphous light eruption
   W. Herpes gestationalis

II. **Skin conditions associated with pustules:** A *pustule* is a raised lesion filled with an exudate, such that is appears white or yellow.
   A. Acne
   B. Hand-foot-mouth disease
   C. Acropustulosis of infancy
   D. Abscess/folliculitis
   E. Kerion: often has pustules within boggy red nodules
   F. Congenital candidiasis
   G. Pustular melanosis
   H. Herpes simplex and herpes zoster (varicella-zoster)
   I. Miliaria pustulosis
   J. Pustular psoriasis
   K. Dyshidrotic eczema: pompholyx
   L. Palmoplantar pustulosis
   M. Subcorneal pustulosis (Sneddon-Wilkinson disease)

III. **Papulosquamous skin lesions:** A *papular lesion* is a solid raised area, usually less than 1 cm in diameter, with distinct borders. *Papulosquamous disorders* describe skin lesions with red, pink, or violaceous papules that have an accompanying scale.
   A. Psoriasis
   B. Eczema/nummular eczema
   C. Seborrheic dermatitis
   D. Contact dermatitis
   E. Candida dermatitis (may present with collarette of scale on pink papule)
   F. Tinea corporis
   G. Ichthyosis
   H. Lupus
   I. Dermatomyositis
   J. Pityriasis rosea
   K. Pityriasis rubra pilaris
   L. Parapsoriasis
   M. Lichen planus
   N. Keratosis pilaris
   O. Histiocytosis syndromes
   P. PLEVA (pityriasis lichenoides et varioliformis acuta; Mucha-Haberman)
   Q. Secondary syphilis
   R. Scabies

IV. **Red lesions (not including lesions listed previously: *Papulosquamous lesions* include erythema with scale. In early stages, however, scale may not be present.)**
 A. Viral exanthems: may be red or pink and can include any variety of macular (*not* raised, by definition), petechial (*not* raised), urticarial, morbilliform, pustular, papular, ulcerative, as well as vesicular
  1. Viruses include adenoviruses, enterovirus, especially coxsackie, rubella, rubeola, echoviruses, reoviruses, Epstein-Barr virus, cytomegalovirus, human herpesvirus types 6 and 7 (roseola or exanthem subitum), parvovirus B19 (fifth disease or erythema infectiosum)
 B. Rickettsial illnesses
  1. Rocky Mountain spotted fever
  2. Q fever
  3. Typhus
  4. Rickettsialpox
 C. Scarlet fever and scarlatiniform exanthems (look like scarlet fever, but cause is viral, often adenovirus or enteroviruses, especially coxsackie)
 D. Urticaria
 E. Insect bites
 F. Cellulitis/erysipelas
 G. Erythema multiforme
 H. Erythema toxicum
 I. Miliaria rubra
 J. Erythema marginatum (rash associated with rheumatic fever)
 K. Juvenile arthritis
 L. Erythema annulare
 M. Angiofibroma
 N. Angioedema
 O. Tinea versicolor (although more often hypopigmented or hyperpigmented and not red)
 P. Acne
 Q. Atopic dermatitis (usually with scale)
 R. Diaper dermatitides: *Candida,* contact, psoriatic, seborrheic
 S. Lupus panniculitis
 T. Kawasaki syndrome
 U. Trauma
 V. Sunburn
 W. Hemangioma
 X. Contact dermatitis
 Y. Erythema (chronicum) migrans (early rash of Lyme disease)
 Z. Pyogenic granuloma
AA. Secondary syphilis

Author: **Lynn C. Garfunkel, M.D.**

SORE THROAT

■ DEFINITION

Any painful sensation localized to the mouth, pharynx, or surrounding tissues. Most cases of sore throat are caused by infections.

■ DIFFERENTIAL DIAGNOSIS

I. Infectious causes
A. Upper respiratory viruses
B. Group A streptococcus
C. Herpes gingovostomatitis
D. Enteroviruses
E. Mononucleosis/Epstein-Barr virus
F. *Mycoplasma pneumoniae*
G. *Neisseria gonorrhoeae*
H. Peritonsillar abscess
I. Retropharyngeal abscess
J. Epiglottitis
K. Diphtheria

II. Foreign body

III. Irritants/ingestion
A. Dry air
B. Allergens
C. Caustic substances
D. Postnasal discharge

IV. Referred pain
A. Dental problems
B. Cervical adenitis
C. Otitis media

Author: **Jeffrey Kaczorowski, M.D.**

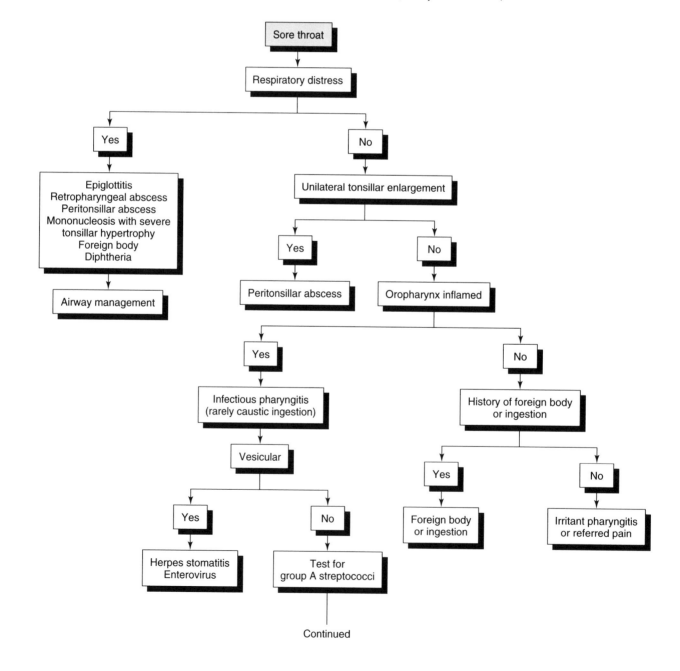

Continued

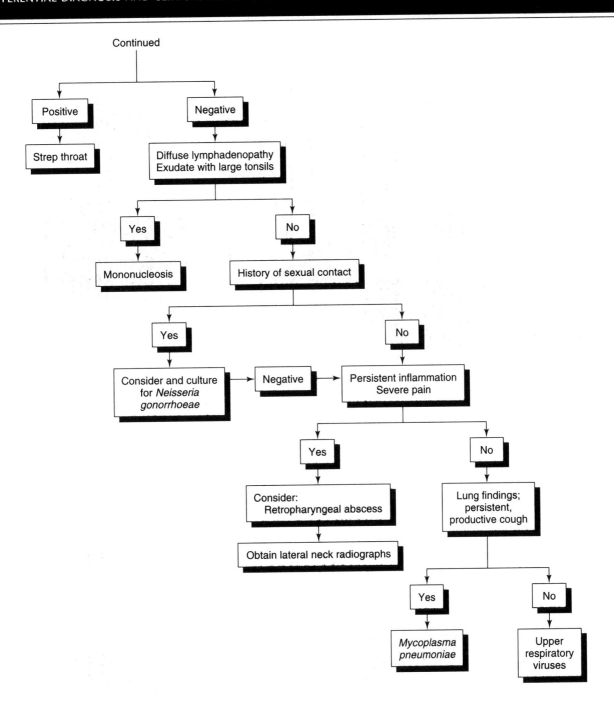

SPLENOMEGALY

■ DEFINITION

The spleen may be palpable in premature infants and some newborns. Otherwise, a palpable spleen should be considered enlarged. This chapter considers only isolated splenomegaly. For hepatosplenomegaly, see the section "Hepatomegaly/Hepatosplenomegaly."

■ DIFFERENTIAL DIAGNOSIS

I. **Infectious**
   A. Viral
      1. Epstein-Barr virus
      2. Cytomegalovirus
      3. Herpes simplex virus
      4. Enteroviruses
      5. Varicella-zoster virus
      6. Human immunodeficiency virus
   B. Bacterial
      1. Sepsis
      2. Endocarditis
      3. Tuberculosis
      4. Splenic abscess
      5. Brucellosis
   C. Parasites
      1. Malaria
      2. Schistosomiasis
      3. Others
   D. Fungal
      1. Histoplasmosis
   E. Rickettsial
      1. Rocky Mountain spotted fever

II. **Trauma/splenic laceration**

III. **Hemolytic anemia**
   A. Intrinsic red blood cell defects
      1. Hemoglobinopathies
      2. Membrane abnormalities
      3. Enzyme defects
   B. Extrinsic
      1. Immune
      2. Physical
      3. Chemical

IV. **Splenic sequestration (sickle cell disease)**

V. **Neoplasms**
   A. Leukemia
   B. Lymphoma
   C. Splenic tumor

VI. **Collagen vascular disease**
   A. Systemic lupus erythematosus
   B. Juvenile rheumatoid arthritis

VII. **Portal hypertension (obstruction of the portal vein or its branches)**
   A. Portal vein thrombosis
      1. Omphalitis
      2. Umbilical vein catheterization
   B. Cirrhosis
   C. Extrinsic compression

Author: **Jeffrey Kaczorowski, M.D.**

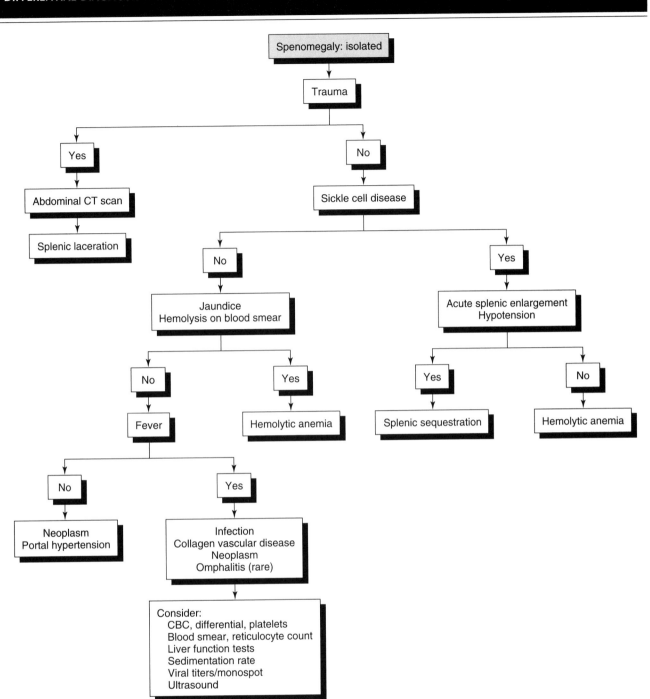

CBC, Complete blood count; CT, computed tomography.

STRIDOR AND STERTOR

■ DEFINITION

Stridor is a harsh, continuous noise most often heard during inspiration. *Stertor* is heavy, snoring-type breathing during inspiration. Stridor generally results from obstruction of the laryngeal or tracheal airways. Stertor comes from the nasopharynx or oropharynx.

■ DIFFERENTIAL DIAGNOSIS

I. Nasopharynx
  A. Congestion
  B. Foreign body
  C. Polyp
  D. Congenital anomalies
    1. Choanal atresia
    2. Dermoid cyst
    3. Encephalocele
  E. Neoplasm
    1. Hemangioma
    2. Angiofibroma
    3. Rhabdomyosarcoma

II. Oropharynx
  A. Enlarged tonsils or adenoids
  B. Infection
    1. Mononucleosis
    2. Peritonsillar abscess
    3. Retropharyngeal abscess
    4. Ludwig's angina
  C. Foreign body
  D. Poor tone/poor swallowing
  E. Congenital anomalies
    1. Micrognathia
    2. Macroglossia
    3. Thyroglossal duct cyst or lingual thyroid
  F. Neoplasms
    1. Hemangioma
    2. Lymphangioma
    3. Rhabdomyosarcoma

III. Larynx
  A. Infection
    1. Croup
    2. Epiglottitis
  B. Laryngospasm
    1. Anaphylaxis
    2. Angioneurotic edema
    3. Hypocalcemia
  C. Foreign body
  D. Congenital anomalies
    1. Laryngomalacia
    2. Laryngeal web
    3. Laryngocele
    4. Laryngeal cleft
    5. Subglottic stenosis
  E. Vocal cord paralysis
  F. Traumatic intubation
    1. Laryngeal or subglottic edema
    2. Subglottic stenosis
  G. Neck trauma
  H. Neoplasms
    1. Laryngeal papilloma
    2. Hemangioma
    3. Lymphangioma/cystic hygroma

IV. Trachea
  A. Infection
    1. Bacterial tracheitis
    2. Laryngotracheobronchitis
  B. Foreign body
  C. Congenital anomalies
    1. Tracheomalacia
    2. Tracheal ring, web, or cyst
    3. Tracheal stenosis
    4. Tracheoesophageal fistula
    5. Vascular anomalies
  D. Traumatic intubation or tracheostomy leading to tracheal stenosis
  E. Neoplasms
    1. Papilloma
    2. Hemangioma
    3. Lymphangioma/cystic hygroma
    4. Neoplasm of adjacent structure (thyroid, thymus, or esophagus)
    5. Mediastinal tumor

Author: **Jeffrey Kaczorowski, M.D.**

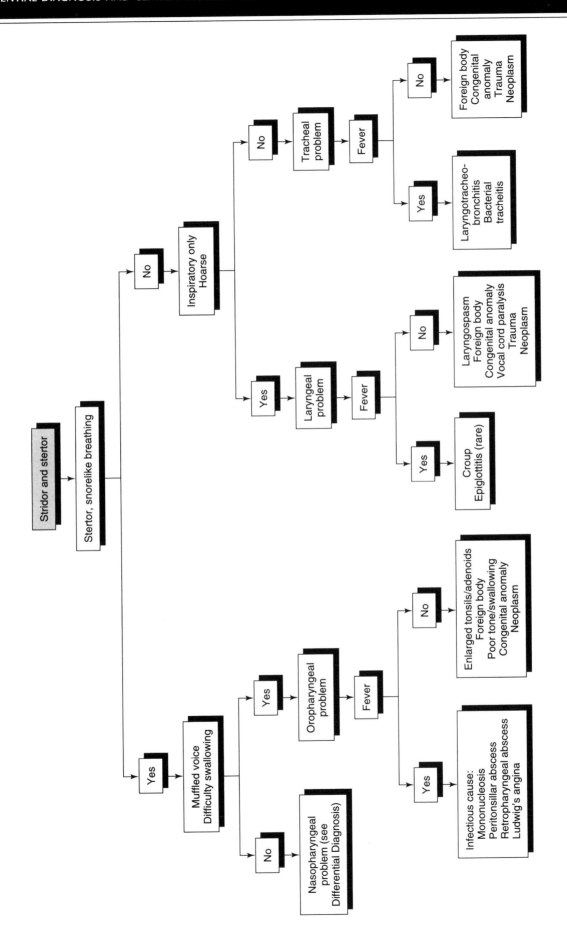

SYNCOPE

■ DEFINITION

A transient, usually sudden, loss of consciousness caused by inadequate delivery of blood, oxygen, or glucose to the brain. Also referred to as *fainting*.

■ DIFFERENTIAL DIAGNOSIS

I. Vasovagal (common faint) syncope

II. Postural or orthostatic syncope

III. Cardiac disorders
A. Structural
1. Severe left or right outflow tract obstructions (aortic or pulmonic stenosis)
2. Hypertrophic cardiomyopathy
3. Pulmonary hypertension
4. Hypoxemic attack with tetralogy of Fallot ("tet spell")
B. Arrhythmias
1. Prolonged QT syndrome
2. Bradyarrhythmias associated with second- or third-degree heart block
3. Tachyarrhythmias, including supraventricular tachycardia, ventricular tachycardia, and ventricular fibrillation

IV. Respiratory disorders
A. Hyperventilation
B. Breath-holding spell
C. Coughing or tussive syncope (often associated with asthma or pertussis)

V. Metabolic causes
A. Hypoglycemia
B. Anemia

VI. Psychologic causes
A. Acute stress
B. Hysteria

VII. Other
A. Micturition syncope
B. Hair-grooming syncope

Loss of consciousness lasting more than several seconds should raise suspicion for a seizure rather than a syncopal episode. Differentiation between a seizure and syncope may be difficult; Table 1-2 reviews some characteristics that may be helpful in differentiating the two.

Author: **Jeffrey Kaczorowski, M.D.**

TABLE 1-2 Differential Diagnosis of Syncope and Seizure

	SYNCOPE	SEIZURE
History	May include anxiety, hyperventilation, fasting, illness, prolonged standing	Prior seizures, febrile illness
Period of unconsciousness	Usually several seconds	Often several minutes or longer
Tonic-clonic movements	Generally absent; occasionally seen if unconsciousness is of longer duration	Often present
Incontinence	Usually absent	Often present
Confusion after event	Usually absent	Marked, except with febrile seizures

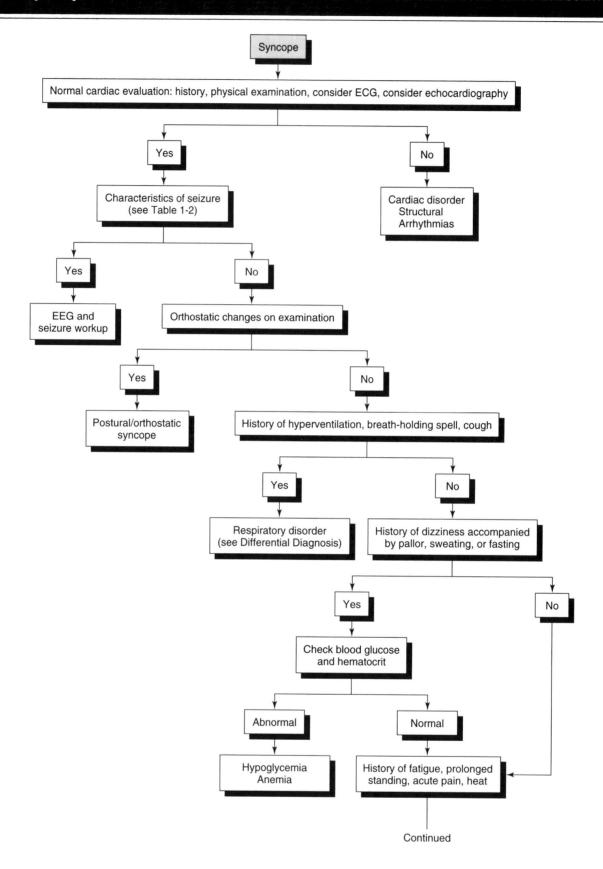

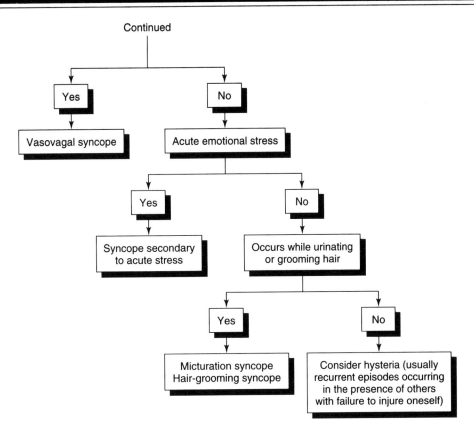

ECG, Electrocardiogram; EEG, electroencephalogram.

TACHYCARDIA

■ DEFINITION

A heart rate greater than the upper limit of normal for age (see Table 1-3).

■ DIFFERENTIAL DIAGNOSIS

I. Fever

II. Dehydration

III. Anxiety/fear/strong emotion

IV. Exercise

V. Anemia

VI. Congestive heart failure

VII. Hypoglycemia

VIII. Hyperthyroidism

IX. Pheochromocytoma

X. Drugs/toxins
   A. Caffeine
   B. Tobacco
   C. Albuterol
   D. Pseudoephedrine
   E. Antihistamines
   F. Cocaine
   G. Amphetamines
   H. Antidepressants
   I. Organophosphates
   J. Antiarrhythmics
   K. Others

XI. Intrinsic cardiac arrhythmias
   A. Supraventricular tachycardia
      1. Wolff-Parkinson-White syndrome
      2. Other reentrant atrial tachycardias
      3. Ectopic atrial focus
      4. Nodal tachycardia
      5. Congenital heart disease
         a. Ebstein's anomaly
         b. Single ventricle
      6. Postoperative cardiac repair
      7. Drugs
   B. Ventricular tachycardia
      1. Prolonged QT syndrome
      2. Myocarditis
      3. Acute rheumatic fever
      4. Hypertrophic cardiomyopathy
      5. Myocardial ischemia/infarction
      6. Congenital heart disease
      7. Postoperative cardiac repair
      8. Drugs
      9. Metabolic
         a. Hyperkalemia
         b. Hypocalcemia

Author: **Jeffrey Kaczorowski, M.D.**

TABLE 1-3   Normal Heart Rate—Birth to 13 Years and Older

AGE	NORMAL HEART RATE (BEATS/MIN)
Birth	110-160
6 mo-1 yr	100-140
2-3 yr	90-110
4-5 yr	80-100
6-8 yr	70-100
9-12 yr	70-90
≥13 yr	55-80

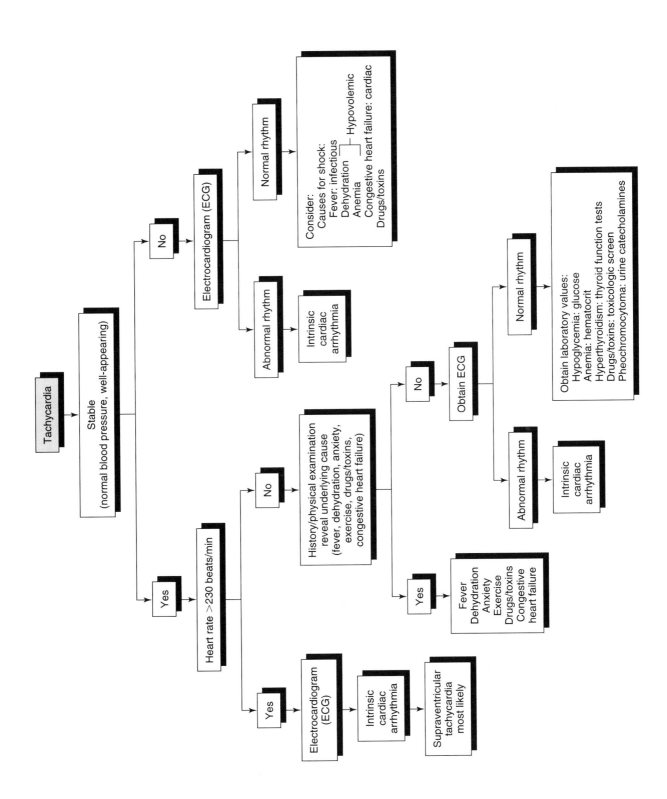

TORTICOLLIS

■ DEFINITION

Literally "twisted neck," with head tilt being the predominant finding and often accompanied by neck stiffness. Torticollis is caused by contraction or contracture of muscles of neck that causes the head to be tilted to one side. Usually, the head is tilted toward, and the chin is rotated away from the affected side when the sternocleidomastoid (SCM) muscle is in spasm. (Also see "Torticollis" in Part II.)

I. Congenital
  A. Muscular—SCM muscle hematoma with scarring, presumably from birth trauma
  B. Vertebral anomaly—hemivertebrae or other vertebral segmentation abnormalities
    1. Klippel-Feil syndrome—decreased number and fusion of cervical vertebrae
  C. Intrauterine positional abnormality, perhaps leading to shortening of SCM muscle
  D. Congenital nystagmus
    1. Spasmus mutans—usually presents before 6 months with head bobbing, head tilt, and nystagmus

II. Infectious
  A. Retropharyngeal, or less commonly peritonsillar, cellulitis or abscess
  B. Cervical adenopathy or adenitis
  C. Vertebral osteomyelitis
  D. Pneumonia (in particular upper lobe disease)
  E. Tuberculosis

III. Ocular
  A. Cranial nerve (CN) palsies, especially CN IV: head tilts to allay diplopia
  B. Nystagmus

IV. Trauma
  A. Neck muscle spasm resulting from primary muscle (SCM) injury or vertebral injury
  B. Myositis or fibromyositis—spasm (draft on neck, wry neck) or inflammation of SCM muscle
  C. Cervical spine injury
    1. Fracture
    2. Subluxation
    3. Dislocation
      a. Dislocation/subluxation more common with bony dysplasias (i.e., achondroplasia)
      b. Ligamentous laxity (i.e., trisomy 21)
  D. Clavicle fracture

V. Tumors
A. Posterior fossa tumor
B. Eosinophilic granuloma—may involve vertebrae
C. Osteoid osteoma—nighttime pain, relieved by aspirin
D. Intraspinal tumor

VI. Movement disorders (in which a part of the picture may involve torticollis)
A. Dystonia
   1. Dystonia musculorum deformans
   2. Kernicterus
   3. Wilson's disease (hepatolenticular degeneration)
B. Dystonic reactions (oculogyric crisis)
   1. Phenothiazines
      a. Antidepressants—chlorpromazine, droperidol, fluphenazine, haloperidol, thioridazine, trifluoperazine
      b. Antiemetics—prochlorperazine (Compazine), trimethobenzamide (Tigan)
      c. Motility agents—metoclopramide (Reglan)
   2. Sandifer syndrome—gastroesophageal reflux with dystonic-like movements; presumably, in response to discomfort of esophagitis, patient tries to reposition to relieve pain, which leads to writhing movements

VII. Miscellaneous
A. Juvenile arthritis
B. Fibrodysplasia ossificans progressiva
C. Ligamentous laxity
D. Poliomyelitis
E. Cerebral palsy

Author: **Lynn C. Garfunkel, M.D.**

VAGINAL BLEEDING

■ DEFINITION

Vaginal bleeding is normal during the immediate neonatal period (secondary to maternal hormone withdrawal) and during menstruation. *Menstruation* is the periodic shedding of endometrial tissue and blood that accompanies puberty in girls. Menstrual bleeding can be categorized as normal or excessive. Menstrual patterns in the first 2 years after menarche (onset of menses) vary widely. In general, a menstrual period is considered excessive if it lasts longer than 8 days or more than eight pads/tampons are soaked per day at the peak of the cycle. Periods generally occur every 21 to 34 days.

■ DIFFERENTIAL DIAGNOSIS

Vaginal Bleeding before Menarche

I. Physiologic bleeding in the neonate

II. Trauma
   A. Accidental
   B. Sexual abuse
   C. Scratching
      1. Pinworms

III. Foreign body

IV. Vulvovaginitis
   A. Group A β-hemolytic streptococci
   B. *Shigella*
   C. *Neisseria gonorrhoeae*
   D. *Candida*

V. Urethral prolapse

VI. Exogenous estrogens

VII. Precocious puberty

VIII. Tumor
   A. Papilloma
   B. Adenocarcinoma
   C. Others

Vaginal Bleeding after Menarche

I. Normal menstruation

II. Trauma
   A. Accidental
   B. Sexual abuse
   C. Scratching
      1. Pinworms

III. Foreign body

IV. Dysfunctional uterine bleeding

V. Vulvovaginitis
   A. *Neisseria gonorrhoeae*
   B. Group A β-hemolytic streptococci
   C. *Shigella*
   D. *Candida*

VI. Cervicitis or pelvic inflammatory disease
   A. *Neisseria gonorrhoeae*
   B. *Chlamydia trachomatis*

VII. Pregnancy related
   A. Ectopic pregnancy
   B. Spontaneous abortion
   C. Placenta previa
   D. Abruptio placenta

VIII. Contraceptive use
   A. Oral contraceptives
   B. Medroxyprogesterone injection
   C. Intrauterine device

IX. Bleeding disorder
   A. von Willebrand disease
   B. Idiopathic thrombocytopenic purpura

X. Hypothyroidism

XI. Tumor
   A. Papilloma
   B. Adenocarcinoma
   C. Others

Author: Jeffrey Kaczorowski, M.D.

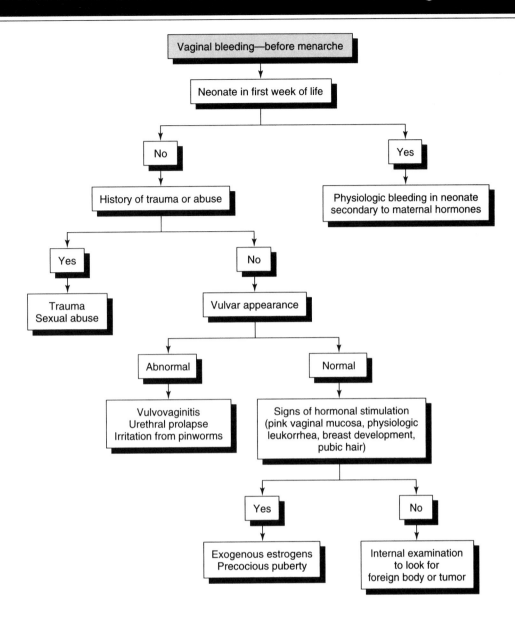

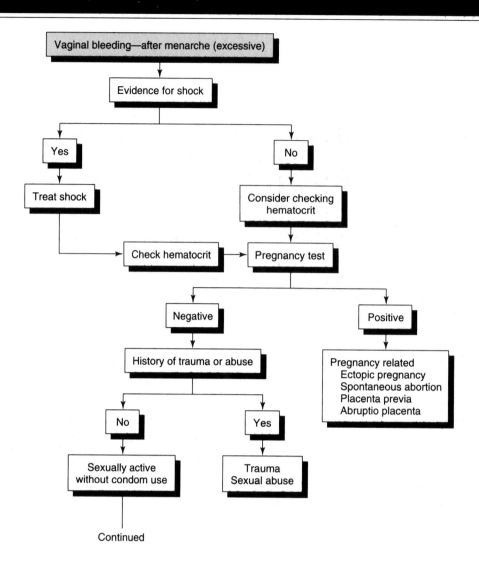

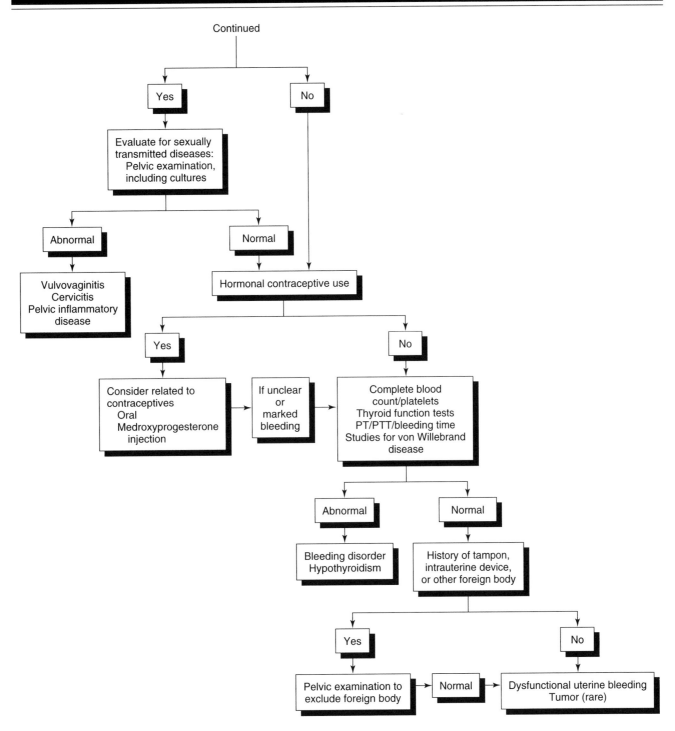

PT, Prothrombin time; PTT, partial thromboplastin time.

VAGINAL DISCHARGE

■ **DEFINITION**

Vaginal discharge can be normal during the first month of life and periodically after puberty. This discharge, termed *physiologic leukorrhea,* is stimulated by maternal or pubertal estrogens; it is not associated with pain or irritation. Any vaginal discharge after the neonatal period in the prepubertal child or discharge accompanied by discomfort is abnormal.

■ **DIFFERENTIAL DIAGNOSIS**

Vaginal Discharge before Puberty

I. Physiologic leukorrhea in the neonate

II. Noninfectious vulvovaginitis
   A. Poor hygiene
   B. Chemical irritation
      1. Soaps and detergents
      2. Bubble baths

III. Infectious vulvovaginitis
   A. Nonsexually transmitted
      1. Pinworms
      2. Group A streptococcus
      3. *Haemophilus influenzae*
      4. *Shigella* species
      5. *Gardnerella vaginalis*
   B. Sexually transmitted
      1. *Neisseria gonorrhoeae*
      2. *Chlamydia trachomatis*
      3. *Trichomonas vaginalis*
      4. Herpes simplex

IV. Foreign body

V. Smegma

VI. Genitourinary malformations

Vaginal Discharge after Puberty

I. Physiologic leukorrhea

II. Noninfectious vulvovaginitis
   A. Poor hygiene
   B. Chemical irritation
      1. Soaps and detergents
      2. Bubble baths

III. Infectious vulvovaginitis
   A. Not sexually transmitted
      1. *Candida albicans* (yeast)
      2. *Gardnerella vaginalis*
   B. Sexually transmitted
      1. *Neisseria gonorrhoeae*
      2. *Chlamydia trachomatis*
      3. *Trichomonas vaginalis*
      4. Herpes simplex

IV. Cervicitis or pelvic inflammatory disease
   A. *Neisseria gonorrhoeae*
   B. *Chlamydia trachomatis*

V. Foreign body

Author: **Jeffrey Kaczorowski, M.D.**

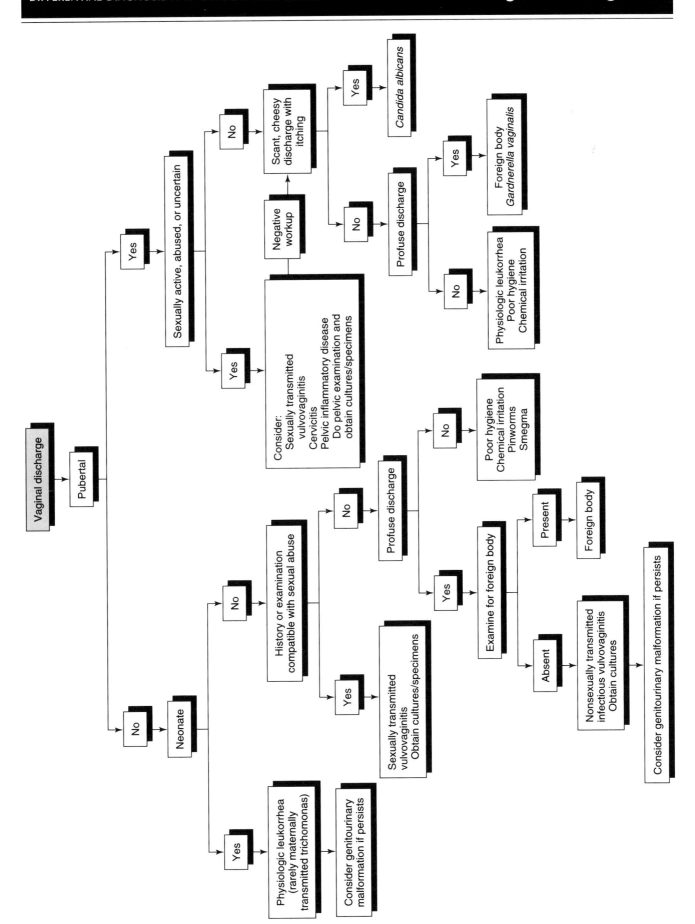

VOMITING AND REGURGITATION

■ **DEFINITION**

Vomiting is the forceful expulsion of stomach contents through the mouth. *Regurgitation* is the nonforceful expulsion of stomach or esophageal contents from the mouth. The differential diagnosis of vomiting and regurgitation varies according to the child's age.

■ **DIFFERENTIAL DIAGNOSIS**

Newborn (Birth to Several Weeks)

I. **Normal variation (normal regurgitation, or "spitting up")**

II. **Obstructive gastrointestinal causes**
   A. Esophageal obstruction
      1. Esophageal atresia/stenosis
      2. Tracheoesophageal fistula
      3. Esophageal web
      4. Vascular rings
      5. Hiatal hernia
      6. Other congenital esophageal abnormalities
   B. Gastric obstructions
      1. Pyloric stenosis
      2. Antral web
      3. Gastric duplication
      4. Gastric atresia
      5. Gastric volvulus
      6. Lactobezoar (*lacto* = milk; *bezoar* = concretion in stomach)
   C. Small intestine obstructions
      1. Duodenal atresia/stenosis
      2. Malrotation with or without volvulus
      3. Annular pancreas
      4. Preduodenal portal vein
      5. Meconium ileus
      6. Jejunoileal atresia/stenosis
      7. Enteric duplications
   D. Large intestine obstructions
      1. Colonic atresia/stenosis
      2. Hirschsprung's disease
      3. Imperforate anus
      4. Meconium plug
      5. Enteric duplication

III. **Nonobstructive gastrointestinal causes**
   A. Overfeeding
   B. Excessive air swallowing or poor burping
   C. Gastroesophageal reflux
   D. Formula allergy or intolerance
   E. Necrotizing enterocolitis or perforation

IV. **Infectious causes**
   A. Sepsis
   B. Meningitis

V. **Neurologic**
   A. Increased intracranial pressure (ICP)
      1. Intracranial hemorrhage
      2. Hydrocephalus
      3. Cerebral edema
   B. No increased ICP
      1. Kernicterus

VI. **Endocrine**
   A. Congenital adrenal hyperplasia

VII. **Metabolic**
   A. Amino acid disorders, including urea cycle disorders
   B. Organic acid disorders
   C. Carbohydrate metabolism disorders, including galactosemia

VIII. **Renal**
   A. Obstructive uropathy
   B. Renal insufficiency/failure

Infant (Several Weeks to 1 Year)

I. **Normal variation (normal regurgitation, or "spitting up")**

II. **Obstructive gastrointestinal causes**
   A. Esophageal obstruction (generally acquired as opposed to congenital causes of obstruction noted in previous section)
      1. Foreign body
      2. Esophageal stricture secondary to esophagitis
      3. Retroesophageal abscess
   B. Gastric obstructions
      1. Pyloric stenosis
      2. Bezoar/foreign body
      3. Gastric volvulus
   C. Small intestine obstructions
      1. Malrotation with or without volvulus
      2. Intussusception
      3. Incarcerated inguinal hernia
      4. Meckel's diverticulum complications
      5. Meconium ileus equivalent
      6. Adhesions (after surgery)
      7. Intramural hematoma
      8. Neoplasms (polyps or lymphoma)
      9. Pancreatic pseudocyst

D. Large intestine obstructions
   1. Hirschsprung's disease
   2. Intussusception
   3. Meconium plug
   4. Adhesions (after surgery)
   5. Neoplasms (polyps, lipomas, fibromas, or lymphoma)

III. **Nonobstructive gastrointestinal causes**
   A. Overfeeding
   B. Excessive air swallowing or poor burping
   C. Gastroenteritis
   D. Gastroesophageal reflux
   E. Formula allergy or intolerance
   F. Celiac disease
   G. Gastritis
   H. Peritonitis
   I. Paralytic ileus

IV. **Infectious causes**
   A. Sepsis
   B. Meningitis
   C. Pneumonia
   D. Pyelonephritis/urinary tract infection
   E. Pertussis
   F. Hepatitis

V. **Neurologic**
   A. Increased ICP
      1. Intracranial hemorrhage
      2. Brain tumor
      3. Hydrocephalus
      4. Cerebral edema

VI. **Endocrine**
   A. Adrenal insufficiency
   B. Hypercalcemia

VII. **Metabolic**
   A. Amino acid disorders
   B. Organic acid disorders
   C. Carbohydrate metabolism disorders

VIII. **Renal**
   A. Obstructive uropathy
   B. Renal insufficiency/failure

IX. **Drugs/toxins**

Child (Older Than 1 Year) and Adolescent

I. **Obstructive gastrointestinal causes**
   A. Esophageal obstruction
      1. Foreign body
      2. Esophageal stricture secondary to esophagitis
      3. Retroesophageal abscess
   B. Gastric obstructions
      1. Bezoar
   C. Small intestine obstructions
      1. Malrotation with or without volvulus
      2. Intussusception
      3. Incarcerated inguinal hernia
      4. Meckel's diverticulum complications
      5. Meconium ileus equivalent
      6. Adhesions (after surgery)
      7. Intramural hematoma
      8. Neoplasms (polyps or lymphoma)
      9. Pancreatic pseudocyst
   D. Large intestine obstructions
      1. Hirschsprung's disease
      2. Intussusception
      3. Meconium plug
      4. Adhesions (after surgery)
      5. Neoplasms (polyps, lipomas, fibromas, or lymphoma)

II. **Nonobstructive gastrointestinal causes**
   A. Gastroenteritis
   B. Appendicitis
   C. Peptic ulcer disease
   D. Pancreatitis
   E. Celiac disease
   F. Gastritis
   G. Peritonitis
   H. Paralytic ileus

III. **Infectious causes**
   A. Group A streptococcal pharyngitis
   B. Meningitis
   C. Pneumonia
   D. Pyelonephritis/urinary tract infection
   E. Hepatitis
   F. Sepsis

IV. Neurologic
  A. Increased ICP
    1. Brain tumor
    2. Intracranial hemorrhage
    3. Cerebral edema
    4. Hydrocephalous/VP shunt malfunction
  B. No increased ICP
    1. Migraine
    2. Motion sickness

V. Endocrine
  A. Diabetic ketoacidosis
  B. Adrenal insufficiency

VI. Metabolic
  A. Amino acid disorders
  B. Organic acid disorders
  C. Carbohydrate metabolism disorders

VII. Renal
  A. Obstructive uropathy
  B. Renal insufficiency or failure

VIII. Drugs/toxins

IX. Pregnancy

X. Psychologic disorders
  A. Anxiety
  B. Bulimia

XI. Other
  A. Abdominal migraine
  B. Abdominal epilepsy
  C. Cyclic vomiting
  D. Reye's syndrome

Author: **Jeffrey Kaczorowski, M.D.**

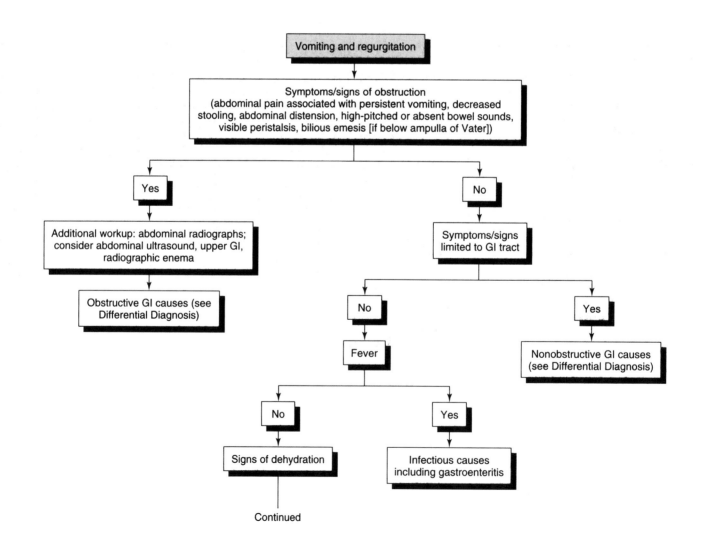

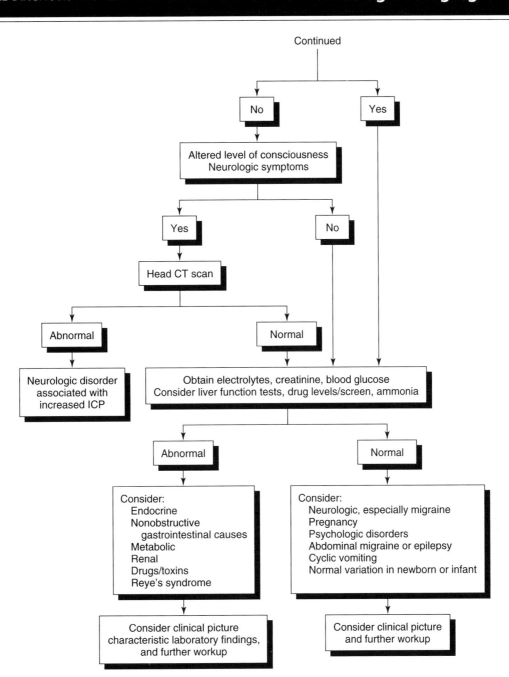

CT, Computed tomography; GI, gastrointestinal; ICP, intracranial pressure.

WHEEZING

■ DEFINITION

A continuous, high-pitched sound that is classically heard during expiration but that may be heard during inspiration as well. It is almost always caused by lower airway (small bronchi or bronchioles) obstruction but rarely may be caused by obstruction of the bronchi or trachea. Remember, "all that wheezes is not asthma," but much of it is.

■ DIFFERENTIAL DIAGNOSIS

I. Asthma

II. Bronchiolitis

III. Anaphylaxis

IV. Foreign body

V. Gastroesophageal reflux

VI. Congenital anomalies
   A. Cystic malformations of the lung
   B. Vascular ring
   C. Tracheoesophageal fistula
   D. Tracheobronchomalacia
   E. Congenital heart disease

VII. Intrinsic lung disease
   A. Cystic fibrosis
   B. Bronchopulmonary dysplasia
   C. α_1-Antitrypsin deficiency
   D. Immotile cilia syndrome
   E. Pulmonary hemosiderosis
   F. B-cell immunodeficiencies

VIII. Mediastinal masses
   A. Lymph nodes
      1. Lymphoma
      2. Leukemia
      3. Tuberculosis
      4. Sarcoidosis
      5. Histoplasmosis
   B. Tumors
      1. Neuroblastoma
      2. Ganglioneuroma
      3. Thymoma
      4. Teratoma

IX. Hysterical or psychogenic wheezing

X. Other
   A. Organophosphate poisoning
   B. Smoke inhalation
   C. Swallowing disorders

Author: **Jeffrey Kaczorowski, M.D.**

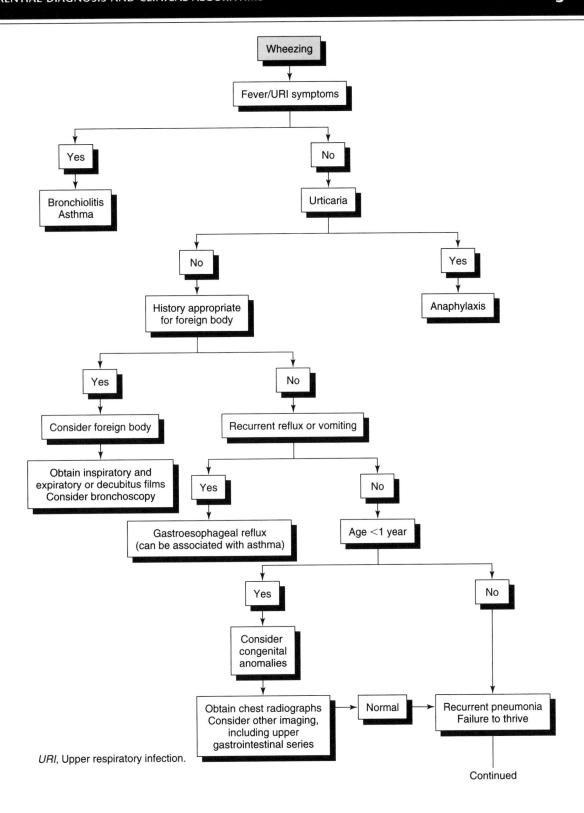

URI, Upper respiratory infection.

Continued

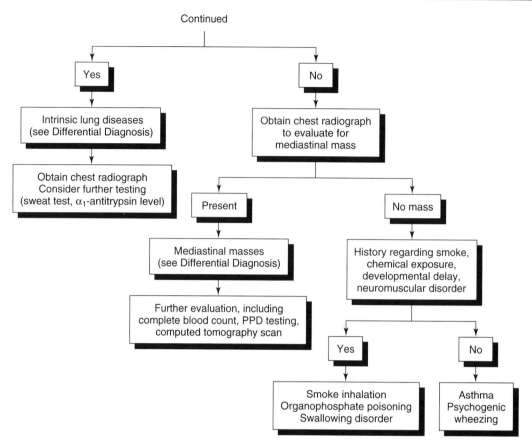

PPD, Purified protein derivative.

PART II

Clinical Disorders

BASIC INFORMATION

DEFINITION

Acetaminophen (*N*-acetyl-*p*-aminophenol) is widely available as a single agent for relief of fever and pain. It is also widely available in combination cold and pain preparations. Both acute and chronic overingestion are associated with gastrointestinal (GI) disturbance and potentially fatal hepatotoxicity.

SYNONYMS

- APAP
- Paracetamol
- Tempra
- Panadol
- Tylenol

ICD-9CM CODE

965.4 Acetaminophen poisoning

ETIOLOGY

- Hepatotoxic effects result from cytochrome P450 metabolism of acetaminophen to a toxic metabolite (acetamidoquinone) that binds irreversibly to liver proteins unless conjugated with endogenous glutathione.
- Centrilobular hepatic necrosis develops if glutathione stores are depleted.
- Other pathways available for APAP metabolism include sulfation (predominant in neonates) and glucuronidation (this pathway is well developed by 3 years of age).

EPIDEMIOLOGY & DEMOGRAPHICS

Most common potentially toxic ingestion in children younger than 6 years of age

- On average, more than 46,000 exposures occur per year.
- Less than 1% of fatalities from acetaminophen toxicity occur in this age group (0 to 6 years).
  1. Reasons for this are not known.
  2. Children younger than 6 years may have increased glutathione synthesis and turnover.

HISTORY

- It is often possible to obtain history of ingestion. As with all potentially toxic exposures, one should inquire specifically about the following:
  1. Time of ingestion
  2. Liquid or tablet form
  3. Exact preparation ingested so that effects of a coingestant may be anticipated
  4. Quantity ingested
  5. Where ingestant was stored
  6. Degree of supervision at time of ingestion
  7. History of prior ingestions

- If acute overingestion history cannot be obtained, inquire about recent routine Tylenol dosing because chronic overingestion of acetaminophen can result in clinical toxicity.
- Generally, an acute ingestion of more than 140 mg/kg in pediatric patients or more than 6 g in adult-sized patients is considered potentially toxic.
  1. Acetaminophen toxicity should be considered in the differential diagnosis when evaluating any patient with anorexia, nausea, and vomiting.
  2. Acetaminophen toxicity should be considered with serum transaminase elevation or other liver function abnormalities (as occurs later in the course).
- Many experts advocate routinely obtaining serum acetaminophen levels on all patients presenting with potentially significant ingestion of any kind because acetaminophen is a common coingestant.

SIGNS & SYMPTOMS

- Initially, many patients may be asymptomatic.
- The first symptoms are anorexia, nausea, and vomiting.
  1. At 24 to 72 hours, patients may develop right upper quadrant pain and serum transaminases may start to rise.
  2. Further clinical evidence of hepatic dysfunction, such as jaundice, excessive bleeding, and encephalopathy, typically develops at 72 to 96 hours.
  3. After 96 hours, the severely toxic patient may develop irreversible hepatic failure.
  4. Ultimate outcome is usually known by 2 weeks after ingestion.
- The clinical picture may be dominated early on by effects of the coingestant (i.e., anticholinergic effects from combination cold preparations) or by respiratory depression from combination pain medications.

DIAGNOSIS

DIFFERENTIAL DIAGNOSIS

- Acute gastroenteritis
- Viral hepatitis
- Other toxic/chemical hepatitis
- Reye's syndrome
- Inborn error of metabolism
- Wilson disease
- α_1-Antitrypsin deficiency

DIAGNOSTIC WORKUP

- Serum acetaminophen level should be determined 4 hours after ingestion. Relationship of initial and subsequent serum levels to time of ingestion should be interpreted according to the well-known Rumack-Matthew nomogram.
  1. Four-hour serum levels between 150 and 200 µg/ml are potentially toxic, and 4-hour levels in excess of 200 µg/ml are probably toxic.
- Serum chemistries, including blood glucose, blood urea nitrogen (BUN), creatinine, and baseline serum transaminases, ammonia, and prothrombin time/partial thromboplastin time (PT/PTT), are useful early on.
- Consider obtaining serum levels of other common coingestants, such as a salicylate (aspirin).
  1. Broad-spectrum urine or serum toxicology screens are of uncertain value in acute management. Evidence of a significant coingestion is usually clinically apparent.
- In cases of potentially toxic ingestion, hepatic function status should be monitored by obtaining serum transaminases and PT/PTT (the PT is primarily affected) at 24 hours after ingestion and periodically thereafter if laboratory abnormality has developed.
  1. Special attention should be given to monitoring hepatic function in patients who are at high risk by virtue of chronic exposure to another potentially hepatotoxic agent (e.g., alcohol).
  2. Clinical and/or laboratory evidence of hepatic dysfunction is usually evident by 48 to 72 hours after ingestion.
- Clinical and laboratory markers of renal function should also be followed because renal failure may develop in the presence or absence of hepatic failure.

THERAPY

- Maintain the airway, assist ventilation if necessary, and support intravascular volume.
- For initial GI decontamination, syrup of ipecac may be given to children who present within 60 minutes of ingestion. Single-dose activated charcoal (dose: 1 g/kg body weight) should be administered early in the course.
  1. Activated charcoal adsorbs acetaminophen effectively in the GI tract.
  2. Many experts believe that it can be given concurrently with the first dose of *N*-acetylcysteine (NAC; see following discussion) with no appreciable loss of NAC activity.

- Vomiting caused by the acute ingestion should be controlled as much as possible because ongoing emesis interferes with administration of appropriate treatment.
  1. Ondansetron and high-dose metoclopramide have both been used with some success to inhibit vomiting.
- While awaiting initial serum level, if significant ingestion is suspected or if the 4-hour level is 150 μg/ml or greater (or if the initial level relative to time of ingestion falls above the *lower* line in the Rumack-Matthew nomogram), specific antidotal therapy with 20% NAC (Mucomyst) is indicated.
  1. NAC decreases the potential for ongoing hepatotoxicity by acting as a glutathione substitute, by enhancing glutathione stores, and by enhancing metabolism by the alternative sulfation pathway.
  2. The initial dose is 140 mg/kg enterally, and complete treatment consists of 17 subsequent enteral doses of 70 mg/kg. Doses are given at 4-hour intervals.
  3. Maximal benefit is derived from NAC if it is administered before the toxic metabolite of acetaminophen accumulates or within 8 to 10 hours of acute ingestion.
     a. It is of diminishing value in protecting against hepatotoxicity if initiated later.
     b. It should still be initiated, even if presentation is delayed beyond 24 hours after ingestion.
- Because of its noxious odor and taste, oral NAC often potentiates ongoing nausea and vomiting in patients who require it. Emesis should be controlled as much as possible with metoclopramide and/or ondansetron.

■ SURGICAL
Hepatic transplantation may be necessary in rare cases. Patients who develop severe acidosis, coagulopathy, or encephalopathy may be candidates for transport to a transplant facility.

■ FOLLOW-UP & DISPOSITION
- All patients with intentional ingestions should receive a psychiatric evaluation once they are medically stable.
- In cases of accidental ingestion, social work consultation is often helpful to assess the degree of supervision in the home.

■ PATIENT/FAMILY EDUCATION
- Parents should be educated about the potential toxicity of acetaminophen (and preparations containing acetaminophen) in the home. These and other medications should be kept locked and out of reach of children, even if they are packaged with child-proof caps.
- Families should be provided with the phone number of the nearest regional poison center.

■ PREVENTION & ANTICIPATORY GUIDANCE
- The danger of accidental poisoning in the home should be discussed routinely at pediatric health supervision visits, beginning at the 6-month visit.
  1. Parents should be instructed to "childproof" the home, including locking all medications and other toxic products out of the reach of children.
  2. Parents should be provided with the phone number of the regional poison center.
  3. Parents should be instructed to call the poison center immediately when they suspect that an inappropriate ingestion may have occurred.
  4. Syrup of ipecac should be administered under the guidance of the regional poison center.

■ REFERRAL INFORMATION
- In general, all patients suspected of having a potentially toxic exposure should be stabilized acutely and then referred to the nearest tertiary care facility with experience in managing critically ill children.
- The nearest regional poison center should be consulted in all cases of intentional or accidental toxic ingestion.

❂ PEARLS & CONSIDERATIONS
- Oral NAC may be better tolerated if given by nasogastric tube or if diluted down to at least 5% by mixing 1 part of the 20% stock formulation with 3 parts cola or juice. The addition of ice may also improve compliance with the regimen.
- Falsely elevated serum levels of acetaminophen may be seen if the patient has also ingested salicylate compounds, cephalosporins, or sulfonamides.

REFERENCES
1. Clark RF et al: The use of ondansetron in the treatment of nausea and vomiting associated with acetaminophen poisoning, *J Toxicol Clin Toxicol* 34:163, 1996.
2. Combination therapy for acetaminophen overdose, *Pediatr News* 33:43, 1999.
3. Mack RB: Introduction, *Pediatr Ann* 25: 12, 1996.
4. Nolan RJ: Poisoning. In Hoekelman RA et al (eds): *Primary pediatric care*, ed 3, St Louis, 1997, Mosby.
5. Olson K (ed): *Poisoning and drug overdose*, Englewood Cliffs, NJ, 1994, Appleton & Lange.
6. Rumack BM, Matthew M: Acetaminophen poisoning and toxicity, *Pediatrics* 55:871, 1975.
7. Smilkstein MJ et al: Efficacy of oral *N*-acetylcysteine in the treatment of acetaminophen overdose: analysis of the National Multicenter Study (1976-1985), *N Engl J Med* 319:1557, 1988.
8. Wright RO et al: Effect of metoclopramide dose on preventing emesis after oral administration of *N*-acetylcysteine for acetaminophen overdose, *J Toxicol Clin Toxicol* 37:35, 1999.

Author: **Kathleen M. Ventre, M.D.**

BASIC INFORMATION

■ DEFINITION
Acne vulgaris is a disorder of the hair follicle and sebaceous gland affecting most people in adolescence or young adulthood.

ICD-9CM CODE
706.1 Acne vulgaris

■ ETIOLOGY
- Causes are multifactorial.
- Androgen production causes increasing sebum levels.
- Obstruction of pilosebaceous follicles is caused by excessive sebum combined with desquamated epithelial cells from follicle.
- *Propionibacterium acnes* proliferates in environment of excessive sebum and follicular cells.
- Inflammation is caused by mediators and chemotactic factors produced by bacteria.

■ EPIDEMIOLOGY
- Most common skin disease, affecting nearly 80% of persons at some time between the ages of 11 and 30 years
- Most prevalent during adolescence, with greater severity in males

■ HISTORY
- Located in areas of highest sebaceous gland concentration; therefore the face, chest, and back are common sites of involvement.
- Ninety-eight percent of patients with acne have facial involvement; a smaller percentage have involvement on back and chest.

■ PHYSICAL EXAMINATION
- Classic lesions are open and closed comedones (blackheads and whiteheads).
  1. Formed by sebum-plugged pilosebaceous follicle
- Inflammatory papules, pustules, and cysts are present.
  1. Develop after proliferation of *P. acnes* in noninflammatory comedones, with rupture of contents into surrounding dermis
- Cystic acne manifests by fluctuant and painful nodules and cysts that heal with postinflammatory pigment changes and scar formation.

DIAGNOSIS

■ DIFFERENTIAL DIAGNOSIS
- Papular scars
- Eosinophilic folliculitis
- Syringomas
- Adenoma sebaceum
- Drug eruption (lithium, corticosteroids)

■ DIAGNOSTIC WORKUP
Diagnosis is usually made on basis of characteristic clinical picture.

THERAPY

■ NONPHARMACOLOGIC
- Wash with mild soap (Dove, Purpose, Neutrogena, Basis) one to two times a day.
- Apply mild moisturizer (Cetaphil, Purpose, Moisturel) as needed.
- Avoid rubbing and scrubbing, which may worsen the condition.

■ MEDICAL
- No single agent addresses all etiologic factors.
- Combination regimens are the mainstay of treatment.
- Benzoyl peroxide is antibacterial and comedolytic.
  1. Available in 1%, 2.5%, 5%, 10% gel, lotion, and wash preparations.
  2. Also available as 5% solution with 3% erythromycin (Benzamycin), which must be refrigerated.
  3. Use one to two times a day.
  4. Side effects include erythema, peeling, and staining clothes.
- Topical antibiotics are antibacterial and antiinflammatory.
  1. Erythromycin solutions include A/T/S, T-Stat, Emgel, Erycette, Erygel, Erystat, Staticin, and Theramycin.
  2. Clindamycin comes as a solution, gel, or lotion (Cleocin T).
  3. Use one to two times per day.
  4. Side effects include erythema, peeling, and drying.
- Topical tretinoin (Retin-A) increases cell turnover in follicle wall and thereby allows expulsion of keratin plugs of microcomedones.
  1. Available as 0.025%, 0.05%, 0.1% cream; 0.01%, 0.025% gel; and 0.025% microsponge gel (Retin-A micro).
  2. Begin with lowest concentration and slowly increase if needed.
  3. Apply small amount (pea-size for full face) every night.
  4. Side effects include transient worsening of acne, irritation, and photosensitivity.
- Systemic antibiotics have an antibacterial and antiinflammatory mechanism of action.
  1. The goal is 2 to 3 months of therapy and then tapering as topical agents are continued.
  2. Tetracycline is administered as 500 mg twice a day (take on empty stomach).
  3. Erythromycin is administered as 500 mg twice a day (stomach upset).
  4. Minocycline is administered as 50 to 100 mg twice a day (hyperpigmentation, autoimmune hepatitis, lupuslike syndrome).
  5. Doxycycline is administered as 50 to 100 mg twice a day (sun sensitivity).
- Hormonal therapy (oral contraceptive pills) may be used.
  1. A low-dose oral contraceptive containing nonandrogenic progestin, such as norgestimate or desogestrel, may be effective (Ortho-Tri-Cyclen).
  2. Treatment for 2 to 4 months is required before any improvement occurs.
- Isotretinoin (Accutane) may be used.
  1. It is indicated for severe nodulocystic acne.
  2. It decreases sebum production.
  3. It decreases "stickiness" of follicular cells.
  4. Side effects include severe teratogen, increased triglycerides, dry skin and mucous membranes, decreased night vision, hyperostosis, and pseudotumor cerebri.
  5. Consult a dermatologist for 16- to 20-week course.

PEARLS & CONSIDERATIONS

■ CLINICAL PEARLS
- The dark color of a blackhead results from oxidized lipids, melanin, and densely packed keratinocytes, not dirt.
- Stress may aggravate acne, but it is not a major primary factor.
- There is no link between acne and diet.
- Strains of *P. acnes* that are less sensitive to antibiotics have become more prevalent.

■ WEBSITES
- American Academy of Dermatology AcneNet: www.derm-infonet.com/acnenet/
- Society for Pediatric Dermatology: www.spdnet.org

REFERENCES
1. DeGroot HE, Friedlander SF: Update on acne, *Curr Opin Pediatr* 10:381, 1998.
2. Leyden JJ: Therapy for acne vulgaris, *N Engl J Med* 336:1156, 1997.
3. Lucky AW: A review of infantile and pediatric acne, *Dermatology* 196:95, 1998.
4. Weiss JS: Current options for the topical treatment of acne vulgaris, *Pediatr Dermatol* 14:480, 1997.
Author: **Susan Haller Psaila, M.D.**

BASIC INFORMATION

■ DEFINITION

Adjustment disorder is comprised of emotional or behavioral symptoms occurring within 3 months of a stressor and lasting no more than 6 months after the stressor or its consequences end.

■ SYNONYM

Situational reaction

ICD-9CM CODES

309.00 With depressed mood
309.2   With anxiety
309.28 Mixed anxiety and depression
309.3   With disturbance of conduct

■ ETIOLOGY

- Adjustment disorder occurs in response to an adverse event or stressor.
- The tendency to such a response may be cultural, familial (both genetic and taught), or situational.

■ EPIDEMIOLOGY & DEMOGRAPHICS

Actual incidence is unknown.

■ HISTORY

Inciting stressor should be evident.

■ PHYSICAL EXAMINATION

Noncontributory

DIAGNOSIS

■ DIFFERENTIAL DIAGNOSIS

- Mood or anxiety disorders caused by a general medical condition
- Mood disorders
  1. May be precipitated by stressor but persist
  2. Bereavement
- Anxiety disorders
- Personality disorder (diagnosed more in older adolescents)

■ DIAGNOSTIC WORKUP

- Patient should have been asymptomatic before specific stressor occurred.
- This condition is often misdiagnosed in misguided hope that condition will be transient.

THERAPY

- Remove stressor and/or change environment.
- Lend vigorous emotional support.
- Initiate brief (2 to 3 weeks) use of benzodiazepines or antihistamines (as sedative).

■ FOLLOW-UP & DISPOSITION

Repeated episodes imply a different diagnosis; suggest family therapy and environmental change.

■ PATIENT/FAMILY EDUCATION

Encourage alternatives to encounter-by-crisis or emergency room visits.

■ PREVENTIVE TREATMENT OR TESTS

Identification of ongoing conditions (e.g., depression) with appropriate treatment

■ REFERRAL INFORMATION

- Referral is usually not required in true adjustment disorder because, by definition, this is an acute situational response.
- Alteration of ongoing, predisposing circumstances may prevent recurrence.

PEARLS & CONSIDERATIONS

■ CLINICAL PEARLS

- Two thirds of adjustment disorder diagnoses occur in patients whose conditions have existed for more than a year.
- Too often, this diagnosis is a measure of the clinician's wish to dismiss troublesome situations in crisis-oriented, unmotivated families.

■ WEBSITES

- Anxiety Disorders Association of America: www.adaa.org
- American Academy of Child & Adolescent Psychiatry: www.aacap.org

REFERENCES

1. Grimes K: Behavioral problems and stress. In Parmelee DX (ed): *Child and adolescent psychiatry,* St Louis, 1996, Mosby.
2. Levine MD, Carey WB, Crocker HC: *Developmental behavioral pediatrics,* ed 3, Philadelphia, 1992, WB Saunders.

Author: **Christopher Hodgman, M.D.**

BASIC INFORMATION

■ DEFINITION
Adrenal insufficiency is the impaired secretion of adrenocorticoid steroid hormones as a result of adrenal dysfunction or lack of adrenocorticotropic hormone (ACTH) from the pituitary. *Addison's disease* is the term used to refer to acquired adrenal insufficiency caused by adrenal gland destruction.

■ SYNONYMS
- Addison disease
- Adrenocorticoid insufficiency

ICD-9CM CODE
255.4 Addison's disease, adrenal insufficiency

■ ETIOLOGY
- Primary (adrenal pathology)
  1. Congenital adrenal hypoplasia
     a. DAX-1 gene deletion or mutation
     b. An X-linked form associated with hypogonadotropic hypogonadism
     c. Sometimes part of contiguous gene deletion syndrome with Duchenne muscular dystrophy and/or glycerol kinase deficiency
  2. ACTH unresponsiveness
     a. Occasionally associated with achalasia and alacrima
  3. Autoimmune
     a. Most common cause in adults
     b. May be isolated but is often associated with one of the following syndromes: autoimmune polyendocrinopathy candidiasis ectodermal dystrophy (APECED) *or* polyglandular autoimmune syndrome (PGA) type I, which is associated with the following:
        (1) Mucocutaneous candidiasis
        (2) Hypoparathyroidism
        (3) Occasionally, type 1 diabetes or hypothyroidism
  4. Adrenoleukodystrophy (ALD)
     a. X-linked disorder in which progressive central demyelination causes neurologic manifestations starting in the late first decade of life
     b. Appears to be a common cause of adrenal insufficiency in children and young adults
  5. Infections include the following:
     a. Tuberculosis
     b. Histoplasmosis
     c. Sarcoidosis
     d. Acute adrenal hemorrhage in meningococcemia (Waterhouse-Friderichsen syndrome)

- Secondary and tertiary (pituitary/hypothalamic) adrenal insufficiencies: caused by ACTH deficiency
  1. Pituitary or hypothalamic tumor
  2. Postoperative or postradiation therapy
  3. Suppression after long-term glucocorticoid use
     a. This is usually not a problem if glucocorticoid therapy is for less than 2 consecutive weeks.

■ EPIDEMIOLOGY & DEMOGRAPHICS
- Not well defined in children
- Incidence of X-linked ALD: 1 per 20,000

■ HISTORY
- The presentation may be acute or chronic.
- Symptoms may include any of the following:
  1. Weakness
  2. Fatigue
  3. Fever
  4. Abdominal pain
  5. Anorexia
  6. Nausea
  7. Vomiting
  8. Easy tanning or frank hyperpigmentation
- Patients may have increased salt craving if they are mineralocorticoid deficient.

■ PHYSICAL EXAMINATION
- General: thin, fatigued appearing
- Vital signs
  1. Orthostatic hypotension
  2. Hypotension or shock
  3. Tachycardia
- Signs of dehydration
  1. Dry mucous membranes
  2. Sunken eyes, fontanelle
  3. Lethargy, skin tenting
  4. Tachycardia
- Skin: hyperpigmentation (primary adrenal failure with subsequent high ACTH levels)
  1. Most obvious around skin creases, nipples, lip borders, and buccal mucosa

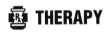

DIAGNOSIS

■ DIFFERENTIAL DIAGNOSIS
- Nonspecific and vague nature makes differential large and variable depending on the presentation.
- Gastrointestinal complaints may suggest inflammatory bowel disease, celiac disease, malignancy, or anorexia nervosa.

■ DIAGNOSTIC WORKUP
- Serum electrolytes and glucose
  1. Low sodium and high serum potassium levels are common if aldosterone deficiency is present.
  2. Acidosis may also be seen.
  3. Hypoglycemia is common.
- Cortisol level (preferably morning sample)
  1. Low serum cortisol (less than 10 µg/dl) on morning sample
- ACTH level
  1. High ACTH level in primary adrenal failure, inappropriately low for cortisol level in secondary (pituitary) hypoadrenalism
- Renin level
  1. High renin level if aldosterone deficiency is present
- ACTH stimulation test: administer 0.25 µg of Cortrosyn IV with cortisol levels at time 0 and 60 minutes
  1. Level should rise to above 15 µg/dl after ACTH stimulation.
- Radiographic studies
  1. Possibly adrenal imaging by computed tomography or magnetic resonance to assess size, consistency, and presence of mass

THERAPY

■ MEDICAL
- Acute (adrenal crisis)
  1. Intravenous (IV) fluids: bolus of normal saline if the patient is hemodynamically unstable; then rehydration rate of normal saline with 5% dextrose
  2. IV glucocorticoids: bolus of 100 mg injectable hydrocortisone (e.g., hydrocortone phosphate via intravenous push), then infusion at 100 mg/m²/day
  3. Mineralocorticoid
     a. Not needed initially because high-dose hydrocortisone effectively replaces mineralocorticoid
     b. Not generally needed in secondary adrenal insufficiency (ACTH deficiency)
- Long-term therapy
  1. Glucocorticoid: hydrocortisone by mouth at 15 to 20 mg/m²/day
  2. Mineralocorticoid: Florinef (9-αfluorocortisol) at 0.05 to 0.20 mg/day
- Stress dosing
  1. Illnesses without vomiting: A three to five times increase in the usual oral dose is needed for the duration of illness (hydrocortisone, approximately 50 mg/m²/day).
  2. Illness with vomiting: Parenteral administration of stress-dose glucocorticoids is needed.

■ **PATIENT/FAMILY EDUCATION**
- Education regarding stress-dose glucocorticoids is imperative.
- All patients should have injectable glucocorticoids at home for emergency dosing if unable to take stress dose by mouth because of vomiting.

■ **PREVENTIVE TREATMENT**
Patients known to have ALD or PGA should be tested for adrenal insufficiency.

■ **REFERRAL INFORMATION**
- All patients with adrenal insufficiency should be referred to an endocrinologist for complete evaluation and initial management.
- Treatment of suspected adrenal insufficiency should *not* be delayed until consultation because fatal adrenal crisis could occur in the interim.

⁝⟡⁝ PEARLS & CONSIDERATIONS

■ **CLINICAL PEARLS**
- Addisonian crisis with hypotension can occur with only glucocorticoid deficiency and thus with relatively normal electrolytes.
  1. Addisonian crisis and need for stress-dose glucocorticoids cannot be ruled out by normal electrolytes.
- All patients should have medical alert bracelet or equivalent to alert medical emergency personal of their condition.
  1. Failure to treat with stress doses promptly during significant trauma or illness is potentially fatal.

■ **WEBSITES**
- National Association of Adrenal Disorders: www.medhelp.org/nadf/

- Support Group and Quarterly Newsletter: http://my.dmci.net/~hoffmanrj/

REFERENCES

1. Adams R, Hinkebein MK, McQuillenn M: Prompt differentiation of Addison's disease from anorexia nervosa during weight loss and vomiting, *South Med J* 91:208, 1998.
2. Agwu JC et al: Tests of adrenal insufficiency, *Arch Dis Child* 80:330, 1993.
3. Jorge P et al: X-linked adrenoleukodystrophy in patients with idiopathic Addison disease, *Eur J Pediatr* 153:594, 1994.
4. New MI, Rapaport R: The adrenal cortex. In Sperling MA (ed): *Pediatric endocrinology*, Philadelphia, 1996, WB Saunders.

Author: **Craig C. Orlowski, M.D.**

BASIC INFORMATION

DEFINITION

HIV infection is caused by the human immunodeficiency virus (HIV), leading to a spectrum of illness from an early asymptomatic latent period to progressive immunologic deterioration and associated opportunistic infections and malignancies. The final stage is acquired immunodeficiency syndrome (AIDS).

ICD-9CM CODES

042 HIV infection or AIDS
795.71 Infant born to HIV-infected mother, not yet diagnosed with certainty by HIV polymerase chain reaction (PCR) or culture assays
V65.44 Code to be used for pretest and posttest counseling

ETIOLOGY

- HIV-1, a human retrovirus, is the major etiologic agent worldwide.
- A related retrovirus, HIV-2, causes a similar illness predominantly in West Africa.
- HIV has a tremendous mutation rate, resulting in significant variation in antigenic reactivity and antiviral resistance of viruses isolated from different individuals and even from within the same individual.

EPIDEMIOLOGY & DEMOGRAPHICS

- General epidemiology
  1. In the United States children account for only 2% of cumulative AIDS cases, but worldwide they account for nearly 25% of cases.
- Modes of transmission
  1. Currently, more than 95% of children with HIV infection acquire the infection from their mother (vertical transmission); transfusion of contaminated blood or clotting factor concentrates is now rarely observed in the United States.
  2. Other modes of transmission, particularly in adolescents, include sexual contact and injecting drug use.
  3. Breastfeeding remains a possible risk for transmission as well.
  4. Remarkably few well-documented cases of HIV transmission have occurred after bites or routine care in hospitals, clinics, or child care settings.
- Risk groups
  1. Infants born to HIV-infected mothers
     a. Risk of infection is 13% to 39% if no antiretroviral therapy delivered to mother and infant.

b. With appropriate therapy, risk is less than 5%.
c. Risk factors for vertical transmission include maternal viral load and degree of immunodeficiency and prolonged rupture of membranes.
  2. Adolescents engaging in unprotected sexual contact or injecting drugs with shared and/or contaminated equipment
- Predominant clinical syndromes (variable, may include all organ systems; antiretroviral therapy may delay onset/modify syndromes)
  1. *HIV-infected infants:* Infants are generally asymptomatic for first few months of life; mean age of onset of symptoms is 1 year, but some remain asymptomatic for more than 5 years. Two categories are recognized:
     a. From 10% to 15% rapidly progress to symptoms by 6 to 12 months; death occurs by 2 to 4 years.
     b. From 85% to 90% have slower progression and survive beyond 5 years.
  2. Common manifestations in infancy include failure to thrive, hepatosplenomegaly, oral candidiasis, and *Pneumocystis carinii* pneumonia between 3 to 6 months of age.
  3. *HIV-infected children:* Common manifestations include generalized lymphadenopathy, hepatosplenomegaly, failure to thrive, oral candidiasis, recurrent diarrhea, parotitis, developmental delay (either static or progressive), recurrent bacterial infections, lymphocytic interstitial pneumonitis, nephropathy, hepatitis, and cardiomyopathy.
  4. Common opportunistic infections include *P. carinii* pneumonia (most common), *Candida* esophagitis, chronic or disseminated cytomegalovirus (CMV), herpes simplex virus (HSV), or varicella-zoster virus (VZV) infections. Rarely, tuberculosis, atypical *Mycobacterium* infections, toxoplasmosis, and cryptococcosis may develop.
  5. Malignancies are uncommon compared with adults with HIV infection, but leiomyosarcomas and lymphomas (especially of the central nervous system or non-Hodgkin's B-cell Burkitt type) occur. Kaposi's sarcoma is rare in children.

HISTORY

Risk factors discussed previously (e.g., infant born to HIV-infected mother, high-risk behaviors, history of opportunistic infections)

PHYSICAL EXAMINATION

Generalized lymphadenopathy, organomegaly, oral thrush, scars from recurrent HSV or herpes zoster infections, chronic infiltrative parotitis, failure to thrive

DIAGNOSIS

DIFFERENTIAL DIAGNOSIS

- Congenital primary immunodeficiency syndromes
- Congenital or early infancy infections (CMV, syphilis, Epstein-Barr virus [EBV], toxoplasmosis)

DIAGNOSTIC WORKUP

- Anemia, neutropenia, and thrombocytopenia are common.
- Progressive loss of total lymphocytes, especially with CD4 lymphopenia, is seen; progressive humoral immune dysfunction occurs, with frequent elevations in serum IgG, IgM, and IgA.
- Children older than 18 months: HIV infection is diagnosed by positive antibody test (enzyme immunoassay confirmed by Western blot).
- Children younger than 18 months: Antibody tests are confounded by transplacental maternal antibody. Diagnosis at this age requires virologic tests such as HIV PCR or culture.
  1. Tests should be performed at 1 month *and* 4 to 6 months of age at a minimum.
  2. Positive results constitute presumptive evidence of infection and should be immediately confirmed by repeat testing.
  3. Two negative virologic tests, one of which are performed at 1 month or older and one of which is performed at 4 months or older, exclude HIV infection with reasonable certainty (95%).
     a. Such children are followed until antibody tests revert to negative (15 to18 months of age) to absolutely exclude infection.
  4. Some experts perform additional PCR tests at less than 1 month of age.
- Several states are implementing routine HIV antibody screening of pregnant women and/or newborns to increase the opportunity for successful interruption of vertical transmission by antenatal therapy; such efforts should be supported.
- Oral counseling and consent should be obtained when HIV antibody tests

II

are performed (some jurisdictions require written consent).

℞ THERAPY

■ MEDICAL

- On the basis of an increasing number of pediatric clinical trials and extrapolation from adult studies, antiretroviral therapy has become the standard of care for HIV-infected children.
  1. Primary care physicians are encouraged to participate actively in the care of HIV-infected children in consultation with specialists who have expertise in the treatment of pediatric HIV infection.
  2. Expert opinions and knowledge about diagnostic and therapeutic approaches are changing rapidly, making frequent consultation crucial.
  3. When possible, enrollment of the HIV-infected child into available clinical trials should be encouraged.
- Therapy is suggested for infected infants younger than 12 months of age, symptomatic (clinically or immunologically) children older than 12 months of age, and often asymptomatic children older than 12 months of age.
- Currently available medications include six nucleoside reverse transcriptase inhibitors (NRTIs) (i.e., zidovudine, didanosine, stavudine, lamivudine, Abacavir, and zalcitabine); three nonnucleoside reverse transcriptase inhibitors (NNRTIs) (i.e., nevirapine, delavirdine, and Efavirenz); and five protease inhibitors (PIs) (i.e., saquinavir, ritonavir, indinavir, nelfinavir, and Amprenavir).
- Generally, a three-drug combination of two NRTIs and one PI, or two NRTIs and one NNRTI, or one drug of each class, is used for maximum effect.
  1. Regimens are adjusted based on virologic suppression, tolerance of adverse effects, and palatability of medications.
- Prophylaxis against opportunistic infections is an important adjunct to antiretroviral therapy.
  1. Beginning at 4 to 6 weeks of age, trimethoprim-sulfamethoxazole (TMP-SMX) should be given to all infants born to HIV-infected women to prevent *P. carinii* disease and should be continued

until HIV infection is excluded by serial negative virologic tests. It is also given throughout the first year of life to children whose infection status remains undetermined and to those children of all ages who are HIV infected and who have advanced immunosuppression (CD4 lymphocyte percentage less than 15%).
  2. Prophylaxis against other organisms, such as atypical mycobacteria, CMV, and *Candida*, are occasionally used for some children with advanced AIDS.
- Appropriate immunization is the third component of pediatric HIV therapy.
  1. In general, live vaccines (e.g., oral poliovirus vaccine [OPV], bacille Calmette-Guérin [BCG]) are contraindicated.
  2. Exceptions include the measles, mumps, rubella (MMR) vaccine, which is indicated for asymptomatic and symptomatic HIV-infected children, except for those who are severely immunocompromised, and the varicella vaccine, which has been shown recently to be safe in asymptomatic and early-stage HIV-infected children.
  3. Killed (inactivated) vaccines such as hepatitis B virus; diptheria, tetanus, acellular pertussis (DTaP); and *Haemophilus influenzae* type B (Hib) conjugate and pneumococcal conjugate vaccines are routinely indicated for all HIV-infected children, as are annual influenza vaccinations and possible pneumococcal polysaccaride vaccinations. Consultation with a pediatric HIV specialist is recommended.

■ PREVENTIVE TREATMENT OR TESTS

- Antiretroviral therapy of HIV-infected women during pregnancy and labor and of the infant for 6 weeks is effective at interrupting vertical transmission.
- HIV-infected women should be counseled *not* to breast-feed their infants (recommendations in developing countries where clean water and formula are not available may differ).
- Safer sex practices, including appropriate use of condoms and avoidance of shared and/or unclean injectable drug apparatus, are effective in preventing HIV infection among adolescents and adults.

- Blood or bloody fluids in hospitals, schools, or child care settings or on athletic fields should be disinfected with freshly diluted household bleach (1:10 to 1:100).

☼ PEARLS & CONSIDERATIONS

■ CLINICAL PEARLS

- Clinical manifestations seen *more often* in pediatric HIV than in adult HIV cases include more rapid progression, more recurrent invasive bacterial infection, occurrence of lymphocytic interstitial pneumonitis, and more frequent progressive encephalopathy.
- Clinical manifestations seen *much less often* in pediatric HIV than in adult HIV cases include cerebral toxoplasmosis, cryptococcal meningitis, CMV retinitis, Kaposi's sarcoma, and TMP-SMX hypersensitivity.

■ WEBSITES

- HIV/AIDS Treatment Service (ATIS): www.hivatis.org; a federal government site sponsored by the Department of Health and Human Services, the Centers for Disease Control and Prevention (CDC), and the National Institutes of Health (NIH); is a continually updated source of approved treatment guidelines for adult and pediatric HIV/AIDS and related topics
- HIV/AIDS Clinical Trials Information Service (ACTIS): www.hivactis.org; sister site of ATIS and provides access to information on ongoing clinical trials for adults and children with HIV/AIDS
- CDC: www.cdc.gov/hiv/hivinfo.htm; HIV/AIDS information site containing several multimedia tools and information resources, including a fax information service and information in Spanish
- *JAMA* HIV/AIDS Information Center: www.ama-assn.org/special/hiv/hivhome.htm; maintained by the editors and staff of *JAMA*; contains news releases, treatment guidelines, drug information, links to other organizations, and patient information
- National Pediatric and Family HIV Resource Center at the University of Medicine and Dentistry at New Jersey: www.pedhivaids.org; contains treatment guidelines, patient educational materials, newsletters, and other information

REFERENCES

1. American Academy of Pediatrics: HIV infection. In *1997 Red Book: Report of the Committee on Infectious Diseases,* ed 24, Elk Grove Village, Ill, 1997, American Academy of Pediatrics.
2. Burns DN, Mofenson LM: Paediatric HIV infection, *Lancet* 354(suppl 2): 1, 1999.
3. Weinberg GA: Human immunodeficiency virus (HIV) infection in children. In Beers MH, Berkow R (eds): *The Merck manual of diagnosis and therapy,* ed 17, Whitehouse Station, NJ, 1999, Merck.
4. Weinberg GA: Pediatric human immunodeficiency virus (HIV) infection. In Mandell GL, Bennett JE, Dolin R (eds): *Mandell, Douglas and Bennett's principles and practice of infectious diseases,* ed 5, Philadelphia, 2000, WB Saunders.

Author: **Geoffrey A. Weinberg, M.D.**

II

BASIC INFORMATION

■ DEFINITION

Acute intoxication is caused by the excessive oral intake of ethyl alcohol.

■ SYNONYMS

• Inebriation
• Drunkenness
• Acute alcoholism
• Alcohol poisoning

ICD-9CM CODES

305.0 Acute intoxication
303.0 With alcoholism
980.9 Acute alcohol poisoning, specify ethyl alcohol
291.4 Pathologic intoxication
303.9 Alcoholism

■ ETIOLOGY

• Accidental ingestion of alcoholic beverages (younger children)
• Accidental overingestion by inexperienced older children and adolescents
• Purposeful intoxication (adolescent binge-drinking, alcohol abuse, alcoholism)

■ EPIDEMIOLOGY & DEMOGRAPHICS

• Ethyl alcohol is widely available in adult beverages; therefore large numbers of children and adolescents are exposed.
• Approximately 80% of ninth- to twelfth-grade students have drunk alcohol at least once, 50% are current drinkers, and 33% are current binge-drinkers (five or more drinks in a row).
• Males are more likely to engage in heavy drinking than females, and whites and Hispanics are more likely to engage in heavy drinking than are African-American students.
• Almost 17% of high school students drink and drive.
  1. More than 36% ride in cars with an intoxicated driver.
  2. Alcohol-related motor vehicle crashes are a leading cause of death among young people.

■ HISTORY

• Accidental injury or trauma
• Concurrent use of illicit drugs or prescription medications
• Associated health-risk behaviors (e.g., drinking and driving, unprotected sex)
• Prior alcohol use or abuse
• Friends who drink and/or use drugs
• Parent or family history of alcohol abuse or alcoholism

■ PHYSICAL EXAMINATION

• Classic physical findings include odor of alcohol on breath, nystag-mus, conjunctival injection, hypore-flexia, ataxia, and orthostatic hypotension.
• Signs and symptoms vary with blood alcohol concentration (BAC, in mg/dl):
  1. BAC lower than 100: incoordination, decreased reflexes, and emotional lability
  2. BAC 100 to 250: slurred speech, ataxia, confusion, nausea, and vomiting
  3. BAC 250 to 400: stupor, unresponsiveness, incontinence, and respiratory depression
  4. BAC higher than 400: hypothermia and death (may occur at lower BAC in children)
• Check carefully for signs of trauma, aspiration, or other drug use.

DIAGNOSIS

■ DIFFERENTIAL DIAGNOSIS

• Head trauma
• Other drug intoxication
• Hypoglycemia
• Sepsis, shock
• Central nervous system infection
• Hepatic encephalopathy
• Any other condition that can cause alteration in mental status

■ DIAGNOSTIC WORKUP

• Laboratory analysis
  1. BAC (see previous listing for interpretation)
  2. Blood and urine toxicology
  3. Serum glucose, blood urea nitrogen (BUN), and electrolytes
  4. Head computed tomography (CT) scan or magnetic resonance imaging (MRI) scan should be considered in the following cases:
     a. Trauma is known or suspected.
     b. Mental status fails to improve during a brief period of observation.

THERAPY

■ NONPHARMACOLOGIC

• Mild alcohol intoxication usually requires observation only.
• Intravenous hydration (10% glucose to prevent hypoglycemia)
• If unresponsive:
  1. Assess integrity of the gag reflex.
  2. Secure the airway if necessary.
  3. Support ventilation.
  4. Perform gastric lavage after airway is secure.
• Consider hemodialysis if hepatic damage is present or BAC is higher than 300 in a comatose patient.

■ MEDICAL

• If ingestion occurred within 2 to 3 hours, administer activated charcoal (30 to 60 g for young children; 60 to 100 g for adolescents) and magnesium sulfate 250 mg/kg.
• Administer naloxone if concurrent drug use is suspected.
• Administer multivitamins, thiamine, and folate if alcoholism is suspected.

■ FOLLOW-UP & DISPOSITION

• Rapid clearing of sensorium is to be expected.
  1. If steady improvement is not seen over the first few hours, patient must be reassessed for other possible causes of altered mental status (e.g., head trauma, drug intoxication).
• Assessment and therapy for substance abuse disorders (see "Patient/Family Education")
• Assessment and therapy for comorbid mental health problems

■ PATIENT/FAMILY EDUCATION

• For an isolated occurrence of intoxication in an adolescent, the physician should emphasize risk reduction.
  1. Provide information and advice about drinking and driving or riding in a car with an intoxicated driver.
  2. Negotiate or "contract" for specific changes in behavior and arrange follow-up.
• For youth with recurrent episodes of intoxication or other alcohol-related problems, physicians should make a referral to an appropriate community treatment program.
  1. Attendance at 12-step support meetings (e.g., Alcoholics Anonymous [AA]) should be encouraged.
  2. Youth should be accompanied by an adult "temporary sponsor."
     a. Call the AA central service number listed in the local telephone directory.

■ PREVENTIVE TREATMENT OR TESTS

• According to the American Medical Association's Guidelines for Adolescent Preventive Services, every adolescent should be screened for alcohol and drug use as part of routine care.
• One way of accomplishing this is with the following CRAFFT test:
  C Have you ever ridden in a **CAR** driven by someone (including yourself) who was "high" or had been using alcohol or drugs?
  R Do you ever use alcohol or drugs to **RELAX**, feel better about yourself, or fit in?

A   Do you ever use alcohol or drugs while you are **ALONE**?

F   Do you ever **FORGET** things you did while using alcohol or drugs?

F   Do your family or **FRIENDS** ever tell you that you should cut down on your drinking or drug use?

T   Have you ever gotten into **TROUBLE** while you were using alcohol or drugs?

*   *Two or more "yes" answers suggests a significant problem.*

■ REFERRAL INFORMATION

Physicians should be familiar with treatment resources in their own community. For most adolescents, outpatient counseling is the appropriate initial treatment.

☼ PEARLS & CONSIDERATIONS

■ CLINICAL PEARLS

BAC may be estimated by calculating serum osmolal gap (serum osmolality [$2 \times$ Na + BUN/2.8 + glucose/18]); then estimating BAC of 100 mg/dl for every 22 to 25 osmolal gap increment.

■ WEBSITES

*   Alcoholics Anonymous: www.alcoholics-anonymous.org/
*   National Center for Alcohol and Drug Information (NCADI): www.health.org/index.htm

REFERENCES

1. American Academy of Pediatrics, Committee on Substance Abuse: Tobacco, alcohol, and other drugs: the role of the pediatrician in prevention and management of substance abuse, *Pediatrics* 101:125, 1998.
2. Henretig F et al: Toxicologic emergencies. In Fleisher G, Ludwig S (eds): *Textbook of pediatric emergency medicine*, ed 2, Baltimore, 1988, Williams & Wilkins.
3. Kleinschmidt K, Delaney K: Ethanol. In Haddad L, Winchester J, Shannon M (eds): *Clinical management of poisoning and drug overdose*, Philadelphia, 1997, WB Saunders.
4. Knight J: Substance use, abuse, and dependency. In Levine M, Carey W, Crocker A (eds): *Developmental-behavioral pediatrics*, Philadelphia, 1999, WB Saunders.
5. Knight JR et al: A new brief screen for adolescent substance abuse, *Arch Pediatr Adolesc Med* 153:591, 1999.
6. Morality trends and leading causes of death among adolescents and young adults—United States, 1979-1988, *MMWR Morbid Mortal Week Rep* 42:459, 1993.
7. Youth risk behavior surveillance—United States, 1997, *MMWR Morbid Mortal Week Rep* 47:1, 1998.

Author: **John R. Knight, M.D.**

II

BASIC INFORMATION

DEFINITION

Allergic bronchopulmonary aspergillosis (ABPA) is a hypersensitivity pulmonary disease occurring in individuals with asthma or cystic fibrosis; it is characterized by transient pulmonary infiltrates, reversible airway obstruction, eosinophilia, and evidence of hypersensitivity to *Aspergillus fumigatus*, a fungus.

SYNONYMS

- ABPA
- Bronchopulmonary aspergillosis
- Allergic aspergillosis

ICD-9CM CODE

518.6 ABPA

ETIOLOGY

- Ubiquitous *A. fumigatus* spores are inhaled and trapped in obstructed airways with impaired clearance.
- Colonization is helped by small spore size and temperatures at which *A. fumigatus* grows.
- High colonization rate of *A. fumigatus* is seen in patients with asthma or cystic fibrosis (CF).
- Continuous source of antigenic stimulation leads to both type I IgE-mediated and type III immune complex–mediated hypersensitivity reactions.

EPIDEMIOLOGY & DEMOGRAPHICS

- Present in 8% to 11% of patients with CF
- Occurs in 6% to 20% of adults with asthma; rare in pediatric patients with asthma
- Reported from most countries of the world

HISTORY

- Medical history of asthma, atopy, or CF
- Episodic wheezing of increasing frequency or severity
- Possibly fever, weight loss, anorexia, dyspnea, malaise, chest pain, fatigue, or hemoptysis

PHYSICAL EXAMINATION

- Generalized airway obstruction with wheezes and rhonchi is present.
- Signs of hyperaeration (e.g., barrel chest, prolonged expiratory phase) are observed.
- Localized crackles may be heard.
- Digital clubbing is present in those with more severe disease.

DIAGNOSIS

DIFFERENTIAL DIAGNOSIS

- Lung diseases caused by *A. fumigatus*: invasive aspergillosis, aspergilloma, IgE-mediated asthma from *A. fumigatus* sensitivity, and hypersensitivity pneumonitis caused by *A. fumigatus*
- Bacterial, fungal, viral, tuberculous, or eosinophilic pneumonia
- Inadequately controlled asthma
- CF

DIAGNOSTIC WORKUP

- Major diagnostic criteria
  1. Episodic reversible bronchial obstruction (by history and pulmonary function testing)
  2. Peripheral blood eosinophilia (more than 500 cells/mm^3) (*Note:* Eosinophilia is one of the best measures of disease activity.)
  3. Immediate type 1 skin reactivity to *A. fumigatus* antigen
  4. Precipitating antibodies to *A. fumigatus* antigen (by double gel diffusion technique of Ouchterlony)
  5. Elevated serum IgE level (more than 1000 IU/ml) (only a fraction against *A. fumigatus*) (*Note:* This factor is a good reflection of disease activity.)
  6. History of pulmonary infiltrates (see following discussion)
  7. Central bronchiectasis by chest radiograph or chest computed tomography (CT) scan
  8. Specific IgE and IgG antibodies to *A. fumigatus* (by radioallergosorbent test [RAST], enzyme-linked immunosorbent assay [ELISA])
- Minor criteria
  1. *A. fumigatus*–positive sputum cultures
  2. History of expectorating brown sputum plugs that contain hyphae of *A. fumigatus*
  3. Arthus (late) skin reaction to *A. fumigatus* antigen
  4. Sputum smear (expectorated or by bronchoscopy) with septate hyphae and eosinophils
- Chest radiograph findings
  1. Transient or migratory opacities
  2. Upper lobe predominance
  3. Ring shadows
  4. Atelectasis of a segment, lobe, or entire lung
  5. Central bronchiectasis
  6. Hyperinflation, bronchial mucoid impaction, and/or tram-line shadows
  7. Gloved-finger shadows
  8. Fibrosis

- Five stages
  1. Stage I (acute): symptoms, chest radiograph and laboratory findings
  2. Stage II (remission): clearing of infiltrates; decline in IgE for 6 months after steroids
  3. Stage III (exacerbation): new infiltrates and more than twofold rise in IgE
  4. Stage IV (corticosteroid-dependent asthma)
  5. Stage V (fibrotic end stage): irreversible obstructive and restrictive defects

THERAPY

NONPHARMACOLOGIC

- Avoidance of farm buildings, barns, stables, silos, and compost heaps where *A. fumigatus* is prevalent
- Airway clearance with chest physiotherapy and postural drainage

MEDICAL

- Systemic corticosteroids are the treatment of choice for acute-stage disease and exacerbations.
- Prednisone should be given at a dosage of 0.5 mg/kg/day for 2 weeks, then an alternate-day regimen should be used for 3 to 6 months.
- Useful adjunct therapies include itraconazole, inhaled steroids, and possibly cromolyn sodium.
- Allergen immunotherapy has no role with *Aspergillus* species.

FOLLOW-UP & DISPOSITION

- Serial total serum IgE should be monitored monthly for the first year.
  1. Total serum IgE falls by 35% or more within 2 months after treatment with systemic steroids.
  2. Total serum IgE antibodies and blood eosinophil count best reflect disease activity.
- Serial chest radiographs should be taken every 3 to 4 months for 2 years, then every 6 to 12 months.

PATIENT/FAMILY EDUCATION

- The prognosis is good if diagnosed early, before severe lung destruction.
  1. Death occurs from end-stage fibrotic lung disease in the presence of cor pulmonale.
- Symptoms are not always reliable indicators of disease activity or pulmonary infiltrates.
- Serial prospective evaluation may be indicated to confirm or exclude ABPA.

■ REFERRAL INFORMATION

Diagnosis can be difficult; most cases require referral to a pediatric pulmonologist or allergist.

☼ PEARLS & CONSIDERATIONS

■ CLINICAL PEARLS
- This condition may be the initial presentation of CF.
- Early diagnosis and treatment are essential to prevent pulmonary fibrosis and insufficiency.
- Overlap of symptoms and radiographic findings in ABPA and CF make the diagnosis difficult.
- A clue to ABPA in CF is that infiltrates progress despite antibiotics and resolve with steroid therapy.

■ WEBSITE
Dr. Koop: www.drkoop.com/adam/peds/top/000070.html

REFERENCES

1. Brueton MJ et al: Allergic bronchopulmonary aspergillosis complicating cystic fibrosis in childhood, *Arch Dis Child* 55:348, 1980.
2. Greenberger PA: Allergic bronchopulmonary aspergillosis, *J Allergy Clin Immunol* 74:645, 1984.
3. Laufer P et al: Allergic bronchopulmonary aspergillosis in cystic fibrosis, *J Allergy Clin Immunol* 73:44, 1984.
4. Simmonds EJ, Littlewood JM, Evans EG: Cystic fibrosis and allergic bronchopulmonary aspergillosis, *Arch Dis Child* 65:507, 1990.
5. Slavin RG, Gottlieb CC, Avioli LV: Allergic bronchopulmonary aspergillosis, *Arch Intern Med* 146:1799, 1986.

Author: **Barbara Chini, M.D.**

II

BASIC INFORMATION

■ DEFINITION

A symptom complex of nasal congestion, rhinorrhea, sneezing, and nasal itching resulting from inflammation of the mucosal lining of the nose and contiguous mucosal membranes, usually occurring in temporal relationship to an airborne allergen exposure

■ SYNONYMS

- Hay fever
- Rose fever

ICD-9CM CODE

477.9 Allergic rhinitis

■ ETIOLOGY

- Airborne allergens (e.g., pollens, cat dander, dust mites) contact the respiratory mucosa in a susceptible patient who has had IgE sensitization to the antigen or antigens.
- Immediate phase
  1. This results from allergen contact with IgE on mucosal mast cells or basophils.
  2. This leads to cell degranulation and release of mediators.
     a. Preformed mediators (e.g., histamine)
     b. Preformed but slowly eluted mediators (e.g., heparin, trypsin)
     c. Newly synthesized mediators (e.g., leukotrienes, prostaglandins)
  3. These mediators increase vascular permeability, tissue edema, and begin cellular recruitment.
- Late phase
  1. This phase occurs 4 to 24 hours after mast cell activation.
  2. Cellular infiltration plays a more significant role and produces nasal obstruction that is less responsive to antihistamines and decongestants.

■ EPIDEMIOLOGY & DEMOGRAPHICS

- Allergic rhinitis is a disease predominantly occurring in childhood (mean onset, 10.6 years).
- It is very common, with prevalence rates of 10% in those younger than 12 years and 20% to 30% among adolescents.
- Although racial differences have been reported, migration studies suggest that environmental factors play a more important role.
  1. A 17% prevalence of allergic rhinitis among children born to parents without allergic rhinitis
  2. A 26% prevalence in children with one parent with allergic rhinitis
  3. A 52% prevalence rate in children with both parents with allergic rhinitis

■ HISTORY

- Typical symptoms are sneezing, nasal itching, nasal congestion, clear rhinorrhea, and palatal itching.
- These symptoms can coexist with ocular symptoms of itching, tearing, and redness.
- Pattern and chronicity is seasonal, perennial, or episodic.
- This can be associated with specific triggers:
  1. Indoor: dust mites and animal dander
  2. Outdoor: molds and pollens
  3. Nonallergic triggers: cigarette smoke can also exacerbate symptoms
- Significant risk factors are a personal and family history of allergic disorders.

■ PHYSICAL EXAMINATION

- External examination: allergic facies
  1. Allergic shiners: infraorbital dark skin discoloration
  2. Allergic crease: a transverse nasal crease caused by rubbing and pushing the tip of the nose upward to relieve obstruction and itching
  3. Puffy eyelids
- Examination of the interior of the nose
  1. Clear, watery discharge
  2. Pale, edematous mucosa
     a. Nasal turbinates may completely occlude the nasal passages.
     b. Examination after placement of topical nasal decongestant drops is needed to exclude nasal polyps and other abnormalities.
- Conjunctival injection
- Examination of the lungs: may show wheezing (asthma is a comorbid condition)
- Examination of skin: may show eczema

DIAGNOSIS

■ DIFFERENTIAL DIAGNOSIS

- Vasomotor rhinitis (irritant rhinitis)
- Nonallergic rhinitis with eosinophilia (NARES syndrome)
- Acute infectious rhinitis
- Acute and/or chronic sinusitis
- Anatomic abnormalities
  1. Septal deviation
  2. Hypertrophic turbinates
  3. Nasal polyps
  4. Adenoidal adenopathy
  5. Foreign bodies
  6. Choanal atresia or stenosis
  7. Nasal tumors (benign and malignant)
  8. Cerebrospinal rhinorrhea
- Hormonal (e.g., hypothyroidism)

■ DIAGNOSTIC WORKUP

- Diagnosis is based on history and physical examination, along with response to therapy.
- There are no diagnostic laboratory tests.
- IgE may be elevated.
- Nasal smears often show eosinophils.

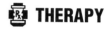

THERAPY

■ NONPHARMACOLOGIC

Involves environmental controls
- Pollens
  1. Keep windows closed and air conditioners on automatic.
- Molds
  1. Dehumidification
  2. Avoidance of outdoor sources such as mowing the lawn or raking leaves
- House dust mites
  1. Enclose mattresses and pillowcases in allergen-proof materials.
  2. Wash bed linens in hot water (above 130° F).
     a. Caution with water temperatures in homes with young children because of scalding risks.
  3. Avoid bedroom carpeting.
- Animals
  1. Remove pets shedding dander and hair from home or isolate (less optimal) from patient.
  2. Eliminate cockroach, mice, or rat infestations.
- Irritants
  1. Eliminate exposure to cigarette smoke, perfumes, chalk dust, and other irritating materials.

■ MEDICAL

- Oral antihistamines effectively reduce rhinorrhea, sneezing, itching, and ocular symptoms.
  1. They have little effect on nasal congestion.
  2. Nonsedating antihistamines, although more costly, are preferred over sedating antihistamines because they pose little risk of performance impairment.
- Decongestants, alone or in combination with antihistamines, can effectively reduce congestion.
  1. Side effects of oral decongestants include nervousness, insomnia, and appetite loss.
  2. Topical decongestants are effective, but prolonged use (more than 3 days) can lead to rebound congestion.
- Intranasal corticosteroids are the most effective agents to control sneezing, rhinorrhea, nasal itching, and congestion.
  1. Concerns have arisen over the potential to affect childhood growth.

2. Medication should be used at the lowest possible dosage for the shortest duration possible.
3. Heights should be monitored.
- Intranasal cromolyn spray is less effective than intranasal corticosteroids but is associated with few side effects.
   1. Recommended frequent dosing (three to four times a day) adversely affects adherence.
- Other therapies include the following:
   1. Nasal saline washes
   2. Intranasal antihistamines
      a. Astelin for children 12 years and older
      b. Has bitter taste and can cause drowsiness
   3. Intranasal anticholinergic agents
      a. Ipratropium 0.03% for children 6 years and older
      b. Helpful for the rhinorrhea component of allergic rhinitis
- For severe cases of allergic rhinitis, a one-time short course of oral corticosteroids (e.g., prednisone 1 mg/kg/day for 3 days) may provide more immediate relief and improve effectiveness of other therapies.
- Immunotherapy (e.g., hyposensitization, allergy shots) may modify disease.
   1. Effective treatment options are available for selected patients with moderate to severe symptoms lasting several months of the year and/or for those who are unresponsive to other treatment options, including both environmental control and pharmacotherapy.
   2. Vaccine is based on a careful patient history and results of allergy testing.
   3. Allergy injections should be given only in an appropriately equipped office with a physician immediately available to treat anaphylactic reactions.
   4. Patients should stay in office 30 minutes after the injection or injections.
      a. Patients should be instructed to report any adverse reactions.
      b. Report changes in chronic medication use—the use of β-blocking agents can intensify anaphylactic reactions.

■ PATIENT/FAMILY EDUCATION
- Education of parents and patients about symptoms and triggers of allergic rhinitis
- Environmental control of allergens and irritants
- Appropriate use of medications
   1. In particular, patients (or parents) should be shown and be able to demonstrate correct use of prescribed nasal inhalers.
- Expected results and precautions for allergy immunotherapy

■ PREVENTIVE TREATMENT
- Lifelong responsiveness to aeroallergens appears to ultimately be determined early in life.
- Proposed strategies of prevention include the following:
   1. Identification of high-risk infants before or after birth
   2. Avoidance of infant exposure to food allergens
      a. Breastfeeding for at least 4 to 6 months
      b. Maternal lactation with no eggs, cows' milk, or peanuts
      c. Supplementation or weaning with a hypoallergenic formula
      d. Delay of solid foods for 6 months and then adding least allergenic food first
      e. For high-risk foods such as eggs, peanuts, and fish, waiting until 2 to 3 years of age before introducing
   3. Early avoidance of aeroallergens by environmental control measures (as noted previously)

■ REFERRAL INFORMATION
- Consider referral to an allergist for patients with prolonged manifestations or allergic rhinitis that impair functioning or quality of life, contribute to comorbid conditions like sinusitis, and/or require prolonged use of medications or unsatisfactory response to them.
- Elucidation of allergic rhinitis triggers and more extensive patient education can be helpful.

☼ PEARLS & CONSIDERATIONS

■ CLINICAL PEARLS
- Adequate examination of the nasal airway in active allergic rhinitis may require placement of topical decongestants a few moments before examination.
- For nasal inhaler use, providing instructions to the patient with a sample inhaler may improve the patient's technique and adherence to the regimen. Some patients prefer "dry" inhalers over "wet" ones and vice versa.

■ WEBSITES
- American Academy of Allergy, Asthma, and Immunology: www.aaaai.org
- American College of Allergy, Asthma, and Immunology: www.acaai.org
- Asthma and Allergy Foundation of America (AAFA): www.aafa.org
- National Institutes of Allergy and Infectious Diseases (NIAID): www.niaid.nih.gov/factsheets/allergyr.htm

REFERENCES
1. Björkstén B, Kjellman NIM, Zeiger RS: Development and prevention of allergic disease in childhood. In Middleton E et al (ed): *Allergy: principles and practice,* St Louis, 1998, Mosby.
2. Dykewicz MS et al: Diagnosis and management of rhinitis: complete guidelines of the Joint Task Force on Practice Parameters in Allergy, Asthma, and Immunology, *Ann Allergy Asthma Immunol* 81:478, 1998.
3. Newachek PW, Stoddard JJ: Prevalence and impact of multiple childhood chronic illnesses, *J Pediatr* 124:40, 1994.
4. Wright AL, et al: Epidemiology of physician-diagnoses allergic rhinitis in childhood, *Pediatrics* 94:895, 1994.

Author: **Thomas J. Fischer, M.D.**

II

BASIC INFORMATION

DEFINITION
In the setting of a recent gain in altitude, headache plus at least one of the following symptoms: fatigue and/or weakness, nausea and/or vomiting and/or anorexia, dizziness and/or light-headedness, or difficulty sleeping.

SYNONYMS
- High-altitude sickness
- Acute mountain sickness (AMS)
- Mountain illness
- Altitude mountain sickness

ICD-9CM CODE
993.2 Other and unspecified effects of high altitude

ETIOLOGY
- Rapid exposure to hypobaric, hypoxic conditions
- Made worse by a poor hypoxic ventilatory response (HVR)—hyperventilation to maintain adequate arterial oxygen saturation

EPIDEMIOLOGY & DEMOGRAPHICS
- Approximately 20% of people who rapidly reach 2400 meters (8000 feet) from sea-level develop acute mountain sickness (AMS).
- Children are affected more than adults.
- The development or degree of AMS is not predicted by physical condition.
- AMS is more likely the higher the altitude and the faster the altitude is achieved.
- Patients with blunted HVR are more likely to develop AMS than those with brisk HVR.

HISTORY
- Rapid ascent from sea-level to high altitude, usually more than 2400 meters (8000 feet)
- Symptoms occurring 12 to 24 hours after altitude reached
  1. Subside in 2 to 7 days
- Symptoms include the following:
  1. Headache
  2. Weakness
  3. Fatigue
  4. Gastrointestinal symptoms (nausea, vomiting, anorexia)
  5. Dizziness
  6. Light-headedness
  7. Difficulty sleeping

PHYSICAL EXAMINATION
- Tired appearing
  1. Dyspnea with exertion but none at rest
  2. Lungs clear
  3. Normal neurologic examination

- High-altitude pulmonary edema (HAPE), a life-threatening condition
  1. Pronounced tachypnea
  2. Dyspnea at rest
  3. Rales
  4. Wheezes
  5. Severe cough
  6. Cyanosis
- High-altitude cerebral edema (HACE), life-threatening
  1. Ataxia
  2. Confusion
  3. Severe headache

DIAGNOSIS

DIFFERENTIAL DIAGNOSIS
- Carbon monoxide poisoning
- Post–alcohol intoxication headache (hangover)
- Early HAPE or HACE
- Influenza
- Vertigo
- Other causes of headache, respiratory distress, and fatigue

DIAGNOSTIC WORKUP
Based primarily on history and physical examination

THERAPY

NONPHARMACOLOGIC
- Stop ascent
- If symptoms are mild or tolerable, remain at present altitude until symptoms stop.
- If symptoms are severe or intolerable, descend until symptoms stop.

MEDICAL
- Nonsteroidal antiinflammatory drugs (NSAIDs) are given for headache.
- Acetazolamide 125 to 250 mg twice a day lessens symptoms in adults.
  1. Effectiveness in children is unknown.
- If symptoms of HAPE:
  1. Supplemental oxygen
  2. Nifedipine (effectiveness in children unknown)
  3. Hyperbaric chamber if available
  4. Descend at least 610 meters (2000 feet) and continue descent until symptoms stop
- If symptoms of HACE:
  1. Supplemental oxygen
  2. Dexamethasone (dose for pediatric HACE unknown)
  3. Hyperbaric chamber if available
  4. Descend at least 610 meters (2000 feet) and continue descent until symptoms stop

COMPLEMENTARY & ALTERNATIVE THERAPIES
- Gingko biloba
  1. Decreased incidence of and milder AMS symptoms
  2. Dosing: 120 mg orally twice per day beginning 5 days before ascent and continuing at altitude
  3. Not studied in children

FOLLOW-UP & DISPOSITION
Watch for symptoms of HAPE or HACE over 1 to 3 days after presentation of AMS.

PATIENT/FAMILY EDUCATION
- Stop ascent if symptoms of AMS develop.
- Ascend gradually.
- Watch for cough, wheezes, sputum production, and ataxia.
- If history of AMS in past, attain altitude slowly.

PREVENTIVE TREATMENT
- Attain altitude slowly.
- In adults, take acetazolamide 125 to 250 mg twice a day 1 to 2 days before going to altitude and continue for 48 hours after attaining altitude.
  1. Decreases incidence of AMS
  2. Effectiveness in children unknown

REFERRAL INFORMATION
Anyone with evidence of HAPE or HACE should be referred to a tertiary center for support.

PEARLS & CONSIDERATIONS

CLINICAL PEARLS
- Physical condition does not predict development of AMS.
- Oxygen desaturations during sleep increase the likelihood of developing AMS.
  1. Try to sleep at lower altitudes.
  2. Follow the old mountaineering adage: "climb high, sleep low."
- In general, once above 2400 meters (8000 feet), climb about 300 meters (1000 feet) per day.
  1. Acclimate for 1 to 2 days for each ascent of 600 meters (2000 feet).
- Denver is at 1610 meters (5280 feet) above sea-level; the top of Mt. McKinley is 6200 meters (20,320 feet); the top of Mt. Everest is 8850 meters (29,028 feet).

WEBSITES
- General information on AMS from healthanswers.com: www. healthanswers.com/cente...d=men's+ health&filename=000133.htm
- High-altitude medicine.com

REFERENCES

1. Carpenter T, Niermeyer S, Durmowicz A: Altitude-related illness in children, *Curr Probl Pediatr* 28:181, 1998.
2. Harris MD et al: High-altitude medicine, *Am Fam Physician* 57:1907, 1998.
3. Krieger B, de la Hoz RE: Altitude-related pulmonary disorders, *Crit Care Clin* 15:265, 1999.
4. Maakestad K et al: Ginko biloba reduces incidence and severity of acute mountain sickness (abstract). Proceedings of Wilderness Medical Society Summer Conference. Park City, Utah, August 2000.
5. Peacock A: Oxygen at high altitude, *Br Med J* 317:1063, 1998.

Author: **Matthew W. Richardson, M.D.**

II

BASIC INFORMATION

■ DEFINITION
- Ambiguity of the external genitalia occurs either when a female fetus is virilized or when a male fetus is undervirilized during sexual differentiation in the first trimester.
- *Female pseudohermaphroditism* refers to masculinization of the external genitalia in a patient with a female karyotype from exposure to abnormally elevated levels of androgens.
  1. If exposure occurs before the twelfth fetal week, fusion of the labioscrotal folds and formation of a urogenital sinus occur.
     a. In severe cases, the urethra may traverse the phallus.
     b. The external genitalia may look like those of a male infant with severe hypospadias and undescended testes.
  2. If exposure occurs after the twelfth fetal week, only clitoral hypertrophy will occur.
- *Male pseudohermaphroditism* occurs when the genitalia of a male infant are undervirilized.

■ SYNONYMS
- Ambiguous genitalia
- Disorders of sex differentiation

ICD-9CM CODES
255.2   Congenital adrenal hyperplasia (CAH)
257.8   Androgen insensitivity—testicular feminization
253.2   Hypopituitarism
752.51 Cryptorchidism
752.61 Hypospadias

■ ETIOLOGY
Multiple etiologies, based on karyotype and sex steroid abnormalities (see "Differential Diagnosis")

■ EPIDEMIOLOGY & DEMOGRAPHICS
- The incidence of the most common form of CAH, 21-hydroxylase deficiency, is approximately 1 in 15,000.
  1. Autosomal recessive inheritance
  2. Three fourths of affected children have severe salt wasting.
- Other disorders are exceedingly rare.
  1. Certain forms of CAH are described in Yupik Eskimos and in the Dominican Republic.
  2. Androgen insensitivity is X-linked

■ HISTORY
- There is no history because this diagnosis is usually made at birth.
- The patient may have positive family history (previously affected siblings).
- Rule out maternal androgen use.

■ PHYSICAL EXAMINATION
- Measure the size of the clitoris or phallus.
  1. The normal-term newborn phallus is 35 ± 7 mm long and 11 ± 2 mm wide.
  2. The maximum normal size of the clitoris is 3 to 4 mm breadth and less than 10 mm long.
- Note vaginal opening location and degree of posterior fusion of the labioscrotal folds.
  1. The ratio of distance between the clitoris and posterior vaginal fourchette over the distance between the clitoris and anus is normally greater than 0.5 mm. If less, suspect masculinization.
- Note the location of the urogenital sinus (urethral opening).
- Note the presence or absence of gonadal tissue in the labioscrotal folds or inguinal region.
  1. Palpation of tissue generally denotes testes, not ovaries.
  2. Palpable gonads suggests a diagnosis of male pseudohermaphroditism.
- Note asymmetry of labioscrotal folds.
  1. Seen in disorder of testicular differentiation rather than androgen insensitivity or defective sex steroid synthesis
- Note the rugation and pigmentation of the scrotal skin.
  1. Seen in CAH
- Inspect for other phenotypic abnormalities.
  1. Craniofacial anomalies (i.e., cleft lip and/or palate) may suggest midline defects.
  2. Midline defects are seen with pituitary hypoplasia or aplasia.

DIAGNOSIS

■ DIFFERENTIAL DIAGNOSIS
- Dependent on genetic sex
- Differential diagnosis of female pseudohermaphroditism—XX genotype
  1. Multiple congenital anomalies
     a. Midline defects
     b. Prune-belly syndrome
     c. Bladder extrophy
  2. Excessive fetal androgens: CAH
  3. Exogenous androgens: oral progestins (e.g., 17-ethinyl testosterone, danazol)
  4. Excessive maternal androgens: ovarian or adrenal tumors
- Differential diagnosis of male pseudohermaphroditism—XY genotype
  1. Disorders of testicular differentiation
  2. Abnormalities of placental or fetal gonadotropins

3. Defective gonadal and adrenal sex steroid synthesis
4. End-organ resistance and defective androgen action

■ DIAGNOSTIC WORKUP
- Female pseudohermaphroditism
  1. Karyotype: 46,XX
  2. 17-OH progesterone and androstenedione levels very elevated in CAH
  3. Urogenital sinogram to outline the urogenital sinus
  4. Pelvic and abdominal ultrasound to show presence of uterus and to look for hyperplastic adrenal glands
- Male pseudohermaphroditism
  1. Palpable gonads
  2. Karyotype: 46,XY
  3. Adrenal and gonadal steroid levels, testosterone, and dihydrotestosterone
     a. Elevated adrenal precursors (pregnenolone, 17-OH pregnenolone, DHEA, or androstenedione) and low gonadal testosterone may be indicative of defective gonadal and adrenal sex steroid synthesis.
     b. Elevated testosterone and low dihydrotestosterone are indicative of 5α-reductase deficiency.
     c. Normal to elevated levels of testosterone may be consistent with androgen insensitivity.
  4. Luteinizing hormone and follicle-stimulating hormone: low in hypopituitarism

THERAPY

■ NONPHARMACOLOGIC
- One of few pediatric endocrine emergencies
  1. Rapid decision should be made with experienced team (pediatrician, endocrinologist, urologist, geneticist) regarding gender decision.
- Ongoing psychologic support for the family to deal with the implications of genital abnormalities

■ MEDICAL
Therapy depends on cause and decision regarding gender rearing.
- Female pseudohermaphroditism from CAH
  1. Oral glucocorticosteroids; cortisol 20 mg/M² /day divided three times a day
  2. Mineralocorticoid; fludrocortisone 0.1 mg/day

- Male pseudohermaphroditism
  1. Consider a testosterone treatment trial: 25 mg monthly for three doses to induce penile growth

SURGICAL

- Female pseudohermaphroditism
  1. Feminizing genitoplasty
     a. Surgical reduction clitoroplasty (not resection)
     b. Vaginoplasty
     c. Repair of the urogenital sinus
- Male pseudohermaphroditism (one of the following)
  1. Repair of the hypospadias; resection of chordee and orchidopexy
  2. Surgical construction of a female-appearing perineum and removal of gonads

FOLLOW-UP & DISPOSITION

- Avoid determining the sex of rearing before an accurate diagnosis is reached.
- Provide full support (medical and psychologic) for adaptation to and development of chosen sex of rearing.
- Physicians who care for children who have ambiguous genitalia must appreciate the family's cultural, religious, and psychologic needs.

PATIENT/FAMILY EDUCATION

In CAH, educate family about the need for increased (three to five times normal) doses of glucocorticoids during stress, including minor illnesses (e.g., fever, diarrhea, upper respiratory infection).

PREVENTIVE TREATMENT OR TESTS

- For CAH, prenatal diagnosis and therapy are available but still experimental.
- In several states, newborn screening for detection of CAH is practiced.

REFERRAL INFORMATION

Care should be coordinated with a pediatric endocrinologist and a pediatric urologist.

☼ PEARLS & CONSIDERATIONS

CLINICAL PEARLS

- In salt-wasting CAH, electrolyte abnormalities first occur at about 1 week of age, with hyperkalemia. Hyponatremia occurs by 2 to 3 weeks of age, and addisonian shock occurs at 4 to 5 weeks of age.
- With vomiting in the 2- to 5-week-old child, be sure to think about salt-wasting CAH. If the electrolytes show hyponatremia and hyperkalemia, CAH is the likely diagnosis.

WEBSITES

- Androgen Insensitivity Syndrome Support Group (AISSG): www.medhelp.org/www/ais/
- Intersex Society of North America: www.isna.org
- The Magic Foundation: www.magicfoundation.org/cah.html
- The National Organization of Rare Diseases: www.rarediseases.org/

REFERENCES

1. Anhalt H, Neely EK, Hintz RL: Ambiguous genitalia, *Pediatr Rev* 17:213, 1996.
2. Warne GL, Zajac JD: Disorders of sexual differentiation, *Endocrinol Metab Clin North Am* 27:945, 1998.
3. Zaontz MR, Packer MG: Abnormalities of the external genitalia, *Pediatr Clin North Am* 44:1267, 1997.
Author: **Nicholas Jospe, M.D.**

II

BASIC INFORMATION

DEFINITION
Amblyopia is reduced visual acuity (after correcting for refractive error) in a structurally normal eye, which is defined as 20/40 or worse or a two-line difference between the eyes.

SYNONYMS
- *Not* strabismus
- Lazy eye

ICD-9CM CODE
368.00 Amblyopia

ETIOLOGY
Abnormal visual experience early in life, such as strabismus, uncorrected refractive error, or deprivation/occlusion in the visual axis (e.g., cataract, droopy eyelid), which leads to cortical suppression of vision from affected side, presumably to avoid diplopia

EPIDEMIOLOGY
- Primary cause of unilateral reduced vision in children
- From 2% to 4% of children in North America affected

HISTORY
- Reduced vision
- Normal-appearing eye
- Strabismus possible (either as the cause of amblyopia or as the effect from poor vision and failure to fixate)

PHYSICAL EXAMINATION
- Reduced vision (in an infant, demonstrated by objection to covering the "good" eye)
- Normal globe anatomy
- Strabismus possible

DIAGNOSIS

DIFFERENTIAL DIAGNOSIS
- Uncorrected refractive error (need for glasses)
- Ocular or visual pathway lesion accounting for reduced vision

THERAPY

- Identify the cause (i.e., refractive error, strabismus, deprivation, or occlusion).
- If the cause is refractive, give glasses and occlude the good eye to force the amblyopic eye to fixate and develop vision. (Occlusion therapy includes patching, cycloplegic drops, or fogging optical devices.)
- If the cause is strabismus, treat with glasses, occlusion, and/or surgery.
- If the cause is deprivation or optical interference, provide a clear visual pathway (e.g., extract cataract, lift a ptotic lid).

FOLLOW-UP & DISPOSITION
- Determined by the eye care provider
- Dependent on the child's age, diagnosis, severity of amblyopia, and method of treatment

PATIENT/FAMILY EDUCATION
- Most cases of amblyopia are correctable.
- Early detection yields the best prognosis.
- After age 7 to 9 years, amblyopia is almost always irreversible.

PEARLS & CONSIDERATIONS

CLINICAL PEARLS
- Amblyopia is often not detected because children "peek" during the eye examination given by the primary care provider or school.
- Although amblyopia is the leading cause of reduced vision in children, it can be reversible in most cases.
- Early detection is the key to a favorable prognosis.

WEBSITE
Yahoo! Health: http://health.yahoo.com/health

REFERENCES
1. Friendly DS: Amblyopia: definition, classification, diagnosis, and management considerations for pediatricians, family physicians, and general practitioners, *Pediatr Clin North Am* 34:6, 1987.
2. Rubin SE, Nelson LB: Amblyopia diagnosis and management, *Pediatr Clin North Am* 40:4, 1993.
Author: **Kristina Lynch-Guyette, M.D.**

BASIC INFORMATION

■ DEFINITION
- Amenorrhea is the absence of menses; it is divided into primary and secondary.
- Primary amenorrhea is defined as follows:
  1. Absence of menarche by age 16 years in presence of normal pubertal development
  2. Absence of menarche by age 14 years in absence of normal pubertal development
  3. Absence of menarche 2 years after completion of sexual maturation
- Secondary amenorrhea is defined as follows
  1. Absence of menstruation for at least three cycles or at least 6 months in females who have already established menstruation

■ ICD-9CM CODE
626.0 Amenorrhea

■ ETIOLOGY
Amenorrhea is a symptom of central nervous system dysfunction, ovarian dysfunction, genital tract abnormality, or pregnancy.

■ EPIDEMIOLOGY
- Median age of menarche in the United States is 12.77 years.
- Approximately 95% to 97% of females reach menarche by 16 years of age.

■ HISTORY
- Menstrual history (menarche, last menstrual period, previous menstrual pattern)
- Events surrounding onset of amenorrhea
  1. Athletic training
  2. Weight loss or gain
  3. Depression
  4. Stress
- Reproductive history
  1. Pubertal development
  2. Sexual activity
  3. Contraceptive use
  4. Gynecologic or obstetric procedures
  5. Pregnancies: outcomes, complications
- General medical history
  1. Endocrine or metabolic disorders
  2. Galactorrhea
  3. Medications (hormonal contraception, tricyclic antidepressants, phenothiazines)
  4. Substance use
  5. Headaches, visual changes
  6. Past and present medical illness
  7. Previous radiation or chemotherapy

- Family history
  1. Age of mother and sister(s) at menarche
  2. Autoimmune disorders
  3. Endocrine disorders (diabetes, thyroid)
  4. Congenital anomalies
  5. Infertility
  6. Menstrual dysfunction

■ PHYSICAL EXAMINATION
- Growth parameters, growth pattern, pubertal spurt
- Stigmata of Turner syndrome or anorexia nervosa
- Hair distribution; quality of skin, hair, and nails
  1. Hirsutism and acne may indicate androgen excess.
  2. Dry skin and pitted nails may indicate hypothyroidism.
  3. *Acanthosis nigricans* indicates insulin resistance.
  4. Hypertrichosis or excessive vellus hair occurs with anorexia nervosa.
  5. Scant pubic and axillary hair may indicate androgen insensitivity.
- Funduscopic examination, gross visual fields, examination of cranial nerves
- Palpation of thyroid
- Breast examination to elicit galactorrhea
- Abdominal examination for masses
- Complete neurologic examination (including sense of smell)
- Pelvic examination with assessment of the following:
  1. External genitalia for pubic hair, hymenal opening, clitoral size
  2. Vaginal mucosa for assessment of estrogenization
  3. Vaginal patency
  4. Visualization of cervix
- Bimanual examination with rectovaginal examination for masses

🔬 DIAGNOSIS

■ DIFFERENTIAL DIAGNOSIS
- Pregnancy
- Hormonal contraception
- Hypothalamic
  1. Chronic or systemic illness
  2. Eating disorder
  3. Hypothalamic pituitary axis immaturity
  4. Infiltration (hemochromatosis)
  5. Isolated gonadotropin-releasing hormone deficiency
  6. Kallmann's syndrome (defects in olfaction)
  7. Obesity
  8. Strenuous exercise
  9. Stress
  10. Substance abuse
  11. Tumor (craniopharyngioma)

- Pituitary
  1. Hypopituitarism
  2. Infiltration (hemochromatosis)
  3. Infarction (Sheehan's syndrome, sickle cell disease)
  4. Tumor (prolactinoma)
- Adrenal
  1. Congenital adrenal hyperplasia (classic, nonclassic)
- Ovarian
  1. Agenesis (46,XX)
  2. Dysgenesis (Turner syndrome [45,XO] or variant with abnormal X chromosome)
  3. Hyperandrogenic chronic anovulation (formerly called *polycystic ovary syndrome*)
  4. Premature ovarian failure (autoimmune, chemotherapy, radiation)
  5. Tumor
- Uterus, cervix, vagina
  1. Agenesis (Mayer-Rokitansky-Kuster-Hauser syndrome)
  2. Androgen insensitivity syndrome (testicular feminization)
  3. Imperforate hymen
  4. Synechiae (Asherman's syndrome)
  5. Transverse vaginal septum
- Other
  1. Endocrinopathies (thyroid disease, Cushing's syndrome)
  2. Prader-Willi syndrome
  3. Laurence-Moon-Biedl syndrome

■ DIAGNOSTIC WORKUP
- A pregnancy test is essential.
- A pelvic ultrasound may be helpful in defining anatomy.
- It is helpful to divide the laboratory evaluation into adolescents with the following characteristics:
  1. Absent breast development with absent uterus
  2. Absent breast development with normal uterus
  3. Normal breast development with absent uterus
  4. Normal breast development with normal uterus
- For absent breast development with absent uterus:
  1. Evaluation includes karyotype, luteinizing hormone (LH), follicle-stimulating hormone (FSH), progesterone, and 17α-hydroxyprogesterone.
  2. Differential diagnosis includes vanishing testes syndrome or enzyme block (17,20-desmolase defect).
- For absent breast development with normal uterus:
  1. Evaluation should include FSH, LH, and karyotype.
  2. Differential diagnosis includes gonadal dysgenesis, hypothalamic/pituitary disorder, or a genetic defect in ovarian steroid production.

II

3. A low or normal FSH suggests a hypothalamic or pituitary abnormality, and a careful neuroendocrine evaluation is in order.
4. A high FSH and normal blood pressure suggest a genetic disorder or gonadal dysgenesis such as Turner syndrome.
5. A high FSH with hypertension suggests a 17α-hydroxylase deficiency. This is confirmed by an elevated progesterone, low 17α-hydroxyprogesterone, and an elevated serum deoxycorticosterone.
- For normal breast development with absent uterus:
  1. Evaluation includes karyotype and testosterone level.
  2. Differential diagnosis includes androgen insensitivity or müllerian agenesis.
     a. A patient with androgen insensitivity will have XY karyotype with normal *male* levels of testosterone.
     b. A patient with müllerian agenesis will have XX karyotype with normal *female* levels of testosterone.
- For normal breast development with normal uterus:
  1. Evaluation includes thyroid-stimulating hormone (TSH), prolactin, and pregnancy test.
     a. A normal prolactin level rules out prolactinoma. Elevated levels or symptoms of visual changes *require magnetic resonance imaging* to exclude prolactinoma.
  2. Differential diagnosis includes vaginal outlet obstruction or disturbance in hypothalamic/pituitary axis.

3. If physical examination reveals androgen excess, the evaluation should also include serum DHEA-S, hydroxyprogesterone (17-OHP), and testosterone levels.
4. If TSH and prolactin are normal and the patient is not pregnant, a progesterone challenge should be performed.
   a. Withdrawal bleeding after the challenge indicates chronic anovulation with estrogen production.
   b. No response suggests ovarian failure or hypothalamic dysfunction; FSH, LH, and estradiol levels should be performed.
   c. A high FSH suggests ovarian failure, and a karyotype and evaluation for autoimmune disease should be performed.
   d. A low or normal FSH should demand a search for risk factors of hypothalamic dysfunction, such as chronic disease, eating disorder, or strenuous exercise.

THERAPY

Varies depending on cause of amenorrhea
- Patients with hyperandrogenic chronic anovulation benefit from combined oral contraceptives.
- Patients who are hypoestrogenic and anovulatory because of hypothalamic suppression (e.g., anorexia, exercise) should be given calcium and oral contraceptives to reduce the long-term risks of osteoporosis.

- Patients with Turner syndrome or ovarian failure require hormonal replacement therapy beginning with gradually increasing doses of estrogen and a progestational agent.

PEARLS & CONSIDERATIONS

CLINICAL PEARLS
- Pregnancy is the most common cause of secondary amenorrhea; thus, regardless of sexual history reported, a pregnancy test is essential.
- Turner syndrome is the most common cause of primary amenorrhea.

REFERENCES
1. Braverman P, Sondheimer S: Menstrual disorders, *Pediatr Rev* 18:17, 1997.
2. Emans SJ: Delayed puberty and menstrual irregularities. In Emans SJ, Laufer MR, Goldstein DP (eds): *Pediatric and adolescent gynecology,* ed 4, Philadelphia, 1998, Lippincott-Raven.
3. Pletcher JR, Slap GB: Menstrual disorders, *Pediatr Clin North Am* 46:505, 1999.
4. Prose C, Ford C, Lovely L: Evaluating amenorrhea: the pediatrician's role, *Contemp Pediatr* 15:83, 1998.
5. Rosenfeld RL: The ovary and female sexual maturation. In Sperling MA (ed): *Pediatric endocrinology,* Philadelphia, 1996, WB Saunders.
Author: **Stephanie Sansoni, M.D.**

BASIC INFORMATION

■ DEFINITION

- *Anal fissure (fissure-in-ano):* superficial linear disruption of the anal epithelium around the anal verge, often leading to local pain and bleeding
- *Fistula-in-ano:* persistently patent tract originating in the crypt of Morgagni at the anal valves and terminating at the perianal skin; often the secondary consequence of draining a perianal or perirectal abscess
- *Perianal abscess:* abscess formed from an infection within the crypt of Morgagni, presenting on the perianal skin; initial and often persistent communication to the anus results in enteric organism infection
- *Perirectal abscess:* uncommon in children; present as perirectal collections but do not communicate with a fistula-in-ano

ICD-9CM CODES

565.1 Fistula-in-ano
565.0 Anal fissure
566.0 Perianal abscess, perirectal abscess

■ ETIOLOGY

- Anal fissure (tearing of mucosal surface with passage of hard, large stool)
- Anal fistula
  1. The primary factor responsible for the formation of perirectal abscesses and subsequent fistula-in-ano is infection of the crypt of Morgagni.
     a. This is located at the base of the anal valves, at the inferior margin of the anal columns.
     b. When these crypts become infected, the infection extends superficially and points to the perianal skin.
- Abscess
  1. Bacterial (usually enteric) and inflammatory collection of fluid in perianal or perirectal areas

■ EPIDEMIOLOGY & DEMOGRAPHICS

- Anal fissure
  1. Fissures are almost always seen in infants and young children.
  2. This is the most common cause of rectal bleeding in infants.
  3. Associated factors include constipation and large, hard stools.
  4. Inflammatory bowel disease must be excluded in chronic or recurrent cases.
- Abscesses and fistulas
  1. Almost always occur within first year of life
  2. Rare in older children and adolescents

■ HISTORY

- Anal fissure
  1. Painful defecation and rectal bleeding
  2. Most often in infants
  3. Stool retention
  4. Constipation causing pain, with further retention and hardening of the stools, increased stool size (leads to perpetuation of the fissure)
  5. Small amount of blood on stool surface common
  6. Significant rectal bleeding uncommon
- Fistula
  1. Recurrent drain and close cycle
- Abscess
  1. Perianal abscess presents with rectal pain
  2. Pain on defecation

■ PHYSICAL EXAMINATION

- Anal fissure
  1. Superficial mucosal break
  2. Most often in posterior location
  3. Because of rectal pain, fissure may not be visualized
  4. Bleeding on examination uncommon
- Abscesses and fistulas
  1. Erythema at the anal opening
  2. Painful examination with tender mass under erythema
  3. Abscess and indurated fistula usually palpable
- Fistula
  1. Punctate opening at old abscess site
  2. Looks like a pimple at site
  3. May have minor degree of local inflammation

DIAGNOSIS

■ DIFFERENTIAL DIAGNOSIS

- Constipation with painful defecation
- Hemorrhoids (uncommon in pediatrics)
- Buttock impetigo, cellulitis, or folliculitis
- Diaper dermatitis, especially perianal with group A β-hemolytic streptococcus
- If recurrent or if multiple tracts seen, should consider inflammatory bowel disease (IBD), chronic granulomatous disease (CGD), immune dysfunction

■ DIAGNOSTIC WORKUP

- Clinical diagnosis
- If underlying disease, consider the following:
  1. Barium enema or endoscopy for IBD
  2. Neutrophil studies for CGD
  3. T- and B-cell studies for immunodeficiencies

THERAPY

■ NONPHARMACOLOGIC

- Anal fissure
  1. Dietary manipulation to increase bulk and looseness of stool
- Abscesses and fistulas
  1. Initial surgical care with sitz baths after drainage

■ MEDICAL

- Anal fissure
  1. Treatment to avoid constipation generally leads to local healing.
- Abscesses and fistulas
  1. Incision and drainage is followed by sitz baths.
  2. A short (3- to 5-day) course of antibiotics is given when cellulitis or induration is significant.

■ SURGICAL

- Anal fissure
  1. Usually, no surgical repair is necessary.
- Abscesses and fistulas
  1. Drain the abscess.
  2. This is done under local anesthesia when the superficial abscess has softened.
  3. More complex or poorly developed abscesses require operative drainage.
  4. A short course of antibiotics after incision and drainage is often required.

■ FOLLOW-UP & DISPOSITION

- Half of cases resolve without further intervention.
- Half form a fistula tract along the communication from the crypt to the anal skin (fistula-in-ano).
- These fistulas are superficial and require operative excision under general anesthesia.
  1. The offending crypt is easily identified and excised, as is the entire tract.
  2. The tract is left open and heals through granulation in the course of days to several weeks.
- Sphincter involvement is rare; continence is not disturbed.
- Recurrence is uncommon.
- When the abscesses are recurrent, multiple tracts are seen, or healing is not forthcoming after drainage, IBD, CGD, or immune dysfunction should be sought.

■ PATIENT/FAMILY EDUCATION

Bowel habits allowing for soft, easily passed stool to avoid fissuring and painful defecation

■ REFERRAL INFORMATION

In general, infants and children with possible abscess and/or fistula should be referred to general pediatric surgeons.

II

☼ PEARLS & CONSIDERATIONS

■ CLINICAL PEARLS

- Perirectal abscesses are one of three types of abscesses that require drainage, despite lack of fluctuance

as they enlarge (others are breast and brain).
- Consider enema or imaging study (magnetic resonance imaging or computed tomography) if in doubt.

REFERENCES

1. Ashcraft KW: Acquired anorectal disorders. In Holder TM, Ashcraft KW (eds): *Pediatric surgery,* ed 3, Philadelphia, 2000, WB Saunders.
2. Keighley MRB, Williams NS: *Surgery of the anus, rectum and colon,* ed 2, London, 1997, WB Saunders.

Author: **Frederick Ryckman, M.D.**

■ OVERVIEW DEFINITION

Anemias of erythroid failure are progressive anemias resulting from the failure of the erythroid marrow. This section focuses on conditions with selective erythroid failure (i.e., Diamond-Blackfan syndrome, transient erythropenia of childhood, erythroid aplastic crises, and a few others), rather than on general marrow failure associated with granulocytopenia and/or thrombocytopenia.

Diamond-Blackfan Syndrome

BASIC INFORMATION

■ DEFINITION

Diamond-Blackfan syndrome is congenital pure red cell aplasia that usually presents at birth or soon thereafter.

■ SYNONYMS

- Congenital hypoplastic anemia
- Erythrogenesis imperfecta
- Chronic congenital aregenerative anemia
- Josephs-Diamond-Blackfan anemia

■ ICD-9CM CODE

284.0 Constitutional aplastic anemia

■ ETIOLOGY

Diamond-Blackfan syndrome is a progressive, severe aplastic anemia of unknown origin.

■ EPIDEMIOLOGY

- Approximately 500 cases have been reported.
- Fifty percent of children are diagnosed by 2 months of age, 75% are diagnosed by 6 months, and 90% by 1 year of age.
- Familial occurrence, with both autosomal-dominant and autosomal-recessive patterns, is described in approximately 20% of patients, suggesting a genetic basis for the disease.

■ HISTORY

Consistent with anemia
- Poor feedings
- Easy fatigue
- Pallor
- Lethargy or fretfulness

■ PHYSICAL EXAMINATION

Also consistent with anemia
- Increased heart rate
- Systolic murmur
- Pallor
- Congenital abnormalities (in approximately 30% of patients), including dysmorphic facies, defects of the upper extremities, and short stature

DIAGNOSIS

■ DIFFERENTIAL DIAGNOSIS

Children most commonly present with profound anemia within the first 2 to 6 months of age.
- Transient erythropenia of childhood (TEC)
- Iron deficiency anemia
- Aplastic crises in patients with hemolytic anemias
- Aplastic anemia
- Congestive heart failure
- Other anemias (e.g., chronic disease, hemolytic)

■ DIAGNOSTIC WORKUP

- The blood film reveals macrocytosis, anisocytosis, teardrop cells, and marked reticulocytopenia (less than 0.5%).
- The red cells have elevated fetal hemoglobin (HbF), increased expression of the "i" antigen, and elevated adenosine deaminase.
- White blood cell and platelet counts are usually normal.
- Marrow evaluation reveals erythroid hypoplasia or total erythroid aplasia.

THERAPY

■ MEDICAL

- Glucocorticoids are the mainstay of therapy.
  1. Initial dosage of prednisone is 2 mg/kg/day.
  2. Repeated blood transfusions with iron chelation may be needed for glucocorticoid-resistant patients.
- The anemia is progressive and usually requires repeated transfusions if drug therapy is not administered.
- Other therapies include danazol (attenuated androgen), 6-mercaptopurine, cyclophosphamide, and hematopoietic growth factors, but their value is not established and response is uncommon.
- Bone marrow transplantation may be considered for patients who do not respond to glucocorticoids.

■ FOLLOW-UP & DISPOSITION

- The patients with the best prognosis are those who respond well to glucocorticoid therapy (approximately 50%).
- Fifteen percent of patients undergo spontaneous remission.
- An elevated risk of leukemia and other cancers is present.

PEARLS & CONSIDERATIONS

■ CLINICAL PEARLS

The diagnosis of Diamond-Blackfan syndrome is very unlikely if the reticulocyte percentage is higher than 0.5%.

Transient Erythroblastopenia of Childhood

BASIC INFORMATION

■ DEFINITION

Transient erythroblastopenia of childhood is a severe, transient hypoplastic anemia.

■ ICD-9CM CODE

284.0 Constitutional aplastic anemia

■ ETIOLOGY

An uncommon disease of unknown origin that results in acquired erythroid marrow failure

■ EPIDEMIOLOGY

- More than 600 cases have been reported.
- This disease affects previously healthy children at 6 months to 5 years of age. The mean age of presentation is 2 years of age.
- A history of a preceding viral illness is often present.
- Patients do not have congenital anomalies as in Diamond-Blackfan syndrome, and there is no evidence for toxic, immune, or specific viral causes.

■ HISTORY

- Pallor
- Fatigue
- Vague change in activity and/or feeding

■ PHYSICAL EXAMINATION

Usually normal except for pallor and signs of anemia (e.g., elevated heart rate, systolic flow murmur)

DIAGNOSIS

■ DIFFERENTIAL DIAGNOSIS

- Other forms of hypoplastic or aplastic anemia (aplastic anemia, Diamond-Blackfan syndrome)
- Other forms of anemia (hemolytic, megaloblastic)
- Marrow infiltration diseases (leukemia, tuberculosis, human immunodeficiency virus)

II

■ DIAGNOSTIC WORKUP
- Children slowly develop a normochromic, normocytic anemia with marked reticulocytopenia.
  1. The mean hemoglobin level is 6.0 g/dl; the reticulocyte count is usually below 0.5%.
  2. The white blood cell and platelet counts are normal in most cases.
     a. A small percentage of patients (20%) have mild neutropenia.
- Bone marrow films contain fewer red blood cell precursors.
- No specific diagnostic test is available. In contrast to Diamond-Blackfan anemia, HbF levels and adenosine deaminase levels are normal.

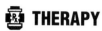 **THERAPY**

■ NONPHARMACOLOGIC
- Watchful waiting is appropriate if no signs of congestive heart failure, respiratory distress, or growth failure are present.
- Spontaneous remission usually occurs within months.

■ MEDICAL
- Red blood cell transfusions may be required for children with severe anemia in the absence of signs of early recovery.
- Glucocorticoid therapy is not helpful.

■ FOLLOW-UP & DISPOSITION
Recurrence of the disease is rare.

☼ PEARLS & CONSIDERATIONS

■ CLINICAL PEARLS
Although TEC and Diamond-Blackfan syndrome can have similar presentations, patients with TEC are usually older than 1 year of age.

Erythroid Aplastic Crisis

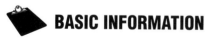 **BASIC INFORMATION**

■ DEFINITION
Erythroid aplastic crisis is characterized by a relative failure of red blood cell production.

ICD-9CM CODES
284.9 Aplastic
284.8 Aplastic—acquired

■ ETIOLOGY
- Severe anemia occurs most commonly in patients with hemolysis who acquire viral infections (particularly parvovirus B19) that cause erythroid marrow suppression.
- In hemolytic anemias, the red cell life span can be less than 20 days (normal is 120 days), leading to a precipitous decrease in hemoglobin concentration if red cell production is suppressed for several days.
- Transient erythroid marrow failure can occur in any person infected with parvovirus or similar viruses, but it has little clinical effect if the red cell life span is normal.

■ EPIDEMIOLOGY
- Aplastic crises should be considered in all children with chronic hemolysis (e.g., sickle cell disease, hereditary spherocytosis) who are evaluated for febrile illnesses.
  1. Children with the shortest red cell life spans are at highest risk for aplastic crisis.

■ HISTORY
- Severe anemia can occur abruptly in patients with hemolysis and can be life-threatening.
- Acute onset of pallor and/or fatigue often occurs, especially in patients with known hemolytic disease.
- Fever is common, as is history of a recent febrile illness.
- Usually, no history of jaundice is elicited.

■ PHYSICAL EXAMINATION
- Signs of anemia
  1. Tachycardia
  2. Pallor
  3. Heart murmur
- Rarely, an enlarged spleen (unless concomitant splenic sequestration)

▲ DIAGNOSIS

■ DIFFERENTIAL DIAGNOSIS
See corresponding sections on Diamond-Blackfan Syndrome and Transient Erythroblastopenia of Childhood.

■ DIAGNOSTIC WORKUP
- The hallmark of the diagnosis is a decrease in the baseline reticulocyte count.
- Bone marrow evaluation may reveal giant proerythroblasts and a paucity of erythroid precursors compatible with parvovirus infection.
- Bone marrow recovery follows shortly after antiparvovirus antibodies are detectable in the serum.

- Viral DNA may be detectable by polymerase chain reaction (PCR) technique.

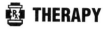 **THERAPY**

■ NONPHARMACOLOGIC
If hemodynamically stable, the patient may be observed for signs of deterioration.

■ MEDICAL
Transfusions may be needed for severe anemia in patients with chronic hemolysis until erythropoiesis is restored.

■ FOLLOW-UP & DISPOSITION
- The erythroid aplasia caused by parvovirus is usually transient; recovery typically occurs within 1 to 2 weeks.
- Provide the usual follow-up of a patient with hemolytic disease.

■ PATIENT/FAMILY EDUCATION
- Patient and parents should understand that acute changes in appetite and/or activity may represent anemia.
- Fever, a concern for patients with sickle cell disease because of the risk of sepsis, is also a concern for aplastic crises in children with hemolytic anemias.

Other Diseases of Erythroid Failure
- *Hormone deficiencies:* Thyroid, glucocorticoid, testosterone, and growth hormone deficiencies may result in normochromic, normocytic anemias with a decreased reticulocyte percentage.
- *Congenital dyserythropoietic anemia:* This includes inherited and sometimes congenital marrow disorders that result in faulty red cell production and anemia with a low reticulocyte count.
- *Acquired pure red cell aplasia:* Isolated erythroid failure can be associated with immune diseases, thymoma, collagen vascular diseases, drugs, viruses, and malnutrition.

■ WORKUP & TREATMENT
Same as for other forms of anemia, with treatment for specific diseases if elucidated

REFERENCES
1. Krijanovski OI, Sieff CA: Diamond-Blackfan anemia, *Hematol Oncol Clin North Am* 11:1061, 1997.
2. Nathan DG, Orkin SH (eds): *Nathan and Oski's hematology of infancy and childhood,* ed 5, Philadelphia, 1998, WB Saunders.
Authors: **Jill S. Halterman, M.D., M.P.H., and George B. Segel, M.D.**

BASIC INFORMATION

DEFINITION
Iron deficiency anemia is caused by insufficient iron for the normal formation of hemoglobin.

ICD-9CM CODE
280.9 Iron deficiency anemia, unspecified

ETIOLOGY
- Iron deficiency may be caused by insufficient dietary intake, iron loss from gastrointestinal (GI) or other bleeding, or rarely, chronic intravascular hemolysis and urinary iron loss.
- Dietary iron deficiency is common in infants from 9 to 24 months of age because stores of iron are depleted during a period of accelerated growth.
- Adolescent girls also may develop iron deficiency because of poor dietary intake in conjunction with high iron requirements related to rapid growth and menstrual blood loss.
- Blood loss must be considered in every child with iron deficiency anemia, particularly in the older child who is less likely to have inadequate dietary intake.
  1. The most common location for blood loss is the GI tract.
  2. Rarely, iron loss may result from bleeding into the lungs (idiopathic pulmonary hemosiderosis or Goodpasture's syndrome) or urinary bleeding.

EPIDEMIOLOGY
- Iron deficiency is the most prevalent hematologic disorder in childhood.
- It affects approximately 5% to 10% of infants.
- Infants who develop dietary iron deficiency often consume large amounts of cow's milk as well as foods not supplemented with iron.
  1. Excessive intake of cow's milk impairs adequate intake of other foods rich in iron.
  2. Proteins in the cow's milk may cause bleeding from irritation of the lining of the GI tract in infants.
- Infants consuming breast milk are somewhat less susceptible to iron deficiency anemia because iron is absorbed more efficiently from human milk than from cow's milk.

HISTORY
- If anemia develops slowly, few symptoms other than pallor may be apparent.
- When anemia is severe (hemoglobin of less than 5 g/dl), symptoms of irritability, anorexia, and exertional intolerance may occur, reflecting the systemic effects of iron deficiency.
- Pica is sometimes present, including consumption of laundry starch, ice, and soil clay.
- Iron deficiency with or without concomitant anemia impairs growth and intellectual development in children.

PHYSICAL EXAMINATION
- Tachycardia
- Pallor
- Irritability
- Systolic murmur
- Growth failure
- Developmental delay

DIAGNOSIS

LABORATORY EVALUATION
- Body iron stores are depleted, as reflected by a low serum ferritin.
  1. Normal is 35 ng/ml.
  2. Less than 10 ng/ml indicates iron deficiency.
- A decrease in serum iron follows: less than 30 µg/dl.
- Iron-binding capacity is increased: greater than 350 µg/dl.
- Subsequently, the percentage of iron saturation falls to less than 15%.
- Accumulation of heme precursors results in an elevated free erythrocyte protoporphyrin.
- As iron deficiency progresses, the mean corpuscular volume (MCV) falls below 75 fL/cell, the hemoglobin content decreases, and the red blood cell (RBC) becomes deformed.
- Iron deficiency alters RBC size unevenly, leading to an elevated red cell distribution width (RDW).
- The Mentzer index (MCV/RBC) occasionally is used to help distinguish iron deficiency from thalassemia trait.
  1. Iron deficiency: greater than 13
  2. Thalassemia: less than 13
- The reticulocyte percentage is typically normal or slightly elevated.
- Thrombocytosis may occur with platelet counts greater than 500,000/mm³.

DIFFERENTIAL DIAGNOSIS
Iron deficiency anemia must be distinguished from other forms of hypochromic, microcytic anemias.
- Lead poisoning
  1. Elevated lead levels
  2. High free erythrocyte protoporphyrin
- β-Thalassemia trait
  1. Elevated hemoglobin A_2
  2. Mentzer index less than 13
- Anemia of chronic inflammatory disease
  1. Decreased serum iron and iron-binding capacity
  2. Normal or increased ferritin

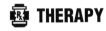 **THERAPY**

NONPHARMACOLOGIC
Cow's milk intake should be limited to less than 16 oz/day in young children.

MEDICAL
- Ferrous salts (6 mg/kg elemental iron in three divided doses for infants and children) should be administered orally until the hemoglobin and hematocrit levels are normal.
  1. Iron is better absorbed if given between meals.
  2. Juices containing ascorbic acid increase iron absorption.
  3. Cow's milk and tannins in tea decrease iron absorption.
- Therapy should be continued for an additional 1 to 2 months after the hemoglobin and hematocrit levels are normal to replete iron stores.
- Parenteral iron (available as iron dextran either intramuscularly or intravenously) is available but rarely indicated. It must be administered with careful observation for local and/or systemic allergic reactions.
- Transfusions should be reserved for profoundly anemic children.
  1. If needed, transfusions should be given slowly.
  2. Diuretics or exchange transfusions should be considered to prevent hypervolemia with cardiac compromise.

PEARLS & CONSIDERATIONS

CLINICAL PEARLS
- A "trial of iron therapy" may be defensible in infants younger than 2 years of age, when dietary iron

II

deficiency is common. In children older than 2 years, dietary iron deficiency is less likely the cause of iron deficiency; therefore further evaluation is needed.

- Poor response to oral iron therapy may represent problems with compliance, poor absorption, continuing unrecognized blood loss, or an incorrect diagnosis.
- Black stools are observed soon after the initiation of iron therapy and can serve as an index of compliance with iron therapy.
- Iron deficiency increases the rate of uptake of both iron and lead from the GI tract. Therefore iron deficiency and lead intoxication often occur together.
- Dietary iron deficiency can be prevented in most children by avoiding excessive cow's milk consumption.

REFERENCES

1. Booth IW, Aukett MA: Iron deficiency anemia in infancy and early childhood, *Arch Dis Child* 76:549, 1997.
2. Nathan DG, Orkin SH (eds): *Nathan and Oski's hematology of infancy and childhood,* ed 5, Philadelphia, 1998, WB Saunders.
3. Provan D: Mechanisms and management of iron deficiency anemia, *Br J Hematol* 105(suppl 1):19, 1999.

Authors: **Jill S. Halterman, M.D., M.P.H., and George B. Segel, M.D.**

BASIC INFORMATION

■ DEFINITION

Megaloblastic anemias are those associated with delayed nuclear maturation in bone marrow and blood macrocytes. The characteristic finding in the marrow is the delay of nuclear maturation compared with cytoplasmic maturation. The following discussions include folate and vitamin B_{12} deficiencies.

Folic Acid Deficiency
ICD-9CM CODE
281.2 Folate deficiency anemia

■ ETIOLOGY & EPIDEMIOLOGY

- Body stores of folic acid are small in comparison to daily requirements; therefore deficiency may result relatively quickly from inadequate folate intake or poor folate absorption.
- Folate requirements are greatest per kilogram in newborn infants, young children, and pregnant and lactating women.
- Other groups with increased folate requirements are those with malabsorption syndromes, premature infants, children receiving chronic antiepileptic therapy, and children with chronic hemolysis with or without anemia.
- Whereas human and cow's milk provide adequate amounts of folic acid, goat's milk contains very little folic acid. Children consuming large amounts of goat's milk likely will become folic acid deficient without supplementation of their diet.
- In adolescents and adults, chronic alcoholism and inadequate diet may result in folic acid deficiency.

DIAGNOSIS

■ CLINICAL MANIFESTATIONS/ LABORATORY EVALUATION

- Children who typically present with a macrocytic anemia may have irritability and poor weight gain.
- Mild folate deficiency can be detected by a decrease in red cell folate.
- In more severe deficiency, laboratory evaluation reveals a macrocytic anemia with a mean corpuscular volume (MCV) greater than 100 fL per cell, hypersegmented granulocytes on the blood film, and a low serum folate (less than 3 ng/ml; normal, 5 to 20 ng/ml), in addition to low red cell folate.

- Granulocytopenia and thrombocytopenia also may be present.
- Total plasma homocysteine level is increased above normal in most patients with folate deficiency.
- Marrow examination reveals megaloblastic maturation.
- Concomitant vitamin B_{12} deficiency must be ruled out because treatment with folic acid may mask the diagnosis of B_{12} deficiency by correcting the hematologic findings. Such children would remain at risk for the neurologic manifestations of vitamin B_{12} deficiency.

THERAPY

■ TREATMENT

- Dietary insufficiency should be corrected to provide adequate folate intake.
- Treatment is initiated with physiologic quantities of folate (50 to 100 μg/day) and monitoring of the reticulocyte percentage.
- Reticulocytosis should occur after the first week of treatment if folate deficiency is present.
- Therapy consists of 1 mg/day of folic acid.
- Larger amounts of folate (5 mg/day) may be needed for children with malabsorption.

Vitamin B_{12} Deficiency
ICD-9CM CODE
281.1 Vitamin B_{12} deficiency anemia

■ ETIOLOGY & EPIDEMIOLOGY

- Body stores of vitamin B_{12} are relatively large, and daily requirements are low.
  1. Vitamin B_{12} is also present in many foods, making dietary deficiency very rare.
  2. However, dietary deficiency may be seen in vegans (who consume no milk, eggs, or animal products) because vegetables do not contain vitamin B_{12}.
- Newborn infants whose mothers are deficient in vitamin B_{12} may develop severe B_{12} deficiency in the first few weeks of life.
  1. The most common cause of vitamin B_{12} deficiency in infants is maternal vitamin B_{12} deficiency.
- Inborn errors of vitamin B_{12} metabolism also can cause inadequate B_{12} availability in newborns and infants.

- Vitamin B_{12} combines with intrinsic factor produced by parietal cells in the stomach and is absorbed in the terminal ileum.
- Deficiency in older children and adolescents may stem from the following:
  1. Surgery or diseases involving the stomach or terminal ileum
  2. Congenital lack of intrinsic factor
  3. Pernicious anemia (rare)
  4. Human immunodeficiency virus infection

DIAGNOSIS

■ CLINICAL MANIFESTATIONS

- Children may present with irritability, anorexia, and listlessness.
- Neurologic manifestations can precede megaloblastic changes and anemia and include the following:
  1. Ataxia
  2. Paresthesias
  3. Hyporeflexia
  4. Clonus
  5. Coma
- Neurologic problems can become irreversible if not treated promptly and adequately.
- Newborns may manifest failure to thrive and slowed development even without anemia and macrocytosis.

■ LABORATORY EVALUATION

- Granulocytopenia and thrombocytopenia may occur, particularly with more prolonged vitamin deficiency.
- The blood film demonstrates oval macrocytes and multilobar neutrophils and occasional pancytopenia.
- Serum B_{12} levels are typically less than 100 pg/ml, but this finding alone is not specific for vitamin B_{12} deficiency.
- Elevated serum levels of methylmalonic acid and total homocysteine, in conjunction with low serum levels of the vitamin, provide evidence of functional B_{12} deficiency.
- Children with juvenile pernicious anemia may have detectable antibodies to intrinsic factor or parietal cells and a positive Schilling test (correction of vitamin B_{12} malabsorption with administration of oral radiolabeled vitamin B_{12} and intrinsic factor).

II

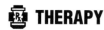 **THERAPY**

■ **TREATMENT**
• Initial subcutaneous injections of 1000 µg/day of vitamin B_{12} for 7 days and then 100 µg subcutaneously weekly for 1 month are given to replete body stores.

• Maintenance therapy is administered with either monthly subcutaneous injections of 100 µg of vitamin B_{12} or oral vitamin B_{12} 1 to 2 µg/day.

■ **PROGNOSIS**
• Some neurologic abnormalities improve rapidly with therapy.
• The anemia associated with vitamin B_{12} deficiency should resolve 1 to 2 months after initiation of therapy.

REFERENCES
1. Nathan DG, Orkin SH (eds): *Nathan and Oski's hematology of infancy and childhood,* ed 5, Philadelphia, 1998, WB Saunders.
2. Rosenblatt DS, Whitehead VM: Cobalamin and folate deficiency: acquired and hereditary disorders in children, *Semin Hematol* 36:19, 1999.
Authors: **Jill S. Halterman, M.D., M.P.H., and George B. Segel, M.D.**

BASIC INFORMATION

■ DEFINITION
Most animal bites are from dogs, cats, or rodents, and most are minor enough to not require medical attention. However, an animal bite is medically significant when the cosmetic appearance of the wound or infection is an issue.

■ ICD-9CM CODE
879.8 Open wound

■ ETIOLOGY
- The most common perpetrators of animal bites are rodents, followed by dogs and then cats.
- Aggressive breeds of dogs, like the pit bull, are often responsible for bite wounds.

■ EPIDEMIOLOGY & DEMOGRAPHICS
- Animal bites tend to occur most often in warm climates or during warm seasons.
- Young children are the most common victims.
- Victims are more likely to be male.
- Approximately 7000 animal bites were reported to the American Association of Poison Control Centers in 1997.

■ HISTORY
- A bite wound victim often can identify the specific animal involved.
- The time elapsed since the injury is an important factor in infection control and wound closure.

■ PHYSICAL EXAMINATION
- The location and type of wound is important not only for cosmetic purposes but also with regard to underlying structural damage.
- Assess the wound for internal injury with the body part in the same position in which it was bitten.
  1. For example, a hand laceration inflicted with the digits flexed may hide a tendon injury if examined only in the extended position.
- Search for underlying structural damage.
  1. Dog bites are most commonly associated with significant occult injury.
  2. Arterial injury may occur with extremity bites.
  3. Skull fracture may occur with scalp bites.

DIAGNOSIS

■ DIAGNOSTIC WORKUP
- The diagnosis of an animal bite is usually made based on information from history and physical examination alone.
- All dog scalp bites should be investigated radiologically for a skull fracture.

THERAPY

■ NONPHARMACOLOGIC
Irrigation and debridement

■ MEDICAL
- Medical therapy is directed toward infection control.
- Antibiotic prophylactic therapy is directed against *Pasteurella multocida* and *Staphylococcus aureus*.
  1. All cat bites should be treated with amoxicillin/clavulanate.
  2. Dog bites that are more than 12 hours old, difficult to clean, in the hand or foot, or in a particularly infection-susceptible patient require amoxicillin/clavulanate therapy.
  3. Penicillin-allergic patients can be given doxycycline for a cat bite or both clindamycin and trimethoprim-sulfamethoxazole for a dog bite as alternatives.
- Update the patient's tetanus status.
- Consider the need for rabies prophylaxis.

■ SURGERY
- Fresh nonpuncture wounds can be sutured.
- Tendon or vascular repair may be needed.
- Plastic surgery repair may be needed for cosmetically challenging injuries.

■ FOLLOW-UP & DISPOSITION
- Most patients can be treated as outpatients. Those with extensive injury may require hospitalization and long-term cosmetic follow-up.
- Follow-up in 48 hours is useful to check for infection.
- Follow-up may be indicated for the psychologic effects of extensive injuries.

■ PATIENT/FAMILY EDUCATION
- Issues surrounding the prevention of animal bites include the following:
  1. Keep young children away from pets.
  2. Choose breeds of dogs that are good with children to be family pets.
  3. Supervise all children around pets.
  4. Train pets to be obedient.
- Signs of infection include the following:
  1. Erythema, warmth, increasing pain, tenderness
  2. Fever, red streaks

■ REFERRAL INFORMATION
Extensive bites or bites in areas where tendonous injury is possible, such as the hand or foot, may require surgical consultation.

PEARLS & CONSIDERATIONS

■ CLINICAL PEARLS
- Do not forget to search for occult injury.
- Infection control is crucial for a good result.
- Consider cosmetic issues.

■ WEBSITE
Mayo Clinic: www.mayohealth.org/mayo/firstaid/htm/fa2b.htm

REFERENCES
1. Goldstein EJ: New horizons in the bacteriology, antimicrobial susceptibility and therapy of animal bite wounds, *J Med Microbiol* 47:95, 1998.
2. Litovitz TL et al: 1997 Annual Report of the American Association of Poison Control Centers Toxic Exposure Surveillance System, *Am J Emerg Med* 16:443, 1998.
3. Rosekrans MD: Animal bites: a summertime hazard, *Cont Ped* 10:23, 1993.
Author: **Robert Freishtat, M.D.**

II

BASIC INFORMATION

■ DEFINITION
An ankle sprain is an injury to the ankle caused by a sudden twisting motion that stretches and/or tears the supporting ligaments.

■ SYNONYMS
- Wrenched or turned ankle
- Sprained ankle
- Twisted ankle

ICD-9CM CODE
845.0 Sprain, ankle

■ ETIOLOGY
- A traumatic event, such as twisting or rapidly rotating about the talar and/or subtalar joints
  1. Causes the ankle joint to move outside its normal range of movement
  2. Causes supporting ligaments to stretch and/or tear

■ EPIDEMIOLOGY
- More than 2 million people in the United States injure their ankles every year.
- The average individual experiences two to three ankle injuries during his or her lifetime.
- Ankle sprains account for 12% of all injuries seen in emergency departments.
- In the athletic population, ankle injuries are the most common injury, accounting for 15% of all musculoskeletal injuries.
  1. Basketball has the highest incidence of ankle sprains (40% of all their injuries), followed by football, volleyball, soccer, and cross-country running.
- Most ankle injuries occur in people 21 to 30 years old.
  1. Injuries in younger age groups tend to be more serious.
- Of all ankle injuries, 85% are ankle sprains.
  1. Five percent are eversion injuries,
  2. Ten percent involve the syndesmosis.
- Sports with the highest ankle sprain injury rates emphasize jumping, cutting, or running on uneven ground.

■ HISTORY
- Time since injury
- Ability to bear weight immediately and later
  1. Able to continue the game?
  2. Able to walk off the field?
- Mechanism of injury
  1. A lateral ankle sprain occurs with the foot in plantar-flexion with an inversion force applied. The patient describes "rolling" foot under.

2. A deltoid sprain occurs with the foot in dorsiflexion with an eversion force applied, such as when a wrestler tries to get a wider stance on the mat.
3. A syndesmosis injury occurs when the foot is forcibly rotated, such as in football when a player falls on top of the ankle of another player who is lying prone.
- Was a "pop" or "snap" heard?
- Site of initial pain and swelling
- Skin integrity
- History of previous injury and treatment

■ PHYSICAL EXAMINATION
- It is best to examine the patient as soon as possible after the injury.
  1. Pain, swelling, and ecchymosis increase with time, making examination more difficult.
- Inspect for swelling, ecchymosis, and deformity.
- Assess neurovascular integrity.
- Range of motion may be limited because of pain; attempt active and passive assessment of the following six cardinal movements:
  1. Dorsiflexion
  2. Dorsiflexion with inversion and eversion
  3. Plantar-flexion
  4. Plantar-flexion with inversion and eversion
- Palpate the following areas that are most often injured during ankle trauma:
  1. Entire length of the fibula
  2. Malleoli
  3. Base of the fifth metatarsal
  4. Navicular
  5. Peroneal tendons behind the lateral malleolus
  6. Anterior, medial, and lateral joint lines
  7. Achilles tendon
- Point tenderness or crepitation may be indicative of a fracture.
- Palpate ankle ligaments.
  1. The anterior talofibular ligament (ATFL) is palpated two finger-breadths anteroinferior to the lateral malleolus.
  2. The calcaneofibular ligament (CFL) is palpated two finger-breadths inferior to the lateral malleolus.
  3. The posterior talofibular ligament (PTFL) is palpated posteroinferior to the posterior edge of the lateral malleolus.
- The anterior drawer test is performed as follows:
  1. Place the patient's ankle in a neutral position with the knee flexed at 90 degrees.
  2. Place one hand 3 inches above the ankle joint to stabilize the tibia-fibula.
  3. Grip the heel with the other hand to apply anterior force.

4. If there is greater than a 5-mm difference from the uninjured side, this is indicative of an incompetent ATFL ligament.
- The talar tilt test is performed with the patient and examiner in the same position as the anterior drawer test.
  1. The hand that cups the heel applies an inversion force in both neutral and 20-degree plantar-flexion.
  2. If the head of the talus is felt laterally, ATFL and CFL incompetence are present.
- To test the tibiofibular syndesmosis, perform the following actions:
  1. Interlace the fingers together behind the distal third of the calf.
  2. Use the heels of the hands to squeeze the tibia and fibula together.
  3. If there is a tear in the syndesmosis or a fibula fracture, the patient will experience pain with both squeeze and release of squeeze.
- Assess ability to bear weight/walk.
- Perform modified Romberg test to evaluate balance and proprioception.
  1. Have patient balance on injured leg with eyes closed.

DIAGNOSIS

■ DIFFERENTIAL DIAGNOSIS
- Fractures
  1. Fifteen percent of all ankle injuries have an associated fracture.
  2. Prepubescent children are at risk for physeal injury because the ligaments are stronger than the physis at this age.
  3. Be suspicious of prepubescent "ankle sprains."
- Peroneal tendon injuries
  1. The patient experiences point tenderness behind the lateral malleolus and pain on dorsiflexion.
  2. Achilles tendinitis or rupture consists of local tenderness, crepitus, and pain on passive dorsiflexion and resisted plantar-flexion.
  3. The patient may hear a "pop" and notice weakness on plantar-flexion.
  4. If the tendon is completely ruptured, the foot will not plantar-flex when the calf is squeezed (positive Thompson's test).

■ DIAGNOSTIC WORKUP
Indications for an ankle radiograph (also see Part III, Figure 3-56) are as follows, known as the "Ottawa Rules":
- Pain in the area of the malleoli *and* one of the following:
  1. Inability to bear weight (four steps)
  2. Bony tenderness at the posterior edge of the distal tibia or fibula

- A foot radiograph is necessary if there is pain in the area of the midfoot *and* one of the following:
  1. Inability to bear weight (four steps)
  2. Bony tenderness of the navicular or the base of the fifth metatarsal
- For mild to moderate ankle sprains, stress films are usually unnecessary.
  1. Prolonged pain and dysfunction after a typical healing period may indicate the need for stress radiographs to rule out ligamentous rupture.
     a. The anterior drawer test is performed as lateral views are taken. (The test is considered abnormal if anterior subluxation of the talus is greater than 6 mm.)
     b. The talar tilt test is performed as the mortise view is taken. (Any talar tilt of more than 5 degrees is considered abnormal.)
- Arthroscopy, computed tomography (CT), and magnetic resonance imaging (MRI) may be useful in the evaluation of persistent chronic ankle pain after an acute sprain.
  1. MRI may be especially useful if a double ligament tear is suspected and surgery is being considered.

▩ THERAPY

■ TREATMENT PRINCIPLES
PRICEMMS, an extension of RICE
- **P** = Protection from further injury by the following means:
  1. Air stirrup allows dorsi and plantar-flexion and limits inversion and eversion.
  2. Stirrups should be used continuously during the initial phases of healing.

- **R** = Relative rest
  1. Do nothing that hurts.
  2. Use crutches if needed.
- **I** = Ice is effective as long as there is swelling. Cold should be applied for at least 20 minutes, four times a day.
- **C** = Compression dressings are most useful in the first 48 to 72 hours.
  1. Do not obstruct distal venous return.
  2. Use an elastic wrap bandage, Unna boot, or air stirrup.
- **E** = Elevation should be initiated, optimally above the level of the heart.
- **M** = Medications (analgesics and antiinflammatory agents) should be instituted.
- **M** = Mobilization should start after an initial 24- to 72-hour period of rest.
  1. Active plantar-flexion and dorsiflexion—ankle pumps
  2. Writing the alphabet in the air with the big toe—alphabets
  3. Rising up on toes and lower heel back down—heel raises
  4. Cast immobilization of sprained ankles to increase short-term disability
- **S** = Strength training of the peroneal and gastrocnemius muscles should start as soon as possible to minimize deconditioning.

■ FOLLOW-UP & DISPOSITION
- A grading system for ankle ligament injuries is based on the degree of injury of each ligament and helps predict the return to full activities (Table 2-1).
- The goal of rehabilitation is to regain full strength, range of motion, and proprioception while minimizing the loss of cardiovascular fitness.
- Isometric exercises used to strengthen the peroneals involve

pushing the lateral aspect of the forefoot against a fixed surface.
  1. Exercises using a series of rubber bands of graduated strengths provide isotonic exercises for strengthening dorsiflexors and evertors.
- Range of motion incorporates "ankle pumps" and "alphabets."
- A progressive walking program should be initiated once 10 toe raises have been accomplished.
  1. Walk on a circular track for 20 minutes per day.
  2. Then walk the curved portion and jog the straight portion.
  3. Then jog the entire track.
- Proprioceptive retraining is achieved by standing on one foot with and then without support.
  1. The next step is balancing with eyes closed with and without support.
  2. When balance is maintained for 2 to 3 minutes, proprioception is recovered.
- Once the athlete is ready to return to practice, he or she should start with simple drills and progress to no restrictions.
- All exercises should be performed with a protective brace because this support improves proprioceptive feedback.
  1. The benefit of ankle taping decreases rapidly with exercise.
  2. The Aircast Stirrup, by reducing ankle inversion, decreases the incidence of ankle sprains and may be preferred over taping.
  3. High-top sneakers significantly increase the passive resistance to inversion and may be advisable for children predisposed to ankle sprains.

■ PATIENT/FAMILY EDUCATION
See "Follow-up & Disposition."

TABLE 2-1   Ankle Sprain Grading

SEVERITY	PATHOLOGY	SIGNS AND SYMPTOMS	DISABILITY	STRESS EXAMINATION
Grade 1	Ligament stretch	Minimal swelling, small area of tenderness, little or no hemorrhage, minimal decreased range of motion	Little or no limp with walking, difficulty hopping, expected recovery 7-10 days with rehabilitation	Normal
Grade 2	Partial ligament tear	Moderate swelling, more generalized tenderness, some hemorrhage, decreased range of motion	Limping with walking, unable to hop/run/toe raise, expected recovery 2-4 wk with rehabilitation	Anterior drawer and Talar tilt tests may be positive or negative
Grade 3	Complete ligament tear	Diffuse swelling, diffuse tenderness, evident hemorrhage, pronounced decreased range of motion	Unable to bear weight, expected recovery 5-10 wk with rehabilitation	Anterior drawer and Talar tilt tests positive

■ **REFERRAL INFORMATION**

Orthopedic consultation should be considered for all patients with third-degree ankle sprains.

☼ **PEARLS & CONSIDERATIONS**

■ **CLINICAL PEARLS**

- The Ottawa Rules offer guidelines for when ankle radiographs are necessary.
- Be very suspicious of prepubescent ankle sprain.
- The essential elements for the management of ankle sprains may be remembered by the use of the mnemonic *PRICEMMS* (protection, rest, ice, compression, elevation, medication, mobilization, strengthening).

■ **WEBSITES**

- MedScope: www.medscope.com
- MDConsult: www.Mdconsult.com
- WebMD: www.webmd.com

REFERENCES

1. Adamson C, Cymet T: Ankle sprains: evaluation, treatment, rehabilitation, *Md Med J* 46:530, 1997.
2. Bennett WF: Lateral ankle sprains. Part I: anatomy, biomechanics, diagnosis, and natural history, *Ortho Rev* 23:381, 1994.
3. Bennett WF: Lateral ankle sprains. Part II: acute and chronic treatment. *Ortho Rev* 23:504, 1994.
4. Chorley J, Hergenroeder A: Management of ankle sprains, *Pediatr Ann* 26: 56, 1997.
5. Eiff M, Smith A, Smith G: Early mobilization verses immobilization in the treatment of lateral ankle sprains, *Am J Sports Med* 22:83, 1994.
6. Fallat L, Grimm D, Saracco J: Sprained ankle syndrome: prevalence and analysis of 639 acute injuries, *J Foot Ankle Surg* 37:280, 1998.
7. Kuwada G: Current concepts in the diagnosis and treatment of ankle sprains, *Clin Podiatr Med Surg* 12:653, 1995.
8. Pigman E et al: Evaluation of the Ottawa clinical decision rules for the use of radiography in acute ankle and midfoot injuries in the emergency department: an independent site assessment, *Ann Emerg Med* 24:41, 1994.
9. Shapiro M et al: Ankle sprain prophylaxis: an analysis of the stabilizing effects of braces and tape, *Am J Sports Med* 22:78, 1994.
10. Shrier I: Treatment of lateral collateral ligament sprains on the ankle: a critical appraisal of the literature, *Clin J Sports Med* 5:187, 1995.
11. Stiell IG et al: Implementation of the Ottawa ankle rules, *JAMA* 271:827, 1994.
12. Stiell IG et al: The "real" Ottawa ankle rules, *Ann Emerg Med* 27:103, 1996.

Author: **Marc S. Lampell, M.D., F.A.A.P., F.A.C.E.P.**

BASIC INFORMATION

DEFINITION
- Anorexia nervosa is the refusal to maintain body weight over a minimum necessary for height.
  1. In early adolescence, anorexia nervosa can exist without a history of weight loss; instead, there is a failure to achieve expected weight gain during a period of growth.
- This disorder is characterized by intense fear of weight gain.
- These patients have a distorted body image.
- In postmenarchal females, amenorrhea (absence of three consecutive menstrual cycles) occurs.
  1. In the first 1 to 2 years after menarche, healthy adolescents may have periods of amenorrhea for longer than 3 months.

The use of strict criteria may preclude the diagnosis of anorexia nervosa in early stages.

SYNONYMS
- Eating disorder
- Anorexia

ICD-9CM CODES
307.1 Anorexia nervosa
307.50 Eating disorder, not otherwise specified

ETIOLOGY
Combination of factors, including the following:
- Genetic (increased rates of eating disorders in first- and second-degree relatives)
- Neurochemical (serotonin imbalance may contribute in some cases)
- Psychodevelopmental (low self-esteem, anxiety, depression, family conflict)
- Sociocultural (societal emphasis on thinness)

EPIDEMIOLOGY & DEMOGRAPHICS
- Prevalence: 0.5% among 15- to 19-year-old females in the United States
  1. Third most common chronic illness among adolescent females
  2. Significantly larger number with important subclinical forms
- Gender: more than 90% female
- Socioeconomic status: occurs in all ethnic groups and socioeconomic classes in United States
  1. More common among Caucasians
  2. More common in industrialized countries
- Typical age at onset: during adolescence or young adulthood
  1. Increasingly more common in younger children

HISTORY
- Weight loss or failure to gain weight
- Restrictive intake (careful review of dietary intake)
- Excessive exercise
- Purging (i.e., self-induced vomiting; use of ipecac to induce vomiting; use of laxatives, diuretics, or appetite suppressants)
  1. Purging with or without binge eating may exist in anorexia nervosa.
- Amenorrhea
- Other possible physical symptoms: fatigue, cold intolerance, abdominal discomfort, constipation, headaches, and syncope
- Distorted body image, intense fear of weight gain
- Low self-esteem, anxiety, depression, irritability
- History of family conflict, family history of eating disorders

PHYSICAL EXAMINATION
- Weight and height: calculation of appropriateness of weight for height, age, and sex.
  1. Body mass index (BMI) = Weight (kg) ÷ Height (m)^2 (Compare against reference data.)
  2. Percentage of ideal body weight (%IBW): Weight ÷ IBW (estimate of IBW for postmenarchal females: 100 pounds at 5 feet plus 5 pounds per inch over 5 feet)
- Vital signs: hypotension, bradycardia, hypothermia, orthostatic pulse changes
- Skin: dry, lanugo, alopecia, calluses or abrasions over the knuckles secondary to self-induced vomiting
- Head and neck: parotid gland enlargement, dental enamel erosion caused by vomiting
- Extremities: acrocyanosis, decreased capillary refill, edema, loss of muscle mass

OTHER MEDICAL COMPLICATIONS
- Cardiovascular: mitral valve prolapse, arrhythmia, ipecac-induced cardiomyopathy
- Gastrointestinal: constipation, delayed gastric emptying, mild elevations of liver function tests, esophagitis, hematemesis (including Mallory-Weiss tears)
- Endocrine: growth retardation and short stature, delayed puberty
- Skeletal: osteopenia
- Neurologic: peripheral neuropathy, cortical atrophy

DIAGNOSIS

DIFFERENTIAL DIAGNOSIS
- Inflammatory bowel disease
- Diabetes mellitus

- Thyroid disease
- Neoplastic disease

DIAGNOSTIC WORKUP
- Diagnosis is primarily based on history from patient and family.
- Laboratory data varies based on degree of malnutrition and presence or absence of purging.
  a. Laboratory tests in anorexia nervosa are often normal.
  b. There is no confirmatory laboratory test.
  1. Serum electrolytes, glucose, and renal function tests
     a. Hypokalemic, hypochloremic metabolic alkalosis (associated with vomiting)
     b. Hyponatremia
     c. Blood urea nitrogen elevated (dehydration) or low (low protein intake)
     d. Low blood glucose
  2. Complete blood count and erythrocyte sedimentation rate
     a. Mild anemia, leukopenia, thrombocytopenia, low sedimentation rate
  3. Electrocardiogram
     a. Prolonged QTc interval, T-wave abnormalities, low voltage, conduction defects

THERAPY

NONPHARMACOLOGIC
- Interdisciplinary approach (biologic, nutritional, psychosocial)
  1. Biologic: medical and nutritional stabilization
     a. Weight gain to within appropriate range of 90% to 110% IBW
     b. Correction of complications of malnutrition and purging
     c. Close monitoring of weight, vital signs, and physical examination
  2. Nutritional: education about nutrition and caloric intake
     a. Structured meal planning to establish healthy patterns of eating
     b. Identification of events that trigger abnormal eating behaviors
  3. Psychosocial: combination of individual, group, and/or family treatment
- Indications for hospitalization
  1. Presence of significant malnutrition
  2. Physiologic evidence of medical compromise
     a. Vital sign instability
     b. Dehydration
     c. Significant electrolyte disturbances

3. Acute food refusal or rapid weight loss
4. Failure of outpatient treatment
5. Medical or psychiatric emergencies

■ MEDICAL

- Antidepressant medication should be prescribed for coexisting depression (selective serotonin reuptake inhibitors, such as fluoxetine, paroxetine)
  1. Psychopharmacologic agents have not been effective in reducing the primary symptoms of anorexia nervosa during the acutely malnourished state.
  2. Fluoxetine may help stabilize recovery in patients with anorexia nervosa who have regained to more than 85% IBW.
- Treatment of amenorrhea with estrogen/progestin must be individualized.
  1. Studies have yet to determine the effect of estrogen on bone density in anorexia nervosa.
- Supplementation with calcium (1000 to 1500 mg/day) and a multivitamin, including vitamin D (400 IU/day), should be provided.

■ FOLLOW-UP & DISPOSITION
See "Therapy."

■ PATIENT/FAMILY EDUCATION
- Education should be developmentally appropriate for both age and psychosocial development.
- Education and involvement of parents and family members are essential.
- Confidentiality is very important.

■ PREVENTIVE TREATMENT
Early recognition of risk factors (see "Etiology & Epidemiology") and symptoms is important to prognosis.

■ REFERRAL INFORMATION
- Referral to an interdisciplinary treatment team (i.e., adolescent medicine specialist, mental health provider, and nutritionist) with expertise in managing adolescents with eating disorders is extremely helpful in providing the broad treatment necessary.
- Communication among members of the treatment team is essential.

☼ PEARLS & CONSIDERATIONS

■ CLINICAL PEARLS
- Ninety percent IBW should be established as the initial goal weight, based on probable return of menstrual function.

- Patients with anorexia nervosa who are taking oral contraceptive pills may have a "false sense" of health because they have monthly menstrual bleeding even at low weights.
- Many patients with anorexia nervosa consider their eating disorder to be a helpful "coping mechanism"; therefore they can be resistant to treatment. Acknowledging this conflict can be beneficial.

■ WEBSITE
Academy for Eating Disorders: www.acadeatdis.org

■ SUPPORT GROUPS
Many cities have support groups available for patients with anorexia nervosa.

REFERENCES
1. Becker AE et al: Eating disorders, *N Engl J Med* 340:1092, 1999.
2. Kreipe RE, Dukarm CP: Eating disorders in adolescents and older children, *Pediatr Rev* 20:410, 1999.
3. Society for Adolescent Medicine: Eating disorders in adolescents: a position paper of the Society for Adolescent Medicine, *J Adolesc Health* 16:476, 1995.
Author: **Carolyn Piver Dukarm, M.D.**

BASIC INFORMATION

■ DEFINITION
Antibiotic-associated diarrhea is the presence of diarrhea (defined as three mushy or watery stools per day or a significant increase in the frequency and/or looseness of stools above baseline) either during or after the administration of antibiotics.

■ SYNONYMS
- Antibiotic-associated colitis
- *Clostridium difficile*–associated diarrhea/colitis
- Pseudomembranous colitis

ICD-9CM CODE
008.45 Pseudomembranous colitis

■ ETIOLOGY
- Antibiotic-associated diarrhea can be related to a number of factors.
  1. Suppression or altered composition of normal intestinal flora can lead to the following:
     a. Functional disturbances, including colonic carbohydrate metabolism, which can result in an osmotic diarrhea, and metabolism and absorption of bile acids, which are potent secretory agents in the colon
     b. Overgrowth of pathogenic microorganisms, including *C. difficile,* other potential pathogens (rarely), toxin-producing gram-negative organisms, *Candida,* and *Staphylococcus aureus*
  2. Direct effects of the antibiotic include the following:
     a. Allergic and toxic effects on intestinal mucosa: Neomycin directly damages small bowel mucosa.
     b. Pharmacologic effects on motility: Erythromycin acts as a motilin receptor agonist and stimulates gastroduodenal contractions.
- Usually caused by growth of *C. difficile.*
  1. Gram-positive, anaerobic, spore-forming bacterium
     a. Spores allow the organism to survive for weeks to months.
  2. Produces an enterotoxin (toxin A) and a cytotoxin (toxin B), which cause mucosal damage and inflammation in the colon
  3. Can cause a spectrum of disease ranging from mild to severe:
     a. Diarrhea
     b. Self-limited colitis
     c. Pseudomembranous colitis
     d. Toxic megacolon and fulminant colitis
  4. Antimicrobial agents that predispose to *C. difficile* diarrhea and colitis
     a. Frequent: cephalosporins, penicillins (amoxicillin, ampicillin), and clindamycin
     b. Infrequent: tetracyclines, sulfonamides, erythromycin, chloramphenicol, trimethoprim, and quinolones
     c. Rarely or never: parenteral aminoglycosides, bacitracin, metronidazole, and vancomycin

■ EPIDEMIOLOGY & DEMOGRAPHICS
- Diarrhea is often associated with antibiotic use and can develop anywhere from 2 hours to 8 to 10 weeks after antibiotic use (usually 4 to 9 days).
- The incidence differs with antibiotics and ranges from 5% to 38%.
- Approximately 10% to 20% of cases of antibiotic-associated diarrhea are related to toxigenic *C. difficile.*
  1. It is acquired by the oral-fecal route.
  2. From 1% to 3% of healthy adults are asymptomatic carriers compared with 25% to 60% of healthy neonates and infants (up to 12 months of age).
     a. Infants may lack the intestinal membrane receptor for the toxin.
  3. It may occur without antibiotic exposure in immunosuppressed patients and patients with inflammatory bowel disease.
  4. It is one of the most common nosocomial infections in hospital practice.
  5. It is isolated in 95% to 100% of patients with pseudomembranous colitis.
  6. The risk is related to the type of antibiotic, length of treatment, and number of antibiotics used.

■ HISTORY
- Diarrhea after exposure to antibiotics (within 2 hours to 2 to 3 months)
- Other symptoms vary
  1. Simple antibiotic-associated diarrhea
     a. Mild watery diarrhea with mucus but no blood
     b. Mild crampy abdominal pain
  2. Nonpseudomembranous colitis (often *C. difficile*)
     a. Watery diarrhea with or without visible blood
     b. Malaise, nausea, and anorexia
     c. Possible low-grade fever
  3. Pseudomembranous colitis (*C. difficile*)
     a. Similar but more severe symptoms
     b. Diarrhea usually bloody and may actually contain pseudomembranes
  4. Fulminant colitis/toxic megacolon (*C. difficile*)
     a. Severe and diffuse abdominal pain
     b. Bloody diarrhea
     c. If an ileus develops, may be no stool output
     d. High fever and chills

■ PHYSICAL EXAMINATION
- Physical findings also vary.
  1. Simple antibiotic-associated diarrhea
     a. Unremarkable
     b. May have mild abdominal tenderness
  2. Nonpseudomembranous colitis
     a. Abdominal tenderness
     b. Low-grade fever
     c. Hemoccult-positive stools
  3. Pseudomembranous colitis
     a. Similar findings but abdominal tenderness may be more pronounced and fever higher
     b. Hemoccult-positive stools
  4. Fulminant colitis/toxic megacolon
     a. Toxic appearing with high fever, evidence of dehydration or shock
     b. Abdominal distension with significant tenderness with or without peritoneal signs
     c. Hemoccult-positive stools

DIAGNOSIS

■ DIFFERENTIAL DIAGNOSIS
- Simple antibiotic-associated diarrhea
  1. Infectious diarrhea
     a. Bacterial
     b. Viral
     c. Parasitic *(Giardia)*
  2. Lactose intolerance
  3. Milk protein sensitivity (infants and toddlers)
  4. Postenteritis enteropathy
- Colitis (mild to severe)
  1. Infectious diarrhea
     a. Bacterial (enteric pathogens): *Salmonella, Shigella, Yersinia, Campylobacter, Escherichia coli* O157:H7
     b. Parasites (entamoeba histolytica)
  2. Inflammatory bowel disease
  3. Henoch-Schönlein purpura
  4. Hirschsprung's enterocolitis (usually infants)
  5. Allergic colitis (infants)

■ DIAGNOSTIC WORKUP
- Stool studies should include the following:
  1. Stool hemoccult
  2. *C. difficile* toxin, preferably both A and B

II

3. Stool culture for enteric pathogens
4. Stool for *E. coli* O157:H7 in the appropriate setting
5. Stool for ova and parasite
- Stool test for *C. difficile:*
  1. Although stool can be cultured for *C. difficile*, the conditions are strict, and outside of research studies, this is not a reliable test.
  2. Toxin assays are currently the diagnostic test of choice to determine the presence of *C. difficile* in the setting of antibiotic-associated diarrhea.
     a. Enzyme immunoassays to toxin A and B are fairly sensitive (70% to 90%) and very specific (99% to 100%). False-negative results do occur.
     b. The cytotoxin assay to detect toxin B is more sensitive (94% to 100%) but takes longer to perform, is more expensive, and requires a tissue culture facility.
     c. Studies in children suggest that assay for only one of the two toxins can result in a missed diagnosis.
- In the setting of mild signs and symptoms, negative stool studies:
  1. Trial of lactose-free diet or lactose tolerance test (breath hydrogen test)
- In the setting of more severe signs and symptoms:
  1. Complete blood count with differential, erythrocyte sedimentation rate
  2. Electrolytes and albumin
  3. Kidney, ureter, and bladder study
     a. Toxic megacolon: a dilated colon, greater than 7 cm in greatest diameter
- Sigmoidoscopy/colonoscopy is usually performed in the presence of persistent symptoms with negative stool studies.
  1. Can document the presence of colitis and make the diagnosis of pseudomembranous colitis
     a. Raised yellow plaques from 2 to 10 mm in size scattered over colorectal mucosa, usually in the rectosigmoid, although may be limited to the proximal colon
  2. Performed with extreme caution in cases of toxic megacolon and fulminant colitis

℞ THERAPY

■ NONPHARMACOLOGIC
- General measures (simple antibiotic-associated diarrhea)
  1. If the child is still taking the antibiotic, discontinue the medication or change to an antibiotic less likely to cause diarrhea, if possible.
  2. Avoid lactose, excessive poorly soluble carbohydrates (e.g., fructose, sorbitol), and excessive dietary fibers (vegetables such as cabbage, carrots, peas) while symptomatic.
  3. Functional disturbances related to antibiotic use are usually self-limited.

■ COMPLIMENTARY & ALTERNATIVE THERAPIES
- Probiotics have been used both during and after antibiotic use to prevent or ameliorate antibiotic-associated diarrhea.
  1. Lactobacillus GG 1 to 2 capsules daily (1 capsule = 10 billion colony-forming units)
  2. Live culture yogurt (if tolerated); not always tolerated by lactose-deficient children

■ MEDICAL
- If *C. difficile*–positive diarrhea persists after the antibiotic is discontinued or symptoms are moderate to severe, consider the following:
  1. Metronidazole 20 mg/kg/day (up to 500 mg/dose) orally divided three times daily for 7 to 14 days
     a. First-line treatment of choice (inexpensive, effective)
     b. Side effects: nausea, vomiting, metallic taste, alcohol intolerance
     c. Secreted in bile and colon, so can be used intravenously (although not as effective as orally)
  2. Vancomycin 5 mg/kg/dose (up to 125 mg/dose) four times daily for 7 to 14 days
     a. May be slightly more effective than metronidazole but is significantly more expensive
     b. Side effects: few
     c. Indicated for patients who are intolerant or fail to respond to metronidazole and those with severe pseudomembranous colitis
     d. Not as effective as metronidazole intravenously
     e. Predisposes to development of vancomycin-resistant enterococcus
  3. Another alternative: bacitracin (up to 25,000 U/dose) divided four times daily for 7 to 14 days (However, this medication is expensive and less effective than metronidazole or vancomycin.)
- Recurrent (relapsing) *C. difficile* infection
  1. First relapse: repeat 10- to 14-day course of antibiotic
     a. Antibiotic resistance does not occur, so the same antibiotic can be used again.
     b. This can be followed with a course of lactobacillus GG.
  2. Second relapse: vancomycin for 7 to 14 days, followed by a taper over 2 to 3 weeks
- Overgrowth of other organisms
  1. Treat based on sensitivities, if available.
  2. *Candida:* Give nystatin (250,000 to 1,000,000 units) orally three or four times a day

■ SURGICAL
- Toxic megacolon or fulminant colitis may require surgical intervention.
- Subtotal colectomy with temporary ileostomy is performed in the following settings:
  1. Persistent toxicity despite aggressive medical therapy
  2. Perforation

■ PREVENTION
- Antibiotics should be used judiciously.
- Universal precautions should be followed with hospitalized/institutionalized patients.
- Lactobacillus GG during antibiotic use may decrease the incidence.

■ REFERRAL INFORMATION
- Infants and children should be referred to a gastroenterologist for the following:
  1. Evidence of moderate-severe colitis (systemic signs and symptoms)
  2. Recurrent *C. difficile*
  3. Negative stool tests and persistent diarrhea

■ PATIENT/FAMILY EDUCATION
- Avoid unnecessary use of antibiotics.
- Mild diarrhea during and after antibiotic exposure may respond to simple dietary manipulations and use of probiotics.
  1. Avoid excessive lactose, carbohydrates (juices), and some fiber-containing foods.
- Avoid alcohol while taking metronidazole.

☼ PEARLS & CONSIDERATIONS

■ CLINICAL PEARLS
- Avoid unnecessary use of antibiotics, particularly in children with a history of antibiotic-associated diarrhea.
- Use the antibiotic with the narrowest spectrum or those less frequently associated with diarrhea.
- Consider using probiotics (lactobacillus GG) in patients with a history of antibiotic-associated diarrhea.

- The diagnosis of *C. difficile* may be missed in children if the laboratory does not measure both toxin A and B. If the index of suspicion is high enough and other causes have been ruled out, consider an empiric trial of metronidazole.

- *C. difficile* may be present in neonates and infants up to 1 year of age without causing disease.

REFERENCES

1. Kader HA et al: Single toxin detection is inadequate to diagnose *Clostridium difficile* diarrhea in pediatric patients, *Gastroenterology* 115:1329, 1998.
2. Kelly CP, LaMont JT: *Clostridium difficile* infection, *Ann Rev Med* 49:375, 1998.
3. Vanderhoof JA et al: Lactobacillus GG in the prevention of antibiotic-associated diarrhea in children, *J Pediatr* 135:564, 1999.

Author: **M. Susan Moyer, M.D.**

BASIC INFORMATION

■ DEFINITION
α_1-Antitrypsin deficiency is an inherited autosomal-recessive liver and lung disease caused by mutant type Z α_1-antitrypsin (α1ATZ) protein. This deficiency leads to both liver dysfunction and emphysema.

ICD-9CM CODE
277.6 α_1-Antitrypsin deficiency

■ ETIOLOGY
- Liver disease is caused by the accumulation of abnormally folded α_1-antitrypsin protein within hepatocytes.
  1. Patients may also have an alteration in the endoplasmic reticulum protein degradation pathway.
- Lung disease (pulmonary emphysema) is caused by uninhibited proteolytic destruction of the connective tissue backbone of the lung.

■ EPIDEMIOLOGY & DEMOGRAPHICS
- PiZZ homozygotes are seen in 1 in 1600 to 1 in 2000 live births in Northern Europe and the United States.
- This is the most common genetic cause of liver disease in children and pulmonary emphysema in adults.
- From 10% to 15% of all PiZZ homozygotes develop clinically significant liver disease during the first 20 years of life.
- Liver disease may present in infancy (most common), childhood, or adulthood.
- Clinically significant pulmonary dysfunction does not occur until adulthood.

■ HISTORY
- Persistent jaundice as infant
- Feeding difficulties
- Poor growth
- Easy bleeding and bruising
- Pruritus
- Melena
- Chronic cough, particularly with a history of smoking or parental smoking

■ PHYSICAL EXAMINATION
- Jaundiced, particularly as infant
- Hepatomegaly with or without splenomegaly
- Ascites with advanced liver disease
- Mild signs of obstructive lung disease possible as a teenager and may progress
  1. Increased anteroposterior diameter of chest
  2. Prolonged expiratory phase
  3. Clubbing
  4. Hyperresonant
  5. Poor air exchange

DIAGNOSIS

■ DIFFERENTIAL DIAGNOSIS
- Other causes of neonatal jaundice (see "Jaundice/Hyperbilirubinemia" in Part I)
- Chronic hepatitis
  1. Viral
  2. Autoimmune
  3. Drug-induced hepatitis
  4. Wilson disease in older children and teenagers

■ DIAGNOSTIC WORKUP
- Liver function tests
  1. Modest elevation of transaminases
  2. May have elevated conjugated bilirubin
- Abnormal prothrombin time with more advanced liver disease
- Decreased serum albumin with progression of liver failure
- α_1-Antitrypsin phenotype
  1. Altered migration of the abnormal α1ATZ protein in isoelectric-focusing gels confirms diagnosis
- Liver biopsy
  1. Characteristic positive periodic acid–Schiff test
  2. Diastase-resistant globules in liver cells
- Pulmonary function testing (PFT)
  1. PFT abnormalities precede clinically significant symptoms.
  2. Abnormalities of DL_{CO} are seen: decreased diffusion capacity as alveolar surface area is lost.
  3. Abnormal FEV_1/vital capacity (VC)% is seen by 18 years of age.
- Abdominal ultrasound
  1. As a baseline assessment for evidence of portal hypertension
  2. To rule out (very rare) an intrahepatic mass

THERAPY

■ NONPHARMACOLOGIC
- Liver disease: primarily supportive
  1. Nutritional support, including fat-soluble vitamins
- Lung disease
  1. Avoidance of cigarette smoking *and* avoidance of passive smoke exposure delays progression of emphysema.

■ MEDICAL
- Medical management should be provided for complications of cirrhosis:
  1. β-Blockers for esophageal varices
  2. Diuretics for ascites
- α_1-Antitrypsin protein replacement therapy may delay progression of lung disease in adults.
  1. Not yet demonstrated in a well-controlled trial

■ SURGICAL
- Endoscopic therapy for esophageal varices
- Liver or lung transplant for organ failure
  1. Liver transplant: 5-year survival of 80% (pediatric data)
  2. Lung transplant: 5-year survival of 50% (adult data)

■ FOLLOW-UP & DISPOSITION
- From 10% to 15% of all PiZZ homozygotes followed prospectively from birth have clinically significant liver disease at 18 years of age.
- Up to one third of pediatric patients followed in gastrointestinal referral centers may ultimately require liver transplantation 5 to 10 years after diagnosis.
- Patients should be followed by a pediatric gastroenterologist with periodic laboratory work.
  1. Abdominal ultrasounds should be taken as needed to evaluate for portal hypertension or intrahepatic mass if increasing hepatosplenomegaly is present.
- Significant pulmonary dysfunction is unlikely during childhood.
- Progressive emphysema, cirrhosis, and/or hepatocellular carcinoma may occur during adulthood.

■ PATIENT/FAMILY EDUCATION
- Cigarette smoking and passive smoke significantly accelerate the progression of lung disease.
- Signs and symptoms of progressive liver disease (i.e., poor growth, gastrointestinal bleeding, and ascites) should be reviewed.
- Children may experience progression of liver disease requiring liver transplantation.
- Living-related liver transplantation is increasingly being used.
- Relatives with unexplained liver or lung disease should be evaluated.

■ PREVENTIVE TREATMENT OR TESTS
Avoidance of smoking and passive smoke

■ REFERRAL INFORMATION
- All patients should be referred to a pediatric gastroenterologist.
- Older teenagers should also be referred to a pulmonologist for initial evaluation of pulmonary function, as well as counseling regarding the utility of replacement therapy as adults.

☼ PEARLS & CONSIDERATIONS

■ CLINICAL PEARLS

- The α1ATZ level in blood may be transiently elevated as a positive acute-phase protein; always determine the phenotype.
- α1ATZ phenotype should be included in the evaluation of every patient with unexplained liver disease.
- MZ heterozygotes may also be at risk for progressive liver disease, particularly in the setting of concurrent viral or autoimmune hepatitis (M is the normal phenotype).

- Immunize all patients with chronic liver disease against hepatitis A and B because these infections may precipitate liver failure in patients with chronic liver disease.

■ SUPPORT GROUP

Alpha-1-Antitrypsin Deficiency, Alpha1 National Association, 8120 Pennsylvania Ave. S., Suite 549, Minneapolis, MN 55431, 800-521-3025; email: julie@alpha1.org; website: www.kumc.edu/gec/support/alpha1.html

REFERENCES

1. Perlmutter DH: Alpha-1-antitrypsin deficiency, *Semin Liver Dis* 18:217, 1998.
2. Piitulainen E, Sveger T: Effect of environmental and clinical factors on lung function and respiratory symptoms in adolescents with alpha₁-antitrypsin deficiency, *Acta Paediatr* 87:1120, 1998.
3. Suchy FJ (ed): *Liver disease in children*, St Louis, 1994, Mosby.
4. Sveger T, Eriksson S: The liver in adolescents with alpha₁-antitrypsin deficiency, *Hepatology* 22:514, 1995.

Author: **Lee A. Denson, M.D.**

II

BASIC INFORMATION

DEFINITION
- *Separation anxiety disorder:* anxiety symptoms caused by separation from parents or loved ones
- *Generalized anxiety disorder (overanxious disorder):* excessive and unrealistic worry about past or future events and behavior
- *Reactive attachment disorder:* disturbance of social relatedness, either inhibited or disinhibited
- *Social phobia:* excessive anxiety in social or performance situations
- *Simple or specific phobias:* irrational or excessive fear of a specific object or situation, associated with avoidance behavior and functional or social impairment
  1. Common phobias involve fear of animals, blood, dark, fire, germs or dirt, heights, insects, small or closed spaces, snakes, spiders, strangers, or thunder.
- *Selective mutism:* failure to speak in specific social situations (e.g., school) and ability to speak in other situations (e.g., home)
- *Panic disorder:* recurrent spontaneous episodes of panic that are associated with physiologic and psychologic symptoms

SYNONYMS
- Separation anxiety disorder
  1. School phobia
  2. School avoidance
- Generalized anxiety disorder
  1. Overanxious disorder
- Social phobia
  1. Avoidant disorder

ICD-9CM CODES
309.21 Separation anxiety disorder
300.02 Generalized anxiety disorder
313.89 Reactive attachment disorder
300.12 Social phobia
300.29 Specific phobia
313.23 Selective mutism
300.01 Panic disorder without agoraphobia
300.21 Panic disorder with agoraphobia

ETIOLOGY
- Neurotransmitters, including GABA, serotonin, and norepinephrine, are associated with anxiety phenomena in the central nervous system
- Genetic predispositions are evident
  1. Family history of anxiety disorder, depression, alcoholism, or somatization disorder is a risk factor
  2. Family history is also associated with earlier onset and increased severity

EPIDEMIOLOGY & DEMOGRAPHICS
- High prevalence of anxiety disorders, but often unrecognized and undertreated
- One-year prevalence of anxiety disorder: 15.4%
  1. Prevalence rate is based on parent and child interviews.
  2. Simple phobia, separation anxiety disorder, and overanxious disorder were the most prevalent, with rates of 9.2%, 4.1%, and 4.6%, respectively.
- Demographic profiles
  1. Separation anxiety disorder
     a. Younger children
     b. Lower socioeconomic status
     c. Single-parent families
  2. Reactive attachment disorder
     a. Insecure attachment is a risk factor.
  3. Overanxious disorder and social phobia
     a. Female gender
     b. Caucasian
     c. Middle- and upper-class families

HISTORY
- Children who are passive, shy, and fearful and who avoid new situations are more likely to exhibit anxiety.
- Increased tension is felt in the throat.
- "Behavioral inhibition to the unfamiliar" is an enduring, temperamental trait.
- Separation anxiety:
  1. Bedtime difficulties, including refusal to go to sleep and insistence on sleeping with parents
  2. Abdominal pain
     a. The pattern of abdominal pain associated with separation anxiety disorder often involves pain on Sunday night, on Monday morning, or at the end of a school vacation.
  3. Excessive worry about harm befalling loved one
  4. Nightmares
  5. Anticipatory anxiety with separations
- General anxiety:
  1. Extremely self-conscious
  2. Requires excessive reassurance
  3. Unable to relax
  4. Headaches
  5. Abdominal pain
  6. Muscle tension
  7. Sleep problems
- Reactive attachment disorder:
  1. Associated with maternal anxiety or depression
  2. Grossly pathologic care
  3. Chaotic environment

- Social phobia:
  1. Fears humiliation or embarrassment
  2. Exhibits avoidance or inability to function
- Simple or specific phobias:
  1. Often recognizes own irrational fear

PHYSICAL EXAMINATION
- Usually normal despite complaints of abdominal pain or headache
- Increased heart rate
- Pupillary dilation

DIAGNOSIS

DIFFERENTIAL DIAGNOSIS
- Separation anxiety disorder
  1. This type of anxiety overlaps with depression in one third of cases.
  2. School refusal (i.e., truancy) is not associated with anxiety about leaving loved ones or home.
  3. Medical causes for recurrent abdominal pain should be considered.
- Generalized anxiety
  1. Medical causes, including hyperthyroidism, excessive catecholamine, hypoglycemia, and cardiac arrhythmias
  2. Medication reactions
  3. Overuse of caffeine or other stimulants; common in adolescents
- Reactive attachment disorder
  1. Normal developmental variations must be considered. Indiscriminate acceptance of strangers is common until about 8 months.
  2. Autistic and retarded children may display disturbed social relatedness.
  3. Failure to thrive may have a medical cause associated with malnutrition and metabolic disturbance compromising mood and social relatedness.
- Social phobia
  1. In schizophrenia and other psychotic disorders, individuals do not recognize their fears as unreasonable or excessive.
- Simple phobia
  1. Developmentally normal fears
  2. Other anxiety disorders
- Panic disorder
  1. Physiologic cause for autonomic flooding (must be evaluated)
  2. Catecholamine excess or hyperthyroidism
  3. Real fears resulting from trauma (i.e., family stressors, abusive relationship, sibling abuse, unsafe neighborhood or school)

■ DIAGNOSTIC WORKUP

- Developmental, medical, school, social, and family histories, often lead to the appropriate diagnosis.
- Diagnostic interviews are generally used by psychologists.
  1. K-SADS—Schizophrenia and Affective Disorders Scale for Children: a semistructured clinical diagnostic interview tool
  2. DICA—Diagnostic Interview for Children and Adolescents: a semistructured clinical diagnostic interview tool
  3. DISC—Diagnostic Interview Scale for Children: a structured clinical diagnostic interview
  4. ADIS IV-C/P—Anxiety Diagnostic Interview Scale for Children and Parents: a semistructured clinical diagnostic interview tool
- The following clinician rating scales are available.
  1. Hamilton Anxiety Rating Scale
  2. Anxiety Rating for Children—Revised
- Parent or self-report instruments include the following:
  1. State-Train Anxiety Inventory for Children
  2. Children's Manifest Anxiety Scale
- If history or physical examination is suggestive, may need to consider workup for the following:
  1. Hypoglycemia
  2. Hyperthyroidism
  3. Cardiac arrhythmias
  4. Caffeinism
  5. Pheochromocytoma
  6. Seizure disorders
  7. Migraine
  8. Central nervous system disorders
  9. Medication reactions
- As part of the workup, usually screen for misdiagnosed or comorbid psychiatric disorders, including mood disorders, attention deficit/hyperactivity disorders, substance abuse, and eating disorders.
- Laboratory:
  1. Correlates of behavioral inhibition include the following:
     a. Elevated cortisol
     b. Elevated catecholamine levels

💊 THERAPY

■ NONPHARMACOLOGIC

- In infants and preschool children, the clinician should attend to parents whose anxiety, losses, and traumatic experiences may affect attachment relationships.
- Behavioral programs for separation anxiety disorder should include a plan for return to school as soon a possible.
  1. Generally, home tutoring is contraindicated.

2. Behavioral techniques such as systematic desensitization, extinction, exposure, and response prevention may be helpful.
- Family interventions, and often family therapy, are critical in treating separation anxiety disorder.
- Cognitive-behavioral therapy integrates behavioral approaches and cognitive techniques.
- Individual therapy is more effective when combined with pharmacologic intervention (see following discussion).
- For social phobia and selective mutism, group therapy with peers may promote social skills, peer involvement, and age-appropriate assertiveness.
- A panic attack diary, which describes the number, intensity, and type of panic attacks, will allow the clinician to evaluate triggers and plan for effective and focused intervention.

■ MEDICAL

- Separation anxiety disorder
  1. Earlier investigations showed effectiveness of imipramine in treating school phobia, recent studies have not replicated positive results.
  2. Small doses of short-acting benzodiazepines may be part of multimodal treatment plan for anxiety.
  3. Selective serotonin receptor inhibitors (SSRIs) may be effective when used in multimodal treatment.
- Generalized anxiety disorder
  1. Little research has been done about the role of pharmacotherapy.
  2. Anecdotal reports suggest possible role for SSRIs or buspirone.
- Reactive attachment disorder
  1. No role for pharmacotherapy has been defined.
- Social phobia
  1. Pharmacotherapy has not been well studied in children and adolescents.
  2. There is some evidence for usefulness of SSRIs or buspirone in treating social anxiety.
- Panic disorder
  1. Pharmacotherapy has not been well studied in children and adolescents.
  2. Some studies show effectiveness of benzodiazepines and SSRIs.
     a. SSRIs may cause worsening of panic-anxiety when treatment is initiated.
     b. Low initial dosages (5 mg of Prozac, 10 mg of Paxil) may protect against this.
     c. A high percentage (almost 50% of adults) show a significant treatment response to placebo, suggesting the need for psycho-

therapeutic approach and multimodal treatment.
- Benzodiazepines in children and adolescents: controversial
  1. Psychopharmacology consultation should be considered.
  2. Problems with benzodiazepine use include dependency, sedation, memory dysfunction, disinhibition, ataxia, and drug interactions.

■ FOLLOW-UP & DISPOSITION

- Anxiety disorders are recurrent.
- Medication should be tapered slowly, and ongoing consultation and therapy will help identify risks of decompensation.

■ PATIENT/FAMILY EDUCATION

- Use of medication in combination with behavioral, individual, and family therapy is more effective than either alone.
- Parents and caregivers should be educated about the signs of recurrence and ways of identifying stressors.
- Cognitive-behavioral techniques may prevent recurrence.
- Education and consultation for school personnel is valuable.

■ REFERRAL INFORMATION

Psychopharmacologic consultations, behavioral treatment, and family therapy are important because there is a high risk of recurrence in anxiety disorders and the treatment course is often extended.

☼ PEARLS & CONSIDERATIONS

■ CLINICAL PEARLS

- Successful treatment of school phobia requires family therapy interventions.
  1. Pharmacotherapy alone is rarely helpful.
  2. Home tutoring is generally contraindicated.
- Cognitive-behavioral therapy with a trained practitioner has been shown to be effective for a range of anxiety disorders.
- Adolescents who receive inadequate treatment for anxiety disorders may resort to self-medication and substance abuse.

■ WEBSITES

- American Academy of Child and Adolescent Psychiatry: www.aacap.org
- Anxiety Disorders Association of America (ADAA) Home Page: www.adaa.org
- NIMH Anxiety Disorders Education Program: www.nimh.nih.gov/anxiety/index.htm

■ SUPPORT GROUPS

The ADAA (see website) lists support groups by region and state.

REFERENCES

1. American Academy of Child and Adolescent Psychiatry: AACAP practice parameters, *J Am Acad Child Adolesc Psychiatry* 36:69S, 1997.
2. American Psychiatric Association: *Diagnostic and statistic manual,* ed 4, Washington, DC, 1994, American Psychiatric Association.
3. Bernstein G et al: Anxiety disorders in children and adolescents: a review of the past 10 years, *J Am Acad Child Adolesc Psychiatry* 35:1110, 1996.
4. Kutcher S (ed): *Child & adolescent psychopharmacology news,* New York, 1996-2000, Guilford Press (quarterly newsletters with reviews of research).
5. Lewis M (ed): *Anxiety disorder: child and adolescent psychiatry,* ed 2, Baltimore, 1996, Williams & Wilkins.
6. Werry JS, Aman MG: *Practitioner's guide to psychoactive drugs for children and adolescents,* ed 2, New York, 1999, Plenum Medical Book Company.

Author: **Stuart Loeb, M.D.**

BASIC INFORMATION

■ DEFINITION
- Acute appendicitis: inflammation of the vermiform appendix
- Chronic appendicitis: chronic inflammatory changes of the vermiform appendix thought to be a possible factor in chronic recurrent abdominal pain (*Note:* Many surgeons are unsure how often this occurs.)
- Perforated appendicitis: perforation of the vermiform appendix; perforated appendicitis may result in the formation of a localized periappendiceal abscess with an appendiceal mass, or generalized peritonitis
- Gangrenous appendicitis: acute appendicitis or perforated appendicitis accompanied by gangrene of the vermiform appendix

■ SYNONYMS
- "Appy"
- Perityphlitis

ICD-9CM CODES
541 Appendicitis
540 Perforation, peritonitis

■ ETIOLOGY
- Acute appendicitis, the most common appendiceal disorder, is most often initiated by proximal luminal obstruction.
  1. Often, luminal obstruction is the result of fecalith or inspissated enteric material forming an impaction at the appendiceal orifice.
  2. Lymphoid hyperplasia is also an important cause of luminal obstruction in children.
  3. Obstruction of the luminal orifice leads to elevated luminal pressure, which eventually exceeds capillary venous pressure, resulting in mucosal ischemia and infarction. This also results in decreased bacterial clearance from the appendiceal lumen with subsequent bacterial overgrowth, inflammation, infection, infarction, and pain.
  4. Protracted obstruction may result in perforation.
- Other causes of appendicitis include the following:
  1. Foreign bodies
  2. Bacterial infections, including *Yersinia*
  3. *Salmonella* and *Shigella*
  4. Parasitic infections, most commonly pinworms
  5. Tumors, most commonly a mucocele or carcinoid

■ EPIDEMIOLOGY & DEMOGRAPHICS
- No particular demographics are associated with appendicitis.
- Appendicitis occurs somewhat more often in boys than in girls.
- Peak incidence is 10 to 12 years of age.

■ HISTORY
- The history often is misleading when diagnosing acute appendicitis.
- The classic history of 24 to 36 hours of pain starting in the periumbilical area and localizing to the right lower quadrant is often absent.
- Classically, the child with appendicitis has a low-grade fever and lower abdominal pain, usually greater in the right lower quadrant than in the left.
- The child is anorexic and may be nauseated or have a history of vomiting.
- A low-lying or pelvic appendix can produce diarrhea, dyschezia, or pelvic pain in female patients.
- None of these symptoms is universal or diagnostic of appendicitis.
- A history of more than a few days' duration should alert the clinician to the possibility of a perforated appendix or an appendiceal abscess.
- Children younger than 3 years of age often present with perforated appendicitis.
  1. The higher increase in morbidity in young children, including higher incidence of perforation, is thought to be secondary to the difficulty in making diagnosis and later surgery.
  2. Young children may be unable to communicate symptoms effectively.
  3. Appendicitis may present as general abdominal pain and fever and be mistaken for viral gastroenteritis.

■ PHYSICAL EXAMINATION
- The child may be lethargic and lying on the stretcher with his or her knees bent in an attempt to decrease peritoneal irritation.
  1. All pediatric surgeons have seen children who look well and still have appendicitis.
- Low-grade fever is common.
- A child with appendicitis has tenderness in the right lower quadrant, usually with rebound tenderness.
- Such a child may exhibit a number of peritoneal signs:
  1. Rovsing's sign: pain in the right lower quadrant when pressing on the patient's left and releasing suddenly

  2. Obturator sign: pain after internal rotation of the flexed thigh
  3. Psoas sign: pain on passive extension of the right hip
  4. Jump sign: pain in the right lower quadrant upon jumping and landing on the heels
- Rectal examination may reveal inflammation in the right lower quadrant or a mass in the pelvis if the patient has a pelvic abscess low enough to be palpated.
- The physical examination is the most important aspect in diagnosing appendicitis, and proficiency in making this diagnosis improves with increasing experience.

DIAGNOSIS

■ DIFFERENTIAL DIAGNOSIS
- Porphyria
- Trauma
- Cholecystitis
- Ectopic pregnancy
- Ovarian torsion
- Ruptured ovarian cyst
- Constipation
- Crohn's disease
- Henoch-Schönlein purpura
- Intussusception
- Meckel's diverticulitis
- Pancreatitis
- Pelvic inflammatory disease
- Primary peritonitis
- Urinary tract infection
- Renal lithiasis
- Viral gastroenteritis

■ DIAGNOSTIC WORKUP
- In some centers, clinical pathways for right lower quadrant pain exist for children older than 3 years of age.
  1. These pathways attempt to minimize unnecessary laboratory and radiographic studies and were developed so that a unified approach to patients with suspected appendicitis occurs.
- Abdominal radiographs are ordered only for suspected free intraperitoneal air or bowel obstruction, a palpable mass, or suspected renal stones or gallstones.
- Ultrasound is ordered in postpubertal females with pelvic pain or in patients with suspected gallstones.
  1. More often than not, the appendix is not visualized and a negative ultrasound does not exclude, and may in fact cloud, the diagnosis of appendicitis.
  2. Ultrasound is a useful diagnostic tool for imaging the pelvic organs in the adolescent female patient and can help in the diagnosis of a ruptured ovarian cyst, an ovarian mass, or ovarian torsion.

II

- Complete blood counts (CBCs) are ordered only when there is suspicion of a perforation or abscess.
- In general, many surgeons will request a CBC as well as a urinalysis (to rule out a urinary tract infection or renal stone). Others prefer abdominal radiographs to look for an appendicolith, which has a high association with perforated appendicitis, or evidence of constipation with a full colon.
- Computed tomography (CT) has sensitivities of greater than 95% reported in the adult literature.
  1. The sensitivity in children is probably somewhat less because of less well-developed fat planes in the retroperitoneum and abdominal wall.
  2. CT does expose the patient to a significant amount of radiation but may be a useful diagnostic adjunct in cases in which the diagnosis may be questionable.
  3. In the case of perforated appendicitis, CT scanning is probably the most sensitive test to diagnose an intraabdominal abscess.

THERAPY

■ SURGICAL
- For acute appendicitis:
  1. Acute, nonperforated appendicitis is best treated with prompt appendectomy.
  2. Morbidity of this operation remains quite low, with wound infection and intraabdominal abscess formation being the most common postoperative complications.
  3. Children are given a dose of antibiotics preoperatively, usually a second-generation cephalosporin, and 1 or 2 doses postoperatively and are allowed to eat ad lib postoperatively.
  4. Most patients with uncomplicated appendicitis are discharged on postoperative day 1.

- Recently, many surgeons have chosen to perform their appendectomies laparoscopically.
  1. The benefits of this approach are mostly cosmetic, although in the young menstruating patient, laparoscopy allows for inspection of the pelvic organs.
  2. Some studies have shown a higher incidence of pelvic and intraabdominal abscess formation with the laparoscopic approach.
- For perforated appendicitis:
  1. Treatment for perforated appendicitis is also surgical.
  2. Some institutions have advocated intraperitoneal drainage for all cases of perforated appendicitis, but this has not been universally accepted.
  3. Postoperatively, these patients often have a prolonged ileus, requiring nasogastric tube decompression, and can be febrile for many days.
  4. Postoperative culture of the febrile patient with perforated appendicitis is unnecessary.
  5. Broad-spectrum intravenous antibiotics are initiated preoperatively and continued postoperatively at least until discharge, with some authors advocating a 7-day course and others switching the patient to oral antibiotics on discharge.
  6. An elevation in white blood cell count should raise the suspicion of an intraperitoneal abscess and may warrant a CT scan.

■ FOLLOW-UP & DISPOSITION
- There usually are no significant risks for uncomplicated appendicitis.
- Patients with perforated appendix and/or peritonitis have a long-term increased risk of bowel obstruction and adhesions.

■ REFERRAL INFORMATION
Appendicitis is a surgical disease, and as such, pediatric or general surgeons should be consulted for treatment.

PEARLS & CONSIDERATIONS

■ CLINICAL PEARLS
- The best clinical pearl for the practicing pediatrician is that the diagnosis missed is the diagnosis not considered.
- A child with abdominal pain and fever should raise the suspicion for appendicitis.
- If there is any question about the diagnosis, prompt surgical consultation should be requested.

REFERENCES
1. Ein SH: Appendicitis. In Ashcraft KW et al (eds): *Pediatric surgery*, ed 3, Philadelphia, 2000, WB Saunders.
2. Fishman SJ et al: Perforated appendicitis: prospective outcome analysis for 150 children, *J Pediatr Surg* 35:923, 2000.
3. Horwitz JR et al: Should laparoscopic appendectomy be avoided for complicated appendicitis in children? *J Pediatr Surg* 32:1601, 1997.
4. Rao PM et al: Effect of computed tomography of the appendix on treatment of patients and use of hospital resources, *N Engl J Med* 338:141, 1998.
5. Rice HE et al: Results of a randomized trial comparing prolonged intravenous antibiotics to sequential intravenous/oral antibiotics for children with perforated appendicitis, *J Pediatr Surg* (in press).
6. Warner BS et al: An evidence-based clinical pathway for acute appendicitis decreases hospital duration and cost, *J Pediatr Surg* 33:1371, 1998.
7. Wong ML et al: Sonographic diagnosis of acute appendicitis in children, *J Pediatr Surg* 29:1356, 1994.
Authors: **Mark Arkovitz, M.D., and Frederick Ryckman, M.D.**

BASIC INFORMATION

■ DEFINITION
Infectious and septic arthritis refers to microbial invasion of synovial space, typically with bacteria in acute septic arthritis and rarely fungi or mycobacteria.

■ SYNONYMS
- Acute suppurative pyoarthrosis
- Infectious arthritis
- Acute septic arthritis

ICD-9CM CODES
711.0 Septic
711.9 Infectious

■ ETIOLOGY
- The synovial space may become infected by (1) hematogenous seeding, (2) local spread from adjacent infection, or (3) trauma or surgical infection.
- Synovial fluid cushions and nourishes the avascular cartilage of the joint.
- The rich capillary network of the synovial membrane produces synovial fluid.
  1. This network is the port of entry for bacteria.
  2. Bacterial hyaluronidase decreases the viscosity and function of synovial fluid.
  3. Bacterial endotoxin stimulates the release of cytokines.
  4. Cytokines stimulate the release of proteolytic enzymes.
  5. This eventually leads to pressure necrosis from accumulation of purulent fluid.
- Infants have blood vessels that connect metaphysis and epiphysis, so it is not uncommon for osteomyelitis in this age group to rupture into the joint, causing septic arthritis.
- Hips and shoulders are at risk for extension of osteomyelitis into septic arthritis because the joint capsule overlies the metaphysis in the femur and humerus.
- Predisposing factors for infectious arthritis include the following:
  1. Trauma
  2. Joint surgery
  3. Joint injections
  4. Hemoglobinopathies
  5. Immunodeficiency
  6. Intravenous drug use
  7. Juvenile arthritis
- Bacterial causes
  1. *Staphylococcus aureus* is the most common, followed by group A streptococcus and *Streptococcus pneumoniae*.
  2. *Haemophilus influenzae* is becoming extremely rare since the introduction of immunization.
  3. Other causes include *Neisseria gonorrhoeae* (neonates, sexually active adolescents), gram-negative bacteria, *Salmonella* (about 1% of all cases, more common with sickle cell disease), *Kingella kingae*
  4. Causes in neonates include *S. aureus,* group A β-hemolytic streptococcus, gram-negative enteric organisms, methicillin-resistant *Staphylococcus aureus* (MRSA)

■ EPIDEMIOLOGY & DEMOGRAPHICS
- The incidence is estimated at 5.5 to 12 cases per 100,000 individuals.
- The peak incidence occurs in children younger than 3 years of age.
- Males are affected twice as often as females.
- Lower extremities (knees, hips, ankles) account for 80% of infections.
- More than 90% of infections are monoarticular.

■ HISTORY
- Fever, malaise, and arthralgias are present.
- Some patients report a recent upper respiratory infection (URI) or local soft tissue infection.
- Neonates are described as having poor feeding, irritability, or limb pseudoparalysis.
- Children have pain, limp, and refusal to walk.
- Usually, the onset is more acute than that seen with osteomyelitis.

■ PHYSICAL EXAMINATION
- Local erythema, warmth, and swelling are present.
- Tenderness is noted with passive joint motion; decreased range of motion is seen.
- Joint is held in position of comfort (abduction, external rotation for hip).
- In infants, swelling and erythema may not be present; may only have systemic signs:
  1. Fever
  2. Irritability
  3. Decreased or absent movement of the affected limb or joint

DIAGNOSIS

■ DIFFERENTIAL DIAGNOSIS
- Toxic synovitis
- Juvenile arthritis
- Rheumatic fever
- Leukemia
- Henoch-Schönlein purpura
- Legg-Calvé-Perthes
- Slipped capital femoral epiphysis
- Villonodular synovitis
- Ulcerative colitis
- Bacterial endocarditis
- Reactive arthritis; can follow a variety of infectious agents:
  1. *Borrelia burgdorferi*
  2. *Chlamydia*
  3. *Mycoplasma*
  4. Viral hepatitis A and B, rubella, human immunodeficiency virus, mumps, parvovirus B19, enterovirus, herpes
  5. Sterile inflammatory arthritis in association with infection at a distant site
  6. Reiter's syndrome, which occurs after intestinal infection with *Salmonella, Shigella, Yersinia, Campylobacter*
  7. May or may not have fever; can be monoarticular or oligoarticular
  8. Knees and ankles most commonly affected
  9. Culture only way to differentiate between septic and reactive arthritis
  10. Synovial leukocyte count (may be helpful)
- Gonococcal arthritis: hematogenous spread of infection leading to fever, chills, maculopapular rash with petechiae, tenosynovitis, and migratory polyarthralgia.
  1. Polyarthritis is seen in 50% of patients.
  2. Knees, elbows, ankles, wrists, and the small joints of hands and feet all may be affected.
  3. Arthritis can be reactive or septic.
  4. Synovial culture is positive in 25% to 35%; blood culture is positive in 20%; genital culture is positive in 80%.
- Lyme arthritis: occurs several weeks to months after infection with spirochete *B. burgdorferi*
  1. Most cases occur in the Northeast, with lower frequency in the upper Midwest, and less common in northern California.
  2. Acute, oligoarticular arthritis (knees) may be seen.
  3. This arthritis is episodic, lasting days, and may occur without prior symptoms.
  4. Treat with oral amoxicillin or doxycycline (for patients older than 8 years).
- Viral arthritis: most common viruses—rubella, parvovirus B19, hepatitis B
  1. More common in adults than in children
  2. Often arthralgia more than arthritis, migratory, lasts for 1 to 2 weeks, resolves without residual disease
  3. Symmetric joints of the hand in rubella and hepatitis B

- Mycobacterial arthritis: unusual in North America and Europe
  1. Joint infection from reactivation and hematogenous spread
  2. Slowly progressive monoarthritis, usually knee and hip
  3. History of exposure, positive purified protein derivative
- Fungal arthritis: rare
  1. Risk factors: immunodeficiency, malignancy
  2. Chronic monoarticular arthritis

■ DIAGNOSTIC WORKUP

- Joint aspiration should be done without delay if diagnosis is suspected.
  1. Aspirate should be sent for Gram stain, aerobic and anaerobic culture, cell count with differential, synovial glucose and comparative blood glucose, and mucin clot test.
  2. Median synovial fluid leukocyte count is 40,000 to 50,000 white blood cells (WBCs)/mm^3
     a. 75% to 90% neutrophils
     b. Sensitivity and specificity: 90% for WBC counts higher than 40,000/mm^3.
  3. Glucose concentration is often decreased (30% of blood value), but also seen in rheumatoid joint and acute rheumatic fever.
  4. Joint culture is positive in 50% to 60% of cases.
- Blood work includes the following:
  1. Complete blood count (CBC) with differential (may be elevated with left shift)
  2. Erythrocyte sedimentation rate (ESR) (usually elevated, but nonspecific; returns to normal in about 4 weeks) or C-reactive protein (CRP) (elevated, returns to normal more quickly than ESR, secondary rise may be a warning sign of return of infection)
  3. Blood cultures: 30% positive
- Imaging includes the following:
  1. Radiograph: increased joint space or soft tissue swelling
     a. May see subluxation of femoral head, especially in neonate
  2. Ultrasound: modality of choice to identify fluid and guide aspiration
  3. Scintigraphy: increased tracer uptake, less focal and less intense than with osteomyelitis
  4. Computed tomography (CT) and magnetic resonance imaging

(MRI) scans: do not differentiate septic from nonseptic arthritis
  a. MRI is highly sensitive for early detection of joint fluid.
  b. MRI is superior to CT in outlining soft tissue.

■ THERAPY

■ MEDICAL

- Joint aspiration is followed by parenteral antimicrobial therapy for 3 to 4 weeks.
- Empiric coverage should include a β-lactamase–resistant penicillin or a first-generation cephalosporin.
  1. Cefuroxime is a useful alternative (covers *H. influenzae*).
  2. If MRSA or pneumococcus is suspected or the patient has penicillin or cephalosporin allergy, administer vancomycin.
  3. For neonates, a β-lactamase–resistant penicillin in combination with an aminoglycoside, or alternately a third-generation cephalosporin, is suggested.
  4. For children with sickle cell anemia, a third-generation cephalosporin (ceftriaxone or cefotaxime) and antistaphylococcal therapy (nafcillin) are used.
  5. Parenteral treatment with abtriaxone or afotaxime for 7 to 14 days is indicated for gonococcal arthritis.
  6. For immunocompromised hosts, ceftazidime or ticarcillin-clavulanate with an aminoglycoside are chosen.
- Antibiotic therapy should be narrowed once the organism and sensitivities are identified.
- Oral therapy can be instituted when the patient's condition has stabilized and compliance can be ensured (oral antibiotics given in two to three times usual doses).
- Direct infusion of antibiotics into the joint is not helpful; some antibiotics may even increase the inflammatory response.

■ SURGICAL

- Open drainage is indicated if the hip joints (and some suggest shoulders) are involved.
- If large amounts of fibrin, tissue debris, or loculation are present, surgical drainage is needed.
- If the patient is not improving with medical treatment in 3 days, drainage may be needed.

■ FOLLOW-UP & DISPOSITION

- Acute treatment follow-up
  1. Serial ESR, CRP, or CBC
  2. Serial bactericidal titers of at least 1:8
  3. Adverse drug reaction monitoring
- Long-term follow-up for residual effects
  1. Poor outcome
     a. Leg length discrepancy
     b. Limitation of motion
     c. Chronic pain
     d. Need for secondary surgical procedures
  2. Important predictors of poor outcome
     a. Duration of symptoms longer than 7 days before treatment
     b. Age younger than 1 year
     c. Infection of hip or shoulder

■ PATIENT/FAMILY EDUCATION

Stress the need for strict compliance and follow-up.

■ REFERRAL INFORMATION

Early orthopedic consultation is critical for diagnosis and management.

PEARLS & CONSIDERATIONS

■ CLINICAL PEARLS

- A Gram stain of joint fluid is particularly important.
  1. Joint fluid is bacteriostatic, and organisms may not grow in culture.
  2. Approximately 30% of joint cultures are sterile despite other findings consistent with a septic joint.
- Preceding URI is particularly common in septic arthritis caused by *H. influenzae* and *K. kingae*.

REFERENCES

1. Krogstad P, Smith AL: Osteomyelitis and septic arthritis. In Feigin R, Cherry J (eds): *Pediatric infectious diseases*, Philadelphia, 1998, WB Saunders.
2. Shetty AK, Gedalia A: Septic arthritis in children, *Rheum Clin North Am* 24: 287, 1998.
3. Sonnen GM, Henry NK: Pediatric bone and joint infections: diagnosis and management, *Pediatr Clin North Am* 43:933, 1996.
Author: **Emma Hughes, M.D.**

BASIC INFORMATION

■ DEFINITION

Aspiration pneumonia is pneumonia resulting from aspiration of materials and/or chemicals foreign to the tracheobronchial tree, either from above (e.g., aspiration of foreign bodies) or from below (e.g., gastroesophageal reflux [GER] with aspiration).

■ SYNONYMS

- Aspiration syndromes
- Aspiration lung injury
- Chemical pneumonitis
- Bacterial aspiration pneumonia

ICD-9CM CODES

507.0 Aspiration pneumonia or pneumonitis
997.3 Aspiration acid pulmonary syndrome

■ ETIOLOGY

- Congenital anomalies of the palate and upper respiratory tract
- Swallowing disorders from anatomic or mechanical causes
- Disorders of esophageal motility
- Decreased lower esophageal sphincter (LES) pressure
- Delayed gastric emptying
- Depressed level of consciousness

■ EPIDEMIOLOGY & DEMOGRAPHICS

- Silent aspiration is common, even in normal individuals. However, the incidence of GER-related respiratory illness in infants and children is unknown.
- GER with aspiration may cause acute and/or chronic chemical injury to the lung.
- Craniofacial anomalies, with associated swallowing dysfunction, increase risk of aspiration.
- Aspiration occurs in 16% to 80% of children who are endotracheally intubated.
- Neuromuscular deficits or weakness of bulbar musculature increases risk.
  1. Depressed level of consciousness (from drug overdose, general anesthesia, head trauma, seizures, central nervous system infection)
  2. Immaturity or increased age
  3. Vocal cord paralysis
  4. Various neurologic conditions (e.g., cerebral palsy, increased intracranial pressure, muscular dystrophy, Werdnig-Hoffmann disease).
- As many as 50% of cases of aspiration pneumonia are associated with subsequent bacterial infection.

- The mortality rate after aspiration of gastric contents is high.
  1. Immediate death: 16%
  2. Death as the disease progresses: 24%
  3. Stabilization and recovery: 60%

■ HISTORY

- Irritability, colic, Sandifer syndrome, abdominal pain, or heartburn
- Nighttime/recumbent episodes of wheezing, cough, or respiratory distress
- Frequent regurgitation or vomiting
- Coughing, gagging, or choking with feeds by mouth or via nasogastric tube
- Apnea or apparent life-threatening event
- Failure to thrive
- Recurrent pneumonia
- Stridor or hoarseness
- Anemia secondary to hematemesis or melena

■ PHYSICAL EXAMINATION

- Respiratory distress (e.g., dyspnea, cyanosis, tachypnea, acute bronchospasm)
- Fever
- Orotracheal suctioning of gastric contents
- Localized erythema or inflammation of tracheobronchial tree on bronchoscopy

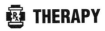

DIAGNOSIS

■ DIFFERENTIAL DIAGNOSIS

- Acute or chronic sinobronchitis
- Airways hyperreactivity without aspiration
- Reflex laryngospasm without aspiration

■ DIAGNOSTIC WORKUP

- Chest radiograph
  1. Airspace disease or interstitial infiltrates in the basilar or superior segments of the lower lobes
  2. In the posterior segments of the upper lobes when supine
  3. Atelectasis or obstructive pneumonitis
  4. Possible visible aspirated substance on the roentgenogram
- Upper gastrointestinal (GI) series with fluoroscopy
  1. To evaluate anatomic defects (e.g., vascular ring, tracheoesophageal fistula [TEF], pulmonary sling)
  2. To observe for esophageal dysmotility
  3. To assess deglutition and/or aspiration into the larynx or trachea
- Gastroesophageal scintiscan (milk scan) with technetium-99m sulfur

colloid mixed with milk or formula given orally
  1. To detect radioactivity in the lung fields, which indicates aspiration
- Bronchial washings
  1. To detect food fibers or particles
  2. To evaluate quantitative lipid-laden macrophages (The lipid-laden macrophage index correlates with the degree of chronic lung disease in children.)
- Manometry to measure esophageal motility and sphincter pressures

THERAPY

■ NONPHARMACOLOGIC

- Direct therapy at the underlying condition.
- Alter feeding techniques (e.g., thickened feeds; frequent, smaller feeds; continuous tube feedings instead of bolus feedings).
- Alter position (e.g., feeding only when upright, laying down in semi-upright position, prone position for infants).
- Provide adequate oxygen and/or ventilatory support.
- Provide good pulmonary toilet.

■ MEDICAL

- Prokinetic drugs: agents with cholinergic activity, which improve sphincter tone and increase esophageal motility and gastric emptying
  1. Metoclopramide
  2. Bethanecol
- Acid modifiers: reduce gastric acidity and decrease the release of gastric secretions
  1. Histamine$_2$-receptor antagonists: cimetidine, ranitidine, famotidine, nizatidine
  2. Proton pump inhibitors: omeprazole, lansoprazole
- Antibiotics: broad spectrum to cover enteric gram-negative bacilli, anaerobic, and gram-positive organisms
  1. Second- or third-generation cephalosporins, clindamycin, or penicillin G

■ SURGICAL

- Bronchoscopy: to remove particulate matter in the tracheobronchial tree
- Antireflux surgery:
  1. Nissen or Thal fundoplication in patients with GER alone
  2. Gastrostomy tube placement with fundoplication in patients with oral or pharyngeal dysphagia
  3. Fundoplication and pyloroplasty in patients with GER and delayed gastric emptying

■ FOLLOW-UP & DISPOSITION

- Fewer than one third of infants and children undergoing antireflux surgery experience side effects from the surgical procedure.
  1. Inability to vomit or burp: 28%
  2. Gas bloating: 36%
  3. Slow eating: 32%
  4. Choking on some solids: 25%
- Approximately 9% require reoperation ("slipped" wrap or disrupted fundoplication, incisional hernia or dehiscence, hiatal hernia, and bowel obstruction).
- A 1.3% fatality rate results from the surgical procedure.
- Pneumonia recurs in up to 40% of patients and appears to be highest in children with profound neurologic disability.

■ PATIENT/FAMILY EDUCATION

- Good oral hygiene should be encouraged, especially in neurologically disabled patients.
- Early recognition and treatment prevent progression to chronic lung disease and permanent damage.
  1. Interstitial pulmonary fibrosis
  2. Bronchiectasis
  3. Bronchiolitis obliterans
  4. Complications
     a. Adult respiratory distress syndrome
     b. Hypovolemia
     c. Sepsis
     d. Death
- The most favorable outcome and the lowest morbidity are achieved when surgery is postponed until the patient is adequately nourished.

■ PREVENTIVE TREATMENT

- Early recognition and modification of factors that place patients at high risk are important.
- Good oral hygiene and antibiotic treatment of upper respiratory bacterial infections can decrease the risk of complications in aspiration.
- Craniofacial abnormalities, vascular ring or sling, or TEF should be surgically corrected.
- Patients scheduled for anesthesia and surgery should fast preoperatively.
- Preoperative use of H_2-blockers and prokinetic drugs may reduce risk of aspiration pneumonitis in patients with this history.
- Oversedation, excessive analgesia, and obtundation should be avoided to help maintain the tone and function of the LES and the protective laryngeal closing reflex.
- Patients intubated with uncuffed endotracheal tubes should be suctioned frequently.
- For dysphagic patients, chin lowering as a postural technique will help eliminate aspiration resulting from delayed pharyngeal swallow or reduced airway closure.
- Maintain mechanically ventilated and bedridden patients in a semirecumbent or upright position to reduce gastric aspiration.

■ REFERRAL INFORMATION

- Patients should be referred to appropriate subspecialists for workup and management when necessary.
  1. Gastroenterologist
  2. Pulmonologist
  3. Otolaryngologist
  4. Pediatric surgeon
  5. Nutritionist
  6. Speech pathologist
  7. Respiratory therapist

☼ PEARLS & CONSIDERATIONS

■ CLINICAL PEARLS

- A high index of suspicion should be maintained in light of chronic cough or wheeze, nighttime symptoms, recurrent pneumonias, and failure to thrive.
- Adequate nutritional rehabilitation in malnourished patients improves the surgical outcome.
- Strict nothing-by-mouth orders and a program of respiratory care during nutritional rehabilitation in preparation for surgery prepares patients' lungs in best possible and healed condition because persistent cough can disrupt surgical fundoplication.

REFERENCES

1. Collins KA et al: The cytologic evaluation of lipid-laden alveolar macrophages as an indicator of aspiration pneumonia in young children, *Arch Pathol Lab Med* 119:229, 1995.
2. Colombo JL, Sammut PH: Aspiration syndromes. In LM Taussig et al (eds): *Pediatric respiratory medicine,* St Louis, 1999, Mosby.
3. Faubion WA Jr, Zein NN: Gastroesophageal reflux in infants and children, *Mayo Clin Proc* 73:166, 1998.
4. Langston C, Pappin A: Lipid-laden alveolar macrophages as an indicator of aspiration pneumonia (letter to editor), *Arch Pathol Lab Med* 120:326, 1996.
5. Lomotan JR, George SS, Brandstetter RD: Aspiration pneumonia: strategies for early recognition and prevention, *Postgrad Med* 102:225, 1997.
6. Platzker AG: GER and respiratory illness. In Chernick V, Kendig EL Jr (eds): *Disorders of the respiratory tract in children,* ed 5, Philadelphia, 1990, WB Saunders.

Author: **Eulalia R. Cheng, M.D.**

BASIC INFORMATION

■ DEFINITION

Asthma is a chronic inflammatory disorder of airways leading to airway hyperresponsiveness to a variety of stimuli. This hyperresponsiveness manifests as airflow obstruction, which is often reversible spontaneously or with treatment. The inflammation also leads to recurrent respiratory symptoms, including wheezing, breathlessness, chest tightness, and cough.

■ SYNONYMS

- Reactive airway disease (RAD)
- Wheezy bronchitis

ICD-9CM CODES

- 493.0   With hay fever
- 493.1   Intrinsic (late onset)
- 493.9   Asthma
- 493.91 With status asthmaticus

■ ETIOLOGY

- Genetic predisposition
  1. Genetic markers on chromosomes 5, 11, and 14 associated with atopy and asthma
- Structural predisposition
  1. Wheezing in early life (younger than 6 years of age) and in young boys associated with decreased measures of lung function compared with children who do not wheeze
- Inflammation and airway hyperresponsiveness: final pathway
  1. Mast cells, eosinophils, T lymphocytes, macrophages, neutrophils, and epithelial cells all have a role in producing proinflammatory cytokines and chemokines.
  2. Constituent cells of airway (i.e., fibroblasts, endothelial cells, and epithelial cells) also produce cytokines and chemokines.
  3. Modulation of smooth muscle tone, vascular permeability, neuronal activity, and mucus secretion is orchestrated by cell mediators.

■ EPIDEMIOLOGY & DEMOGRAPHICS

- Asthma prevalence is estimated at 5% to 6% of children 0 to 4 years of age and 7% to 10% of children 5 to 14 years of age.
- Nearly 5 million children younger than 18 years have been diagnosed with asthma.
- In 1994, more than 3 million office visits, 500,000 emergency department visits, and 165,000 hospitalizations occurred as a result of asthma in children younger than 14 years of age.
- Approximately 30% of all children wheeze by age 3 years; only one third

of these children have persistent symptoms up to age 6.
- High-risk populations include the following:
  1. Minority (especially African Americans)
  2. Inner-city dwellers
  3. Premature or low-birth-weight children (irrespective of bronchopulmonary dysplasia history)
- Predisposing factors include the following:
  1. Personal or family history of atopy
  2. Passive smoke exposure
  3. Exposure to maternal tobacco smoke in utero
  4. Male gender (in early childhood)
  5. Maternal history of asthma

■ HISTORY

- The patient has a history of recurrent respiratory symptoms (cough, wheeze, difficulty breathing, chest tightness) that are often worse at night.
- Symptoms occur or worsen in the presence of the following:
  1. Exercise
  2. Viral infections
  3. Animals with fur or feathers
  4. House-dust mites
  5. Molds
  6. Smoke (tobacco, wood)
  7. Pollen
  8. Changes in weather
  9. Strong emotional expression
  10. Airborne chemicals or dusts
  11. Menses

■ PHYSICAL EXAMINATION

- Hyperexpansion of thorax
- Wheezing during normal breathing or prolonged expiratory phase during forced maneuvers
- Symptomatic relief following bronchodilator use
- Consideration of alternative diagnosis of evidence of clubbing, nasal polyps, or stridor

DIAGNOSIS

■ DIFFERENTIAL DIAGNOSIS

- Large airway obstruction or compression
  1. Foreign body
  2. Mediastinal mass
  3. Laryngotracheomalacia, tracheal stenosis, or bronchostenosis
  4. Vascular rings or slings
- Large and small airway involvement
  1. Aspiration (either primary or secondary)
  2. Cystic fibrosis
  3. Gastroesophageal edema
  4. Pulmonary edema
- Other
  1. Recurrent lower respiratory

infection secondary to immune dysfunction
  2. Vocal cord dysfunction
  3. Psychogenic cough
  4. Allergic rhinitis and/or sinusitis
  5. Hyperventilation syndrome
  6. Hypersensitivity pneumonitis
  7. Bronchiolitis obliterans

■ COMPLICATING & COMORBID CONDITIONS

- Gastroesophageal reflux
- Rhinitis and sinusitis
- Allergic bronchopulmonary aspergillosis
- Exposure to inhalant allergens or irritants
- Aspirin or sulfite sensitivity

■ DIAGNOSTIC WORKUP

- Detailed medical history
- Pulmonary function studies, including spirometry
  1. Documentation of airflow obstruction and/or reversibility useful for diagnosis
     a. Reversible airflow obstruction (at rest, with exercise, or following bronchoprovocation) as measured by spirometry
  2. Bronchoprovocation with methacholine or exercise challenge
  3. Peak flow measurements not recommended for initial evaluation because of wide variability in normative values and results
- History- or examination-directed evaluations
  1. Chest x-ray
     a. Hyperinflation
     b. Peribronchial cuffing
     c. Patchy atelectasis (also common)
  2. Allergy testing
     a. May identify particular allergens for directed environmental control or avoidance
  3. pH probe and/or barium swallow to rule out gastroesphageal reflux or aspiration
  4. Possibly bronchoscopy in young children to rule out structural abnormalities
- Asthma specialist referral
  1. Goals of therapy not being met (see following discussion)
  2. Diagnostic assistance
  3. Educational support
  4. Nonstandard or exceptional therapy indicated
  5. Asthma severe or life-threatening

THERAPY

- Goals of therapy should be achieved in all asthmatics.
  1. Prevent chronic and troublesome symptoms.

II

2. Maintain normal or near-normal pulmonary function.
3. Maintain normal activity levels.
4. Prevent recurrent exacerbations.
5. Minimize adverse effects from therapy.
6. Meet patient's and family's expectations for care.

■ NONPHARMACOLOGIC

• Environmental control
• Irritant and allergen avoidance
• Adjunctive therapy
  1. Bioregulation and self-hypnosis
  2. Psychologic counseling

■ MEDICAL

• Stepwise approach recommended
  1. Amount and frequency of therapy are dictated by asthma symptoms and severity.
  2. Generally, initiate at a higher level to establish prompt control and then step down.
• Review of written asthma action plan for acute and chronic intervention; regular revision if necessary
• Acute, home-based management
  1. Begin scheduled β_2-agonist therapy with first onset of exacerbation.
     a. Action plan should include when to contact physician if insufficient relief is obtained.
  2. Corticosteroids should be given.
     a. Initiation of double-dose inhaled corticosteroids at first onset of symptoms may be useful.
     b. Short-term oral bursts may be necessary to control moderate symptoms associated with viral infection or exposure to an irritant.
• Chronic
  1. Inhaled corticosteroids
     a. This is first-line therapy for patients with persistent symptoms.
     b. Multiple strengths, formulations, and dosing schedules are available.
        (1) Multiple delivery devices also available (metered-dose inhaler, breath-actuated).
        (2) Choose those that are most acceptable to patient.
     c. Monitor patients closely for adverse side effects, which include the following:
        (1) Oral candidiasis: Encourage patients to rinse and spit following each dose; risk reduced with spacer use.
        (2) Dysphonia: Use of spacer device has not been shown to decrease the occurrence of dysphonia.
            Some evidence suggests that Turbuhaler inhaler decreases

prevalence as a result of different positioning of vocal cords during inhalation.
        (3) Altered linear growth: Shown to diminish growth velocity in early puberty with catch-up growth achieved in late puberty, even if patient remains on inhaled corticosteroids during that time.
            No difference is noted in adult height between corticosteroid users and nonuser asthmatics (*Journal of Asthma* 36:15, 1999).
        (4) Cataracts: Rare in children. Occur primarily in patients with high-dose inhaled and frequent systemic corticosteroid bursts
        (5) Adrenal suppression: Although clinical symptoms of adrenal insufficiency have not been reported in children taking inhaled corticosteroids alone, some adrenal axis suppression can be identified in patients taking high-dose inhaled steroids (especially in conjunction with other forms of corticosteroid use). The clinical relevance of this finding is not clear.
  2. Inhaled mast-cell stabilizers (i.e., cromolyn or nedocromil)
     a. Useful in infants because of safety profile
     b. Alternative to short-acting β_2-agonists before activity in patients with exercise-induced symptoms
  3. Inhaled β_2-agonists
     a. Short-acting agents may be used on as-needed basis.
        (1) Daily use may indicate need to increase chronic therapy.
     b. Long-acting agents may be considered for those with nighttime symptoms or as an adjunct to antiinflammatory therapy.
  4. Oral β_2 agonists
     a. These long-acting oral agents may be useful for those with nighttime symptoms or those unable to master inhaler technique.
  5. Leukotriene-receptor antagonists
     a. Role as first-line agent still unclear
     b. Available in oral formulation for children older than 6 years of age

c. Useful as corticosteroid-sparing agent
  6. Theophylline
     a. Low-dose chronic therapy may be considered as a corticosteroid-sparing agent
     b. May be useful for patients with nighttime symptoms or those unable to master inhaler technique
  7. Immunosuppression
     a. Not indicated for most asthmatic children but may be useful in subgroup with concurrent allergic rhinitis

■ FOLLOW-UP & DISPOSITION

• Frequent (i.e., monthly) follow-up is necessary until control is maintained.
• Once under good control, semiannual visits are needed to review goals and reinforce education, as well as to consider step-down therapy.
• Risk factors for death from asthma include the following:
  1. History of sudden severe exacerbations
  2. Prior intubation or intensive care unit admission for asthma
  3. Two or more hospitalizations, or three or more emergency care visits for asthma in the past year
  4. Hospitalization or emergency care visit for asthma within the past month
  5. Use of more than two canisters per month of inhaled short-acting β_2-agonist
  6. Current use of systemic corticosteroids or recent withdrawal from systemic corticosteroids
  7. Difficulty perceiving airflow obstruction or its severity
  8. Comorbidity, as from cardiovascular diseases
  9. Serious psychiatric disease or psychosocial problems

■ PATIENT/FAMILY EDUCATION

• Reinforce frequently.
• Establish partnership between parents, patients, and provider for asthma management and role of medications.
• Develop acute action plan.
• Ensure proper techniques for inhaled

medications (spacers should be encouraged for all age groups).
- Review techniques for self-monitoring (symptom recognition or peak flow monitoring).
- Discuss environmental control measures and precipitant avoidance.
- Review cultural beliefs and practices associated with asthma.

☼ PEARLS & CONSIDERATIONS

■ CLINICAL PEARLS
- Chronic antiinflammatory therapy may also be useful for patients with exercise-induced asthma poorly controlled with bronchodilator use before exercise.
- Peak flow monitoring is technique dependent.
  1. Need to establish personal baseline when well.
  2. Zones are based on personal best, and plan is based on zone.
     a. Green: 80% to 100% of personal best peak flow; continue daily medication
     b. Yellow: 60% to 80% of personal best peak flow; step up therapy as instructed
     c. Red: less than 60% of personal best peak flow; contact physician
- With acute exacerbation, the patient may need to increase the dose of inhaled short-acting β_2-agonist from 2 puffs to 4 to 6 puffs to provide adequate relief.
  1. Be very specific in action plan to prevent overuse of medication.

- For elective surgery:
  1. Maximize control, which may include short course of systemic corticosteroids.
     a. Stress-dose hydrocortisone may be indicated for patients receiving recent systemic corticosteroids.
     b. Once control is achieved, attempt to reduce the dose.

■ WEBSITES
- American Medical Association: www.ama-assn.org/special/asthma/treatmnt/treatmnt.htm; *JAMA* asthma information center/treatment center; provides summary of clinical guidelines, treatment updates, practice parameters, and drug information
- Asthma in America: www.asthmainamerica.com; up-to-date overview of asthma in the United States; includes information in clear outline form that is appropriate for patient handouts; easy hyperlink to 1998 NHLBI practical guidelines; list of resources for families
- National Heart, Lung, and Blood Institute (NHLBI): www.nhlbi.nih.gov/guidelines/asthma/asthgdln.htm; actual copy of most recent NHLBI asthma guidelines

■ SUPPORT GROUPS
- Allergy and Asthma Network/Mothers of Asthmatics (www.aanma.org)
- Asthma and Allergy Foundation of America (www.aafa.org)

REFERENCES
1. Barnes PJ, Pedersen S, Busse WW: Efficacy and safety of inhaled corticosteroids: new developments, *Am J Respir Crit Care Med* 157:S1, 1998.
2. Brooks AM, McBride JT: The asthma specialist: when and why to refer the pediatric patient, *Pediatr Ann* 28:55, 1999.
3. Li JTC, Reed CE: What role for immunotherapy in managing allergic asthma? *J Respir Dis* 13:1735, 1992.
4. Mannino DM et al: Surveillance for asthma—United States 1960-1995, *MMWR Morb Mortal Wkly Rep* 47:1, 1998.
5. National Asthma Education Program Expert Panel: Report II. Guidelines for the diagnosis and management of asthma, Bethesda, Md, National Institutes of Health, National Heart, Lung and Blood Institute, NIH Publication No. 97-4051, April 1997.
6. Sigman K, Mazer B: Immunotherapy for childhood asthma: is there a rationale for its use? *Ann Allergy Asthma Immunol* 76:299, 1996.
7. Szilagyi PG, Kemper KJ: Management of chronic childhood asthma in the primary care office, *Pediatr Ann* 28:43, 1999.
8. Taylor WR, Newacheck PW: Impact of childhood asthma on health, *Pediatrics* 90:657, 1992.
9. Yoos HL, McMullen A: Symptom monitoring in childhood asthma: how to use a peak flow meter, *Pediatr Ann* 28:31, 1999.

Author: **Ann Marie Brooks, M.D.**

II

BASIC INFORMATION

■ DEFINITION
Atopic dermatitis is an inherited inflammatory skin disorder often found in association with asthma or allergic rhinitis.

■ SYNONYM
Eczema

ICD-9CM CODE
691.8 Atopic dermatitis and related conditions

■ ETIOLOGY
- Although the cause is unknown, both genetic and environmental factors play a role.
- Immune dysfunction exists in patients with atopic dermatitis (AD), but whether it is the cause or effect of the disease has not been determined.
- Food allergens in some patients have been found to be an exacerbating factor.
- Aeroallergens, such as trees and grass pollens, play an important role in the exacerbation of AD.
- Both immediate hypersensitivity skin tests and delayed-type hypersensitivity patch tests are often positive in patients with AD.

■ EPIDEMIOLOGY
- Up to 75% of all patients have a positive family history of atopic disease.
- Sixty percent of children with AD manifest their disease in the first year of life.
- No racial differences are noted in children manifesting disease.

■ HISTORY
- The clinical picture varies with the age of the patient and disease severity.
- Pruritus is a hallmark of the disease.
- Associated clinical findings include xerosis, ichthyosis vulgaris, keratosis pilaris, allergic shiners (orbital hyperpigmentation), Dennie-Morgan folds (atopic pleats), hyperlinear palms or soles, and susceptibility to recurrent cutaneous infections (bacterial, viral, and fungal).

■ PHYSICAL EXAMINATION
INFANTS
- Infants usually present with acute dermatitis.
- Intensely pruritic erythematous papules and vesicles that become excoriated and exudative are observed.
- Lesions are distributed over the scalp, forehead, cheeks, trunk, and extensor extremities.
- The diaper area is usually spared.
OLDER CHILDREN
- A more subacute presentation is common.
- Excoriated erythematous scaling papules and plaques located on the wrists, ankles, and antecubital and popliteal fossae are observed.
- The hands and feet are commonly involved, with dryness, cracking, and scaling.
- Chronic changes secondary to repeated rubbing and scratching include lichenification with skin that is thickened and has prominent skin markings.
- Perifollicular accentuation is common in patients with dark skin.

DIAGNOSIS

■ DIFFERENTIAL DIAGNOSIS
- Seborrheic dermatitis
- Psoriasis
- Tinea corporis
- Nummular dermatitis
- Irritant or allergic contact dermatitis
- Scabies (especially in infants)
- Histiocytosis X
- Wiskott-Aldrich syndrome

■ DIAGNOSTIC WORKUP
The diagnosis is usually made on the basis of a characteristic clinical picture, as well as a family and personal history of atopy.

THERAPY

■ NONPHARMACOLOGIC
- Mild soaps (e.g., Dove, Tone, Purpose, Basis) or a soap substitute (e.g., Cetaphil) should be used once or twice a day.
- Emollients (e.g., Vaseline petroleum jelly, Aquaphor ointment, Theraplex emollient, Eucerin cream) should be used two to three times per day.
- In general, creams or ointments are preferred.
- Bathing (5 to 10 minutes in lukewarm water) is fine as long as damp skin is moisturized with creams or ointments immediately after bathing.
- Irritants such as detergents and solvents and fabrics such as wool or nylon should be avoided.

■ MEDICAL
- Choose the mildest topical steroid that can control the disease.
- Most patients can be controlled with low-potency topical corticosteroids applied twice a day to individual areas for several weeks.
- Use stronger, nonfluorinated low-potency to midpotency ointments during flare-ups.
- Reduce corticosteroid potency as the disease is controlled.
- Sedating antihistamines (e.g., hydroxyzine, cyproheptadine, diphenhydramine) may help children sleep and prevent itching during sleep.
- Secondary bacterial infection can be present during flare-ups.
  1. *Staphylococcus aureus* colonizes the skin of more than 95% of patients with AD.
  2. Treat superinfections with appropriate systemic antibiotics for 7 to 14 days.
- Patients with severe or extensive disease should be referred to a dermatologist.

PEARLS & CONSIDERATIONS

■ CLINICAL PEARLS
More than 75% of children with AD improve by adolescence.

■ WEBSITES
- American Academy of Dermatology: www.aad.org
- National Eczema Association for Science and Education: www.eczema-assn.org
- The National Eczema Society: www.eczema.org
- Society for Pediatric Dermatology: www.spdnet.org

REFERENCES
1. Kim HJ, Honig PJ: Atopic dermatitis, *Curr Opin Pediatr* 10:387, 1998.
2. Knoell KA, Greer KE: Atopic dermatitis, *Pediatr Rev* 20:46, 1999.
3. Krafchik BR: Treatment of atopic dermatitis, *J Cutan Med Surg* 3:16, 1999.
Author: **Susan Haller Psaila, M.D.**

BASIC INFORMATION

DEFINITION
A direct communication between the right and left atria, most commonly in the region of the fossa ovalis, with normally connected pulmonary veins. Sinus venosus defects lie outside of the confines of the fossa ovalis near the superior vena cava and are always associated with abnormal connection of the right pulmonary veins to the right atrium.

SYNONYMS
- Secundum atrial septal defect
- Fossa ovalis atrial defect

ICD-9CM CODE
745.5 Ostium secundum–type atrial septal defect

ETIOLOGY
- Secundum atrial defects are caused by defective development of the septum secundum or excessive resorption of the septum primum.
- Sinus venosus defects are caused by unroofing of the right pulmonary veins.

EPIDEMIOLOGY & DEMOGRAPHICS
- Common, accounting for 7% to 10% of congenital cardiac malformations
- Incidence: 1 in 1500 live births
- Male:female ratio: 1:2
- Usually sporadic
- Spontaneous closure: 40% to 50% of defects detected in early infancy; closure by 2 years of age
- Familial occurrence: Holt-Oram syndrome (atrial defect with upper limb deformities, cardiac conduction abnormalities) with autosomal-dominant inheritance
- Often an integral (and at times a necessary) component of complex congenital cardiac malformations
- From 25% to 30% of individuals with an otherwise normal heart have a probe patent foramen ovale, not considered an atrial defect

HISTORY
- The patient is usually asymptomatic, although endurance may be limited in retrospect after closure.
- Uncommonly, fatigue, dyspnea upon exertion, or recurrent lower respiratory infections are reported.
- The patient is usually small in stature, but true failure to thrive is rare.
- The disease is commonly detected in early childhood but may be identified in infancy.
- In untreated patients, late atrial arrhythmias, such as atrial fibrillation, congestive heart failure, or pulmonary vascular obstructive disease, may ensue in an unpredictable fashion.

PHYSICAL EXAMINATION
- Height and weight are often below normal.
- Precordial activity is increased.
- Grade I to III/VI systolic pulmonary flow murmur is noted at the upper left sternal border.
- A persistent wide split of the second heart sound with a pulmonary closure sound of normal intensity is present.
- If pulmonary blood flow is at least twice systemic flow, a soft middiastolic murmur related to relative tricuspid stenosis is audible at the lower left sternal border.

DIAGNOSIS

DIFFERENTIAL DIAGNOSIS
- Functional pulmonary flow murmur
- Pulmonary valve stenosis
- Primum atrial septal defect

DIAGNOSTIC WORKUP
- Electrocardiogram
  1. Frontal plane QRS axis to the right
  2. RSR′ pattern in V_1, V_3R (right ventricular volume load)
  3. Mild right atrial enlargement
  4. Mild PR prolongation
  5. May be normal in 5% of patients
- Chest roentgenogram
  1. Mild cardiomegaly
  2. Right atrial and ventricular and main pulmonary artery enlargement
  3. Increased pulmonary blood flow
- Echocardiography
  1. Visualization of the defect in the region of the fossa ovalis
  2. Visualization of the pulmonary venous connections
  3. Color and pulsed Doppler documentation of flow across the defect, usually left-to-right
  4. Right atrial and ventricular and main pulmonary artery enlargement
  5. Exclusion of associated anomalies

THERAPY

NONPHARMACOLOGIC
Because many atrial septal defects (ASDs) close spontaneously, observation alone may be sufficient.

MEDICAL
- None are appropriate for ASD.
- Other associated congenital cardiac malformations and/or congestive heart failure may predispose patients with an ASD to arrhythmias, requiring medical treatments.

SURGICAL
- If a hemodynamically significant defect is present at age 2 years or older, closure should be performed at 2 to 4 years of age to prevent late problems such as arrhythmias, heart failure, or pulmonary vascular disease.
- Closure can be accomplished surgically with a very low mortality and morbidity rate.
- Alternatively, closure with a catheter-inserted device may be feasible.
- Sinus venosus defects require baffling or redirection of the right pulmonary veins to the left atrium on cardiopulmonary bypass.

FOLLOW-UP & DISPOSITION
- The outlook after closure is highly favorable, with a normal life expectancy.
- From 2% to 7% of patients experience late atrial arrhythmias, perhaps less with earlier closure (2 to 3 years of age).
- An increase in exercise endurance and growth are common after atrial defect closure.

PATIENT/FAMILY EDUCATION
Contact the cardiologist if palpitations or syncope occur.

REFERRAL INFORMATION
Children with a suspected atrial defect should be referred to a cardiologist.

PEARLS & CONSIDERATIONS

CLINICAL PEARLS
- If the second heart sound split in a newborn or young infant is "too easy" to detect, consider an atrial defect, even in the absence of a murmur.
- For isolated atrial defects, bacterial endocarditis prophylaxis is not necessary preoperatively or 6 months or more after surgery unless a patch was used in the repair.

II

■ SUPPORT GROUPS

Local Helping Hearts and other parental organizations are available to provide support and information.

REFERENCES

1. Bricker T et al: Dysrhythmias after atrial septal defect repair, *Tex Heart Inst J* 13:203, 1986.
2. Campbell M: The natural history of atrial septal defects, *Br Heart J* 32:820, 1970.
3. Ghisla RP et al: Spontaneous closure of isolated secundum atrial septal defects in infants: an echocardiographic study, *Am Heart J* 109:1327, 1985.
4. Murphy JG et al: Long-term outcome after surgical repair of isolated atrial septal defects, *N Engl J Med* 323:1645, 1990.
5. Rome JJ et al: Double-umbrella closure of atrial septal defects, *Circulation* 82: 751, 1990.

Author: **J. Peter Harris, M.D.**

BASIC INFORMATION

■ DEFINITION
Complete atrioventricular (AV) canal defect is an embryonic cardiovascular malformation caused by the failure to separate the common AV orifice into the mitral and tricuspid valves and the failure to close the atrial and ventricular (inlet) septums. Less severe variants of AV canal include a primum atrial septal defect (partial AV canal), an inlet or posterior ventricular septal defect, and a cleft mitral valve. Unbalanced AV canals are developmentally related but are not discussed further here.

■ SYNONYMS
- AV canal defects
- AV septal defects
- Endocardial cushion defects
- Canal defects

ICD-9CM CODE
745.69 Atrioventricular canal–type ventricular septal defect

■ ETIOLOGY
- The developmental hallmarks of AV canal defects include the following:
  1. Maldevelopment of the endocardial cushions that guard the embryonic AV orifice
  2. Failure to close the atrial and ventricular septums
  3. Malformation of the anterior leaflet of the mitral valve
- During normal cardiac development, the endocardial cushion containing extracellular matrix is invaded by cardiac fibroblasts in response to several growth factors.
  1. Cardiac fibroblasts form the AV valve leaflets via a process called *ectomesenchymal transformation.*
  2. Abnormalities in the extracellular matrix are believed to be responsible for the pathogenesis of AV canal defects.
- The frequent association of trisomy 21 and AV canal defects implicates a genetic locus on chromosome 21; however, other loci are likely to be important as well.

■ EPIDEMIOLOGY & DEMOGRAPHICS
- Congenital cardiovascular malformations have an incidence of 8 per 1000 live births.
- This spectrum of defects accounts for 2% to 4% of all congenital cardiovascular malformations.
- Other commonly associated congenital cardiovascular lesions include the following:
  1. Patent ductus arteriosus (PDA)
  2. Secundum atrial septal defects (ASDs)
  3. Ventricular septal defects (VSDs)
  4. Tetralogy of Fallot (TOF)
- Approximately 40% of children born with an AV canal have trisomy 21 or Down syndrome.
  1. Trisomy 21 has an incidence of approximately 1 in 700 to 800 live births.
- Approximately 40% of children with trisomy 21 have a congenital heart defect.
  1. AV canal is the most common (approximately 40%) congenital heart defect.
- The typical child with trisomy 21 and AV canal has a complete and balanced defect.
  1. These patients are excellent candidates for complete surgical repair.
- AV canals associated with normal karyotypes include the following:
  1. Seen in the heterotaxia syndromes
     a. Asplenia and polysplenia
     b. Right and left atrial isomerism
     c. With heterotaxia: other thoracoabdominal abnormalities, such as the number, location, and function of splenic tissue and malrotation of the gut, must be determined
        (1) More complex and unbalanced
        (2) More difficult surgical repair
- The Ellis-van Creveld syndrome is associated with common atrium, which is a variant of AV canal.

■ HISTORY
- The child is usually asymptomatic at birth, unless severe AV regurgitation is present.
- With the normal neonatal decrease in pulmonary vascular resistance, progressive congestive heart failure (CHF) typically occurs from pulmonary overcirculation.
- The child has feeding difficulties and failure to thrive.
- Respiratory infections are common.

■ PHYSICAL EXAMINATION
- Children with AV canal defects may exhibit stigmata of trisomy 21 (see the section "Down Syndrome [Trisomy 21]").
- A holosystolic regurgitant murmur from AV valve regurgitation is usually present.
  1. The grade of the holosystolic regurgitant murmur ranges from I-II/VI with mild AV regurgitation to III-IV/VI with severe AV regurgitation.
  2. The location of the murmur depends on whether the source is right-sided AV regurgitation (most intense at the left lateral sternal border) or left-sided AV regurgitation (most intense at the apex with radiation to the back).
- With the development of CHF, the following occurs:
  1. Poor weight gain, tachypnea, and tachycardia
  2. Possible hyperdynamic precordium, with a thrill at the left lower sternal border
  3. Possible middiastolic rumble and a gallop rhythm
  4. Hepatomegaly

🔬 DIAGNOSIS

■ DIFFERENTIAL DIAGNOSIS
- Lesions with left-to-right shunts, such as ASD, VSD, PDA, or acyanotic TOF
- Lesions with significant AV valve regurgitation, such as Ebstein's malformation or congenital mitral regurgitation

■ DIAGNOSTIC WORKUP
- Electrocardiography
  1. A right and superior (northwest) QRS frontal plane axis is characteristic of AV canal defects.
  2. First-degree AV block (prolonged PR interval) is often seen.
  3. Right ventricular hypertrophy or right bundle branch block is often encountered.
- Chest radiography
  1. Cardiomegaly and increased pulmonary vascular markings from CHF are often seen.
- Echocardiography
  1. Two-dimensional echocardiography delineates all of the critical anatomic components for the medical and surgical management of AV canals.
     a. The size of the AV valve orifices and how evenly they are committed to each ventricular mass
     b. Chordal insertion of the AV valves
     c. Size of each ventricle
  2. Color-flow Doppler echo is important in quantifying AV regurgitation.
  3. Prenatally, AV canals can be readily diagnosed by fetal echocardiography in the four-chamber view.
     a. Prenatal genetic counseling and testing for trisomy 21 should be considered.

II

THERAPY

■ MEDICAL
- Most infants require CHF therapy.
  1. Digitalis
  2. Diuretics
     a. Potassium homeostasis must be preserved using a potassium-sparing agent or potassium.
  3. Afterload reduction

■ SURGICAL
- Presently, all infants with AV canal undergo repair in infancy.
- If corrective repair is not possible, palliation with a pulmonary arterial band limits CHF and protects the pulmonary bed from pulmonary hypertension.
- Unrepaired:
  1. CHF can cause significant morbidity and mortality during infancy.
  2. An unrepaired AV canal will develop progressive pulmonary hypertension and irreversible pulmonary vascular obstructive disease (PVOD).
     a. PVOD causes right-sided heart failure and polycythemia from progressive cyanosis and is invariably fatal.
- Important factors for the repair of AV canals include the following:
  1. Degree of AV regurgitation
  2. Relative size of the AV valves and their spatial relationship to the ventricles
  3. Location of the AV valve chordae insertion into the ventricles
- With favorable anatomy, primary repair is often performed in infancy without the need for further surgery.
  a. Primary repair can be achieved with either a one- or two-patch technique.

■ FOLLOW-UP & DISPOSITION
- Prolonged postoperative ventilation may be required.
  1. Resolve significant pulmonary overcirculation.
  2. Reestablish adequate calories from preoperative cachexia.
- Rarely, distortion of the AV valves from the surgical repair results in increased AV regurgitation requiring further repair of the AV valve.
  1. This aspect is more critical for the newly created mitral valve because of the elevated pressures in the left ventricle compared with those of the right ventricle.
- Rarely, postoperative mitral regurgitation induces a hemolytic anemia from mechanical shearing of the regurgitant red blood cells striking the left side of the atrial patch.
- Postoperative third-degree (complete) heart block is seen less often today but may require permanent pacemaker implantation.

■ PATIENT/FAMILY EDUCATION
- With trisomy 21, appropriate genetic counseling is needed.
- Preoperative counseling includes the following:
  1. Management of CHF
  2. Discussion of the anatomic factors that are critical to the requisite surgical repair
  3. Operative morbidity and mortality risks
     a. The risks for an uncomplicated AV canal are presently quite low.
- Postoperative counseling includes the following:
  1. Cessation of anticongestive (CHF) therapy
  2. Potential long-term complications of arrhythmias and AV valve dysfunction

✷ PEARLS & CONSIDERATIONS

■ WEBSITES
- Loyola University, Stritch School of Medicine: www.meddean.luc.edu/lumen/MedEd/GrossAnatomy/thorax0/Heart_Development/PersistentAV.html
- Network Access Services: www.nas.com/downsyn/

REFERENCES
1. Apfel HD, Gersony WM: Clinical evaluation, medical management and outcome of atrioventricular canal defects, *Prog Pediatr Cardiol* 10:129, 1999.
2. Daebritz S, del Nido PJ: Surgical management of common atrioventricular canal, *Prog Pediatr Cardiol* 10:161, 1999.
3. Levine JC, Geva T: Echocardiographic assessment of common atrioventricular canal, *Prog Pediatr Cardiol* 10:137, 1999.
4. Kertesz NJ: The conduction system and arrhythmias in common atrioventricular canal, *Prog Pediatr Cardiol* 10:153, 1999.

Author: **Peter N. Bowers, M.D.**

BASIC INFORMATION

■ DEFINITION
A behavioral syndrome characterized by developmentally inappropriate levels of inattention and/or hyperactivity and impulsivity that interfere significantly with function

■ SYNONYMS
- ADD
- AD/HD, combined type
- AD/HD, predominantly inattentive type
- AD/HD, predominantly hyperactive-impulsive type
- AD/HD, not otherwise specified

ICD-9CM CODES
314.0 AD/HD
314.01 AD/HD, combined type
314.00 AD/HD, predominantly inattentive type
314.01 AD/HD, not otherwise specified

■ ETIOLOGY
- Genetic
  1. Accounts for up to 80% of the variance
  2. Probably polygenic inheritance
- Neurologic
  1. Thought to represent dysfunction of prefrontal cortex, basal ganglia, cerebellum
- Neuropsychology
  1. Disorder of executive function leading to disinhibition
- Environmental
  1. "Goodness of fit" between environment and individual will affect severity of symptoms

■ EPIDEMIOLOGY & DEMOGRAPHICS
- Most common significant behavior disorder in children
- From 4% to 6% of school-age children have combined type; another 2% to 3% have inattentive type.
- The incidence is reportedly higher in lower socioeconomic status groups.
- The male:female ratio is approximately 3:1.
- Persists into adolescence and adulthood in up to 70% of patients.

■ HISTORY
Diagnostic criteria from *Diagnostic and Statistical Manual of Mental Disorders,* fourth edition, 1994, American Psychiatric Association
- Signs must occur often and be present for at least 6 months to a level that is maladaptive and inconsistent with the child's developmental level.
- Symptoms must cause impairment in social, academic, or occupational functioning.
- Some symptoms must have been present before 7 years of age.
- Symptoms must be causing impairment in two or more settings.
- Symptoms do not occur exclusively as part of another disorder.

■ PHYSICAL EXAMINATION
- Physical examination is usually normal.
- Patients may have increased incidence of "soft" neurologic signs (e.g., synkinesia, overflow, disinhibition, motor clumsiness).
- Careful assessment of developmental status should be undertaken.
- Symptoms may not be evident in medical setting,

- Attention should be paid to hearing, vision, dysmorphic features, cutaneous markers of neurologic disorders, and neurologic abnormalities.

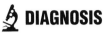

DIAGNOSIS

■ DIFFERENTIAL DIAGNOSIS
- Several other conditions may have similar behavioral manifestations.
- More than 50% of individuals have comorbid conditions.

■ DIAGNOSTIC WORKUP
- There is no single diagnostic test.
- Diagnosis is clinical and based on the following factors:
  1. History (preferably from multiple observers)
  2. Collaboration with schools to screen for learning disability or cognitive delay
  3. Developmental assessment with appropriate referrals for suspected delay
  4. Physical examination
  5. School, parent, and student rating scales and questionnaires to ascertain that symptoms are outside normal range and to screen for other disorders
  6. Psychosocial assessment
  7. Laboratory assessment only as indicated by history and physical
     a. Electroencephalographic (EEG) and neuroimaging studies are not part of routine assessment.
     b. In preschool children, check hematocrit and lead level.

TABLE 2-2 Diagnostic Criteria for Attention Deficit/Hyperactivity Disorder

Inattention (Six or More of the Following)
1. Fails to give close attention to details or makes careless mistakes in schoolwork, chores, or other tasks.
2. Has difficulty sustaining attention to tasks, chores, or duties.
3. Does not seem to listen when spoken to directly.
4. Does not follow through on instructions and fails to finish schoolwork, chores, or duties.
5. Has difficulty organizing tasks and activities.
6. Avoids, dislikes, or is reluctant to engage in tasks that require sustained mental effort.
7. Loses things necessary for tasks or activities.
8. Is easily distracted by extraneous stimuli.
9. Is forgetful in daily activities.

Hyperactivity and Impulsivity (Six or More of the Following)
1. Fidgets with hands or feet or squirms in seat.
2. Leaves seat in classroom or in other situations in which remaining seated is expected.
3. Runs about or climbs excessively in situations in which it is inappropriate (in adolescents and adults may be limited to restlessness).
4. Has difficulty playing or engaging in leisure activities quietly.
5. Is "on the go" or acts as if "driven by a motor."
6. Talks excessively.
7. Blurts out answers before questions have been completed.
8. Has difficulty awaiting turns.
9. Interrupts or intrudes on others.

AD/HD, combined type: six or more symptoms from each list.
AD/HD, predominantly inattentive type: six or more symptoms from Inattention list.
AD/HD, predominantly hyperactive-impulsive type: six or more symptoms from Hyperactivity-Impulsivity list.

TABLE 2-3 Differential Diagnosis and Common Comorbid Conditions

Medical Conditions

Seizure disorder
Sensory impairment
Iron deficiency
Hyperthyroid or hypothyroid
Traumatic brain injury
Substance abuse
Medication side effect
Sleep disorder
Tourette's syndrome
Neurodegenerative disorders
Fetal alcohol and drug exposure

Environmental Conditions

Social chaos
Mental illness in family
Substance abuse in family
Violence/abuse
Inappropriate educational setting

Developmental Conditions

Developmental delay
Mental retardation
Pervasive developmental disorders
Language disorders
Giftedness
Learning disabilities

Emotional Conditions

Anxiety
Depression
Mood disorders
Posttraumatic stress disorder
Oppositional defiant disorder
Conduct disorder
Mania
Adjustment reaction

℞ THERAPY

■ NONPHARMACOLOGIC

- Parents and patients should be educated about the disorder.
- Parents and teachers should be trained in specific behavior management techniques for impulsive and inattentive children.
- The environment should be modified, including educational interventions.
  1. Children usually can be managed in the regular education setting.
- Some children may benefit from social skills training.
- Some families may benefit from family therapy.
- Dietary interventions are of no proven benefit.
- Intervention should be implemented for comorbid conditions.

■ MEDICAL

- Multiple studies overwhelmingly demonstrate that medication intervention is the single most effective strategy for managing AD/HD.
- Medication management is indicated for specific target symptoms.
- Medication management remains effective for adolescents and adults.
- Primary care physician should refer to developmental pediatrician, child neurologist, or child psychiatrist when the following conditions exist:
  1. There is diagnostic confusion.
  2. First-line interventions are not beneficial.
  3. Combinations of medications are necessary.
  4. The prescriber is not familiar with the medication.

- Medications, listed in order of prevalence and importance, are as follows:
  1. Stimulant medications: methylphenidate, dextroamphetamine, mixed amphetamine salts, pemoline
     a. These are first-line medications.
     b. If side effects occur with one stimulant, try another.
     c. Pemoline is not recommended for first-line therapy because of reported hepatic toxicity.
  2. α-Adrenergic agents: clonidine, guanfacine
     a. Watch for sedation and hypotension.
     b. Some controversy exists about use in combination with stimulants.
     c. Sudden discontinuation can result in rebound hypertension.
  3. Antidepressants: not often prescribed by primary care provider
     a. Tricyclic antidepressants
        (1) Potential for cardiac toxicity
        (2) Must measure blood levels
        (3) Most authorities recommend electrocardiographic monitoring
     b. Novel antidepressants (Bupropion)
     c. Selective serotonin reuptake inhibitor medications usually for comorbid conditions (e.g., anxiety, obsessive-compulsive disorder, depression)

■ FOLLOW-UP & DISPOSITION

This is a chronic disorder that requires ongoing assessment and intervention. Ongoing needs include the following:

- Medication management
- Monitoring of educational achievement
- Monitoring of social progress
- Monitoring of family functioning
- Ongoing surveillance for other comorbid conditions
- Referrals as indicated

■ PATIENT/FAMILY EDUCATION

- The most common cause of AD/HD is genetic.
- The condition is lifelong in up to 70% of people.
- The patient and family must learn strategies to manage the symptom complex.
- Manifestations and symptoms change over time.
- The severity of symptoms varies dramatically in different environments.

■ REFERRAL INFORMATION

- Many children with AD/HD, especially those with comorbid conditions, are referred to a developmental pediatrician, a child neurologist, or a child psychiatrist.
- Other subspecialty referrals may include those to a clinical psychologist, educational specialist, and/or speech and language pathologist.

☼ PEARLS & CONSIDERATIONS

■ CLINICAL PEARLS

- In very young children with symptoms of AD/HD, a thorough developmental assessment is imperative.
- The effect of stimulant medication is not paradoxical and does not stop at puberty.
- As with other chronic conditions, numerous nontraditional interventions are without proven efficacy.

■ WEBSITES

- Children and Adults with Attention Deficit Disorder (CHADD): www.chadd.org
- National Attention Deficit Disorder Association: www.add.org

■ SUPPORT GROUPS

- CHADD has many local chapters throughout the United States. Information can be obtained from their website.
- Many communities and some schools have local support groups. School psychologists, school social workers, developmental pediatricians, child neurologists, and child psychiatrists often are aware of local resources.

REFERENCES

1. Dunne JE: Attention-deficit/hyperactivity disorder and associated childhood disorders, primary care, *Clin Office Practice* 26:350, 1999.
2. Miller KJ, Castellanos FX: Attention deficit/hyperactivity disorders, *Pediatr Rev* 19:373, 1998.
3. Practice parameters for the assessment and treatment of children, adolescents, and adults with attention deficit/hyperactivity disorder, *J Am Acad Child Adolesc Psychiatry* 35:855, 1997.

Author: **Ellen Gellerstedt, M.D.**

II

BASIC INFORMATION

■ **DEFINITION**

A developmental disorder characterized by a qualitative impairment in social reciprocity, a qualitative impairment in communication, and repetitive behaviors. The Autism Spectrum includes five disorders: (1) autism in which stringent criteria are met; (2) Asperger's syndrome in which there is normal early language and normal cognition; (3) Rett syndrome in which there is loss of language and hand use; (4) disintegrative disorder in which the symptoms start later in childhood; and (5) pervasive developmental disorder, which is not otherwise specified when the criteria for the other disorders in this category are not met.

■ **SYNONYMS**

• Autism spectrum disorders
• Pervasive developmental disorders (PDDs)

ICD-9CM CODES
299.0 Autism
299.8 Asperger's syndrome, PDD

■ **ETIOLOGY**

• The cause is unknown.
• The evidence for a genetic etiology is strong; concordance in identical twins is greater than 60% for autism and greater than 90% if symptoms, but not the complete disorder, are included.
• Pathologic findings are varied but include the following:
  1. Hypoplasia of cerebellar vermis
  2. Decreased numbers of Purkinje cells in the cerebellum
  3. Increased cell packing in the limbic system
  4. Hypoplasia of cranial nerve nuclei
• This condition can be associated with fetal exposure to infectious agents (e.g., rubella) or teratogens (e.g., thalidomide, valproic acid, ethanol).
• Immunologic factors are under investigation.
• Psychologic construct: Theory of Mind—cannot understand that other people have a different point of view, which is necessary for communication and social reciprocity.

■ **EPIDEMIOLOGY & DEMOGRAPHICS**

• This condition may affect as many as 1 in 750 to 1 in 1000 people; older studies cite numbers of 4 to 5 in 10,000.
  1. Question of increasing prevalence versus better detection and broader definition
• There is a male predominance.

• Up to 70% of people with autism also have mental retardation.
• In Asperger's syndrome, cognition is normal.

■ **HISTORY**

One fourth to one third of autistic children lose language skills in the second year of life.
• Infancy: decreased eye contact, language delays, acts like deaf, repetitive behaviors
• Early childhood: insistence on routine, lack of pretend play, repetitive behaviors
• Later childhood/adolescence: problems with peer interactions

■ **PHYSICAL EXAMINATION**

• Generally nondysmorphic
• May be associated with tuberous sclerosis, Möbius' syndrome, and Joubert's syndrome, among others
• May be comorbid with other disorders that cause mental retardation (e.g., Fragile X, Down syndrome)
• May have clumsiness, mild hypotonia

🔬 **DIAGNOSIS**

■ **DIFFERENTIAL DIAGNOSIS**

• Mental retardation with stereotyped behaviors
• Sensory impairment
• Epileptic aphasia
• Tourette's disorder
• Obsessive-compulsive illness
• Childhood schizophrenia

■ **DIAGNOSTIC WORKUP**

• Diagnosis is made by history and clinical presentation, applying DSM-IV criteria.
• Diagnosis is supported by valid assessment measures.
  1. Autism Diagnostic Interview—Revised
  2. Autism Diagnostic Observation Schedule-G
  3. Childhood Autism Rating Scale
  4. PDD Screening Test
  5. Autism Behavior Checklist
• Testing should include cognitive, language, and hearing assessments.
• An electroencephalogram (optional) is suggested when there has been a loss of skills, variability in behavior, or seizures.
  1. Twenty-five percent of people with autism have a seizure.
• Assessment of the underlying cause is based on history, family history, examination, and presence or absence of mental retardation.
• Popular complementary approaches include immune, nutritional, and allergic assessments that have not yet been scientifically investigated.

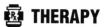 **THERAPY**

■ **NONPHARMACOLOGIC**

• The mainstay of therapy involves educational interventions, behavioral therapy, and speech therapy.
• Multiple service models are available; little outcome data exist, though, except for strict behavioral programs.
• Children with language and higher cognitive abilities need social skills and pragmatic language training in inclusive environments.

■ **MEDICAL**

• Inattention, impulsivity, and motor hyperactivity may respond to stimulant medications or clonidine, as in attention deficit/hyperactivity disorder.
• Selective serotonin reuptake inhibitors may decrease aggression, self-injury, and obsessions.
• Neuroleptics (e.g., haloperidol) and atypical neuroleptics (e.g., risperidone) may decrease aggression, stereotyped behaviors, and self-injury.
• Medication should be used only as an adjunct to a behavioral program.

■ **COMPLEMENTARY & ALTERNATIVE THERAPIES**

Mentioned here are a variety of complementary therapies that have been tried, with no scientific evidence for success:
• Casein-free and gluten-free diet
• Auditory integration training
• Vitamin B_6 with magnesium
• Dimethylglycine
• Antiyeast agents
• Intravenous secretin, which has been given to thousands of children based on a case series
  1. Multiple double-blind controlled trials could not detect any benefit in autism.

■ **FOLLOW-UP**

• Medication monitoring requires input from school personnel and parents.
• The efficacy of intervention needs to be monitored. School reassessment should be conducted every 3 years for formal testing. Response to the program must be reevaluated more often.

■ **PATIENT/FAMILY EDUCATION**

• The recurrence risk is 3% to 7% unless a specific cause is known.
• Cognitive assessment is difficult in very young children with PDD and may not be predictive of later intellectual potential.
• Obtaining disorder-specific educational programs may require significant parental advocacy.

■ REFERRAL INFORMATION

- 0 to 3 years of age: early intervention program
- 3 to 21 years of age: school district committee on special education
- Confirmation of the diagnosis by a child psychologist, developmental/behavioral pediatrician, child neurologist, or child psychiatrist familiar with the disorder

☼ PEARLS & CONSIDERATIONS

■ CLINICAL PEARLS

- It is possible to have a few symptoms of the disorder without meeting the diagnostic criteria. This is called the *broader autistic phenotype.*
- Symptoms in toddlers include absence of pointing to show interest, absence of pretend play, and decreased eye gaze to regulate social interaction, especially with language delays. Many people with PDD, and all people with Asperger's syndrome, have normal intelligence. They may seem professorial as children.

■ WEBSITES

- Autism Society of America: www.autism-society.org
- ARI for complementary therapies: www.autism.com/ari

■ SUPPORT GROUPS

- The Autism Society of America provides information and has local chapters in most cities.
- There are many local groups and groups with special interests, such as ASPEN for Asperger's syndrome.

REFERENCES

1. American Psychiatric Association: *Diagnostic and statistical manual IV,* Washington, DC, 1994, American Psychiatric Association.
2. Bauer S: Autism and the pervasive developmental disorders. Part 1, *Pediatr Rev* 16:130, 1995.
3. Bauer S: Autism and the pervasive developmental disorders. Part 2, *Pediatr Rev* 16:168, 1995.
4. Clinical practice guideline, the guideline technical report, autism/pervasive developmental disorders: assessment and intervention for young children (age 0-3 years), Albany, 1999, NY State Department of Health, NY Publ. No. 4217.
5. Rapin I: Autism, *N Engl J Med* 337:97, 1997.

Author: **Susan Hyman, M.D.**

II

BASIC INFORMATION

■ DEFINITIONS

- *Bacteremia:* the presence of bacteria in the blood in the absence of clinical evidence of sepsis or focal infection
- *Sepsis:* the presence of bacteria in the blood *and* signs of systemic response to infection, such as tachycardia, tachypnea, decreased organ perfusion, and/or shock
- *Fever:* a rectal temperature of higher than 38.0° C (100.4° F)
- *Fever of uncertain source* (FUS): an acute febrile illness in which the cause of the fever is not apparent after careful history and physical examination
- *Well-appearing child:* is playful, smiles, interacts easily, consolable; no signs of dehydration; good peripheral perfusion with warm, pink extremities; no evidence of respiratory distress
- *Ill-appearing child:* is irritable, crying, less playful but still responsive to caregiver, may have poor feeding, briefly smiles
- *Toxic-appearing child:* is irritable; not easily consolable; poor interaction even with caregivers; lethargic or unresponsive; weak; signs of severe dehydration; poor perfusion with mottled and/or cool extremities; weak pulse; signs of respiratory distress
- *Serious bacterial infection* (SBI): bacteremia, meningitis, pneumonia, urinary tract infection, cellulitis, bone and joint infection, and enteritis

ICD-9CM CODES
790.7 Bacteremia
038.9 Sepsis
780.6 Fever

■ ETIOLOGY

- Most common causes of bacteremia and sepsis by age
  1. Age younger than 2 months
     a. Group B streptococcus
     b. *Escherichia coli*
     c. *Listeria monocytogenes*
     d. *Enterococcus*
     e. *Staphylococcus* species
     f. *Salmonella* species
  2. Age 2 to 36 months
     a. *Streptococcus pneumoniae*
     b. *Neisseria meningitidis*
     c. Group A streptococcus (*Streptococcus pyogenes*)
     d. Salmonella species
     e. *Haemophilus influenzae* type B (rare if immunized)

■ EPIDEMIOLOGY & DEMOGRAPHICS

- Fever accounts for approximately 15% of all visits to the pediatrician, and most of these visits are for children younger than 3 years of age.
- Fever is most common in children older than 2 months of age.
- The peak incidence of fever for children younger than 3 years of age is November to March.
- A second peak incidence occurs between July and September for infants younger than 2 months of age, most likely because of enterovirus outbreaks.
- In febrile infants younger than 2 months of age, the incidence of SBI is 8% to 10%; the incidence of bacteremia is 2% to 4%.
- For febrile children between 2 and 36 months of age:
  1. The incidence of bacteremia is 3% to 5% (for temperatures greater than or equal to 39° C).
  2. The incidence of SBI is less than 3% chance if the child appears well but greater than 90% chance if the child is toxic appearing.
  3. Risk for bacteremia increases with increasing temperature above 39° C.
  4. *Pneumococcus* accounts for more than 90% of bacteremias, with the highest incidence before age 2 years.

■ HISTORY

- It is essential to determine the child's risk for bacteremia and sepsis.
  1. Age
  2. Height and duration of documented temperature
  3. Underlying chronic illness or immunodeficiency
  4. Ill contacts and exposure to known infectious pathogens
  5. Current community epidemics (e.g., influenza, enterovirus)
  6. Illness-specific symptoms, including cough, bloody diarrhea, dysuria, ear pain, emesis
  7. Activity level, ability to be consoled, interaction
- For infants younger than 2 months of age, the following increase the likelihood of SBI:
  1. Prematurity—less than 37 weeks' gestation
  2. Prior hospitalizations and/or prior antibiotic therapy
  3. Hospitalized longer than mother after delivery
  4. Unexplained hyperbilirubinemia

■ PHYSICAL EXAMINATION

- Make the child as comfortable as possible to maximize the possibility of finding an abnormality; examine the child in the caregiver's lap if possible.
  1. Vital signs
     a. Height of fever
     b. Tachypnea, retractions, grunting, flaring
     c. Tachycardia and widened pulse pressure may be early signs of sepsis
     d. Blood pressure and evidence for postural hypotension
  2. General appearance
     a. Interactive behaviors
     b. Alertness
     c. Response to caregiver
     d. Eye contact
     e. Irritability
     f. Peripheral perfusion
     g. Color—pink, cyanosis
     h. State of hydration
  3. Skin
     a. Petechiae, purpura (*N. meningitidis*)
     b. Vesicles (herpes simplex virus, varicella)
     c. Pustules, soft tissue warmth and redness
     d. Umbilical irritation (omphalitis)
  4. Head and neck
     a. Anterior fontanelle
     b. Head circumference
     c. Meningismus
     d. Red, bulging, nonmobile tympanic membranes
     e. Pharyngeal irritation
     f. Lymphadenopathy
  5. Cardiorespiratory
     a. Heart murmur associated with hyperactive precordium ("warm" shock)
     b. Focal rhonchi, wheezes, crackles, decreased breath sounds
  6. Abdominal/genitourinary
     a. Masses
     b. Signs of rigid abdomen (bowel perforation, appendicitis)
     c. Anal abscess
  7. Orthopedic
     a. Range of motion of all joints, especially hips, shoulders, wrists
     b. Note pain with extension and flexion and warmth and/or tenderness to palpation of joints
  8. Neurologic
     a. Responsiveness, lethargy
     b. Confusion (older child)
     c. Gait disturbance
     d. Kernig's and Brudzinski's signs

🔬 DIAGNOSIS

■ DIFFERENTIAL DIAGNOSIS
- Acute viral syndrome: more common than bacterial disease (most common are respiratory syncytial virus, rotavirus, and enteroviruses)
- Systemic herpes simplex infection
- Cardiac disease: congestive heart failure, endocarditis
- Bronchopulmonary dysplasia with secondary infection
- Immunodeficiency
- Acute surgical abdomen: malrotation with obstruction, appendicitis

■ DIAGNOSTIC WORKUP— LABORATORY TESTS
Low-risk criteria for SBI include the following:
- White blood cell (WBC) count: 5000 to 15,000 cells/mm³
- Absolute band form count: less than 1500/mm³
- Band:neutrophil ratio: less than 0.2
- Urinalysis
  1. Less than 10 WBCs per high-power field (×40) on microscopic examination of spun urine sediment
  2. No organisms seen on Gram stain (obtain urine by bladder catheterization or bladder tap only)
- Lumbar puncture
  1. No organisms on Gram stain
  2. No pleocytosis (varies by age)
- Stool smear: less than 5 WBCs per high-power field (×40) on microscopic examination of a stool smear (only if history of diarrhea)
- Blood, urine, cerebrospinal fluid (CSF) cultures for bacterial pathogens
- Consider viral cultures
- Consider chest radiograph if signs and symptoms of lower respiratory tract disease

■ DIAGNOSTIC WORKUP
- Younger than 2 months of age
  1. All should have complete history, thorough physical examination, and complete blood count (CBC) and urinalysis as a minimum.
  2. Some clinicians do a lumbar puncture (LP) for all infants younger than 4 weeks of age and for selected infants between 4 and 8 weeks of age.
  3. Ill- or toxic-appearing child:
     a. *Is not at low risk* for SBI: Do complete history, physical examination, and laboratory evaluation.
  4. Well-appearing child:
     a. If negative history, nonfocal physical examination, *and* all laboratory tests (low-risk criteria) are normal, at *low risk* for SBI (some clinicians include

infants with only otitis media in this risk group).
     b. If at least one abnormality in history, physical examination, or laboratory tests is found, *not at low risk* for SBI.
- 2 to 36 months of age
  1. Ill- or toxic-appearing child:
     a. Do CBC, urinalysis, and LP, and consider chest radiograph, especially for those with WBC counts greater than 20,000 cells/mm³.
     b. Blood, urine, and CSF cultures for bacterial pathogens
  2. Well-appearing child, nonfocal examination, *and* temperature less than 39° C:
     a. No laboratory evaluation
  3. Well-appearing child *and* temperature higher than 39° C:
     a. Blood culture all or blood culture those with WBC counts greater than 15,000 or less than 5000 cells/mm³.
     b. Perform urine cultures for all girls younger than 2 years of age and all boys younger than 6 months of age.
     c. Perform an LP, especially with abnormal findings on physical examination.
     d. Consider a stool culture if bloody diarrhea is present.
     e. Consider chest radiograph, especially if the WBC count is greater than 20,000 cells/mm³.
     f. Consider viral cultures as warranted by history or physical examination.

℞ THERAPY

Depends on risk assessment, ability of caregivers to continue to reassess the child, and ability of primary care physician to follow up with family

■ NONPHARMACOLOGIC
- Younger than 2 months of age
  1. Ill- or toxic-appearing child/not low risk for SBI:
     a. Admit. Provide supplemental therapies as needed, including oxygen and intravenous hydration. Consider intensive care unit (ICU) monitoring for clinical signs of early sepsis.
  2. Low risk for SBI:
     a. Admit all younger than 30 days of age.
     b. Consider home management for 31 to 60 days of age if excellent outpatient follow-up can be ensured.

- 2 to 36 months of age
  1. Ill- or toxic-appearing child:
     a. As previously described for ill- or toxic-appearing infants younger than 2 months of age
  2. Well-appearing child:
     a. Home observation with plan to return for evaluation by primary physician if persistent fever at 24 to 48 hours or deteriorating clinical condition

■ MEDICAL
- Younger than 2 months of age
  1. Ill- or toxic-appearing child/not low risk for SBI:
     a. Use gentamicin with ampicillin intravenously (IV) for infants younger than 2 weeks of age.
     b. Consider either ceftriaxone or cefotaxime with ampicillin for children older than 2 weeks of age.
     c. Ampicillin sodium
        (1) 100 to 200 mg/kg/day IV divided into 6-hour doses if not meningitis
        (2) 200 to 400 mg/kg/day IV divided into 6-hour doses for meningitis
     d. Gentamicin
        (1) 3 mg/kg/dose IV every 24 hours if younger than 1 month of age
        (2) 2.5 mg/kg/dose IV every 12 hours if older than 1 month of age
     e. Ceftriaxone
        (1) 50 mg/kg/dose IV every 24 hours if not meningitis; every 12 hours for meningitis; avoid in jaundiced infant
     f. Cefotaxime
        (1) 50 mg/kg/dose IV every 8 hours if not meningitis; every 6 hours for meningitis
  2. Low risk for SBI:
     a. Consider intravenous antibiotics (see previous section) for all inpatients younger than 30 days of age while awaiting bacterial culture results.
     b. Home management
        (1) Observation alone without antibiotics *or* observation with once-daily ceftriaxone 50 mg/kg/dose intramuscularly
        (2) Reevaluation within 24 hours
     c. Blood, urine, and CSF cultures for bacterial pathogens before administration of antibiotics
- 2 to 36 months of age
  1. Ill- or toxic-appearing child:
     a. Ceftriaxone 50 mg/kg/dose IV

every 12 hours or cefotaxime 50 mg/kg/dose IV every 6 hours
  b. Acetaminophen 15 mg/kg/dose every 4 to 6 hours for temperature control and irritability
2. Well-appearing child, nonfocal examination, temperature lower than 39° C:
  a. No antibiotics
  b. Acetaminophen 15 mg/kg/dose every 4 to 6 hours for temperature control and irritability
3. Well-appearing child, nonfocal examination, temperature greater than or equal to 39° C:
  a. Empiric antibiotic therapy for all *or* for those children who also have WBC counts less than 5000 or higher than 15,000 cells/mm³
  b. Amoxicillin 60 to 100 mg/kg/day divided into three daily doses, or
  c. Ceftriaxone 50 to 75 mg/kg/dose intramuscularly once daily (maximum dose, 1 to 2 g/24 hr)
  d. Strong consideration of obtaining CSF culture before beginning antibiotics is recommended

■ FOLLOW-UP & DISPOSITION
• Younger than 2 months of age
  1. All infants managed at home should have phone or visit follow-up with the responsible physician within 24 hours of initial presentation, regardless of the use of antibiotics.
  2. Infants initially treated with antibiotics may discontinue therapy after 48 hours if all cultures are negative for bacterial pathogens.
  3. If a bacterial pathogen is recovered from any culture, the infant is reexamined, repeat cultures for bacteria are obtained, and the infant is admitted and begun on intravenous antibiotics (see section on therapy, not low-risk infant) pending repeat culture results.

• 2 to 36 months of age
  1. Follow-up by phone or visit with primary care provider is necessary within 24 to 48 hours.
  2. If febrile at time of follow-up and cultures are negative for bacterial pathogens, do complete physical examination and continue observation if no new findings.
  3. If febrile at time of follow-up and blood culture is positive, do complete physical examination to look for new focus of infection and for the following:
    a. *N. meningitidis* or *H. influenzae* type B
      (1) Admit.
      (2) Repeat blood culture.
      (3) Obtain CSF culture.
      (4) Consider chest radiograph.
      (5) Begin intravenous ceftriaxone or cefotaxime (follow therapy guidelines for ill-appearing child, age 2 to 36 months).
    b. *S. pneumoniae:*
      (1) If child is ill appearing or febrile, follow previous plan for *N. meningitidis* bacteremia.
      (2) If child is well appearing and afebrile and no changes are noted on physical examination, repeat blood culture, continue present outpatient therapy, and follow up within next 24 hours.

■ PATIENT/FAMILY EDUCATION
• Medical staff should instruct caregivers in the proper use and reading of a rectal thermometer.
• Caregivers should know to call the physician for temperatures greater than or equal to 38.0° C in all infants younger than 2 months of age and for temperatures greater than or equal to 39° C in older children, particularly those between 2 and 24 months of age.
• Caregivers should be educated regarding the signs and symptoms to look for that may indicate impending serious illness. They also need to

be able to reach medical attention by phone or car as quickly as possible.

■ REFERRAL INFORMATION
• Most febrile children are managed by primary care physicians, but a referral to an infectious diseases consultant may be warranted when the clinical presentation and/or course are unusual.
• Other subspecialty referrals may be desired if a specific abnormality is found.
  1. Many infants with posterior urethral valves or urinary reflux after acute pyelonephritis are referred to a urologist.

☼ PEARLS & CONSIDERATIONS

■ CLINICAL PEARLS
• Antibiotics are not a substitute for careful observation and follow-up of the young child with FUS.
• A young infant at low risk for SBI may need to be hospitalized if close observation, easy access to medical care, or follow-up with a responsible physician cannot be ensured.
• Bacterial resistance to antibiotics is increasing, and the decision to use antibiotics in a febrile child needs to be based more and more on the clinician's ability to identify febrile children at risk for SBI.

■ WEBSITE
Children's Hospital Medical Center of Cincinnati: www.chmcc.org; FUS—outpatient evaluation and management for children 2 months to 36 months of age; FUS—in infants 60 days of age or younger

REFERENCES
1. Jaskiewicz JA, McCarthy CA: Evaluation and management of the febrile infant 60 days of age or younger, *Pediatr Ann* 22:477, 1993.
2. McCarthy PL: Fever, *Pediatr Rev* 19: 401, 1998.
Author: **Julie Jaskiewicz, M.D.**

BASIC INFORMATION

■ DEFINITION
Balantitis is an inflammation of the glans penis or clitoris.

■ SYNONYMS
- Balanoposthitis: Inflammation includes prepuce.
- Zoon's balanitis plasmacellularis: Inflammatory cells are predominantly plasma cells.
- Balanitis xerotica obliterans (BXO): Inflammation is characterized by submucosal edema, fibrosis, and little cellular component. Grossly, aggressive scarring and a pale plaque are present.
- Balanitis circinata: Inflammation grossly appears as a reddened papular ring.

ICD-9CM CODE
607.1 Balanitis

■ ETIOLOGY
- Infectious
  1. *Candida albicans*
  2. β-Hemolytic streptococci (groups A and B)
  3. *Bacteroides* species
  4. *Gardnerella vaginalis*
  5. *Chlamydia trachomatis*
  6. Tuberculosis
  7. Herpes simplex virus
  8. *Trichomonas vaginalis*
  9. *Amoeba enterocolitica*
  10. Scabies
- Dermatoses
  1. Psoriasis
  2. Lichen planus
  3. Seborrheic dermatitis
  4. Contact dermatitis
- Miscellaneous
  1. Erythema multiforme exudativum (Stevens-Johnson syndrome)
  2. Fixed drug eruption
  3. Ankylosing spondylitis
  4. Reiter's syndrome

■ EPIDEMIOLOGY & DEMOGRAPHICS
- Peak age: 2 to 4 years balanoposthitis; 9 to 11 years BXO
- Incidence: 3% balanoposthitis in uncircumcised males by age 18 years
- Diabetes: 11% in adults presenting with balanoposthitis

■ HISTORY
- Redness and/or swelling of the glans penis
- Pain
- Dysuria
- Preputial or urethral discharge
- Inability to retract previously reducible foreskin
- Prior episodes in less than 1%

■ PHYSICAL EXAMINATION
- Focal or global erythema of glans
- Discharge, swelling, erythema, or fissures of prepuce (balanoposthitis)
- Inguinal adenopathy

DIAGNOSIS

■ DIFFERENTIAL DIAGNOSIS
- Reddened glans
  1. Chemical burn (ammonia, detergents)
  2. Trauma
  3. Insect bite
  4. Condyloma acuminatum
  5. Erythroplasia of Queyrat
  6. Chancre/chancroid
- Preputial swelling
  1. Paraphimosis (prolonged retraction of the uncircumcised prepuce, which results in distal edema)
  2. Angioedema
  3. Lymphedema
  4. Leukemic infiltration

■ DIAGNOSTIC WORKUP
- The diagnosis is made on clinical grounds and based on characteristic appearance or the presence of lesions at other sites (e.g., mouth, conjunctiva, skin, anus).
- Urinalysis, including a glucose screen, is obtained.
- Cultures are done as needed.
- Gram stains of discharge or epithelial scrapings may direct therapy.
- Cultures should be sent of discharge or biopsy material to refine treatment.
- Biopsy may be warranted in atypical, unresponsive, or persistent lesions. Urethral involvement should lower the threshold for early biopsy (BXO).
- Specific testing for conditions in the differential diagnosis should be performed as warranted.

THERAPY

■ NONPHARMACOLOGIC
- Balanitis
  1. Observe the patient.
  2. Eliminate exposure.
  3. Administer sitz baths.
- Balanoposthitis
  1. Observe the patient.
  2. Eliminate exposure.
  3. Administer sitz baths.
  4. *Rare:* Irrigate with saline solution between prepuce and glans.

■ MEDICAL
- Balanitis
  1. Topical triamcinolone or nystatin, *and/or*
  2. Oral trimethoprim-sulfamethoxazole or cephalexin
- Balanoposthitis
  1. Amoxicillin-clavulanic acid

■ SURGICAL
- Balanoposthitis
  1. Dorsal slit to provide drainage as adjunct to antibiotics is rarely indicated.

■ FOLLOW-UP & DISPOSITION
- Follow the patient for 24 to 48 hours to ensure a response in balanoposthitis.
- Remainder of follow-up depends on the cause.

■ PATIENT/FAMILY EDUCATION
- Most episodes are self-limited and do not recur.
- A single episode of balanoposthitis does not warrant mandatory circumcision.
- The foreskin should never be retracted forcibly because fissures may represent portals of entry for infection.

■ REFERRAL INFORMATION
All lesions that persist, recur, or involve the urethra mandate evaluation by a pediatric urologist.

PEARLS & CONSIDERATIONS

■ CLINICAL PEARLS
- Thirty percent to forty percent of preputial discharge cultures are sterile.
- Oatmeal baths are a soothing adjunct and are often therapeutic.
- Infections should be congruent with the child's reported sexual activity, or possible abuse should be considered.
- In sexually active patients, consider latex allergy or spermicidal agent as causes.

REFERENCES
1. Langer JC, Coplen DE: Circumcision and pediatric disorders of the penis, *Pediatr Clin North Am* 45:801, 1998.
2. Rickwood AMK: Medical indications for circumcision, *BJU Int* 83:45, 1999.
3. Waugh MA: Balanitis, *Dermatol Clin* 16:757, 1998.
Authors: **Robert A. Mevorach, M.D., Ronald Rabinowitz, M.D., and William C. Hulbert, M.D.**

II

BASIC INFORMATION

■ **DEFINITION**

Blepharitis is a spectrum of acute and chronic inflammation of the eyelids.

■ **SYNONYMS**
- Meibomitis
- Chalazia
- Seborrheic blepharitis
- *Staphylococcus* blepharitis

ICD-9CM CODE
373.00 Blepharitis—unspecified

■ **ETIOLOGY**
- Myriad, including acute infection of bacteria such as *Staphylococcus aureus, Propionibacterium acnes,* and *Streptococcus epidermidis*
- Demodex folliculorum, which may act as a vector for bacteria
- Seborrhea

■ **EPIDEMIOLOGY & DEMOGRAPHICS**

More commonly a disease of adults but can be seen in pediatric population

■ **HISTORY**
- Nonspecific ocular discomfort (burning, irritation, and itching)
- Red eye
- Tearing
- Ocular discharge, which may occur in cycles

■ **PHYSICAL EXAMINATION**
- Red, thickened eyelids
- Dry crusting on the lid
- Acute hordeolum (or stye)
- Occasionally conjunctivitis or corneal ulceration

 DIAGNOSIS

■ **DIFFERENTIAL DIAGNOSIS**
- Acute or chronic conjunctivitis
- Contact dermatitis
- Preseptal cellulitis
- Sebaceous cell carcinoma (usually adults)

■ **DIAGNOSTIC WORKUP**

The diagnosis is usually made on physical examination.

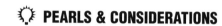 **THERAPY**

■ **NONPHARMACOLOGIC**
- Lid hygiene
- Warm compresses

■ **MEDICAL**
- Topical antibiotic ointment (e.g., erythromycin) is applied to the lids.
- Topical antibiotic and a steroid combination ointment are used for resistant or severe cases.
- Oral antibiotic may be necessary.

■ **FOLLOW-UP & DISPOSITION**
As needed

■ **PATIENT/FAMILY EDUCATION**

Blepharitis is often a chronic disorder with periods of exacerbation requiring daily maintenance of nonpharmacologic therapy.

✿ **PEARLS & CONSIDERATIONS**

May be seen commonly with rosacea and Down syndrome

REFERENCES
1. American Academy of Ophthalmology: *Pediatric ophthalmology and strabismus,* section 6, Basic and Clinical Science Course, Orlando, 1998-1999, American Academy of Ophthalmology.
2. Eliason JA: Blepharitis: overview and classification. In Krachmer JH, Mannis MJ, Holland EJ (eds): *Cornea,* St Louis, 1997, Mosby.

Author: **Anna F. Fakadej, M.D., F.A.A.O.**

BASIC INFORMATION

DEFINITION
Botulism is a neuroparalytic illness characterized by symmetric, descending, flaccid paralysis of motor and autonomic nerves caused by intoxication with botulinum toxin. Three forms of the disease are recognized: (1) Classic botulism is caused by the ingestion of preformed botulinum toxin in contaminated foods; (2) infant botulism is caused by colonization of the gastrointestinal (GI) tract with the organism *Clostridium botulinum,* followed by absorption of the neurotoxin produced in the GI tract; (3) wound botulism follows contamination of a wound with spores from *C. botulinum,* followed by production and absorption of the toxin from the wound.

SYNONYM
Sausage poisoning

ICD-9CM CODE
005.1 Botulism

ETIOLOGY
C. botulinum, an anaerobic, spore-forming, gram-positive bacillus that produces a lethal neurotoxin

EPIDEMIOLOGY & DEMOGRAPHICS
- A median of 100 cases of botulism are reported in the United States per year; 70% are infant botulism.
- Wound botulism increased in 1995 and 1996 primarily among injecting drug users (possibly associated with black tar heroin).
- Recent foodborne botulism outbreaks have been associated with both restaurant- and home-prepared foods, including homemade salsa, potatoes baked in foil, cheese sauce, garlic in oil, sautéed onions, and salted or fermented fish.
- Infant botulism is occurring with increased frequency in California, Utah, and southern Pennsylvania.
- Most cases of infant botulism occur in children between 2 and 6 months of age.
- Infant botulism occurs equally among males and females throughout the year.

HISTORY
- Patients with foodborne botulism initially can present with GI disturbances such as nausea, vomiting, diarrhea, and abdominal pain, followed by neurologic symptoms.
- The most common neurologic symptoms are dry mouth, blurred vision, diplopia, dysphonia, dysphagia, cranial nerve paralysis, and descending muscle weakness, including the muscles of respiration.
- The symptoms of wound botulism are similar to foodborne botulism except the GI complaints are absent.
- Constipation, poor feeding or cry, progressive weakness or floppiness, and decreased spontaneous movements are the most common symptoms reported in infant botulism.
- Prior ingestion of honey is reported in 15% of cases of infant botulism.

PHYSICAL EXAMINATION
- Patients are afebrile, with diminished spontaneous movements and motor responses to stimuli.
- Ptosis, paralysis of the extraocular muscles, decreased pupillary constriction and corneal reflexes, impaired gag and swallow reflexes, and limb weakness in a proximal-to-distal pattern with decreased respiratory effort may all be present.
- Deep tendon reflexes may be decreased or absent in a descending distribution.
- Autonomic dysfunction may include dry mucous membranes, fluctuations in pulse and blood pressure, urinary retention, and alterations in skin color.

DIAGNOSIS

DIFFERENTIAL DIAGNOSIS
- Myasthenia gravis
- Guillain-Barré syndrome
- Eaton-Lambert syndrome
- Poliomyelitis
- Stroke syndrome
- Hypothyroidism
- Drug or heavy metal poisoning
- Paralytic shellfish poisoning or puffer fish ingestion
- Werdnig-Hoffmann syndrome
- Tick paralysis
- Sepsis

DIAGNOSTIC WORKUP
- Electromyography demonstrating a pattern termed *BSAP* (brief, small, abundant motor-unit potentials) is characteristic of botulism and can be completed rapidly.
- The diagnosis is confirmed by detection of the neurotoxin in the serum or stool or by the isolation of *C. botulinum* from feces.

THERAPY

NONPHARMACOLOGIC
Supportive care, including ventilatory and nutritional support, are the mainstays of treatment.

MEDICAL
- Trivalent equine antitoxin given intravenously as one vial (7500 IU of type A, 5500 IU of type B, and 8500 IU of type E antitoxins) to adult patients who have had symptoms of botulism for less than 24 hours has been shown to decrease hospital stay and mortality.
- Trivalent equine antitoxin is the only licensed product for use in the treatment of botulism, but it is not recommended for use in infants.
- Human botulism immune globulin is currently being tested for use in infant botulism and is available under a Treatment Investigational New Drug protocol from the California Department of Health Services (510-540-2646).

FOLLOW-UP & DISPOSITION
- Prolonged hospitalization (5 to 6 weeks) for supportive care is typical.
- One retrospective review found a fatality rate of 10% to 15% in patients who received antitoxin therapy, compared with 46% in untreated adult patients.
- The case:fatality ratio in infant botulism is less than 2% of hospitalized patients.
- The long-term prognosis is excellent, with gradual full recovery if the diagnosis is made promptly with institution of supportive care, and complications of hospitalization can be avoided.

PATIENT/FAMILY EDUCATION
- Infants should not be fed honey because of the risk of botulism.
- There is no known person-to-person transmission of botulism.

PREVENTIVE TREATMENT
Avoid feeding infants honey and Karo syrup.

REFERRAL INFORMATION
Patients with botulism need to be monitored closely and transported to a pediatric center, where airway and ventilatory support can be instituted.

PEARLS & CONSIDERATIONS

CLINICAL PEARLS
With suspected botulism, use aminoglycoside antibiotics with caution because these medications can potentiate neuromuscular blockade and precipitate respiratory decompensation.

■ WEBSITES

- Centers for Disease Control and Prevention: www.cdc.gov/ncidod/diseases/foodborn/botulism.htm
- Virginia Department of Health: www.vdh.state.va.us/epi/botulism.htm

REFERENCES

1. Glatman-Freedman A: Infant botulism, *Pediatr Rev* 17:185, 1996.
2. McKee KT et al: Botulism in infancy, *Am J Dis Child* 131:857, 1977.
3. Schreiner MS, Field E, Ruddy R: Infant botulism: a review of 12 years' experience at the Children's Hospital of Philadelphia, *Pediatrics* 87:159, 1991.
4. Shapiro RL, Hatheway C, Swerdlow D: Botulism in the United States: a clinical and epidemiologic review, *Ann Intern Med* 129:221, 1998.

Author: **Mary Caserta, M.D.**

BASIC INFORMATION

■ DEFINITION

Acute brain injury is accidental or inflicted trauma to the head resulting in the following:

- Mild head injury: Glasgow Coma Scale (GCS) score of 13 or 14 or a traumatically induced physiologic disruption of brain function, as manifested by one of the following:
  1. Any period of loss of consciousness (LOC)
  2. Any loss of memory for events immediately or before the accident
  3. Any alteration in mental state at the time of the accident
  4. Focal neurologic deficits, which may or may not be transient
- Moderate head injury: GCS score of 9 to 12
- Severe head injury: GCS score of 8 or less and coma lasting 6 hours or more

■ SYNONYMS

- Traumatic brain injury
- Closed head injury
- Intracranial injury

ICD-9CM CODES

854   Brain injury
959.01   Head injury
851-854 Intracranial hemorrhage

■ ETIOLOGY

- Approximately 95% of traumatic brain injuries in children are closed head injuries.
- Penetrating brain injuries
- Shaken baby syndrome or shaken impact syndrome
- Primary injury: focal, diffuse, closed head injury or penetrating injury that occurs at the time of impact
- Secondary injury: cascade of biochemical and physiologic events within the brain that contribute to diffuse brain swelling, anoxia, and/or ischemia with further tissue loss or damage

■ EPIDEMIOLOGY & DEMOGRAPHICS

- Approximately 100,000 to 200,000 new head injuries occur in children each year.
- The population incidence is 193 to 367 per 100,000.
- The two peak periods are early childhood (younger than 5 years of age) and middle to late adolescence.
- Up to the age of 5 years, males and females are affected equally; after the age of 5 years, male predominance ranges from 2:1 to 4:1.
- In infants, toddlers, and young children, assaults/child abuse and falls account for 50% of injuries; 20% are motor vehicle related in children 0 to 4 years of age.

1. Younger children more commonly sustain pedestrian or bicycle-related injuries.
- Most injuries in older children and adolescents are motor vehicle related.
  1. Falls and assaults/abuse account for less than 20% of injuries in older children.
  2. Adolescents are more typically injured as passengers in motor vehicles.
  3. Older children and adolescents also sustain sports or recreational injuries, as well as penetrating injuries.
- The highest rate of injuries is reported among the those in the lower socioeconomic classes.
- Focal injuries, such as subdural, epidural, and intracerebral hematomas, occur in 15% to 20% of children, with a higher incidence in children younger than 4 years of age.
- Skull fractures occur in 5% to 25% of children and are associated with epidural hematomas 40% of the time.
- Ten percent to fifteen percent of children hospitalized with head trauma have a severe head injury; of these, the mortality rate is approximately 33% to 50%, with most survivors having permanent deficits.

■ HISTORY

- The source is usually clear; it is more important to define the extent of injury.
- Accidental: Someone witnessed involvement in motor vehicle accident, high fall, or sports injury.
- Nonaccidental or abuse:
  1. Suspicious "falls" or injuries not explained by proposed history
  2. Penetrating injuries caused by gunshot wound or stabbing
- Alteration in mental status, such as behavior changes, irritability, or lethargy, is seen.
- Neurologic abnormalities, such as headache, visual abnormalities, gait abnormalities, or weakness, are present.
- Emesis occurs.
- Patient experiences LOC.

■ PHYSICAL EXAMINATION

- Altered GCS score
- Abnormal cranial nerve examination; abnormal pupillary light reflex, eye position, or eye movements
- Abnormal motor, sensory, or reflex examination
- Lacerations, abrasions, or hematomas about head and scalp
- Depressed skull fracture by palpation
- Otorrhea, rhinorrhea, Battle's sign, or raccoon eyes
- Retinal hemorrhages with suspected abuse

DIAGNOSIS

■ DIFFERENTIAL DIAGNOSIS

- Especially in the infant and toddler, differentiating between accidental and inflicted injury
- Anoxic or hypoxic encephalopathy
- Ruptured arteriovenous malformation or aneurysm
- Postictal phase
- Meningoencephalitis

■ DIAGNOSTIC WORKUP

- Adequately resuscitate (ABCs [airway, breathing, and circulation]), with particular attention directed toward assessing and securing an airway and ensuring adequate ventilation and circulation.
- Stabilize the cervical spine.
- Conduct a brief neurologic examination, including assigning a GCS score.
- Once the patient is stabilized, perform a thorough neurologic examination.
- If a cervical spine injury is possible based on the mechanism of injury, evaluate the cervical spine with anteroposterior, lateral, and open-mouth x-ray views.
  1. Maintain cervical spine immobilization until cleared radiographically and no tenderness to palpation is present over cervical spine.
  2. Additional flexion/extension views may need to be obtained to evaluate for ligamentous injury.
- For mild head injury:
  1. No additional evaluation is necessary if the patient did not experience LOC or amnesia, has a GCS score of 15, has no focal deficits, and has no palpable skull fracture. Discharge home with written instructions for the parents about how to evaluate the child.
  2. With brief LOC (shorter than 5 minutes), amnesia, GCS score of 13 or 14, impaired alertness or memory, or palpable depressed skull fracture, evaluate with computed tomography (CT) scan. If no intracranial disease is present, may discharge home with written instructions for the parents about how to evaluate the child.
  3. If the child experiences LOC for more than 5 minutes, posttraumatic seizures, or focal neurologic deficits or an intracranial lesion is seen on CT scan, the child should be admitted for observation.
- For moderate head injury:
  1. Children with GCS scores of 9 to 12, focal neurologic deficits, or

intracranial disease on CT scan have the potential for deterioration and should be observed closely in an intensive care unit (ICU) setting; obtain neurosurgical evaluation.

- For severe head injury:
  1. CT scan of head and immediate neurosurgical evaluation should be obtained, with close observation in an ICU setting.
- In cases of child abuse:
  1. Initial evaluation of head with CT should be performed to rule out immediate surgical hematomas, but then magnetic resonance imaging (MRI) scan of head, which is superior in determining traumatic hematomas of varying ages, should be performed.
  2. Conduct a skeletal survey to evaluate for fractures of varying ages, posterior rib fractures, or metaphyseal fractures of long bones.
  3. Perform an ophthalmologic evaluation of the retina.
  4. Thoroughly examine the skin for bruises, burns, and other traumatic lesions.

THERAPY

■ NONPHARMACOLOGIC
- Mild or moderate head injury
  1. Closely observe the patient, with frequent neurologic evaluations.
- Severe head injury
  1. Place intracranial monitor if GCS score is less than 8 and monitor intracranial pressures (ICP).
  2. Maintain cerebral perfusion pressure (CPP = Mean arterial pressure – ICP) at 50 mm Hg or more in infants and young children and at *at least* 70 mm Hg in older children and adolescents.
  3. Keep head midline.
  4. Elevate the head of bed 30 to 45 degrees.
  5. Initiate controlled ventilation to maintain a $Paco_2$ of 32 to 35 mm Hg.
  6. Maintain adequate oxygenation (Pao_2 between 90 and 100 mm Hg); avoid hypoxia.
  7. Maintain normal blood pressure; avoid hypotension.
  8. Intermittently drain cerebrospinal fluid to lower ICP and maintain adequate CPP.
  9. Avoid noxious stimuli.
  10. Prevent hyperthermia and add a cooling blanket if antipyretics are ineffective.
  11. In some centers, jugular venous oxygen saturations are monitored continuously with a fiberoptic catheter to detect possible brain ischemia.
  12. Studies are under way to evaluate

the benefits of mild hypothermia (32° to 34° C).

■ MEDICAL
- Mild or moderate head injury
  1. No medical therapy is available, except possible use of an anticonvulsant if a focal lesion is present.
- Severe head injury
  1. Sedatives, including propofol, benzodiazepines, narcotics, may be given.
  2. Nondepolarizing muscle relaxants can be used for intubation and occasionally as needed if sedatives alone are unable to blunt the effects of noxious stimuli.
  3. Osmotic diuretics (mannitol) can be used to reduce brain edema if the patient is hemodynamically stable (0.25 to 0.5 g/kg given every 2 to 6 hours to increase serum osmolarity to between 290 and 305 mOsm).
  4. Loop diuretics (furosemide 1 mg/kg) may be effective to reduce transient intravascular volume increase that follows mannitol infusion.
  5. Isotonic fluids can be used to restore and maintain adequate perfusion and blood pressure.
  6. Pressor support (e.g., dopamine, norepinephrine) can be initiated if unable to maintain adequate CPP.
  7. Anticonvulsants (e.g., dilantin, phenobarbital) can be used to prevent early posttraumatic seizures.
  8. Antipyretics may be administered.
  9. Lidocaine (1 mg/kg; maximum, 6 mg/kg/24 hr) should be given intravenously or intratracheally, or thiopental or pentobarbital (1 mg/kg intravenously) may be given to blunt the increase in ICP associated with tracheal suctioning.
  10. High-dose barbiturates have been used to decrease brain metabolism when the ICP cannot be controlled and thus CPP cannot be maintained by other means.

■ SURGICAL
Surgical evacuation of large epidural or subdural hematomas

■ FOLLOW-UP & DISPOSITION
- Mild to moderate head injuries
  1. If discharged home, specific written instructions should be given to the caregiver.
- Severe head injuries
  1. Transfer the patient to a specialized, multidisciplinary rehabilitation program as soon as the patient is medically stable.

- For children with neurologic or psychiatric deficits, enroll children in specialized school or early childhood development/stimulation programs
- Sports injuries
  1. Grade 1 concussion: no LOC; amnesia lasting less than 30 minutes
     a. First concussion: Return to play if asymptomatic at rest and on exertion for 1 week.
     b. Second concussion: Return to play in 2 weeks after asymptomatic for 1 week.
     c. Third concussion: Terminate season; may return to play next season if asymptomatic.
  2. Grade 2 concussion: LOC less than 5 minutes; amnesia longer than 30 minutes but less than 24 hours
     a. First concussion: Return to play after asymptomatic at rest and on exertion for 1 week.
     b. Second concussion: No play for a minimum of 1 month; may return to play then if asymptomatic for 1 week; consider terminating the season.
     c. Third concussion: Terminate season; may return to play next season if asymptomatic.
  3. Grade 3 concussion: LOC for 5 minutes or longer or amnesia longer than 24 hours
     a. Transport to hospital for evaluation.
     b. First concussion: No play for a minimum of 1 month; may then return to play if asymptomatic for 1 week.
     c. Second concussion: Terminate season; may return to play next season if asymptomatic.
  4. If neurosurgery needed, no contact or collision sports
- Abuse/assault
  1. Notify appropriate authorities.

■ PATIENT/FAMILY EDUCATION & PREVENTIVE TREATMENT
- Use child-restraint devices appropriately in motor vehicles; place children in the back seat.
- Obey speed limits.
- Use sports equipment, especially helmets, appropriately.
- Enforce and follow all sports rules.
- Provide adequate adult supervision.
- Provide information about parenting classes and support services for those at risk for child abuse.
- Fire arm legislation to decrease availability of guns should be advocated.

■ REFERRAL INFORMATION
Children with head injuries and residual cognitive, motor, speech, or behavioral deficits should be referred to a neurologist or neuropsychologist.

☼ PEARLS & CONSIDERATIONS

■ CLINICAL PEARLS

- Preventive measures are the only way to eliminate primary brain injuries. All therapies are focused only at preventing secondary brain injuries.
- Postinjury cerebral edema usually peaks at 24 to 48 hours and gradually resolves over 3 to 4 days.
- Seventy percent of all pediatric trauma deaths occurring within 48 hours of hospital admissions are the result of head injuries.
- Isolated, brief, immediate post-traumatic seizures occurring within seconds of impact require no therapy.
- The severity of head injury outcome is related directly to the duration and degree of coma.
- Children as a group have a better outcome than adults; however, children younger than 7 years of age fare worse, partly because of a higher incidence of child abuse and the functions of the developing brain. Disruption or damage to the centers for acquiring or interpreting new stimuli may adversely affect the child's ability to acquire new and higher functions.
- Children younger than 4 years of age at the time of severe head injury are unlikely to be able to work independently outside of a structured environment.

■ WEBSITES

- Brain Injury Association, Inc.: www.biausa.org/
- National Safe Kids Campaign: www.safekids.org/
- The Pediatric Critical Care Medicine Website: http://anes01.wustl.edu/All-Net/english/neurpage/trauma/head-2html

■ SUPPORT GROUPS

- National Head Injury Foundation
- Brain Injury Association, Inc.

REFERENCES

1. Adelson PD, Kochanek PM: Head injury in children, *J Child Neurol* 13:2, 1998.
2. Cantu RC: Return to play guidelines after a head injury, *Clin Sports Med* 17: 45, 1998.
3. Goldstein B, Powers KP: Head trauma in children, *Pediatr Rev* 15:213, 1994.
4. Schutzman SA: Injury—head. In Fleisher GR, Ludwig S (eds): *Textbook of pediatric emergency medicine*, ed 3, Baltimore, 1993, Williams & Wilkins.

Author: **Karen S. Powers, M.D.**

II

BASIC INFORMATION

DEFINITION

Brain tumors result from an uncontrolled proliferation of cells derived from neural tissue or structural, supportive (glial) tissue within the brain. There are many types of brain tumors. Most are localized growths, but some disseminate throughout the central nervous system (CNS), and in rare instances spread outside the CNS.

SYNONYMS

- Brain cancer
- CNS malignancy

ICD-9CM CODE
239.6 CNS tumor

ETIOLOGY

- Unknown in most cases
- Increased incidence in children with neurofibromatosis types I and II, Gardener's syndrome (Turcot's syndrome), tuberous sclerosis, and Li-Fraumeni syndrome
- Increased incidence after cranial irradiation
- Environmental causes (e.g., power lines, cellular phones, chemical exposures) possible (these have been investigated, but none have been proven to cause brain tumors)

EPIDEMIOLOGY & DEMOGRAPHICS

- The incidence is 34 cases per 1 million children per year. Approximately 1500 children younger than 15 years of age are diagnosed annually in the United States.
- The most common age at diagnosis is 5 to 10 years, but the disease can occur at any age.
- Brain tumors are the second most common pediatric malignancy; they are the most common pediatric solid tumors.
- Sixty percent are posterior fossa tumors; 40% are supratentorial (15% midline, 25% cerebral).
- Major brain tumor types include the following:
  1. Astrocytoma (50%)
     a. Low-grade: low-grade astrocytoma, ganglioglioma, and optic glioma
     b. High-grade: brainstem glioma, anaplastic astrocytoma, and glioblastoma multiforme
  2. Medulloblastoma (20%)
  3. Ependymoma (10%)
  4. Other (20%)
     a. Low-grade: craniopharyngioma and oligodendroglioma
     b. High-grade: lymphoma, supratentorial primitive neuroectodermal tumor (PNET), CNS atypical teratoid/rhabdoid

tumor, choroid plexus carcinoma, and germ cell tumor

HISTORY

- General
  1. Signs and symptoms are often related to hydrocephalous.
  2. Signs and symptoms are often nonfocal.
  3. Headaches, vomiting, and lethargy are common.
  4. Ten percent of children present with seizures.
  5. When focal findings develop in children, they are often related to balance, vision, and facial movements.
- Infants and toddlers
  1. Irritability
  2. Developmental delay or plateau
  3. Vomiting
- School-age children and adolescents
  1. Headaches
  2. Vomiting
  3. Double vision
  4. Lethargy
  5. Decline in school performance
  6. Moodiness

PHYSICAL EXAMINATION

- Focal deficits uncommon, particularly in infants and toddlers
- Lethargy
- Papilledema
- Infants and toddlers
  1. Widened or delayed closure of fontanelles
  2. Abnormal increase in head circumference
  3. Decreased upward gaze
- School-age children and adolescents
  1. Poor balance and coordination
  2. Dysconjugate gaze
  3. Nystagmus
  4. Facial weakness
  5. Focal motor or sensory deficits

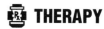 **DIAGNOSIS**

DIFFERENTIAL DIAGNOSIS

- Migraine headache
- Brain abscess or arteriovenous malformation
- Hydrocephalous from other causes
- Depression or other psychologic disorder

DIAGNOSTIC WORKUP

- Magnetic resonance imaging (MRI) with gadolinium is the best imaging study.
- Computed tomography (CT) with contrast can be used if MRI is not available.
- MRI of the spine and lumbar puncture (LP) for cerebrospinal fluid (CSF) cytologic examination should be taken for patients with tumors that can disseminate throughout the CNS

(e.g., ependymoma, medulloblastoma). LP should be done with caution because of the risk of herniation and should be done only after consultation with a neurosurgeon or neurologist.
- Laboratory studies are generally not helpful in making the diagnosis.
  1. Serum and CSF β-human chorionic gonadotropin (β-HCG) and α-fetoprotein (AFP) should be obtained in patients with pineal region or suprasellar tumors to assess the possibility of a CNS germ cell tumor.

THERAPY

SURGERY

- A complete resection improves the prognosis for almost all types of brain tumors.
- Involvement of a skilled pediatric neurosurgeon is essential.
- Ventriculoperitoneal (VP) shunt placement is sometimes necessary.
- Children with more than 95% resection of low-grade astrocytoma, ganglioglioma, and oligodendroglioma need no further therapy.

RADIATION

- Focal external beam radiation is used for children 5 years of age or older who have brainstem glioma, symptomatic optic glioma, anaplastic astrocytoma, glioblastoma, ependymoma, or partially resected craniopharyngioma, as well as for children with symptomatic, incompletely resected, or progressive low-grade astrocytoma.
- Craniospinal radiation is used for children with medulloblastoma, supratentorial PNET, and children with CNS germ cell tumor not receiving chemotherapy.
- Delayed and/or dose-reduced radiation is appropriate for children younger than 5 years of age who are being treated initially with chemotherapy.
- Stereotactic radiosurgery (or gamma knife) is focused, single-dose irradiation for previously irradiated children with local recurrences smaller than 4 cm in diameter.

CHEMOTHERAPY

- Chemotherapy is indicated for children with medulloblastoma, supratentorial PNET, anaplastic astrocytoma, glioblastoma multiforme, and CNS germ cell tumors.
- It is indicated for children younger than 5 years of age who have any of the tumor types except completely resected low-grade astrocytoma, ganglioglioma, or oligodendroglioma.

- Active agents include nitrosoureas, procarbazine, vincristine, VP-16, *cis*-platinum, carboplatin, and cyclophosphamide.
- New promising agents include irinotecan, temozolomide, and thalidomide.
- Toxicity includes hair loss, myelosuppression, hearing loss, and infertility.

■ FOLLOW-UP & DISPOSITION
- Cure rates are as follows:
  1. Completely resected low-grade tumors (e.g., astrocytoma): 90% to 95%
  2. Medulloblastoma, ependymoma: 70% to 80%
  3. Brain tumors in children younger than 3 years of age: 20% to 60%
  4. High-grade astrocytoma (e.g., anaplastic, glioblastoma): 20% to 30%
  5. Brainstem glioma, atypical teratoid tumor: 0% to 20%
- Serial MRI is often performed during treatment and for several years after treatment to assess the response to therapy and the possibility of recurrence.
- The greatest likelihood of recurrence of high-grade tumors is within 2 to 3 years of diagnosis; low-grade tumors are less likely to recur but can recur at any time.

- Careful, coordinated follow-up by a team, including a pediatric neurosurgeon, radiation oncologist, pediatric oncologist, neurologist, social worker, teacher, and late-effects specialist, is essential throughout the initial evaluation, treatment, and follow-up period.
- The late effects of radiation and chemotherapy depend on the child's age and dose and location of radiation.
  1. Hearing loss
  2. Growth failure
  3. Delayed puberty
  4. Intellectual deficits

■ PATIENT/FAMILY EDUCATION
- Brain tumors are complex diseases requiring careful, coordinated care by many subspecialists and support care personnel.
- Opinions among physicians may differ because many cases are complicated and unique.
- Most children with brain tumors are cured. The treatment strategy is designed to maximize cure rates and minimize long-term toxicity.
- There is a high likelihood of long-term toxicity.

■ REFERRAL INFORMATION
- Children should be referred promptly to a pediatric neurosurgeon, pediatric radiation oncologist, and pediatric oncologist/neurooncologist.
- Future therapy will be directed at more selective tumor kill and less long-term toxicity and will include antiangiogenic therapy, gene therapy, and differentiation therapy.

☼ PEARLS & CONSIDERATIONS

■ CLINICAL PEARLS
The pattern of symptoms over time (e.g., headaches, poor school performance, emesis) is far more telling than the findings at a single physician visit.

■ WEBSITES
- National Brain Tumor Foundation: www.braintumor.org
- Pediatric Brain Tumor Foundation: www.ride4kids.org

REFERENCE
1. Heideman RL, Packer RJ, Albright CA et al: Tumors of the central nervous system. In Pizzo PA, Poplack DG (eds): *Principles and practice of pediatric oncology,* Philadelphia, 1997, Lippincott-Raven.
Author: **David N. Korones, M.D.**

II

BASIC INFORMATION

■ DEFINITION
- Nipple trauma: blistering, cracking, bruising, and/or bleeding of nipple associated with breastfeeding
- Breast infection
  1. Mastitis: infection of lobule of breast and cellulitis of overlying skin
  2. Monilial infection of the epidermis of the nipple and surrounding areola
- Obstructed duct: plugging of a collecting duct in the breast
- Engorgement: increased vascularity and accumulation of milk in the breast; may involve the whole breast or the areola

■ SYNONYMS
- Nipple trauma
- Nipple confusion
- Nipple bruising
- Nipple injury resulting from breastfeeding
- Monilial infection (yeast or candidal infection)

ICD-9CM CODES
611.0 Mastitis, breast infection, nipple infection, yeast infection of nipple, yeast infection of breast
611.70 Sore nipple/breast pain
675.00 Infection of nipple
611.79 Engorgement of breast
675.9 Yeast infection/infection of breast with nipple
676.30 Plugged duct/absence of milk secretion

■ ETIOLOGY
- Nipple trauma
  1. Improper latch (poor positioning of infant at breast) may be associated with the following:
     a. Maternal nipple abnormalities or engorgement
     b. Short frenulum or other oral motor abnormalities in infant
  2. Improper detachment techniques
  3. Overly eager baby
  4. Improper breast pump use
- Breast infection
  1. Monilial
     a. Colonization of the maternal breast with yeast from mouth or diaper area of the infant
     b. Predisposition to yeast overgrowth because of antibiotic use in mother or infant
  2. Mastitis
     a. Infection with *Staphylococcus aureus, Escherichia coli,* rarely *Streptococcus* species
     b. Infection after nipple trauma
     c. May be associated with milk stasis, failure to resolve an obstructed duct or engorgement, or poor drainage of an area of

the breast after breast biopsy or surgery
- Obstructed ducts
  1. Breasts overly full
     a. Early lactogenesis with missed or irregular feedings
     b. Poor positioning with ineffective nursing and poor breast emptying
     c. Inadequate letdown
     d. Engorgement
  2. Poor drainage of an area of the breast
     a. External pressure on breast (poorly fitting bra)
     b. Previous breast surgery

■ EPIDEMIOLOGY & DEMOGRAPHICS
- Nipple trauma
  1. Increased prevalence is seen with flat or inverted nipples (approximately 10% of women).
  2. Increased incidence occurs when infants have a short frenulum or oral motor problems.
  3. Most women experience some minimal irritation of the nipples in the first 1 to 2 weeks of breastfeeding that resolves as the nipple adjusts to breastfeeding.
- Mastitis
  1. Occurs in approximately 2% to 3% of women, with the highest incidence in the early postpartum weeks.
  2. Recurrent mastitis is often associated with delayed or inadequate treatment.
     a. Sometimes associated with an area of the breast that drains poorly (e.g., previous surgery)
  3. Abscess formation in a small proportion of women (approximately 4% to 5% of those with mastitis) is often associated with delayed or inadequate treatment.

■ HISTORY
- Nipple trauma
  1. Nipple pain occurs with breastfeeding, lasting throughout the entire feeding.
  2. Trauma is sometimes associated with a vigorous nursing style in the infant.
     a. Appropriate frequency (8 to 12 times per day in the neonate)
     b. Appropriate interpretation of need to feed (Is the infant frantic by the time mother feeds?)
  3. If milk transfer is affected, the infant may not gain weight appropriately.
     a. Neonate should gain 15 to 30 g/day after milk increases in quantity.
     b. Lactogenesis usually occurs by 3 days postpartum.

c. Infant may have feeding-related jaundice.
     d. Lack of urine and stool output may be seen (fewer than six to eight voids and three to four stools per day in neonate).
  4. History of delayed breastfeeding after birth and use of supplemental feedings.
  5. Exposure to artificial nipples such as pacifier use or bottle-feeding.
- Breast infection
  1. Yeast
     a. Stinging, burning pain radiating throughout the breast during and between feedings
     b. Thrush, monilial diaper rash in the infant; yeast vaginitis in the mother
     c. Antibiotic use in the mother or infant
  2. Mastitis
     a. Fever, malaise, nausea, and flulike symptoms
     b. Failure to resolve a plugged duct
     c. History of breast surgery
     d. Poor emptying of breast
        (1) Use of bras with stays
        (2) Engorgement
        (3) Refusal to nurse
- Obstructed duct
  1. Soreness of breast localized to one area with a lump
  2. Mother afebrile without systemic symptoms
- Engorgement
  1. Generalized soreness of entire breast
  2. Missed feedings
  3. Breasts that are hard and warm to touch; shiny and transparent skin
  4. Possible difficulty with latching on
  5. Supplemental feeding of infant
  6. Low-grade fever

■ PHYSICAL EXAMINATION
- Nipple trauma
  1. Observation of breastfeeding to assess technique and infant attachment to the breast (Fig. 2-1)
  2. Cracked, bruised, or blistered nipples
  3. Coexisting problems
     a. Mastitis (see following discussion)
     b. Contact dermatitis: red, irritated, dry nipple
     c. Engorgement: bilateral fullness of breasts with increased vascularity and warmth; skin may be transparent and shiny, and nipple may appear flat if areolar engorgement is prominent
     d. Tight frenulum: heart-shaped appearance of infant's tongue; when he or she attempts to extend tongue, it will not

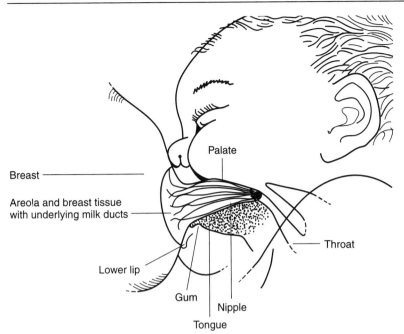

Fig. 2-1 Correct attachment (latch-on) at the breast includes: 1) newborn's nose close to or touching the breast while it breathes through the nasolabial folds; 2) rooting by the infant to move in and grasp the areola well behind the nipple, forming a teat; 3) tongue moving forward beyond the lower gum, cupped and forming a trough, then removing milk from the lactiferous sinuses by peristaltic waves; 4) the jaw moving down, creating a negative pressure gradient that facilitates transfer of the milk into the oral cavity. Illustration by Marcia Smith. (From Powers NG, Slusser W: Breastfeeding update 2: Clinical lactation management, *Pediatr Rev* 18:151, 1997.)

extend over lower alveolar ridge of gum line
- Breast infection
  1. Monilial
     a. Nipple may look normal or be shiny and red with satellite lesions around nipple.
     b. Thrush or monilial diaper rash may be seen in the infant.
  2. Mastitis
     a. Wedge-shaped area of redness that is tender, full, and warm to touch
     b. Maternal temperature 101° F or higher
- Obstructed duct
  1. Tender lump in breast
  2. No evidence of cellulitis (area is not red, indurated, or warm to touch)
  3. Mother well, afebrile without systemic symptoms
- Engorgement
  1. Breasts are hard and warm to touch; skin is shinny and transparent.
  2. Increased vascularity of breast is seen.
  3. Low-grade fever is possible.

DIAGNOSIS

■ DIFFERENTIAL DIAGNOSIS
- Nipple trauma
  1. Negative pressure on ductules with initial latch and suckling often occurs before the development of full lactation (produces temporary discomfort with attachment and initial suckling).

2. Contact dermatitis is caused by use of soaps, astringents, creams, nipple shields, or plastic bra liners.
3. Plugged duct.
4. Monilial infection.
5. Nipple trauma often coexists with other breastfeeding problems.
   a. Mastitis may result from nipple trauma with subsequent infection.
   b. In engorgement, the infant is unable to latch because of engorged areola.
   c. With a short frenulum or other oral motor abnormality, the infant cannot properly position tongue for breastfeeding.
- Breast infection
  1. Monilial infection
     a. Contact dermatitis
     b. Other causes of nipple trauma
  2. Mastitis
     a. Plugged duct
     b. Engorgement
     c. Breast tumor
- Obstructed duct
  1. Mastitis
  2. Engorgement
  3. Breast tumor
- Engorgement
  1. Mastitis
  2. Plugged duct
  3. Breast tumor

■ DIAGNOSTIC WORKUP
- Usually not needed because diagnosis is made during observation of breastfeeding and physical examination of the mother and infant
- Laboratory tests
  1. Scrape and culture of tender or

deeply cracked nipples for bacteria and yeast
   a. Culture may be positive for *S. aureus*
   b. Yeast culture positive, KOH prep may show hyphae indicative of monilia
2. Milk analysis if suspect mastitis
   a. Midstream culture, Gram stain, and white count
   b. Usually positive for *S. aureus*
      (1) Gram stain of milk: may show gram-positive cocci in clusters
      (2) In mastitis: more than 10^6 white blood cells (WBCs)/ml and more than 10^3 bacteria/ml
      (3) In milk stasis without infection: less than 10^6 WBCs/ml and less than 10^3 bacteria/ml

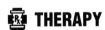 **THERAPY**

■ NONPHARMACOLOGIC
- Nipple trauma
  1. Ensure that positioning at breast is correct.
     a. The infant's head is in line with the body, and the head is well supported.
     b. The mother supports her breast while breastfeeding.
     c. The infant's mouth is open wide, lips are flanged outward, lips are 1 to 1.5 inches from base of nipple, and infant's tongue extends over lower gum line.

d. Audible swallowing is heard from the infant (suck, swallow, pause).
2. Instruct mother about proper detachment.
   a. Break suction with finger before removing the infant from the breast.
3. Encourage short, frequent feedings (8 to 12 per day is normal in early weeks).
   a. Begin with the least sore nipple to help with letdown on the more painful side.
   b. If the mother is unable to put the infant to her breast because of pain, instruct her to begin breast pumping to maintain the milk supply until breastfeeding can be resumed.
4. Discontinue use of pacifier and bottle feeding.
   a. If the infant requires continued supplements, the use of a supplemental nursing system or cup feeding should be considered.
5. Discontinue use of any soaps, creams, and/or ointments if contact dermatitis is an aggravating factor.
6. Express milk and rub it into nipple after breastfeeding, then air dry nipples.
7. Consider referral to a community health nurse (with special training in lactation), or for infants with problems such as short frenulum or oral motor problems, suggest consultation with a lactation consultant or an occupational therapist.
8. Suggest community support groups.
   a. WIC (Women, Infants, and Children) peer counselors
   b. La Leche League
9. If nipple trauma is associated with inverted or flat nipples, the mother may benefit from using something to draw out the nipple before attempting to attach the infant.
   a. Breast shells may be worn inside the bra between feedings.
   b. Use of a pump can help draw out the nipple.
10. If trauma is associated with mastitis, see following discussion.
11. If trauma is associated with engorgement:
    a. Milk expression (by hand or pump) before attaching the infant helps in allowing proper latch (especially if the areola is engorged).
       (1) Massage and application of warm packs to the breast may aid in beginning expression.

(2) Frequent breastfeedings are essential to prevent reengorgement.
(3) Cold packs can be applied to breast after feeding.

- Breast infection
  1. Monilial infection
     a. Air dry nipples.
     b. Avoid plastic liners on nursing pads and change pads frequently.
     c. Sterilize items that come in contact with the infant's mouth (e.g., pacifiers, bottle nipples).
  2. Mastitis
     a. Infant may continue to nurse.
     b. Begin with the least sore breast.
     c. Ensuring adequate emptying of the infected breast, applying warm packs, and massaging the breast before feeding may help.
     d. Ensure that the mother rests adequately because stress and fatigue are often precipitating factors.
     e. Ensure that the mother's bra does not have underwires or stays that inhibit drainage of one aspect of the breast.
- Obstructed duct
  1. Begin frequent and effective nursing on the affected breast.
  2. Apply moist, hot packs to the area before nursing.
  3. Massage the area before nursing.
  4. Alter nursing positions to encourage better drainage of the area.
     a. Position infant so that baby's sucking is directed toward the occluded duct.
- Engorgement
  1. Begin frequent and effective nursing.
  2. Hand express or pump to relieve areola engorgement so that infant can attach.
  3. Massage and apply warm packs to the breast before nursing to enhance letdown.

■ MEDICAL
- Nipple trauma
  1. Administer a mild analgesic, such as aspirin, ibuprofen, or acetaminophen.
  2. If area is dry, consider using an ointment, such as purified lanolin or A & D ointment. Routine use of ointments is not recommended.
  3. Deeply cracked nipples with positive *S. aureus* cultures should be treated with oral antibiotics to prevent the development of mastitis, which occurs in approximately 25% of patients.
     a. After bacterial and fungal infections have been ruled out, severely affected nipples may respond to 1% cortisone ointment or a synthetic corticoid (halobetasol propionate 0.05%

or mometasone furoate 0.1%) rubbed into the nipple and areola after each breastfeeding session (2 days is usually adequate).
- Breast infection
  1. Monilial infection
     a. Prescribe nystatin oral suspension for the infant and nystatin cream for the mother.
     b. Treat for 7 to 10 days.
     c. For resistant cases, consider oral fluconazole in the mother and baby.
  2. Mastitis should be treated for 10 to 14 days with antibiotics that are effective against *S. aureus*.
     a. Dicloxacillin is a safe and effective antibiotic.
     b. Poor compliance with the full course of antibiotics often leads to abscess formation.
     c. If mastitis is bilateral, consider streptococcal infection.
- Obstructed duct or engorgement
  1. Administer a mild analgesic, such as aspirin, ibuprofen, or acetaminophen.

■ SURGICAL
- Sore nipples secondary to a short frenulum in the infant: Some surgeons recommend frenulum release in the infant to allow correct tongue positioning, but *this procedure is very controversial*.
- Abscess formation with mastitis requires surgical drainage.

■ FOLLOW-UP & DISPOSITION
- Uncomplicated nipple trauma
  1. Follow up within 2 to 3 days to assess resolution of pain, nipple healing, and infant well-being.
  2. Condition may require more frequent visits if associated with poor weight gain in infant or feeding-related jaundice.
- Plugged duct
  1. Follow up by telephone within 24 hours to assess resolution.
  2. If maternal systemic symptoms develop, consider progression to mastitis.
- Engorgement or mastitis
  1. Follow up within 24 hours.
  2. Assess improvement in symptoms, response to antibiotics (mastitis), and infant well-being (hydration).

■ PATIENT/FAMILY EDUCATION
- Basic physiology of lactation:
  1. Supply follows demand for milk from infant.
  2. Frequent feedings are the norm (8 to 12 per day in the early weeks of breastfeeding).
  3. Effective and frequent emptying of the breast is essential to maintaining the milk supply and

avoiding milk stasis, which can lead to engorgement, plugged ducts, and mastitis.
- Expect six to eight wet diapers and a minimum of three to four yellow, seedy stools per day to ensure that infant is getting adequate amounts of milk.
- Systemic symptoms, fever, malaise, nausea, or redness of breast indicates mastitis.

■ PREVENTIVE TREATMENT
- Provide patient education in the hospital about proper attachment and detachment.
- Initiate on-demand, frequent breastfeedings.
- Avoid pacifiers and non–medically indicated supplemental feedings.

☼ PEARLS & CONSIDERATIONS

■ WEBSITES
- Academy of Breastfeeding Medicine (ABM): cwebber@applmeapro.com
- Baby Friendly Hospital Initiative, USA: www.aboutus.com/a100/bfusa
- La Leche League International (LLLI): www.lalecheleague.org/
- National Center for Education in Maternal Child Health: www.ncemch.org/databases/pdfs/ord
- San Diego County Breastfeeding Co.: www.breastfeeding.org (They maintain an updated listing of Internet sites with breastfeeding information.)

■ SUPPORT GROUPS
- La Leche League International
- WIC peer support programs

Both groups provide mother-to-mother support for breastfeeding women.

REFERENCES
1. Lawrence RA: *Breastfeeding: a guide for the medical profession,* ed 5, St Louis, 1999, Mosby.
2. Riordan JM, Auerbach KG: *Breastfeeding and human lactation,* Boston, 1993, Jones and Bartlett.
3. Work Group on Breastfeeding: Breastfeeding and the use of human milk, *Pediatrics* 100:1035, 1997.

Author: **Cynthia Howard, M.D., M.P.H.**

II

BASIC INFORMATION

■ DEFINITION

- Breastfeeding jaundice is an abnormal unconjugated hyperbilirubinemia during the first week of life resulting from decreased enteral intake and increased enterohepatic circulation of bilirubin. There is no associated increase in bilirubin production. It is a sign of failure to establish adequate breastfeeding.
- Breastmilk jaundice is a normal extension of physiologic jaundice of the newborn (normally occurring unconjugated hyperbilirubinemia in the first week of life). It begins after the fifth day of life and continues for several weeks. It is believed to be caused by an inhibitor of conjugation present in human milk.

■ SYNONYMS

Breastfeeding jaundice is also termed *lack of breastmilk jaundice*. Infants, whether breastfed or formula fed, will become jaundiced with inadequate caloric intake.

ICD-9CM CODES

774.39 Breastmilk jaundice
774.6 Breastfeeding jaundice (physiologic jaundice) in term infants
774.2 Breastfeeding jaundice (physiologic jaundice) in preterm infants

■ ETIOLOGY

- Breastfeeding jaundice
  1. Lack of adequate caloric intake (lack of breastmilk)
  2. Increased enterohepatic circulation of bilirubin because of lack of stool volume
- Breastmilk jaundice is believed to be caused by an inhibitor of conjugation present in human milk. Suggested substances include the following:
  1. β-Glucuronidase
  2. Pregnanediol
  3. Free fatty acids
  4. Steroids

■ EPIDEMIOLOGY & DEMOGRAPHICS

- Physiologic jaundice
  1. Occurs in 65% of newborns.
  2. Classically, bilirubin rises from 1.5 mg/dl in cord serum to 5 to 6 mg/dl on the third day of life, declining to normal levels by the second week of life.
     a. Asian infants have a more rapid rise in bilirubin levels, with peak values of 8 to 12 mg/dl on days four to five.
     b. Approximately 2% of term Asian newborns attain levels of more than 20 mg/dl in contrast to 1% in white and black infants during the first week of life.
  3. Bilirubin is a potent antioxidant and peroxyl scavenger that may help the newborn avoid oxygen toxicity.
- Breastmilk jaundice
  1. At 5 to 6 days of age, bilirubin concentrations decline more rapidly in artificially fed infants than in breastfed infants (Fig. 2-2).
  2. In breastfed infants, concentrations either rise, remain stable for several days, or gradually decline.
  3. Previously believed to affect less than 1% of all breastfed infants, breastmilk jaundice has now been shown to affect 10% to 30% of infants during the second to sixth weeks of life.
     a. One study demonstrated that one third of 12- to 21-day-old healthy, thriving breastfed infants had bilirubin levels higher than 1.5 mg/dl and another one third had levels higher than 5 mg/dl and were clinically icteric.
     b. Two thirds of normal breastfed infants may be expected to have prolonged indirect hyperbilirubinemia up to 12 weeks of age.
  4. Maximal levels vary from 10 to 30 mg/dl (172 to 516 µmol/L).
  5. If nursing is interrupted for 24 to 48 hours, the bilirubin level falls precipitously and will not rebound to the same level when nursing is resumed.
- Breastfeeding jaundice
  1. Breastfed infants (9%) are more likely than formula-fed infants (2%) to have a bilirubin level greater than 13 mg/dl (224 µmol/L) and are more likely (2% versus 0.3%) to attain levels greater than 15 mg/dl (258 µmol/L).
  2. The pathogenesis appears to be decreased enteral intake and increased enterohepatic circulation.
  3. Under normal circumstances, with optimal breastfeeding initiation, frequency, and support, there are no significant differences in the serum bilirubin concentrations of breastfed and artificially fed infants during the first 4 to 5 days of life (see Fig. 2-2).
  4. A breastfed infant with a high bilirubin level caused by breastfeeding jaundice may go on to have breastmilk jaundice.

■ HISTORY

- Pregnancy information
  1. Blood group and type
  2. Serology
  3. Race and ethnic origin

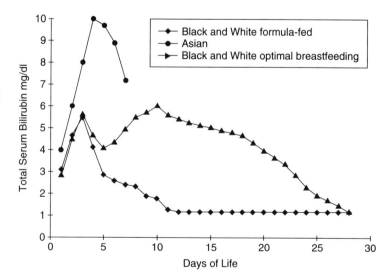

Fig. 2-2 A synthesized representation of the typical patterns of neonatal jaundice in black and white formula-fed infants (◆), black and white optimally breastfed infants (▶) during the first 28 days of life, and Asian infants, both breastfed and formula-fed (●), during the first 7 days of life. (From Gartner LM: *Pediatr Rev* 15:423, 1994.)

4. Illness during pregnancy
5. Medications during pregnancy
6. History of anemia or jaundice in family; previous siblings with jaundice
- Birth history
  1. Premature rupture of membranes
  2. Vacuum extraction or forceps delivery
  3. Type of delivery—vaginal versus cesarean section
  4. Oxytocin induction
  5. Medications or anesthetics for labor
  6. Apgar score
- Age when jaundice first noted
- Vomiting
- Frequency, volume, and type of feeding
- Number of stools and voids noted
- Drugs given to the infant
- Breastfeeding jaundice
  1. The role of inadequate caloric intake makes assessment of breastfeeding adequacy essential.
  2. Breastfeeding jaundice may be associated with the following:
     a. Delayed initiation of feedings
     b. Exposure to pacifiers (substitution of sucking on pacifier for need to feed)
     c. Insufficient maternal milk supply (e.g., inadequate glandular tissue, breast-reduction surgery, maternal thyroid disease, Sheehan's syndrome)
     d. Excessive infant weight loss (more than 8% from birth)
     e. Poor latch and ineffective suckling
     f. Associated maternal nipple trauma
     g. Fussy, irritable, hungry infant
     h. Decreased output, fewer than six to eight voids per day, fewer than three to four stools per day (may report continued meconium stools on days 4 to 5)
     i. Inadequate suckling in premature infant or infant with another condition that inhibits ability to suckle (e.g., poor tone in infant with Down syndrome)
        (1) The relative risk of a bilirubin level in excess of 13 mg/dl (224 µmol/L) is four times higher in a 37-week-gestation infant as compared with 40-week-gestation infant.
- Breastmilk jaundice
  1. Infants are well and have successfully established breastfeeding.
  2. At 5 to 7 days of age, the following should be positive:
     a. Weight loss from birth less than 5% to 7%
     b. Mother reports that breastmilk supply has increased in quantity (leaking, breast fullness,

audible swallowing during feeds)
  c. Infant weight gain should be 15 to 30 g/day.
  d. Feeding 10 to 12 times per day.
  e. No water or formula supplements
  f. Adequate time at breast (untimed on-demand feedings, at least 10 minutes per breast)
  g. Satisfied baby (feedings often terminated by sleep)
  h. Adequate hydration, voids (six to eight per day) and stools (yellow and seedy, minimum of three to four per day)

■ PHYSICAL EXAMINATION
- General assessment
  1. In breastfeeding jaundice, the infant may be irritable and difficult to console or sleepy and difficult to arouse.
  2. In breastmilk jaundice, the infant should be well appearing, have normal activity, and be alert.
- Infant weight
  1. In breastfeeding jaundice, weight loss from birth may be more than 8% or weight gain is inadequate (less than 15 to 30 g/day after 5 days of age).
  2. In breastmilk jaundice, weight gain is adequate (15 to 30 g/day).
- Hydration
  1. Infants with breastfeeding jaundice may be dehydrated.
     a. Dry mucous membranes, sunken fontanelle, poor skin turgor, and tenting
  2. Infants with breastmilk jaundice should be well hydrated.
     a. Moist mucous membranes, normal fontanelle, and normal skin turgor
- Assessment of jaundice
  1. Clinical progression of jaundice from face to trunk to extremities with increasing levels of bilirubin
     a. Facial jaundice is usually appreciated at a bilirubin level of 5 mg/dl (86 µmol/L).
     b. Infant will be jaundiced to abdomen (approximately 10 mg/dl).
     c. Infant will be jaundiced to distal extremities (approximately 15 mg/dl).
- Breastfeeding assessment
  1. Direct observation of breastfeeding is essential.
     a. Proper positioning and attachment at the breast (see Fig. 2-2).
     b. Audible swallowing
     c. Adequate time at breast (minimal of 10 minutes per side)
     d. Prefeeding and postfeeding weight to determine milk intake

- Other pertinent aspects of examination
  1. No hepatosplenomegaly is present.
  2. The infant has normal color and lack of ruddiness or paleness (rule out polycythemia or anemia associated with hemolysis).
  3. Both breastfeeding and breastmilk jaundice may be worsened by other causes of exaggerated physiologic jaundice in the newborn.
     a. Bruising and/or cephalohematoma
     b. Prematurity

🔬 DIAGNOSIS

■ DIFFERENTIAL DIAGNOSIS
See "Diagnostic Workup"

■ DIAGNOSTIC WORKUP
- Bilirubin—direct and indirect
  1. Indirect hyperbilirubinemia is present in both breastfeeding and breastmilk jaundice.
- Mother and infant's blood type (to rule out ABO disease), direct and indirect Coombs' test
- Maternal prenatal antibody screen (to rule out Rh disease and other blood group sensitization)
- Syphilis serology of cord blood
- Urine for reducing substances (to rule out galactosemia)
- Hemoglobin, blood smear, reticulocyte count (to rule out polycythemia and hemolysis, as well as red blood cell membrane abnormalities)
- Consideration of assay if indicated by history to rule out enzyme deficiencies such as glucose-6-phosphate dehydrogenase deficiency (G6PD) and pyruvate kinase
- Consideration of serum electrolytes if infant appears dehydrated
  1. Potential hypernatremia, elevated blood urea nitrogen (BUN), and creatinine in breastfeeding jaundice
- Consideration of need to evaluate for sepsis
- Consideration of evaluating electrolytes on maternal milk
  1. Sodium may be elevated in breastfeeding jaundice if milk volume has decreased because of poor removal (involution of glandular tissue) or in cases of insufficient glandular tissue.

💊 THERAPY

■ NONPHARMACOLOGIC
- Breastfeeding jaundice
  1. Ensure adequate breastmilk intake (observation of nursing is essential, see "Physical Examination").

TABLE 2-4 Recommendations for Management of Hyperbilirubinemia in the Healthy Term Newborn (Total Serum Bilirubin Concentrations)

AGE (IN HR)	CONSIDER PHOTOTHERAPY*	IMPLEMENT PHOTOTHERAPY	IMPLEMENT EXCHANGE TRANSFUSION IF PHOTOTHERAPY FAILS†	IMPLEMENT EXCHANGE TRANSFUSION
≤24‡	≥10 mg/dl (171 µM/L)	≥15 mg/dl (257 µM/L)	≥20 mg/dl (342 µM/L)	≥20 mg/dl (342 µM/L)
25-48	≥13 mg/dl	≥18 mg/dl (220 µM/L)	≥25 mg/dl (428 µM/L)	≥30 mg/dl (513 µM/L)
49-72	≥15 mg/dl (257 µM/L)	≥20 mg/dl (342 µM/L)	≥25 mg/dl (428 µM/L)	≥30 mg/dl (513 µM/L)
>72	≥17 mg/dl (291 µM/L)	≥22 mg/dl (376 µM/L)	≥25 mg/dl (428 µM/L)	≥30 mg/dl (513 µM/L)

Reprinted with permission from Provisional Committee on Quality Improvement, American Academy of Pediatrics. Practice Parameter: The management of hyperbilirubinemia in the healthy term newborn. *Pediatrics* 92:558, 1994.
From Gartner LM: *Pediatr Rev* 15:430, 1994.
*Phototherapy at these total serum bilirubin concentrations is a clinical option, meaning that the intervention is available and used on the basis of the individual clinical judgment.
†Failure of phototherapy is defined as failure of the bilirubin level to stabilize or decline by at least 1 to 2 mg/dl within 4 to 6 hours in infants exposed to intensive phototherapy.
‡It is recognized that the total serum bilirubin concentrations at 24 hours of age may not represent a healthy infant. Management of these infants requires investigation into the cause of hyperbilirubinemia, such as hemolytic disease.

2. If milk transfer is inadequate, infant should be supplemented.
3. Use a supplemental nursing system for best results.
4. Supplement preferably with pumped breastmilk and alternatively with formula.
5. Pump every 2 hours to maintain or enhance breastmilk supply until infant can be fully breastfed.
6. Begin frequent breastfeeding (every 2 to 2.5 hours, 8 to 12 times per day)
7. Consider consultation with a certified lactation specialist.
8. Close follow-up is important to ensure correction of hyperbilirubinemia and successful establishment of lactation.
• Breastmilk jaundice
   1. Do *not* discontinue breastfeeding.
   2. Management options include the following:
      a. Continue breastfeeding with observation.
      b. Supplement breastfeeding with formula.
      c. Temporarily interrupt breastfeeding for 24 to 36 hours, with formula substitution.
      d. If breastfeeding is interrupted, be sure to have mother pump breast to maintain milk supply. Bilirubin will decrease and will not attain previous values with the reinstitution of breastfeeding.

■ **MEDICAL**
• Consider phototherapy (Table 2-4).
• Management options, depending on the level of bilirubin, include the following:
   1. Continue breastfeeding and administer phototherapy.
   2. Supplement breastfeeding with formula and administer phototherapy.
   3. Temporarily interrupt breastfeeding for 24 to 36 hours with formula substitution and phototherapy.
   4. If breastfeeding is interrupted, have mother pump breast to maintain milk supply.
• Follow closely to assess bilirubin levels, hydration, adequate feeding, and weight gain.

■ **FOLLOW-UP & DISPOSITION**
• Breastfeeding jaundice
   1. If phototherapy is not indicated, the infant should be followed every 1 to 2 days, depending on level of bilirubin, to assess jaundice, hydration, adequate feeding, and weight gain.
• Breastmilk jaundice
   1. After bilirubin has peaked and infant is otherwise well (with bilirubin less than 12 mg/dl), infant can be followed per usual well-child routine.

■ **PATIENT/FAMILY EDUCATION**
• Basic physiology of lactation:
   1. Ensure proper positioning, attachment, and detachment.
   2. Breastmilk supply follows demand; encourage on-demand, frequent breastfeedings (8 to 12 per day).
   3. Avoid pacifiers and non–medically indicated supplemental feedings.
   4. Expect six to eight wet diapers and three to four yellow, seedy stools per day to ensure that infant is getting adequate amounts of milk.

■ **PREVENTIVE TREATMENT OR TESTS**
• Breastfeeding jaundice
   1. Provide patient education in the hospital about proper positioning, attachment, and detachment.
   2. Encourage early initiation and frequent opportunities to breastfeed.
   3. Avoid non–medically indicated supplemental feedings.
   4. Avoid pacifiers.

■ **REFERRAL INFORMATION**
• Lactation consultants (certified by the international board of lactation consultants [IBCLC]) can be helpful in managing lactation problems that may lead to breastfeeding jaundice.
• Consider early referral for the following problems:
   1. Maternal nipple or breast abnormalities

2. Maternal illness, stress, and/or fatigue
3. Maternal anxiety about breastfeeding
4. Multiple births
5. Infants with special needs (e.g., premature infants, those with Down syndrome)

☼ PEARLS & CONSIDERATIONS

■ CLINICAL PEARLS
- Infant bruising at birth, gestational age less than 37 weeks, maternal illness, or breast and nipple abnormalities may increase the risk of exaggerated physiologic hyperbilirubinemia.
- In these mother-infant dyads, attention to breastfeeding management, including early consultation with a lactation consultant, may help prevent breastfeeding jaundice.

■ WEBSITES
- Academy of Breastfeeding Medicine (ABM): cwebber@applmeapro.com
- American Academy of Pediatrics: www.aap.org/family/jaundice; treating jaundice in healthy newborns

- La Leche League International (LLLI): www.lalecheleague.org/
- San Diego County Breastfeeding Company: www.breastfeeding.org; an updated list of Internet sites with breastfeeding information

■ SUPPORT GROUP
The La Leche League International and WIC (Women, Infants, and Children) peer support programs provide mother-to-mother support for breastfeeding women.

REFERENCES
Standard
1. Lawrence RA: *Breastfeeding: a guide for the medical profession,* ed 5, St Louis, 1999, Mosby.
2. De Carvalho M, Robertson S, Klaus M: Fecal bilirubin excretion and serum bilirubin concentrations in breastfed and bottle-fed infants, *J Pediatr* 107: 786, 1985.
3. De Carvalho M, Klaus MH, Merkatz RB: Frequency of breastfeeding and serum bilirubin concentration, *Am J Dis Child* 136:737, 1982.
4. Gartner LM: Neonatal jaundice, *Pediatr Rev* 15:422, 1994.
5. Gartner LM: On the question of the relationship between breastfeeding and jaundice in the first 5 days of life, *Sem Perinatol* 18:502, 1994.
6. Maisels MJ, Newman TB: Kernicterus in otherwise healthy, breastfed term newborns, *Pediatrics* 95:730, 1995.
7. Martinez JC, Maisels MJ, Otheguy L et al: Hyperbilirubinemia in the breastfed newborn: a controlled trial of four interventions, *Pediatrics* 92: 470, 1993.

Practice Guidelines
1. American Academy of Pediatrics, Provisional Committee for Quality Improvement and Subcommittee on Hyperbilirubinemia Practice Parameter: Management of hyperbilirubinemia in the healthy term newborn [published erratum appears in *Pediatrics* 95:458, 1995] (see comments), *Pediatrics* 92:558, 1994.
2. Work Group on Breastfeeding: Breastfeeding and the use of human milk, *Pediatrics* 100:1035, 1997.

Author: **Cynthia Howard, M.D., M.P.H.**

II

BASIC INFORMATION

DEFINITION
Bulimia nervosa consists of episodic binges (large amounts of food and drink ingested in a brief period) followed by self-deprecating thoughts and a fear of gaining weight that result in behaviors intended to rid the body of the effects of the binge, including fasting and/or exercising (nonpurging subtype), vomiting, laxative or diuretic use (purging subtype).

SYNONYMS
Bulimia, although the term strictly applies to binge eating/drinking

ICD-9CM CODES
783.6   Polyphagia
307.51 Bulimia

DSM-IV CODE
307.51 Bulimia nervosa

ETIOLOGY
- Specific etiologic source is unknown; triggers vary for individual patients.
- Several risk factors may play a role in the onset of bulimia nervosa. These factors can include, but are not limited by, the following:
  1. Being female; if male, more likely athletic
  2. Familial predisposition, may be partially genetic
  3. Individual personality ("borderline") traits
  4. Societal thin ideal
  5. History of sexual abuse
  6. Overweight

EPIDEMIOLOGY & DEMOGRAPHICS
- Prevalence of bulimia nervosa in adolescents has increased during the past 50 years
- Approximately 90% to 95% of patients affected are female. Males are more likely to have bulimia nervosa than anorexia nervosa.
- Bulimia is more likely to develop in the late teens and early twenties, slightly later than anorexia nervosa.
- It is estimated that bulimia occurs in 1% to 2% of adolescents and young women, although various symptoms and a milder version of the disorder occur in 5% to 10% of young women.
- Most girls and women with eating disorders are white, although in recent years, the disorder has been increasing in minority women.

HISTORY
- Usually preceded by dieting behaviors

- Presence of negative feelings regarding body image and weight
- Personal and/or family history of substance abuse
- Personal history of sexual abuse

PHYSICAL SIGNS
- Salivary gland enlargement
- Subcutaneous and subconjunctival hemorrhage
- Chronic throat irritation
- Fatigue and muscular pain
- Loss of dental enamel without apparent cause
- Weight variations (as much as 10-kg fluctuation)
- Fluid and electrolyte imbalances (especially hypochloremic, hypokalemic metabolic alkalosis)
- Calluses and scars over the proximal interphalangeal joint (Russell sign) as a result of repetitive stimulation of the gag reflex
- Serious cardiac and/or skeletal muscle problems possible in individuals who regularly use syrup of ipecac to induce vomiting
- Menstrual irregularity or amenorrhea

AFFECTIVE SIGNS
- Change in mood (depressive symptoms or depression)
- Severe self-criticism
- Strong need for approval from others
- Self-esteem related closely to body weight
- Interpersonal relationship difficulties (either too close or too distant) and impulsivity

DIAGNOSIS

- Medical disorders or syndromes associated with weight fluctuation or vomiting can usually be ruled out by taking a detailed history focused on weight control methods (e.g., binge eating, fasting, vomiting, laxative or diuretic use, exercise).
- Psychiatric disorders should also be ruled out (e.g., depression, schizophrenia).
- A detailed physical examination is required, with special emphasis on cardiovascular stability and electrolyte status.
- There are no diagnostic laboratory studies.

DIFFERENTIAL DIAGNOSIS
- Anorexia nervosa
- Eating disorder, not otherwise specified (NOS)
- Kleine-Levin syndrome
- Depressive disorders
- Borderline personality disorder

DIAGNOSTIC WORKUP
- Comprehensive history and physical examination focused on weight-control methods are essential.
  1. Determine the relationship of moods to weight control.
  2. This is useful to detect physiologic status and any underlying physical and/or psychiatric disorders.
- Additional assessments should include nutritional and psychologic evaluations.

THERAPY

NONPHARMACOLOGIC
- Psychotherapy
  1. Cognitive-behavioral therapy is the most effective mode of treatment.
  2. It incorporates food diaries, self-control techniques, self-edification of affect and situations that provoke bingeing behavior, and positive reinforcement.
  3. This treatment also focuses on assisting the patient in changing his or her thoughts about eating, self-perceptions, and weight gain.
  4. Group, family, and interpersonal and insight-oriented therapies may also be useful.
- Additional treatment(s)
  1. Highly structured meal plans with regularly scheduled times to eat three to five times daily.
  2. Medical monitoring of physical health to validate seriousness of the condition and to enable early treatment of medical complications

PSYCHOPHARMACOLOGIC
- Most selective serotonin reuptake inhibitors (SSRIs) reduce the symptoms of bulimia nervosa, including in those who are not depressed clinically.
  1. Fluoxetine is the only SSRI approved by the U.S. Food and Drug Administration (FDA) for this purpose.
  2. SSRIs may be especially helpful for patients who have major depression, those who have significant obsessive-compulsive or anxiety symptoms, or patients who do not respond to other treatments.

PATIENT/FAMILY EDUCATION
- Biologic and emotional consequences of the disorder, as well as benefits from establishing a highly structured daily schedule, should be discussed.
- Patients should be given realistic information regarding treatment, resolution, and relapse.

■ PREVENTIVE TREATMENT

Participation in programs that promote healthy eating and activity habits, as well as positive self-esteem and weight acceptance

■ REFERRAL INFORMATION

- Referral to a mental health provider is imperative to effective treatment.
- Patients with eating disorders require an interdisciplinary approach to health care.
  1. The primary members of the team should include the primary care provider, an eating disorder specialist, a dietitian, and a counselor or therapist.
  2. Additional members could include a social worker and necessary medical consultants (e.g., dentist, gastroenterologist, cardiologist).

☼ PEARLS & CONSIDERATIONS

■ CLINICAL PEARLS

- Patients with bulimia nervosa often have an overwhelming sense of shame and guilt in addition to low self-esteem. Therefore they need an unusual amount of nonjudgmental support and encouragement from the professionals working with them.
- Focusing on the immediate medical consequences of their weight-control methods may help patients change their behaviors, especially if engaging in healthy alternative behaviors causes them to feel better (e.g., less tired, less cold, less weak, less fatigued).
- Because patients with bulimia nervosa have often experienced boundary transgressions in interpersonal relationships, they need care providers who are consistent and caring but who do not attempt to be controlling in their interactions.

■ WEBSITES

- American Academy of Child and Adolescent Psychiatry: www.aacap.org
- Eating Disorders Awareness and Prevention, Inc.: http://members.aol.com/edapinc/
- National Eating Disorders Organization: www.laureate.com
- National Institute of Mental Health: www.nimh.nih.gov/home.htm

REFERENCES

1. American Psychiatric Association: *Diagnostic and statistical manual of mental disorders,* ed 4, Washington, DC, 1994, American Psychiatric Association.
2. Steiner H, Lock J: Anorexia nervosa and bulimia nervosa in children and adolescents: a review of the past 10 years, *J Am Acad Child Adolesc Psych* 37:352, 1998.
3. Wolraich MI, Felice ME, Drotar D (eds): *The classification and adolescents mental diagnoses in primary care, diagnostic and statistical manual for primary care (DSM-PC),* Child and Adolescent Version, Elk Grove Village, Ill, 1996, American Academy of Pediatrics.

Authors: **Kathryn Castle, Ph.D., and Richard E. Kreipe, M.D.**

II

BASIC INFORMATION

■ DEFINITION
This is an infection caused by *Campylobacter jejuni;* it includes both diarrheal and systemic illnesses.

■ SYNONYM
Bacterial enterocolitis

ICD-9CM CODE
008.5 Bacterial enterocolitis

■ ETIOLOGY
Aerobic, motile, curve-shaped gram-negative rod

■ EPIDEMIOLOGY & DEMOGRAPHICS
- In the United States:
  1. *C. jejuni* is the most common cause of bacterial diarrhea.
  2. The peak ages of illness occur in children younger than 5 years old and in individuals 15 to 29 years old.
  3. *Campylobacter* infection occurs throughout the year, with outbreaks common in summer and early fall.
- *C. jejuni* causes acute enteritis after tissue invasion at the terminal ileum and colon.
- Sources of *C. jejuni* are undercooked poultry, unpasteurized milk, untreated water, and young household pets with diarrhea (e.g., puppies, kittens, hamsters, birds).
- The mode of transmission is ingestion of contaminated foods or water, fecal-oral spread, or direct contact with animal feces.

■ HISTORY
- The incubation period is 1 to 7 days.
- Acute onset of enteric illness occurs 2 to 4 days after exposure.
- Symptoms include diarrhea with visible or occult blood, crampy abdominal pain, malaise, and fever.
- Associated symptoms include vomiting, malaise, myalgia, and headache,

■ PHYSICAL EXAMINATION
- Abdominal pain in any quadrant
- Blood-streaked stools or hematochezia

DIAGNOSIS

■ DIFFERENTIAL DIAGNOSIS
- Bacterial diarrhea is also caused by *Salmonella, Shigella, Vibrio parahaemolyticus,* or invasive *Escherichia coli.*
- The clinical presentation may mimic appendicitis, ulcerative colitis, or Crohn's disease.

■ DIAGNOSTIC WORKUP
- Stool culture of *C. jejuni* may have to be specifically requested because growth of this organism requires selective media.
- The white blood cell (WBC) count can be normal or elevated, and the differential shows a left shift.
- A mild elevation in alanine aminotransferase and alkaline phosphatase is present in 25% of patients.
- Bacteremia is uncommon and occurs primarily in immunocompromised children.

THERAPY

In general, diarrheal episodes are mild and self-limited.

■ NONPHARMACOLOGIC
Symptomatic treatment is oral rehydration.

■ MEDICAL
- Antibiotic treatment shortens the convalescent period from 2 to 3 weeks to 2 to 3 days and helps prevent relapse of infection.
- A macrolide is the drug of choice. Erythromycin, azithromycin, and clarithromycin are all acceptable choices. The duration of treatment is 5 to 7 days.
- Alternative antibiotic choices are clindamycin, tetracycline for children 8 years and older, and fluoroquinolone for children 18 years and older. The duration of treatment is 5 to 7 days.
- If systemic illness is present, gentamicin, imipenem, or cefotaxime should be administered pending antibiotic-susceptibility results.

■ FOLLOW-UP & DISPOSITION
- Children are contagious for 2 to 3 days after antibiotic treatment is administered. Children not treated with antibiotics can shed *C. jejuni* in the stool for up to 5 to 7 weeks.
- Immunocompromised children may have prolonged, relapsing diarrheal episodes or extraintestinal infections, which include cholecystitis, urinary tract infection, pancreatitis, and meningitis.
- Complications are reported mainly in adolescents and young adults.
  1. Guillain-Barré syndrome results in neurologic symptoms that occur 1 to 3 weeks after diarrheal illness.
  2. Reactive arthritis is reported in 2% to 3% of individuals with *C. jejuni* enteritis.
     a. Arthritis typically involves multiple large joints.
     b. Onset of arthritis ranges from 3 to 40 days after diarrhea occurs. Joint symptoms usually resolve after 1 to 21 days without sequelae.
     c. An erythrocyte sedimentation rate (ESR) is elevated, but fever and leukocytosis are not usually present. Approximately 50% of patients are positive for HLA-B27.
     d. Synovial fluid is always sterile.
  3. Reiter's syndrome is reported in 2% to 3% of individuals with *C. jejuni* enteritis.
  4. Erythema nodosum is rare, but a few case reports have been noted in the literature.
  5. Septic arthritis is rare and is reported mainly in immunocompromised persons.

■ PATIENT/FAMILY EDUCATION
- Exclusion from child care/preschool
  1. Children should be kept home until 2 days after beginning antibiotic treatment or until they are asymptomatic, whichever is shorter.
  2. Because asymptomatic carriage is uncommon, a stool culture is not necessary unless a child is symptomatic.
- Hospitalized persons
  1. For non–toilet-trained persons, implement contact precautions for the duration of the illness.
- Occupational precautions
  1. Exclude symptomatic food-handlers, hospital employees, and child care personnel until symptoms resolve completely.
  2. Infected individuals may return to work as long as they are asymptomatic.
     a. Specific guidelines regarding the duration of an asymptomatic period before returning to work have not been outlined.
     b. A symptom-free period for 24 hours occurring after the start of antibiotic treatment is a reasonable time frame.
     c. Erythromycin eradicates *C. jejuni* from the stool within 2 to 3 days.
        (1) May not be symptom free until 3 to 4 days after beginning treatment with this antibiotic

■ PREVENTIVE TREATMENT
- Advise careful handwashing, especially after changing diapers and before food preparation.
- Cook all poultry thoroughly.
  1. Internal meat temperature should reach 170° F for breast meat and 180° F for thigh meat.

☼ PEARLS & CONSIDERATIONS

■ CLINICAL PEARLS

- Onset of diarrhea less than 16 hours after food exposure is more likely caused by *Staphylococcus aureus, Bacillus cereus,* or *Clostridium perfringens.*
- In developing countries, secretory diarrhea caused by *C. jejuni* is a more common presentation than inflammatory diarrhea.

■ WEBSITE

Foodborne Diseases Active Surveillance Network: www.cdc.gov/ncidoc/dbmc/foodnet

REFERENCES

1. *Campylobacter* infections. In Pickering LK (ed): *2000 Red Book: Report of the Committee on Infectious Diseases,* ed 25, Elk Grove Village, Ill, 2000, American Academy of Pediatrics.
2. Blaser MJ: *Campylobacter jejuni* and related species. In Mandell GL, Bennett JE, Dolin R (eds): *Principles and practices of infectious diseases,* ed 5, Philadelphia, 2000, Churchill Livingstone.
3. Ellis ME et al: *Campylobacter colitis* associated with erythema nodosum, *Br Med J* 285:937, 1982.
4. Johnsen K et al: HLA-B27 negative arthritis related to *Campylobacter jejuni* enteritis in three children and two adults, *Acta Med Scand* 214:165, 1983.
5. Michaels MG: *Campylobacter.* In Donowitz LG (ed): *Infection control in the child care center and preschool,* ed 4, Philadelphia, 1999, Lippincott Williams & Wilkins.
6. Peterson MC: Rheumatic manifestations of *Campylobacter jejuni* and *C. fetus* infections in adults, *Scand J Rheumatol* 23:167, 1994.
7. Ruiz-Palacios GM: *Campylobacter jejuni.* In Long SS, Pickering LK, Prober CG (eds): *Principles and practice of pediatric infectious diseases,* Edinburgh, London, 1997, Churchill Livingstone.

Author: **Lucia H. Lee, M.D.**

II

BASIC INFORMATION

DEFINITION

Diaper dermatitis is a superficial cutaneous infection caused by *Candida albicans* that results in a typical erythematous, vesiculopustular rash in the perineal area.

SYNONYMS

- Napkin thrush
- Skin thrush

ICD-9CM CODES

112.1 Candidiasis of vulva/vagina
112.2 Candidiasis of other urogenital sites
691.0 Diaper dermatitis

ETIOLOGY

- *C. albicans* is the predominant fungus responsible for candidal dermatitis.
- Acquisition occurs when the neonate contacts infected vaginal mucosa during passage through the birth canal.
- Gastrointestinal and fecal colonization occur as a result of transmission and lead to skin infection in the perineal area.
- Oropharyngeal candidiasis is often seen before the development of candidal diaper dermatitis.

EPIDEMIOLOGY & DEMOGRAPHICS

- The overall incidence among immunocompetent infants is high.
- Seventy-five percent of cases of neonatal candidal diaper dermatitis occur in the first week of life.
- The peak prevalence in young infants is during the second to fourth months of life.

HISTORY

Specific complaint of a red rash in the diaper area that has been unresponsive to barrier or lubricant diaper creams

PHYSICAL EXAMINATION

- Maceration of the anal mucosa and perianal skin is the first clinical sign.
- Perineal skin examination reveals erythematous, scaly papules that coalesce to characteristic well-defined weeping, eroded lesions with a scalloped border.
- The rash is evident in the intertriginous folds.
- Additional satellite vesicopustules extending beyond the intertriginous area are classic.
- African-American infants may exhibit marked hypopigmentation of lesions.

DIAGNOSIS

DIFFERENTIAL DIAGNOSIS

The diagnosis is usually obvious, especially if intertriginous involvement and satellite lesions are evident; however, the differential diagnosis for this rash is extensive and includes the following:

- Irritant dermatitis
- Psoriasis
- Seborrhea dermatitis
- Histiocytosis X (Letterer-Siwe disease)
- Nutritional abnormalities (zinc and biotin deficiencies)
- Bullous impetigo
- Congenital syphilis

DIAGNOSTIC WORKUP

- Ninety percent of patients will have *C. albicans* detected in their feces.
- KOH (potassium hydroxide) preparation (10% to 20% solution) of a lesion may reveal classic budding yeast with hyphae or pseudohypha.
- Routine stool culture or KOH preparations are unnecessary in the typical patient.

THERAPY

NONPHARMACOLOGIC:

- Prevention of moist, macerated skin is helpful in decreasing *C. albicans* virulence.
- Other helpful techniques include the following:
  1. Frequent diaper changes
  2. Air drying of infected perineal skin
  3. Avoidance of soap or alcohol-containing preparations in the perineal area (these damage the barrier properties of skin)
  4. Use of disposable paper diapers

MEDICAL

- Topical antifungal therapy is indicated.
  1. All agents demonstrate clinical cure rates of 80% to 90%.
  2. Most studies that evaluated the efficacy of these agents have methodologic shortcomings.
  3. Nystatin should be applied to the affected area at least three to four times per day for 2 days after the rash has cleared.
  4. Miconazole (2% cream) should be applied twice daily for 5 to 10 days.
  5. Clotrimazole (1% cream or lotion) should be applied twice daily for 5 to 10 days.
- Concomitant use of an oral antifungal agent may eradicate oral and gastrointestinal colonization.
  1. Supportive evidence for this approach is limited.

PEARLS & CONSIDERATIONS

CLINICAL PEARLS

- Cornstarch powder should be avoided because it is an excellent medium for *Candida*.
- Living *C. albicans* does not penetrate healthy tissues; therefore epidermal damage seen with candidal diaper dermatitis is caused by irritant yeast products and toxins that filter into inflamed skin after the organisms die and disintegrate. Once the inflammation has reached a peak, the KOH preparation will not reveal the organism.
- Beyond the neonatal period, *C. albicans* is a normal constituent of the intestinal flora.

REFERENCES

1. Edwards JE: *Candida* species. In Feigin RD, Cherry JD (eds): *Textbook of pediatric infectious diseases*, Philadelphia, 1998, WB Saunders.
2. Hoppe JE: Treatment of oropharyngeal candidiasis and candidal diaper dermatitis in neonates and infants: review and reappraisal, *Pediatr Infect Dis J* 16:885, 1997.

Author: **Kate Tigue, M.D.**

BASIC INFORMATION

■ DEFINITION
Oropharyngeal *Candida* is an infection of the oral mucosal surfaces secondary to *Candida albicans,* a fungus.

■ SYNONYM
Thrush

ICD-9CM CODES
771.7 Newborn thrush
112.0 Thrush

■ ETIOLOGY
- *Candida* species of fungi, especially *C. albicans,* is responsible for oropharyngeal candidiasis.
- Transmission of *C. albicans* to the infant occurs by two main methods:
  1. Acquisition from infected maternal vaginal mucosa during passage of the infant through the birth canal
  2. Acquisition during breast-feeding from the skin of the mother's breasts or hands or from imperfect sterilization of the babies' feeding bottles and nipples
- Nosocomial transmission occurs in 7% of neonates.
- Immaturity of neonatal and infant host defenses and incomplete establishment of normal orointestinal flora allow *C. albicans* to act in a pathogenic manner.

■ EPIDEMIOLOGY & DEMOGRAPHICS
- Overall incidence among immunocompetent infants is high.
- Thirty-five times more common in neonates of infected than noninfected mothers.
  1. From 25% to 35% of pregnant women infected with *Candida* are asymptomatic.
- Incubation period is 4 to 14 days.
- Oropharyngeal candidiasis is rare in the first week of life, and peak prevalence of colonization occurs in the second to fourth weeks of life.

■ HISTORY
- White spots or plaques in the mouth or on the gums, inner cheeks, palate, or tongue
- Inconsistent history of poor feeding or discomfort with feeding

■ PHYSICAL EXAMINATION
- Pearly white, irregular patches are seen on the mucosal surfaces, including the buccal mucosa, tongue, gums, and inner lips.
- Involvement of the soft palate, fauces, uvula, and tonsils is seen less commonly.
- Candidal diaper dermatitis (erythematous, scaly plaques involving the intertriginous areas with satellite lesions) may also be seen because oral candidal infection leads to gastrointestinal colonization and subsequent infection in most cases (see the section "*Candida,* Diaper Dermatitis").

DIAGNOSIS

■ DIFFERENTIAL DIAGNOSIS
The diagnosis is usually clinically apparent with little else in the differential diagnosis.

■ DIAGNOSTIC WORKUP
- Although positive culture rates in infants with oropharyngeal candidiasis approach 100%, routine fungal cultures are not indicated.
- Persistent thrush that is unresponsive to appropriately administered therapy should prompt consideration of immunosuppression and human immunodeficiency virus (HIV) infection, and serologic testing should be performed.

THERAPY

■ NONPHARMACOLOGIC
- Sterilization of all nipples and pacifiers is required to eliminate colonization with *C. albicans.*
- Careful handwashing is necessary to decrease transmission between mother and infant as well as to decrease nosocomial transmission.

■ MEDICAL
- Treatment modalities include oral antifungal agents with limited or no absorption from the gastrointestinal tract (i.e., Gentian violet, nystatin, amphotericin B, miconazole, and clotrimazole) and agents that are readily absorbed (i.e., flucytosine, ketoconazole, fluconazole, and itraconazole).
- In general, treatment of oropharyngeal candidiasis in infants without an underlying medical condition should center around the nonabsorbed drugs.
  1. Gentian violet (methylrosaniline) was first introduced in 1925 for the treatment of thrush and has moderate efficacy.
     a. The aqueous solution appears to be well tolerated, but prolonged use results in mucosal irritaton and ulceration.
     b. Gentian violet acts only in the mouth and will not eradicate *C. albicans* from the gastrointestinal tract.
     c. An obvious drawback to its use is the tendency to stain tissues and clothing.
  2. Nystatin is a polyene antifungal agent with broad antifungal activity.
     a. It is fungistatic against *C. albicans* and is fungicidal at higher concentrations.
     b. It can be used topically and orally with few harmful reactions.
        (1) Prolonged oral use may lead to nausea and vomiting.
     c. What constitutes an effective dose remains controversial.
        (1) 100,000 to 200,000 units three to five times per day
        (2) 1,000,000 units four or more times per day in severe cases
     d. One drawback is its inability to maintain contact with the infected mucosa.
     e. Clinical cure rates are 80% to 90%.
  3. Amphotericin B is an additional polyene antifungal agent with broad-spectrum antifungal activity.
     a. Recently commercially available in the United States as an oral suspension
     b. More active than nystatin against *C. albicans* in vitro
     c. 100 mg (1 ml) orally four times daily
        (1) Excellent or good therapeutic response in 86% of patients
     d. Systemic absorption of oral Amphotericin B is low.
  4. Miconazole is a first-generation imidazole antifungal agent.
     a. It is more active against *C. albicans* in vitro than nystatin.
     b. Miconazole oral gel (20 mg/g) is commercially available in many countries but not yet in the United States.
     c. The recommended dosage for infants is 25 mg four times per day.
        (1) The gel adheres well to oral mucosa.
        (2) Clinical cure rates of 96% to 100% have been reported.
  5. Clotrimazole is another first-generation imidazole derivative.
     a. It is used topically for vaginal and skin infections secondary to yeasts
        (1) May have a role in treatment of oropharyngeal candidiasis in infants
     b. Clotrimazole suppositories inserted into the tip of a slit

pacifier three to four times daily has been recommended.

(1) Clotrimazole has not been scientifically studied.

(2) In some countries, the agent is available as oral troches, but use in infants is limited because of its association with elevated liver enzymes.

6. Fluconazole is a fungistatic agent taken orally and absorbed well.

a. Cure rates for fluconazole are greater than those for nystatin, but relapse rates are comparable.

b. Fluconazoles not well studied in infants younger than 6 months old.

c. The suggested dosage is 3 to 6 mg/kg/day in a single dose for 14 days.

☼ PEARLS & CONSIDERATIONS

■ CLINICAL PEARLS

• In breast-fed infants with oropharyngeal candidiasis, do not forget to treat mother with topical antifungal on her breasts to eliminate transmission.

• Nystatin suspension contains high amounts of sucrose to mask its bitter taste.

1. High osmolality makes administration to premature infants inadvisable.

2. Amphotericin B does not contain sucrose and is tasteless.

REFERENCES

1. Feigin RD, Cherry JD: *Textbook of pediatric infectious diseases,* Philadelphia, 1998, WB Saunders.

2. Hoppe JE: Treatment of oropharyngeal candidiasis and candidal diaper dermatitis in neonates and infants: review and reappraisal, *Pediatr Infect Dis J* 16:885, 1997.

Author: **Kate Tigue, M.D.**

BASIC INFORMATION

■ **DEFINITION**
Dilated cardiomyopathy is dilation of the heart associated with cardiac dysfunction caused by myocardial disease. The other classes of cardiomyopathy include hypertrophic and restrictive.

■ **SYNONYMS**
- Cardiomyopathy
- Dilated cardiomyopathy
- Idiopathic dilated cardiomyopathy

ICD-9CM CODES
425.4 Idiopathic (encompasses all types)
Specific types of cardiomyopathy may be coded with extensions by cause (if known).

■ **ETIOLOGY**
The cause may be known or unknown, and any patient at any point in time may show characteristics of any given physiologic classification (e.g., hypertrophic cardiomyopathy progressively becomes dilated).
- Idiopathic: no cause identified, most common
- Primary myocardial
  1. Diseases related to energy creation or utilization abnormalities: fatty acid transport defects, carnitine deficiency, abnormalities in glucose utilization, defects in protein metabolism, mitochondrial dysfunction
  2. Disorders of lysosomal enzymes: mucopolysaccharidoses, mucolipidoses, glycoproteinoses, ceramidase deficiency, sphingomyelin lipidoses, glucosylceramide lipidoses, gangliosidosis
- Secondary myocardial
  1. Viral infections: Coxsackie A and B virus, echovirus, adenovirus, Epstein-Barr virus, cytomegalovirus, varicella-zoster virus, mumps, hepatitis B virus
  2. Septicemia
  3. Postmyocarditis
  4. Acquired immunodeficiency syndrome
  5. Nutritional: thiamin deficiency (beri-beri), protein deficiency (kwashiorkor), niacin deficiency (pellagra), selenium deficiency
  6. Endocrine: hypothyroidism, pheochromocytoma, hypoglycemia
  7. Neuromuscular: Duchenne's muscular dystrophy
  8. Autoimmune: systemic lupus erythematosus
  9. Drugs and toxins: radiation therapy, chemotherapy, catecholamines
  10. Other: Turner syndrome, Kawasaki disease, rheumatic fever, epidermolysis bullosa

■ **EPIDEMIOLOGY & DEMOGRAPHICS**
The true incidence and prevalence are not known, although epidemiologic studies are being completed.

■ **HISTORY**
- This condition may present as sudden death and be found incidentally by autopsy.
- Nonspecific history of recurrent respiratory illness is reported.
  1. Later found to be secondary to congestive heart failure producing pulmonary edema
- In infants and small children, pallor, lethargy, irritability, tachypnea, and sweating with feeding are seen.
- Poor growth occurs.
- Older children may manifest respiratory (reactive or obstructive airway disease) or gastroenterologic (early satiety, pain, nausea, vomiting) symptoms and easy fatigability.
- From 10% to 20% of patients present with high-grade arrhythmia.
- Syncope may occur or be a presenting symptom.
- Neurologic or seizure disorder may be reported.
- A nonspecific acute febrile illness may have occurred within 3 months of development of symptoms.

■ **PHYSICAL EXAMINATION**
- Signs of congestive heart failure: tachypnea, tachycardia, diaphoresis, pallor
- Hypotension or shock, poor peripheral perfusion
- Hepatomegaly and occasionally jugular venous distension
- Wheezing or crackles on lung auscultation
- Muffled or poor-quality heart sounds with S_3 or S_4
- Apical systolic murmur of mitral regurgitation

🔬 **DIAGNOSIS**

■ **DIFFERENTIAL DIAGNOSIS**
- Pericarditis
- Structural heart disease

■ **DIAGNOSTIC WORKUP**
- Chest radiograph may show enlarged cardiac silhouette or pulmonary venous congestion
- Electrocardiogram
  1. Nonspecific ST-T wave changes, in particular, inversion of the T waves and ST-segment depression, particularly in the precordial leads, but may occur throughout
  2. Diminished voltage, particularly in limb leads, or evidence for left ventricular hypertrophy
  3. Prolongation of the QT interval
  4. High-grade arrhythmia: ventricular ectopy
- Echocardiogram
  1. This is an accurate, rapid, and widely used technique for initial evaluation and monitoring of left ventricular function.
  2. Thin-walled, enlarged left ventricle with global dyskinesis is seen.
  3. Look for left ventricular thrombus secondary to poor cardiac contractility.
- Blood tests
  1. Nonspecific indicators for inflammation, such as leukocytosis and elevation of the sedimentation rate
  2. Mild or no elevation of the cardiac isoenzymes or troponin I or T
  3. Bacterial, viral, fungal cultures
  4. Serum electrolytes, blood urea nitrogen, and creatinine
  5. Human immunodeficiency virus antibody
  6. Thyroid studies
  7. Vitamin B and selenium levels
  8. Carnitine
- Cardiac catheterization evaluates myocardial function and hemodynamics.
  1. Look for structural problems, such as anomalous left coronary artery.
- Endomyocardial biopsy
  1. Cell counts
  2. Hematoxylin and eosin (H&E) stains
  3. Polymerase chain reactions to Coxsackie and adenoviruses (causes of myocarditis, which may culminate in dilated cardiomyopathy)
     a. Myocarditis may have a better prognosis.
     b. May affect listing for transplantation.
  4. Mitochondrial analysis

💊 **THERAPY**

■ **NONPHARMACOLOGIC**
If possible, place the patient on a low-salt diet and fluid restriction.

■ **MEDICAL**
- Anticongestive therapy: Digoxin and diuretics are still the mainstay of treatment.
- Afterload reduction: Angiotensin-converting-enzyme inhibitors are used.

II

- Support of myocardium and circulation in an acute care setting may be necessary.
  1. Inotropic or pressor support
  2. Intubation to reduce afterload on the heart
- Anticoagulants: Aspirin, warfarin, heparin, or low-molecular-weight heparin may be given.

■ **SURGICAL**
- Cardiac transplantation is considered when medical therapy has failed.
- Left ventricular-assist devices or extracorporeal membrane oxygenation may be necessary while awaiting transplantation

■ **FOLLOW-UP & DISPOSITION**
- The natural history of cardiomyopathy is not well known and is variable.
- Some patients are followed for years while taking anticongestive medications.
  1. Some may show spontaneous resolution of their disease.

2. Some have relentless progression despite maximal therapy.
- Patients who undergo cardiac transplantation are followed closely for the remainder of their lives.

■ **PATIENT/FAMILY EDUCATION**
- Educate the patient and family about familial occurrence of cardiac disease and sudden death.
- Infants and children with dysmorphology or genetic syndromes should undergo cardiac evaluation.
- Infants and children with known neuromuscular disease should be followed by a cardiologist.

■ **REFERRAL INFORMATION**
Regular follow-up with a cardiologist is important.

☼ PEARLS & CONSIDERATIONS

■ **WEBSITES**
- Boston University: www.bu.edu/cohis/cardiovasc/heart/c_diltd.html

- drkoop.com: www.drkoop.com/adams/peds/top/000147.html
- Health Answers: www.healthanswers.com/database/ami/converted/000168.html
- MedWeb Plus: www.medwebplus.com/subjects/Discussion_groups/Myocardial_Disease.html

REFERENCES
1. Chan DP, Allen HD: Dilated cardiomyopathy. In Emmanoillides GC et al (eds): *Heart disease in infants, children and adolescents: including the fetus and young adult,* Baltimore, 1995, Williams & Wilkins.
2. Colan SD et al: Cardiomyopathies. In Fyler DC (ed): *Nadas' pediatric cardiology,* Philadelphia, 1992, WB Saunders.
Author: **Michelle A. Grenier, M.D.**

BASIC INFORMATION

■ DEFINITION

A cataract is an opacity of the lens, which may be present at birth or evolve over time.

■ ICD-9CM CODE

743.30 Cataract—congenital, unspecified

■ ETIOLOGY

- In an otherwise healthy child, a cause may be elusive.
- Common causes include the following:
  1. Intrauterine infection
     a. TORCH (toxoplasmosis, rubella, cytomegalovirus, or herpes)
     b. Varicella-zoster virus
  2. Chromosomal abnormalities
     a. Hereditary—autosomal dominant is most common
     b. Down syndrome, trisomy 13, trisomy 15, Lowe syndrome, Marfan's syndrome
  3. Metabolic syndromes
     a. Galactosemia, Fabry's disease, homocystinuria

■ EPIDEMIOLOGY & DEMOGRAPHICS

For bilateral cataracts:
- One third are inherited, usually in an autosomal-dominant fashion but can be autosomal recessive or X-linked.
- One third are associated with other disorders, either chromosomal abnormalities or metabolic disorders.
- One third have an unknown cause.

■ HISTORY

- Visual function
  1. Does infant turn to face?
  2. Does infant track?
  3. Do eyes move together?
  4. Do eyes align?
  5. Are eyes symmetric?
- Family history of cataracts in childhood
- Medications or illegal substances used during pregnancy
- Infections during pregnancy

■ PHYSICAL EXAMINATION

- Assess visual function.
  1. Test tracking and fixation if nonverbal.
  2. If older and verbal, use acuity testing.
  3. *Test each eye separately,* and be diligent to observe for peeking.
- Observe alignment. If any abnormality is present, suspect visual impairment.
- A thorough newborn examination may lead to a constellation of physical findings that suggest a chromosomal abnormality or metabolic disorder.
- Development of cataracts during childhood may be familial, and examination of parents and siblings may be helpful.
  1. Look for a familial pattern or physical findings such as aniridia.
  2. Childhood cataracts may be associated with use of medications (e.g., corticosteroids) or systemic diseases of childhood (e.g., juvenile rheumatoid arthritis).

DIAGNOSIS

- The diagnosis is usually made on physical examination; often seen during well-child examinations. Shining a bright direct ophthalmoscope into both eyes:
  1. Look for bright symmetric red reflex.
  2. Any shadow or dark spot in the red reflex suggests a cataract or other lens abnormality.
- Look for associated physical findings of various genetic syndromes and metabolic disorders.

THERAPY

- Treatment for visually significant cataracts is surgical removal of the lens and sometimes implantation of an intraocular lens.
- Surgical intervention should be undertaken within the first 6 to 8 weeks of life for congenital cataracts.
- Visual rehabilitation may include use of aphakic spectacles or contact lenses.
- Diligent evaluation of visual acuity should be continued.
- Management of amblyopia should be initiated, if necessary.

■ FOLLOW-UP & DISPOSITION

- Infants and children who are believed to have decreased vision and/or a cataract should be immediately referred to an ophthalmologist for a complete evaluation.
- Children with a history of cataracts should have follow-up by an ophthalmologist for amblyopia and the development of other ocular disorders, such as glaucoma.

■ PATIENT/FAMILY EDUCATION

- Family members must be informed that visual prognosis is guarded, even if the cataract is successfully removed.
  1. Family members must be involved with careful follow-up and management of visual development.
- Development of amblyopia is a real concern until at least 8 or 9 years of age.
- Other ocular disorders, such as glaucoma, occur with greater frequency in children with cataracts.

PEARLS & CONSIDERATIONS

Cataracts can occasionally be caused by trauma, and in children with other signs of trauma, child abuse should be suspected.

■ SUPPORT GROUPS

- National Association of Parents of the Visually Impaired, 800-562-6265
- National Association for the Visually Handicapped, 22 West 21 St., New York, NY 10010, 212-889-3141

REFERENCES

1. Childhood cataracts and other pediatric lens disorders. In *Pediatric ophthalmology and strabismus*, Basic and Clinical Science Course, San Francisco, 1998-1999, American Academy of Ophthalmology.
2. Lambert S: Lens. In Taylor D (ed): *Pediatric ophthalmology*, ed 2, Boston, 1997, Blackwell Science.
3. Robb RM: Congenital and childhood cataracts. In Albert DM, Jakobiec FA (eds): *Principles and practice of ophthalmology*, Philadelphia, 1994, WB Saunders.

Author: **Anna F. Fakadej, M.D., F.A.A.O.**

II

BASIC INFORMATION

■ DEFINITION
Cat-scratch disease (CSD) is a subacute to chronic regional lymphadenitis syndrome that occurs after cutaneous, ocular, or mucous membrane inoculation in a person who has contact with a cat.

■ SYNONYM
Cat-scratch fever

■ ICD-9CM CODE
078.3 Cat-scratch disease

■ ETIOLOGY
Bartonella henselae, a fastidious, pleomorphic, gram-negative bacillus

■ EPIDEMIOLOGY & DEMOGRAPHICS
- There are 22,000 to 24,000 cases per year in the United States (9.3 per 100,000 population).
- Approximately 2000 patients are hospitalized per year in the United States (0.77 to 0.86 per 100,000 hospital discharges).
- Distribution is worldwide, but it is most prevalent in warm and humid climates.
- The incidence is more common in fall and winter (60% of cases identified from September to January).
- Fifty percent of patients are younger than 15 years of age.

■ HISTORY
- The person has had contact with a cat, especially kittens.
- A papule or pustule at the site of the scratch precedes the appearance of regional lymphadenopathy by 1 to 6 weeks in 60% to 93% of patients.
- Patients may have constitutional symptoms, including fatigue (30%), headache (14%), anorexia or weight loss (15%), or sore throat (9%).

■ PHYSICAL EXAMINATION
- Gradual enlargement of a single, tender lymph node is observed in 80% of patients (20% have multiple node enlargement).
- Most nodes (80%) are between 1 to 5 cm in size and appear on the head, neck, or upper extremity.
- A papule or pustule at a distal site is drained by the enlarged node.
- Fever is usually absent or low grade (10% with temperature higher than 39° C)
- From 10% to 15% of nodes spontaneously suppurate, but most resolve over 2 to 6 months.

- Atypical presentations include encephalopathy with seizures, hepatosplenic granulomas, multiple bone lesions, or Parinaud's oculoglandular syndrome (conjunctival granuloma with ipsilateral preauricular adenopathy).

🔬 DIAGNOSIS

- Initially, a clinical diagnosis is based on appropriate symptoms and a history of exposure to a cat or kitten.
- The diagnosis is confirmed by serology.

■ DIFFERENTIAL DIAGNOSIS
- Bacterial adenitis
- Infectious mononucleosis
- Toxoplasmosis
- *Mycobacteria* infection
- Cytomegalovirus infection
- Lymphoma/malignancy

■ DIAGNOSTIC WORKUP
- Serologic diagnosis is the test of choice (indirect immunofluorescence assay or enzyme immunoassay) with a positive titer of more than 1:64 for immunoglobulin G (IgG) or more than 1:20 for immunoglobulin M (IgM).
- Lymph node biopsy reveals scattered granulomas with central necrosis and abscess formation.
- Routine culture and Gram stain of *B. henselae* are very technically difficult.
- Polymerase chain reaction test is available for research only.

℞ THERAPY

■ NONPHARMACOLOGIC
Local care, including the application of moist heat to an enlarged node or nodes

■ MEDICAL
Azithromycin 10 mg/kg on day 1 then 5 mg/kg on days 2 to 5 decreases lymph node size faster than a placebo.

■ SURGICAL
A few patients require needle aspiration for drainage and relief of symptoms or complete removal of the involved node or nodes.

■ FOLLOW-UP & DISPOSITION
Gradual and spontaneous resolution of lymphadenopathy over 2 to 6 months is the rule.

■ PATIENT/FAMILY EDUCATION
- Approximately 28% of cats have evidence of past or present infection with *B. henselae.*
- Cat infection is correlated with fleas.
- There is no known person-to-person transmission of CSD.

■ REFERRAL INFORMATION
Children can be cared for by their primary care pediatrician or a pediatric infectious diseases expert.

⚙ PEARLS & CONSIDERATIONS

■ CLINICAL PEARLS
- Examine the web spaces between the fingers for an inoculation papule in a patient with lymphadenopathy of the upper extremity.
- Always consider CSD in the differential diagnosis of seizures, encephalopathy, or combative behavior and inquire about a history of cat contact while examining the patient closely for an inoculation papule or lymphadenopathy.

■ WEBSITES
- Association of State and Territorial Directors of Health Promotion and Public Health Education: www. astdhpphe.org/infect/catscratch.html (for health professionals)
- ParentsPlace.com: www.parentsplace. com/expert/pediatrician/general/qa/ 0,3459,1011,00.html (for parents)

REFERENCES
1. Bass JW, Vincent JM, Person DA: The expanding spectrum of *Bartonella* infections: II, cat-scratch disease, *Pediatr Infect Dis J* 16:163, 1997.
2. Bass JW et al: Prospective randomized double blind placebo-controlled evaluation of azithromycin for treatment of cat-scratch disease, *Pediatr Infect Dis J* 17:447, 1998.
3. Carithers HA: Cat-scratch disease: an overview based on a study of 1,200 patients, *Am J Dis Child* 139:1124, 1985.
4. Jackson LA, Perkins BA, Wenger JD: Cat scratch disease in the United States: an analysis of three national databases, *Am J Public Health* 12:1707, 1993.
5. Klein JD: Cat scratch disease, *Pediatr Rev* 9:348, 1994.
6. Margileth AM: Antibiotic therapy for cat-scratch disease: clinical study of therapeutic outcome in 268 patients and a review of the literature, *Pediatr Infect Dis J* 11:474, 1992.
Author: **Mary Caserta, M.D.**

BASIC INFORMATION

■ DEFINITION
Celiac disease is permanent intestinal intolerance to dietary gluten (wheat gliadin and related proteins), which produces a characteristic mucosal lesion in the proximal small bowel in genetically susceptible individuals.

■ SYNONYMS
- Gluten-sensitive enteropathy
- Celiac sprue
- Nontropical sprue

ICD-9CM CODE
579 Celiac disease

■ ETIOLOGY
- Interaction with cereal proteins, including wheat, rye, and barley, is toxic to the small bowel mucosa. The toxicity of oats is controversial.
- Genetically, the strongest association of celiac disease is with the HLA class II D region markers (chromosome 6).
- Other environmental factors may play a role.
  1. Breastfeeding (has protective effect)
  2. Type and amount of cereals introduced
  3. Infective (particularly viral) factors
- The result of interaction of the toxic proteins in susceptible individuals is immunologically mediated damage to the small bowel mucosa, resulting in malabsorption.
- The target antigen has been identified as tissue transglutaminase (TTG), which is also the endomysial antigen recognized by the anti-endomysial IgA antibody (see "Diagnostic Workup").

■ EPIDEMIOLOGY & DEMOGRAPHICS
- The prevalence of symptomatic celiac disease is 1 in 1000 live births, ranging from 1 in 250 to 1 in 4000.
- The incidence is higher in Europe than in the United States, even among individuals with similar genetic backgrounds.
  1. Countries with the highest incidence are Sweden, the British Isles, and Italy.
- Celiac disease can be clinically silent; therefore the prevalence may be underestimated.
  1. Results of serologic screening of healthy blood donors in the United States suggest that the prevalence is actually similar to that in Europe.
- There also appears to be varied prevalence by age as well as by geography. This may be related to environmental factors such as infant feeding practices, lower antigenicity of formulas, and later introduction of gluten.
  1. Probably changes clinical presentation, not incidence
- Symptoms usually present between 1 and 5 years of age, but there is considerable variation in the age of onset.
- Prevalence appears to be slightly higher in women than in men.
- There is a strong association with dermatitis herpetiformis.
- A higher incidence exists in children with Down syndrome and IgA deficiency.
- A higher frequency of other autoimmune disorders occurs in individuals with celiac disease.
  1. Thyroid disease, Addison's disease, type 1 diabetes mellitus
  2. Pernicious anemia, autoimmune thrombocytopenia
  3. Sarcoidosis
  4. Alopecia
- Celiac disease is also associated with an increased risk of small bowel lymphomas.

■ HISTORY
- The presentation varies considerably, and the disease can be clinically silent.
- The classic history in an infant or toddler is onset of diarrhea (malabsorptive stools), irritability, anorexia, and poor weight gain after the introduction of cereals into the diet.
  1. Malabsorptive stools (steatorrhea) are bulky, foul smelling, greasy, "float in toilet."
- History in childhood is that of intermittent abdominal discomfort, variable stool pattern (from diarrhea to constipation), short stature, joint pains, and delayed puberty.
- Ethnic background is typically Western European.
- A family history of celiac disease may be reported.
- For associated conditions with an increased incidence of celiac disease, see "Epidemiology & Demographics."

■ PHYSICAL EXAMINATION
- Evidence of malnutrition
  1. Crossing weight and then height percentiles
  2. Muscle wasting in the extremities and buttocks
  3. Abdominal distension
  4. Finger clubbing
- Short stature

DIAGNOSIS

■ DIFFERENTIAL DIAGNOSIS
- Cystic fibrosis
- Postenteritis enteropathy
- Food protein allergies (milk, soy, wheat)
- Chronic giardiasis

■ DIAGNOSTIC WORKUP
- Serologic studies are excellent screening tests for celiac disease.
  1. Antigliadin antibodies (IgA, IgG)
  2. Antireticulin antibodies (IgA)
  3. Antiendomysial antibodies (IgA)
  4. Anti-TTG antibodies (IgA): not yet widely commercially available
- IgG antigliadin is more sensitive but less specific (can have false-positive results).
- IgA antibodies are more specific but less sensitive (can have false-negative results).
- Quantitative IgA should also be obtained because there is an increased incidence of IgA deficiency in association with celiac disease and IgA antibodies are the most specific serologic test. Coincident IgA deficiency would invalidate these tests.
- Small bowel biopsy while ingesting wheat products is still recommended.
  1. Villous atrophy, crypt hyperplasia, inflammatory cell infiltration of the lamina propria, intraepithelial lymphocytes
- A typical biopsy, along with a clinical response to a gluten-free diet, is required to make the diagnosis of celiac disease.
- Repeat biopsy after initiating a gluten-free diet is considered necessary only if complete clinical remission does not occur.
- Other potential laboratory abnormalities include the following:
  1. Iron deficiency anemia
  2. Low serum carotene
  3. Elevated transaminases
  4. Increased fecal fat (qualitative and quantitative)

THERAPY

- Gluten-free diet is essential (lifelong).
- Some children may have other secondary dietary protein intolerances, particularly to milk and/or soy, and these may need to be restricted for a period as well.
- Attention must be paid to the child's overall nutritional state until the intestinal mucosa has healed and malabsorption has been corrected.

II

■ REFERRAL INFORMATION

- All patients should be referred to a (pediatric) gastroenterologist to confirm the diagnosis with an intestinal biopsy.
- Seeking a nutritionist with experience in gluten-free diets as a resource to families is recommended.

■ PATIENT/FAMILY EDUCATION

- This is a lifelong condition, and the diet should be adhered to even when the patient is asymptomatic.
- Strict adherence to a gluten-free diet decreases the incidence of the following conditions:
  1. Small bowel lymphomas
  2. Nutritional deficiencies
  3. Other autoimmune disease
- The mortality rate for individuals diagnosed with celiac disease in childhood and who adhere to appropriate dietary restrictions appears to be similar to the general population.

✺ PEARLS & CONSIDERATIONS

■ CLINICAL PEARLS

- Celiac disease can be clinically silent, so a high index of suspicion must be maintained in the appropriate setting.
- Laboratory screening for celiac disease consists of quantitative IgA, antigliadin (IgA, IgG), and antiendomysial (IgA) antibodies.
  1. A quantitative IgA should always be obtained, along with serologies.
- Screening serologic tests are excellent, but small bowel biopsy is still needed for definitive diagnosis.

■ SUPPORT GROUPS

Celiac Sprue Association/USA, Inc., 402-558-0600; fax: 402-558-1347; email: celiacs@csaceliacs.org; website: csaceliacs.org. Local support groups can also be identified.

REFERENCES

1. Hill I et al: The prevalence of celiac disease in at-risk groups of children in the United States, *J Pediatr* 136:86, 2000.
2. Murray JA: The widening spectrum of celiac disease, *Am J Clin Nutr* 69:354, 1999.
3. Victoria JC: Antibodies to gliadin, endomysium and tissue transglutaminase for the diagnosis of celiac disease, *J Pediatr Gastroenterol Nutr* 29:571, 1999.

Author: **M. Susan Moyer, M.D.**

BASIC INFORMATION

■ DEFINITION

- *Cellulitis* refers to a group of infections of the subcutaneous tissue, with an additional involvement of the dermis. Other superficial infections of the epidermis, such as impetigo, folliculitis, furunculosis, and hidradenitis, do not fall under the rubric of cellulitis.
- Erysipelas is a specific form of superficial cellulitis caused by group A β-hemolytic streptococci.
- Cellulitis is classified by body area: periorbital, orbital, buccal, extremity, and so forth.
- Periorbital (preseptal) cellulitis is an infection of the soft tissues superficial to the orbital septum. It does not involve the eye or the orbital contents.

ICD-9CM CODE
682.9 Cellulitis and periorbital cellulitis

■ ETIOLOGY

- Cellulitis is generally associated with previous skin trauma, such as scratches, insect bites, or lacerations, but the inoculation site may be small and often overlooked.
- The most common etiologic agents are *Staphylococcus aureus*, group A β-hemolytic streptococcus, *Streptococcus pneumoniae*, and *Haemophilus influenzae* type B (HIB) (declining incidence with routine childhood immunization).
- *Pseudomonas aeruginosa* and other gram-negative bacilli may be present in immunocompromised patients.
- Buccal cellulitis in neonates may be caused by *H. influenzae* or group B streptococcus.
  1. Group B streptococci may cause a facial cellulitis in infants that is associated with fever, poor feeding, irritability, and facial or submandibular swelling.
- Periorbital cellulitis is caused by bacterial infection from bacteremia, extension from paranasal sinusitis, or extension from a localized eyelid infection.
  1. The most common pathogens include *S. aureus, S. pneumoniae, Streptococcus pyogenes* (group A), and anaerobes. *H. influenzae* can also be a pathogen.
- Cat-bite cellulitis is most often caused by *Pasteurella multocida* and *S. aureus.*

■ EPIDEMIOLOGY & DEMOGRAPHICS

- The most common cause of cellulitis in children is a trauma-induced skin lesion with secondary bacterial infection.
- Both cellulitis and periorbital cellulitis from hematogenous spread have declined since the advent of the HIB vaccine.
- Most patients with periorbital cellulitis are younger than 5 years old.
- Ninety-five percent of periorbital cellulitis is unilateral.

■ HISTORY

- History of local trauma (e.g., abrasion, insect sting) may be reported.
- Red, painful, and expanding area with a poorly defined border is observed.
- Malaise, fever, and chills may be present.
- More than 75% of patients with periorbital cellulitis are febrile.
- For periorbital cellulitis, the patient sometimes has a history of trauma to the affected eye, with or without evidence of local wound infection.
- It is important to obtain an immunization history because a child who has received his or her second HIB vaccine more than 1 week before infection is unlikely to have HIB disease.

■ PHYSICAL EXAMINATION

- Erythema, warmth, tenderness, and edema are noted. Tenderness is usually marked.
- Regional lymphadenopathy is common.
- Lymphangitic streaking may extend from distal extremity lesions.
- In periorbital cellulitis, the eyelid is swollen, red, and tender, and it may have a violaceous hue.
  1. Proptosis, decreased eye movement, and pain on movement are absent in periorbital cellulitis.
  2. In periorbital cellulitis, fever is present 75% of the time, otitis occurs in 25% of patients younger than 2 years old, and signs of local trauma or infection occur in 33% of cases.
  3. The eyelid must be retracted to rule out the presence of a foreign body.

DIAGNOSIS

■ DIFFERENTIAL DIAGNOSIS

- Infectious: erysipelas, impetigo, staphylococcal scalded skin syndrome, folliculitis, furunculosis, hidradenitis, septic emboli (endocarditis, *Neisseria meningitidis*)
- Traumatic contusions
- Contact dermatitis
- Popsicle panniculitis
- Allergic swelling, angioedema
- Periorbital swelling with retinoblastoma, metastatic neuroblastoma, rhabdomyosarcoma, or rupture of a dermoid cyst
- Insect bite with local reaction

■ DIAGNOSTIC WORKUP

- Obtain a blood culture and complete blood count (CBC), and consider aspiration of the central, most inflamed area most likely to yield the etiologic agent; in erysipelas, the advancing margin is distinct and more likely to yield a pathogen. (Use a 20- or 22-gauge needle on a 3-ml syringe.)
- The blood culture is usually negative with *Staphylococcus* and *Streptococcus* infections but positive with HIB infection.
- Because cellulitis may extend to and involve subjacent structures, it can be associated with osteomyelitis or septic arthritis. Radiographs or joint aspirations should be obtained as deemed appropriate.
- In periorbital cellulitis, bacteremia typically occurs in children younger than 2 years of age, with a white blood cell (WBC) count greater than $15,000/mm^3$.
- Lumbar puncture is indicated in children younger than 1 year of age with periorbital cellulitis if any suspicion of meningitis exists or if the child has an inadequate HIB vaccine status.
- Computed tomography scans of the orbits should be done if orbital cellulitis is a concern.
- Cultures of conjunctival or nasopharyngeal swab specimens are not helpful in periorbital cellulitis.

THERAPY

■ MEDICAL

- Empiric therapy is usually initiated before laboratory results are available.
- Coverage for both *Staphylococcus* and *Streptococcus* should be administered with an antistaphylococcal penicillin or a first-generation cephalosporin.
- In immunocompromised patients, efforts should be made to identify an etiologic agent.
  1. Empiric coverage for *Pseudomonas* and enteric gram-negative organisms
  2. Aminoglycoside plus third-generation cephalosporin
- If *H. influenza* is suspected (i.e., hematogenous dissemination in an unvaccinated child), an appropriate agent such as cefotaxime or cefuroxime should be used.
- In periorbital cellulitis, antibiotics should be β-lactamase resistant and cover *H. influenzae* as well as *Staphylococcus* and *Streptococcus.*
  1. If patients are nontoxic and have no signs of orbital involvement, they may be followed as outpatients after a dose of a parenteral third-generation cephalosporin.

II

2. If follow-up cannot be ensured, admission is mandatory.

■ SURGICAL

Deeper infections or suspected abscesses may need to be surgically drained.

■ FOLLOW-UP & DISPOSITION

- Improvement should occur rapidly.
- Complications of periorbital cellulitis may occur with direct extension to the orbit or with development of bacteremia accompanied by sepsis or meningitis.
- Periorbital infections should be seen daily until clinical resolution is evident and blood cultures are negative at 48 hours.

■ PATIENT/FAMILY EDUCATION

Improvement should occur in 24 to 48 hours.

■ PREVENTIVE TREATMENT

- Good local wound care for skin abrasions and injuries can prevent many cases of cellulitis.

- All wounds should be cleansed with soap and water and covered with a clean, dry cloth or bandage.

■ REFERRAL INFORMATION

- An ophthalmology evaluation is indicated if any question of orbital involvement exists.
- Hospitalization is necessary for orbital cellulitis.

PEARLS & CONSIDERATIONS

■ CLINICAL PEARLS

- Cellulitis tends to occur on the extremities because of its association with trauma.
- HIB infection is rare in this era of HIB vaccination.
- Eczema may predispose patients to recurrent infections.
- *P. aeruginosa* can cause toe web infections, green nail syndrome, and otitis externa.

- Infections of the malar region of the face may be confused with lupus erythematosus.
- Blistering distal dactylitis is an uncommon form of cellulitis in children caused by *S. pyogenes* involving the volar fat pads of the distal phalanx.
- Up to 80% of cat bites become infected and should be treated at the first sign of erythema.

REFERENCES

1. Feigin RD, Cherry JD: *Textbook of pediatric infectious diseases,* ed 3, Philadelphia, 1992, WB Saunders.
2. Moschella SL, Hurley HJ: *Dermatology,* ed 3, Philadelphia, 1992, WB Saunders.
3. Powell KR: Orbital and periorbital cellulitis, *Pediatr Rev* 16:163, 1995.

Author: **Frank Magill, M.D.**

BASIC INFORMATION

■ DEFINITION

Cerebral palsy (CP) is a group of disorders of movement and posture caused by a nonprogressive lesion of the developing brain. Clinical features change over time, although the lesion does not (Table 2-4).

■ SYNONYMS

- CP
- Spastic diplegia
- Spastic paraplegia
- Spastic hemiplegia
- Spastic quadriplegia

ICD-9CM CODES

343.0 Diplegic
343.1 Hemiplegic
343.2 Quadriplegic
343.3 Monoplegic
343.8 Other specified infantile cerebral palsy
343.9 Infantile cerebral palsy, unspecified

■ ETIOLOGY

- Unknown in many cases
- Risk factors
  1. Preterm delivery (less than 32 weeks) or low birth weight (less than 2001 g)
  2. Intraventricular hemorrhage and periventricular leukomalacia
  3. Significant perinatal asphyxia: low 15- or 20-minute Apgar score
  4. Head trauma in infancy or early childhood
     a. Stroke
     b. Intracranial bleeding
     c. Shaken baby syndrome
  5. Near-drowning, asphyxia, hypoxemia, smoke inhalation
  6. Infection
     a. Perinatal: toxoplasmosis, rubella, cytomegalovirus (CMV) or herpes (TORCH)
     b. Neonatal meningitis
     c. Childhood meningitis and encephalitis
  7. Multiple gestation
  8. Genetic predisposition of unknown inheritance pattern
  9. Hyperbilirubinemia historically more common

■ EPIDEMIOLOGY & DEMOGRAPHICS

- Prevalence is 1.5 to 2.5 per 1000 live births.
- Incidence is up to 5 children per 1000 live births.

■ HISTORY

- Delayed or deviant acquisition of motor milestones (gestation corrected)
- Handedness before 12 months (Infants do not typically cross midline to reach object before 12 months.)
- Toe walking
- Abnormal movements
- No regression of milestones
- Parental concern
- History of a risk factor

■ PHYSICAL EXAMINATION

- Persistent primitive reflexes or delay in acquisition of protective responses (Table 2-5)

TABLE 2-4 Types of Cerebral Palsy

PYRAMIDAL (MOTOR CORTEX, INTERNAL CAPSULE, CORTICAL SPINAL TRACT)	EXTRAPYRAMIDAL (BASAL GANGLIA, THALAMUS, SUBTHALAMIC NUCLEUS, CEREBELLUM)
Spastic diplegia: LE involvement greater than UE involvement	Athetoid: slow, writhing movements
Spastic hemiplegia: unilateral involvement	Chorea: quick, jerky movements
Spastic paraplegia: LE only	Choreoathetoid: combination of above
Spastic quadriplegia: involvement of all extremities	Ataxic: tremor, wide-based gait
	Hypotonic: floppy
	Dystonic: lead pipe rigidity with movement

LE, Lower extremity; *UE*, upper extremity.

TABLE 2-5 Normal Reflex Development and Loss

REFLEX	1 mo	2 mo	3 mo	4 mo	6 mo	9 mo	12 mo	15 mo	18 mo	24 mo	36 mo
Palmar grasp	+	+	+/–	+/–	0	0	0	0	0	0	0
ATNR	+	+	+/–	+/–	0	0	0	0	0	0	0
Moro	+	+	+/–	+/–	0	0	0	0	0	0	0
Rooting	+	+	+	+	+	+/–	0	0	0	0	0
Neck righting	0	0	0	+/–	+/–	+	+	+	+	+	+
Parachute	0	0	0	0	+/–	+	+	+	+	+	+
Landau	0	0	0	0	0	+	+	+	+	+/–	0

ATNR, Asymmetric tonic neck reflex.

- Asymmetry in neurologic examination
- Tone: increased, decreased anterior scarf sign, lead pipe rigidity
- Fluctuation in tone during first year of life
- Deep tendon reflexes (DTRs) (brisk = long tract sign); may not be increased early in life
- Toe walking
- Persistent fisting after 3 months of age
- Log-roll: babies should roll segmentally
- Scissoring of the lower extremities after 2 months

DIAGNOSIS

■ DIFFERENTIAL DIAGNOSIS
- A progressive disorder of the neurologic system
- Normal variant (e.g., toe walking)

■ DIAGNOSTIC WORKUP
- CP is difficult to diagnose before 1 year of age and in some cases before 2 years.
- Diagnosis is based on the history and physical examination.

- A brain magnetic resonance imaging (MRI) scan can be normal or can show evidence of hypoxic insult.
  1. Scarring, gliosis
  2. Periventricular leukomalacia
- Metabolic workup is necessary if ataxic form is present and MRI and birth history are unrevealing.
  1. Type 1 glutaric aciduria
  2. Propionic acidemia
  3. Some forms of 3-methylglutaconic aciduria
- Skull radiograph or computed tomography scan in microcephalic children may show calcifications with congenital CMV infection.
- A hearing test should be performed.
- The child should be evaluated by an ophthalmologist.
- An electroencephalogram should be taken if seizures are suspected.
- If in utero stroke is suspected, consider a workup for coagulopathy.

THERAPY

■ PREVENTIVE TREATMENT
- Prevention of preterm delivery and low birth weight may lead to some decrease.

- Continued efforts to vaccinate against infection and prenatally acquired infections are ongoing.
- Continued monitoring and intervention for jaundice are helpful.
- It is unknown how to prevent most cases.
- For further treatment, follow-up, and referral considerations, see Table 2-6.

PEARLS & CONSIDERATIONS

■ WEBSITES
- American Academy for Cerebral Palsy and Developmental Medicine: www.links2go.com/mor/
- United Cerebral Palsy: www.UCPA.org

REFERENCES
1. Eicher P, Batshaw M: Cerebral palsy, *Pediatr Clin North Am* 40:537, 1993.
2. Gage J: Cerebral palsy, *Curr Probl Pediatr* Feb:71, 1998.
3. Kuba KCK, Leviton A: Cerebral palsy, *N Engl J Med* 330:188, 1994.
4. Taft L: Cerebral palsy, *Pediatr Rev* 16:411, 1995.
Authors: **Nancy E. Lanphear, M.D., and Susan Wiley, M.D.**

TABLE 2-6 Associated Complications with Specific Treatment and Follow-Up/Referral by System

SYSTEM	COMPLICATIONS	TREATMENT	FOLLOW-UP/REFERRAL
Musculoskeletal	Subluxed/dislocated hips	Surgical	Orthopedic surgeon
	Spasticity/contractures/pain	ROM exercises, casting, orthotics, appropriate seating devices, surgical tendon releases, antispasticity medications (including Botox, baclofen pump), dorsal rhizotomy	Physical therapist, occupational therapist, orthopedic surgeon, psychiatrist, neurosurgeon
	Scoliosis	Bracing, surgical intervention	Orthopedic surgeon
	Mobility issues	Bracing, wheelchair	Physical therapist
Ophthalmologic	Strabismus	Patching, eye drops, glasses, surgery	Ophthalmologist
	Refractive errors	Glasses	
	Visual field defects		Local association for the blind
	Cortical visual impairment	Therapy through early intervention for visual impairments	
Gastrointestinal	GER with or without recurrent aspiration pneumonia	Acid reduction and promotility agents, surgical antireflux procedure	Gastroenterologist or pediatric surgeon if needed
	Constipation	Dietary fiber, bowel program, laxatives, suppositories, enemas	Gastroenterologist if needed

GER, Gastroesophageal reflux; *ROM,* range of motion.

TABLE 2-6 **Associated Complications with Specific Treatment and Follow-Up/Referral by System—cont'd**

SYSTEM	COMPLICATIONS	TREATMENT	FOLLOW-UP/REFERRAL
Gastrointestinal—cont'd	Growth and nutrition (feeding difficulties, poor suck/swallow coordination, tonic bite, hyperactive gag, tongue thrust)	Follow growth on CP grid, dietary supplements, sometimes G-tube feeds	Occupational therapist, nutritionist if needed
Neurologic	Seizures (30%, 50% in hemiplegic CP)	Antiepileptic medications, seizure precautions	Pediatric neurologist
	Learning disabilities (motor planning, visuospatial difficulties)	Educational interventions	Multifactored developmental evaluation, IEP
	AD/HD	Behavioral modification, medication management	Developmental pediatrician, pediatric psychologist, IEP
	Mental retardation	Educational interventions	Multifactored developmental evaluation, IEP
	Communication disorders	Augmentative communication devices, signing, picture boards	Speech and language therapist knowledgeable in CP
	Oral-motor dyspraxia (affects communication and drooling)	Antidrooling medications, antidrooling surgical procedures	Pediatric ENT for surgical intervention, speech and language therapist
Dental	Malocclusion	Regular brushing and flossing	Dentist
	Caries		
Hearing	Hearing loss in 10%	Aggressive treatment of OM, hearing aids	Audiologist, speech language pathologist, pediatric ENT
Skin	Skin breakdown if poor nutrition, unable to shift weight	Prevention! Improve nutrition, frequent turning, well-fitted wheelchair, cushion for pressure areas, appropriate bedding	If severe, plastic surgeon
Social	Family adjustments to a child with a disability, financial burdens, estate planning, advocacy for child and family, minimal respite services, peer interactions, independent living options	Multidisciplinary approach to maximize functional and independent outcomes	Counseling, SSI, MCH funding, early intervention, preschool disabilities, BVR, county board of MRDD, local parent support groups, therapeutic recreation program

AD/HD, Attention deficit/hyperactivity disorder; *BVR*, Bureau of Vocational Rehabilitation; *CP*, cerebral palsy; *ENT*, ear, nose, throat surgeon; *IEP*, individualized education plan; *MCH*, maternal-child health; *MRDD*, mental retardation and developmental disabilities; *OM*, otitis media; *SSI*, supplemental security income.

BASIC INFORMATION

■ DEFINITION

- A cerebrovascular accident (CVA), or stroke, is a syndrome characterized by the rapid onset, usually over minutes to hours, of neurologic symptoms such as hemiparesis, sensory abnormalities, or aphasia.
- Any vascular insult resulting in a focal neurologic deficit lasting longer than 1 hour is a CVA.
- Subtypes of stroke include hemorrhagic and ischemic.

■ SYNONYMS

- Stroke
- Hypoxic-ischemic brain injury

ICD-9CM CODE

436 Acute, but ill-defined, cerebrovascular disease; includes cerebrovascular accident and stroke

■ ETIOLOGY

- Causes of CVA include hemorrhage and focal or diffuse ischemia.
- All types of CVAs result in inadequate delivery of substrate (glucose and oxygen) to neurons, with resultant neuronal cell death.
- There are multiple conditions that can predispose to CVA in the pediatric population
  1. Hemorrhagic stroke
     a. Vascular malformations
        (1) Arteriovenous malformation
        (2) Galen's vein
        (3) Hereditary hemorrhagic telangiectasia
        (4) von Hippel-Lindau disease
        (5) Intracranial aneurysms
        (6) Moyamoya disease
        (7) Sturge-Weber syndrome
        (8) Brain tumors
        (9) Leukemia
     b. Neoplasm
     c. Head trauma
     d. Coagulopathy
        (1) Disseminated intravascular coagulation (DIC)
        (2) Idiopathic thrombocytopenic purpura
        (3) Clotting factor deficiencies
        (4) Afibrinogenemia
        (5) Vitamin K deficiency
        (6) Anticoagulation therapy (heparin, warfarin)
        (7) Platelet defects
        (8) Hemolytic uremic syndrome
        (9) Herpes simplex encephalitis
        (10) Mycotic aneurysm
        (11) Bacterial, mycotic meningoencephalitis
        (12) Tuberculous meningitis
     e. Systemic disorders
        (1) Hypertension
        (2) Hepatic failure
        (3) Aplastic anemia
        (4) Sickle cell disease
     f. Drugs
        (1) Cocaine
        (2) Amphetamines
     g. Genetic disorders
        (1) Ehlers-Danlos syndrome (type IV)
        (2) Neurofibromatosis
        (3) Tuberous sclerosis
        (4) Polycystic kidney disease ("adult" type)
        (5) Hereditary neurocutaneous angiomatosis
        (6) Fabry's disease
  2. Ischemic stroke
     a. Cardiac
        (1) Congenital heart disease with right-to-left shunt
        (2) Rheumatic heart disease
        (3) Prosthetic heart valve
        (4) Atrial myxoma
        (5) Cardiomyopathy
        (6) Myocardial infarct
        (7) Arrhythmia
     b. Infection
        (1) Meningitis
        (2) Encephalitis
        (3) Systemic: rubella, mycoplasma
     c. Inflammatory
        (1) Systemic lupus erythematosus
        (2) Polyarteritis nodosa
        (3) Takayasu's disease
        (4) Inflammatory bowel disease
     d. Vasculopathy
        (1) Migraine
        (2) Subarachnoid hemorrhage
     e. Trauma
     f. Hematologic disorders/hypercoagulable states
        (1) Sickle cell disease, sickle-C disease
        (2) Protein C or S deficiency
        (3) Antithrombin III deficiency
        (4) Dysfibrinogenemia
        (5) Antiphospholipid antibodies
        (6) Polycythemia
        (7) Thrombotic thrombocytopenic purpura
        (8) Hemolytic uremic syndrome
     g. Metabolic
        (1) Homocystinuria
        (2) Fabry's disease
        (3) Mitochondrial encephalomyelopathies
        (4) Organic acidemias
        (5) Glutaric aciduria type II
        (6) Sulfite oxidase deficiency
        (7) Hypoglycemia
     h. Familial lipid disorders
     i. Drugs and toxins
        (1) Cocaine
        (2) Amphetamines
        (3) Oral contraceptives
        (4) Radiation therapy
        (5) L-asparaginase
     j. Other systemic disorders
        (1) Leukemia
        (2) Dehydration
        (3) Nephrotic syndrome

■ EPIDEMIOLOGY & DEMOGRAPHICS

- The incidence in children is 2.5 per 100,000 population per year.
- Male:female ratio is equal.
- Approximately 45% of CVAs in children are hemorrhagic; 55% are ischemic.
- Incidence in African-American population is increased secondary to sickle cell disease.

■ HISTORY

In search for a cause, ask for the following:
- History suggestive of vascular malformations
  1. Chronic or new headaches
  2. Changes in vision, school performance, and/or motor activity (e.g., clumsiness)
- Coagulopathy or hemoglobinopathy
- Febrile illness
- Trauma
- Underlying medical diagnoses such as neurocutaneous syndromes
- Hypertension, kidney disease, heart disease, or metabolic disease
- Paresthesias or anesthesia with or without headache
- Drug use, especially cocaine

■ PHYSICAL EXAMINATION

- Evaluation of head and neck for possible nidus of infection
- Heart examination with emphasis on evaluation of potential source of paradoxical embolus
- Skin examination for manifestations of neurocutaneous disorders, vasculitides, or evidence of trauma
- Neurologic examination to help localize the lesion
- Pupillary examination for miotic pupil and ptosis on contralateral side to hemiparesis, which suggests Horner's syndrome

🔬 DIAGNOSIS

■ DIFFERENTIAL DIAGNOSIS

- Hemiplegic migraine
- See "Etiology" for multiple types of stroke

■ DIAGNOSTIC WORKUP

- Computed tomography scan
  1. Can detect hemorrhagic infarct early
  2. May miss ischemic stroke in first 12 hours
- Magnetic resonance imaging to detect ischemic or hemorrhagic stroke early in course

- Echocardiogram to rule out structural heart disease
- Electrocardiogram to evaluate for arrhythmia or underlying conduction defects
- Blood work
  1. Complete blood count
  2. Erythrocyte sedimentation rate
  3. Coagulation studies (prothrombin time/partial thromboplastin time, bleeding time, protein S, protein C, antithrombin III, factor V Leiden)
  4. Blood glucose
  5. Electrolytes and urea nitrogen
- Remainder of diagnostic evaluation: should be undertaken after a detailed history to focus on the more likely causes

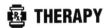

THERAPY

■ NONPHARMACOLOGIC
- Supportive care, paying close attention to the ABCs (airway, breathing, and circulation)
  1. Airway: If the stroke involves the brainstem, the patient may lose airway-protective reflexes and require endotracheal intubation.
  2. Breathing: The patient may have respiratory depression associated with CVA.
  3. Circulation: Special attention must be paid to circulation to avoid hypotension or rapid changes in blood pressure; avoid hyperglycemia in fluid resuscitation.
  4. Avoid hyperthermia.

■ MEDICAL
- Depends on cause
- May need antihypertensives, antibiotics, blood transfusion or exchange transfusion, or factor or platelet replacement

■ SURGICAL
- Rarely required
- May involve surgical evacuation of large hemorrhagic infarct or tumor debulking if associated with significant increase in intracranial pressure or mass effect

■ FOLLOW-UP & DISPOSITION
- Pediatric neurology and neurosurgery should be consulted.
- Remainder of follow-up depends on cause discovered in the workup.

■ PREVENTIVE TREATMENT
- Some evidence in adults that daily aspirin use decreases risk of recurrence
- Doppler echo of brain in patients with sickle cell disease to assess risk of stroke
  1. Early and recurrent exchange transfusion for those at risk of stroke

PEARLS & CONSIDERATIONS

■ WEBSITE
National Institute of Neurological Disorders and Stroke www.ninds.nih.gov/patients/stroke

REFERENCES
1. Trescher WH: Ischemic stroke syndromes in childhood, *Pediatr Ann* 21: 374, 1992.
2. Pavlakis SG, Gould RJ, Zito JC: Stroke in children, *Adv Pediatr* 38:151, 1991.
Author: **Robert Englander, M.D., M.P.H.**

II

BASIC INFORMATION

■ DEFINITION
Mucopurulent cervicitis (MPC) is a sexually transmitted disease (STD) syndrome that is characterized by a mucopurulent discharge from an inflamed cervix.

■ SYNONYMS
- Cervicitis
- Endocervicitis
- MPC

ICD-9CM CODES
616.0 Nonspecific
099.53 Chlamydial
098.15 Gonococcal
098.35 Chronic
131.09 *Trichomonas*

■ ETIOLOGY
- It is common that no infectious cause is identified.
- If the pathogen is identified:
  1. Most commonly caused by *Chlamydia trachomatis* and/or *Neisseria gonorrhoeae*
  2. Less commonly caused by herpes simplex virus or *Trichomonas vaginalis*
- Persistent cases during adolescence are most likely the result of noncompliance with treatment or reinfection from an untreated partner.

■ EPIDEMIOLOGY & DEMOGRAPHICS
- MPC is most common during adolescence.
- Sexual abuse is a consideration for females 12 years of age or younger.
- Complications include the following:
  1. Pelvic inflammatory disease (PID) and its sequelae (see the section "Pelvic Inflammatory Disease")
  2. Chronic pelvic pain
  3. Perihepatitis (Fitz-Hugh-Curtis syndrome)
  4. Increased risk of human immunodeficiency virus (HIV) transmission and infection

■ MEDICAL HISTORY
- Vaginal discharge
- Vaginal itching
- Irregular vaginal bleeding, especially after sexual intercourse
- Dyspareunia
- Lower abdominal pain—must consider pelvic infection

■ PHYSICAL EXAMINATION
- Purulent or mucopurulent discharge from cervical os
- Easily induced endocervical bleeding (i.e., friability)
- Edema and erythema of the zone of ectopy on cervix
- Signs of possible upper genital tract or pelvic infection: lower abdominal tenderness, cervical motion tenderness, and/or adnexal tenderness
- Right upper quadrant tenderness—must consider perihepatitis

DIAGNOSIS

■ DIFFERENTIAL DIAGNOSIS
- Vaginitis
- Endometritis
- PID
- Inflamed ectropion-columnar epithelial cells on area surrounding cervical os
- Foreign body

■ DIAGNOSTIC WORKUP
- "Swab test" is positive if yellow cervical exudate is visualized on a white cotton-tipped swab specimen.
- Gram stain of endocervical mucus specimen to evaluate for an increased number of polymorphonuclear leukocytes is not recommended for the following reasons:
  1. Has not been standardized
  2. Has a low positive-predictive value
  3. Is not available in many clinical settings
- DNA amplification tests and cultures are available to test for *C. trachomatis* and *N. gonorrhoeae* (see section discussing *C. trachomatis* and *N. gonorrhoeae*).
  1. Cervical specimens and first-void urine specimens can be used for DNA amplification tests.
- Tests for *Trichomonas vaginalis*, bacterial vaginosis, and vulvovaginal candidiasis are done to rule out vaginitis (see sections discussing vaginitis and trichomoniasis).
- Additional tests may be done to rule out syphilis and HIV coinfection.

THERAPY

■ TREATMENT PRINCIPLES
Empiric treatment for *C. trachomatis* and *N. gonorrhoeae* infection is recommended by the Centers for Disease Control and Prevention (CDC) in populations at high risk for infection, treatment noncompliance, and poor follow-up, such as adolescents (see the sections discussing *C. trachomatis* and *N. gonorrhoeae*).

■ MEDICAL
The CDC recommends the following regimens:
- Recommended regimens for *C. trachomatis* (one of the following):
  1. Azithromycin 1 g orally in a single dose
  2. Doxycycline 100 mg orally twice a day for 7 days
- Recommended regimens for *N. gonorrhoeae*:
  1. Treatment for *C. trachomatis* PLUS one of the following:
     a. Cefixime 400 mg orally in a single dose
     b. Ceftriaxone 125 mg intramuscularly in a single dose
     c. Ciprofloxacin 500 mg orally in a single dose
     d. Ofloxacin 400 mg orally in a single dose
- Treatment regimens for trichomonas and herpes simplex virus are outlined in their respective sections.

■ FOLLOW-UP & DISPOSITION
- See the sections discussing *C. trachomatis* and *N. gonorrhoeae*.
- Patients should return for diagnostic laboratory test results.
- Abstinence is recommended until therapy is completed.
- Notification, examination, and treatment of sex partners are essential.
- Partner notification is often the responsibility of the provider and patient because of a lack of resources at health departments.

PEARLS & CONSIDERATIONS

■ CLINICAL PEARLS
- Awareness of consent laws applying to minors and patient confidentiality rights for STD services in the state is important.
- HIV-infected patients should receive standard treatment.
- Counseling messages for STD prevention should be provided.

■ WEBSITES
- Adolescent-appropriate STD information websites: www.iwannaknow.org; www.itsyoursexlife.com

- American Social Health Association (ASHA) for patient information brochures, STD Hotline telephone number (800-783-9877), online STD information: www.ashastd.org
- Centers for Disease Control and Prevention, Division of STD Prevention: www.cdc.gov/nchstp/dstd/dstdp.html
- ETR Associates for patient information brochures: www.etr.org; 831-438-4060
- National STD Hotline: 800-227-8922

REFERENCES

1. Centers for Disease Control and Prevention: 1998 guidelines for treatment of sexually transmitted diseases, *MMWR Morb Mortal Wkly Rep* 47: RR-14, 1998.
2. Holmes KK, Stamm WE: Lower genital tract infections in women. In Homes KK et al (eds): *Sexually transmitted diseases,* ed 3, New York, 1999, McGraw-Hill.

Authors: **Gale R. Burstein, M.D., M.P.H., and Sheryl A. Ryan, M.D.**

II

BASIC INFORMATION

■ DEFINITION

Child abuse is a nonaccidental injury of a child by a caretaker. Most states add other factors to the legal definition, such as the caretaker's age and the nature of the injury. In general, the injuries include bruises, lacerations, blunt trauma, fractures, shaking, and poisoning. The complex syndromes, such as Munchausen syndrome by proxy, may be included.

■ SYNONYMS

- Child maltreatment
- Battered child syndrome
- Shaken infant syndrome (shaken baby)

ICD-9CM CODES

995.5 Child abuse—general
V62.83 Nonparent
V61.22 Parent
V61.21 Victim
995.51 Emotional abuse
995.55 Multiple forms
995.54 Physical abuse
995.51 Psychologic abuse
995.52 Child neglect—nutritional
995.55 Shaken infant syndrome
995.53 Sexual abuse
An ICD-9CM code is often used for the type of injury, with a "V" code of V71.8 (observation for suspected condition) if nonaccidental injury is suspected.

■ ETIOLOGY

- The causes of child abuse are numerous and complex.
- It is customary to consider the social risk factors in the parent/caretaker, as well as characteristics of the child.
- Caretaker risk factors include the following:
  1. Young
  2. Single
  3. Economic stress—acute and chronic
  4. Poor impulse control
  5. Abused as a child
  6. Substance abuse problem
  7. Lack of social and/or emotional support
  8. Low socioeconomic status
- Child risk factors include the following:
  1. Premature infant
  2. Developmental disability
  3. Physical disability
  4. Chronic medical condition
  5. Autistic
  6. Attention deficit/hyperactivity disorder or other behavioral problems
  7. Colicky infant

■ HISTORY

- In evaluation of an injured child, considerations include the following:
  1. The type of injury and circumstances surrounding the injury
  2. How medical care was obtained
- These elements are important when deciding whether an injury may have been inflicted or nonaccidental.
- The types of injuries that are regarded as high risk for being child abuse can be divided into the following categories:
  1. Bruises
  2. Burns
  3. Fractures
  4. Head injuries
  5. Thoracic injuries
  6. Abdominal injuries
  7. Dental injuries
- In taking the history, consider the following questions to determine whether there are high-risk indicators for abuse:
  1. Do the findings fit the history based on the age and development of the child?
  2. Was medical care sought promptly?
  3. Was supervision at the time of injury adequate?
  4. Is the appearance/hygiene of the parent(s) appropriate for circumstances?
  5. Is the behavior of the child appropriate?
  6. Is there evidence of substance abuse?
  7. Is the injury a burn?
  8. Is the injury a human bite?
  9. Does the injury involve the cheeks, ears, neck, chest, back, abdomen, buttocks, or genitalia?
  10. Are there any inconsistencies in the parent or child's story?

■ PHYSICAL EXAMINATION

- Pay attention to the oral cavity, looking for mouth lesions and/or broken teeth.
- Look closely behind the ears for bruising.
- Examine for bruises, lacerations, or abrasions on the neck.
- Carefully examine the inner surfaces of the arms and legs for bites, bruises, and/or burns.
- Inspect the buttocks for bruises and/or abrasions.
- Examine the external genitalia for any abnormalities.
- Determine the type of lesion. The diagnosis of child abuse depends on the type of injury. Each of the most common types of injuries is discussed as follows, with high-risk and low-risk patterns described.
  1. Bruises
     a. High risk
        (1) Behind the ears

        (2) Cheeks
        (3) Neck
        (4) Chest
        (5) Abdomen
        (6) Back (see the following discussion)
        (7) Inner surfaces of extremities
        (8) Genital area
        (9) Any bruise with a "pattern"
     b. Low risk
        (1) Bony prominences surrounding the eye
        (2) Nose
        (3) Chin
        (4) Spinous processes of the back
        (5) Bony prominences of the hip
        (6) Bony prominences of the extremities
  2. Burns
     a. High risk
        (1) Immersion burns: These include burns in a "stocking-glove" pattern or any burn with a sharp demarcation between the injured and noninjured skin. The back and buttocks may also be burned in this way. Flexion creases may be spared.
        (2) Contact burns: These are burns that reflect the shape of the object used. Examples are those made from an iron, curling iron, radiator, heating grate, or cigarette.
        (3) Full-thickness burns: Like immersion burns, these burns are more apt to be inflicted.
        (4) Burns to the inner surfaces of the arms, legs, dorsum of the hand, the torso, or genitals are more likely to be inflicted.
     b. Low risk
        (1) Partial-thickness burns
        (2) Hot liquid spills down the shoulder or head or down the arm/torso with splash marks
        (3) Burns to the palm/fingertips
  3. Fractures
     a. High risk
        (1) Any fracture in a child who is not ambulatory
        (2) Metaphyseal "corner," "chip," or "bucket handle" fractures
        (3) Transverse or oblique/spiral fractures of the humerus, femur, or tibia in a young child
        (4) Femur fracture in a child younger than 1 year old

(5) Rib fractures
(6) Skull fractures with a history of a low-velocity or short-distance fall
(7) Scapular fractures
(8) Sternal fractures
(9) Spinous process fractures
(10) Vertebral body fractures
(11) Multiple fractures
(12) Fractures of different ages
b. Low risk
(1) Long-bone shaft fractures in ambulatory children
(2) Linear skull fractures with appropriate history
(3) Clavicle fractures
4. Thoracic/abdominal injuries
a. Injuries to the internal organs of the chest, abdomen, and pelvis are extremely rare in common childhood injuries.
b. Any injury to these organs in the absence of a long-distance fall or high-velocity accident warrants suspicion of child abuse.
c. Internal injuries seen in abuse include the following:
(1) Esophageal tear
(2) Pharyngeal injury
(3) Pulmonary contusion
(4) Duodenal hematoma
(5) Liver laceration
(6) Splenic laceration
(7) Pancreatic injury
(8) Mesenteric tear
5. Oral injuries
a. These injuries are uncommon but sometimes result from rough feeding or deliberate injury by a caretaker.
(1) Cuts to the inside of the mouth in a child with no teeth
(2) Frenulum tears
(3) Bruising inside the mouth

🔬 DIAGNOSIS

■ DIFFERENTIAL DIAGNOSIS
- Making the diagnosis of child abuse involves a complete history, knowledge of risk factors, and a complete physical examination.
- Laboratory and radiographic studies may be required to explain possible medical conditions that mimic abuse.
- For bruises
  1. Ehlers-Danlos syndrome
  2. Phytophotodermatitis
  3. Coagulation factor deficiencies
  4. von Willebrand syndrome
  5. Henoch-Schönlein purpura
  6. Thrombocytopenia
  7. Vitamin K deficiency
  8. Rocky Mountain spotted fever
  9. Syphilis

  10. Sepsis with disseminated intravascular coagulation
  11. Traditional healing practices (e.g., coining)
  12. Birthmarks
- For burns
  1. Herpes simplex
  2. Epidermolysis bullosa
  3. Bullous impetigo
  4. Cellulitis
  5. Staphylococcal scaled skin syndrome
  6. Erysipelas
  7. Diaper dermatitis
  8. Traditional healing (e.g., cupping)
- For fractures
  1. Accidental trauma
  2. Osteogenesis imperfecta
  3. Syphilis
  4. Scurvy
  5. Ricketts
  6. Hyperparathyroidism
  7. Menkes' syndrome
  8. Toxicity from medications (e.g., methotrexate)
  9. Schmidt and Schmidt-like metaphyseal chondroplasia
  10. Jansen-type metaphyseal dysostosis
  11. Malignancy
  12. Caffey's disease

■ DIAGNOSTIC WORKUP
- This varies with the type of abuse suspected.
- Fractures: skeletal survey if the child is 3 years old or younger and specific radiographs as indicated by physical examination
  1. Skeletal survey
     a. May show high risk or multiple fractures; may be normal
     b. Unexpected results: findings consistent with bone diseases would guide the workup
- Bruises
  1. Skeletal survey if the child is 3 years old or younger to evaluate for other signs of current and/or past trauma
  2. Coagulation studies and complete blood count
     a. Expect to be normal
     b. Coagulopathy: possible in severe head trauma, resulting from intracranial bleeding
     c. Hematocrit: may be abnormally low if bleeding is present
     d. Other abnormalities: see "Differential Diagnosis" for bruising
- Burns: skeletal survey if the child is 3 years old or younger
- Thoracoabdominal trauma: as per fractures and bruises
- Oral trauma: as per fractures plus dental consult, if indicated
- Shaken infant syndrome: as per fractures and bruises plus head computed tomography (CT) scan and

retinal examination, ideally done with dilation by a pediatric ophthalmologist
1. Head CT
   a. Bleeding is usually evident in the shaken infant.
   b. If CT scan is normal, other diagnoses (metabolic or infectious) should be considered.
2. Retinal examination
   a. Hemorrhages in the shaken infant, but may be normal
- In addition to any of the aforementioned tests, the following are required:
  1. Previous medical records must be investigated.
  2. A social worker and specialists relevant to the child's problem should be consulted.
  3. Consultations with a child abuse expert or forensic pediatrician may be needed.
  4. It is important to rule out any medical condition that may explain the child's signs and symptoms before making a diagnosis of child abuse.
  5. The child who may be at risk for abuse must be protected.
  6. If the diagnosis of child abuse is being considered, the medical provider must be sure that the child remains safe until the investigation (medical and psychologic) is done.
  7. Providing safety involves a referral to an appropriate child protective agency.
  8. The child in question and any other children at risk in the home will be legally protected.
  9. These pieces of information are often necessary before child abuse can be diagnosed.
  10. The agency also performs a psychosocial assessment and investigates the home environment.

Shaken Infant Syndrome
- This form of abuse is also known as *shaken baby syndrome* and *shaken impact syndrome*.
- The caretaker may strike the baby's head against an object during the shaking; even a pillow will cause a significant increase in acceleration force.
- Other forms of trauma may occur; thus this may be more appropriately called *nonaccidental injury of infancy*.
- The presentation is often similar to that of an infant with a severe infectious or metabolic illness, including the following:
  1. Apnea
  2. Altered mental status
  3. Shock
  4. Seizures
  5. Vomiting

6. Head or extremity bruising or swelling
7. Full fontanel
- Often, findings are not present on the initial examination.
- These infants often require aggressive resuscitation on presentation.
- As the workup progresses, the absence of metabolic or infectious causes leads to the suspicion of abuse and prompts evaluation.
- Some, but not necessarily all, of the following elements of the diagnosis should be present:
  1. Intracranial hemorrhage
  2. Retinal hemorrhage (may require dilated examination)
  3. Skull fracture
  4. Rib fractures, particularly posterior
  5. Extremity fractures, particularly metaphyseal fractures

■ DIFFERENTIAL DIAGNOSIS
- No disease has all of the elements of shaken infant syndrome.
- Glutaric aciduria type I can cause subdural fluid collections.
- Coagulopathies can cause abnormal bleeding.
- Retinal hemorrhages can be from birth; however, those usually resolve by 1 month of age.
- Severe trauma, such as a motor vehicle crash, may cause similar injuries.

Munchausen Syndrome by Proxy
- The caretaker (most often the mother) inflicts injury on a child, causing symptoms of illness, or she fabricates or exaggerates symptoms.
- Both scenarios lead to diagnostic studies, therapy, and often, hospitalization.
- The diagnosis requires a team of physicians, nurses, social workers, and often, legal counsel.
  1. Must either prove that the caretaker is inflicting injury *or*
  2. Arrange to temporarily remove the child from the mother, thereby observing resolution of symptoms (see the section "Munchausen Syndrome by Proxy")

℞ THERAPY

■ NONPHARMACOLOGIC
- The medical provider must make referrals to the appropriate agencies, which investigate the possibility of child abuse and determine a safe place for the child.
  1. The agencies must know the extent of the injury and the medical likelihood that the injuries were nonaccidental.
  2. They can determine placement of the child and the need for involvement of other agencies, such as law enforcement.

■ MEDICAL & SURGICAL
The medical and surgical therapies are directed at the child's injuries.

✧ PEARLS & CONSIDERATIONS

■ PEARLS
- The diagnosis of child abuse has important medical, legal, and social consequences, and it should involve a team with medical, legal, and social expertise.
- A medical provider's suspicion of abuse is sufficient to warrant a referral to the appropriate agency; it obligates the provider to ensure the safety of the child.

■ WEBSITES
- American Academy of Pediatrics: www.aap.org; type "child abuse" in the search box
- American Professional Society on the Abuse of Children: www.apsac.org
- National Clearinghouse on Child Abuse and Neglect Information: www.calib.com/nccanch

REFERENCES
1. Krugman SD, Wissow LS, Krugman RD: Facing facts: child abuse and pediatric practice, *Contemp Pediatr* 15:131, 1998.
2. Reece RM: *Child abuse: medical diagnosis and management*, Malvern, Pa, 1994, Lea & Febiger.
3. Woelfle J, Kreft B, Emons D et al: Subdural hemorrhage as an initial sign of glutaric aciduria type A: a diagnostic pitfall, *Pediatr Radiol* 26:779, 1996.
Author: **Ann Lenane, M.D.**

BASIC INFORMATION

■ DEFINITION

Chlamydia trachomatis infections are clinical syndromes caused by an obligate intracellular sexually transmitted genital pathogen that causes symptoms that resemble those of infections caused by *Neisseria gonorrhoeae*.

■ SYNONYM

Chlamydia

ICD-9CM CODE

099.41 *Chlamydia trachomatis* urethritis
099.5 *Chlamydia trachomatis* venereal disease

■ ETIOLOGY

- A sexually transmitted infection during adolescence
- Vertical transmission from mother to infant during infancy

■ EPIDEMIOLOGY & DEMOGRAPHICS

- *C. trachomatis* infections are the most common bacterial sexually transmitted disease (STD) during adolescence.
- Sexual abuse is a consideration for transmission in girls younger than 12 years old.
- The disease is asymptomatic in both males and females in many cases.
- Complications include the following:
  1. Reiter's syndrome and increased risk of human immunodeficiency virus (HIV) transmission and infection
  2. Proctitis (in persons participating in anal intercourse)
  3. Conjunctivitis (from autoinoculation and perinatal infection)
  4. Pelvic inflammatory disease and its sequelae (see the section "Pelvic Inflammatory Disease"), chronic pelvic pain, and perihepatitis (Fitz-Hugh-Curtis syndrome) (in females)
  5. Epididymitis (in males)
  6. Pneumonitis in infants

■ HISTORY

- May have no history suggestive of genital or rectal inflammation
- Complaints of mucopurulent cervicitis (MPC), including vaginal discharge or pruritus, irregular vaginal bleeding, dyspareunia (see the section "Mucopurulent Cervicitis")
- Complaints of urethritis, including urethral discharge or pruritus, dysuria, urinary frequency, and burning with urination (see the section "Urethritis")
- Complaints of endometritis or salpingitis, including lower abdominal pain (see the section "Pelvic Inflammatory Disease")
- Complaints of proctitis, including anorectal pain, tenesmus, and rectal discharge

■ PHYSICAL EXAMINATION

- Signs of mucopurulent cervicitis (mucopurulent cervical discharge, cervical friability; see the section "Mucopurulent Cervicitis")
- Signs of urethritis (mucoid or purulent urethral discharge; see the section "Urethritis")
- Signs of endometritis or salpingitis (lower abdominal tenderness, cervical motion tenderness, and adnexal tenderness; see the section "Pelvic Inflammatory Disease")
- Signs of proctitis (rectal discharge and rectal examination tenderness)
- Signs of conjunctivitis (conjunctival erythema and discharge)

■ DIFFERENTIAL DIAGNOSES

- Infection by another sexually transmitted pathogen, especially *N. gonorrhoeae* and herpes simplex virus (see the sections "Mucopurulent Cervicitis" and "Urethritis")
- Foreign body
- Other infectious and autoimmune causes of proctitis

■ DIAGNOSTIC WORKUP

- Cell culture for *C. trachomatis* (cervical, urethral, and rectal specimens)
  1. This test was previously the gold standard, but it is technically cumbersome and costly, with relatively low sensitivity.
  2. It is currently the only test legally admissible as evidence for sexual abuse.
- Nonculture chlamydial tests: cervical and urethral specimens
  1. Enzyme immunoassay
  2. Direct fluorescent antibody
  3. DNA probe
  4. DNA amplification tests (also approved for urine specimens)
- DNA amplification tests (the most sensitive and specific test available)
  1. Cervical, first-void urine, and urethral specimens
- Urine leukesterase test on first-void urine (relatively insensitive and not specific for *C. trachomatis* urethritis)
- Serologic tests (not recommended for diagnosis of acute *C. trachomatis* infections because of poor sensitivity and specificity)
- Tests for *Trichomonas vaginalis,* bacterial vaginosis, and vulvovaginal (to rule out vaginitis; see the section "Vaginitis")
- Serologic test for syphilis and HIV (because of high risk of STD/HIV coinfection)

THERAPY

The Centers for Disease Control and Prevention's recommended regimens are as follows:

- Standard regimens (one of the following):
  1. Azithromycin 1 g orally in a single dose
  2. Doxycycline 100 mg orally twice a day for 7 days
- Alternative regimens (one of the following):
  1. Erythromycin base 500 mg orally four times a day for 7 days
  2. Erythromycin ethylsuccinate 800 mg orally four times a day for 7 days
  3. Ofloxacin 300 mg orally twice a day for 7 days
- Indications for pregnancy (one of the following):
  1. Erythromycin base or ethylsuccinate at recommended regimens *or* at half the dose for twice the duration of therapy
  2. Amoxicillin 500 mg orally three times a day for 7 days
  3. Azithromycin at recommended regimens
- Contraindications during pregnancy:
  1. Doxycycline
  2. Ofloxacin
  3. Erythromycin estolate
  4. Azithromycin (safety and efficacy in pregnant and lactating women is not established, although preliminary data indicate that it may be safe and effective)
- Indications for children:
  1. Weight less than 45 kg: erythromycin base 50 mg/kg/day orally divided into four doses daily for 10 to 14 days (effectiveness is 80%; second course of therapy may be required)
  2. Weight 45 kg or more but age younger than 8 years: azithromycin 1 g orally in a single dose
  3. Age older than 8 years: azithromycin 1 g orally in a single dose or doxycycline 100 mg orally twice a day for 7 days
- Indications for infants
  1. Ophthalmia neonatorum: erythromycin 50 mg/kg/day orally, divided into four doses daily for 10 to 14 days
     a. A strong association exists between erythromycin and a subsequent increased incidence of infantile hypertrophic pyloric stenosis.
     b. Monitoring at delivery rather than prophylactic treatment is recommended for infants who are born to women with *C. trachomatis* infection.

II

■ FOLLOW-UP & DISPOSITION
- Testing for "reinfection" 3 to 6 months after treatment recommended for adolescents
- "Test of cure"
  1. Not recommended less than 3 weeks after treatment with doxycycline or azithromycin
  2. Recommended more than 3 weeks after treatment with erythromycin
- Management of sex partners
  1. Notification, examination, and treatment of sex partners is essential.
  2. Partner notification often becomes the provider and patient responsibility because of a lack of resources at health departments.

☼ PEARLS & CONSIDERATIONS

■ SPECIAL CONSIDERATIONS
- Awareness of consent laws regarding minors and patient confidentiality rights for STD services in the state
- Standard treatment for HIV-infected patients
- Monitoring of infants born to *Chlamydia*-infected mothers
- Suspected child abuse (see the section "Child Abuse")
- Developmentally appropriate counseling messages for STD prevention, especially consistent, correct condom use

■ CLINICAL PEARLS
Any change in menses (i.e., heavier or lighter menstrual flow, worse cramping, or a change in the timing of menses [occurring earlier or later in the expected cycle]) may indicate STD infection in the sexually active female and should prompt the clinician to perform screening tests.

■ WEBSITES
Health care provider information:
- Centers for Disease Control and Prevention, Division of STD Prevention, www.cdc.gov/nchstp/dstd/dstdp.html

Patient information:
- American Social Health Association (ASHA) for patient information brochures, STD hotline telephone number, online STD information, 800-783-9877, www.ashastd.org
- ETR Associates for patient information brochures, 831-438-4060, www.etr.org
- Adolescent-appropriate STD information websites: www.iwannaknow.org, www.itsyoursexlife.com
- Adolescent-appropriate STD information hotline: National STD Hotline, 800-227-8922

REFERENCES
1. American Academy of Pediatrics: Chlamydial infections. In Peter G (ed): *1997 Red Book: report of the Committee on Infectious Diseases,* ed 24, Elk Grove Village, Ill, 1997, American Academy of Pediatrics.
2. Centers for Disease Control and Prevention: 1998 Guidelines for treatment of sexually transmitted diseases, *MMWR Morb Mortal Wkly Rep* 47:RR-14, 1998.
3. Centers for Disease Control and Prevention: Hypertrophic pyloric stenosis in infants following pertussis prophylaxis with erythromycin—Knoxville, Tennessee, 1999, *MMWR Morb Mortal Wkly Rep* 48:1117, 1998.
4. Holmes KK, Stamm WE: Lower genital tract infections in women. In Holmes KK, Sparling PF, Mardh PA, et al (eds): *Sexually transmitted diseases,* ed 3, New York, 1999, McGraw-Hill.
5. Schachter J: Biology of *Chlamydia trachomatis.* In Holmes KK, Sparling PF, Mardh PA, et al (eds): *Sexually transmitted diseases,* ed 3, New York, 1999, McGraw-Hill.

Authors: **Gale R. Burstein, M.D., M.P.H., and Sheryl A. Ryan, M.D.**

BASIC INFORMATION

■ DEFINITION

Cholelithiasis, or gallstones, are made of varying combinations of cholesterol, calcium salts, and protein. Stones may be found in the gallbladder or in the cystic, common, or intrahepatic bile ducts. *Cholecystitis,* or inflammation of the gallbladder, may be chronic or acute, acalculous or secondary to obstruction caused by stones in the neck of the gallbladder or in the cystic or common bile duct. *Hydrops* of the gallbladder is acute distention without gallstones or inflammation. *Choledochal cysts* are congenital cystic dilations of the extrahepatic biliary tract. *Cholangitis* is inflammation/infection of the bile ducts.

■ SYNONYMS

Cholelithiasis
- Gallstones
- Gallbladder stones
- Choledocholithiasis (common duct stones, usually seen with gallstones)

ICD-9CM CODES
574.2   Cholelithiasis
574.5   Choledocholithiasis
575.10 Cholecystitis
576.1   Cholangitis
782.3   Hydrops
751.69 Choledochal cyst

■ ETIOLOGY
- Cholelithiasis
  1. Two major classifications of cholelithiasis: predominantly pigment stones and predominantly cholesterol stones
  2. Pigment stones: 70% to 80% of cases in children
     a. Black pigment stones predominantly pigment polymer and calcium salts with less than 10% cholesterol
        (1) Develop in up to 60% of patients with sickle cell disease
     b. Brown pigment stones predominately calcium bilirubinate, calcium fatty acid soaps, and less than 30% cholesterol
  3. Cholesterol stones: 15% of pediatric patients with cholelithiasis
     a. More than 50% cholesterol in content
     b. Caused by the relative imbalance of too little bile salt and lecithin with too much cholesterol
  4. Other/unknown: 10% to 20%
- Acalculous cholecystitis—uncommon
  1. Associated with infection or other systemic illness
     a. Streptococci: groups A and B
     b. Gram-negative organisms: *Escherichia coli, Salmonella, Shigella*
     c. Leptospira interrogans
     d. Parasites: ascaris, *Giardia*
  2. May be associated with trauma
  3. Associated with systemic vasculitis: Kawasaki disease, periarteritis nodosa, others
- Cholecystitis: may also occur secondary to obstruction by gallstone (calculous cholecystitis) in neck of gallbladder or in cystic or common bile duct
- Hydrops of the gallbladder: may be temporally associated with infections such as scarlet fever and leptospirosis as well as Kawasaki disease
- Choledochal cyst: cause unknown

■ EPIDEMIOLOGY & DEMOGRAPHICS
- Cholelithiasis is often seen with underlying conditions.
  1. Black pigment stones are associated with the following:
     a. Hemolytic diseases (40% to 50%)
     b. Sepsis
     c. Serious medical illness with biliary stasis
     d. Hepatobiliary diseases
     e. Gastrointestinal disorders
        (1) Necrotizing enterocolitis
        (2) Malabsorption, ileal diseases, previous intestinal resection
        (3) Total parenteral nutrition (TPN) in premature infants or chronic TPN in older patients
     f. Congenital heart disease
  2. Brown pigment stones are seen predominantly in Asia.
     a. Associated with parasitic infections
  3. Cholesterol stones are usually associated with the following:
     a. Obesity
     b. Pregnancy
- Spontaneous resolution of stones in infants has been reported.
- Obese female patients with a family history of gallstones are more likely to have cholesterol stones.
  1. Small bile acid pool size is related and may be causative in cholesterol stone development.
  2. Very high incidence is seen in the Pima Indian population.
- Approximately 10% to 15% of patients with cholelithiasis will develop pancreatitis.
- Cholecystitis as a complication of cholelithiasis is less common in children than in adults and is often chronic.
- Choledochal cysts occur in 1 in 13,000 to 1 in 15,000 persons in Western civilization.
  1. Females outnumber males.
  2. Two thirds of patients present before 10 years of age.
- Primary sclerosing cholangitis is a rare, progressive disorder with inflammation and fibrosis of the biliary duct and eventual cirrhosis.
  1. Not further discussed here

■ HISTORY
- Cholelithiasis
  1. Usually asymptomatic
  2. Colicky, recurrent abdominal pain
  3. Right upper quadrant (RUQ) abdominal pain
  4. Irritability in infants
  5. Jaundice
  6. Acholic stools
  7. Fatty food intolerance
  8. Personal history positive for hemolytic anemia, malabsorption or bowel stasis, or systemic illness
  9. Family history positive for gallstones, especially in obese female patients with no other predisposing factors
- Cholecystitis
  1. RUQ pain
  2. Nausea, vomiting
  3. Fever
  4. In chronic cholecystitis, may have intolerance to fatty foods
- Hydrops of the gallbladder
  1. Crampy abdominal pain
  2. Nausea, vomiting
  3. Fever
  4. Jaundice
- Choledochal cyst
  1. Acholic stools
  2. Jaundice
  3. Epigastric pain
  4. Vomiting
  5. Failure to thrive
  6. Irritability

■ PHYSICAL EXAMINATION
- Cholelithiasis
  1. Asymptomatic in most
  2. Jaundice, especially with obstruction or in hemolytic diseases
  3. Tender RUQ if infection is present
  4. Obesity
  5. Pregnant or recent childbirth
- Cholecystitis
  1. Shallow breathing
  2. Tenderness or mass in RUQ
  3. Positive Murphy's sign
     a. Inflamed gallbladder is palpated by pressing the fingers under the rib cage; deep inspiration causes pain when the gallbladder is forced down to touch the fingers.
  4. Jaundice
  5. Fever
- Hydrops of the gallbladder
  1. Distended gallbladder may be palpable.
- Choledochal cyst
  1. Infants often present with jaundice.
  2. Hepatomegaly.
  3. Abdominal pain.
  4. Fewer than one third of patients will have a palpable abdominal mass.

II

5. Classic triad of abdominal pain, jaundice, and palpable mass is seen in less than 20% of patients.
6. Portal hypertension and ascites may be found in the presence of underlying cirrhosis from chronic obstruction.

DIAGNOSIS

■ DIFFERENTIAL DIAGNOSIS
Aside from differentiating these disorders from each other, the differential diagnoses of RUQ pain and/or jaundice include other liver and biliary tract diseases and other abdominal processes.
- Hepatitis
- Cirrhosis
- Hepatocellular tumor, other liver tumor (primary or metastatic)
- Biliary atresia, paucity of bile ducts (syndromic, nonsyndromic)
- Biliary duct obstruction (idiopathic, posttraumatic, pancreatic compression)
- Caroli's disease
- Peptic ulcer disease
- Acute gastroenteritis
- Fitz-Hugh-Curtis syndrome
- Pneumonia and/or empyema

■ DIAGNOSTIC WORKUP
- Ultrasound is the single best test for helping define gallbladder and bile duct abnormalities.
  1. Stones are easily visualized, with and without dilation of the bile ducts.
     a. The most sensitive and specific test for cholelithiasis and bile duct dilation
  2. Thick-walled gallbladder is seen with cholecystitis.
  3. Ultrasound confirms a large gallbladder in hydrops.
  4. Choledochal cysts are easily visualized.
- Mildly elevated bilirubin, alkaline phosphatase, and transaminases are common with symptomatic stones, cholecystitis, and choledochal cysts.
- Complete blood count demonstrates leukocytosis with cholecystitis.

- Inability to visualize the gallbladder with hepatobiliary scintigraphy suggests acute cholecystitis.
- Cholangiogram (usually endoscopic retrograde cholangiopancreatography [ERCP]) is often used to localize obstruction and stones and to define the anatomy and extent of cysts. Stones in the common bile duct can also be removed endoscopically.

THERAPY

■ MEDICAL
- The treatment for most gallbladder disease in children is surgery.
- Lithotripsy or dissolution therapy can be tried for those at high surgical risk.
  1. Dissolution therapy does not work well with pigment stones.
- Antibiotic coverage, especially for acalculous cholecystitis, is recommended.
  1. Piperacillin and an aminoglycoside, *or*
  2. Unasyn
- Antiinflammatory therapy for the primary disorder will presumably resolve noninfectious forms of acalculous cholecystitis.

■ SURGICAL
- Patients with symptomatic cholelithiasis and cholecystitis usually require cholecystectomy.
  1. Performance of nonemergent cholecystectomy is encouraged.
  2. Morbidity and mortality are higher with emergent than with elective surgery.
  3. Most can be done laparoscopically.
- Children with stones secondary to an underlying hemolytic disorder (e.g., sickle cell disease) should undergo cholecystectomy, even if asymptomatic.
- Patients with asymptomatic stones or hydrops may not need surgery.
  1. Treatment of the underlying disease usually leads to resolution of hydrops of the gallbladder.

2. If stones become symptomatic, cholecystectomy is indicated.
- A choledochal cyst requires excision.
  1. Roux-en-Y hepaticojejunostomy is usually done.
  2. The abnormal ducts may have malignant potential.

■ FOLLOW-UP & DISPOSITION
- Patients with underlying disorders need to be followed closely, both for complications and for recurrences.

■ REFERRAL INFORMATION
- Pediatric gastroenterologist involvement is imperative; surgeons will need to be consulted for cholecystectomy or choledochal cyst excision and repair.

PEARLS & CONSIDERATIONS

■ CLINICAL PEARLS
- Gallbladder disease is uncommon in children but should be considered in the appropriate clinical setting.
- Ultrasound is the diagnostic screening test of choice for gallbladder disease.
- The etiology of cholelithiasis in pediatrics is evolving; a smaller percentage of stones are related to hemolysis.

REFERENCES
1. Heubi JE, Lewis LG, Pohl JF: Diseases of the gallbladder in infancy, childhood and adolescence. In Such FJ, Sokol RJ, Balistreri WF (eds): *Liver disease in children,* Philadelphia, 2001, Lippincott Williams & Wilkins.
2. McEvoy C, Suchy F: Biliary tract disease in children, *Pediatr Clin North Am* 43:75, 1996.
3. Miyano T, Yamataka A: Choledochal cysts, *Curr Opin Pediatr* 9:283, 1997.
4. Shaffer EA: Gallbladder disease. In Walker WA et al (eds): *Pediatric gastrointestinal disease: pathophysiology, diagnosis, management,* ed 3, Philadelphia, 2000, BC Decker.
Author: **Lynn C. Garfunkel, M.D.**

BASIC INFORMATION

■ DEFINITION
Chronic fatigue syndrome (CFS) is profound fatigue of greater than 6 months' duration that causes significant functional disability and is unexplained after a comprehensive medical and psychologic evaluation. The 1994 revised Centers for Disease Control and Prevention case definition (see following discussion) allows the coexistence of nonmelancholic depression and anxiety disorders and requires a minimum of four additional physical symptoms.

■ SYNONYMS
- Chronic fatigue and immune dysfunction syndrome
- Postviral fatigue syndrome
- Myalgic encephalomyelitis
- Chronic Epstein-Barr virus syndrome
- Neuromyasthenia
- Akureyri disease
- Royal Free disease

ICD-9CM CODE
780.71 Chronic fatigue syndrome

■ ETIOLOGY
- The cause is unknown.
- Prominent theories include the following:
  1. Persistent latent viral infection
  2. Subtle immune system activation
  3. Orthostatic intolerance
  4. Decreased corticotropin-releasing hormone secretion
  5. Sleep disorder
  6. Atypical depression
  7. Somatoform disorder

■ EPIDEMIOLOGY & DEMOGRAPHICS
Scant pediatric data exist.
- Adult population-based studies estimate the prevalence of CFS-like illness at 200 to 2800 per 100,000, with a 3:1 female:male ratio.
- CFS appears to be rare in childhood, with increasing prevalence in adolescence, estimated from 23 to 116 per 100,000 with a 2.5:1 female:male ratio.
- Studies in referred populations suggest that CFS is increased in the Caucasian population, with no consistent trend in socioeconomic status.

■ HISTORY
- In approximately two thirds of cases, onset follows an apparent acute viral illness; one third may develop insidiously.
- The clinical course is persistent in approximately half of cases and intermittent in the other half, with remissions and relapses of several months' duration.
- In addition to profound, disabling fatigue, common symptoms, in descending order, include headache, exercise intolerance, sore throat, difficulty concentrating, insomnia, hypersomnia, myalgia, generalized weakness, and arthralgia.
- Functional disability usually impairs all spheres of activity, and decreased school performance and marked absenteeism are often dramatic.

■ PHYSICAL EXAMINATION
- The initial examination is generally unremarkable.
- Growth and development, as well as pubertal progression, are unaffected.
- Although common in adults with CFS, more than a few fibromyalgia tender points are not usually found in adolescents.
- Despite the reported sensation of cervical adenopathy and sore throat, otolaryngologic examination usually is normal.
- Supine-to-standing blood pressure measurements usually do not reveal orthostatic changes.
- Mental status examination usually is normal.

DIAGNOSIS

Revised case definition for the Chronic Fatigue Syndrome (International Chronic Fatigue Syndrome Study Group, 1994):
- Clinically evaluated, unexplained, persistent, or relapsing fatigue that meets the following criteria:
  1. Of new or definite onset
  2. Associated with a substantial reduction in previous levels of occupational, educational, social, or personal activities
  3. Not the result of ongoing exertion
  4. Not substantially reduced by bed rest
- Concurrent occurrence of four or more of the following symptoms, all of which must have persisted or recurred for at least 6 months and must not have predated the fatigue:
  1. Substantially impaired short-term memory or concentration
  2. Sore throat
  3. Tender cervical or axillary adenopathy
  4. Myalgias
  5. Polyarthralgias
  6. Headache of a new type, pattern, or severity
  7. Unrefreshing sleep
  8. Postexertional malaise lasting longer than 24 hours
- The following conditions *exclude* an individual from the diagnosis:
  1. Any active medical condition that may explain symptoms
  2. Any past or current diagnosis of a major depressive disorder with psychotic or melancholic features, bipolar affective disorders, schizophrenia, delusional disorders, dementias, anorexia nervosa, and bulimia nervosa
  3. Alcohol or substance abuse
  4. Severe obesity
- The following conditions do *not* exclude the diagnosis:
  1. Any condition defined primarily by symptoms that cannot be confirmed by laboratory tests, including fibromyalgia, anxiety disorders, somatoform disorders, nonpsychotic or nonmelancholic depression, neurasthenia, and multiple chemical sensitivity disorder

■ DIFFERENTIAL DIAGNOSIS
- Occult systemic disease (e.g., cardiopulmonary disorder, hypothyroidism, Addison's disease, connective tissue disease, neoplasm, renal failure, inflammatory bowel disease)
- Significant psychosocial stress in family, peer, school, or community relationships
- Depression, anxiety, somatoform disorder
- Drug and alcohol abuse
- Sleep disorder
- Malingering (appears to be unusual)

■ DIAGNOSTIC WORKUP
- Conduct a comprehensive history, review of systems, and physical examination.
- Obtain a confidential psychosocial history from the adolescent and parent separately.
- Complete a selected laboratory evaluation, including complete blood count, acute-phase reactant, thyroid-stimulating hormone, electrolytes, blood urea nitrogen, creatinine, lactate dehydrogenase, alanine aminotransferase (ALT), aspartate aminotransferase (AST), and urinalysis.
  1. Unless specifically suggested by the history and physical examination, other laboratory studies, such as antinuclear antibodies, viral titers, immunoglobulins, and cortisol, are rarely useful in establishing the diagnosis of CFS in adolescence.
  2. Cardiovascular tilt-table testing may be useful in patients with symptoms suggestive of orthostatic intolerance.

THERAPY

- There is no specific therapy for CFS.
- Treatment should be aimed at target symptoms.

■ NONPHARMACOLOGIC

- Cognitive-behavioral therapy may improve coping and decrease functional disability.
- Sleep hygiene (e.g., routine, consistent sleep rituals) to minimize napping and normalize sleep-wake cycles is important.
- A graduated exercise program may enhance activity level.
- A gradual return to normal activity and school attendance is indicated.

■ MEDICAL

- Analgesics and antiinflammatory agents may be useful for headache, arthralgia, and myalgia.
- Salt, mineralocorticoids, peripheral vasoconstrictors, and selective serotonin reuptake inhibitors may ameliorate symptoms of orthostatic intolerance.
- Antidepressants may be indicated for associated anxiety and depression.

■ FOLLOW-UP

Regular follow-up to monitor functional status and promote return to normal activity is indicated.

■ PATIENT/FAMILY EDUCATION

- There is no evidence that the disorder is progressive or degenerative.
- Although prospective studies are few, it appears that most adolescents with CFS improve within 6 months to 2 years.

■ REFERRAL INFORMATION

- Unless there is evidence of a specific disorder, multiple medical subspecialty consultations are rarely useful.
- With significant functional disability and/or associated anxiety or depressive symptoms, a mental health consultation is indicated.

☼ PEARLS & CONSIDERATIONS

■ CLINICAL PEARLS

- Although fatigue is a common complaint in anxiety and depression, many adolescents with CFS do not meet the criteria for psychiatric disorders.
- When present with CFS, it may be difficult to ascertain whether anxiety and depression are primary or secondary conditions.
- Many adolescents with CFS and their parents believe that the disorder is often not validated by others as a true medical condition and may be defensive and resistant to discussion regarding the role of psychosocial factors and stress.
- Nevertheless, psychological factors are common in adolescent CFS and may play an important role in precipitation or maintenance of the disorder.

■ WEBSITES

As with many unexplained disorders associated with significant disability, multiple alternative explanations of CFS pathogenesis have been proposed and many unproven therapies are espoused; websites often reflect this variance.

- Centers for Disease Control and Prevention: www.cdc.gov/ncidod/diseases/cfs/cfshome.htm
- The CFIDS Association of America, Inc.: www.cfids.org

■ SUPPORT GROUPS

- It is not at all clear that CFS is the same disorder in adolescents and adults.
- Because of significantly different developmental stage and subsequent life issues, adult CFS support groups generally are not appropriate for adolescents.

REFERENCES

1. Carter BD et al: Psychological symptoms in chronic fatigue and juvenile rheumatoid arthritis, *Pediatrics* 103: 975, 1999.
2. Jordan KM et al: Chronic fatigue syndrome in children and adolescents: a review, *J Adolesc Health* 22:4, 1998.
3. Komaroff AL, Buchwald DS: Chronic fatigue syndrome: an update, *Ann Rev Med* 49:1, 1998.
4. Marshall GS: Report of a workshop on the epidemiology, natural history and pathogenesis of chronic fatigue syndrome in adolescents, *J Pediatr* 134: 395, 1999.

Author: **Mark Smith, M.D.**

BASIC INFORMATION

■ DEFINITION
Cleft lip/palate is incomplete closure of the lip and/or palate.

■ ICD-9CM CODE
749.2 Cleft palate with cleft lip, unspecified

■ ETIOLOGY
- Both cleft lip and cleft palate can be associated with genetic syndromes (approximately 30% to 40%).
- Nonsyndromic cleft lip and/or palate have a multifactorial cause, being partly genetic and partly environmental.
- Pedigree analysis suggests two genetic forms of nonsyndromic palatal clefting:
  1. Cleft lip with or without palate
  2. Cleft palate only

■ EPIDEMIOLOGY & DEMOGRAPHICS
- The incidence is about 1 in 700 Caucasians, 1 in 500 in Asians, and 1 in 2500 in African Americans.
- Minor variations exist among different races.
- See "Patient/Family Education."

■ HISTORY
- Usually recognized at birth
- May be prenatally diagnosed by ultrasound
- Occasionally family history of clefting

■ PHYSICAL EXAMINATION
- Cleft lip can be unilateral or bilateral, complete or incomplete, and it is usually accompanied by nasal and maxillary flattening of the affected side.
- Cleft palate is broadly classified into V-shaped or U-shaped cleft, affecting the soft and/or hard palate.
  1. V-shaped clefts generally represent primary malformation.
  2. U-shaped clefts represent interference with palatal closure by the tongue.
     a. Seen in Pierre Robin sequence
     b. Micrognathia and/or retrognathia common
- The extent of palatal clefting can vary between complete clefting of palate, alveolar ridge, and lip to that involving the secondary palate only.
- Bifid uvula, submucous cleft palate, and midline furrowing of the palate are the mildest but most common manifestations of palatal clefting.
- Notching of vermilion with lip crease is a mild form of cleft lip.
- Hypernasal speech is caused by velopharyngeal insufficiency.

- Multiple dental abnormalities, such as malocclusion or inhibition of tooth eruption caused by alveolar clefting, are also seen.
- Because clefting may be associated with a genetic syndrome, a careful, comprehensive physical examination should be performed, looking for other minor anomalies.
  1. Lip-pits seen in patients with cleft lip suggest the van der Woude syndrome, an autosomal-dominant trait.
  2. The velocardiofacial syndrome, which consists of a conotruncal heart defect, velopharyngeal insufficiency or clefting, facial characteristics, long tapering fingers, and behavioral abnormalities, is often caused by a deletion of chromosome 22q.

DIAGNOSIS

■ DIFFERENTIAL DIAGNOSIS
- Amniotic band disruption sequence can cause facial clefting that does not follow the usual landmarks of labial or palatal fusion.
- Pseudocleft of the upper lip, which is seen in some genetic syndromes (e.g., orofaciodigital syndromes), is a slight median indentation or clefting of the upper lip that usually does not extend beyond the vermilion border.
- For clefting in patients with a high likelihood of a syndrome association because of the presence of other congenital anomalies, the differential diagnosis should be considered within the context of these other anomalies.

■ DIAGNOSTIC WORKUP
- Evaluation of feeding and respiratory competence of primary concern in the newborn infant
- A cleft-craniofacial team evaluative approach for future surgical and non-surgical interventions
- Speech and language evaluation
- Hearing evaluation
- Genetic evaluation for a possible syndrome association as indicated
  1. Chromosomal analysis is indicated if other congenital anomalies are identified.

THERAPY

■ NONPHARMACOLOGIC
- Special nipples are available to help with feeding.
  1. Children with cleft palate are not able to achieve a negative-pressure suck.

2. Special squeeze bottles help manually dispense milk or formula intraorally.
- Infants with the Pierre Robin sequence may have respiratory obstruction caused by micrognathia and glossoptosis. Prone positioning often helps alleviate this difficulty.
- All children with cleft lip and/or palate can benefit from nasoalveolar molding, which helps align the lip and alveolar elements before surgical correction of the clefts.

■ SURGICAL
- Staged correction of clefts can be managed by plastic surgery, with cleft lip repair occurring around 3 months and cleft palate repair at about 9 months.
- Hearing loss often requires myringotomy tube placement.
- Children with severe Pierre Robin sequence and respiratory obstruction can benefit from tongue-lip adhesion surgery.

■ FOLLOW-UP & DISPOSITION
- Monitoring growth and development for late-developing signs of a genetic syndrome (e.g., retinal detachment or degenerative arthritis in Stickler syndrome)
- Monitoring for conductive hearing loss caused by recurrent otitis media
- Continued speech and language evaluation and therapy
- Monitoring for multiple dental and orthodontic problems caused by inherent midface growth deficiency

■ PATIENT/FAMILY EDUCATION
- For nonsyndromic cleft lip or palate, the chance for the parents who have one affected child to have additional children with clefting is on the order of 3% to 5% for each pregnancy.
- This recurrence risk is higher for families in which the affected child has a more severe manifestation (e.g., recurrence risk is higher for families with bilateral cleft lip versus unilateral cleft lip).
- The recurrence risk increases significantly to 10% to 15% if the parents have two affected children.
- For syndromic clefting, the recurrence risk depends on the pattern of inheritance for the particular syndrome.

■ PREVENTIVE TREATMENT
- Several prenatal environmental exposures, such as alcohol, cigarette smoking, or valproate, are associated with an increased risk for clefting, but in no case is the risk greater than 5%.
- Some reports suggest the association of poor prenatal nutrition (e.g.,

folate deficiency) with an increased risk of clefting, but these theories are difficult to prove. Good prenatal care should be provided to all pregnant women.
- Prenatal diagnosis for some forms of syndromic cleft lip and/or palate is available.

■ REFERRAL INFORMATION
- All patients should be referred to a craniofacial team consisting of the following specialists:
  1. Plastic surgeons
  2. Otolaryngologists
  3. Speech pathologists
  4. Dentists, orthodontists, oral surgeons, and prosthodontists
  5. Geneticists
  6. Pediatricians

- Craniofacial teams certified by the American Cleft Palate Association can be found on their website.

☼ PEARLS & CONSIDERATIONS

■ CLINICAL PEARLS
- The presence of lip-pits suggests the van der Woude syndrome, which has an autosomal-dominant pattern of inheritance.
- Growth hormone deficiency is sometimes seen in children with cleft lip and/or palate and may require growth hormone replacement therapy.
- Cleft lip and/or palate seen in individuals with hypertelorism or hypotelorism suggests a more extensive midline defect (e.g., Opitz syndrome or holoprosencephaly, respectively).
- Hypernasal voice, with or without obvious palatal cleft, should raise the suspicion of velocardiofacial syndrome, and a fluorescence in situ hybridization study for a chromosome 22q deletion should be considered.

■ WEBSITE
American Cleft Palate Association: www.cleft.com/cpf/cpffrm.html

REFERENCE
1. Tewfik TL, Der Kaloustian VM: *Congenital anomalies of the ear, nose and throat,* Cary, NC, Oxford University Press, 1997.

Authors: **Joseph Losee, M.D., and Chin-To Fong, M.D.**

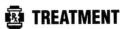
 BASIC INFORMATION

■ DEFINITION
Clubfoot is a complex deformity of the foot with hindfoot equinus (plantar-flexion) and varus (turned inward) and forefoot adduction of varying severity.

■ SYNONYM
Talipes equinovarus

ICD-9CM CODE
754.70 Talipes, unspecified

■ ETIOLOGY
The major categories of clubfeet include the following:
- Postural: caused by intrauterine molding ("cramped quarters")
- Idiopathic: most common (the subject of this section)
- Neurogenic: spina bifida, tethered spinal cord, arthrogryposis
- Syndromic: diastrophic dwarfism, Freeman-Sheldon syndrome, Smith-Lemli-Opitz syndrome

■ EPIDEMIOLOGY & DEMOGRAPHICS
- The incidence is 1 in 1000 for Caucasians and higher for Pacific Islanders.
- The incidence among males is greater than among females (2:1).
- The disease is bilateral in 30% to 50% of cases.
- Multifactorial inheritance:
  1. The risk of having a subsequent child with a clubfoot if the first child was a boy is 1 in 40; if the first child was a girl, the risk is 1 in 16.
  2. The risk of having a subsequent child with a clubfoot if a parent has a clubfoot is 1 in 4.

■ PHYSICAL EXAMINATION
- The deformity is evident at the time of the neonatal examination (occasionally, the diagnosis is suggested by prenatal ultrasound).
- Careful examination of the entire child is necessary to rule out syndromic or neurologic feet.
- The clubfoot is smaller than its counterpart and cannot be held in a corrected position.
- The ankle is in equinus (plantar-flexion).
- The hindfoot is in equinus and varus, and the Achilles tendon is contracted.
- Forefoot supination and metatarsus adductus are present, and a cavus component may also be present.
- The calf is atrophic.
- Leg length discrepancy is often present.

🔬 DIAGNOSIS

- The differential diagnosis is not in doubt except to rule out neurologic or syndromic clubfeet.
- Radiographs:
  1. Radiographs are of limited value early.
     a. Ossification of tarsal bones may be delayed.
     b. Ossification centers may be eccentrically positioned.
  2. Anteroposterior, lateral, and dorsiflexion lateral radiographs measure residual deformity.
  3. Ultrasound, computed tomography scan, and magnetic resonance imaging scan have limited use at this time.

💊 TREATMENT

- The goal is to obtain a normal-looking, painless, flexible, plantigrade foot.
- Nonoperative:
  1. Serial manipulation with immobilization in either an above- or below-knee cast
  2. Satisfactory results in approximately 20% of cases
- Operative:
  1. Achilles tendon lengthening
  2. Posteromedial (plantar) lateral release
  3. Age 3 to 12 months
  4. Satisfactory results in more than 80% of cases
  5. Residual deformity may require additional surgery (e.g., tendon transfers, osteotomy, triple arthrodesis)

■ FOLLOW-UP & DISPOSITION
Periodic examinations and radiographs are necessary to follow growth and development.

REFERENCES
1. Carroll NC: Clubfoot: what have we learned in the last quarter century? *J Pediatr Orthop* 17:1, 1997.
2. Cooper DM, Dietz FR: Treatment of idiopathic clubfoot: a thirty-year follow-up note, *J Bone Joint Surg* 77A: 1477, 1995.
3. Thompson GH, Simons GW II: Congenital *Talipes equinovarus* (clubfoot) and *Metatarsus adductus*. In Drennan JC (ed): *The child's foot and ankle*, New York, 1992, Raven.
Author: **Dennis R. Roy, M.D.**

II

BASIC INFORMATION

DEFINITION
- Coarctation of the aorta is an obstructing shelf-like lesion arising from the posterolateral aortic wall opposite the aortic end of the ductus arteriosus or ligamentum arteriosum as a result of localized thickening of the aortic media protruding into the vessel lumen.
- It is often associated with narrowing of the proximal descending thoracic aorta and poststenotic dilation of the distal descending thoracic aorta.

SYNONYMS
- Coarc
- Aortic coarctation
- Tubular or isthmus hypoplasia, stenosis, narrowing

ICD-9CM CODE
747.1 Coarctation of the aorta (preductal; postductal)

ETIOLOGY
- Unknown but attributed to disturbed prenatal arterial flow patterns at the junction of the proximal descending thoracic aorta (isthmus), patent ductus arteriosus, and postductal descending thoracic aorta
- Often with a relatively rapid obstructive exacerbation as the ductus arteriosus closes in the neonatal period

EPIDEMIOLOGY & DEMOGRAPHICS
- The disease accounts for approximately 7% of congenital heart disease.
- Incidence is 15 per 100,000 live births.
- Male predominance is seen.
- It is the most common cause of congestive heart failure in acyanotic infants in the first 2 weeks of life.
- Associated lesions include bicuspid aortic valve in 50% to 85% of patients, and ventricular septal defects and mitral valve anomalies in more complex coarctation malformations.
- Coarctation is found in 15% of patients with Turner syndrome.
- Berry aneurysms in the circle of Willis may occur in up to 10% of patients, with the greatest risk of rupture in late adulthood.
- There is a 90% mortality by age 50 in untreated patients because of early cardiogenic shock in the neonatal period and later aortic rupture or dissection, endocarditis, congestive heart failure, and intracranial hemorrhage.

HISTORY
- Two presentations are commonly seen:
  1. Congestive heart failure and cardiogenic shock in the neonatal period
  2. Heart murmur, systemic hypertension, and decreased lower extremity pulses in later infancy or childhood
- In the early presentation, infants usually have a history of progressively worsening feeding, tachypnea, pallor, diaphoresis, lethargy, diminishing urine output, and grunting.
- Rarely, young infants may be asymptomatic.
- Older infants and children are usually asymptomatic, but complaints of leg discomfort with running (possible claudication variant), headaches, and epistaxis may be elicited.

PHYSICAL EXAMINATION
- Symptomatic neonates commonly exhibit signs of congestive heart failure, including tachypnea, retractions, grunting, pallor, diaphoresis, tender hepatomegaly, a gallop rhythm, and a single accentuated second heart sound.
- If cardiogenic shock is present, all of the pulses are diminished, with lower and upper extremity hypotension.
- Physical findings in older infants and children are more characteristic, with a clear-cut disparity between upper and lower extremity pulses and blood pressures.
  1. Blood pressure in the legs is often unobtainable.
  2. Distal lower extremity pulses are commonly absent, and diminished femoral pulses lag behind the brachial pulses.
  3. Upper extremity pulses are vigorous.
- If a bicuspid aortic valve is present, an ejection click is heard between the lower left sternal border and the apex.
  1. Typically, a systolic bruit is audible over the midleft back and the upper left sternal border.
  2. If a systolic ejection murmur is heard at the upper right sternal border, aortic stenosis is present.
- Collateral vessels (branches off the subclavian arteries feeding the intercostal arteries in a retrograde direction, thereby enhancing aortic flow below the coarctation) are often, but not invariably, palpable along the inferolateral border of the scapula in children but not in young infants.
- Short stature, webbed neck, shield chest, cubitus valgus, and neonatal nonpitting edema of the dorsae of the hands and feet suggest Turner syndrome.

DIAGNOSIS

DIFFERENTIAL DIAGNOSIS
- Early presentation: other causes of cardiogenic shock in the neonatal period
  1. Hypoplastic left heart syndrome
  2. Critical aortic stenosis
  3. Myocarditis
  4. Cardiomyopathies
- Older infant/child: abdominal coarctation

DIAGNOSTIC WORKUP
- Electrocardiogram
  1. Right ventricular (RV) hypertrophy or RV dominance in neonates
  2. Normal or left ventricular (LV) hypertrophy in children
  3. Occasionally left atrial enlargement
- Chest roentgenogram
  1. Cardiomegaly, pulmonary venous congestion in neonates
  2. Normal or LV enlargement in children
  3. Three sign (prestenotic and poststenotic dilation of the descending aorta): may be seen in the upper left mediastinum in children
  4. Rib notching: rare in children younger than 5 years of age
- Echocardiography
  1. Useful for identifying the coarctation, ductus arteriosus, associated lesions, and ventricular function
- Cardiac catheterization: not usually necessary unless atypical features are present or if a balloon angioplasty is being considered

THERAPY

MEDICAL (FOR NEONATES WITH CARDIOGENIC SHOCK)
- Prostaglandin E_1 infusion to maintain ductal patency, thereby reducing LV afterload and improving subdiaphragmatic blood flow
- Dopamine or dobutamine to improve LV function, which may bring out an upper-lower extremity pulse discrepancy
- Intubation/mechanical ventilation

SURGICAL
Surgical intervention is the definite therapy.
- After initial stabilization, symptomatic neonates should undergo repair within 2 to 3 days.
- Asymptomatic infants and children should undergo repair by 4 years of age.

- If upper extremity hypertension persists or if LV dysfunction or severe ventricular hypertrophy develops, repair should be undertaken immediately.
- Types of repair include subclavian flap, patch aortoplasty, and extended aortic arch anastomoses in neonates and infants and end-to-end beveled anastomoses in older children. At some centers, balloon aortoplasty of the native coarctation is undertaken.

■ FOLLOW-UP & DISPOSITION
- Patients with coarctation require lifelong follow-up and infective endocarditis prophylaxis.
- Late problems include systemic hypertension, coarctation recurrence, endocarditis, aortic dilation-dissection-rupture, dilated cardiomyopathy with ventricular dysfunction, and intracranial hemorrhage.
- Recoarctations are usually treated with a balloon valvuloplasty.

■ PATIENT/FAMILY EDUCATION
Explain the need for follow-up and endocarditis prophylaxis.

■ REFERRAL INFORMATION
All patients with suspected or proven coarctation should be referred to a pediatric cardiologist.

☼ PEARLS & CONSIDERATIONS

■ CLINICAL PEARLS
- The most likely cause in an infant presenting at 8 to 12 days of age in cardiogenic shock is an aortic coarctation.
- In the presence of shock, an inotropic agent is often necessary to bring out the pulse and blood pressure disparity between the upper and lower extremities.
- The treatment of coarctation is surgical, not medical.
- Hypertension is an indication for surgical intervention.
  1. Persistent preoperative hypertension is unlikely to resolve after repair.
- Femoral pulses may be adequate at newborn discharge if the aortic end of the ductus is still open.

- Vigorous distal lower extremity pulses rule out an important coarctation.

■ SUPPORT GROUPS
Helping Hearts (a local-based organization) and other parental organizations are available to provide support and information.

REFERENCES
1. Ing FF et al: Early diagnosis of coarctation of the aorta in children: a continuing dilemma, *Pediatrics* 98:378, 1996.
2. Kimball TR et al: Persistent hyperdynamic cardiovascular state at rest and during exercise in children after surgical repair of coarctation of the aorta, *J Am Coll Cardiol* 24:194, 1994.
3. McNamara DG: Coarctation of the aorta: difficulties in clinical recognition, *Heart Dis Stroke* 1:202, 1992.
4. Ward KE et al: Delayed detection of coarctation in infancy: implication for timing of newborn follow-up, *Pediatrics* 86:972, 1990.
Author: **J. Peter Harris, M.D.**

II

BASIC INFORMATION

■ DEFINITION
Coccidioidomycosis is a pulmonary or disseminated infection caused by the fungus *Coccidioidomycosis immitis,* which is endemic to the southwestern United States.

■ SYNONYMS
- San Joauqin Fever
- Valley Fever

ICD-9CM CODES
114.9 Coccidioidomycosis
114.0 With pneumonia
114.3 Disseminated

■ ETIOLOGY
- Coccidioidomycosis immitis is a fungus that grows in soil, primarily under arid conditions.
- The life cycle consists of two stages: saprophytic (vegetative) and parasitic (tissue).
  1. Saprophytic phase: The fungus exists as a mycelium with septate hyphae; subsequently spores, called *arthroconidia,* form, which become airborne.
  2. The spores deposit in the aveolae, starting the parasitic phase.
  3. Parasitic phase: Arthroconidia form spherules that enlarge until they rupture, releasing endospores.
     a. In turn, the endospores may reenter the parasitic phase by forming spherules.
     b. In cavities or dressings, endospores may form mycelium, thus reentering the saprophytic phase.
- Arthroconidia (spores) become airborne through disruption of the soil, most commonly by windstorms, farming, or construction.

■ EPIDEMIOLOGY & DEMOGRAPHICS
- It is endemic to the southwestern United States: western Texas, New Mexico, Arizona, and California.
  1. Seen in those with recent travel to these areas
- Approximately 100,000 cases per year (less than 0.5% of which are extrapulmonary) are reported.
- It is most commonly seen in summer and fall, when dispersion of spores is increased because of the dry weather conditions.
- Primary pulmonary infection has no predilection for any particular age, sex, or race.
- Disseminated infection is seen more commonly in immunocompromised hosts, infants, Filipinos (100 times risk compared with Caucasians), Hispanics, African Americans (10 times risk), and pregnant women.

- Immunosuppressed patients may experience reactivation at a distant time.
- No direct person-to-person transmission occurs because growth in humans occurs in the tissue phase, which is noninfective. However, conversion to the mycelial (transmissible) phase may occur in wound dressings or casts.

■ HISTORY
- Incubation period: mean of 10 to 16 days (range of less than 1 week to 1 month)
- Primary infection
  1. Approximately 60% have an upper respiratory infection or no symptoms; 40% have flulike symptoms or pneumonia.
  2. Symptoms include fatigue (77%), cough (64%), pleuritic chest pain (53%), dyspnea (17%), rash (50% of children, less common in adults), and arthritis.
  3. Early-onset rash is erythematous maculopapular, later (3 days to 3 weeks) erythema multiforme and nodosum are seen.
- Disseminated disease (less than 0.5% of primary infection)
  1. Skin: verrucous granuloma on nasolabial fold
  2. Bones and joints: chronic osteomyelitis of the vertebrae, tibia, metatarsals, and skull; may present with pain and/or limp
  3. Meningitis
     a. Meningitis may occur with acute infection or up to 6 months later.
     b. Granulomatous and suppurative basilar meningitis with or without parenchymal involvement may be seen.
     c. Children often have no meningeal signs and/or symptoms; they may have focal deficits or headache.
     d. Without treatment, the mortality approaches 90% in 12 months.

■ PHYSICAL EXAMINATION
- Elevated respiratory rate
- Signs of consolidation on lung examination
- Disseminated disease as listed previously
  1. Leg, feet, skull, or back pain; limp or gait abnormalities
  2. Osteomyelitis, which may lead to tenderness or refusal to bare weight
  3. Meningeal signs such as nuchal rigidity
  4. Erythema nodosum and erythema multiforme (especially in children)

DIAGNOSIS

■ DIFFERENTIAL DIAGNOSIS
Includes bacterial or viral pneumonia, histoplasmosis, sarcoidosis, lung carcinoma, tuberculosis, and all other causes of meningitis

■ DIAGNOSTIC WORKUP
- Eosinophilia on complete blood count
- Elevated erythrocyte sedimentation rate
- Chest roentgenogram: bronchopneumonic infiltrate with hilar lymphadenopathy
- Cavitation or nodules (5%)
- Empyema and fistulas (rare)
- Bone roentgenograms: lytic lesion, 60% to 90% of which are solitary
- Bone scan: will show chronic osteomyelitis changes
- If meningeal involvement, lumbar puncture results will have cerebrospinal fluid (CSF) pleocytosis with mononuclear cells, eosinophils, elevated protein, and low glucose
- Skin test
  1. Positive result can be seen as early as 2 days, but 90% are positive by 2 weeks.
  2. If negative after 1 month of symptoms, latent dissemination may be more likely.
  3. Skin testing is unreliable in immunocompromised patients and those living in endemic areas, unless recent conversion can be documented.
  4. Use 1:10 dilution in those with erythema nodosum because of the exaggerated cell-mediated immune response.
- Serology (90% will have positive immunoglobulin G [IgG] or immunoglobulin M [IgM] response after symptomatic primary infection)
  1. IgM is positive in 50% by 1 week, 90% by 2 to 3 weeks. Response wanes over time, with only 10% positive by 5 months.
  2. IgG is positive in 50% to 90% by 3 months.
  3. False-positive results occur with blastomycosis or noncoccidiodal pulmonary illness.
  4. Patients with meningeal disease may not have positive titers except in CSF.
  5. IgG titers greater than 1:16 to 1:32 usually indicate disseminated infection.
  6. Titers of antibodies can be used to monitor disease response.
- Pathology
  1. A definite diagnosis can be made from seeing spherules in tissue biopsy or body fluid.
  2. Culture is more sensitive than direct examination but requires

either DNA probes or conversion to readily identifiable spherules by animal inoculation.
- Yield from pleural and spinal fluid and blood low
- Only one third of CSF cultures positive; direct examination almost 100% negative
- Bronchial washing: cytology yields 33%

⚕ THERAPY

■ NONPHARMACOLOGIC
Because 90% of primary nondisseminated pulmonary infections are self-limited, watchful waiting usually is appropriate.

■ MEDICAL
- Primary infection: indications to treat
  1. Continuous fever for more than 1 month, extensive or progressive pulmonary disease, high risk for dissemination (negative skin test with positive serology; high IgG titers greater than 1:16; immunocompromised, human immunodeficiency virus [HIV]-positive, Filipino patients), pregnant women, infants
  2. Amphotericin B followed by oral azoles for 1 month to 1 year
- Nonmeningeal disseminated disease: lesions outside of the thorax
  1. Requires treatment with amphotericin 7.5 mg/kg for mild disease;

up to 100 mg/kg for severe disease (usual range is 15 to 45 mg/kg; adult maximum dose, 1 to 2.5 g total; pediatric maximum dose, undefined) for 2-3 months
  2. No comparative studies with ketoconazole, itraconazole, or fluconazole but all are associated with a high relapse rate (up to 37%); treat at least few months after resolution of symptoms or 1 year of therapy
- Meningitis
  1. Intrathecal amphotericin should be given.
  2. Children may develop obstructive hydrocephalus.
  3. Azoles may be effective but are associated with high relapse rates (up to 75%) and require treatment for at least 1 year and perhaps lifetime.

■ SURGICAL
May be indicated for pulmonary cavitary lesions persistent for more than 1 year

☀ PEARLS & CONSIDERATIONS

■ CLINICAL PEARLS
- Coccidioidomycosis is endemic to the southwestern United States or those with travel to this area.
- No person-to-person transmission occurs.
- Most primary infections are asymptomatic.

- Around 90% of primary infections will have positive IgG or IgM titers.
- High IgG titers (greater than 1:16 to 32) are associated with dissemination.
- Dissemination is seen in high-risk groups: Filipino, pregnant, HIV-positive, and immunosuppressed patients, as well as infants.
- In meningitis, serum IgG may be negative but CSF IgG usually is positive.
- Titers can be followed to monitor response to therapy.
- Reactivation of primary infection may occur, especially in HIV-positive or immunocompromised host.

REFERENCES
1. American Academy of Pediatrics. Coccidioidomycosis. In Pickering LK (ed): *2000 Red Book: report of the Committee on Infectious Diseases,* ed 25, Elk Grove Village, Ill, 2000, American Academy of Pediatrics.
2. Galgiani JN: Coccidioidomycosis: a regional disease of national importance—rethinking approaches for control, *Ann Intern Med* 130:293, 1999.
3. Shehab ZM: Coccidioidomycosis. In Feigin RD, Cherry JD (eds): *Pediatric infectious disease,* Philadelphia, 1998, WB Saunders.
4. Stevens DA: Coccidioidomycosis, *N Engl J Med* 332:1077, 1995.
Author: **Jeffrey H. Lee, M.D.**

II

BASIC INFORMATION

■ DEFINITION
Colic is intense, inconsolable crying or fussiness in otherwise healthy infants. It occurs during the first 3 months of life, for 3 hours or more per day, on 3 days or more per week, and it lasts for more than 3 weeks.

■ SYNONYMS
- Excessive infant crying
- Persistent crying in infancy
- Paroxysmal fussing in infancy

ICD-9CM CODE
789.0 Colic

■ ETIOLOGY
- No convincing evidence exists for any discrete cause, although many have been proposed, including the following:
  1. Abdominal pain or "gassiness"
  2. Hunger
  3. Lactose intolerance, cow's milk protein allergy
  4. Reflux or esophagitis
- Some researchers have suggested that caregivers for colicky infants lack knowledge in recognizing infant cues.
  1. Caregiver lacks adaptive ability to respond to infant appropriately.
  2. Caregiver rapidly becomes frustrated because responses are unsuccessful in soothing infant.
- Other researchers propose a developmental phenomenon as the infant learns self-calming techniques with transition to sleep.
- It is most likely a multifactorial phenomenon involving interactions between the infant, caregiver, and environment.
- Colicky infants tend to be more sensitive, irritable, intense, and/or less adaptable.

■ EPIDEMIOLOGY & DEMOGRAPHICS
- Occurs in 10% to 25% of infants
- No gender, racial, or socioeconomic status differences
- Unrelated to food allergy, infant feeding practices, parental age, or parental education level

■ HISTORY
- Parents: exhausted and frustrated in caring for colicky infants
- Infants: younger than 4 months old with intense crying for 3 hours or more per day, 3 days or more each week
- Crying often at the same time each day—late afternoon and evening
  1. These infants also cry more than nonaffected babies throughout the day.

- Flexing or drawing up legs
- Arching
- Reddened face
- Struggling
- Passing flatus often
- Infants described as difficult or intense reactors
- Mothers of colicky infants: increased incidence of postpartum depression

■ PHYSICAL EXAMINATION
A comprehensive physical examination is important to rule out organic disease; the examination is generally negative.

DIAGNOSIS

■ DIFFERENTIAL DIAGNOSIS
- Hunger
- Neglect
- Cow's milk protein intolerance or allergy (with symptoms beginning at a mean age of 13 weeks)
- Infection
- Trauma, including nonaccidental
- Failure to thrive
- Constipation
- Ingestion
- Intussusception
- Corneal abrasion
- Supraventricular tachycardia

■ DIAGNOSTIC WORKUP
- Thorough history and physical examination are essential.
- Typical clinical findings are seen in an infant of the appropriate age.
- The diagnosis is typically one of exclusion and can often be confirmed only after the condition has run its characteristic course.

THERAPY

Be aware that colic may impair the relationship between parents and infant and often places the infant at increased risk for abuse.

■ NONPHARMACOLOGIC
- The condition is time-limited.
  1. Crying peaks at 6 weeks of age.
  2. It decreases and resolves by 3 to 4 months of age.
- Parent counseling in behavioral management for infant is the only intervention consistently shown to be of benefit.
- Regardless of approach, supportive listening to parents is essential. Individualize the following approaches:
  1. Support appropriate parenting techniques.
  2. Encourage positive feelings toward infant.
  3. Restore confidence.
  4. Dispel guilt.

- Provide reassurance that colic does not result from pain or disease.
- Acknowledge severe stress that affects family as a result of colic.
  1. Discuss parental support systems.
  2. Review the means for parents to deal with stress and obtain respite.
  3. Ensure that adequate parental sleep is being achieved.
- Observe infant crying and parental responses, if possible, to direct behavioral treatment strategy.
- Avoid the impression that you know how to calm the infant or possess better skills than parents.
- Environmental strategies include the following:
  1. Swaddling
  2. "White" noise or background noise
  3. Pacifiers
  4. Increased carrying
  5. Automobile rides
  6. Strolling
  7. Swings or bouncers
- Behavioral strategies include the following:
  1. Crying episodes escalate quickly and can sometimes be averted if parents intervene rapidly.
  2. One study suggests that crying signals a need, not pain.
     a. Offer infant feeding, sucking, sleep, stimulation, or holding.
     b. Try tactics to meet one of these needs for 5 minutes.
     c. Change to alternative strategies to address the next need if unsuccessful.
  3. Feed on demand.
  4. Burp the infant in the upright position.
  5. Place in positions that apply pressure to the abdomen—across the knees.

■ MEDICAL
- Some physicians approach this condition by prescribing a succession of medications, often with the goal of giving parents "something to do" until colic runs its course.
  1. However, this approach may encourage parents to believe that something is wrong with the baby, and they may despair each time a new treatment fails.
  2. Simethicone is probably the only harmless medication.
  3. Dicyclomine hydrochloride (Bentyl) was previously widely used but was later found to be associated with apnea, coma, and death.
  4. Other drugs that are no longer recommended for colic include hyoscyamine sulfate (Levsin), diphenhydramine (Benadryl), phenobarbital, and paregoric.

■ ALTERNATIVE & COMPLEMENTARY THERAPIES

In one double-blind study, herbal tea containing extracts from chamomile, vervain, licorice, fennel, and balm mint was more effective than a placebo in decreasing colic symptoms.

■ FOLLOW-UP & DISPOSITION

- Colic may impair the relationship between parents and infant and may place the infant at increased risk for abuse.
- Studies suggest that mothers view children who were colicky in a different manner even up to age 3. Focus on establishing a positive parent-child relationship.
- Poor infant attachment may result.
- Behavior problems in school have been suggested to result from colic; however, further study of this theory is needed.

■ PATIENT/FAMILY EDUCATION

- It is essential to recognize that parents often feel overwhelmed by endless crying and at times may be clinically depressed.
- Parents often feel guilt and anxiety, and lack confidence in their parenting skills.
- Education and reassurance are as important to treatment as addressing infant or environmental factors.

■ PREVENTIVE TREATMENT

One study suggests that beginning prophylactic carrying at 3 weeks of age reduces subsequent colic.

■ REFERRAL INFORMATION

Parents may need to be referred to their primary care physician or counseling services if significant symptoms of depression or anxiety are recognized.

☼ PEARLS & CONSIDERATIONS

■ WEBSITES

Hundreds of websites offer advice and support for colicky and crying infants. Many provide substantial misinformation and should be used with caution. Consider the following sites for useful, reliable information:

- drkoop.com: www.drkoop.com
- drpaula.com: www.drpaula.com
- Nightime Pediatric Clinics, Inc.: www.nightimepediatrics.com

■ SUPPORT GROUP

CRY-SIS (tel., 0171-404-5011 UK)

REFERENCES

1. Carey WB: The effectiveness of parent counseling in managing colic (commentary), *Pediatrics* 94:333, 1994.
2. Fleisher DR: Coping with colic, *Contemp Pediatr* 15:144, 1998.
3. Lehtonen LA, Rautava PT: Infantile colic: natural history and treatment, *Curr Probl Pediatr* 26:79, 1996.
4. Wessel MA et al: Paroxysmal fussing in infancy, sometimes called "colic," *Pediatrics* 14:421, 1954.
5. Wolke D, Gray P, Meyer R: Excessive infant crying: a controlled study of mothers helping mothers, *Pediatrics* 94:322, 1994.

Author: **Michael Visick, M.D.**

BASIC INFORMATION

DEFINITION
Congenital adrenal hyperplasia (CAH) is any of several related conditions caused by decreased activity of one of multiple adrenal cortex enzymes involved in the biosynthetic pathways of cortisol, resulting in overstimulation of the adrenal cortex and, in most forms, hyperandrogenism.

SYNONYMS
- Adrenogenital disorder
- CAH
- Classic CAH (21-hydroxylase deficiency)

ICD-9CM CODE
255.2 Adrenogenital disorders, congenital adrenal hyperplasia

ETIOLOGY
- From 90% to 95% of cases of CAH are caused by an autosomal-recessive deficiency of the enzyme 21-hydroxylase.
  1. This enzyme deficiency leads to the decreased efficiency of cortisol production, resulting in pituitary overstimulation of the adrenal gland.
  2. Subsequently, there is an increase in concentration of precursors, such as 17-hydroxyprogesterone, proximal to the step involving the defective enzyme.
  3. The increased concentrations of precursors result in increased androgen production.
  4. The enzymatic defect may also decrease the production of the mineralocorticoid aldosterone.
- Other, rare forms of CAH include the following:
  1. 11-hydroxylase deficiency (3% of CAH)
  2. 3-β-hydroxysteroid dehydrogenase deficiency

EPIDEMIOLOGY & DEMOGRAPHICS
- Classic 21-OH deficiency found in 1 per 12,000 to 1 per 15,000 births
- Much higher in select populations (e.g., Aleut Eskimos)

HISTORY
There are three characteristic presentations.
- Salt-losing male infant
  1. Infant is well at birth and during the first week.
  2. During the second to fourth weeks of life, the infant develops vomiting with increasing lethargy, poor weight gain, and dehydration.
- Female infant
  1. Ambiguous genitalia are noted at birth (see "Physical Examination").
- Non–salt-losing male
  1. The child is normal in infancy and early childhood.
  2. Then, there is an increased rate of linear growth and signs of androgen activity, such as pubic hair growth or adult body odor.

PHYSICAL EXAMINATION
Based on characteristic presentations and gender described under "History"
- Salt-losing male infant
  1. Hyperpigmentation of areolae and scrotum
  2. Enlarged penis, usually not detected before salt-losing crisis
  3. During salt losing crisis, lethargy and signs of dehydration and, potentially, shock
- Female infant
  1. Ambiguous genitalia are characterized by clitoral enlargement and midline posterior labial fusion present at birth.
  2. Occasionally, clitoral size may be severe enough to mimic bilaterally cryptorchid male.
- Non–salt-losing male
  1. Signs of increased androgen activity include the following:
     a. Pubic hair
     b. Axillary hair
     c. Skin oiliness, acne
     d. Accelerated linear growth
  2. Notably, testes are prepubertal size.

DIAGNOSIS

DIFFERENTIAL DIAGNOSIS
- Salt-losing male infant
  1. Other causes for dehydration and acidosis include the following:
     a. Acute gastroenteritis
     b. Sepsis
     c. Vomiting caused by elevated intracranial pressure (e.g., meningitis, intracranial hemorrhage)
     d. Renal tubular acidosis
     e. Metabolic disease resulting in acidosis
  2. This condition is sometimes confused with pyloric stenosis because of age at presentation and vomiting.
- Female infant
  1. Other causes for ambiguous genitalia include the following:
     a. Partial androgen insensitivity
     b. Prenatal androgen exposure
     c. Ovotestes
     d. Virilizing tumor
- Non–salt-losing male
  1. Other causes for hyperandrogenism include the following:
     a. Central precocious puberty
     b. Adrenal tumor
     c. Exogenous androgens

DIAGNOSTIC WORKUP
- Adrenal steroid levels
  1. 17-Hydroxyprogesterone (17-OHP) and androstenedione are usually sufficient to make the diagnosis, especially in the infant.
  2. Marked elevation in 17-OHP (often elevated 100 times normal) with increased androstenedione is noted.
- Adrenocorticotropic hormone (ACTH) stimulation test with 17-OHP levels before and 60 minutes after 0.25 mg of synthetic ACTH (e.g., Cortrosyn) may be helpful in less obvious cases
- Serum electrolytes
  1. Hyponatremia, hyperkalemia, and acidosis, which may be severe, in mineralocorticoid deficient infant
  2. May be normal in non–salt-losing older child
- Bone age
  1. Especially helpful in noninfant presentations
  2. Should expect to see significant advancement over chronologic age
- Ultrasound and chromosomal analysis in infants with ambiguous genitalia (see the section "Ambiguity of the External Genitalia")

THERAPY

NONPHARMACOLOGIC
- Infants often benefit from added dietary salt.
  1. This is *not* sufficient for treatment, however.

MEDICAL
- Glucocorticoid replacement
  1. Usually, hydrocortisone at 10 to 25 mg/m^2/day divided into two to three doses during growing years
  2. Equivalent (glucocorticoid) dose as dexamethasone once daily sufficient in adults
- For salt-wasters, also need mineralocorticoid replacement
  1. Usually as 9-αfluorohydrocortisone (Florinef) at 0.1 mg/day initially in addition to glucocorticoid replacement
- During salt-losing crisis
  1. Normal saline infusion
  2. Calcium gluconate (protects against cardiac arrhythmia)

3. Potassium binder and/or insulin and glucose infusion to lower potassium and/or sodium bicarbonate to lower potassium and treat acidosis

■ SURGICAL
- Urologic consultation is imperative in the newborn period for the female with ambiguous genitalia.
- Surgical reconstruction of genitalia in females is usually done in the first year or two of life, although there is some controversy regarding timing.

■ FOLLOW-UP & DISPOSITION
- Every 3 to 6 months
  1. Perform a physical examination and carefully document height and pubertal status.
  2. Adrenal steroid determinations are necessary to adjust glucocorticoid dose.
     a. Androstenedione should be kept in normal range for age.
     b. 17-OHP should be between 500 and 1000 ng/dl (several times normal).
- Every year: bone age determination indicated to assess linear growth and bone maturation

■ PATIENT/FAMILY EDUCATION
- Stress-dose glucocorticoids are critical with physiologic stress; failure to use stress doses can result in shock and death.
  1. Glucocorticoid dose should be increased three to five times the normal daily dosage.

2. Patients/parents should have injectable form of glucocorticoid available at home.

■ PREVENTIVE TREATMENT
- Newborn state screening tests, done in some states, may reduce the incidence of salt-losing crisis in affected infant boys.
- Intrauterine treatment of the female fetus affected by CAH via administration of dexamethasone to the mother may ameliorate genital ambiguity.

■ REFERRAL INFORMATION
All patients with classic CAH should be evaluated and have therapy overseen by pediatric endocrinologist, if possible.

☼ PEARLS & CONSIDERATIONS

■ CLINICAL PEARLS
- Some cases of hirsutism and amenorrhea in adult women may be caused by "late-onset" CAH.
- Hypothalamic maturation caused by excessive androgen exposure as a result of undertreatment or nontreatment may result in true central precocious puberty.
- Controversial data suggest that behavioral effects may occur in girls as

a result of prenatal androgen exposure associated with CAH.

■ WEBSITES
- American Academy of Family Physicians: www.aafp.org/afp/990301ap/1190.html
- The Endocrine Society: 216.205.53.178/endo/pubrelations/patientInfo/cah.cfm
- Johns Hopkins Pediatric Endocrinology: www.med.jhu.edu/pedendo/cah/
- The MAGIC Foundation: www.magicfoundation.org/cah.html
- University of Maryland Medicine: umm.drkoop.com/conditions/ency/article/000411.htm
- WebMD Health: my.webmd.com/content/asset/adam_disease_adrenogenital

REFERENCES
1. Frias J et al: Technical report: congenital adrenal hyperplasia, *Pediatrics* 106: 1511, 2000.
2. Levine LS: Congential adrenal hyperplasia, *Pediatr Rev* 21:159, 2000.
3. New MI, Rapaport R: The adrenal cortex. In Sperling MA (ed): *Pediatric endocrinology*, Philadelphia, 1996, WB Saunders.
4. Pang S: Congenital adrenal hyperplasia, *Endocrinol Metab Clin North Am* 26: 853, 1997.

Author: **Craig Orlowski, M.D.**

II

BASIC INFORMATION

■ DEFINITION
Congenital diaphragmatic hernia (CDH) is a diaphragmatic defect resulting from failure of the posterolateral portion of the diaphragm to develop, usually involving the foramen of Bochdalek, resulting in herniation of abdominal contents into the chest cavity. This leads to varying degrees of pulmonary hypoplasia.

■ SYNONYMS
- Diaphragmatic hernia
- D-hernia
- Congenital hernia of the diaphragm

ICD-9CM CODE
756.6 Congenital diaphragmatic hernia

■ ETIOLOGY
- Most cases are sporadic; an autosomal-recessive variant has been described.
- Approximately 40% are associated with anomalies: chromosomal, genitourinary, renal, cardiac, central nervous system

■ EPIDEMIOLOGY
- Prevalence of 1 per 3000 live births
- Up to 50% mortality even with aggressive support

■ HISTORY
- Prenatal: Polyhydramnios, lack of stomach bubble, and loops of intestine are seen in the chest during ultrasound.
- Patients are at high risk for pneumothorax with positive-pressure ventilation because of pulmonary hypoplasia.
- Respiratory distress may occur in the delivery room; mild symptoms may delay the diagnosis.

■ PHYSICAL EXAMINATION
- Respiratory distress
- Decreased left-sided breath sounds (90% of hernias are left sided)
- Heart sounds shifted to right
- Scaphoid abdomen

DIAGNOSIS

■ DIFFERENTIAL DIAGNOSIS
- Pneumothorax
- Cystic adenomatoid malformation
- Bronchogenic cyst
- Congenital lobar emphysema

■ DIAGNOSTIC WORKUP
- Chest radiograph: Stomach or liver herniation carries a worse prognosis.
- Arterial blood gas: The degree of hypercarbia is related to the severity of pulmonary hypoplasia.
- Cardiac ECHO is used to evaluate for persistent pulmonary hypertension.
- Perform evaluation of chromosomes and other organs if clinical suspicion exists.

THERAPY

- In delivery room
  1. If positive-pressure ventilation is required, make every effort to provide it through endotracheal tube to minimize intestinal distension; place nasogastric tube to decompress stomach.
- In nursery
  1. Take steps to avoid persistent pulmonary hypertension. Maintain thermoneutral environment; minimize stress; target normal pH, Pao_2, $Paco_2$; and avoid overdistension of the lungs.
  2. Place Replogle on low intermittent suction.
  3. Establish arterial and venous access.
- Surgical repair once stable (potentially while receiving extracorporeal membrane oxygenation [ECMO])

■ FOLLOW-UP & DISPOSITION
- Most patients have long-term gastroesophageal reflux and intestinal motility problems.
- Follow growth parameters closely for evidence of failure to thrive.
- If infant survives neonatal period, chronic lung disease usually improves with time.
- Ongoing neurodevelopmental assessment is essential.
- Reherniation is a risk in first few months.
- There is a low index of suspicion for volvulus with vomiting illness.

■ PATIENT/FAMILY EDUCATION
- Explain signs and symptoms of volvulus and the need for immediate intervention if present.
- Discuss intestinal motility and gastroesophageal reflux management.

PEARLS & CONSIDERATIONS

■ REFERRAL INFORMATION
- Prenatal consult with neonatology and pediatric surgery
- Plan delivery at perinatal center with intensive care support services

■ WEBSITES
- March of Dimes: www.modimes. org/HealthLibrary2/FactsFigures/ descrip.htm
- Texas Pediatric Surgical Associates: www.pedisurg.com/PtEduc/ Congenital_Diaphragmatic_ Hernia.htm

REFERENCES
1. Glick PL, Irish MS, Holm BA: New Insights into the pathophysiology of CDH, *Clin Perinatol* 23:625, 1996.
2. Katz AL, Wiswell TE, Baumgart S: Contemporary controversies in the management of CDH, *Clin Perinatol* 25: 219, 1998.
3. Kays WD et al: Detrimental effects of standard medical therapy in CDH, *Ann Surg* 230:340, 1999.
4. Weber TR et al: Improved survival in CDH with evolving therapeutic strategies, *Arch Surg* 133:498, 1998.
Author: **Patricia Chess, M.D.**

BASIC INFORMATION

■ DEFINITION

Congestive heart failure (CHF) is the heart's inability to generate enough output to meet the metabolic demands of the body.

■ SYNONYMS

- CHF
- Heart failure
- Pump failure

ICD-9CM CODE

428.0 Congestive heart failure

■ ETIOLOGY

- Imposition of an excessive workload
  1. Volume-overload lesions: ventricular septal defects, atrial septal defects, truncus arteriosus, patent ductus arteriosus, aortopulmonary window, atrioventricular canal, arteriovenous malformation, single ventricle physiology
  2. Pressure-overload lesions: valvar stenosis, coarctation of the aorta, hypoplastic left heart syndrome
- Imposition of a normal workload on damaged myocardium
  1. Myocarditis
  2. Asphyxia
  3. Cardiomyopathy
  4. Iron overload: seen with most chronic hemolytic anemias, including β-thalassemia
- Secondary heart failure
  1. Renal disease (either via toxin, such as blood urea nitrogen [BUN], or volume, or both)
  2. Hypertension
  3. Thyroid disease (myocardial injury)
  4. Sepsis (myocardial injury)
  5. Sickle cell anemia (volume overload)
- Differs for each age group:
  1. In utero: anemia, arrhythmias, volume overload, myocarditis
  2. Neonates: myocardial dysfunction, heart muscle abnormalities, pressure overload, volume overload, arrhythmias, myocarditis
  3. Infants: volume overload, heart muscle abnormalities, secondary heart disease, myocarditis
  4. Children: palliated congenital heart disease, atrioventricular valve regurgitation, rheumatic fever, myocarditis, heart muscle abnormalities, bacterial endocarditis, secondary causes

■ EPIDEMIOLOGY & DEMOGRAPHICS

- Depends on the prevalence of the underlying disease states

■ HISTORY

- In the neonatal period, CHF is associated with asphyxia, sepsis, and hypoglycemia; the infant is floppy, lethargic, and pale with or without respiratory compromise and refuses to feed.
- Infants may be irritable, diaphoretic, pale, lethargic, or tachypneic; refuse to feed; and have a history of wheezing.
- If CHF is chronic, children fail to gain weight and height may be stunted despite what appears to be appropriate intake.
- Children may have dyspnea, particularly on exertion, tachypnea, orthopnea, and less energy than their peers.
- Children may also have a history of facial puffiness, excessive sweatiness, pallor, and lost interest in surroundings.
- Children may have abdominal pain, nausea, and vomiting with eating.

■ PHYSICAL EXAMINATION

- Recognized in the fetus by echocardiography as hydrops
- Tachypnea and tachycardia
- Diaphoresis
- Pallor
- Crackles and wheezes on lung examination
- Peripheral edema (less common)
- Pulses and blood pressure sometimes diminished
- Cardiomegaly
  1. Impulse quiet with cardiac muscle disease
  2. Impulse hyperdynamic with volume-overload or atrioventricular valve regurgitation
- Third heart sound
- Pulsus alternans: an alteration in pulses from weak to strong that is thought to be secondary to the inability of the myocardium to complete recovery from each contraction
- Pulsus paradoxus: a fall in blood pressure greater than 10 mm Hg on inspiration and a rise on expiration (rarely useful in pediatrics, however)

DIAGNOSIS

■ DIFFERENTIAL DIAGNOSIS

- Primarily respiratory illness
  1. Pneumonia or pneumonitis, where clinical and radiology findings may be similar to those of pulmonary edema seen with CHF
  2. Primary gastroenterologic illness, such as gastroenteritis, which causes nausea and vomiting and is seen in a patient with CHF and hepatomegaly
  3. The aforementioned two must be differentiated.
- Infectious disease states, such as viral syndromes, which may cause hepatosplenomegaly and may be confused with the hepatosplenomegaly of CHF

■ DIAGNOSTIC WORKUP

- Chest radiograph will likely show cardiomegaly with hilar "fullness," representing pulmonary edema (when the capillary pressures exceed 20 to 25 mm Hg), resulting in Kerley B lines.
- Urinalysis: There may be proteinuria and high specific gravity secondary to diminished renal perfusion.
- Serum sodium is elevated.
- Serum BUN and creatinine are elevated.
- Liver transaminases may be elevated because of hepatocellular dysfunction secondary to congestion.
- Electrocardiographic changes are relatively nonspecific.
  1. If CHF is chronic, volume- or pressure-overload ventricular hypertrophy with or without a ventricular strain pattern may be seen.
- Echocardiogram may reveal the following:
  1. Structural heart disease, myocardial dysfunction, or functional disease
  2. Occasionally, volume-overload states (this is best done by clinical assessment, however)

THERAPY

■ NONPHARMACOLOGIC

- Reduce physical activity.
- Initiate a low-sodium, fluid-restricted diet.

■ MEDICAL

- Digitalis increases contractility; although its role has been questioned periodically, it is still the first-line therapy.
- Diuretic therapy is important for CHF.
  1. Begin with furosemide and add or use any combination of bumetadine, ethacrynic acid, thiazides, spironolactone, and/or acetazolamide.
- Vasodilators for afterload reduction include nitroprusside, hydralazine, enalapril, enalaprilat, and captopril.
- Inotropic agents include dopamine, dobutamine, epinephrine, norepinephrine, and isoproterenol.
- Combination inotropic agents and vasodilators include amrinone and milrinone.

■ SURGICAL

- CHF is a medical condition that may resolve with surgical intervention in correction or palliation of complex structural heart disease.
- Left ventricular assist devices may be temporary bridges to cardiac transplantation.
- Extracorporeal membrane oxygenation may sustain life while a "curative process" is occurring (i.e., resolution of sepsis or an acute pulmonary disease).

■ FOLLOW-UP & DISPOSITION

Depends on the cause of CHF but requires long-term surveillance by a cardiologist

■ PATIENT/FAMILY EDUCATION

Parents need to be educated about the constellation of symptoms associated with CHF.

■ PREVENTIVE TREATMENT OR TESTS

The role of such biomarkers as the cardiac dioponing is being explored for confirmation of the diagnosis of heart disease.

■ REFERRAL INFORMATION

Regular follow-up with a primary care provider should be maintained, and a cardiologist should be contacted if deemed necessary.

○ PEARLS & CONSIDERATIONS

■ CLINICAL PEARLS

- "All that wheezes is not asthma."
- Diuretic therapy may assist in patients who cannot (or will not) maintain fluid- and sodium-restricted diets; serum electrolytes must be followed closely and supplemented as necessary.
- Increasing caloric density assists in appropriate growth in children with high-energy needs caused by CHF.

REFERENCES

1. Freed MD: Cardiomyopathies. In Fyler DC (ed): *Nadas' pediatric cardiology,* St Louis, 1992, Mosby.
2. Talner NS: Heart failure. In Emmanouilides GC et al (eds): *Heart disease in infants, children, and adolescents: including the fetus and young adult,* Baltimore, 1995, Williams & Wilkins.

Author: **Michelle A. Grenier, M.D.**

BASIC INFORMATION

■ **DEFINITION**

Conjunctivitis is any inflammatory condition of the membranes that line the eyelids or exposed surface of the sclera.

■ **SYNONYMS**

- Pink eye
- Red eye

ICD-9CM CODES

372.0   Acute/allergic
372.01 Chronic
077.99 Viral
077.98 Chlamydial
098.40 Neonatal

■ **ETIOLOGY**

- Infectious
  1. Viral: adenovirus (most common viral cause), Coxsackie virus, herpes simplex virus (HSV), varicella-zoster virus, Epstein-Barr virus, rubeola, rubella, mumps, enteroviral
  2. Bacterial: *Haemophilus influenzae* (most common bacterial cause), streptococcal, pseudomonal, *Moraxella*, staphylococcal, *Staphylococcus epidermitis, Neisseria gonorrhoeae*
  3. Chlamydial: *Chlamydia trachomatis*
- Allergic: hayfever conjunctivitis (pollens, molds, fungi, dust, foods), vernal conjunctivitis
- Chemical/toxic: ophthalmologic medications, work/environmental exposures, cosmetics
- Foreign body: contact lenses, other foreign bodies
- Idiopathic
- Other: graft-versus-host disease, Stevens-Johnson syndrome, Reiter's syndrome, Kawasaki disease

■ **EPIDEMIOLOGY & DEMOGRAPHICS**

- Most common acute condition of the eye seen by pediatricians
- Neonate
  1. Occurs in 1.6% to 12% of all newborns
  2. Ophthalmia neonatorum
     a. Acute: chemical (silver nitrate), chlamydial, bacterial, or rarely, viral (without other nonocular manifestations)
- Infant
  1. Chlamydial, bacterial
  2. Secondary to obstructed lacrimal duct
- Children
  1. Bacterial pathogen twice as likely as viral
  2. *H. influenzae:* 40% to 50%
  3. *Streptococcus pneumoniae:* 10% to 15%

4. *Moraxella Catarrhalis:* 8%
5. Adenovirus: 20% to 30%
- Allergic
  1. Hayfever conjunctivitis
  2. Vernal: childhood

■ **HISTORY**

- Viral: acute onset, often associated with upper respiratory symptoms or other systemic complaints (e.g., adenoviral pharyngoconjunctival fever), unilateral or bilateral
- Bacterial: acute or hyperacute onset, morning crusting common, unilateral or bilateral
- Allergic: usually bilateral, itching is hallmark
  1. Hayfever conjunctivitis: acute onset, short duration, many recurrences
  2. Vernal conjunctivitis: onset at age 3 to 12 years
     a. More common in warm climates
     b. Onset usually in spring
     c. Often associated with history of atopy, rhinitis, or sinusitis
  3. Atopic keratitis
  4. Giant papillary conjunctivitis
- Chemical/toxic: medication history, work-related exposures, cosmetics
- Dry eyes: antidepressant use, collagen vascular diseases
- Foreign body: unilateral
- Time of onset: especially important in neonatal conjunctivitis
  1. In first 24 hours of life: chemical most likely
  2. Between 2 and 5 days of life: gonococcal (later onset if prophylaxis given)
  3. Between 5 and 23 days of life: chlamydial

■ **PHYSICAL EXAMINATION**

- Pattern of the conjunctivitis
  1. Papillary: allergic but nonspecific
  2. Follicular: adenoviral, chlamydial, topical medication, HSV
- Viral
  1. Conjunctival injection
  2. Watery or serous discharge
  3. Preauricular adenopathy
  4. Bilateral or unilateral
  5. Associated rashes
  6. If associated with pharyngitis: adenovirus
  7. If vesicles or corneal ulceration: HSV keratoconjunctivitis possible cause
- Bacterial
  1. Conjunctival injection
  2. Chemosis
  3. Mucopurulent or purulent discharge
  4. No preauricular adenopathy (except *N. gonorrhoeae*)
  5. Often associated with otitis media (*H. influenzae*)

- Allergic
  1. Serous or mucoid discharge: often very stringy
  2. Ocular itching
  3. Conjunctival injection
  4. With or without photophobia
  5. Hayfever conjunctivitis: mild conjunctival swelling, upper more than lower eyelid
  6. Vernal: more severe injection than hayfever conjunctivitis; large papillary response of upper lid or perilimbal corneal opacifications
  7. Atopic keratitis: lower lid papillary response more than upper lid
- Must examine ears for otitis media.
- Complete a physical examination to look for systemic disorders.

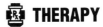 **DIAGNOSIS**

■ **DIFFERENTIAL DIAGNOSIS**

- Keratitis: inflammation of the cornea caused by infection, trauma (contact lens use), ultraviolet radiation exposure
- Uveitis: anterior uveitis (iritis, iridocyclitis) is inflammation of iris and ciliary muscle; usually an autoimmune reaction
- Scleritis: focal or diffuse scleral inflammation, usually autoimmune
- Episcleritis: focal inflammation of deep subconjunctival (episcleral) tissues, autoimmune
- Acute glaucoma: medical emergency caused by blockage of aqueous humor outflow leading to a sudden elevation in intraocular pressure; uncommon in pediatrics

■ **DIAGNOSTIC WORKUP**

- The diagnosis is usually made based on history and physical examination.
- Conjunctival culture and scraping with Gram stain is taken in neonates.
  1. Must rule out gonococcal and chlamydial disease.
- Culture and Gram stain may be helpful in other selected individuals.
- Many eosinophils (Giemsa stain) in eye discharge may indicate allergic etiology.
- High serum and tear immunoglobulin E (IgE) is seen in vernal conjunctivitis and atopic keratitis.

THERAPY

■ **NONPHARMACOLOGIC**

- Apply warm or cool compresses to eye.
- Avoid the irritant or allergen.

■ MEDICAL

- Antibiotic therapy is necessary to help prevent sight-threatening complications of gonococcal and chlamydial conjunctivitis.
- With other bacterial causes, topical antibiotic treatment hastens resolution of symptoms and prevents secondary cases, although most cases will resolve without specific antibiotic therapy.
- If systemic antibiotic treatment is used, topical treatment is not necessary.
- In neonates, the specific antibiotic is based on culture results and clinical suspicion.
  1. Gonococcal: ceftriaxone or cefotaxime for 1 to 7 days
  2. Chlamydial: systemically administered erythromycin (eliminates nasopharyngeal carriage and possibly subsequent pneumonia)
  3. Staphylococcal and streptococcal: topical ophthalmologic antibiotic preparation (drops or ointment)
  4. Allergic conjunctivitis: topical ophthalmologic antihistamine or mast cell stabilizer (Oral antihistamine may be appropriate for some.)

■ PATIENT/FAMILY EDUCATION

- Good handwashing technique should be taught and used in family and day-care setting.
- The rapid spread and high contagiousness of infective conjunctivitis should be explained and understood.
- Known irritants or allergens should be avoided, if possible.

■ PREVENTIVE TREATMENT

- Neonatal prophylaxis (1% silver nitrate or 0.5% erythromycin or 1% tetracycline)
- All equally effect for prophylaxis of gonorrheal eye infections
- Helpful in reducing chlamydial ophthalmic infections
- Good handwashing practice in families, in day-care settings, and for individuals with upper respiratory infections

■ REFERRAL INFORMATION

- Referral to a pediatric ophthalmologist should be considered if the patient has blurred vision that does not improve with blinking, severe pain, or photophobia.
- Patients with HSV infections or other agents that produce corneal ulcerations should also be referred to a pediatric ophthalmologist.

☼ PEARLS & CONSIDERATIONS

■ CLINICAL PEARLS

- One fourth of patients have associated otitis media at the time of diagnosis, and another one fourth develop otitis media if treated with a topical antibiotic.
- Outside the neonatal period, conjunctivitis is often self-limited (7 to 10 days); antibiotic therapy helps hasten the amelioration of symptoms and prevents secondary cases caused by spread.

REFERENCES

1. Gigliotti F: Acute conjunctivitis, *Pediatr Rev* 16:203, 1995.
2. Gigliotti F et al: Etiology of acute conjunctivitis in children, *J Pediatr* 98:531,1981.
3. Gigliotti F et al: Efficacy of topical therapy in acute conjunctivitis in children, *J Pediatr* 104:623, 1984.
4. Morrow GL, Abbott RL: Conjunctivitis, *Am Fam Physician* 57:735, 1998.
5. Weber CM, Eichenbaum JW: The red eye: differentiating viral conjunctivitis from other, common causes, *Postgrad Med* 101:185, 1997.

Author: **Eric Ingerowski, M.D.**

BASIC INFORMATION

DEFINITION

Constipation is hard, infrequent stool that is usually painful to pass. Failure to empty the lower colon with each bowel movement is another definition. According to the Clinical Practice Guidelines, "delay or difficulty in defecation, present for two or more weeks and sufficient to cause significant distress to the patient." Encopresis is fecal soiling as a result of stool leaking around a distended rectum that has decreased sensation.

SYNONYMS

- Constipation
  1. Idiopathic constipation
  2. Functional fecal retention
  3. Fecal withholding
- Encopresis
  1. Soiling
  2. Fecal soiling

ICD-9CM CODES

564.0 Constipation, neurogenic
306.4 Constipation, psychogenic
787.6 Encopresis

ETIOLOGY

- Several theories regarding constipation are as follows:
  1. Diminished relaxation of internal anal sphincter and active contraction of external anal sphincter during defecation
  2. Decreased awareness of rectal distention
  3. Increased threshold volume of distention
  4. Decreased ability to evacuate rectal content
  5. Possible right-sided colonic dysfunction in severe constipation
- No data are available to confirm or refute that these dysfunctions predate clinical findings.
- Usually, no underlying organic or psychiatric problem is present.
- Symptom, not a disease, with contributions caused by the following:
  1. Low-fiber diet
  2. Decreased fluid intake
  3. Medication
  4. Withholding (i.e., not wanting to defecate at school)
  5. Inappropriate toilet training

EPIDEMIOLOGY & DEMOGRAPHICS

- Twenty-five percent present before 1 year of age.
- Peak occurs at 2 to 4 years; the incidence is higher in males than in females.
- Up to 10% of all children experience this problem, most without an associated abnormality.
- Encopresis is three to six times more common in boys.
- Constipation accounts for 3% of general pediatric and 25% of pediatric gastroenterologist visits.

HISTORY

- Meconium passage: if late, may indicate primary colonic problem (i.e., Hirschsprung's disease)
- Perinatal illnesses, especially necrotizing enterocolitis (NEC), which may lead to stricture development
- Character of stools should be assessed: consistency, caliber, volume, frequency
  1. Stool patterns should be assessed at birth and in the first 24 hours, early infancy, later infancy, and childhood.
  2. Small pellets indicate incomplete evacuation.
  3. Massive stools indicate infrequent stooling with functional retention.
  4. Narrow-caliber stools, especially with abdominal distention, may indicate the following:
     a. Hirschsprung's disease
     b. Stenosis
     c. Ectopic anus
- Perianal disorders (e.g., fissure, dermatitis, abscess)
- History of sexual or physical abuse
- Prior surgery
- Laxative abuse
- Tolerance of early feeding
- Transitions and bowel habits
  1. Breast-to-bottle milk transition may change stool.
  2. Introduction of cow's milk is the most common cause of constipation.
  3. Strained foods-to-table foods transition may change stool.
  4. Home care-to-day care transition may change stool.
  5. Diaper-to-toilet training transition is the most common time for withholding.
- Other medical issues
  1. Hospitalizations
  2. Allergies
  3. Coarse, dry hair
  4. Cold or heat sensitivity
  5. Recurrent otitis
- Developmental history
- Social history
- Family history of bowel habits and problems
- Family history of thyroid disease, myopathies, Hirschsprung's disease, or cystic fibrosis

PHYSICAL EXAMINATION

- Fever, anorexia, nausea, vomiting, poor weight gain, and weight loss all indicate organic disorder.
- Growth parameters and velocity must be measured.
- A thorough neurologic examination should be conducted because children with primary neurologic or myopathic abnormalities (e.g., cerebral palsy, muscular dystrophy, discitis) have abnormal stool patterns.
  1. Cremasteric reflex
  2. Anal wink
  3. Tone, strength, deep tendon reflexes
- Abdominal distention
- Bowel sounds
- Perineal examination for acute infections (candidal, group A streptococcal)
- Anal tags, fissures
- Anal placement: assess for normal location
  1. Ectopic anterior displacement of anus
     a. This is one of the most common and underdiagnosed anatomic causes of constipation.
     b. Female anus-fourchette:coccyx-fourchette ratio of less than 0.34 is abnormal.
     c. Male anus-scrotum:coccyx-scrotum ratio of less than 0.46 is abnormal.
- Rectal examination
  1. The anal canal should relax, although it may be initially tight on examination.
  2. Dilated ampulla, especially if filled with stool, indicates retention.
  3. Assess for fecal and other masses.
  4. Hemorrhoids are rare in children.
  5. Perirectal ulcers, fistulas, abscess, and strictures are associated with Crohn's disease.
  6. May palpate internal fissures.
- Back and spine examination
  1. Dimple
  2. Hair tufts

COMPLICATIONS

- Gastrointestinal (GI)
  1. Encopresis
     a. Fecal soiling occurs from leakage around formed stool in dilated, insensitive rectum.
     b. It may be the first recognized problem in chronic constipation.
  2. Overflow diarrhea
  3. Abdominal pain
  4. Abdominal distention
  5. Anal fissure or rectal bleeding
  6. Rectal prolapse
  7. Megacolonrectum
- Urologic
  1. Urinary tract infection
  2. Enuresis
  3. Pelviocaliceal dilation
- Behavioral
  1. Depression
  2. Low or poor self-esteem
  3. Association with host of behavioral and developmental difficulties
     a. Attention deficit/hyperactivity disorder

II

b. Oppositional defiant disorder
c. Obsessive-compulsive disorder
d. Anxiety
e. Developmental delay/mental retardation

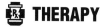 DIAGNOSIS

■ DIFFERENTIAL DIAGNOSIS
- Malnutrition
- Dehydration
- Cow's milk protein reaction (questionably an allergic reaction)
- Electrolyte abnormality
  1. Hyponatremia
  2. Hypercalcemia
  3. Hypokalemia
- Cystic fibrosis
- Hirschsprung's disease
- Hypothyroidism
- Diabetes mellitus (DM):neuropathy of colon, seen as a late complication of DM
- Structural abnormality
  1. Perianal abscess, fistula, hemorrhoid
  2. Rectal prolapse: rule out cystic fibrosis
  3. Rectal ectasia
  4. Anterior ectopic anus
- Neuromuscular disease with constipation as a common feature
  1. Cerebral palsy
  2. Muscular dystrophy
  3. Multiple sclerosis
  4. Myelomeningocele
- Chronic intestinal pseudoobstruction
  1. Diarrhea is more common because of bacterial overgrowth.
  2. Pseudoobstruction is divided into two main types:
     a. Neuropathic
     b. Myopathic
- Medications
  1. Anticholinergics (i.e., atropine, scopolamine, hyoscyamine)
  2. Antidiarrheal agents (i.e., diphenoxylate, loperamide, paregoric)
  3. Cholestyramine
  4. Bismuth
  5. Tricyclic antidepressants
  6. Anticonvulsants
  7. Opiate narcotics
  8. Antihistamines
  9. Some chemotherapeutic agents
  10. Nonsteroidal antiinflammatory drugs
  11. Iron supplements
  12. Calcium channel blockers

■ DIAGNOSTIC WORKUP
- Most children without suspicions on history or physical examination do not need an extensive workup.
- Perianal injury caused by sexual abuse leads to pain on defecation and constipation.

- Organic causes must be excluded.
  1. If suspicions arise on physical examination or history, may suggest the following:
     a. Thyroid studies to rule out hypothyroidism
     b. Electrolytes, calcium, and magnesium to rule out abnormality
     c. Urinalysis and urine culture
     d. Abdominal flat plate to show excessive stool or obstruction
     e. Barium enema to rule out Hirschsprung's disease and stenosis (especially post-NEC)
     f. Lumbosacral spine imaging to rule out tumor, discitis, or other spinal or canal abnormalities
  2. Anorectal manometry may be useful and usually requires gastroenterology referral.
  3. Rectal biopsy may be done in patients suspected of having Hirschsprung's disease.

℞ THERAPY

■ NONPHARMACOLOGIC
- Explain to parents that their child is experiencing pain with defecation; this is usually not willful misbehavior.
- The goal of therapy is to remove the association of pain, anxiety, and negative attributes with stooling and soiling.
- Diet guidelines are as follows:
  1. High-fiber diet should be initiated according to the following equation:
     a. Age (in years) + 5 (or 6) = Number of grams of fiber per day
  2. Good fluid intake, especially juices with high osmotic load, should be ensured.
     a. Absorbable and nonabsorbable carbohydrates soften stool.
     b. Sorbitol (in prune, pear, and apple juices) increases the frequency and water content of stool.
- Behavioral modification calendars and stickers are useful adjuncts.
  1. Regular, unhurried time on toilet
  2. Stooling pattern/consistency diary
  3. Reward system
- Relaxation treatment and biofeedback can be used.
  1. Must be at least 5 years old to participate and cooperate effectively
  2. Painless and risk free

■ MEDICAL
- The three phases of constipation care are as follows:
  1. Empty the rectum thoroughly.
  2. Sustain rectal clearing and restore normal tone.
  3. Wean from medical interventions.

- Disimpaction may be required before initiation of maintenance therapy.
  1. Any one of the following types of enemas can be used, if necessary, every 6 to 12 hours for 1 to 2 days or every 24 hours for 2 to 4 days:
     a. Saline
     b. Mineral oil
     c. Phosphate
     d. Phosphate and mineral oil (3:1)
     e. Milk and molasses (3 ounces milk and 3 ounces molasses, 1 to 2 ounces mineral oil)
  2. Oral disimpaction is also possible.
     a. Mineral oil (1 ounce per year of age twice a day for 2 to 3 days, maximum 8 ounce/dose)
     b. Polyethylene glycol electrolyte solution (10 to 40 ml/kg/hr for 12 to 36 hours often given in hospital by nasogastric tube)
- Maintenance phase may need to continue for months.
  1. Daily loose stool is goal.
     a. Stool should be loose so that defecation occurs without pain.
     b. Stool should be loose so that the child cannot withhold and the rectum empties completely.
  2. Osmotic cathartics or lubricants alone or in combination may be used.
     a. Lactulose: 1 to 3 ml/kg/day, one to two times per day
     b. Milk of magnesia: 1 to 2 ml/kg/day, one to two times per day
        (1) May mix with juice, milk, cereal, or anything
     c. Sorbitol: 1 to 3 ml/kg/day
     d. Mineral oil: 1 to 4 ml/kg, one to two times per day
        (1) Less palatable; mix with juice
        (2) Lipoid pneumonia if patient aspirates
- Once normal, soft stools are achieved daily for 1 month, may decrease dose 25% monthly for several months.
  1. If defecation continues without constipation, continue to decrease dose.
  2. If constipation recurs, return to previous dose that led to soft, daily stool.
- If cathartics or lubricants are not successful, may add or substitute with bulk agents or stimulants.
  1. Bulk-forming agents increase the nonabsorbable contents and increase movement through the GI tract. May also be used as maintenance.
     a. Psyllium, age-based dosing: 1.25 to 7.5 g/dose orally one to three times per day
     b. Malt soup extract: ½ to 2 tsp per 8 ounces liquid, one to two times per day
  2. Stimulants or irritants allow the GI tract to respond to distention

more quickly. Use briefly, as rescue agents, for 2 to 4 days when necessary.
   a. Senna: 10 to 20 mg/kg/dose at bedtime
   b. Bisacodyl: 1 to 3 5-mg tablets per day (0.3 mg/kg/day) or 0.5 to 1 10-mg suppository per day
3. Lubricants soften feces.
   a. Mineral oil
   b. Docusate 40 to 50 mg per day divided one to four times per day
4. Hyperosmotic agents increase volume.
   a. Glycerine suppository
   b. Lactulose
   c. Polyethylene glycol 17 g in 8 ounces of fluid every day, for a maximum of 2 weeks
   d. Magnesium (hydroxide or citrate); age-based dosing

■ FOLLOW-UP & DISPOSITION
Significant involvement by phone or in office is needed to ascertain success and compliance with therapy.

■ PATIENT/FAMILY EDUCATION
- If stool is hard, it hurts to defecate, and it is important to indicate this to parents and patient.
- One needs to achieve soft to runny stool daily to twice daily to avoid pain association.
- *Short term* means months of therapy, especially in toddler.

■ PREVENTIVE TREATMENT
- Appropriate guidance for diet
- Appropriate guidance for toilet training
- Early treatment for new-onset constipation

■ REFERRAL INFORMATION
- Pediatric gastroenterologist if unsuccessful or question of other causes
- Pediatric surgeon if not a functional problem

⚙ PEARLS & CONSIDERATIONS

■ CLINICAL PEARLS
- Discuss with parents (and child if old enough) to explain pain and long-term therapy.
- Too often, parents use too little medication for too short a time.

■ WEBSITES
- Medinfo: medinfo.co.uk/conditions/constipation.html
- National Institute of Digestive Disorders: www.niddk.nih.gov/health/digest/pubs/whyconstr/whyconst.htm
- Wellness Web: www.wellweb.com/index/qconstip.htm

■ SUPPORT GROUP
International Foundation for Functional Gastrointestinal Disorders, P.O. Box 1786, Milwaukee, WI 53217, 414-964-1799.

REFERENCES
1. Abi-Hanna A, Lake AM: Constipation and encopresis, *Pediatr Rev* 19:23, 1998.
2. Baker S et al: Constipation in infants and children: evaluation and management, *J Pediatr Gastroent Nutr* 29:612, 1999.
3. Dantenhahn LW, Blumenthal BI: Functional constipation: a radiologist's perspective, *Pediatr Ann* 28:304, 1999.
4. Guerrero RA, Cavender CP: Constipation: physical and psychological sequelae, *Pediatr Ann* 28:312, 1999.
5. Hatch T: Encopresis and constipation in children, *Pediatr Clin North Am* 35:257, 1988.
6. Love JR, Parks BR: Movers and shakers: a clinician's guide to laxatives, *Pediatr Ann* 28:307, 1999.
7. Nowicki MJ, Bishop PR: Organic causes of constipation in infants and children, *Pediatr Ann* 28:293, 1999.
8. Parker PH: To do or not to do? That is the question, *Pediatr Ann* 28:280, 1999.

Author: **Lynn C. Garfunkel, M.D.**

II

BASIC INFORMATION

■ **DEFINITION**
Contact dermatitis is an acute or relapsing skin disorder whose hallmarks are pruritus and skin inflammation caused by some offending agent; two subtypes are primary irritant and allergic.

■ **SYNONYMS**
• Diaper dermatitis
• Rhus dermatitis

ICD-9CM CODE
692.9 Contact dermatitis

■ **ETIOLOGY**
• Irritant: There is a direct toxic effect to the skin, thought to be related to the concentration and duration of the exposure as well as the underlying skin integrity. No immune response is involved.
• Allergic: Exposure to a particular antigen mediates a delayed hypersensitivity (type IV) immunologic response. The antigen penetrates the skin, is processed by cutaneous (Langerhans) macrophages, and presented to the T lymphocytes, which circulate throughout the system.

■ **EPIDEMIOLOGY & DEMOGRAPHICS**
• The exact incidence in children is unknown but is thought to represent approximately 20% of all dermatitis in children.
• Nearly 50% of all infants will have diaper dermatitis; onset is usually between 9 and 12 months of age.
• Irritant: Common offending agents include saliva, urine, and feces.
• Allergic: The most common offending agent is poison ivy or oak (Rhus dermatitis). Other common agents are nickel, topical medications, soaps, and latex.
• Allergic reactions generally occur about 1 week after the primary exposure (sensitization phase). Subsequent exposures occur within hours because of memory of the T lymphocytes.

■ **HISTORY**
• History taking should be guided by the age of patient and location of rash.
• History of known exposure is often difficult to elicit and requires thoughtful questioning.

■ **PHYSICAL EXAMINATION**
• Discrete areas of erythema corresponding to the area of skin exposed is seen.

• Vesiculation, oozing, and erythematous papules may be present, particularly in acute allergic dermatitis.
• In diaper dermatitis, confluent erythema is present on maximal exposure areas, sparing the inguinal folds. More severe forms may be associated with erosions and blister formation and possibly secondary infection.
• Chronic exposure in allergic and irritant contact reactions leads to lichenification (thickening) of the skin.
• "Id" reaction
  1. Secondary, generalized pruritic eruption consisting of fine, erythematous papules
  2. Caused by more generalized sensitivity in a person with a localized allergic contact reaction
• Phytophotodermatitis
  1. Develops from exposure to lime or lemon juice, carrot, or celery followed by exposure to sunlight
  2. Redness, blistering, or hyperpigmentation (may be confused with abuse.)

🔬 **DIAGNOSIS**

■ **DIFFERENTIAL DIAGNOSIS**
• Atopic dermatitis
• Nummular dermatitis
• Tinea corporis
• Herpes simplex
• Impetigo
• Seborrheic dermatitis
• Psoriasis
• Langerhans cell histiocytosis (rare)

■ **DIAGNOSTIC WORKUP**
• Irritant: based on history and clinical findings, with particular attention to distribution of rash (e.g., chronic erythema of the lips and perioral area: liplicker's dermatitis)
• Allergic
  1. History and clinical findings
  2. Patch testing: uses prepackaged antigens applied to skin's surface and reexamined in 48 to 72 hours for inflammation
     a. Adult testing reagents are used.
     b. High false-positive rate occurs in children with active lesions.
• Indications for patch testing
  1. Refractory atopic dermatitis
  2. Recurrence of acquired dermatitis after response to steroid therapy
  3. Atopic dermatitis requiring systemic therapy
  4. Worsening nonatopic dermatitis in potential sites for contact allergen

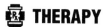 **THERAPY**

■ **NONPHARMACOLOGIC**
• Removal of offending agent, if possible
• Cool compresses
• Diaper dermatitis
  1. Keep diaper area dry with very frequent diaper changes (every several hours).
  2. Use an occlusive barrier, such as zinc oxide, to protect skin.
  3. Avoid use of plastic or rubber pants.
  4. When the child is soiled, rinse skin with warm water but minimize soap and diaper wipe use. (Some caregivers find that a spray bottle works well to minimize insult to the skin.)

■ **MEDICAL**
• Topical corticosteroids
  1. Usually mid to high potency is required.
  2. Low potency is indicated for the face, axilla, and groin.
  3. Apply twice a day for 5 to 7 days.
• Oral diphenhydramine for antipruritic effect, comfort management
• Systemic steroids
  1. May be required if more than 10% to 15% body surface involvement
  2. Prednisone 2 mg/kg/day for 7 days followed by a 7-day taper
     a. Longer courses (2 to 3 weeks) of systemic therapy are often required for allergic (Rhus) dermatitis because of persistence of immunologic response.
     b. Increased incidence of relapse occurs with short courses of therapy.
  3. Apply mild hydrocortisone 1% cream twice a day for several days.
  4. Use a generous amount of antifungal cream if rash persists for more than 3 days because candidal colonization is common.

■ **FOLLOW-UP & DISPOSITION**
May want to follow up in 1 to 2 weeks to assess child's response to therapy.

■ **PATIENT/FAMILY EDUCATION**
• For diaper dermatitis, emphasize the importance of therapeutic measures and the need to decrease contact of urine and feces with skin.
• Emphasize use of topical steroids for short periods only (less than 2 weeks) for contact dermatitis.

■ **REFERRAL INFORMATION**
Refer to dermatologist if patch testing is indicated.

☼ PEARLS & CONSIDERATIONS

■ CLINICAL PEARLS

- Consider a contact reaction whenever a rash is localized to the face, hands, or feet.
- With diaper dermatitis, always consider the possibility of superinfection, particularly with *Candida,* and consider adding nystatin or clotrimazole cream to the treatment regimen.
- Cloth diapers (versus disposable) may actually increase the severity of the dermatitis.
- Topical therapy rules of thumb: Use cream on wet lesions, gels on scalp, and ointments on dry and lichenified lesions.

REFERENCES

1. Eichenfield LF, Friedlander SF: Coping with chronic dermatitis, *Contemp Pediatr* 15:53, 1998.
2. Friedlander SF: Contact dermatitis, *Pediatr Rev* 19:166, 1998.
3. Weston WL, Lane AT, Morelli JG: *Color textbook of pediatric dermatology,* St Louis, 1996, Mosby.

Author: **Kristen Smith Danielson, M.D.**

BASIC INFORMATION

DEFINITION

A corneal abrasion is a superficial deepithelialization of the cornea, usually secondary to trauma or chemical, thermal, or ultraviolet light exposure.

ICD-9CM CODE

918.1 Corneal abrasion

ETIOLOGY

- Trauma
  1. Young children: sand, dirt, or other foreign bodies
  2. Teens: sports impact, contact lens wear, or foreign bodies
- Chemical: contact lens solution
- Ultraviolet radiation: exposure to welding arc
- Thermal
  1. Young children: cigarette burns
  2. Teens: curling iron burns

EPIDEMIOLOGY & DEMOGRAPHICS

- Corneal abrasions account for 10% of new patients seeking medical attention in emergencies rooms for eye problems.
- Corneal abrasions are common in young adults, especially in those who work on cars.

HISTORY

- Usually a history of exposure with at least one of the following:
  1. Intense ocular pain
  2. Redness
  3. Light sensitivity
  4. Copious tearing
  5. In nonverbal children: only history may be inconsolable irritability

PHYSICAL EXAMINATION

- Relief is obtained with topical anesthesia.
- Irregular epithelium is noted on slit-lamp examination.
- Fluorescein dye may stain the abraded area and can be seen with cobalt blue light or Wood's lamp.

DIAGNOSIS

DIFFERENTIAL DIAGNOSIS

- Corneal ulcer
- Occult ruptured globe
- Uveitis
- Congenital glaucoma

DIAGNOSTIC WORKUP

Thorough physical examination, including visual acuity

THERAPY

NONPHARMACOLOGIC

- Patching of the affected eye
  1. Small abrasions may not require patching.
     a. Maintaining a patch is a challenge.
     b. There is a risk of deprivation amblyopia.

MEDICAL

- Broad-spectrum antibiotic solution or ointment
- Artifical tears

FOLLOW-UP & DISPOSITION

- The abrasions should heal within 2 to 3 days.
- The patient should be followed until corneal abrasion heals and visual acuity returns to baseline.

REFERRAL INFORMATION

- Referral is indicated if visual acuity does not return to baseline or if healing is not seen within 4 to 5 days.
- An uncommon complication is recurrent erosion syndrome, which is an intermittent deepitheliazation of a previously abraded area.

PEARLS & CONSIDERATIONS

CLINICAL PEARLS

Corneal abrasion is in the differential diagnosis of the inconsolable child.

REFERENCES

1. Hamill MB: Corneal injury. In Krachmer JH, Mannis MJ, Holland EJ (eds): *Cornea,* St Louis, 1997, Mosby.
2. Wilson ME et al: Ocular trauma in childhood. In *Pediatric ophthalmology and strabismus,* San Francisco, 1998-1999, American Academy of Ophthalmology.
Author: **Anna F. Fakadej, M.D., F.A.A.O.**

BASIC INFORMATION

■ DEFINITION
Cor pulmonale is right-sided heart failure or significant right ventricular hypertrophy (RVH) secondary to pulmonary hypertension. It usually implies that the pulmonary hypertension is secondary to pulmonary parenchymal disease, airway obstruction, or hypoventilation syndromes rather than secondary to left-sided heart failure, congenital heart disease, or primary pulmonary hypertension syndromes. (See the section "Pulmonary Hypertension" for descriptions of pediatric primary pulmonary hypertension or pulmonary hypertension secondary to left-sided heart disease or congenital heart disease.)

ICD-9CM CODE
416.9 Cor pulmonale

■ ETIOLOGY
- Cystic fibrosis
- Chronic interstitial pneumonitis, including human immunodeficiency virus (HIV) infection
- Obstructive apnea
- Primary hypoventilation
- Muscular dystrophies
- Thoracic dystrophies
- Sickle cell anemia with recurrent pulmonary infarction
- Bronchopulmonary dysplasia/chronic lung disease after prematurity

■ EPIDEMIOLOGY & DEMOGRAPHICS
Much more rare in children than in adults, in whom chronic obstructive pulmonary disease and emphysema are common causes

■ HISTORY
- History of underlying diseases as mentioned under "Etiology"
- Dyspnea
- Fatigue and exercise intolerance
- Syncope

■ PHYSICAL EXAMINATION
- Prominent right ventricular impulse on precordial palpation
- Loud, narrowly split or single second heart sound
- Pulmonary artery ejection click
- Jugular venous distention
- Edema or ascites (rare)
- Cyanosis and clubbing in severely hypoxemic patients (e.g., cystic fibrosis)

◢ DIAGNOSIS

■ DIFFERENTIAL DIAGNOSIS
- Chronic lung disease may cause similar symptoms even without pulmonary hypertension or its secondary cardiac effects.
- Primary cardiac disorders, especially right-sided congenital heart disease or unrepaired cyanotic heart disease, may have similar clinical signs and symptoms.
  1. Severe RVH in pulmonic valve stenosis
  2. Eisenmenger complex

■ DIAGNOSTIC WORKUP
- Electrocardiogram usually shows RVH.
- Chest radiography may suggest RVH or show enlarged central pulmonary arteries. Chronic pulmonary parenchymal disease is suspected from radiographic findings (e.g., cystic fibrosis).
- Echocardiogram confirms RVH and may demonstrate pulmonary hypertension without congenital heart disease.
- Pulmonary function testing and oximetry may show abnormalities of primary lung disease.
- Polysomnography may diagnose sleep apnea/obstructive apnea.
- Testing for HIV infection may be warranted if clinical signs of interstitial pneumonitis are present.
- Neurologic examination or consultation may demonstrate muscular or skeletal dystrophies.
- Cardiac catheterization is only rarely required to demonstrate pulmonary hypertension/RVH.

℞ THERAPY

■ MEDICAL
- Therapy is directed toward primary lung disease.
- Supplemental oxygen to correct hypoxia can decrease pulmonary hypertension and allow abnormal RVH to regress.
- Aggressive pulmonary toilet and antibiotics may improve right-sided heart failure in serious chronic parenchymal disease, such as cystic fibrosis.
- Home ventilator treatment may be needed in some patients with muscular or thoracic dystrophies when signs of right heart failure occur.
- Primary cardiac medication, such as digoxin, is often prescribed, but studies proving its benefit are lacking.
- Vasodilators have limited use in the pulmonary diseases listed here.

■ SURGICAL
- Hypoventilation or obstructive apnea must be effectively treated even if a tracheostomy is necessary.
- Nitric oxide and other primary pulmonary vasodilator therapy are discussed in the section "Pulmonary Hypertension."

■ FOLLOW-UP & DISPOSITION
- Periodic echocardiography
  1. Look for changes in pulmonary hypertension or right ventricular size and function after treatment of pulmonary disease or airway obstruction.

■ PATIENT/FAMILY EDUCATION
- Right-sided heart failure signs are secondary to the pulmonary process. Cardiac disease is not the major problem, and treatment is directed at pulmonary or ventilatory problem.
- Cardiac effects usually are reversible if the primary disease process causing pulmonary hypertension can be effectively treated.

■ REFERRAL INFORMATION
- Most children with cor pulmonale need subspecialty referral appropriate to the primary pulmonary process.
- Pediatric pulmonology referral is necessary for most children, with otolaryngologic consultation if there is obstructive apnea, neurology if there is muscular dystrophy, and hematology for sickle cell disease.

☼ PEARLS & CONSIDERATIONS

■ CLINICAL PEARLS
- Adenotonsillar hypertrophy and sleep obstruction should be investigated even in patients who may have another reason for pulmonary hypertension (e.g., sickle cell patients with past pulmonary infarctions).
- Sleep obstruction is common, can coexist with other diseases, and is additive in its deleterious effect on pulmonary vascular resistance.
- Obstructive apnea and hypoventilation are common in children with trisomy 21 and other syndromic diagnoses in which midfacial hypoplasia and other abnormalities in the growth and development of the facial, oral, pharyngeal, and hypopharyngeal structures may be present.

■ WEBSITE
Kuppersmith R: Pediatric obstructive sleep apnea, 1996: www.bcm.tmc.edu/oto/grand/121996.html

REFERENCES
1. Lefaivre JF et al: Down syndrome: identification and surgical management of obstructive sleep apnea, *Plast Reconstr Surg* 99:629, 1997.
2. Perkin RM, Downey R III, Macquarrie J: Sleep-disordered breathing in infants and children, *Respir Care Clin North Am* 5:395, 1999.
Author: **David Hannon, M.D.**

BASIC INFORMATION

■ DEFINITION
Costochondritis is inflammation of the costal cartilages associated with pain. If associated with fusiform swelling, redness, and warmth of the joint, it is called *Tietze's syndrome.*

■ SYNONYM
Chest wall syndrome

ICD-9CM CODE
733.6 Costochondritis

■ ETIOLOGY
- Exact cause unclear
- Most often idiopathic
- Associated with excessive exercise or a preceding viral respiratory illness

■ EPIDEMIOLOGY & DEMOGRAPHICS
- Approximately 20% of pediatric patients presenting with chest pain are found to have costochondritis.
- This percentage increased to 80% when the study was isolated to adolescent girls.
- Tietze's syndrome generally occurs in patients in their late teens to early twenties.
  1. Has been described in young children
  2. No sex predominance

■ HISTORY
- Sharp pain in anterior chest wall that may radiate to back or upper abdomen
- May last for several months
- Varies in intensity and quality
  1. May be dull, sharp, or pleuritic
  2. May be mild to severe
- Tends to be unilateral

■ PHYSICAL EXAMINATION
- Pain can be clinically reproduced by palpation at local site or movements of the arm and shoulder.
  1. Tietze's at right sternoclavicular or second sternochondral junction
  2. Costochondritis at left second to fourth costochondral junction
- Vital signs may show evidence of mild tachypnea, tachycardia, and systolic hypertension, depending on the level of the patient's pain and anxiety.
- Oxygen saturation is normal.
- Distortion of local soft tissues defines Tietze's syndrome.

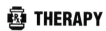

DIAGNOSIS

■ DIFFERENTIAL DIAGNOSIS
- Chest wall
  1. Common
     a. Herpes zoster
     b. Trauma
     c. Muscular strain (especially associated with cough)
     d. Xiphodynia
     e. Breast development
  2. Rare
     a. Myositis
     b. Osteomyelitis
     c. Precordial catch
     d. Slipping rib syndrome
     e. Bone tumors
     f. Connective tissue disorders
     g. Intercostal neuritis
     h. Fibromyalgia
- Visceral
  1. Common
     a. Asthma
     b. Pneumonitis
     c. Esophagitis/gastroesophageal reflux
     d. Mitral valve prolapse
     e. Pneumothorax
     f. Sickle cell crisis
  2. Rare
     a. Pleurodynia
     b. Pleuritis
     c. Myocarditis
     d. Myocardial ischemia
     e. Pulmonary embolism
- Miscellaneous
  1. Psychogenic
  2. Hyperventilation

■ DIAGNOSTIC WORKUP
- Diagnosis is made with thorough historical and physical clues.
  1. Chest radiograph may be obtained if classic findings are not present to rule out the presence of visceral disease.
- If swelling is present, may proceed with biopsy to rule out tumor.
  1. Increased cartilage and lack of inflammatory changes are characteristic of Tietze's syndrome.

THERAPY

■ NONPHARMACOLOGIC
Rest

■ MEDICAL
Antiinflammatory medications

■ FOLLOW-UP & DISPOSITION
- Treatment is symptomatic.
- Patient must be reassured and encouraged to rest.

REFERENCE
1. Coleman WL: Recurrent chest pain in children, *Pediatr Clin North Am* 31: 1007, 1984.

Author: **Ann Marie Brooks, M.D.**

BASIC INFORMATION

■ DEFINITION
Croup is a syndrome of respiratory distress caused by subglottic narrowing characterized by hoarseness, inspiratory stridor, and a barklike cough.

■ SYNONYM
Laryngotracheobronchitis

■ ICD-9CM CODE
464.4 Croup

■ ETIOLOGY
- Parainfluenza type 1 (most common)
- Parainfluenza types 2 and 3
- Respiratory syncytial virus
- Influenza A and influenza B
- Adenovirus types 1 through 4, 7, 8, 11, 14, and 21
- Rhinovirus
- Coxsackie types A9 and B4
- Echovirus types 4, 11, and 21
- Infrequently, *Mycoplasma pneumoniae*

■ EPIDEMIOLOGY & DEMOGRAPHICS
- Primarily affects children ages 6 months to 3 years
- Peaks at age 2 years
- Predominance in fall and winter
- Spread via person-to-person contact, or by large droplets and contaminated nasopharyngeal secretions
- Incubation period of 2 to 4 days.

■ HISTORY
- Prodrome of upper respiratory tract symptoms for 1 to 2 days
- Hoarse voice, cry
- Barky, hoarse cough (seallike quality)
- Respiratory difficulty, noisy breathing common
- Fever usually less than 39° C
- Thorough history to narrow diagnosis
  1. Trauma
  2. Previous intubation
  3. Cough associated with oral intake
  4. Cough or choking after playing with small toys

■ PHYSICAL EXAMINATION
- Vital signs:
  1. Increased respiratory rate, often with elevated pulse and temperature
- General appearance is not toxic, although if severe airway narrowing is present, the child may be in significant respiratory distress.
  1. Is the patient's preferred position "sniffing dog" or tripod position?
     a. Indicates imminent airway obstruction
     b. Distinctly unusual in croup (seen with epiglottitis)

- The Leipzig et al. croup scoring system is based on the degree of following symptoms:
  1. Stridor
  2. Sternal retractions
  3. Dyspnea
  4. Tachypnea
  5. Cyanosis
- Many scoring systems exist, but in general, the classifications are as follows:
  1. Mild croup: normal color, normal mental state, air entry with stridor audible only with stethoscope, and no retractions
  2. Moderate croup: normal color, audible stridor, mild to moderate retractions, and slightly diminished air entry in an anxious child
  3. Severe croup: cyanotic, loud stridor, significant decrease in air entry, and marked retractions in a highly anxious child
  4. Imminent respiratory failure would be heralded by the disappearance of retractions and stridor in a child with severe croup.

DIAGNOSIS

■ DIFFERENTIAL DIAGNOSIS
- Spasmodic croup
- Foreign body
- Epiglottitis
  1. Rare
  2. Toxic infant
  3. Muffled voice or not talking
- Bacterial tracheitis
  1. High fever, toxic appearance
  2. May follow irritation of trachea or be seen in patients with underlying immunocompromise
- Peritonsillar or retropharyngeal abscess
- Vocal cord dysfunction: acute onset lasts minutes to hours, usually in older child or adolescent
- Tracheomalacia
- Trauma (i.e., burns, laryngeal fracture)
- Neoplasm
- Vascular ring
- Angioneurotic edema: often with hives or edema or seen with generalized allergic reaction
- Tracheal hemangioma/vocal cord papilloma
- Psychogenic stridor
- Hypocalcemic tetany
- Diptheria (rare)

■ DIAGNOSTIC WORKUP
- Radiographs of the neck can serve as a diagnostic aid.
  1. The classic "steeple sign" associated with viral croup demonstrates narrowing of the laryngeal air column 5 to 10 mm below the vocal cords.

  2. Sensitivity is 93% and specificity 92% for the diagnosis of viral laryngotracheitis.
- Appropriate airway management should never be delayed for the sake of obtaining a radiographic study.
- Endoscopy should be reserved for children with an atypical course or when an underlying anatomic abnormality, bacterial tracheitis, epiglottitis, or foreign body is highly suspected.
- Isolation of the virus by culture or antigen detection can also be used for specific viral cause.

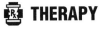

THERAPY

■ NONPHARMACOLOGIC
- There is no substitute for close observation and frequent reassessment.
- The child should be kept as calm and comfortable as possible, often in the parents' arms.
- Cool mist tents are not recommended because they can increase the child's anxiety and obstruct the caretaker's view. The cold night air or steam from the shower are generally effective.

■ MEDICAL
- Nebulized epinephrine (0.5 ml of 2.25% solution in normal saline) is given to patients with stridor at rest, in those with associated with reduced air entry, and/or for those with retractions.
- Patients should be observed for at least 2 hours after treatment to monitor for recurrent symptoms before discharge from clinical setting.
- Dexamethasone 0.6 mg/kg orally or intramuscularly as a single dose or every 8 to 12 hours for three doses may be used and may prevent hospital admission.
  1. Nebulized budesonide is as effective as oral dexamethasone, but its cost remains prohibitive.
- Children with the following circumstances should be hospitalized:
  1. Significant respiratory distress unresponsive to or requiring more than two nebulized epinephrine treatments
  2. Long distance from clinical setting
  3. Lack of appropriate home setting for outpatient management
- Droplet isolation precautions should be observed in inpatient hospital settings.
- Occasionally, oxygen and rarely intubation are needed for respiratory failure caused by obstruction.

■ PROGNOSIS

Most patients recover completely within 2 to 4 days and do not require hospitalization.

■ PREVENTIVE TREATMENT

- No vaccine is currently available.
- Influenza vaccine may prevent some cases.
- Antiviral therapy could be administered for acute influenza.
- Good handwashing technique should be practiced.

■ PATIENT/FAMILY EDUCATION

- Review the signs and symptoms of respiratory distress.
- Parents should be aware that symptoms may continue to flare at night for 2 to 3 days after initiating acute management.
- Home mist, the benefits of the cool night air, and the importance of adequate hydration should be emphasized.

■ COMPLICATIONS

- Bacterial tracheitis
  1. Caused by secondary infection with *Staphylococcus aureus, H. influenzae, Streptococcus pneumoniae, Moraxella catarrhalis,* or *Streptococcus pyogenes.*
     a. After several days of typical croup symptoms, patients present with increasing toxicity, fever, drooling, increased secretions, and increased respiratory effort.
     b. White blood count elevation with left shift is noted.
     c. Blood cultures are generally negative.
     d. Lateral neck film may demonstrate cloudiness of tracheal air column or scalloping of tracheal wall (membranous croup).
     e. Management includes aggressive antibiotic usage and often intubation for airway stabilization.

☼ PEARLS & CONSIDERATIONS

■ CLINICAL PEARLS

- Croup is the most common cause of stridor in children.
- In children younger than 2 years old, be sure to rule out foreign body aspiration.

■ WEBSITE

KidsHealth: www.kidshealth.org/parent/common/croup.html

REFERENCES

1. Battaglia JD: Severe croup: the child with fever and upper airway obstruction, *Pediatr Rev* 7:227, 1986.
2. Croup. In Hay WW Jr (eds): *Current pediatric diagnosis and treatment,* Stamford, Conn, ed 12, 1995, Appleton & Lange.
3. Hall C, Hall W: Croup. In Hoekelman RA (ed): *Primary pediatric care,* ed 3, St Louis, 1997, Mosby.
4. Kaditis AG, Wald ER: Viral croup: current diagnosis and treatment, *Contemp Pediatr* 16:139, 1999.
5. Kaditis AG, Wald ER: Viral croup: current diagnosis and treatment, *Pediatr Infect Dis J* 17:827, 1998.
6. Kairys SW, Olmstead EM, O'Connor GT: Steroid treatment of laryngotracheitis: a meta-analysis of the evidence of randomized trials, *Pediatrics* 83:683, 1989.
7. Leipzig B et al: A prospective randomized study to determine the efficacy of steroids in treatment of croup, *J Pediatr* 94:194, 1979.
8. Roberts GW et al: Repeated dose inhaled budesonide versus placebo in the treatment of croup, *J Paediatr Child Health* 35:170, 1999.
9. Zwerdling R: Inflammatory diseases of the upper airway. In Dershewitz RA (ed): *Ambulatory pediatric care,* ed 3, Philadelphia, 1999, Lippincott Williams & Wilkins.

Authors: **Mary Anne Jackson, M.D., and Heather Vahle, M.D.**

BASIC INFORMATION

DEFINITION
Cryptorchidism is failure of the testis to completely descend into the scrotum. The term is derived from the Greek words *kryptos* and *orchis,* meaning "hidden testis."

SYNONYMS
- Undescended testis
- Incompletely descended testis

ICD-9CM CODE
752.51 Undescended testis

ETIOLOGY
- The cause is uncertain, but it probably results from multiple factors, including the following:
  1. Improper gubernacular (fetal cord that attaches to the testis) traction
  2. Abnormal intraabdominal pressure
  3. Epididymal differentiation and maturation abnormalities
  4. Improper attachment of gubernaculum testis
  5. Hormonal impairment
     a. Androgen deficiency
     b. Decreased luteinizing hormone-releasing hormone
- Traumatic dislocation of testis
  1. Straddle injury
- Surgical dislocation of testis
  1. Surgeon snags spermatic cord in hernia repair or does not pex testis correctly.

EPIDEMIOLOGY & DEMOGRAPHICS
- Incidence is related to gestational age because testes descend late in fetal growth.
  1. It occurs in up to 30% of preterm infants.
  2. The incidence is 1 in 33 term newborns.
  3. A less than 1% incidence is seen after age 6 months.
- Five percent of cases are nonpalpable.
- Distribution is 65% right, 25% left, and 10% bilateral.
- Approximately 80% of cases are obvious at birth, whereas 20% present later in childhood.
- It is associated with many central nervous system anomalies, including the following:
  1. Myelomeningocele
  2. Hydrocephalus
  3. Anencephaly
  4. Hypopituitarism
- It is associated with abdominal wall defects such as prune-belly syndrome.
- Increased incidence occurs in premature infants and small-for-gestational-age (SGA) babies.

- Increased familial incidence (10% of siblings) is observed.
- Increased incidence of testicular malignancy is present in maldescended testes.
- Increased risk exists for impaired fertility in those with undescended testes.
- Increased incidence occurs in multiple malformation syndromes, including chromosomal anomalies and single gene defects.

HISTORY
- This condition is usually noted on physical examination.
- It is not associated with pain, tenderness, or discomfort in most cases.
- Many malformation syndromes, chromosomal abnormalities, and neurologic defects are associated with maldescended testes, including the following:
  1. Aarskog syndrome
  2. de Lange's syndrome
  3. Kallmann's syndrome
  4. Klinefelter syndrome
  5. Laurence-Moon-Biedl syndrome
  6. Noonan-Opitz-Frias syndrome
  7. Prader-Willi syndrome
  8. Robinow's syndrome
  9. Rubinstein-Taybi syndrome
  10. Smith-Lemli-Opitz syndrome
  11. Trisomy 21

PHYSICAL EXAMINATION
- It is important to have the following conditions present during examination:
  1. Warm environment
  2. Relaxed patient in the frogleg position
  3. Warm examiner's hands
- Examine patients carefully, especially those with risk factors listed in "Epidemiology"
- Examine genitalia for other abnormalities (e.g., hypospadias).

DIAGNOSIS

DIFFERENTIAL DIAGNOSIS
- Ectopic testes—will never descend
- Retractile testes
- Anorchia (lack of testes)
- Atrophic testis
- Ambiguous genitalia
  1. Genetic female with androgen excess
  2. Genetic male with androgen insensitivity

DIAGNOSTIC WORKUP
- The diagnosis is made on physical examination.
- Ultrasonography is rarely helpful in localizing testes.
- Computed tomography can help localize testes and/or evaluate testes but is rarely necessary.

- Endocrine evaluation should be performed in patients with bilateral nonpalpable testes who are chromosomal males (testosterone, dihydrotestosterone, luteinizing hormone [LH], and follicle-stimulating hormone [FSH]).
  1. Elevated LH and FSH with low or absent testosterone indicate nonfunctioning or absent testes or an intersex disorder.
  2. Elevated testosterone occurs with androgen insensitivity.
- A human chorionic gonadotropin (hCG) stimulation study should be conducted for bilateral nonpalpable testes; after stimulation, measure testosterone, LH, and FSH.
  1. If testosterone is elevated, testes are present.
  2. If no testosterone is detected and LH and FSH are elevated, no functioning testes exist.
- Inhibin test
  1. This test is not widely available.
  2. No inhibin indicates no functioning testes.
  3. Inhibin presence indicates functional testicular tissue.
  4. May be a more sensitive marker than testosterone.

THERAPY

PHARMACOLOGIC
Therapeutic hCG stimulation for bilateral nonpalpable testes:
- To bring testes down and potentially avoid surgery
- To stretch cord structure in preparation for surgery

SURGICAL
- Open inguinal and abdominal incisions to manage most undescended testes
- Laparoscopy in selected instances of older boys with nonpalpable undescended testes

FOLLOW-UP & DISPOSITION
- The primary care physician should perform interval physical examinations throughout childhood and puberty.
- Follow pubertal testicular growth for possible atrophy.
- Instruct the patient to conduct monthly testicular self-examinations beginning in teens to look for malignancy.

PATIENT/FAMILY EDUCATION
- Pubertal testicular self-examination
- Pubertal education regarding fertility potential
- Pubertal education regarding malignant potential

■ REFERRAL INFORMATION
- All boys with cryptorchidism should be referred to a pediatric urologist.
  1. If bilateral nonpalpable, refer at birth.
  2. If unilateral at birth, refer at 3 to 6 months.
  3. If highly retractile or late presentation of cryptorchidism, refer at that time.
- Endocrinologists are usually involved in cases that are complicated by either ambiguous genitalia or micropenis to rule out and manage enzyme defects (and hormonal deficiencies).

☼ PEARLS & CONSIDERATIONS

■ CLINICAL PEARLS
- Ultrasound is rarely helpful for this condition.
- Because of the potential for late presentation of cryptorchidism, all boys should have confirmation of testicular location at intervals throughout childhood and puberty.

■ WEBSITE
Society for Pediatric Urology: www.spu.org

REFERENCES
1. Bogaert GA, Kogan BA, Mevorach RA: Therapeutic laparoscopy for intra-abdominal testes, *Urology* 42:182, 1993.
2. Rabinowitz R, Hulbert WC: Late presentation of cryptorchidism: the etiology of testicular re-ascent, *J Urol* 157:1892, 1997.
3. Rajfer J et al: Hormonal therapy of cryptorchidism, *N Engl J Med* 314:466, 1986.
4. Scorer CG: The descent of the testis, *Arch Dis Child* 39:605, 1964.
Authors: **Ronald Rabinowitz, M.D., William C. Hulbert, M.D., and Robert A. Mevorach, M.D.**

BASIC INFORMATION

■ DEFINITION

- Cystic fibrosis (CF) is an inherited, multisystem disease of exocrine gland function that is primarily characterized by the following:
  1. Diffuse obstruction and chronic infection of the airways
  2. Poor digestion resulting from exocrine pancreatic insufficiency
- Although multiple organ systems are affected, progressive lung destruction (bronchiectasis) is the major cause of morbidity and mortality in those affected with CF.

ICD-9CM CODES
518.89 Cystic fibrosis—pulmonary
277.00 Cystic fibrosis—pancreatic

■ ETIOLOGY

- The basic defect is an abnormality of chloride transport by apical membrane epithelial cells.
- The responsible gene is located on the long arm of chromosome 7 at position 7q31 and codes for the protein CFTR (CF transmembrane conductance regulator).
- More than 700 gene mutations are known.
- The most prevalent mutation of CFTR is the deletion of one phenylalanine residue at amino acid 508, or DeltaF508.
- DeltaF508 mutation is usually associated with poorer overall prognosis.
- Genetic heterogenicity occurs and may partially account for the wide spectrum of disease severity and rate of progression.
  1. Individual genotype poorly predicts pulmonary disease progression.
- The patient is unable to clear mucous secretions easily.
  1. Inadequate water in mucous secretions ("sticky mucus")
  2. Persistent infection of the lower respiratory airways
  3. Increased salt content of sweat most commonly accounts for clinical signs, symptoms, and disease progression

■ EPIDEMIOLOGY & DEMOGRAPHICS

- Most common lethal inherited disorder among Caucasians
- Autosomal-recessive inheritance
- Estimated incidence: 1 per 3500 Caucasians; 1 per 17,000 African Americans; 1 per 80,000 Native Americans

■ HISTORY

- A family history for CF or early deaths from unexplained respiratory and/or gastrointestinal disease may be reported.

- CF most often presents in early childhood with persistent respiratory illness (50%), malnutrition and poor growth (40%), diarrhea (30%), or a combination of these.
- Multiple organ systems are affected.
- Signs and symptoms may vary widely by age.
  1. Infancy
     a. Meconium ileus at birth (15%)
     b. Rectal prolapse
     c. Steatorrhea
     d. Obstructive jaundice
     e. Bronchiolitis/recurrent wheezing
     f. Chronic cough, often productive
     g. Hyponatremia
     h. Hypoproteinemia
     i. Salty "taste"
  2. Childhood
     a. Steatorrhea
     b. Bowel obstruction
     c. Recurrent pneumonia/wheezing
     d. Chronic productive cough, occasional hemoptysis
     e. Nasal polyps
     f. Chronic sinusitis
     g. Skeletal system: digital clubbing, joint stiffness and/or pain, long bone pain
  3. Adolescence/adulthood
     a. Chronic lung disease; hemoptysis; bronchiectasis
     b. Cor pulmonale
     c. Skeletal system: digital clubbing, joint stiffness and/or pain, long bone pain
     d. Glucose intolerance; diabetes mellitus
     e. Biliary cirrhosis, focal
     f. Distal intestinal obstructive syndrome (previously called *meconium ileus equivalent*)
     g. Gallstones
     h. Pulmonary hypertrophic osteoarthropathy
     i. Cyanosis, late
     j. Azoospermia

■ PHYSICAL EXAMINATION

- Respiratory system
  1. Chronic cough, wheezing, diminished breath sounds (especially in young infants)
  2. Barrel-chest deformity
  3. Use of accessory muscles for respiration; tachypnea
  4. Cyanosis
  5. Acute absence of breath sounds—pneumothorax (2% to 10%)
  6. Chronic rhinitis, nasal congestion
  7. Nasal polyps, especially with mouth breathing, widening of the nasal bridge
- Gastrointestinal system
  1. Poor weight gain
  2. Rectal prolapse
  3. Abdominal distention, diffuse tenderness

  4. Loss of subcutaneous fat, muscle
  5. Edema, hepatomegaly (particularly in infants)
  6. Splenomegaly
- Reproductive system
  1. Absence or atresia of vas deferens
  2. Testicular hernia, hydrocele, undescended testes (incidence higher in males with CF than in general population)
  3. Delayed puberty, both male and female
- Skeletal system
  1. Swelling and effusion and stiffness (primarily ankles, wrists, and knees) are consistent with pulmonary hypertrophic osteoarthropathy.
  2. Digital clubbing may be seen.
- Other
  1. Acrodermatitis enteropathica
  2. Enlarged submaxillary glands
  3. Bulging fontanelle (may be presenting sign in infants with vitamin A deficiency)

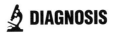

DIAGNOSIS

■ DIFFERENTIAL DIAGNOSIS

CF should be considered when evaluating a wide variety of clinical situations, particularly chronic pulmonary illness and failure to thrive.
- Differential (not inclusive):
  1. Immunodeficiency
  2. Immotile cilia syndrome
  3. Chronic reactive airways disease
  4. Bronchiectasis
  5. Malabsorption syndromes
  6. Protein-calorie malnutrition
  7. Vitamin deficiency
- Non-CF conditions that produce elevated sweat electrolytes:
  1. Ectodermal dysplasia
  2. Hypothyroidism
  3. Malnutrition
  4. Adrenal insufficiency

■ DIAGNOSTIC WORKUP

- Confirmatory diagnosis is made by documentation of elevated sweat chloride content (greater than 60 mEq/L) during the quantitative pilocarpine iontophoresis sweat test (Gibson-Cooke) in a patient with typical features of CF.
- The following are suggestive, but not diagnostic alone.
  1. Measures of exocrine pancreas function
     a. 72-hour fecal fat measurement (less than 5% of dietary fat excreted normally; higher in CF)
     b. Stool for fecal elastase-1: not widely available; very low levels in CF
  2. Chest roentgenogram abnormalities (nonspecific)
  3. Evidence of obstruction on pulmonary function testing

4. Culture of *Staphylococcus aureus* and/or mucoid forms of *Pseudomonas aeruginosa* from sputum very strongly suggestive of CF
- Newborn screening uses immunoreactive trypsinogen, which is confirmed by a positive sweat test and DNA testing.
  1. Controversial

THERAPY

- CF is uniformly fatal, but life span is significantly increasing and appears to be linked to early and aggressive management of the disease.
- Treatment plans must be individualized to account for age and type and severity of symptoms.

■ NONPHARMACOLOGIC

- Hospitalize all newly diagnosed patients to facilitate verification of diagnosis, to provide education for family, and to determine baseline disease status.
- Multidisciplinary team should include a nurse, respiratory therapist, social services advisor, dietitian, psychologist, and physician.
- Maintain hydration, particularly in hot environment and during ongoing losses.
- Perform chest physiotherapy daily to assist with mucous clearing.

■ MEDICAL

- Primarily directed at respiratory and nutrition support
- Inhalation therapy: bronchodilators (before and after chest physiotherapy), aerosolized antibiotics, human recombinant DNase
- Antibiotics
  1. Oral: Use at first sign of increasing lower respiratory tract symptoms.
     a. Cover *S. aureus*, nontypeable *Haemophilus influenzae*, and *P. aeruginosa*

b. Amoxicillin, ciprofloxacin, clindamycin
  2. Intravenous: Use when limited response to oral and inhalation therapy and when symptoms are worsening.
     a. Usually, two antibiotics are necessary to cover suspected pathogens.
     b. Medications can be given through central venous access at home.
  3. Antiinflammatory (corticosteroids): Use in both chronic reactive airways disease and allergic bronchopulmonary aspergillosis.
  4. Nutrition:
     a. Pancreatic enzymes are replaced.
     b. Fat-soluble vitamin deficiency: Replace vitamins A, D, E, and K by supplementation.
     c. Increased caloric need requires increased intake of high-calorie foods.
  5. Immunizations: Schedule should be maintained, with special attention to rubeola, pertussis, and yearly influenza vaccinations.

■ SURGICAL

- Complications of progressive CF may require surgical intervention.
  1. Lobectomy for chronic, recalcitrant atelectasis
  2. Bronchial artery embolization for recurrent hemoptysis
  3. Thoracotomy tube insertion/ closed thoracotomy with sclerosis for recurrent pneumothorax
  4. Lung transplantation for end-stage lung disease
     a. Referral requires FEV_1 less than 30% predicted

■ FOLLOW-UP & DISPOSITION

- Frequent outpatient visits following an initial diagnosis and hospitalization are essential.

- Patients should be seen by the multidisciplinary team every 3 or 4 months. As the disease progresses, more frequent appointments may be necessary.

■ REFERRAL INFORMATION

In addition to the multidisciplinary team, patients may require consultation with experts in gastroenterology, rheumatology, and surgery.

PEARLS & CONSIDERATIONS

■ CLINICAL PEARLS

- Although most common in Caucasians, CF is also seen in African-American and Native American populations
- Patients may present with predominantly respiratory or gastrointestinal symptoms.
- Patients may present with right upper lung collapse, failure to thrive, or hyponatremic dehydration.

■ WEBSITES

- Cystic Fibrosis Foundation: www.cff.org/
- CysticFibrosis.com: www.cysticfibrosis.com/

REFERENCES

1. Boat TF: Cystic fibrosis. In Behrman RE (ed): *Nelson textbook of pediatrics*, ed 16, Philadelphia, 2000, WB Saunders.
2. MacLusky I: Cystic fibrosis for the primary care pediatrician, *Pediatr Ann* 22:541, 1993.
3. Wilmott RW, Fiedler MA: Recent advances in the treatment of cystic fibrosis, *Pediatr Clin North Am* 41:431, 1994.

Author: **Julie Jaskiewicz, M.D.**

BASIC INFORMATION

DEFINITION
Cytomegalovirus (CMV) infections are ubiquitous. Most primary CMV infections are asymptomatic, particularly in children. Primary CMV infections can be symptomatic in the congenitally infected neonate and may manifest as infectious mononucleosis (heterophile negative) in children and adults or as multiorgan disease in the immunocompromised host. Reactivation of latent CMV in immunocompromised individuals most commonly results in retinitis or pneumonitis.

SYNONYMS
- Blueberry muffin baby (not specific for congenital CMV infection)
- Cytomegalic inclusion disease (CID)
- CMV mono

ICD-9CM CODE
078.5 Cytomegaloviral disease

ETIOLOGY
- CMV is an enveloped DNA herpesvirus.
- Horizontal transmission occurs via direct person-to-person contact in saliva, seminal and cervicovaginal fluids, milk, and urine, or via latently infected blood and organs.
- Vertical transmission is via mother-to-child infection occurring in utero.
  1. May occur during both primary and recurrent infections
- Incubation periods are as follows:
  1. Household via horizontal transmission: unknown
  2. After blood transfusion: 4 to 12 weeks
  3. After tissue transplantation: 4 to 16 weeks
- Viral shedding may continue for years after primary infection.
- The infection persists in latent state in blood and organs.
- Presence of CMV immunoglobulin G (IgG) indicates past infection but is not protective against infection; however, humoral immunity modifies the severity of disease (e.g., primary infections are more likely to be symptomatic; neonatal infections occurring as a result of maternal reactivation are rarely symptomatic).

EPIDEMIOLOGY & DEMOGRAPHICS
- The prevalence of CMV antibody increases with age but varies widely based on geographic, socioeconomic, and ethnic backgrounds and on child-rearing practices such as breast-feeding and use of day care.

- Neonatal infections
  1. Transmission rates are 30% to 50% when primary infection occurs during pregnancy.
     a. The congenitally infected neonate is likely to be symptomatic.
  2. Transmission rates are approximately 1% among seropositive or immune pregnant women.
     a. Most infected babies are asymptomatic.
     b. From 10% to 20% will develop sensorineural deafness or mental retardation.
- Perinatal and early childhood infections
  1. Infectious cervicovaginal secretions around the time of delivery transmit infection in more than 50% of patients.
  2. Approximately 50% of infants fed with infectious breast milk become infected.
  3. Shedding rates of 30% to 80% from children in day care have been documented.
     a. Children who are shedding CMV can infect other children and adults in day care and in the home.
- Transmission via blood products (any that contain leukocytes)
  1. In premature infants, infection via blood products may cause shock, lymphocytosis, and pneumonitis.
     a. May hasten progression of bronchopulmonary dysplasia
  2. In those who receive large volumes of blood, transfusion may cause CMV mononucleosis or hepatitis.
- Sexual transmission accounts for increase in seroprevalence during adolescence and early adulthood.
- Transmission in immunosuppressed patients
  1. Can occur via CMV-infected blood products, transplanted bone marrow, or organs
  2. May cause primary infections, reactivation, or reinfection
     a. The highest risk is in CMV-seronegative recipients of latently CMV-infected blood products or organs.
     b. A multitude of manifestations is possible, including pneumonitis, retinitis, hepatitis, gastrointestinal disease, and CMV syndrome.

HISTORY
- Congenital infections
  1. Maternal CMV status
  2. Route of infection: transplacental versus exposure to cervicovaginal secretions
- Other infections
  1. Previous serostatus

  2. Exposure to potentially infectious persons or blood products
  3. Presence and severity of immunosuppression
  4. Duration of immunosuppression

PHYSICAL EXAMINATION
- Severe congenital CMV disease
  1. Intrauterine growth retardation (50%)
  2. Microcephaly (53%)
  3. Chorioretinitis (17% to 41%)
  4. Sensorineural deafness (58%)
  5. Jaundice (67%)
  6. Hepatosplenomegaly (60%)
  7. Petechiae (76%)
  8. Pneumonitis: increased respiratory rate, rales, and cough
- CMV mononucleosis
  1. Fever
  2. Tender hepatomegaly
  3. Tonsillopharyngitis and splenomegaly are rare in contrast to Epstein-Barr virus (EBV) mononucleosis
- In immunocompromised patients: asymptomatic or produce a variety of manifestations
  1. Interstitial pneumonia: fever and dry cough
     a. Progresses to hypoxia
     b. May require assisted ventilation
     c. Occurs most often 1 to 3 months after transplant
  2. Retinitis
     a. Decreased vision or visual field defect
     b. Fluffy white perivascular infiltrates and hemorrhage
  3. CMV syndrome
     a. Fever without other explanation
     b. CMV cultured in blood

DIAGNOSIS

DIFFERENTIAL DIAGNOSIS
- Congenital infections
  1. Toxoplasmosis
  2. Rubella
  3. Herpes simplex
  4. Syphilis
- CMV mononucleosis
  1. EBV
  2. *Toxoplasma gondii*
  3. Viral hepatitis
  4. Acute human immunodeficiency virus infection
  5. Lymphoma, leukemia
- CMV infections in immunocompromised patients
  1. Pneumonitis: *Pneumocystis carinii*, any interstitial pneumonitis
  2. Retinitis: cotton-wool spots, *T. gondii,* syphilis, herpes simplex, varicella-zoster

3. CMV syndrome: the entire spectrum of causes of fever in immunocompromised patients must be considered

■ DIAGNOSTIC WORKUP

- Congenital infections
  1. Infants who have isolation of CMV by culture or detection by electron microscopy from urine within the first 2 weeks of life have congenital CMV infection, regardless of symptoms.
     a. Viral nucleic acid detection methods in this situation are less sensitive.
     b. Positive CMV immunoglobulin M (IgM) in cord blood defines congenital CMV infection.
  2. Negative CMV IgG in cord blood rules out congenital infection.
  3. Positive CMV IgG in cord blood may result from passive transfer of maternal antibodies.
     a. Serial IgG testing at 1, 3, and 6 months is performed to determine resolution or persistence of CMV IgG.
- Perinatal infections
  1. Negative viral culture at birth
  2. Positive viral culture at 2 to 4 months
  3. Persistence of CMV IgG
- Primary infection (beyond perinatal period)
  1. Positive CMV IgG and IgM
  2. Positive viral culture in previously seronegative individual
- Recurrent or reinfection in immunocompromised patients
  1. Because viral shedding may not correlate with clinically significant disease, the diagnosis requires detection of productive infection in the suspected organ.
     a. Detection of CMV in bronchoalveolar lavage (BAL) specimen is achieved by cytologic examination.

b. A positive viral culture is needed to diagnose pneumonitis.
  2. Prospective evaluation of those at high risk is recommended and requires serial testing of blood, and/or urine, and/or BAL specimens.
- Intracerebral calcifications
- Other potential abnormal laboratory tests, including the following:
  1. Elevated alanine aminotransferase (ALT) (83%)
  2. Thrombocytopenia (77%)
  3. Mononucleosis on complete blood count

THERAPY

■ NONPHARMACOLOGIC
Principally supportive

■ MEDICAL
- Treatment of congenital infections: Insufficient data are available to support the routine use of ganciclovir.
- Treatment of CMV infections in immunocompromised patients includes the following:
  1. Pneumonitis: Ganciclovir can be given; the role of CMV hyperimmune globulin is uncertain.
  2. Retinitis: Ganciclovir or foscarnet can be given.
  3. Prophylactic or preemptive therapies (acyclovir, ganciclovir, CMV hyperimmune globulin) have been used with variable or uncertain efficacy.
  4. Ganciclovir is virostatic; therefore maintenance therapy is required for the duration of the immunocompromised state.
  5. Foscarnet deposits in bone, teeth, and cartilage.

■ FOLLOW-UP & DISPOSITION
Congenital infections: Asymptomatic infected infants require close follow-up to detect sensorineural deafness and/or learning problems.

■ PATIENT/FAMILY EDUCATION
Seronegative pregnant women should be taught about the possibility of transmission from children and educated regarding the following:
- Good handwashing practices
- Avoidance of sharing utensils or glassware and kissing on the mouth

■ PREVENTIVE TREATMENT
- Use good handwashing practices in the home, day-care setting, and hospital setting.
- Identify seronegative women early in pregnancy and provide appropriate education.

PEARLS & CONSIDERATIONS

■ WEBSITE
Family Village: www.familyvillage. wisc.edu/lib_cyto.htm

■ SUPPORT GROUP
National Congenital CMV Disease Registry, Texas Children's Hospital, MC3-2371, 6621 Fannin St., Houston, TX 77030-2399; phone: 713-770-4387, fax: 713-770-4330

REFERENCES
1. American Academy of Pediatrics: Cytomegalovirus. In Peter G (ed): *1997 Red Book: report of the Committee on Infectious Diseases,* ed 24, Elk Grove Village, Ill, 1997, American Academy of Pediatrics.
2. Overall JC: Cytomegalovirus. In Feigin R, Cherry J: *Textbook of pediatric infectious diseases,* ed 4, Philadelphia, 1998, WB Saunders.

Author: **Therese A. Cvetkovich, M.D.**

BASIC INFORMATION

■ DEFINITION
Deep venous thrombosis (DVT) is the presence of thrombus within a deep vein, most commonly the iliac, femoral, or popliteal.

■ SYNONYMS
- DVT
- Thromboembolism

ICD-9CM CODE
671.4 Deep venous thrombosis

■ ETIOLOGY
- The main proponents of hypercoagulability are Virchow's triad of the vascular wall, the flow, and the blood contents.
- Conditions that increase risk by damage to the vascular wall include trauma (particularly fractures), tumors, and venous catheter use.
- Conditions that increase risk by changing the blood contents (i.e., hypercoagulable states) include activated protein C resistance; deficiencies of protein C, S, and antithrombin III; antiphospholipid antibodies; dysfibrinogenemia; disseminated intravascular coagulation; pregnancy; and estrogen use.
- Conditions that increase risk by slowing flow include immobilization, tumors, venous stasis, and advanced age (if more sedentary).

■ EPIDEMIOLOGY & DEMOGRAPHICS
- DVT is the third most common cardiovascular disease behind acute coronary syndromes and stroke.
- It affects approximately 2 million Americans per year.
- Nearly 40% of patients with DVT without symptoms of pulmonary embolism (PE) have signs of PE on lung scanning.

■ HISTORY
- Patient reports subacute onset of pain, swelling, and erythema of the affected limb.
- Search for risk factors, especially active cancer, immobility, recent trauma or hospitalization, and family history of DVT.

■ PHYSICAL EXAMINATION
- The traditional Homans' sign (the development of pain in the calf or popliteal region on forceful and abrupt dorsiflexion of the ankle with the knee in a flexed position) is too inaccurate to be relied on.
- More reliable examination points include the following:
  1. Localized tenderness along the distribution of the deep venous system
  2. Thigh and calf swollen (should be measured)
  3. Calf swelling by more than 3 cm when compared with the asymptomatic leg (measured 10 cm below the tibial tuberosity)
  4. Pitting edema in the symptomatic leg only
  5. Dilated superficial veins (nonvaricose) in the symptomatic leg only
  6. Erythema

DIAGNOSIS

■ DIFFERENTIAL DIAGNOSIS
- Cellulitis
- Septic arthritis
- Ruptured Baker's cyst
- Myositis

■ DIAGNOSTIC WORKUP
- Decide based on the history and physical examination whether the patient has a high, moderate, or low pretest probability of disease based on a validated clinical prediction guide.
- The first test of choice is Doppler ultrasonography, with the gold standard of venography being reserved for equivocal cases.

THERAPY

■ NONPHARMACOLOGIC
Elevation of the affected limb

■ MEDICAL
- Once DVT is confirmed, immediate anticoagulation with heparin is indicated to prevent extension or PE.
- Consider searching for a hypercoagulable state.
- Oral anticoagulation with warfarin should be begun the first day because time to adequate anticoagulation (International Normalized Ratio [INR] of 2.0 to 3.0) can take 4 to 7 days.
- Warfarin should be continued for 3 to 6 months for first-time DVT with a known risk factor, and longer (perhaps lifelong) for recurrent DVT or a confirmed hypercoagulable state.

■ SURGICAL
Placement of a vena caval (Greenfield) filter should be reserved for patients with contraindications to anticoagulation or PE despite full anticoagulation.

■ FOLLOW-UP & DISPOSITION
See "Therapy."

■ PATIENT/FAMILY EDUCATION
- Treatment with anticoagulants reduces the incidence of PE to less than 1%.
- The risk of warfarin therapy is major bleeding, with an incidence of 5% per year.
- For those with no risk factors or those not in a hypercoagulable state, the recurrence rate is very low.
- Treatment with oral warfarin necessitates intense education about the risks of bleeding and dietary restrictions.

■ PREVENTIVE TREATMENT
- Early ambulation of hospitalized patients is crucial. There are very few true indications for bed rest in the hospitalized patient.
- Subcutaneous heparin and pneumatic compression stockings have both proven to be effective maneuvers to prevent DVT in high-risk patients. Simple compression stockings are of little value.

■ REFERRAL INFORMATION
If a hypercoagulable state is found, consultation with a hematologist is indicated to direct an adequate anticoagulation level and duration.

PEARLS & CONSIDERATIONS

■ CLINICAL PEARLS
- Treatment with subcutaneous low-molecular-weight heparin (1 mg/kg subcutaneously twice a day) is equally as effective as intravenous unfractionated heparin and does not need any monitoring of activated partial thromboplastin time. It can also be given on an outpatient basis, avoiding hospitalization in appropriate patients.
- DVT of the arm also occurs, usually in association with venous catheters, and should be approached in the same manner as that for the leg because it also has a risk of PE.
- DVT of the leg below the knee has a very low risk of PE. Anticoagulation is reasonable and prevents extension into the proximal leg, where the risk of PE is much higher. Alternatively, taking serial Doppler ultrasounds of the leg to monitor for extension without anticoagulation is also a reasonable clinical approach in the

II

patient at high risk for bleeding on anticoagulants.

REFERENCES

1. Anand SS et al: Does this patient have deep vein thrombosis? *JAMA* 279:1094, 1998.
2. Creager MA, Dzau VJ: Vascular diseases of the extremities. In *Harrison's principles of medicine,* ed 13, New York, 1994, McGraw-Hill.
3. Goldhaber S: Pulmonary embolism, *N Engl J Med* 339:93, 1998.
4. Hyers TM et al: Antithrombotic therapy for venous thromboembolic disease, *Chest* 114(suppl):561S, 1998.
5. Kearon C et al: The role of venous ultrasonography in the diagnosis of suspected deep venous thrombosis and pulmonary embolism, *Ann Intern Med* 129:1044, 1998.
6. Kearon C et al. Noninvasive diagnosis of deep venous thrombosis, *Ann Intern Med* 128:663, 1998.

Author: **Brett Robbins, M.D.**

BASIC INFORMATION

■ DEFINITION
Dehydration is a physiologic disturbance caused by the reduction or translocation of body fluids, leading to hypovolemia.
- Isonatremic or isotonic dehydration
  1. Serum osmolarity 270 to 300 mOsm/L
  2. Serum sodium 130 to 150 mEq/L
- Hyponatremic or hypotonic dehydration
  1. Serum osmolarity less than 270 mOsm/L
  2. Serum sodium less than 130 mEq/L
- Hypernatremic or hypertonic dehydration
  1. Serum osmolarity more than 300 mOsm/L
  2. Serum sodium more than 150 mEq/L
- Severity
  1. Mild: less than 50 ml/kg body fluid loss or less than 5% weight loss
  2. Moderate: 50 to 100 ml/kg body fluid loss or 5% to 10% weight loss
  3. Severe: more than 100 ml/kg body fluid loss or more than 10% weight loss

■ SYNONYMS
- Hypovolemia
- Hypovolemic shock

ICD-9CM CODES
276.5 Volume depletion
785.59 Hypovolemic shock

■ ETIOLOGY
- Decreased intake
  1. Physical restriction
  2. Anorexia
  3. Voluntary cessation: pharyngitis, stomatitis, respiratory distress
- Increased output
  1. Insensible losses: fever, sweating, heat prostration, high ambient temperature, hyperventilation, cystic fibrosis, thyrotoxicosis
  2. Renal losses
     a. Osmotic: diabetic ketoacidosis, acute tubular necrosis, high-protein diet, mannitol
     b. Nonosmotic: diabetes insipidus, sustained hypokalemia/hypercalcemia, sickle cell disease, chronic renal disease, Bartter's syndrome
     c. Sodium losing: congenital adrenal hypoplasia, diuretics, sodium-losing nephropathy, pseudohypoaldosteronism
  3. Gastrointestinal losses
     a. Diarrhea: secretory or nonsecretory
     b. Vomiting: obstructive or nonobstructive

- Translocation of fluids
  1. Burns
  2. Ascites
  3. Intestinal: paralytic ileus, postabdominal surgery
- Hyponatremic dehydration
  1. This is typically seen with diarrhea and vomiting, especially with inappropriate fluid replacement.
  2. It is also seen with excessive salt loss as in congenital adrenal hyperplasia.
  3. The degree of dehydration may be overestimated; will be in shock when only 10% dehydrated.
  4. These patients are the most likely to need immediate circulatory support.
- Hypernatremic dehydration
  1. This is usually associated with winter diarrhea.
  2. Sodium is greater than 150 mEq/L, but total body sodium is depleted.
  3. Hypernatremic dehydration must be distinguished from salt poisoning with dehydration in which total body sodium is increased.
  4. This condition is rarely seen in children older than 2 years of age.

■ EPIDEMIOLOGY & DEMOGRAPHICS
- Diarrhea is the most common cause of dehydration in infants and children and is the leading cause of death worldwide in children younger than 4 years of age.
- In the United States an average of 500 children younger than 5 years of age die each year.
- Another 200,000 children are hospitalized per year in the United States secondary to diarrheal illnesses with dehydration.
- Other common causes include vomiting, stomatitis or pharyngitis with poor intake, febrile illnesses with increased insensible losses and decreased intake, and diabetic ketoacidosis.
- Of all patients with hypernatremic dehydration, 40% to 50% of survivors have some neurologic sequelae, such as the following:
  1. Learning disabilities
  2. Cognitive and/or motor deficits
  3. Behavioral changes
  4. Severely affected: 5% to 10%
  5. Mortality of 10%

■ HISTORY
- Because gastrointestinal losses from diarrhea and vomiting are the most common causes, need information regarding the amount and character of losses
- Any underlying disease such as cystic fibrosis, diabetes, hyperthyroidism, or renal disease
- Weight loss

- Urine output: decrease in number and degree of wet diapers
- Absence of tears
- Character and amount of ingested fluids

■ PHYSICAL EXAMINATION
- Vital signs
  1. Tachycardia: first sign of mild dehydration
  2. Respiratory rate and pattern: with increasing acidosis, develop increased respiratory rate and hyperpneic pattern
  3. Orthostatic changes in older children
  4. Hypotension: late sign of uncompensated severe dehydration
- Weight loss
- Sunken eyes and fontanel
- Dry lips, mucous membranes, absence of tears
- Prolonged capillary refill, cool extremities
- Tenting of skin, except in hypernatremic dehydration
- Older children: generally show signs of dehydration earlier than babies because of their decreased extracellular water
- Hyponatremic dehydration: signs of dehydration are more pronounced and appear earlier
  1. Seizures may occur, especially with rapid decrease in sodium
- Hypernatremic dehydration: signs of dehydration are more subtle and appear later
  1. Lethargic, but excessive irritability when stimulated
  2. Increased muscle tone
  3. Doughy or smooth, velvety skin turgor
  4. Intracranial hemorrhage in 10%
  5. Possible thrombosis of dural sinus
  6. Possible signs of intracranial swelling and seizures with too-rapid rehydration

DIAGNOSIS

■ DIFFERENTIAL DIAGNOSIS
See "Etiology."

■ DIAGNOSTIC WORKUP
- An initial clinical assessment should be made to determine the degree of volume depletion, using weight loss and/or clinical signs, especially to determine whether shock is present.
- Laboratory data include the following:
  1. Hemoconcentration: elevated hemoglobin, hematocrit, plasma proteins
     a. Hemoglobin and hematocrit may be normal with underlying anemia.
  2. Serum sodium: isonatremic, hyponatremic, hypernatremic

3. Alteration in measured or calculated serum osmolarity: isotonic, hypotonic, or hypertonic
4. Serum potassium: hypokalemia with significant stool or gastric losses; hyperkalemia with acidosis or diminished renal function
5. Serum bicarbonate or blood gas determinations
   a. Acidosis occurs with stool losses, tissue catabolism, and diminished renal function.
   b. Alkalosis occurs with protracted vomiting or nasogastric drainage.
6. Glucose: may be low, especially in a young infant who has been poorly tolerating feedings
7. Blood urea nitrogen and serum creatinine elevated
8. Urine specific gravity and osmolarity increased

℞ THERAPY

The goal of therapy is to replace the deficit, provide maintenance fluids, and continue to replace ongoing losses.

■ NONPHARMACOLOGIC
- Consider oral rehydration in patients with mild to moderate dehydration who do not have severe vomiting, who do not have high stool output of more than 20 ml/kg/hr, or who do not have poor compliance.
  1. Initial rehydration fluid should contain 75 to 90 mEq/L of sodium.
     a. Give volume equal to estimated fluid deficit to drink over 4 to 6 hours.
  2. Maintenance solutions should contain 40 to 60 mEq/L of sodium.
  3. Both solutions should have approximately 20 mEq/L of potassium and 2% to 2.5% glucose.

■ MEDICAL
- Patients with moderate or severe dehydration or uncompensated shock require intravascular therapy.
  1. Initial therapy: Restore intravascular volume regardless of serum osmolarity or cause of the dehydration.
     a. Administer 20 ml/kg of isotonic fluid (normal saline or Ringer's lactate) as a rapid intravenous bolus; reassess and repeat until heart rate, perfusion, and blood pressure are improved.
- Deficit water losses are based on the following criteria:
  1. Weight loss: 1 g of water for each gram of weight loss *or*
  2. Physical guidelines: 3% to

5% = dry mucous membranes; 5% to 7% = sunken fontanel, decreased skin turgor; 7% to 10% = sunken eyes, skin tenting, tachycardia; 10% to 15% = shock
- Deficit acute electrolyte losses are 60% extracellular fluid and 40% intracellular fluid.
  1. For every 100 ml of water lost, the following are also lost:
     a. Sodium: 8.4 mEq/100 ml
     b. Potassium: 6.0 mEq/100 ml
     c. Chlorine: 6.0 mEq/100 ml
- Maintenance needs include the following:
  1. Water needs
     a. 100 ml/kg for first 10 kg
     b. 50 ml/kg for second 10 kg
     c. 20 ml/kg for each kg over 20 kg
  2. Electrolyte needs
     a. Sodium: approximately 3.0 mEq/100 ml
     b. Potassium: approximately 2.0 mEq/100 ml
- Base calculations for deficit replacement and maintenance fluids on original "wet" weight.
- Replacement of ongoing losses:
  1. Replace gastric losses with one half normal saline (½NS) plus 10 to 15 mEq/L potassium chloride.
  2. Add bicarbonate with stool or small bowel losses.
  3. Replace cerebrospinal fluid with 0.9% normal saline.
- Isotonic dehydration:
  1. If indicated, give 20 ml/kg of isotonic fluid as a bolus.
  2. Calculate maintenance needs.
  3. Calculate deficit needs (minus fluid and electrolytes given with bolus).
  4. Administer maintenance plus deficit needs over 24 hours (some authors suggest giving half of deficit over 8 hours and other half over remaining 16 hours).
  5. Fluid (water plus electrolytes) often calculates out to be: $D_5$1/3 NS + 40 mEq/L of KCl
- Hypotonic dehydration:
  1. The degree of dehydration may be overestimated; will be in shock when only 10% dehydrated.
  2. These patients are most likely to need immediate circulatory support.
  3. Calculate fluid losses the same as with isotonic dehydration.
  4. Calculate the electrolyte deficit and add it to the maintenance needs (remember to subtract fluid and electrolytes from bolus).
     a. Correct sodium to 130 mEq/L using the following formula: (Desired Na level – Measured Na) × (0.6) × (weight in kg) = mEq Na deficit
     b. If losses are acute, replace over 24 hours.

- Hypertonic dehydration:
  1. Bolus with normal saline or Ringer's lactate as needed.
  2. Avoid electrolyte-free solutions because they are associated with increased complications.
  3. Calculate water maintenance and deficit as before.
  4. Electrolyte replacement:
     a. Total cation (Na or Na + K) should be approximately one half normal solution (70 to 80 mEq/L) initially.
     b. Significant potassium deficit is almost always present; add potassium after patient voids.
     c. No matter what calculating system is used, generally start out with something similar to $D_5$0.2% NS + 40 mEq/L of KCl.
     d. Replace deficit *slowly* over 48 hours: Rate/hr = (Maintenance × 2) + Deficit divided by 48 hours.
     e. *Monitor sodium every 2 to 4 hours and adjust fluids accordingly.*
        (1) Should not correct sodium faster than 10 to 12 mEq/L/ day (0.5 mEq/L/hr).
        (2) Change fluids to D_5W + K if correcting too slowly.
        (3) Change fluids to $D_5$0.45% NS + K if correcting too quickly.
- If seizures or signs of intracranial swelling occurs, treat with 0.5 to 1.0 g/kg of mannitol over 20 minutes.

■ FOLLOW-UP & DISPOSITION
- With hyponatremic or hypernatremic dehydration, to rule out ongoing losses or a chronic condition, reevaluate sodium levels once sodium is corrected and the patient has resumed a normal diet.
- Consider neuropsychiatric testing or neurologic follow-up after hypernatremic dehydration.

■ PATIENT/FAMILY EDUCATION
Provide parents with written instructions of signs, symptoms, home treatment, and when to seek medical attention, especially during gastroenteritis season.

■ PREVENTIVE TREATMENT
Encourage fluids during exercise, high ambient temperatures, vomiting and diarrheal illnesses, and so forth before dehydration occurs.

☼ PEARLS & CONSIDERATIONS

■ WEBSITES
- Drkoop.com: http://drkoop.com/ conditions/encyclopedia/articles/ 004000a/00400025.html

- Health-Center.com: www. healthguide.com/english/family/infant/medical_concepdehydr.htm
- on health: www.onhealth.com/ch1/resource/conditions/item.48191.asp

REFERENCES

1. Adelman RD, Solhaug MJ: Fluid therapy. In Nelson WE et al (eds): *Textbook of pediatrics*, ed 15, Philadelphia, 1996, WB Saunders.
2. Adelman RD, Solhaug MJ: Fluid and electrolyte treatment of specific disorders. In Nelson WE et al (eds): *Textbook of pediatrics*, ed 15, Philadelphia, 1996, WB Saunders.
3. Adelman RD, Solhaug MJ: Principles of therapy. In Nelson WE et al (eds): *Textbook of pediatrics*, ed 15, Philadelphia, 1996, WB Saunders.
4. Cronan KM, Norman ME: Renal and electrolyte emergencies. In Fleisher GR, Ludwig S (eds): *Textbook of pediatric emergency medicine*, ed 3, Baltimore, 1993, Williams & Wilkins.
5. Jospe N, Forbes G: Fluids and electrolytes—clinical aspects, *Pediatr Rev* 17:395, 1996.
6. Liebelt EL: Clinical and laboratory evaluation and management of children with vomiting, diarrhea, and dehydration, *Curr Opin Pediatr* 10:461, 1998.
7. Shaw KN: Dehydration. In Fleisher GR, Ludwig S (eds): *Textbook of pediatric emergency medicine*, ed 3, Baltimore, 1993, Williams & Wilkins.

Author: **Karen Powers, M.D.**

II

BASIC INFORMATION

■ **DEFINITION**
Puberty is considered delayed if there is a lack of secondary sexual characteristics by age 14 years in boys or age 13 in girls.

■ **SYNONYMS**
• Late bloomer
• Constitutional delay
• "Con delay"

ICD-9CM CODE
259.0 Delayed puberty

■ **ETIOLOGY**
Normal variant, cause unknown

■ **EPIDEMIOLOGY & DEMOGRAPHICS**
• Delayed puberty is more often a complaint in boys.
• About 2% of boys are not in puberty by age 14.
• By age 15 years, 0.4% of boys are not in puberty.
• Approximately 50% of patients have a family history of a first- or second-degree relative with late puberty.

■ **HISTORY**
• Chief complaint or associated complaint may be short stature (see the section "Short Stature").
• There is a benign history without any suggestion of chronic systemic illness, gastrointestinal disease, intracranial mass, or hypothyroidism.
• The patient has a history of little or no pubertal development.
• Delayed puberty may be associated with a history of excessive exercise and/or an eating disorder, especially in girls.

■ **PHYSICAL EXAMINATION**
• Delay or lack of secondary sex characteristics is the hallmark.
1. In girls, there is delayed or absent breast development.
2. In boys, there is a lack of testicular enlargement.
a. Less than 4 ml testicular volume *or*
b. Testicular length of less than 2.2 cm
3. In both sexes, there is no pubic hair and no growth acceleration.
• No signs of chronic systemic illness, gastrointestinal disease, intracranial mass, or hypothyroidism are found.

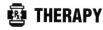 **DIAGNOSIS**

■ **DIFFERENTIAL DIAGNOSIS**
• Permanent hypogonadotropic hypogonadism (permanent lack of gonadotropins)
1. Isolated gonadotropin deficiency
2. Kallmann's syndrome: associated anosmia
3. Gonadotropin deficiency associated with other central nervous system and hypothalamic/pituitary abnormalities such as congenital hypopituitarism, craniopharyngioma, histiocytosis, and others
• Functional hypogonadotropic hypogonadism (transient lack of gonadotropins)
1. Hypothyroidism
2. Weight loss
a. Chronic illness
b. Purposeful dieting
c. Anorexia nervosa
d. Increased physical activity (especially when combined with weight restriction)
3. Chronic disease
• Hypergonadotropic hypogonadism: gonadal failure is associated with elevated gonadotropins
1. Turner syndrome (XO karyotype, girls only): other phenotypic features
2. Klinefelter syndrome (XXY karyotype, boys only): usually have normal start of puberty but may not complete puberty because of testicular fibrosis
3. Other forms of gonadal failure (rare)

■ **DIAGNOSTIC WORKUP**
• Bone age
1. Bone age should be delayed proportional to height.
2. Bone and height age are both delayed compared with chronologic age.
a. For example, a 13-year-old boy with the height of an average 10-year-old and a bone age of 10 years is typical for constitutional delay.
• Screening tests: aimed at ruling out occult disease/conditions
1. All screening tests should be normal for age except hematocrit.
a. Hematocrit will be in the prepubertal to early pubertal range.
2. Complete blood count (CBC) and sedimentation rate should be normal.
3. Urinalysis, electrolytes, and renal function tests should be normal.

• Thyroid function tests (free T_4 and thyroid-stimulating hormone [TSH])
1. Normal thyroid tests are expected in constitutional delay.
2. Low free T_4 with elevated TSH indicates primary hypothyroidism.
• Insulin-like growth factor (IGF)-I/somatomedin-C (screen for growth hormone deficiency)
1. Abnormally low free T_4 and IGF-I/somatomedin-C (adjusted for pubertal stage) may indicate pituitary or hypothalamic abnormalities.
• Morning testosterone (in boys)
1. Testosterone levels should be in the prepubertal to early pubertal range.
2. Morning testosterone level of more than 20 ng/dl indicates good probability of onset of puberty in the next year.
• Gonadotropins (luteinizing hormone [LH] and follicle-stimulating hormone [FSH])
1. Low (i.e., prepubertal) gonadotropin levels are expected in constitutional delay.
2. Elevated gonadotropins indicate gonadal failure and in girls should prompt chromosomal analysis for Turner syndrome.
• Abnormality of any screening test (except those noted): should direct evaluation toward specific system

🔏 **THERAPY**

■ **NONPHARMACOLOGIC**
• Weight gain is important for those with anorexia nervosa or excessive dieting.
• Encourage decrease in extreme exercise routines.

■ **MEDICAL**
Low-dose testosterone (50 to 150 mg intramuscularly every month for 3 to 6 months) may stimulate start of puberty in boys who are peripubertal.

■ **FOLLOW-UP & DISPOSITION**
• Clinical follow-up every 3 to 6 months to document normal height velocity (more than 5 cm per year) and pubertal progression
1. Increase in testicular size is most important.
2. Penis size does not increase significantly in early puberty.
3. Pubic hair growth is also influenced by adrenal androgens.

■ PREVENTIVE TREATMENT

Bone age in a child at risk for delayed puberty may allow for anticipatory guidance.

■ REFERRAL INFORMATION

Referral to pediatric endocrinologist if bone age and height age are not proportional or growth velocity falls below 4 to 5 cm per year

☼ PEARLS & CONSIDERATIONS

■ CLINICAL PEARLS

- Boys often seek evaluation at the time they are in early puberty (determined by testicular size) but do not yet have obvious secondary sex characteristics such as pubic hair.
- Delayed puberty is often associated with a transient "pause" in linear growth just before commencement of puberty.

■ WEBSITES

- American Academy of Family Physicians: www.aafp.org/afp/990700ap/209.html
- House Doctor: www.completediy.com/doctor/i_delayedpub.htm

REFERENCES

1. Kaplowitz P: Delayed puberty in obese boys: comparison with constitutional delayed puberty and response to testosterone therapy, *J Pediatr* 133:745, 1998.
2. Kulin HE: Delayed puberty, *J Clin Endocrinol Metab* 81:3460, 1996.
3. McKeever MO: Delayed puberty, *Pediatr Rev* 21:250, 2000.
4. Saenger P, Sandberg DE: Delayed puberty: when to wake the bugler, *J Pediatr* 133:724, 1998.
5. Styne DM: New aspects in the diagnosis and treatment of pubertal disorders, *Pediatr Clin North Am* 44:505, 1997.

Author: **Craig Orlowski, M.D.**

II

BASIC INFORMATION

■ DEFINITION

Depressive disorders include unpleasant (dysphoric) mood disorders occurring in both medical and psychiatric conditions throughout the life span, with certain symptoms common in children and adolescents.

■ SYNONYMS

- Major depressive disorder: biologic or psychotic depression
- Dysthymia: neurotic depression, chronic depression (at least 1 year in youths)
- Depressive Disorder Not Otherwise Specified: minor, recurrent, brief depression

ICD-9CM CODES

296.2 Major depression
300.4 Dysthymia
311 Depressive Disorder Not Otherwise Specified

■ ETIOLOGY

- Genetic: positive family history
- Biologic: central nervous system neuroamine depletion from the following sources:
  1. Drugs
  2. Infections
  3. Neoplasms
  4. Radiation
- Environment
  1. Losses
  2. Stressors
  3. Emotional trauma

■ EPIDEMIOLOGY & DEMOGRAPHICS

- A family history of mood disorders, anxiety, or substance abuse is common.
- The prevalence is 1% in preschoolers, 2% in school-aged children, 4.7% in adolescents, and 7% in general pediatric patients.
- The gender preference is neutral in childhood, but it is more common in female adolescents.
- No reported racial or ethnic variations exist.
- Family conflict can be a precursor.

■ HISTORY

- Early abuse
- Behavior problems
- New onset of delinquency or substance abuse in a previously happy child
- Mood cycling or volatility before onset of depression
- Symptoms: modified from DSM-IV for children and adolescents
  1. Depressed mood: often bored, irritable, lonely, touchy, difficult to please, dysphoric, and often tearful

2. Poor self-esteem, worthlessness, inappropriate shame and guilt, often feelings of rejection by others (especially peers/schoolmates)
3. Oppositional: often identified as conduct disturbance, which may lift with treatment
4. Sleep disturbances
   a. Some early morning awakening is reported.
   b. Early or middle-of-night sleeplessness is common in children.
   c. Paradoxically prolonged sleep and atypical depression are common in adolescents.
5. Appetite changes
   a. Failure to gain rather than weight loss
   b. Impressive gain caused by driven overeating seen in atypical depression
6. Academic difficulty from poor concentration and motivation
7. Social isolation or "running with a bad crowd"
8. Complaints of headache, stomach ache, sleepiness, loss of energy

■ PHYSICAL EXAMINATION

- Growth delay
- Weight gain or loss
- Bruising if child abuse

DIAGNOSIS

■ DIFFERENTIAL DIAGNOSIS

- Comorbidity with physical and other psychiatric disorders is present in 50% of patients.
- Anxiety is common.
- School refusal is also seen.
- Attention deficit/hyperactivity (AD/HD) disorder may also exist.
- Oppositional disorder is common, often improving with treatment of depression.
- When secondary to conduct disorder, note less family history of mood disorder than when conduct problems are secondary to depression.

■ DIAGNOSTIC WORKUP

- No physical tests (including dexamethasone suppression test, thyroid-stimulating hormone suppression, and rapid eye movement delay) are diagnostic.
- Direct questioning of patient and parent can be aided by self-report.
- Evaluate using the Children's Depression Inventory or Beck Depression Inventory.
- Family history, psychologic testing, and school reports are helpful.

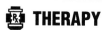

THERAPY

■ NONPHARMACOLOGIC

- Use energetic support and cognitive-behavior therapy for cooperative adolescents.
- Avoid extensive revisiting of symptoms and psychodynamics.
- Either psychotherapy or medication alone is usually less successful than both together.

■ MEDICAL

- Selective serotonin reuptake inhibitors are now first-line treatments in youth.
  1. Fluoxetine is somewhat energizing (give in morning) and well researched.
  2. Paroxetine is somewhat sedating; give at bedtime if sleep is a problem.
  3. Sertraline is sleep and energy neutral; use for depression and anxiety.
- Tricyclic antidepressants are less effective.
  1. Delayed cardiac conduction is a risk and requires electrocardiogram monitoring.
  2. Suicide from overdose is a risk.
- Venlafaxine is useful in depression and AD/HD comorbidity.
- Augmentation with lithium, levothyroxine, or a second antidepressant may be helpful.
- Response to medication may take 4 to 6 weeks or even longer in children.
- Electroconvulsive therapy can be life-saving if other treatments fail.
- Light therapy can be helpful in seasonal affective disorder.

■ FOLLOW-UP & DISPOSITION

The current recommendation is for continued treatment for 1 year after a good response is achieved.

■ PATIENT/FAMILY EDUCATION

- The possibility of recurrence should be stressed to the patient and family.
- Stressing the biologic aspects of depression can allay shame and blame.

■ PREVENTIVE TREATMENT

- Aerobic exercise, promotion of socialization, and pleasurable activities may help.
- Emphasize structure: a regular schedule, good school attendance and part-time and/or summer employment.

■ **REFERRAL INFORMATION**
When a poor response is seen, consult with a child psychiatrist who is experienced in multimodal (including psychopharmacologic) treatment. Telephone and videoconferencing can be useful to aid follow-up.

☼ PEARLS & CONSIDERATIONS

■ **CLINICAL PEARLS**
• An antidepressant that works for a relative is often the best choice.
• An antidepressant that worked for a previous episode should be tried first in recurrences.

• Placebo responses to treatment are common, especially in younger patients.

■ **WEBSITES**
• American Academy of Child and Adolescent Psychiatry: www.aacap.org
• National Depressive and Manic Depressive Association: www.ndmda.org

REFERENCES

1. American Academy of Child and Adolescent Psychiatry: Practice guidelines, *J Am Acad Child Adolesc Psychiatry* 37: 63S, 1998.

2. American Psychiatric Association: *Diagnostic and statistical manual of mental disorders,* ed 4, Washington, DC, 1996, American Psychiatric Association.

3. Kowatch RA et al: Mood disorder. In Parmelee DX (ed): *Child and adolescent psychiatry,* St Louis, 1996, Mosby.

4. Leonard HL et al: Pharmacology of the selective serotonin reuptake inhibitors in children and adolescents, *J Am Acad Child Adolesc Psychiatry* 36:725, 1997.

Author: **Christopher Hodgman, M.D.**

II

BASIC INFORMATION

■ DEFINITION
Seborrheic dermatitis is a subacute or chronic inflammatory disorder confined to the sebaceous gland–rich skin of the head, trunk, and occasionally intertriginous areas.

■ SYNONYMS
- Cradle cap
- Seborrhea
- Dandruff

ICD-9CM CODE
690.10 Seborrheic dermatitis

■ ETIOLOGY
- The cause remains unknown.
- Seborrheic dermatitis coincides with periods of sebaceous gland activity, implicating sebum in pathogenesis.

■ EPIDEMIOLOGY & DEMOGRAPICS
- Seborrheic dermatitis is a common disorder with a bimodal age distribution (early infancy and adulthood).
  1. It may be two separate entities.
  2. Adult disease may begin at puberty.
  3. Equal frequency in seen in both sexes in infancy.
  4. There is no racial predilection.

■ HISTORY
- Pruritus is not a major feature.
- Skin exposed to saliva (perioral and anterior neck crease) is often affected.

■ PHYSICAL EXAMINATION
- The scalp, flexural creases, and diaper area are typically involved.
- Erythematous plaques with sharply defined borders are noted.
- Small erythematous papules with fine scale may be scattered around larger plaques.
- Scalp lesions are thick, yellowish plaques with white scales.

DIAGNOSIS

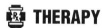

■ DIFFERENTIAL DIAGNOSIS
- Atopic dermatitis
- Psoriasis
- Langerhans cell histiocytosis (Letterer-Siwe)
- *Candida albicans* diaper dermatitis
- Irritant diaper dermatitis
- Acrodermatitis enteropathica

■ DIAGNOSTIC WORKUP
The diagnosis is usually made on the basis of the characteristic clinical picture.

THERAPY

■ NONPHARMACOLOGIC
- Daily shampooing of the scalp and face with mild shampoo is recommended.
- Keratolytic shampoos (containing sulfur or salicylic acid) may be used for thick scales on the scalp.

■ MEDICAL
Mild topical corticosteroids may be given in short courses when dermatitis is unresponsive to shampooing.

PEARLS & CONSIDERATIONS

■ CLINICAL PEARLS
- Severe seborrheic syndrome with generalized exfoliative erythroderma may be seen in a variety of congenital immunodeficiency syndromes.
- Patients with human immunodeficiency virus/acquired immunodeficiency syndrome may have more severe disease, which can be refractive to therapy.

■ WEBSITES
- American Academy of Dermatology: www.aad.org
- Society for Pediatric Dermatology: www.spdnet.org

REFERENCES
1. Hurwitz S: *Clinical pediatric dermatology,* ed 2, Philadelphia, 1993, WB Saunders.
2. Janniger CK: Infantile seborrheic dermatitis: an approach to cradle cap, *Cutis* 51:233, 1993.
3. Williams ML: Differential diagnosis of seborrheic dermatitis, *Pediatr Rev* 7:204, 1986.
Author: **Susan Haller Psaila, M.D.**

BASIC INFORMATION

DEFINITION
Dermatomyositis is a multisystem disease characterized by vascular inflammation, primarily involving the skin and muscle, producing rash and proximal muscle weakness. Additional manifestations of the vasculitis can include esophageal and intestinal dysmotility, myocarditis, conduction abnormalities, alveolitis, interstitial lung disease, arthralgias, arthritis, cutaneous ulcerations, peripheral edema, and calcinosis.

SYNONYMS
- Inflammatory myopathy
- Juvenile dermatomyositis

ICD-9CM CODE
710.3 Dermatomyositis

ETIOLOGY
Several mechanisms have been postulated, and they may all overlap.
- Genetic predisposition is manifested by an increased incidence of HLA-B8 and HLA-DR3 in affected patients.
- Viral-mediated increased antibody titers to Coxsackie B virus and/or Coxsackie B RNA have been detected in the skeletal muscle of some patients.
  1. Influenza and hepatitis B have also been implicated.
- An autoimmune phenomenon is manifested by antinuclear antibodies found in some children, although they are more commonly found in adults.

EPIDEMIOLOGY & DEMOGRAPHICS
- Five to six cases of inflammatory myopathy are reported per 1 million adults and children in the United States.
- Dermatomyositis is the most common inflammatory myopathy of childhood (85% of cases).
- Polymyositis is the second most common inflammatory myopathy of childhood (8% of cases).
- Seventeen percent of all cases occur before adulthood.
- Peak childhood incidence is between 5 and 9 years of age.
- The female:male ratio is 1:1 in children and 2.5:1 in adults.
- The black:white ratio is 1:1 in children and 3:1 in adults.
- Malignancy-associated disease occurs primarily in adults.

HISTORY
- Rapid onset of muscle weakness is reported in half of cases, whereas insidious progression occurs in others.
- Muscle weakness in the proximal extremities and trunk is seen.
  1. Difficulty climbing stairs
  2. Difficulty rising from floor
  3. Awkward gait
- Rash is seen predominantly on the face and hands.
- Photosensitivity is common, with sun exposure producing exacerbation of muscle weakness and rash.
  1. Raynaud's phenomenon
  2. Arthralgias
  3. Extremity swelling

PHYSICAL EXAMINATION
- Heliotropic rash manifests as a violaceous or erythematous rash involving the periorbital area, especially the upper lid.
- Scaling and/or edema of face may be present.
- Gottron's papules are papules or plaques involving the extensor surfaces of joints, particularly the small joints of hands.
- Erythema appears on the malar area, bridge of the nose, and sun-exposed V-area of upper chest and back.
- Proximal muscle weakness is more pronounced than distal weakness.
- Other findings include the following:
  1. Nail bed capillary telangiectasias
  2. Edema of extremities
  3. Calcinosis

DIAGNOSIS

DIFFERENTIAL DIAGNOSIS
- Polymyositis
- Systemic lupus erythematosus
- Mixed connective tissue disease
- Drug-induced myositis
- Hypogammaglobulinemia
- Graft-versus-host disease

DIAGNOSTIC WORKUP
- The clinical diagnosis is based on characteristic skin and muscle findings.
- Supportive laboratory data include elevated creatinine kinase, aspartame transaminase (AST), aldolase, erythrocyte sedimentation rate, and factor VIII antigen.
- Eighty percent of children have no autoantibodies.
  1. Anti–Mi-2 and Anti-nRNP (antinuclear antibodies) are each present in approximately 5% of cases.

- Electromyogram (proximal myopathy) or muscle biopsy (inflammatory infiltrate) may be used to make the diagnosis in some cases.
- Chest radiograph findings indicative of interstitial lung disease or electrocardiogram evidence of conduction abnormalities are present in select cases.

THERAPY

NONPHARMACOLOGIC
- Bed rest for significant muscle weakness
- Aggressive skin care to avoid decubitus ulcers
- Range-of-motion exercises to prevent contractures

MEDICAL
- Corticosteroids are the first-line therapy.
  1. Initially, administer intravenous methylprednisolone 30 mg/kg (maximum of 1 g/day) every 48 hours until evidence of improvement (i.e., normalization of creatinine kinase [CK]) appears.
  2. Then, administer prednisone 2 mg/kg every day.
- Use steroid-sparing agents for nonresponders or patients with significant toxicity.
  1. Methotrexate
  2. Cyclosporine
  3. Hydroxychloroquine
  4. Azathioprine
- Use high-dose intravenous immunoglobulin for refractory cases.

PATIENT/FAMILY EDUCATION
- The clinical course is variable, with monocyclic (lasting up to 2 years), polycyclic, and chronic cases.
- Relapse is uncommon after complete remission.
- Approximately 25% of patients do not respond to steroids, and 25% to 50% develop significant steroid side effects.

PREVENTIVE TREATMENT
Intravenous methylprednisolone may decrease the incidence and severity of calcinosis.

REFERRAL INFORMATION
Rheumatology referral is advised for diagnostic questions and management.

II

☼ PEARLS & CONSIDERATIONS

■ CLINICAL PEARLS

Nail bed capillaries can be examined with immersion oil and an ophthalmoscope at 40+ diopters.

■ WEBSITES

• Arthritis Foundation: www.arthritis.org

• Myositis Association of America: www.myositis.org

REFERENCES

1. Ansell BM: Juvenile dermatomyositis, *Rheum Dis Clin North Am* 17:931, 1991.
2. Callen JP: Dermatomyositis, *Lancet* 355:53, 2000.
3. Klippel JH, Dieppe PA: *Rheumatology*, ed 2, St Louis, 1998, Mosby.
4. Rider LG, Miller FW: Classification and treatment of the juvenile idiopathic inflammatory myopathies, *Rheum Dis Clin North Am* 23:619, 1997.

Author: **Jonathan F. Nasser, M.D.**

BASIC INFORMATION

■ DEFINITION
Developmental dysplasia of the hip (DDH) is an abnormal formation of the hip joint, which occurs prenatally or within the first year of life.

■ SYNONYMS
- Congenital dislocation of the hip
- Congenital dysplasia of the hip
- Congenital disease of the hip

ICD-9CM CODES
755.63 Dysplasia
754.30 Dislocation

■ ETIOLOGY
- Abnormal position of hip is created in association with laxity of the hip joint capsule.
- Femoral head is displaced from acetabulum.
- Changes in alignment lead to bony abnormalities (flattening of the acetabulum, deformation of femoral head) and contractures of hip muscles.

■ EPIDEMIOLOGY & DEMOGRAPHICS
- 1:1000 in population, 1:600 females and 1:4000 in males
- Significant increased risk in breach
- Increased risk in patients with positive family history
- Left (60%) more often than right (20%) and bilateral (20%)
- Increase in Native American, Lapp; decrease in African American, Korean, Chinese
- Older, primiparous mom
- First-born females
- Oligohydramnios
- Increased in patients with metatarsus adductus, clubfoot, hyperextended or dislocated knees, congenital muscular torticollis

■ HISTORY
- Breech (20% of frank breech, 2% footling breech, 0.7% of cephalic presentation)
- Family history (6% risk if one sibling, 12% risk if one parent, 36% risk if one parent and older sibling)
- If missed in infancy, may present with gait abnormalities or pain in second to fourth decade of life

■ PHYSICAL EXAMINATION
- Inner thigh skin fold asymmetry
- Knee height difference: Galeazzi sign
- Abduction limitation: 30 degrees through 75 to 80 degrees and symmetric abduction of hip normal, if less than 50 to 60 degrees abduction, abnormal
- Dynamic instability: positive Barlow (clunking with adduction of thigh while trying to displace femoral head posteriorly) and/or Ortolani (clunking with abduction as femoral head going back into acetabulum)

DIAGNOSIS

■ DIFFERENTIAL DIAGNOSIS
Diagnosis is made on physical examination with little else in the differential diagnosis.

■ DIAGNOSTIC WORKUP
- Ultrasound: before 4 to 6 months; high false-positive rate
  1. Abnormal angles between the acetabulum and ileum on static imaging
  2. Demonstration of hip instability (femoral head moving in and out of acetabular cup) on real time
- Anteroposterior radiograph of hip (after ossification of femoral head, occurs by 4 to 6 months)
  1. Elevation and lateral displacement of femur
  2. Delayed ossification of femoral head
  3. Increased angle between a line that runs through the top of the triradiate cartilages (Hilgenreiner's line) and its intersection with a line that runs parallel to the acetabulum

THERAPY

■ NONPHARMACOLOGIC
- Pavlik harness younger than 6 months
  1. Holds hip in more than 90-degree flexion and abduction of 45 to 60 degrees, allowing movement in "safe" zone
  2. Prohibits dislocation and avoids both adduction and hyper-abduction
     a. Extreme abduction leads to increased risk of avascular necrosis.
  3. Worn constantly for 1 to 3 weeks, with weekly orthopedic checks
  4. Continued for 6 weeks to 9 months
- Closed reduction and immobilization in a spica cast for 6 to 18 months
  1. Cast is changed every 4 to 6 weeks for two to three times.
  2. If unsuccessful, open reduction may be necessary.

■ SURGICAL
- Open reduction for those older than 18 months
  1. Pelvic and femoral osteotomies commonly needed to obtain stable femoral/acetabular relationship.
  2. Rehabilitation takes a long time.
  3. Imperfect repair is common.

■ FOLLOW-UP & DISPOSITION
- The 2000 AAP clinical guidelines suggest screening all breach girls with ultrasound at 6 weeks or radiography at 4 months.
- The guidelines also suggest possible imaging if boy and breach or girl and positive family history.

■ PATIENT/FAMILY EDUCATION
- Eighty percent to ninety-five percent success is achieved for normal hip development when repair is prompt and early.
- Two percent incidence of avascular necrosis (AN) is reported, despite appropriate treatment.
- Long-term results of untreated or unsuccessfully treated DDH include the following:
  1. Early degenerative joint disease or osteoarthritis
  2. Functional disability by the third to fifth decade of life
  3. Pain
  4. Abnormal gait
  5. Leg length discrepancy
  6. Decreased agility

■ REFERRAL INFORMATION
All patients should be referred to an orthopedic surgeon, who will decide therapy and maintain follow-up.

PEARLS & CONSIDERATIONS

■ CLINICAL PEARLS
- The infant must be relaxed at time of examination.
- Barlow and Ortolani are present early (first few months), whereas abduction limitations and knee height abnormalities are noted later.

■ WEBSITES
For parents, information about DDH and Pavlik Harness:
- www.childhosp.bc.ca/childrens/ortho/pavlikharness.html
- www.childhosp.bc.ca/childrens/ortho/CDH.html

II

REFERENCES

1. Aronsson DD et al: Developmental dysplasia of the hip, *Pediatrics* 94:201, 1994.
2. Ballock RT, Richards BS: Hip dysplasia: early diagnosis makes a difference, *Contemp Pediatr* 14:108, 1997.
3. Committee on Quality Improvement, Subcommittee on Developmental Dysplasia of the Hip: Clinical practice guideline: early detection of developmental dysplasia of the hip, *Pediatrics* 105:896, 2000.
4. Donaldson JS, Feinstein KA: Imaging of developmental dysplasia of the hip, *Pediatr Clin North Am* 44:591, 1997.
5. Mooney JF, Emans JB: DDH: a clinical overview, *Pediatr Rev* 16:229, 1995.
6. Novacheck TE: Developmental dysplasia of the hip, *Pediatr Clin North Am* 43:829, 1996.

Author: **Lynn C. Garfunkel, M.D.**

BASIC INFORMATION

■ DEFINITION
Diabetes insipidus (DI) is the inability to concentrate urine, resulting in polyuria (excretion of abnormally large volumes of dilute urine) and polydipsia (large volume of water intake). There are four categories of DI:
- Central (neurogenic, neurohypophyseal, antidiuretic hormone [ADH] responsive): most common type; inadequate secretion of ADH
- Nephrogenic (NDI)
  1. Congenital (vasopressin resistant): very rare; renal insensitivity to antidiuretic effects of vasopressin; normal to slightly elevated ADH levels
  2. Acquired: much more common than congenital; generally less severe and can occur secondary to drugs (e.g., lithium, tetracycline), electrolyte abnormalities (e.g., hypokalemia, hypercalcemia), obstructive uropathy, or systemic disease (e.g., sickle cell anemia)
- Primary polydipsia: occurs because of excessive ingestion of fluids, which may be secondary to abnormal thirst ("thirst thermostat" set abnormally), psychologic dysfunction, or iatrogenic; excessive fluid ingestion suppresses vasopressin release
- Gestational: occurs because of increased metabolism of vasopressin in pregnancy

ICD-9CM CODES
253.5 Diabetes insipidus
253.55 Pituitary
588.1 Nephrogenic, vasopressin resistant

■ ETIOLOGY
- Normally, vasopressin binds to the vasopressin-2 (V_2)receptor located on the principal cells of the collecting duct in the kidney.
- A series of events resulting in transport of aquaporin-2 channels from an intracellular location to the apical membrane of the collecting duct cells is initiated.
- This sequence allows for increased water reabsorption.
- In congenital nephrogenic DI:
  1. X-linked form involves mutation/deletion in V_2 receptor gene and results in one of the following:
     a. Decreased hormone binding, impaired intracellular transport, or coupling to adenylyl cyclase system
     b. Diminished synthesis
     c. Accelerated degradation of the receptor

  2. Autosomal recessive form involves mutation in aquaporin-2 gene.
     a. Impaired trafficking of the water channels
     b. Decreased channel function
  3. Autosomal dominant form also involves mutation in aquaporin-2 gene.
- In acquired nephrogenic DI:
  1. The degree of polyuria generally is not as high as with central or congenital nephrogenic DI.
  2. In hypercalcemia, a concentrating defect may occur if plasma calcium concentration is more than 11 mg/dl; the mechanism of action involves decreased density of aquaporin-2 water channels.
  3. In hypokalemia, a concentrating defect may occur if plasma potassium is chronically below 3 mg/dl; the mechanism of action involves decreased density of aquaporin-2 water channels.
  4. Drugs (e.g., lithium, cidofovir, foscarnet) may lead to impaired water reabsorption; the mechanism of action involves decreased density of aquaporin-2 water channels.
- In central DI, may be caused by one of the following:
  1. Idiopathic
  2. Genetic: can be autosomal dominant or autosomal recessive
  3. Injury to neurohypophysis: most common cause
     a. Head trauma, pituitary surgery, tumor (craniopharyngioma, lymphoma), cerebral anoxia, granulomatous disease (histiocytosis, sarcoidosis), infection (viral or bacterial meningitis, encephalitis)

■ EPIDEMIOLOGY & DEMOGRAPHICS
- The incidence of DI in the general population is estimated at 3 in 100,000.
- The incidence of X-linked NDI is estimated to be 4 in 1 million.
- The transmission of congenital forms can be X-linked, autosomal dominant, or autosomal recessive (see "Etiology").

■ HISTORY
- Symptoms of NDI can occur within the first few weeks of life.
  1. Polyuria and polydipsia
  2. Failure to thrive
  3. Irritability
  4. Constipation
  5. Anorexia
  6. Vomiting
  7. Fever (secondary to dehydration)
  8. Seizures (rare)
     a. May occur during treatment if rehydration occurs too quickly,

with sodium concentrations falling too rapidly
- Symptoms later in childhood
  1. Nocturia
  2. Enuresis
  3. Poor growth, especially if untreated
  4. Malnutrition, secondary to anorexia and/or emesis, which occurs secondary to high volumes of water ingestion
  5. Developmental delay possible as result of repeated bouts of hypernatremic dehydration with or without cerebral edema secondary to overaggressive rehydration
  6. Possible influence on psychosocial development by competing demands for drinking/voiding and playing/learning; hyperactivity and short-term memory problems possible

■ PHYSICAL EXAMINATION
- Growth failure (poor weight gain and poor height velocity)
- Irritability
- Signs of dehydration: dry skin, loss of normal skin turgor, sunken fontanelle, dry mucous membranes, scaphoid abdomen

🔬 DIAGNOSIS

■ DIFFERENTIAL DIAGNOSIS
- Central DI
- Primary polydipsia
- Other acquired forms of concentrating defects or polyuria
  1. Obstructive uropathy
  2. Renal dysplasia
  3. Drug induced (e.g., lithium, tetracycline)
  4. Sickle cell disease
  5. Metabolic (hypokalemia, hypercalcemia)
  6. Protein malnutrition
- Diabetes mellitus

■ DIAGNOSTIC WORKUP
- The diagnosis is suggested by the following:
  1. Polyuria
  2. Specific gravity on first-morning urine of less than 1.010
  3. High serum osmolality associated with low urine osmolality
- The diagnosis is generally made by performing a water deprivation test.
  1. The purpose is to raise serum osmolality to a point where there is sufficient ADH released to maximally concentrate the urine.
  2. If the urine remains dilute at this point, it suggests DI.
  3. If the urine is dilute despite elevated serum osmolality, ADH is given to differentiate central from nephrogenic DI.

II

- Several protocols are available, which involve the following steps:
  1. Conduct the test in a hospital under close observation. If the patient truly has DI, a prolonged period without water can result in dangerous dehydration.
  2. Allow free access to water until early morning, at which point the test is started and the patient is given nothing by mouth (NPO).
  3. At the start of water deprivation, check the patient's weight, vital signs, serum osmolarity (osm) and sodium (Na), and urine osm and specific gravity.
  4. Record time of each void, volume, specific gravity, and osmolality.
  5. Each hour, recheck the patient's weight and vital signs. Calculate the percentage difference in weight from hour 0.
  6. Every 2 hours, recheck the serum osm and Na (and serum blood glucose if patient is an infant).
  7. The test is terminated if urine specific gravity rises to greater than 1.014.
  8. If urine specific gravity remains lower than 1.014, continue the test until serum osm is 295 mOsm/kg or greater, weight loss of 3% to 5% occurs, or urine specific gravity and osm are stable for 2 to 3 hours.
  9. Collect serum osm, Na, urine osm, and specific gravity at the termination of this portion of the test.
  10. The period of water deprivation should not exceed 4 to 6 hours for an infant.
  11. Administer exogenous ADH.
      a. DDAVP should be given intranasally at a dose of 10 µg for infants and 20 µg for older children.
      b. If given intravenously, the suggested dose is one tenth the intranasal dose.
  12. Continue to check serum osm and Na, urine specific gravity and osm, and body weight for 1 to 4 hours.
  13. Patients with central DI will concentrate urine to greater than 450 mOsm/kg in response to the DDAVP. Patients with nephrogenic DI will continue to have very dilute urine after administration of DDAVP.

℞ THERAPY

■ NONPHARMACOLOGIC
- Easy access to water
- Salt (solute) restriction

■ MEDICAL
- Central DI
  1. DDAVP
- Nephrogenic DI
  1. Thiazides with or without amiloride (potassium-sparing diuretic) to reduce the volume of urine output by inducing mild intravascular volume contraction
      a. Hydrochlorothiazide: 2 to 4 mg/kg/day divided twice a day
      b. Amiloride: up to 20 mg/1.73 m^2/day divided twice a day
  2. Indomethacin: to reduce glomerular filtration rate; 2 mg/kg/day divided twice a day
- During an episode of dehydration
  1. The patient may require central line placement to keep up with ongoing urine losses and to replace the deficit.
  2. Need to closely monitor the blood glucose and consider a change to 3% dextrose because patients can become hyperglycemic from high rate of dextrose infusion.
  3. Glycosuria can exacerbate the situation by inducing an osmotic diuresis.
- If DI is caused by a drug, remove the offending agent (e.g., lithium); if it is caused by an electrolyte abnormality, make the appropriate correction.

■ FOLLOW-UP & DISPOSITION
- Close monitoring of electrolytes, especially potassium, should be maintained if the patient is prescribed a thiazide.
- Monitor for side effects of indomethacin: gastrointestinal upset and bleeding; renal function.
- Monitor growth and development.

■ PATIENT/FAMILY EDUCATION
- Review the genetics of the disease with the parents.
  1. With X-linked NDI, unless a new mutation occurred, the mother is a carrier and the father is normal. Half of the male children will be affected, and 50% of female offspring will be carriers.
  2. If the father has NDI (and the mother is normal), all male offspring will be normal and all the female offspring will be carriers.
  3. Conduct perinatal testing for carrier status.

- Severe dehydration can occur quickly, particularly in illnesses associated with vomiting and diarrhea.
- Neurologic sequelae typically occur secondary to repeated bouts of dehydration and overly aggressive rehydration.
- Solute restriction is important in decreasing obligatory water loss.

■ REFERRAL INFORMATION
Most children are referred to a pediatric nephrologist or endocrinologist for evaluation.

⚙ PEARLS & CONSIDERATIONS

■ CLINICAL PEARLS
- A high serum sodium level associated with polyuria in a dehydrated infant suggests a renal concentrating defect.
- Seizures, when they occur, generally occur during too-rapid rehydration.
- Early diagnosis, treatment, and careful rehydration have resulted in a decrease in mental retardation.

■ WEBSITE
NDI Foundation: www.ndif.org

■ SUPPORT GROUPS
- Diabetes Insipidus and Related Disorders (DIARD), 235 North Hibiscus Drive, Miami, FL 33139-5121, 800-434-3508 or 305-538-3904
- The Diabetes Insipidus Foundation, Inc., website: http://diabetesinsipidus.maxinter.net/, email: diabetesinsipidus@maxinter.net
- National Organization for Rare Disorders, Inc., P.O. Box 8923, New Fairfield, CT 06812-8923, website: www.rarediseases.org

REFERENCES
1. Berl T, Kumar S: Disorders of water metabolism. In Johnson RJ, Feehally J (eds): *Comprehensive clinical nephrology,* London, 2000, Mosby.
2. Berl T, Robertson G: Pathophysiology of water metabolism. In Brenner BM, Rector FC (eds): *Brenner and Rector's the kidney,* ed 6, Philadelphia, 2000, WB Saunders.
3. Saborio P, Tipton GA, Chan JC: Diabetes insipidus, *Pediatr Rev* 21:122, 2000.
4. Online Mendelian Inheritance in Man (OMIM) at www3.ncbi.nlm.nih.gov/omim.
5. NDI Foundation at www.ndif.org.
Author: **Ayesa Mian, M.D.**

BASIC INFORMATION

■ DEFINITION

Diabetes mellitus (DM) type 1 is an autoimmune disorder characterized by insulin deficiency resulting from progressive destruction of the insulin-producing β cells of the pancreas. This insulin deficiency leads to hyperglycemia and ketosis. Chronic hyperglycemia is associated with long-term damage, leading to dysfunction of the kidney, eyes, nerves, heart, and blood vessels.

■ SYNONYMS

- Juvenile-onset diabetes mellitus (JODM)
- Insulin-dependent diabetes mellitus (IDDM)
- Type 1 DM

ICD-9CM CODE

250.01 Diabetes mellitus type 1

■ ETIOLOGY

Relative or absolute insulin deficiency

■ EPIDEMIOLOGY & DEMOGRAPHICS

- An incidence of 1.7 affected individuals per 1000 people younger than 20 years has been reported.
- The incidence of type 1 DM is higher in Caucasians than in African Americans and lowest in Asians.
- Diabetes is more prevalent in northern than in southern climates.
- Approximately 13,000 new cases in the United States are diagnosed annually in children.
- Approximately 125,000 individuals younger than 19 years of age have diabetes.

■ HISTORY

- The presentation may be acute with diabetic ketoacidosis (see the section "Diabetic Ketoacidosis").
- The presentation may follow 1 to 3 weeks of polyuria, polydipsia, and/or polyphagia.
- DM may present with new-onset enuresis in a previously continent child.
- The presentation may be an incidental laboratory finding of glucosuria and/or hyperglycemia.

■ PHYSICAL EXAMINATION

- Weight loss possible
- Usually unremarkable unless patient is in diabetic ketoacidosis

⚲ DIAGNOSIS

■ DIFFERENTIAL DIAGNOSIS

- Urinary tract infection
- Diabetes insipidus
- Stress hyperglycemia
- Neurogenic bladder

■ DIAGNOSTIC WORKUP

- Fasting blood glucose higher than 126 mg/dl
- Two-hour post–oral glucose test higher than 200 mg/dl or random glucose higher than 200 mg/dl and symptoms
- Glycosylated hemoglobin higher than normal
- Antibodies to islet cells, glutamate acid decarboxylase, insulin, islet-related autoantigens, and others; these antibodies not used in routine diagnosis of diabetes

℞ THERAPY

■ NONPHARMACOLOGIC

- Begin a diabetic meal plan based either on the diabetic exchange system or the carbohydrate counting system.
  1. The exchange system is based on the American Diabetes Association and American Dietetic Association guidelines for food groups; portion sizes; and carbohydrate, protein, and fat distribution.
     a. The exchange system assigns all foods to one of nine groups.
     b. Carbohydrate, protein, and fat caloric content are given for portion size.
     c. The meal plan is designed for the patient to eat the same number of exchanges from day to day at each meal and snack.
     d. This plan provides consistent carbohydrate, protein, and fat content from day to day.
  2. The carbohydrate counting system is based on the carbohydrate content of all foods.
     a. The goal is to eat a consistent amount of carbohydrates at each meal regardless of the food group.
     b. The carbohydrate counting system requires more guidance to balance protein, carbohydrate, and fat ratios.
     c. The carbohydrate counting system allows more flexibility.
- Psychologic support should be available for the patient and family.

■ MEDICAL

- Insulin: The usual regimen consists of a total daily dose of 0.7 to 1 U/kg/day, divided in two or three doses.
  1. The usual distribution is two thirds of the total daily dose given in the morning.
     a. Two thirds intermediate or long-acting insulin
     b. One third short-acting insulin (regular or Humalog)
  2. The remaining one third of the total daily dose is taken in the evening.
     a. It is divided as one half long-acting and one half short-acting insulin.
     b. The evening dose may be split by giving the short-acting insulin before dinner and the long-acting insulin before bedtime.
- Home blood glucose monitoring is done, with determinations before each meal and at bedtime.
- Urine ketone determination during acute illnesses and with blood sugars higher than 300 mg/dl.

■ FOLLOW-UP & DISPOSITION

- Initial education should be provided regarding diabetes, insulin adjustment, blood glucose, urine ketone monitoring, and meal planning.
- Frequent phone management should occur to review the patient's glucose log and recommend insulin adjustments.
- Usual follow-up is maintained through outpatient pediatric diabetes center visits four times per year.
  1. At each visit, the glucose log is reviewed and recommendations are made for insulin adjustments if needed.
  2. Glycosylated hemoglobin levels should be checked three to four times per year to assess chronic control.
- Phone contact should be maintained for illness management.

■ PATIENT/FAMILY EDUCATION

- The major component of diabetes management is education of patients and their families.
- School personnel (e.g., teachers, nurses, day-care providers) should also be educated regarding diabetes.

■ PREVENTIVE TREATMENT OR TESTS

- An ophthalmologic examination should be performed yearly.
- Thyroid function tests should be performed at the onset of disease and every 2 to 3 years thereafter.
- Urine for microalbuminuria should be checked annually 3 to 5 years after the onset of diabetes.

☼ PEARLS & CONSIDERATIONS

■ CLINICAL PEARLS
- Tight glycemic control significantly reduces the rate of complications.
- During puberty, increases in total daily insulin up to 1.5 U/kg/day are often needed.
- Psychosocial issues of dealing with a chronic disease are the most common cause of difficulties with diabetes care.

■ WEBSITES
- American Diabetes Association: www.diabetes.org/
- Children with Diabetes: www.childrenwithdiabetes.org
- Insulin-Free World Foundation: www.insulin-free.org/main/htm
- Juvenile Diabetes Foundation International: www.jdf.org/index.html

■ SUPPORT GROUPS
- American Diabetes Association
- Juvenile Diabetes Foundation

REFERENCES

1. American Diabetes Association: *Practice guidelines: diabetes care,* vol 22, supplement 1, Clinical Practice Recommendations, 1999.
2. Diabetes Control and Complications Research Group: The effect of intensive diabetes treatment on the development and progression of long-term complications in adolescents with insulin-dependent diabetes mellitus, *J Pediatr* 125:177, 1994.
3. The effect of intensive treatment of diabetes on the development and progression of long-term complications in insulin-dependent diabetes mellitus, *N Engl J Med* 329:977, 1993.
4. Kaufman FR: Diabetes mellitus, *Pediatr Rev* 18:383, 1997.

Author: **Nicholas Jospe, M.D.**

BASIC INFORMATION

DEFINITION
Diabetes mellitus (DM) type 2 is a combination of resistance to insulin action and defective glucose-mediated insulin secretion. Patients are not prone to ketosis under basal conditions, and exogenous insulin is not required for short-term survival.

SYNONYMS
- Type 2 DM
- Non–insulin-dependent diabetes mellitus
- Old-term: adult-onset diabetes mellitus (AODM)

ICD-9CM CODE
250.00 Diabetes type 2

ETIOLOGY
- In Type 2 DM, there is primary insulin resistance with relative insulin deficiency or a predominant secretory defect with insulin resistance.
- Variable interplay exists between genetic and environmental factors.
- The precise genetic factors are unknown and vary among population groups.
- Increasingly, sedentary lifestyles and dietary changes contribute to the increasing prevalence of obesity and type 2 DM.

EPIDEMIOLOGY & DEMOGRAPHICS
- The incidence of type 2 DM is increasing in parallel with the increased prevalence of exogenous obesity.
- Type 2 DM is a polygenic disorder.
  1. Certain minority populations are at a higher risk of both obesity and diabetes.
  2. African Americans, Pima Indians, and Mexican Americans are at high risk for type 2 DM
- Environmental factors are highly associated with type 2 DM.
  1. Increase in sedentary lifestyles
  2. Increased access to high-calorie, high-fat foods

HISTORY
- Symptoms of type 2 DM are subtle because the disease develops and progresses slowly.
- The presentation may follow weeks of polyuria, polydipsia, and polyphagia.
- The presentation may be incidental documentation of glucosuria and/or hyperglycemia.
- The presentation can be diabetic ketoacidosis (DKA).
- Adolescent females may have oligomenorrhea and polycystic ovary syndrome.
- Strong family history for DM and obesity may be reported.

PHYSICAL EXAMINATION
- Obesity is common and usually centripetal.
  1. Body mass index is more than 85% of normal for age and gender.
- Stretch marks may be apparent.
- Acanthosis nigricans may be present on the back of the neck, axilla, and inner thighs.
- Adolescent females may be hirsute.

DIAGNOSIS

DIFFERENTIAL DIAGNOSIS
- Type 1 DM
- Stress hyperglycemia

DIAGNOSTIC WORKUP
- Glycosuria without ketonuria is demonstrated on urinalysis.
- Hyperglycemia is present.
  1. Fasting blood glucose is more than 126 mg/dl.
     a. DKA is possible but much less common than in type 1 DM.
  2. Random glucose is more than 200 mg/dl and symptoms are present.
  3. Two-hour post–oral glucose test is higher than 200 mg/dl.
- Glycosylated hemoglobin is higher than normal.
- Insulin or C-peptide levels are useful when elevated above normal, indicative of insulin resistance.
- Family history of type 2 DM is reported.

THERAPY

NONPHARMACOLOGIC
- Diet to induce weight loss
  1. Even mild weight loss is beneficial for glucose control.
  2. Caloric restriction even before weight loss is beneficial for glucose control.
- Modification of lifestyle to increase exercise

MEDICAL
- Oral agents: These are used in early stages when insulin secretion is still present and may be used alone, in combination, or with insulin.
  1. Long-term safety and efficacy have not been well established in children.
  2. Sulfonylureas stimulate pancreatic insulin secretion and have a direct insulin-sensitizing effect.
     a. They may cause hypoglycemia and weight gain.
     b. Second-generation sulfonylureas, glipizide, glyburide, and glimepiride may be less associated with weight gain.
  3. Biguanides (metformin) inhibit hepatic glucose output.
     a. Enhance insulin sensitivity in liver and muscle
     b. Not associated with hypoglycemia
     c. May also cause some weight loss and gastrointestinal (GI) side effects
     d. Synergistic as glycemic control when used in combination with sulfonylureas
  4. Glucosidase inhibitors (e.g., acarbose) delay digestion of complex carbohydrates.
     a. Decrease the rise in postprandial plasma glucose
     b. Significant GI side effects, such as diarrhea, flatulence, and abdominal distension
  5. Thiazolidinediones are insulin sensitizers.
     a. Troglitazone is the first of these compounds to be available for use with direct insulinomimetic effects as well as insulin-sensitizing actions.
        (1) Hepatotoxicity is a rare, potentially serious complication of troglitazone.
     b. Rosiglitazone and pioglitazone are other recently released compounds that may have less idiosyncratic hepatic response.
- Insulin therapy may be needed in later stages, when β-cell function is lost.
  1. See the section "Diabetes Mellitus Type 1."
  2. Satisfactory glycemic control can usually be obtained with intermediate insulin alone.

FOLLOW-UP & DISPOSITION
- Problems associated with the treatment of children with type 2 DM may be different from those encountered in children with type 1 DM.
  1. Often, control is marked by difficulties with nonadherence to treatment regimen.
     a. Caloric restrictions are difficult to maintain.
  2. The therapeutic intervention is no less intense in presentation.
  3. In type 2 DM, an oral agent, not insulin, is the first line of therapy.
     a. Insulin can be beneficial.
     b. Insulin may be required when oral agents no longer maintain euglycemic state.

PATIENT/FAMILY EDUCATION
- Education is not the same as in type 1 DM.
- Emphasis is on caloric restriction and lifestyle changes.
- Oral pharmacotherapy with hypoglycemic agents is useful; insulin may also be needed.

☼ PEARLS & CONSIDERATIONS

■ CLINICAL PEARLS

- Aggressive intervention with oral agents or insulin is necessary.
  1. Delays complications
  2. Significantly improves outcome
- It may be difficult to establish whether a child with new-onset DM has type 1 or type 2
  1. It is safe to start these patients on insulin.
  2. Switch to oral agents if appropriate.

■ WEBSITE

American Diabetes Association: http://diabetes.org

REFERENCES

1. American Diabetes Association: *Practice guidelines: diabetes care,* vol 22, Supplement 1, Clinical Practice Recommendations, 1999.
2. Dean H: Diagnostic criteria for non-insulin dependent diabetes in youth (NIDDM-Y), *Clin Pediatr* 37:67, 1998.
3. Jones KL: Non-insulin dependent diabetes in children and adolescents: the therapeutic challenge, *Clin Pediatr* 37:103, 1998.
4. Rosenbloom AL, House DV, Winter WE: Non-insulin dependent diabetes mellitus (NIDDM) in minority youth: research priorities and needs, *Clin Pediatr* 37:143, 1998.
5. Rosenbloom AL et al: Emerging epidemic of type 2 diabetes in youth, *Diabetes Care* 22:345, 1999.
6. United Kingdom Prospective Diabetes Study, in *Lancet* 352:837, 1998, and in *Br Med J* 7160:703, 1998.

Author: **Nicholas Jospe, M.D.**

BASIC INFORMATION

Diabetic ketoacidosis (DKA) is a combination of hyperglycemia, ketonemia, acidosis, and dehydration.

■ DEFINITION
DKA is dehydration and acidosis resulting from insulin deficiency (relative or absolute) in a subject with diabetes mellitus type 1 or 2.

ICD-9CM CODE
250.13 Diabetic ketoacidosis

■ ETIOLOGY
- Relative or absolute deficiency of insulin, resulting in uncontrolled hyperglycemia and thus osmotic diuresis with electrolyte, glucose, ketone, and fluid loss
- Hyperglycemia as a result of hepatic and renal overproduction of glucose and muscle underutilization of glucose; ketoacidosis parallels hyperglycemia
- Increased counterregulatory hormones (e.g., cortisol, catecholamines, glucagon, growth hormone)

■ EPIDEMIOLOGY & DEMOGRAPHICS
DKA is three to four times more common in patients with known diabetes than in patients with new-onset diabetes. The mortality rate for DKA ranges from 2% to 5% in developed countries.

■ HISTORY
- DKA may be a presentation of new-onset type 1 diabetes mellitus and, more rarely, type 2 diabetes mellitus.
- DKA ensues after omission of insulin for 24 to 48 hours in a subject with type 1 diabetes mellitus.
- DKA occurs in conjunction with illness and relative underinsulinization.
- Polyuria and polydipsia are seen.
- Abdominal pain is common.
- Vomiting may occur.

■ PHYSICAL EXAMINATION
- Elevated pulse, low blood pressure
- Dry mucosa and lips
- Sunken eyes
- Fruity odor to breath
- Kussmaul's breathing: rapid, deep, nonlabored
- Decreased bowel sounds and tender or rigid abdomen; may simulate peritonitis or acute abdomen
- Mental status examination ranging from normal to comatose

DIAGNOSIS

■ DIFFERENTIAL DIAGNOSIS
- No other metabolic abnormality can account for laboratory and physical examination findings.
- Initial presentation with polyuria or polydipsia may suggest diabetes insipidus.
- Other causes of dehydration and vomiting may be entertained until laboratory values are known.
- Other causes of mental status abnormalities may be suggested until laboratory results are returned.

■ DIAGNOSTIC WORKUP
- Hyperglycemia (normal glucose does not rule out DKA)
- Acidosis: venous blood gas with pH less than 7.2 and P_{CO_2} less than 15 mEq/L
- Ketonemia, ketonuria (urine Acetest)
- Hyperosmolarity mostly caused by hyperglycemia
- Hyperlipidemia
- Electrolyte disturbances
  1. Sodium loss of approximately 10 mEq/kg body weight
     a. Expect a 1.6-mEq/L decrease in serum sodium for every 100-mg/dl increase of glucose concentration.
  2. Chloride loss of 4 mEq/kg
  3. Potassium loss of 5 mEq/kg
     a. Hypokalemia: Usual deficit is 3 to 5 mEq/kg, but therapy and continued losses may exacerbate hypokalemia (nadir at 4 to 12 hours).
- Urinary ketones correlate poorly with degree of serum ketonemia.
  1. Remain positive up to 2 days after successful treatment of DKA
  2. Not useful as a monitor of ongoing therapy

THERAPY

The goal is to restore volume, correct electrolyte deficits, and administer insulin. These steps normalize blood glucose and stop ketoacid production.

■ NONPHARMACOLOGIC
- Clinical monitoring should be maintained every 30 to 60 minutes.
- Laboratory: Glucose should be taken hourly at the bedside; electrolytes and pH should be taken at admission and at 2, 6, 9, 12, 18, and 24 hours.
- Keep a good flowsheet.

■ MEDICAL
- Fluids: bolus with 10 to 20 ml/kg normal saline over 1 hour
- Insulin: 0.1 U/kg/hr using regular insulin or lispro insulin by continuous intravenous infusion
  1. Alternative is 0.3 U/kg intramuscularly every 3 hours.
  2. Avoid the subcutaneous route.
  3. The infusion rate may be doubled if the pH fails to rise within 4 to 6 hours.
  4. If the glucose falls by more than 100 mg/dl/hr, the insulin infusion may be decreased by 30% to 50% and glucose is added to the intravenous fluid.
- Replace fluid over 24 to 48 hours using one half normal saline, combining deficit plus daily maintenance:
  1. Fluid deficit (usually 7% to 10%) = body weight × estimated deficit × 1000 ml.
  2. Daily maintenance = 100 ml/kg for first 10 kg body weight, 50 ml/kg for next 10 kg, and 20 ml/kg over 20 kg.
  3. Do not give more than 4 L/m² over first 24 hours.
  4. Add potassium to the intravenous fluid only after urine output is confirmed and based on potassium in the following ranges:
     a. If serum [K] = 3.0 to 4.0 mEq/L, add 40 mEq/L of potassium (as KCl plus KPO_4).
     b. If [K] = 4.0 to 5.5, add 20 mEq/L of potassium.
     c. If [K] = 5.5 to 6.0, add 10 mEq/L of potassium.
     d. If [K] is greater than 6.0, add no potassium to the intravenous fluids.
  5. Routine use of phosphate supplementation is not recommended.
  6. Add 5% dextrose when serum glucose falls to 250 to 300 mg/dl.
  7. Bicarbonate therapy is not recommended, except possibly with incipient circulatory collapse.

■ FOLLOW-UP & DISPOSITION
- Patients may begin eating when no longer vomiting or complaining of abdominal pain or anorexia.
- Transition by administering appropriate subcutaneous insulin and, 30 minutes later, discontinue intravenous insulin.
  1. Do transition around meal time, using established insulin dose.
  2. Begin new patient on appropriate dose (see section "Diabetes Mellitus Type 1").

■ **PATIENT/FAMILY EDUCATION**
- DKA prevention is the goal when teaching the principles of insulin dosage adjustment, blood glucose and urine ketone monitoring, and "sick day" management skills.
- Analysis of the cause of DKA in a patient with established diabetes may reveal areas of education or care that need to be emphasized.
- Appropriate attention needs to be paid to the psychosocial issues that contribute to loss of control, particularly in adolescent patients.

■ **PREVENTIVE TREATMENT OR TESTS**
- Encourage patients to check for urine ketones when glucose is higher than 300 to 350 mg/dl.
- Ensure prompt contact with provider when urine ketones are detected.

■ **REFERRAL INFORMATION**
Transfer patients in moderate to severe DKA to an intensive care unit or tertiary center for therapy and monitoring of therapy.

⚙ **PEARLS & CONSIDERATIONS**

■ **COMPLICATIONS**
- Persistent acidosis: If [HCO_3] fails to rise after 6 hours, increase the insulin infusion rate.
- Cerebral edema
  1. It occurs hours into treatment and is not heralded by specific signs or symptoms.
     a. Estimated to occur in 0.7% to 1.0% of episodes of DKA.
     b. Mortality is about 70%, and recovery without permanent impairment of function is only 7% to 14%.
  2. Cerebral edema is marked by sudden headache, pupillary, mental status, or vital signs changes.
  3. Mannitol (0.5 to 2.0 g/kg repeated as necessary) is the treatment of choice.

■ **CLINICAL PEARLS**
- DKA is in the differential diagnosis of nonsurgical acute abdomen.
  1. Amylase may be elevated in DKA and is not specific for pancreatitis.
  2. Lipase is more specific for pancreatitis.
- Abdominal pain should dissipate as acidosis resolves; if it does not, suspect an intraabdominal problem.

■ **WEBSITES**
- Insulin-Free World Foundation: www.insulin-free.org
- Children with Diabetes: www.childrenwithdiabetes.org
- American Diabetes Association: www.diabetes.org
- Juvenile Diabetes Foundation International: www.jdf.org

REFERENCES

1. Duck SC, Wyatt DT: Factors associated with brain herniation in the treatment of diabetic ketoacidosis, *J Pediatr* 113: 10, 1988.
2. Harris GD et al: Minimizing the risk of brain herniation during treatment of diabetic ketoacidemia: a retrospective and prospective study, *J Pediatr* 117: 22, 1990.
3. Rosenbloom AL, Hanas R: Diabetic ketoacidosis (DKA): treatment guidelines, *Clin Pediatr* 35:261, 1996.
4. Rosenbloom AL, Schatz DA: Diabetic ketoacidosis in childhood, *Pediatr Ann* 23:284, 1994.

Author: **Nicholas Jospe, M.D.**

BASIC INFORMATION

■ DEFINITION
Discitis is a spectrum of conditions ranging from nonspecific inflammation of the disc space to a florid disc space infection involving the vertebral body.

■ SYNONYMS
- Disc space narrowing
- Inflammation of disc

ICD-9CM CODES
722.93 Lumbar
722.92 Thoracic
722.91 Cervical

■ ETIOLOGY
- The cause is unknown, but it is presumed to be bacterial (usually *Staphylococcus aureus*).
- Blood cultures are positive in less than 30% of patients; biopsy culture specimens are positive in less than 50% of patients.
- Arterial supply to the disc space is via the artery to the vertebral body passing through the endplate into the disc.
- Inflammatory response appears to begin in the endplate and spreads to the disc.

■ EPIDEMIOLOGY & DEMOGRAPHICS
- Discitis is most common in children younger than 5 years of age.
- There is no sex predilection.
- It is not associated with trauma or osteomyelitis or septic arthritis elsewhere in body.
- Antecedent upper respiratory infection or diarrhea often predates onset.
- Discitis most commonly involves the lumbar spine.

■ HISTORY
- The history depends on the age of the child.
  1. Younger than 3 years of age: limp or refusal to walk
  2. From 3 to 7 years of age: abdominal complaints may predominate (e.g., constipation, enuresis)
  3. Older than 7 years of age: back pain is the predominant complaint
- Child prefers to be recumbent.

■ PHYSICAL EXAMINATION
- Irritable, but not acutely ill
- Temperature normal or minimally elevated
- Paravertebral muscle spasm
- Limited motion of spine
- Pain caused by any motion of the spine
- Limited straight leg raising (hamstring spasm)
- No neurologic deficits

DIAGNOSIS

■ DIFFERENTIAL DIAGNOSIS
- Acute pyogenic vertebral osteomyelitis
- Tuberculous spondylitis
- *Salmonella* or *Brucella* spondylitis
- Intervertebral disc space calcification
- Spinal cord tumor
- Appendicitis
- Pyelonephritis

■ DIAGNOSTIC WORKUP
- Elevated erythrocyte sedimentation rate (ESR) (in 80% to 90%), possible leukocytosis
- Blood culture usually negative
- Local biopsy and culture indications
  1. Clinical and radiologic progression despite treatment
  2. Enlarging paravertebral abscess
  3. If organism other than *S. aureus* (i.e., *Salmonella*, *Brucella*) is suspected
- Radiologic tests
  1. Early radiographs normal
  2. Disc space narrowing earliest finding (2 to 3 weeks)
  3. Erosion of vertebral endplates
  4. Vertebral body changes
- ^{99}Tc-bone scan (increased uptake useful for early diagnosis)
- Magnetic resonance imaging to determine extent of involvement of disc space, vertebral body and paravertebral body soft tissue abscess if present (may be useful in early diagnosis)

THERAPY

■ NONPHARMACOLOGIC
- Disorder often indolent and self-limiting, responding to bed rest alone

- Traction
- Body cast or spinal orthosis

■ MEDICAL
- Nonsteroidal antiinflammatory drugs
- Antibiotics (antistaphylococcal)
  1. If systemically ill (fever, increased ESR, increased white blood cell count)
  2. For positive culture
  3. If not responding to immobilization
- Antibiotics may reduce symptoms faster, may lead to earlier resolution
- Antibiotics, if used, intravenously initially, followed by oral for total of 4 to 6 weeks

■ FOLLOW-UP & DISPOSITION
- Immobilization should be continued for 4 to 8 weeks.
- Healing generally occurs by 8 weeks.
- Disc space narrowing may be permanent or proceed onto fusion across the intervertebral disc space.
- Observation for possible spinal deformity is necessary for several years.

■ REFERRAL INFORMATION
Refer to an orthopedist if discitis is suspected in the diagnosis.

PEARLS & CONSIDERATIONS

■ CLINICAL PEARLS
Variability of clinical presentation is related to age.

REFERENCES
1. Crawford AH et al: Diskitis in children, *Clin Orthop* 266:70, 1991.
2. Gabriel KA, Crawford AH: Magnetic resonance imaging in a child who had clinical signs of discitis: report of a case, *J Bone Joint Surg* 70A:938, 1988.
3. Menelaus MB: An inflammation affecting the discitis: intervertebral discs in children, *J Bone Joint Surg* 46B:16, 1964.
4. Payne WK III, Ogilvie JW: Back pain in children and adolescent, *Pediatr Clin North Am* 43:899, 1996.
5. Wenger DR, Bobechko WP, Gilday DL: The spectrum of intervertebral disc space infection in children, *J Bone Joint Surg* 60A:100, 1978.
Author: **Dennis R. Roy, M.D.**

II

BASIC INFORMATION

■ DEFINITION
Disseminated intravascular coagulation (DIC) is an acute or chronic disorder causing thrombosis or hemorrhage, which occurs as a secondary complication of an underlying disease. It is characterized by consumption of coagulation factors caused by intravascular activation of the coagulation sequence, which leads to the formation of thrombi throughout the microcirculation of the body, and secondarily, activation of fibrinolysis.

■ SYNONYMS
- Consumption coagulopathy
- Defibrination syndrome
- DIC

ICD-9CM CODE
286.6 DIC

■ ETIOLOGY
- Thrombin production is a normal response to tissue damage.
  1. Multiple illnesses result in unregulated thrombin production, which leads to widespread microvascular thrombosis.
  2. Thrombin is produced in sepsis and other inflammatory illnesses via cytokines.
     a. Cytokines (i.e., tissue necrotic factor-α [TNF-α]) are generated in response to endotoxin.
     b. Cytokines induce the extrinsic pathway, which results in thrombin production.
- Excess plasmin production is a compensatory mechanism to maintain vascular patency.
  1. Acute presentation
     a. Infection: gram-negative sepsis; gram-positive sepsis, especially with hyposplenism; systemic fungal infection; malaria; viral infections; rickettsial infections
     b. Obstetric: placental separation, amniotic fluid embolism
     c. Trauma: head trauma, burns, heat stroke, lightning strike
     d. Other: transfusion of ABO-incompatible red blood cells, liver disease, snake bites, extensive surgery, malignant hypertension
  2. Chronic presentation
     a. Malignancy: adenocarcinoma, acute promyelocytic leukemia
     b. Obstetric: retained dead fetus syndrome, toxemia
     c. Vascular disease: aortic aneurysm, giant hemangioma, vasculitis

■ EPIDEMIOLOGY & DEMOGRAPHICS
- Most cases occur in the setting of gram-negative sepsis.
  1. From 10% to 20% of patients with gram-negative bacteremia have evidence of DIC.

■ HISTORY & PHYSICAL EXAMINATION
- Hemorrhage is the most common presentation, but microvascular thrombosis is the primary mechanism. The clinician must be attentive to the possibility of DIC as the cause of severe bleeding, thrombosis, or both.
  1. Manifestations of hemorrhage caused by plasmin generation include the following:
     a. Spontaneous bruising
     b. Petechiae
     c. Gastrointestinal bleeding
     d. Respiratory tract bleeding
     e. Persistent bleeding at venipuncture sites
     f. Bleeding at surgical wounds
     g. Intracranial bleeding
     h. Hematuria
  2. Manifestations of thrombosis caused by thrombin generation include the following:
     a. Renal failure
     b. Coma
     c. Liver failure
     d. Respiratory failure
     e. Skin necrosis
     f. Gangrene
     g. Venous thromboembolism
  3. Manifestations of cytokine generation include the following:
     a. Tachycardia
     b. Hypotension
     c. Edema

DIAGNOSIS

■ DIFFERENTIAL DIAGNOSIS
- Thrombotic thrombocytopenic purpura
- Hemolytic uremic syndrome
- Paroxysmal nocturnal hemoglobinuria
- Heparin-induced thrombocytopenia
- Liver disease
- Vitamin K deficiency

■ DIAGNOSTIC WORKUP
Expected results include the following:
- Thrombocytopenia
- Prolonged prothrombin time
- Prolonged activated partial thromboplastin time
- Decreased fibrinogen
- Elevated fibrin degradation products

Other laboratory results include the following:
- Blood smear may reveal red blood cell fragmentation.
- Other tests should be used to determine the degree of renal, liver, and pulmonary impairment.

THERAPY

■ MEDICAL
- Treatment of the underlying process that initiated DIC is essential. Infection, shock, acidosis, and hypoxia require immediate attention.
- Blood components are used if the patient is bleeding or if an invasive procedure is indicated.
  1. Platelets: Give 1 donor unit per 10 kg of body weight when the platelet count is below 50,000.
  2. Fresh frozen plasma (FFP) has more fibrinogen than cryoprecipitate.
     a. Give 15 ml of FFP per kg of body weight.
     b. Cryoprecipitate may be given when FFP cannot maintain fibrinogen concentration.
- Heparin has been effective in children with DIC associated with purpura fulminans and promyelocytic leukemia. Considerable debate exists regarding the use of heparin.
- Infusions of antithrombin and protein C are being studied but are not considered standard.

■ REFERRAL INFORMATION
Hematology referral is recommended for all patients.

PEARLS & CONSIDERATIONS

■ CLINICAL PEARLS
- Platelet count and fibrinogen may be elevated initially in DIC because of inflammation.
- Vitamin K and folate deficiencies may accompany DIC and can be easily corrected.

REFERENCES
1. Baglin T: Disseminated intravascular coagulation: diagnosis and treatment, *Br Med J* 312:683, 1996.
2. Behrman RE, Kliegman RM, Arvin AM: *Nelson textbook of pediatrics*, ed 15, Philadelphia, 1996, WB Saunders.
3. Cotran RS et al: *Robbins pathologic basis of disease*, ed 6, Philadelphia, 1999, WB Saunders.
4. Levi M et al: Pathogenesis of disseminated intravascular coagulation, *JAMA* 270:975, 1993.

Author: **Edgard A. Segura, M.D.**

BASIC INFORMATION

DEFINITION
Down syndrome is a chromosomal disorder characterized by recognizable facial and physical features, associated with mental retardation and medical issues. Historically, it was the first known chromosomal cause of mental retardation and developmental disability.

ICD-9CM CODE
758.0 Down syndrome

ETIOLOGY
- Approximately 95% of cases are secondary to nondisjunction during meiosis, leading to trisomy 21.
- Approximately 4% of cases are secondary to translocation of a portion of an extra 21 to a separate chromosome 14, 21, or 22.
- Approximately 1% of cases show mosaicism, in which some, but not all, of the cells have an extra 21. This occurs after fertilization during mitosis.

EPIDEMIOLOGY & DEMOGRAPHICS
- Down syndrome is the most common chromosomal anomaly associated with mental retardation.
- The current prevalence is at slightly less than 1 per 1000 live births (0.92 per 1000). This was previously slightly higher but has decreased as a result of prenatal diagnosis and the option for termination.
- A higher incidence occurs with increasing maternal age.
  1. The risk is approximately 1 in 2000 at 20 years of age, but 1 in 20 at 45 years of age.
  2. Most infants with Down syndrome are born to women younger than 35 because of a higher rate of pregnancy in this age group.

HISTORY
- Women 35 years of age and older are often offered prenatal diagnosis with confirmation of disorder by chromosomal analysis of the fetus.
- Obstetricians are using blood screening tests ("triple screen") to identify women younger than 35 years of age who are at high risk.
- Identification often occurs in the neonatal period because of the distinctive facial features.

PHYSICAL EXAMINATION
A combination of the following features is found, but not all features are present in each individual:
- Hypotonia
- Diminished Moro reflex
- Hypermobility of joints
- Microcephaly
- Excess skin at the back of the neck
- Flat midfacial area
- Almond-shaped eye with upslanting of the palpebral fissures
- Epicanthal folds
- Brushfield spots or speckling of the irides
- Ears and mouth may appear small
- Wide gap between first and second toes
- Fifth finger clinodactyly with dysplasia of the midphalanx
- Single palmar crease
- Short and broad hands and feet
- Widely spaced nipples
- Cutis marmorata (lacy pattern to skin)

DIAGNOSIS

DIAGNOSTIC WORKUP
Chromosomes obtained from blood from the neonate, or prenatally from amniocentesis, or from chorionic villus sampling

DIFFERENTIAL DIAGNOSIS
- Little else is considered when many of the distinguishing features are present, but isolated features can be present in individuals without chromosomal disorder.
- Individuals with XXXY, XXXXY, and XXXX can present with some of the characteristics.
- Historically, congenital hypothyroidism may have had similar features without all of the related physical features.

ASSOCIATED MEDICAL COMPLICATIONS
- Congenital heart disease (seen in up to 66% of infants with Down syndrome)
  1. Endocardial cushion defect (arterioventricular canal), ventricular septal defect, and atrial septal defect are the three most common defects. Other defects do occur.
  2. Valvular heart disease can occur after 18 years of age.
  3. Prophylaxis to prevent subacute bacterial endocarditis should be prescribed to all children and adults who are at risk because of cardiac defects.
- Ophthalmologic disorders
  1. Refractive errors, strabismus, nystagmus, blepharitis, and tear duct obstruction are most common
- Ear, nose, and throat issues
  1. Hearing loss, including congenital and acquired with conductive, mixed, and sensorineural
  2. Chronic middle ear fluid: may be difficult to visualize because of narrow ear canals
  3. Recurrent sinusitis and upper respiratory infections (common)
  4. Tracheomalacia
  5. Obstructive sleep apnea
- Gastrointestinal issues
  1. Feeding difficulties, secondary to decreased tone and poor coordination of suck/swallow
  2. Gastrointestinal malformations, including atresias, Hirschsprung's disease, and annular pancreas
  3. Constipation
  4. Gastroesophageal reflux
- Dermatologic issues
  1. Atopic dermatitis
  2. Seborrheic dermatitis
  3. Vitiligo
- Dental issues
- Malocclusion and periodontal disease
- Endocrine and growth issues
  1. Hypothyroidism (may be clinically silent)
  2. Short stature and obesity (Specific growth charts have been developed for individuals with Down syndrome, see Part III.)
  3. Rarely diabetes
  4. Primary gonadal deficiency
- Orthopedic issues
  1. Flat feet
  2. Awkward gait
  3. Atlantoaxial instability
- Neurodevelopmental issues
  1. Hypotonia with associated gross motor delay is seen; typical age of walking is 2 years.
  2. Developmental disability with mental retardation is present.
  3. Patients can have dual diagnoses with disorders similar to the general population, such as attention deficit/hyperactivity disorder, oppositional and aggressive behavior, and autistic spectrum disorders.
  4. Plaques and neurofibrillary tangles are seen in the brains of adults with Down syndrome, similar to individuals with Alzheimer's disease. The exact risk for individuals with Down syndrome to develop Alzheimer's disease is still unclear, but the prevalence is higher than in the general population.
- Hematologic issues
  1. Leukemia occurs at a higher rate than in the general population.

THERAPY

- There is no cure for Down syndrome and little prospects that it will be easily treated with gene therapy.

- Medical disorders should be treated as is standard for individuals without Down syndrome.
- Early intervention educational programs beginning in the newborn to 3-year-old population have been shown to improve motor and developmental functioning. Therapy and school programs often include physical, occupational, and speech therapy.
- Preschool programs and individualized educational plans for preschool and school-age children are helpful. Many children with Down syndrome can be integrated into regular education programs with modifications and support.
- Because of the chronic and incurable nature of Down syndrome, families are especially vulnerable to alternative therapies. Scientific studies have not shown benefit from vitamin, mineral, or hormonal injections or cell therapy. The primary care physician should carefully weigh the risks and benefits of all proposed therapeutic suggestions.
- Referral for Supplemental Security Income may be helpful.

■ FOLLOW-UP & DISPOSITION
- Medical guidelines have been published and regularly updated (most recently in 1999) for individuals with Down syndrome (available at www. denison.edu/dsq).
- Initial investigation into clinical symptoms and monitoring for such things as hearing loss, vision, thyroid function, atlantoaxial instability, and heart disease are an important part of anticipatory management in individuals with Down syndrome.

■ REFERRAL INFORMATION
- The primary care physician manages many children with Down syndrome with consultations to such individuals as cardiologists, ophthalmologists, audiologists, otolaryngologists, geneticists, and dentists. In some areas, a consultative clinic for individuals with Down syndrome is available.
- Behavior at times can warrant a referral to a behavioral specialist.
- Other referrals are made as individually necessary.

☼ PEARLS & CONSIDERATIONS

■ CLINICAL PEARLS
- Ensure that information presented is accurate and unbiased by own beliefs in developmental delays and mental retardation.
- It is often best to discuss sensitive issues with both parents present, particularly when discussing the initial diagnosis.
- Individuals with Down syndrome function the same as those without Down syndrome in many ways.

■ WEBSITES
- Growth Charts for Children with Down Syndrome: www. growthcharts.com
- Down Syndrome: Health Issues: www.ds-health.com
- Denison Down Syndrome Quarterly: www.denison.edu/dsq
- National Down Syndrome Society: www.ndss.org
- National Down Syndrome Congress: www.ndsccenter.org

REFERENCES
1. Batshaw ML: *Children with disabilities,* ed 4, Baltimore, 1997, Paul Brookes Publishing.
2. Cohen W: Health care guidelines for individuals with down syndrome, *Down Syndrome Quarterly* 4:1, 1999.
3. Jones KL: *Smith's recognizable patterns of human malformation,* ed 5, Philadelphia, 1997, WB Saunders.
4. Pueschel SM: *Biomedical concerns in persons with down syndrome,* Baltimore, 1992, Paul Brookes Publishing.

Author: **Nancy Lanphear, M.D.**

BASIC INFORMATION

■ DEFINITION
Dysfunctional uterine bleeding (DUB) is excessive, prolonged, and unpatterned endometrial bleeding unrelated to structural or systemic disease.

■ SYNONYMS
- Abnormal uterine bleeding
- Anovulatory bleeding

ICD-9CM CODE
626.8 Dysfunctional uterine bleeding

■ ETIOLOGY
- Anovulatory bleeding is caused by impairment of the hypothalamic-pituitary-ovarian axis.
- Failure of the negative feedback system (follicle-stimulating hormone [FSH] and estrogen) occurs during the follicular phase of the menstrual cycle.
- Failure of FSH levels to decline occurs as a result of continued secretion of estrogen.
  1. Ultimately results in failure of FSH to suppress estrogen
- Persistent estrogen secretion produces an excessively thickened, unstable endometrium with subsequent uncoordinated sloughing.

■ EPIDEMIOLOGY & DEMOGRAPHICS
- Up to 95% of cases of abnormal vaginal bleeding in adolescents are caused by DUB.
- Although many adolescents are anovulatory, most do not develop DUB.

■ HISTORY
- To obtain an accurate menstrual history and to rule out other causes of bleeding
- Detailed menstrual history (e.g., duration, frequency, regularity of menses, dysmenorrhea) and menstrual calendar (calendar with days of spotting and bleeding)
- Age at menarche
- Characteristics of first menses
- History of sexual activity, contraceptive use, and pregnancies (obtained without parental presence)
- Review of systems

■ PHYSICAL EXAMINATION
- Orthostatic pulse and blood pressure
- Signs of androgen excess (indicative of polycystic ovaries)
  1. Hirsutism
  2. Acne
  3. Clitoromegaly
- Pelvic examination with bimanual digital examination or rectoabdominal examination for non–sexually active adolescent
  1. Expect a normal examination in DUB.

2. Rule out foreign body, trauma, infection (including pelvic inflammatory disease), ovarian or uterine mass, and partial obstruction of the genital tract.

🔬 DIAGNOSIS

■ DIFFERENTIAL DIAGNOSIS
- Uterine causes
  1. Pregnancy-related complications
  2. Endometritis (*Chlamydia* and *Neisseria gonorrhoeae*)
  3. Endometrial polyps
  4. Fibroids
  5. Arteriovenous malformation
  6. Intrauterine device
  7. Uterine cancer (rare in adolescents)
- Vaginal causes
  1. Trauma
  2. Foreign body
  3. Vaginitis
  4. Vaginal neoplasm
- Medications
  1. Exogenous hormones
     a. Oral contraceptive agents (OCPs)
     b. Levonorgestrel implant (Norplant)
     c. Depomedroxyprogesterone acetate (Depo-Provera)
  2. Anticoagulants
  3. Platelet inhibitors
  4. Anticonvulsants
  5. Androgens
- Systemic diseases
  1. Endocrine: polycystic ovary syndrome, hypothyroidism, hyperthyroidism, hyperprolactinemia, adrenal disease, ovarian failure, diabetes
  2. Blood dyscrasias: thrombocytopenia, von Willebrand disease, and other clotting disorders
  3. Renal disease, liver disease
  4. Iron deficiency anemia
  5. Endometriosis

■ DIAGNOSTIC WORKUP
- Diagnosis of exclusion!
- Hemoglobin and hematocrit
- Urine or blood pregnancy test
- Remainder of workup: guided by history and physical examination to rule out other suspected causes (i.e., thyroid-stimulating hormone, factor VIII levels and activity, Ristocetin level, platelet count, cervical or vaginal cultures)

℞ THERAPY

■ NONPHARMACOLOGIC
Menstrual calendar (days of bleeding and spotting)

■ MEDICAL
- Guided by hemoglobin and hematocrit and presence of active bleeding
- Hemoglobin 12 mg/dl
  1. Menstrual calendar
  2. Iron supplementation
  3. Reassurance
  4. Reevaluation in 3 to 6 months
- Hemoglobin 10 to 12 mg/dl
  1. Menstrual calendar
  2. Iron supplementation
  3. Hormonal therapy
     a. Low-dose estrogen/progesterone OCP
     b. Intermittent oral progesterone if unable or unwilling to take OCPs
        (1) Medroxyprogesterone acetate 10 mg for 10 to 14 days every month for three to six cycles
        (2) Norethindrone acetate 5 to 10 mg daily for 10 to 14 days
  4. Reevaluation in 3 months with continued, regular follow-up
- Hemoglobin 10 mg/dl; patient asymptomatic with no active bleeding
  1. Menstrual calendar
  2. Iron supplementation
  3. Hormonal therapy
  4. Low-dose estrogen/progestin OCP
  5. Frequent follow-up until hemoglobin and hematocrit normalize, then every 3 to 6 months
- Hemoglobin 10 mg/dl; patient symptomatic (postural blood pressure changes, fatigue, syncope, fainting, dizziness, light-headed) or actively bleeding
  1. Consideration of admission to the hospital
  2. Iron supplementation
  3. Hormonal therapy
     a. High-dose OCP and antiemetic (Lo/Ovral with 30 g ethinyl estradiol, 1 pill four times per day for 4 days, 1 pill three times per day for 3 days, 1 pill two times per day for 2 weeks)
     b. Intravenous conjugated estrogen if unable to tolerate oral medication (25 mg intravenously every 4 hours for two to three doses until the bleeding stops), with the addition of oral progesterone to stabilize the endometrium
  4. Blood transfusions (rarely necessary)
  5. Maintenance therapy
     a. OCPs should be continued for 3 to 6 months.
     b. If the patient is unwilling or unable to take OCPs and iron stores are normal, therapy may be discontinued and the patient's menstrual calendar followed.

II

c. If the patient has a period of more than 6 weeks without menses, give oral medroxyprogesterone acetate (10 mg for 10 to 14 days) to induce withdrawal bleeding.
6. Frequent follow-up

■ SURGICAL
Dilation and curettage is necessary when hemostasis cannot be achieved medically.

■ FOLLOW-UP & DISPOSITION
• See "Therapy."
• Patients with a long history of anovulatory cycles and dysfunctional uterine bleeding have an increased risk of later infertility and endometrial carcinoma.

■ PATIENT/FAMILY EDUCATION
• Adolescents have more variation in menstrual cycle length, with normal duration of from 3 to 7 days and normal blood loss less than 80 ml (average of 30 to 40 ml).
• The interval between menarche and regular, ovulatory periods is associated with age at menarche:
1. Younger than 12 years at menarche: 50% of periods will be ovulatory by 1 year.
2. Between 12 and 13 years: 50% of periods ovulatory by 3 years.
3. Older than 13 years: 50% of periods ovulatory by 4.5 years.
• Most adolescents respond well to treatment, with half of patients having regular menstrual patterns within 4 years of menarche.

■ PREVENTIVE TREATMENT
Administer OCPs.

■ REFERRAL INFORMATION
Consider obstetrician/gynecologist referral for patients with a hemoglobin level of 10 mg/dl who are symptomatic or if uncomfortable with managing.

☼ PEARLS & CONSIDERATIONS

■ CLINICAL PEARLS
• DUB is a diagnosis of exclusion.
• The longer the period of anovulation for an adolescent, the higher the risk for DUB.

• Most adolescents respond well to treatment, with half of patients having regular menstrual patterns within 4 years of menarche.
• Patient estimations of menstrual blood flow tend to be inaccurate.

■ WEBSITE
Women's Health Interactive: www.womens-health.com

REFERENCES
1. Abnormal vaginal bleeding. In Emans SJH et al (eds): *Pediatric and adolescent gynecology*, ed 4, Philadelphia, 1998, Lippincott Williams & Wilkins.
2. Bravender T, Emans SJ: Menstrual disorders, *Pediatr Clin North Am* 46:545, 1999.
3. Cameron IT: Dysfunctional uterine bleeding, *ACOG Tech Bull* 134, 1989.
4. Dealy MF: Dysfunctional uterine bleeding in adolescents, *Nurse Pract* 23:12, 1998.
Author: **Heather Chapman, M.D.**

BASIC INFORMATION

■ DEFINITION
- Primary dysmenorrhea is pain with menses in the absence of a secondary cause.
- Secondary dysmenorrhea is pain with menses that is secondary to other pelvic disease.

■ SYNONYM
Menstrual cramps

■ ICD-9CM CODE
625.3 Dysmenorrhea

■ ETIOLOGY
- The exact cause is unclear.
- There is an association of increased prostaglandin F_2 (PGF_2) and E_2 (PGE_2) levels with symptoms of dysmenorrhea.
- Under the influence of progesterone, PGE_2 and PGF_2 are produced and act locally in the menstrual fluid to cause increased myometrial tone and contractions, vasoconstriction, and then ischemia of the uterine lining.
- PGE_2 also causes hypersensitivity of pain nerve terminals in the myometrium.
- Drugs that inhibit the conversion of arachidonic acid to prostaglandins via the enzyme cyclooxygenase prevent the production of prostaglandins.

■ EPIDEMIOLOGY & DEMOGRAPHICS
- The prevalence of primary dysmenorrhea is estimated to be 50% to 80% of the general population of menstruating females.
- Onset of symptoms occurs within 6 months to 2 years of menarche.
- Prevalence is higher with increasing Tanner stage and increasing age, until 20 years.
- Secondary dysmenorrhea usually occurs later in the reproductive years of women because it is associated with the development of other pathologic conditions.

■ HISTORY
- The most common symptom is crampy lower abdominal pain that may radiate to the back and/or thighs and that ensues with the onset of menses.
- Other symptoms include dizziness, nausea, vomiting, diarrhea, and headache.
- Obtaining a careful menstrual history is important to characterize symptoms.
  1. Onset and frequency of menses
  2. Length and quality of flow
  3. Timing of symptoms as they relate to cycle
  4. Quantify degree of impairment of daily activities

■ PHYSICAL EXAMINATION
- The physical examination is tailored to identify causes of secondary dysmenorrhea.
  1. In absence of physical findings, a diagnosis of primary dysmenorrhea may be made with a consistent history.
- For sexually active adolescents and adolescents 18 years or older, a pelvic examination with speculum is indicated.
- Evaluate for sexually transmitted diseases (*Chlamydia,* gonorrhea, pelvic inflammatory disease [PID]).
- Assess the anatomy of the external and internal genitalia.
- Bimanual examination is indicated to evaluate for the following:
  1. Uterine anomalies
  2. Size and quality of adnexa
  3. Specific areas of tenderness
- In the adolescent who is younger than 18 years and not sexually active, the history is sufficient to try therapy.
- If the patient is unresponsive to therapy, an external genital examination with rectoabdominal bimanual examination are performed.
  1. Palpate the uterus and adnexa to evaluate for tenderness, masses, and congenital anomalies.

DIAGNOSIS

■ DIFFERENTIAL DIAGNOSIS
- Sexually transmitted diseases (*Chlamydia,* gonorrhea, PID)
- Endometriosis
- Genital tract cysts and neoplasms
- Pelvic adhesions
- Obstructing malformations of the uterus or vagina
- Complications of pregnancy
- Intrauterine device

■ DIAGNOSTIC WORKUP
- Laboratory tests
  1. Erythrocyte sedimentation rate should be obtained to evaluate for malignancy or PID.
  2. Cervical cultures should be taken.
- Imaging
  1. Endovaginal or transabdominal ultrasonography is indicated if the history is atypical for primary dysmenorrhea, and further evaluation of anatomic structures is indicated.
  2. Magnetic resonance imaging may also be useful for the same purpose.

THERAPY

■ NONPHARMACOLOGIC
- Education and reassurance
- Well-balanced diet

■ MEDICAL
- Nonsteroidal antiinflammatory drugs (NSAIDs): propionic acids and phenates
  1. Ibuprofen 400 mg orally three to four times per day
  2. Naproxen 500 mg orally then 250 mg orally every 12 hours
  3. Naproxen sodium 550 mg orally then 275 mg orally every 12 hours
  4. Mefenamic acid 500 mg orally then 250 mg orally every 4 to 6 hours
- Oral contraceptives if NSAID regimen is insufficient to control symptoms
- Depomedroxyprogesterone acetate or implantable levonorgestrel if OCPs unrealistic
- Calcium channel blockers; have been tried with some success

■ SURGICAL
Laparoscopy or laparotomy is indicated either when pain persists despite all other interventions or when the history suggests that further evaluation of pelvic anatomy is indicated in addition to physical examination and ultrasonography.

■ FOLLOW-UP & DISPOSITION
- Primary dysmenorrhea: Follow-up should occur after another menstrual cycle has passed to see how effective intervention has been.
- Secondary dysmenorrhea: Follow-up is indicated by the nature of the primary diagnosis.

■ PATIENT/FAMILY EDUCATION
- Medication should be started immediately upon initiation of pain, before it becomes severe.
- NSAIDs are often associated with decreased menstrual flow.
- The benefits of oral contraceptives may not be noticed for two to three cycles.

■ PREVENTIVE TREATMENT OR TESTS
Omega-3-fatty acids, which are found in "fish oil" supplement containing 1080 mg eicosapentaenoic acid, 720 mg docosapentaenoic acid, and 1.5 mg of vitamin E, should be administered in two divided doses per day. Taken daily, this supplement significantly diminishes symptoms as compared with a placebo.

II

■ **REFERRAL INFORMATION**

For patients who are unresponsive to standard approaches, referral to a gynecologist who is familiar with the comprehensive evaluation and treatment for pelvic pain is indicated.

☼ PEARLS & CONSIDERATIONS

■ **CLINICAL PEARLS**

A monthly pain calendar may be useful to identify the cyclic and recurrent nature of pain.

■ **WEBSITES**

- Support-Group.com: www.support-group.com
- The Virtual Lecture Hall: www.vlh.com/courses/06/index.htm

REFERENCES

1. Dysmenorrhea and premenstrual syndrome. In Neinstein LS (ed): *Adolescent health care,* Baltimore, 1996, Williams & Wilkins.
2. Harel Z et al: Supplementation with omega-3 polyunsaturated fatty acids in the management of dysmenorrhea in adolescents, *Am J Obstet Gynecol* 174:1335, 1996.
3. Laugher M, Goldstein D: Dysmenorrhea, pelvic pain, premenstrual syndrome. In Emans SJH, Laugher M, Goldstein D (eds): *Pediatric and adolescent gynecology,* Philadelphia, 1998, Lippincott Raven.
4. Stenchever M: Primary and secondary dysmenorrhea and premenstrual syndrome: etiology, diagnosis, management. In Mishell DR (ed): *Comprehensive gynecology,* St Louis, 1997, Mosby.

Author: **Susan Birndorf, D.O.**

BASIC INFORMATION

■ DEFINITION

An ectopic pregnancy is a fertilized ovum implanted anywhere other than the endometrial lining of the uterine cavity, generally in the fallopian tubes.

■ SYNONYM

Tubal pregnancy

■ ICD-9CM CODE

633.9 Ectopic pregnancy

■ ETIOLOGY

- Tubal damage secondary to inflammation
- Contraceptive devices: intrauterine device (IUD), progesterone therapies
- Prior tubal surgeries or abdominal surgeries, including tubal ligation
- Advanced reproductive technologies (interfere with embryo migration)
- Developmental abnormalities: diethylstilbestrol (DES) exposure

■ EPIDEMIOLOGY & DEMOGRAPHICS

- Incidence: 20 per 1000 pregnancies
  1. Fatality rate is decreasing.
- Sites of ectopic pregnancies
  1. Tubal: 95% to 97%
  2. Cornual, interstitial: 2% to 4%
  3. Ovarian: 0.5%
  4. Cervical: 0.1%
  5. Abdominal: 0.03%
- Chance of recurring ectopic pregnancies: 15% to 25%
- Other risk factors for ectopic pregnancy
  1. History of chlamydia or gonorrhea genital infections or pelvic inflammatory disease (PID)
  2. Tubal surgery
  3. Abdominal surgery
  4. Tubal ligation
     a. Increased risk of ectopic pregnancy during the first 2 years after sterilization
  5. IUD
  6. Infertility treatment: 1.1% to 4.6% risk of ectopic pregnancy
  7. Cigarette smoking: increases risk almost twofold
  8. DES exposure: more than twofold risk
  9. Increasing maternal age

■ HISTORY

- Lower abdominal pain, usually on side of ectopic, in 90% of patients
- Absent or irregular bleeding
  1. Vaginal bleeding is noted in 80% of patients.
  2. Most patients present 6 to 10 weeks after their last menstrual period (LMP)
- Shoulder pain
- Dizziness or syncope
- Urge to defecate
- Breast tenderness
- Nausea

■ PHYSICAL EXAMINATION

- Tachycardia
- Hypotension
- Pelvic mass
- Abdominal or pelvic tenderness
- Ovarian tenderness or mass
- Uterine enlargement (6 to 8 week sized)

🔬 DIAGNOSIS

■ DIFFERENTIAL DIAGNOSIS

- Normal uterine pregnancy
- Abortion
- Ruptured ovarian cyst
- Appendicitis
- Ovarian torsion
- PID
- Gastroenteritis
- Degenerating uterine leiomyoma
- Endometriosis
- Dysfunctional uterine bleeding

■ DIAGNOSTIC WORKUP

- The diagnosis is complicated by the wide spectrum of patient presentations ranging from vaginal spotting to shock.
- Major advances in early detection include β-human chorionic gonadotropin (β-hCG) assays, ultrasound, and laparoscopy.
- Culdocentesis and curettage can also be useful.
- β-hCG determination:
  1. An abnormal pregnancy is indicated by β-hCG not doubling in 48 hours.
     a. A 66% rise in the β-hCG level over 48 hours represents the lower limit of normal for a viable intrauterine pregnancy (IUP).
     b. Fifteen percent of viable IUPs will have less than a 66% rise in 48 hours.
     c. Fifteen percent of ectopic pregnancies will have more than a 66% rise in β-hCG.
  2. The β-hCG is best used early in pregnancy.
     a. It is less reliable after 6 to 7 weeks' gestation.
     b. β-hCG alone does not help distinguish between an ectopic and an abnormal intrauterine pregnancy.
- Ultrasound detects IUP within 5 to 6 weeks of the LMP.
  1. An IUP can be visualized at a β-hCG level above 6500 mIU/ml by transabdominal ultrasound and a level above 1000 to 2000 mIU/ml by a transvaginal ultrasound.
- Culdocentesis confirms the presence of intraabdominal bleeding.
  1. Diagnosis cannot necessarily be determined by culdocentesis.
     a. If nonclotting blood is obtained, the results are positive for intraabdominal bleeding.
        (1) Blood may be present for other reasons, such as ruptured cysts.
        (2) Of patients with suspected ectopic pregnancy, 85% have positive culdocentesis.
     b. If no fluid is obtained, the test is nondiagnostic.
     c. If clotting blood is obtained, the vascular plexus has been aspirated and the test is nondiagnostic.
     d. If ectopic did not rupture, results of culdocentesis may also be nondiagnostic.
- Dilation of the cervical os and curettage of the endometrial lining (D&C) can be a useful tool.
  1. D&C establishes the diagnosis of ectopic pregnancy if chorionic villi are not found in the uterine cavity.
     a. If decidua without chorionic villi are found, this may indicate an ectopic pregnancy.
     b. A completed spontaneous miscarriage may also have decidua only.
- Progesterone level is another diagnostic tool.
  1. The progesterone level cannot necessarily distinguish an IUP from a spontaneous abortion (SAB) or an ectopic pregnancy.
  2. Progesterone level is an adjunct to β-hCG and ultrasound.
     a. A level less than 5 ng/ml indicates a nonviable pregnancy despite the location.
     b. A level greater than 25 ng/ml indicates a normal pregnancy.
     c. A level between 10 and 20 ng/ml is not diagnostic.
        (1) About 50% have an ectopic pregnancy.

💊 THERAPY

■ NONPHARMACOLOGIC

- Less than 25% of ectopic pregnancies resolve without treatment.
- Expectant management is restricted to the following:
  1. Falling β-hCG titers
  2. Ectopic in the fallopian tube, not in the cervix, abdomen, or ovary
  3. No bleeding
  4. No evidence of rupture

II

■ MEDICAL
- Methotrexate, a folic acid antagonist, is used.
  1. Success rates: 67% to 100%
- Methotrexate is used for small, un-ruptured ectopics.
  1. It inhibits dihydrofolic acid reductase and interrupts DNA synthesis.
  2. Complete blood count and platelets, liver function test, creatinine, and β-hCG are drawn on day 0 as a baseline.
  3. Intramuscular methotrexate 50 mg/M^2 is given.
  4. Rhogam is given to Rh-negative women.
  5. β-hCG is repeated on days 4 and 7.
     a. If there is less than a 15% decrease from day 4 to 7, a second dose of methotrexate (50 mg/M^2) is given.
     b. If there is greater than a 15% decrease, continue monitoring of β-hCG every 3 to 4 days.
  6. Approximately 50% of patients have abdominal pain with treatment.
- Evaluate for ruptured ectopic if the patient has abdominal pain.
- Patients are eligible for medical treatment if the following criteria are met:
  1. They are hemodynamically stable
  2. They agree to close outpatient follow-up
  3. They have a small unruptured ectopic
     a. Presence of fetal heart is not a definitive exclusion criteria.
  4. They have a β-hCG that is not decreasing 12 to 24 hours after curettage (if preformed)
  5. There is no evidence of liver or renal disease (transaminases [AST] less than twice normal and creatinine less than 1.5 mg/dl)
  6. There are no other contraindications to methotrexate
     a. Breastfeeding
     b. Liver disease
     c. Overt immunodeficiency
     d. Significant anemia
     e. Peptic ulcer disease

■ SURGICAL
- For tubal ectopic pregnancy
  1. Laparoscopic salpingostomy or salpingectomy is done; minimal surgery is done for resection of pregnancy.
  2. Laparotomy may be necessary.
- For ovarian ectopics
  1. A wedge resection of ovary is indicated.
- For cervical ectopic pregnancy (management is controversial)
  1. D&C is contraindicated.
  2. Methotrexate can be given both systemically or locally.
  3. Uterine artery embolization is often successful and useful for management of hemorrhage.
  4. Hospitalization is often necessary to monitor blood loss.

■ FOLLOW-UP & DISPOSITION
- Patients with a tubal ectopic pregnancy have a 15% to 25% chance of a subsequent ectopic pregnancy.
- Outpatient evaluation of the fallopian tubes by hysterosalpingogram can be helpful after the resolution of the ectopic pregnancy

■ PATIENT/FAMILY EDUCATION
- When waiting for the 48 hours between β-hCG levels to determine the status of the pregnancy, the patient should be given information regarding possible ectopic rupture as well as spontaneous abortion precautions. Reasons to seek urgent medical care include the following:
  1. Increasing abdominal pain
  2. Dizziness or light-headedness
  3. Shoulder pain
  4. Increasing vaginal bleeding
- After methotrexate is given, the patient should stop prenatal vitamins, decrease foods high in folic acid, and abstain from alcohol.

■ PREVENTIVE TREATMENT
- Avoid conditions that scar the fallopian tube.
- Risk factors for sexually transmitted diseases include the following:
  1. Multiple partners
  2. Intercourse without a condom
- Provide early treatment for sexually transmitted diseases.

■ REFERRAL INFORMATION
All patients with suspected ectopic pregnancy should be referred to an obstetrician/gynecologist emergently.

☼ PEARLS & CONSIDERATIONS

■ CLINICAL PEARLS
- In general, complete abortion will have a rapidly falling β-hCG level.
  1. About 50% over 48 hours
  2. β-hCG levels during an ectopic pregnancy rise or plateau
- The majority of ectopic pregnancies have β-hCG levels of less than 6500 mIU/ml.
- In IUPs:
  1. β-hCG is approximately 100 mIU/ml at the time of the missed menses.
  2. β-hCG is 100,000 mIU/ml at 10 weeks (highest).

■ WEBSITES
- Advanced Fertility Center of Chicago: www.advancedfertility.com
- Ectopic Pregnancy Trust: www.ectopic.org.uk
- Estronaut: A Forum for Women's Health: www.estronaut.com

■ SUPPORT GROUP
ParentsPlace.com: www.parentsplace.com/messageboards

REFERENCES
1. ACOG practice bulletin: Medical management of tubal pregnancy. No 3, December 1998, *Int J Gynaecol Obstet* 65:97, 1999.
2. Carson SA, Buster JE: Ectopic pregnancy, *N Engl J Med* 329:1174, 1993.
3. Kadar N, Devore G, Romero R: Discriminatory zone: its use in the sonographic evaluation for ectopic pregnancy, *Obstet Gynecol* 58:156, 1981.
4. Rock J, Damario M: Ectopic pregnancy. In Te Linde RW, Thompson JD (eds): *Te Linde's operative gynecology,* ed 8, Philadelphia, 1997, Lippincott Williams & Wilkins.
5. Stovall TG, Ling FW: Ectopic pregnancy: diagnostic and therapeutic algorithms minimizing surgical intervention, *J Reprod Med* 38:807, 1993.
6. Stovall T, McMord M: Early pregnancy loss and ectopic pregnancy. In Berek JS, Adashi EY (eds): *Novak's gynecology,* ed 12, Philadelphia, 1988, Lippincott Williams & Wilkins.

Author: **Elizabeth K. Cherot, M.D.**

BASIC INFORMATION

■ DEFINITION

Acute viral encephalitis is inflammation of parenchymal brain tissue caused by a virus. It occurs over a relatively short period (days). Viral encephalitis is classified as either primary or postinfectious:

- *Primary viral encephalitis:* resultant of direct viral entry into the parenchymal brain tissue, which produces cortical dysfunction (e.g., rabies, arbovirus, herpes simplex virus [HSV], enterovirus)
- *Postinfectious viral encephalitis:* signs and symptoms of encephalitis; temporally associated with a systemic viral infection; without direct viral invasion of the central nervous system (CNS); likely an immune-mediated demyelination (e.g., associated with measles, with varicella, and after upper respiratory tract infections, particularly influenza)

ICD-9CM CODES
045.0 Polioencephalitis
049.0 Lymphocytic choriomeningitis
049.9 Unspecified nonarthropodborne viral diseases of CNS
052.0 Postvaricella encephalitis
054.3 Herpes simplex encephalitis
055.0 Postmeasles encephalitis
062.2 Eastern equine encephalitis
062.9 Mosquitoborne viral encephalitis, unspecified
063.9 Tickborne viral encephalitis, unspecified

■ ETIOLOGY
See box to the right.

■ EPIDEMIOLOGY & DEMOGRAPHICS
- Routes of CNS viral entry
  1. Hematogenous: most common
     a. Arthropodborne viral disease
  2. Neuronal
     a. HSV
     b. Varicella-zoster virus (VZV)
     c. Rabies
- Antecedent systemic illness: often a 2- to 12-day lag between primary viral infection and postinfectious encephalitis
- Arboviruses: an important worldwide cause of encephalitis
- Human immunodeficiency virus (HIV): likely to become the most common cause of CNS viral infection worldwide
- Japanese encephalitis: most common epidemic infection of the CNS outside the United States
- Enteroviruses: a leading viral cause of neurologic disease in children in the United States; most commonly causes aseptic

DIRECT INFECTION	POSTINFECTION
Togaviridae	Togaviridae
Alphaviruses	Rubivirus
Eastern equine	Rubella
Western equine	Orthomyxoviridae
Venezuelan equine	Influenza
Flaviviridae	Paramyxoviridae
St. Louis	Paramyxovirus
Murray Valley	Mumps
West Nile	Morbillivirus
Japanese	Measles
Dengue	Poxviridae
Tickborne complex	Orthopoxvirus
Bunyaviridae	Vaccinia
La Crosse	Herpesviridae
Rift Valley	Herpesvirus
Toscana	Varicella-zoster virus
Paramyxoviridae	Epstein-Barr virus
Paramyxovirus	
Mumps	
Morbillivirus	
Measles	
Hendra	
Nipah	
Arenaviridae	
Arenavirus	
Lymphocytic choriomeningitis	
Machupo	
Lassa	
Junin	
Picornaviridae	
Enterovirus	
Poliovirus	
Coxsackievirus	
Echovirus	
Hepatitis A	
Reoviridae	
Colorado tick fever	
Rhabdoviridae	
Lyssavirus	
Rabies	
Filoviridae	
Ebola	
Marburg	
Retroviridae	
Human immunodeficiency virus	
Herpesviridae	
Herpesvirus	
HSV-1 and HSV-2	
Varicella-zoster virus	
Herpes B virus	
Epstein-Barr virus	
Cytomegalovirus	
Human herpes virus type 6	
Adenoviridae	
Adenovirus	

HSV, Herpes simplex virus.

meningitis and less commonly causes encephalitis
- Mumps: in areas lacking vaccine, a leading cause of meningoencephalitis

- HSV: most common cause of nonepidemic, sporadic, acute encephalitis in the United States
  1. HSV-2: the leading cause of severe and often fatal encephalitis in neonates

2. HSV-1: most common HSV cause of encephalitis in older children and adults
- Congenital viral infection: associated encephalitis with rubella and cytomegalovirus (CMV)
- Rabies: uncommon in the United States, but a significant worldwide problem
- Reye's syndrome: often follows VZV or influenza infections; epidemiologically related to salicylate use during infection
- Seasonal
  1. Summer: mosquitoborne (arboviruses; West Nile virus)
  2. Spring and summer: tickborne
  3. Late summer and fall: enteroviruses
  4. Winter: lymphocytic choriomeningitis
- Geographic
  1. Arthropodborne encephalitides—highly regional (Eastern equine encephalitis)
     a. Great Lakes and Atlantic and Gulf coast regions
  2. Western equine encephalitis: western states
  3. Japanese encephalitis: Southeast Asia, China, and India
  4. Tickborne encephalitis
     a. Northern Asia and eastern Europe
  5. West Nile virus encephalitis
     a. Northeastern United States
- Age predilections
  1. Neonates are at risk for severe enterovirus and HSV-2 encephalitis.
  2. St. Louis and Western equine encephalitides affect the extremes of age (very young and old).
  3. La Crosse, Eastern, and California encephalitides are clinically present most commonly in children.

■ HISTORY
- Initial site of viral exposure/replication
  1. Respiratory
     a. VZV
     b. Measles
     c. Mumps
  2. Gastrointestinal
     a. Enterovirus
     b. Echovirus
  3. Genital/oropharyngeal
     a. HSV
  4. Subcutaneous
     a. Arthropod-associated diseases
- Recent vaccinations
  1. Rare association with postinfectious encephalitis
     a. Polio
- Medications
  1. Allergic reactions
  2. Drug reactions (e.g., neuroleptic malignant syndrome)

3. Chemotherapy-induced leukoencephalopathy
4. Toxins (pesticides or heavy metals)
- Immune compromise
  1. May be associated with unusual or chronic forms of the common causes of encephalitis
     a. Enterovirus
     b. HSV
     c. Adenovirus
- Exposures
  1. To ill contacts in past 2 to 3 weeks
  2. Animal (herpes B—monkey, Nipah virus—swine, Hendra virus—horse, rabies)
  3. Travel
     a. Prevalent diseases within the community

■ PHYSICAL EXAMINATION
- Fever
  1. The hallmark of viral encephalitis is the acute onset of a febrile illness.
- Altered level of consciousness
  1. Wide variation, from personality change to confusion to coma
  2. Infants: may have screaming spells and abdominal distress
  3. Variably present: meningismus
- Seizures (focal or generalized)
- Neurologic deficit
  1. Cranial nerve deficits
  2. Movement disorders
  3. Ataxia
  4. Increased deep tendon reflexes
  5. Extensor plantar responses
  6. Hemiparesis
- Evaluate
  1. Nasopharyngitis; may signify associated respiratory infection
  2. Enanthem
     a. Enteroviral changes
  3. Exanthem
     a. VZV
     b. HSV
     c. Enterovirus

🔬 DIAGNOSIS

■ DIFFERENTIAL DIAGNOSIS
- Disease processes presenting similarly to encephalitis:
  1. Metabolic diseases: hypoglycemia, uremia, hepatic failure
  2. Toxic disorders: drug ingestion, Reye's syndrome
  3. Mass lesions: tumor and abscess
  4. Intracerebral or subarachnoid hemorrhage
  5. Demyelinating disorders: multiple sclerosis
  6. Seizure conditions: postictal, nonconvulsive seizure
  7. Infectious and postinfectious diseases

■ DIAGNOSTIC WORKUP
- Computed tomography (CT) scan to rule out mass lesions (tumor, abscess) and hemorrhage
- Magnetic resonance imaging to detect subtle, edematous change of early encephalitis
  1. Sensitive indicator of demyelination
  2. Better visualization of the spinal cord
- Single-photon emission CT to localize area of greatest involvement
- Cerebrospinal fluid (CSF) examination: essential (first exclude increased intracranial pressure)
  1. White blood cell (WBC) count: variable pleocytosis; mononuclear cells predominate
  2. Usually 10 to 2000 WBC/mm^3
  3. Red blood cell count (RBC): may see small number of RBCs present (e.g., HSV)
  4. Protein: moderate or no elevation
  5. Glucose: usually in the normal to mildly decreased range
- CSF
  1. Stains (e.g., Gram stain, AFB stain, India ink)
  2. Antigen detection (e.g., cryptococcal, histoplasma)
  3. PCR-HSV, CMV, human herpesvirus type 6 (HHV-6), enteroviruses
  4. Rabies: brain biopsy or corneal smear
  5. Culture: bacteria, fungi, mycobacteria, amoeba, and viruses
  6. Cytology: exclude acutely presenting neural neoplasms
- Viral culture (CSF viral culture is very low yield)
  1. Consider viral culture of blood, feces, or nasopharynx.
- Electroencephalogram, especially in temporal lobe localization of HSV
- Antibodies
  1. Serum and CSF antibodies may be useful retrospectively.
  2. Japanese encephalitis is diagnosed by enzyme-linked immunosorbent assay to IgM antibody
  3. HIV
  4. EBV-VCA (viral capsid antigen), IgG, and IgM

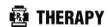 THERAPY

■ MEDICAL
- HSV
  1. Neonates: acyclovir or vidarabine
     a. Similar efficacy
     b. Acyclovir preferred: decreased toxicity, ease of administration
  2. Young children and adults
     a. Acyclovir
- VZV
  1. Acyclovir

- Herpes B virus
  1. Acyclovir
  2. Ganciclovir
- CMV
  1. Ganciclovir
  2. Foscarnet
  3. Cidofovir
- HIV encephalitis
  1. Antiretroviral treatment
- Lassa fever virus
  1. Ribavirin

PEARLS & CONSIDERATIONS

■ CLINICAL PEARLS

- Many infectious and noninfectious illnesses present similarly, with fever and altered mental status. If the clinical scenario warrants, it is often advisable to repeat the lumbar puncture in 24 to 72 hours to define the pattern of CSF change with evolution of the illness.
- Antigen-based diagnostic testing means, such as CSF PCR, will aid in the definitive diagnosis of CNS viral infections.

REFERENCES

1. Griffin DE: Encephalitis, myelitis, and neuritis. In Mandell GL, Bennett JE, Dolin R (eds): *Principles and practice of infectious diseases,* ed 5, Philadelphia, 2000, Churchill Livingstone.
2. Johnson RT: Acute encephalitis, *Clin Infect Dis* 23:219, 1996.
3. Whitley RJ, Kimberlin DW: Viral encephalitis, *Pediatr Rev* 20:192, 1999.

Author: **H. Reid Mattison, M.D.**

BASIC INFORMATION

■ DEFINITION
Infective endocarditis (IE) is an intravascular infection of the endocardium, including valvular structures, or an infection of the endothelium of large blood vessels (endarteritis).

■ SYNONYMS
- Bacterial endocarditis
- Subacute bacterial endocarditis
- Acute bacterial endocarditis

ICD-9CM CODE
421.0 Infective endocarditis

■ ETIOLOGY
- Endocardial or endothelial injury is caused by the following:
  1. A jet lesion from a ventricular septal defect, valvular insufficiency, systemic-to-pulmonary artery shunt, valvular or vascular stenosis
  2. An intravascular catheter
- Both lead to platelet and fibrin deposition to form a nonbacterial thrombotic vegetation (NBTV).
- Circulating microorganisms then adhere to the NBTV, initiating IE and propagation of the vegetation, followed by local invasive damage and distal embolic events.

■ EPIDEMIOLOGY & DEMOGRAPHICS
- *Staphylococcus aureus* and *Streptococcus* species are the most common pathogens.
- Other infective organisms include *Staphylococcus epidermidis*, enterococci, *Candida*, HACEK bacteria (*Haemophilus parainfluenzae* and *aphrophilus, Actinobacillus, Cardiobacterium, Eikenella,* and *Kingella), Coxiella,* and *Brucellae.*
- Culture-negative endocarditis occurs in 5% to 10% of patients, related to prior antibiotic therapy as well as fastidious and slow-growing organisms.
- Pediatric hospital admissions for IE have declined recently.
- Substrates:
  1. Most common
     a. Prosthetic cardiac valves and conduits
     b. Repaired or palliated complex cyanotic congenital cardiac malformations
     c. Systemic-to-pulmonary artery shunts
  2. Less common
     a. Unrepaired congenital malformations
     b. Mitral valve prolapse
     c. Rarely rheumatic heart disease
- In infancy and in immunocompromised patients, venous catheters are a common predisposing factor.
- Minimal to no risk is present in patients with an atrial septal defect or mild pulmonary valve stenosis.

■ HISTORY
- Underlying congenital or acquired cardiovascular lesion or surgery with a predisposition to the formation of NBTVs
- Central venous catheter
- Recent procedure or infection associated with bacteremia
- Fever
- Malaise, weakness, fatigue, poor appetite, weight loss, arthralgias
- Insidious or rapidly progressive onset

■ PHYSICAL EXAMINATION
- Fever: 95% or more
- Splenomegaly: 50%
- Congestive heart failure: 30% to 40%
- Petechiae: 10% to 25%
- Splinter hemorrhages: 10%
- Osler's nodes, Janeway lesions: less than 5%
- Roth spots: very rare
- Major systemic emboli: 15% to 25%
- New or changed murmur: incidence difficult to define
  1. New aortic or mitral insufficiency is significant.
  2. Louder preexisting murmur is not sufficient.

🔬 DIAGNOSIS

■ DIFFERENTIAL DIAGNOSIS
- Acute rheumatic fever
- Rheumatoid diseases
- Collagen vascular disease
- Kawasaki disease
- Sepsis or other infections
- Cardiac myxoma

■ DIAGNOSTIC WORKUP
- Blood cultures, three or more (prior antibiotic therapy reduces the recovery rate of bacteria by 35% to 40%)
- Transthoracic echocardiography (TTE) (sensitivity, 80%)
- Transesophageal echocardiography (TEE) if TTE is negative and endocarditis is strongly considered
- Electrocardiogram
- Chest radiograph
- Complete blood count, sedimentation rate, circulating immune complexes
- Urinalysis
- Duke clinical criteria
  1. Definite IE
     a. Pathologic criteria
        (1) Microorganisms: demonstrated by culture or histology in a vegetation or in a vegetation that has embolized, or in an intracardiac abscess, *or*
        (2) Pathologic lesions: vegetations or intracardiac abscess present, confirmed by histology showing active endocarditis
     b. Clinical criteria using the following definitions:
        (1) Two major criteria, *or*
        (2) One major criterion and three minor criteria, *or*
        (3) Five minor criteria
  2. Possible IE
     a. Findings consistent with IE that fall short of "Definite" but not "Rejected"
  3. Rejected
     a. Firm alternative diagnosis for manifestations of endocarditis, *or*
     b. Resolution of manifestations of endocarditis with antibiotic therapy for 4 days or less, *or*
     c. No pathologic evidence of IE at surgery or autopsy, after antibiotic therapy for 4 days or less
- Definition of terms used in the Duke criteria
  1. Major criteria
     a. Positive blood culture for IE; typical microorganisms consistent with IE from separate blood cultures
        (1) *Viridans streptococci,** *Streptococcus bovis,* or HACEK group, or community-acquired *S. aureus* or enterococci, in the absence of a primary focus, *or*
        (2) Microorganisms consistent with IE from "persistently positive blood cultures," defined as two or more positive cultures of blood samples drawn more than 12 hours apart, *or*
        (3) All three or a majority of four or more separate cultures of blood with first and last sample drawn 1 hour or more apart
     b. Evidence of endocardial involvement
        (1) Positive echocardiogram for IE defined as oscillating intracardiac mass, on valve or supporting structures, or in the path of regurgitant jets, or on implanted material in the absence of an alternative anatomic explanation
        (2) Abscess
        (3) New partial dehiscence of prosthetic valve
        (4) New valvular regurgitation (worsening or changing of preexisting murmur not sufficient)

---

*Includes nutritionally variant strains (*Abiotrophic* species).

2. Minor criteria
   a. Predisposing heart condition or intravenous drug use
   b. Temperature 38.0° C or higher
   c. Vascular phenomena: major arterial emboli, septic pulmonary infarcts, mycotic aneurysm, intracranial hemorrhage, conjunctival hemorrhages, and Janeway lesions
   d. Immunologic phenomena: glomerulonephritis, Osler's nodes, Roth spots, and rheumatoid factor
   e. Microbiologic evidence: positive blood culture, but does not meet a major criterion as noted previously* or serologic evidence of active infection with organism consistent with IE
   f. Echocardiographic findings: consistent with IE but do not meet a major criterion as noted previously

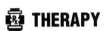

THERAPY

■ NONPHARMACOLOGIC
Nonpharmacologic therapy is inappropriate for IE.

■ MEDICAL
- Prolonged parenteral therapy with bactericidal antibiotics is necessary for complete eradication of the infecting organism.
- Antibiotic sensitivity data are essential for guiding therapy.
- Antibiotic combinations may be synergistic, allowing smaller doses of each drug to be used, thereby reducing toxicity.
- Repeat blood cultures are done after therapy is initiated to document vascular cleansing.
- For acutely ill patients, in whom waiting for culture data before initiating therapy may be very hazardous, an appropriate starting regimen would be a penicillinase-resistant penicillin and an aminoglycoside.
- Early consultation with the pediatric infectious disease service is recommended to determine and guide antibiotic therapy.

■ SURGICAL
Indications for surgery include the following:
- Congestive heart failure unresponsive to medical therapy

---

*Excludes single positive cultures for coagulase-negative staphylococci and organisms that do not cause endocarditis.

- Valvular obstruction
- Prosthetic valve dehiscence
- Uncontrollable infection or relapse
- Fungal endocarditis
- Emboli
- Local invasion
  1. Purulent pericarditis
  2. Papillary muscle/chordal rupture
  3. Sinus of valsalva rupture
  4. Ventricular septal rupture
  5. Heart block

■ FOLLOW-UP & DISPOSITION
- Although home therapy has been proposed for IE, this approach should be reserved for uncomplicated infections with common and sensitive organisms and only after observation in the hospital because of the risk of serious complications, which include the following:
  1. Congestive heart failure, usually related to valvular destruction
  2. Localized suppuration leading to abscess formation
  3. A ventricular septal defect or creation of a fistula
  4. Emboli
  5. Mycotic aneurysms
  6. Conduction and rhythm abnormalities
  7. Purulent pericarditis and/or myocarditis

■ PATIENT/FAMILY EDUCATION
Parents should contact their pediatric practitioner and cardiologist in the presence of persistent fever, even if low grade, and constitutional symptoms.

■ PREVENTIVE TREATMENT
- Prophylaxis
  1. Prophylaxis is indicated for dental, respiratory, gastrointestinal, and genitourinary procedures associated with important bacteremias to kill circulating or adhered bacteria (see Part III, "Endocarditis Prophylaxis").
  2. Only 5% to 20% of IE can be related to prior procedures.
  3. Prophylaxis is generally administered 30 to 60 minutes before a procedure but may be effective up to 2 hours after a procedure.
  4. The regimen for dental or respiratory procedures consists of amoxicillin or clindamycin/azithromycin for penicillin-allergic patients.
  5. Ampicillin plus gentamicin is used for gastrointestinal or genitourinary procedures in high-risk patients (vancomycin plus genta-

mycin in penicillin-allergic individuals). Moderate-risk patients are given amoxicillin or ampicillin (vancomycin, alternatively).
- Lesions not requiring prophylaxis
  1. Native secundum atrial defects
  2. More than 6 months after repair of atrial and ventricular defects and ductus arteriosis without residua
  3. Mitral valve prolapse without regurgitation
  4. Previous Kawasaki disease or rheumatic fever without valvular involvement
- Consultation with the patient's pediatric cardiologist is always appropriate if questions arise concerning prophylaxis

■ REFERRAL INFORMATION
All patients with unexplained fever and lesions, or central venous catheters, which place them at high risk for IE, should be referred back to their cardiologist.

PEARLS & CONSIDERATIONS

■ CLINICAL PEARLS
- Rarely, patients may be afebrile, especially with prior antibiotic therapy.
- The risk of IE in patients with aortic stenosis increases over time.
- Consider taking blood cultures in febrile patients with high-risk lesions (prosthetic valves, shunts, complex congenital malformations, aortic stenosis,) before initiating antibiotic therapy, even if the source of fever is apparent.

REFERENCES
1. Bayer AS et al: Diagnosis and management of infective endocarditis and its complications, *Circulation* 98:2936, 1998.
2. Morris CD, Reller MD, Menashe VD: Thirty-year incidence of infective endocarditis after surgery for congenital heart defect, *JAMA* 279:599, 1998.
3. Pajani AS et al: Prevention of bacterial endocarditis: recommendations by the American Heart Association, *JAMA* 277:1794, 1997.
4. Saiman L, Prince A, Gersony WM: Pediatric infective endocarditis in the modern era, *J Pediatr* 122:847, 1993.
Author: **J. Peter Harris, M.D.**

BASIC INFORMATION

■ DEFINITION
Endometriosis is the presence and growth of endometrial stroma and glands in locations other than the uterine cavity and musculature.

ICD-9CM CODES
617.3 Pelvic peritoneum
617.8 Site specified (lung, bladder, umbilicus, vulva)
617.9 Site unspecified

■ ETIOLOGY
- Most widely proposed and accepted mechanism
  1. Theory of transplanted endometrium by retrograde menstruation
- Theory of deficient cell-mediated immunity
  1. Inability of the immune system to remove refluxed menstrual debris
- Other theories
  1. Theory of transplanted endometrium by vascular, lymphatic, or iatrogenic spread of endometrial cells
  2. Theory of coelomic metaplasia
     a. Embryologically multipotent cells undergo metaplastic transformation into functioning endometrium.
  3. Induction theory
     a. Shed endometrium releases substances that induce undifferentiated mesenchyma to form endometriotic tissue.

■ EPIDEMIOLOGY & DEMOGRAPHICS
- Prevalence is approximately 10% of menstruating adolescents and women.
- Prevalence in adolescents with chronic pelvic pain is approximately 45% to 65%.
- The average age of diagnosis is 25 to 29 years.
- Familial predisposition is recognized.
- Incidence is increased in patients with reproductive tract anomalies, such as müllerian duct abnormalities, or cervical or vaginal obstruction.

■ HISTORY
- Cyclic pelvic pain
- Abnormal uterine bleeding
- Pain with defecation
- Rectal pain with bleeding
- Dyspareunia
- Infertility

■ PHYSICAL EXAMINATION
- Tenderness of pelvic structures
- Tender lymph nodes in the cul-de-sac
- Tender uterosacral ligaments
- Tender, enlarged adnexa if ovary involved
- Fixed and retroverted uterus

DIAGNOSIS

■ DIFFERENTIAL DIAGNOSIS
- Primary dysmenorrhea
- Pelvic inflammatory disease
- Pelvic masses, including fibroids, ovarian neoplasms
- Bowel neoplasm
- Anatomic abnormalities

■ DIAGNOSTIC WORKUP
- Laparoscopy or laparotomy is necessary for definitive diagnosis and staging. Findings include "powder burn" or "chocolate cyst" implants (8 mm to 8 cm) located in the dependent portions of the female pelvis. Less common sites include, but are not limited to, the rectosigmoid, umbilicus, and areas of previous surgery.
- Magnetic resonance imaging is not diagnostic but gives detailed confirmatory information.
- Pelvic ultrasonography is not diagnostic but may help distinguish solid from cystic lesions.
- Measurements of serum proteins: CA-125 is neither sensitive nor specific but may be used to follow response to therapy and progression of disease.

THERAPY

■ MEDICAL
- Danazol is a synthetic steroid with mild androgenic effects that suppresses pituitary-ovarian axis.
  1. Causes anovulation
  2. Causes androgenic side effects, of which deepening of the voice may be irreversible
  3. Results in resolution of implants
  4. Reduces pain up to 6 months after discontinuation of therapy
  5. Does not appear to affect fertility
  6. Usual dosage is 100 to 400 mg orally two times per day for approximately 6 months
- Gonadotropin-releasing hormone analogs do the following:
  1. Produce a state of medical oophorectomy
  2. Reduce pain
  3. Have unknown effect on fertility
  4. Can be given as one of the following:
     a. Leuprolide 3.75 mg intramuscularly every month up to 6 months
     b. Nafarelin 200 to 400 mg intranasally two times per day for 6 months
     c. Goserelin 3.6 mg subcutaneously every 28 days for 6 months
- Continuous low-dose monophasic oral contraceptives produce amenorrhea.
  1. This reduces symptoms by approximately 80%.
  2. The dosage is increased to manage breakthrough bleeding.
- Progestins do the following:
  1. Result in prolonged amenorrhea
  2. Do not appear to affect fertility
  3. Reduce pain
  4. Can be given in one of the following ways:
     a. Medroxyprogesterone acetate 30 mg orally daily
     b. Depomedroxyprogesterone acetate 150 mg intramuscularly every 3 months (maximum dose of 200 mg every month)
- Analgesics:
  1. Naproxen sodium was found to be more helpful than a placebo.

■ SURGICAL
- Conservative
  1. Laparoscopy or laparotomy to remove implants by coagulating, vaporizing, or resecting the lesions while preserving reproductive capacity may be performed.
  2. Presacral neurectomy may also be performed for severe, midline pain.
  3. Length of results varies.
  4. Approximately 25% of patients return for subsequent laparoscopy.
- Definitive
  1. Total abdominal hysterectomy, bilateral salpingo-oophorectomy, and removal of endometriosis lesions may be performed.
  2. This procedure is reserved for advanced and burdensome disease.

■ FOLLOW-UP & DISPOSITION
Patients require close follow-up to ensure proper monitoring of the progression of disease and response to treatment, as well as to ensure appropriate education.

■ PATIENT/FAMILY EDUCATION
- A monthly pain calendar may be useful to identify the cyclic nature of pain.
- When using danazol, need to also use barrier contraception for the first month to avoid the complication of female pseudohermaphroditism in a developing fetus.

■ PREVENTIVE TREATMENT OR TESTS

When the presentation of endometriosis occurs in adolescence, the practitioner should evaluate for congenital outflow obstruction, which may be corrected and allow for less severe disease.

■ REFERRAL INFORMATION

Patients with suspected endometriosis must be managed by practitioners who are familiar with techniques to definitively diagnose and treat this disorder.

✇ PEARLS & CONSIDERATIONS

■ CLINICAL PEARLS

The stage of disease (i.e., the number and extent of lesions) is not related to the severity of symptoms.

■ WEBSITES

- Endometriosis Association: www.endometriosis.org.au/teen.htm
- OBGYN.net: www.obgyn.net

REFERENCES

1. Droegemueller W: Endometriosis and adenomyosis: evaluation, pathology, diagnosis, management. In Mishell DR (ed): *Comprehensive gynecology,* St Louis, 1997, Mosby.
2. Emans SJ: Dysmenorrhea, pelvic pain and premenstrual syndrome. In Emans SJH, Laugher M, Goldstein DP (eds): *Pediatric and adolescent gynecology,* Philadelphia, 1998, Lippincott-Raven.
3. Olive J, Schwartz L: Medical progress: endometriosis, *N Engl J Med* 328:1759, 1993.

Author: **Susan Birndorf, D.O.**

II

BASIC INFORMATION

■ DEFINITION

- Enuresis is the involuntary passage of urine, more often than once a month, in children older than age 5.
- It is considered primary if it has always existed without periods of dryness.
- It is considered secondary if the child had a period of being consistently dry for 6 months before starting to wet again.
- Nocturnal enuresis is wetting that occurs at night.
- Diurnal enuresis is wetting that occurs during the day.

■ SYNONYMS

- Wetting
- Bedwetting

ICD-9CM CODE

788.30 Enuresis

■ ETIOLOGY

- Likely multifactorial
- Genetic
  1. Research suggests autosomal-dominant inheritance with 90% penetrance.
  2. Scandinavian studies suggest linkage to chromosome 13 between q13 and q14.
  3. It is related to defective circadian rhythm of vasopressin production.
     a. Lack normal nocturnal increase in antidiuretic hormone (ADH).
     b. Nocturnal urine production exceeds bladder capacity.
- Other causes
  1. Questionably reduced functional bladder capacity
  2. Questionably sleep disorder (deep sleep versus sleep transitions)
  3. Organic disease
  4. Urinary tract infections
  5. Diabetes (mellitus or insipidus)
  6. Neurogenic bladder
  7. Anatomic abnormalities, such as ectopic ureter
  8. Emotional stress, usually associated with secondary enuresis
  9. Response to abuse

■ EPIDEMIOLOGY & DEMOGRAPHICS

- No clear-cut definition exists across studies.
- In most cases, no clearly identifiable cause can be found.
- In one study using a national database of 10,960 children, bedwetting was reported in 33% of 5-year-olds, 18% of 8-year-olds, 7% of 11-year-olds, and 0.7% of 17-year-olds.
  1. This study did not distinguish primary from secondary enuresis.

- Another study found secondary enuresis in 3% to 8% of children 5 to 12 years old.
- This condition is associated with constipation.
- More than 50% of primary nocturnal enuresis is familial.
- Enuresis is more common in boys and in children living in large, impoverished families.
- Some association with school difficulties has been reported.

■ HISTORY

- Establish whether the enuresis is primary or secondary.
- Document the degree, frequency, and timing of wetting.
- Characterize the urinary stream.
- Document the amount and types of fluid ingested in a day and timing of ingestion.
- Note any signs of illness (e.g., fever, dysuria, polydipsia).
- Constipation and/or encopresis present?
- Any developmental delays?
- Family history of enuresis?
- What has family tried and what are consequences for child?
  1. Is the child kept from participating in peer or family activities because of enuresis?
- How stressed is the family by occurrence?
  1. Are laundry facilities easily accessible?
  2. Are parents angered or frustrated by extra workload?
- Any other stressors, including domestic violence or abuse?

■ PHYSICAL EXAMINATION

- Usually normal
- Blood pressure
  1. If elevated, consider renal disease.
- Abdomen examination looking for masses, constipation
- Genital and urinary tract abnormalities
- Lumbar and sacral spine examination
- Neurologic examination with attention to gait and abdominal, genitourinary, and lower extremity reflexes, strength and sensation

DIAGNOSIS

Made by history, with cause narrowed down by physical examination and workup

■ DIFFERENTIAL DIAGNOSIS

- Urinary tract infection, cystitis
- Diabetes mellitus and insipidus
- Neurogenic bladder
- Ectopic ureter

- Bladder or ureteral fistula
- Chronic constipation

■ DIAGNOSTIC WORKUP

- Urinalysis and urine culture
- Voiding cystourethrogram and bladder/kidney ultrasound if bacteriuria present
- Lumbosacral spine films if cutaneous lumbar or sacral anomalies present
- Magnetic resonance imaging scan of spine if plain films of spine are abnormal or if neurologic examination is abnormal

THERAPY

■ NONPHARMACOLOGIC

- Behavioral modifications, such as avoiding caffeinated beverages and voiding before bed
- Reward systems
- Enuretic alarms: bell and pad system, minialarm (attached to undergarments)
  1. High noncompliance rate
- Combination therapies
- Treatment of constipation if it exists

■ MEDICAL

- Desmopressin acetate (ADH analog)
  1. Reduces nightly urine production.
  2. Discontinuation usually leads to recurrence.
  3. It is often used for symptomatic control of enuresis for special occasions, such as sleepovers.
  4. Begin with 10 μg to each nostril at bedtime, increasing to two sprays to each nostril as needed.
- Imipramine
  1. Offers two beneficial physiologic effects:
     a. Direct anticholinergic action on bladder tone (improved bladder capacity)
     b. Decrease in the depth of sleep during the last third of the night
  2. Discontinuation of use usually leads to recurrent incontinence.
  3. Start with 10 to 25 mg orally at bedtime.
     a. Can increase 10 to 25 mg/dose at 1- to 2-week intervals.
  4. Continue for 2 to 3 months, then taper slowly.

■ COMPLEMENTARY & ALTERNATIVE THERAPY

Some evidence exists for success with imagery therapy.

■ FOLLOW-UP & DISPOSITION

- Monitor for efficacy of intervention and gauging of familial stressors.
  1. Initially, every 3 months

■ PATIENT/FAMILY EDUCATION

- Only about 1% of bedwetting is caused by a disease or other physical problem.
- Caregivers should contact the pediatrician for the following symptoms:
  1. Straining during urination, small/narrow stream of urine, or constant dribbling
  2. Cloudy or pink urine or bloodstains on underpants or pajamas
  3. Daytime as well as nighttime wetting
  4. Dysuria, frequency
- Have the child use the toilet and avoid drinking large amounts of fluid just before bed.
- Protect the bed with a rubber or plastic cover between the sheet and mattress.
- Allow the child to help change wet sheets and covers if the task would not lead to embarrassment.
- Offer a lot of emotional support to children until bedwetting resolves.
- Provide reassurance about the prevalence of the problem and its eventual resolution.
  1. Fifteen percent of children per year with both primary and secondary nocturnal enuresis experience spontaneous resolution.
  2. Persistent nocturnal enuresis may exist in up to 1.5% to 3% of the adult population, according to one reference.

■ REFERRAL INFORMATION

- Children with suspected urologic anomalies should be referred to a urologist.
- Patients having neurologic findings should see a neurologist.
- Psychiatric or counseling referrals are warranted in cases of abuse.

☼ PEARLS & CONSIDERATIONS

■ CLINICAL PEARLS

- Constipation can be a companion problem.
- Older children are embarrassed by this problem and are often shamed or punished by their worn-out parents.
- Approach to resolution is variable based on the cause and family's level of concern.
- Enuresis is associated with increased rates of behavior problems.

■ WEBSITES

- KidsHealth: Kidshealth.org/parent/healthy/enuresis.html
- National Enuresis Society: www.peds.umn.edu/centers/NES
- Travis International: www.travisinternational.com/index.html (e.g., alarms)

REFERENCES

1. Byrd R, Weitzman M: Bed-wetting in US children: epidemiology and related behavior problems, *Pediatrics* 98:414, 1996.
2. Dershewitz RA: *Ambulatory pediatric care,* Philadelphia, 1993, JB Lippincott.
3. Super M, Postlethwaite RJ: Genes, familial enuresis, and clinical management, *Lancet* 350:159, 1997.
4. Tietjen DN, Husmann DA: Nocturnal enuresis: a guide to evaluation and treatment, *Mayo Clin Proc* 71:857, 1996.

Author: **Andree Jacobs-Perkins, M.D.**

BASIC INFORMATION

■ DEFINITION
Epididymitis is inflammation of the epididymis, the coiled tubular structure adjacent and posterior to the testis, which is essential for sperm transport and maturation.

■ SYNONYM
Epididymoorchitis

ICD-9CM CODE
604.90 Epididymitis

■ ETIOLOGY
- Bacterial
  1. Prepubertal: gram-negative coliforms, usually *Escherichia coli*
  2. Postpubertal/sexually active: *Chlamydia trachomatis, Neisseria gonorrhoeae*
  3. Less common: *Mycobacterium tuberculosis, Haemophilus influenzae, Brucellosis,* and cytomegalovirus
- Nonbacterial
  1. Trauma
  2. Autoimmune disease/vasculitis
- Reflux of sterile urine into ejaculatory ducts
  1. May be associated with various manifestations of high-pressure bladder storage or voiding, as in neurogenic or nonneurogenic dysfunctional voiding, and some types of reflux in male infants
  2. Posterior urethral valve obstruction
  3. Straining or lifting with a full bladder

■ EPIDEMIOLOGY & DEMOGRAPHICS
- Up to 50% of cases are associated with a urologic or anorectal structural abnormality, especially if a positive urine culture is obtained.
- Approximately 20% to 60% of cases are associated with a urinary tract infection in non–sexually active children.
- Rare in prepubertal boys

■ HISTORY
- Scrotal pain with gradual onset
- May have referred pain to the ipsilateral inguinal canal or abdomen
- May have fever, dysuria, urgency, and/or frequency
- Rarely, nausea and vomiting
- Urethral discharge possible in sexually active adolescents
- Important to ask about instrumentation and trauma

■ PHYSICAL EXAMINATION
- Patient may have a fever.
- Examine the uninvolved testis first, as a baseline, in both the erect and supine positions.
- There is unilateral testicular pain and tenderness.
- The epididymis is tender and swollen, sometimes to such a degree as to obliterate normal landmarks.
- The testis has a normal lie.
- Cremasteric reflex is usually present.
- It is important to examine the back carefully for signs of occult spinal dysraphism.
- The anus should be examined for signs of anorectal abnormality.

DIAGNOSIS

■ DIFFERENTIAL DIAGNOSIS
- Torsion of spermatic cord (*must be eliminated as a possible diagnosis*)
- Torsion of a testicular or epididymal appendage
- Orchitis
- Testicular neoplasm with or without hemorrhage
- Testicular abscess
- Traumatic hydrocele/hematocele
- Henoch-Schönlein purpura
- Lymphedema
- Scrotal skin inflammation or infection
  1. Cellulitis
  2. Infected sebaceous cyst
- Incarcerated scrotal hernia
- Other intraperitoneal process manifesting in scrotum (e.g., meconium scrotitis)

■ DIAGNOSTIC WORKUP
- Urinalysis may demonstrate pyuria.
- If the physical examination does not rule out testicular torsion, *immediate urologic consultation is imperative.*
- The goal of imaging is to rule out testicular torsion.
  1. Color Doppler ultrasound
     a. This test typically demonstrates an increase in blood flow to the affected epididymis and at least normal or increased blood flow to the testicle compared with the normal side.
  2. Scintigraphy
     a. This test typically demonstrates good flow to the testicles and increased flow to the epididymis.
     b. In the prepubertal child who is afebrile with a normal urinalysis, increased blood flow probably reflects a torsed testicular appendage with surrounding inflammatory response.

- In prepubertal boys:
  1. Urine culture
  2. Radiographic evaluation after therapy for underlying structural abnormalities
  3. Rarely, aspiration of an intrascrotal collection or abscess for culture
- In sexually active adolescents:
  1. Gram stain of urethral exudate
  2. Culture of urethral exudate for *C. trachomatis* and *N. gonorrhoeae*
  3. Evaluation for syphilis and human immunodeficiency virus counseling and testing recommended

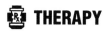

THERAPY

■ NONPHARMACOLOGIC
- Bed rest/scrotal elevation should be used to decrease edema.
- Scrotal support may be helpful.

■ MEDICAL
- Antiinflammatory agents and analgesics
- In prepubertal boys:
  1. Antimicrobial therapy for urinary tract infection (usually gram-negative organisms)
- In sexually active adolescents:
  1. Antimicrobial therapy in accordance with Centers for Disease Control and Prevention guidelines
  2. Treatment of all sexual partners within the past 60 days
- Patients who are systemically ill: may require hospital admission for parenteral antibiotics

■ SURGICAL
Surgical exploration is needed if testicular torsion cannot be ruled out.

■ FOLLOW-UP & DISPOSITION
- The pain and edema usually resolve within 1 week, but the epididymal induration may take several weeks to normalize.
- Obtain a follow-up culture if urinary tract infection is present.

■ PREVENTIVE TREATMENT OR TESTS
- In prepubertal boys, it is important to evaluate for structural abnormalities.
  1. Voiding cystourethrogram and
  2. Intravenous urography or
  3. Ultrasound

■ REFERRAL INFORMATION
A pediatric urologist should be consulted for any child with an acute scrotum.

✹ PEARLS & CONSIDERATIONS

■ CLINICAL PEARLS

Prehn's sign (relief of pain with elevation of the scrotum) is not specific and therefore not useful in the diagnosis of epididymitis.

REFERENCES

1. Kass EJ, Lundak B: The acute scrotum, *Pediatr Clin North Am* 44:1251, 1997.
2. Merlinia E et al: Acute epididymitis and urinary tract anomalies in children, *Scand J Urol Nephrol* 32:273, 1998.
3. Rabinowitz R, Hulbert WC: Acute scrotal swelling, *Urol Clin North Am* 22: 101, 1995.

Authors: **Stephanie Sansoni, M.D., William C. Hulbert, M.D., Ronald Rabinowitz, M.D., and Robert Mevorach, M.D.**

II

BASIC INFORMATION

■ DEFINITION
Epistaxis is hemorrhage from the nose.

■ SYNONYMS
- Nosebleed
- Bloody nose

■ ICD-9CM CODE
784.7 Epistaxis

■ ETIOLOGY
- The nose is a common site for recurrent minor trauma.
- Small vessels that supply the nasal mucosa have little structural support; contraction and hemostasis for an injured vessel are thus limited.
- Nasal mucosa has a rich vascular supply (terminal branches from the internal and external carotid arteries) that forms multiple anastomosis.
- The anterior portion of the nose is the most common site of bleeding in children.
  1. Kiesselbach's plexus in Little's area of the anterior nasal septum, approximately 0.5 cm from the tip of the nose, is a common site of anterior bleeding.
  2. This area is easily irritated by finger manipulation and drying effects of the air.
- Posterior bleeding is more common in the elderly.

■ EPIDEMIOLOGY & DEMOGRAPHICS
- Epistaxis occurs most commonly in the winter months (dry air).
- Children ages 2 to 10 are more commonly affected than adults.
- It may be a presentation of coagulopathy (e.g., von Willebrand disease).

■ HISTORY
- Frequency of occurrence
- Bleeding from one or both nostrils
- Amount and duration of bleeding; ability to stop bleeding with home first aid
- Sensation of blood in back of throat as first awareness of bleeding (more suggestive of posterior bleeding)
- Trauma
- Nose picking
- History of upper respiratory infections and sinusitis
- Allergic rhinitis or chronic nasal discharge
- Bleeding disorder (e.g., easy bruising, bleeding) or family history of bleeding disorder
- Recent surgery
- Nasal obstructive symptoms; progressing obstructive symptoms after trauma or surgery
- Medications

- Exposure to airborne irritants and toxic chemicals, including cigarette smoke
- Cocaine use

■ PHYSICAL EXAMINATION
- Vital signs
- Airway
- Mental status
- Nasal speculum: useful for identifying source of bleeding (anterior versus posterior, right versus left)
- Posterior bleeding usually seen as bleeding along the posterior pharynx
- Inspection of the nose for discharge, trauma, or evidence of foreign body
- Evidence of other hematologic disease (e.g., petechiae, purpura, pallor, hepatosplenomegaly, lymphadenopathy)
- Septal hematoma (a large, soft, red or bluish mass, obstructing one or both nares)

DIAGNOSIS

■ DIFFERENTIAL DIAGNOSIS
- Trauma
  1. Nose picking
  2. Facial trauma
  3. Perforation: usually as a result of chronic erosion, but must consider vasculitis, granulomatous disorder, or lymphoma; cocaine use should be considered in older children
  4. After facial surgery
- Inflammation
  1. Acute respiratory infection, sinusitis, allergic rhinitis; cause nasal lining inflammation
  2. Foreign body: unilateral, foul-smelling discharge typical
- Tumor
  1. Juvenile nasopharyngeal angiofibroma: benign vascular neoplasm in lateral nasopharynx
  2. Malignant neoplasms: rhabdomyosarcoma, lymphoma, midline reticuloses
  3. Polyps (uncommon except in cystic fibrosis)
  4. Meningocele or encephalocele
- Chemical
  1. Airborne irritants and toxic chemicals can cause epistaxis.
  2. Primary or secondary exposure to cigarette smoke can cause epistaxis.
- Blood disorders
  1. von Willebrand disease
  2. Hemophilia
  3. Thrombocytopenia
  4. Leukemia
  5. Sickle cell anemia
  6. Osler-Weber-Rendu disease (hereditary telangiectasis)

- Other
  1. Hypertension: very rare in children
  2. Vicarious menstruation: monthly epistaxis related to monthly vascular congestion coinciding with menses; related to monthly hormonal changes
  3. Septal deviation: nasal dryness and crusting in area of deflection
  4. Septal hematoma: hematoma separates perichondrium from septal cartilage; vascular supply compromised; can progress to necrosis, abscess

■ DIAGNOSTIC WORKUP
- Children with no evidence of significant blood loss, no evidence of systemic disease by history and physical examination, and anterior epistaxis that is easily stopped by local pressure require no laboratory workup.
- Consider coagulation disorder workup for patients with pertinent findings on personal or family history or physical examination. Workup to begin with the following:
  1. Complete blood count and platelet count are obtained to look for anemia.
  2. Prothrombin time, partial thromboplastin time, bleeding time may require further workup pending results.

THERAPY

■ NONPHARMACOLOGIC
- Exert digital compression over the nasal alar and anterior septal area for at least 5 minutes.
- Place a cotton or tissue plug in the nose.
- Bend forward at the waist, which allows blood to flow out of nostrils rather than into the back of the throat.
- Apply anterior nasal packing when local measures are unsuccessful at controlling bleeding.
  1. Petroleum gauze impregnated with antibiotic ointment is inserted into the nares.
  2. It is removed by 72 hours.
  3. Synthetic sponge packs (tampons) may also be used.
  4. There is a risk of toxic shock with both methods.
  5. Patients should receive prophylactic oral antibiotics because of the risk of sinusitis.
     a. Oral antibiotics do not affect the risk of toxic shock.
- Posterior nasal packing is rarely needed in children.
- Remove a foreign body if present.

■ MEDICAL
- Remove clots and apply topical oxymetazoline hydrochloride (Afrin), epinephrine (1:1000), or 4% cocaine to the involved area with a cotton pledget.
  1. Local vasoconstrictors are usually combined with an anesthetic, such as tetracaine or lidocaine.
- Cauterize with silver nitrate.
  1. Both sides of septum should not be cauterized at the same time because of the risk of septal perforation.
- Apply antibiotic cream or ointment to the cauterized area twice daily for 5 days to prevent crusting and infection.

■ SURGICAL
- Septal hematoma: simple aspiration for small hematoma; may require more complicated surgical drainage
- Endoscopic cauterization under general anesthesia
  1. Nasal cavity cleansed and endoscopically examined
  2. Source of bleeding identified
  3. Electrocauterization to appropriate area
- Arterial ligation to decrease arterial blood flow to the bleeding area

■ PREVENTIVE TREATMENT
- Nose picking: Apply antibiotic ointment to inside of nose daily to decrease crust buildup and itching.
- Use buffered nasal saline regularly during transitional weather times (fall to winter, winter to spring).
- Apply petroleum jelly to the inside of the nares twice daily to help maintain moisture of nasal mucosa.
- Use a cool mist vaporizer during the winter, especially with forced-air heating.
- In allergic rhinitis, treatment with an antihistamine-decongestant may be indicated; however, overuse may cause overdrying of the mucosa.

■ REFERRAL INFORMATION
Ear, nose, and throat referrals should be considered for the following:
- Patients with specific local abnormalities, such as tumors, polyps, telangiectasias
- Patients with severe, recurrent, or posterior nasal bleeding

☼ PEARLS & CONSIDERATIONS

■ CLINICAL PEARLS
- Nose picking is the most common cause of epistaxis in children.
- Juvenile nasopharyngeal angiofibroma are found only in pubescent males and are hormonally sensitive.

REFERENCES
1. Alvi A, Joyner-Triplett N: Acute epistaxis: how to spot the source and stop the flow, *Postgrad Med* 99:83, 1996.
2. Culbertson MC, Manning SC: Epistaxis. In Bluestone CD, Stool SE, Scheetz (eds): *Pediatric otolaryngology*, Philadelphia, 1990, WB Saunders.
3. Emanuel J: Epistaxis. In Cummings CW et al (eds): *Otolaryngology: head & neck surgery*, St Louis, 1998, Mosby.
4. Henretig F: Epistaxis. In Fleisher GR, Ludwig S (eds): *Textbook of pediatric emergency medicine*, Baltimore, 1993, Williams & Wilkins.
5. Mulbury P: Recurrent epistaxis, *Pediatr Rev* 12:213, 1991.
Author: **Rachel Budiansky, M.D.**

II

BASIC INFORMATION

DEFINITION
In the normal host, the most common manifestation of Epstein-Barr virus (EBV) infection is infectious mononucleosis (IM). IM is an acute multisystem illness, which is usually self-limited with systemic signs of acute and subacute infection. Acute neurologic disorders may be associated with IM or as a manifestation of primary EBV infection without IM. These disorders include Bell's palsy, aseptic meningitis, encephalitis, Guillain-Barré syndrome, and transverse myelitis. Diseases caused by EBV associated with immunodeficiency include the X-linked lymphoproliferative syndrome, posttransplant lymphoproliferative disorders, B-cell lymphomas, and severe atypical EBV infections. Burkitt lymphoma (in Central Africa and Papua New Guinea) and nasopharyngeal carcinoma (in Southeast Asia) are important EBV-associated diseases outside the United States.

SYNONYMS
- Infectious mononucleosis
- Mono

ICD-9CM CODE
075 Epstein-Barr virus infection

ETIOLOGY
- EBV is an enveloped DNA herpesvirus.
- It is transmitted via saliva, requiring close personal contact.
- The incubation period for IM is 30 to 45 days.
- IM persists in a latent state in B lymphocytes after primary infection.

EPIDEMIOLOGY & DEMOGRAPHICS
- In lower socioeconomic communities, primary infection occurs early in life.
  1. Approximately 80% to 100% of people are seropositive by 3 to 6 years of age.
  2. In this setting, most infections are asymptomatic or produce mildly symptomatic disease (tonsillitis).
- In developed countries, primary infection occurs between the ages of 10 and 30 (particularly among college students), most often manifest as acute IM.
- There is no seasonal pattern.

HISTORY
- IM
  1. Prodrome of fatigue, malaise, myalgia, and headache may last 7 to 14 days.
  2. Acute onset of high fever occurs in some cases.
  3. Common symptoms of acute IM are as follows:
     a. Fever
     b. Sore throat, swallowing difficulty
     c. Malaise
     d. Headache
     e. Myalgia
     f. Sweats
     g. Anorexia
     h. Abdominal pain
     i. Chest pain
     j. Cough
  4. Onset may be insidious.
- Reactivation diseases/syndromes: congenital or acquired immunodeficiency

PHYSICAL EXAMINATION
- Fever is present in more than 90% of cases.
- Lymphadenopathy is present in more than 90% of cases.
- Tonsillopharyngitis is present in 70% of cases.
- Splenomegaly is present in 75% of cases.
- Hepatomegaly is present in 50% of cases.
- Petechial enanthem may occur.
- Lymphadenopathy involves the anterior and posterior cervical chains but may be generalized.
- Traumatic palpation of the spleen must be avoided because of the risk of splenic rupture.
- Maculopapular rashes occur rarely; however, almost all patients given ampicillin develop such rashes.

DIAGNOSIS

DIFFERENTIAL DIAGNOSIS
- Cytomegalovirus
- *Toxoplasma gondii*
- Viral hepatitis
- Leptospirosis
- Rubella
- Acute human immunodeficiency virus infection
- Lymphoma or leukemia

DIAGNOSTIC WORKUP
- Lymphocytosis: relative (more than 50% lymphocytes) and absolute (more than $4500/mm^3$)
- Atypical lymphocytes (Downey cell) on smear
- Hemolytic anemia (rare)
- Abnormal liver function tests in 80% of cases
- Heterophile antibody testing
  1. Paul-Bunnell test and slide agglutination (Monospot) may be positive.
  2. Heterophile antibodies are a nonspecific serologic response to EBV infection.
  3. Repeat testing may be necessary.
     a. Approximately 40% are positive in the first week.
     b. Approximately 80% to 90% are positive by the third week.
  4. These tests are most often negative in infants and children younger than 4 years of age because they do not develop detectable heterophile antibodies during acute EBV infection.
- Specific tests for EBV antibodies (i.e., anti-VCA IgG, anti-VCA IgM, anti-EA, and anti-EBNA) are not usually necessary to diagnose typical IM.
  1. Useful in the diagnosis of heterophile-negative IM, severe or atypical disease, or lymphoproliferative disease
- Rapid test or throat culture for group A β-hemolytic streptococci should be obtained.
  1. Positive in 5% to 25% of patients.

THERAPY

NONPHARMACOLOGIC
- Symptomatic therapy
- Bed rest and limited activity
- Fluids
- No contact sports for splenomegaly

MEDICAL
- Antipyretics and analgesics are given for comfort.
- Corticosteroids: Prednisone 1 mg/kg/day for 7 days is indicated for the following:
  1. Severe tonsillitis and prevention of airway obstruction caused by pharyngeal or laryngeal edema
  2. Acute hemolytic anemia
  3. Neurologic complications
- Antiviral agents such as acyclovir have not demonstrated a clinical benefit in otherwise healthy children.
- Appropriate treatment of positive test for group A β-hemolytic streptococci

■ **FOLLOW-UP & DISPOSITION**
- Symptoms of IM usually last 2 to 4 weeks.
- Organomegaly most often resolves within 1 to 3 months.
- Several months may be required for patient to return to normal sense of wellness.

■ **PATIENT/FAMILY EDUCATION**
Avoid contact sports until splenomegaly has resolved.

■ **PREVENTIVE TREATMENT**
- Kissing is thought to be one mechanism of transmission.

- No specific isolation precautions are necessary other than handwashing and careful handling of oral secretions.
- Blood donation should be deferred in those with recent IM or IM-like illness.

☼ **PEARLS & CONSIDERATIONS**

■ **WEBSITE**
HealthlinkUSA: www.healthlinkusa. com/epstein-barr_virus.htm; contains links to websites, information on treatment and diagnosis, prevention, and support groups

REFERENCES

1. American Academy of Pediatrics: Epstein-Barr infections. In Pickering LK (ed): *2000 Red Book: report of the Committee on Infectious Diseases,* ed 25, Elk Grove Village, Ill, 2000, American Academy of Pediatrics.
2. Sumaya CV: Epstein-Barr virus. In Feigan R, Cherry J: *Textbook of pediatric infectious diseases,* ed 4, Philadelphia, 1998, WB Saunders.

Author: **Therese A. Cvetkovich, M.D.**

II

BASIC INFORMATION

■ DEFINITION
Erythema multiforme is an acute hypersensitivity reaction characterized by distinctive target-shaped skin lesions.

■ SYNONYMS
- Erythema multiforme minor
- EM

ICD9-CM CODE
695.1 Erythema multiforme

■ ETIOLOGY
- Most children with erythema multiforme have preceding herpes simplex virus (HSV) infection.
- Up to 50% have noted herpes labialis infection.
- Controversy exists regarding the role of medications and *Mycoplasma pneumoniae* infection.

■ EPIDEMIOLOGY & DEMOGRAPHICS
- Incidence is unknown but rare in children.
- Of all cases of erythema multiforme, approximately 20% occur in childhood.

■ HISTORY
- Usually, there is no prodrome in childhood erythema multiforme.
- Acute onset of multiple lesions is typical, with most appearing within 24 hours.
- Lesions may itch or burn.
- The disease is self-limited, lasting approximately 2 weeks.
- Heals without scarring.
- HSV lesion usually precedes the onset of erythema multiforme by 3 to 14 days.
- One or two recurrences per year are common.

■ PHYSICAL EXAMINATION
- Initial lesions are dusky red macules or erythematous wheals.

- They progress into target-shaped lesions of concentric zones of color, with duskier areas more centrally located.
  1. Target lesions have a central dusky or purple zone surrounded by a pale edematous ring with a peripheral erythematous margin.
- The lesions are symmetric.
- Most common locations are the dorsum of hands and forearms.
  1. Often found on palms, trunk, neck, and face
- Lesions tend to be grouped, especially around elbows and knees.
- Any part of the lesion may develop vesicles or bullae.
- Discrete oral lesions are present in more than 50% of children with erythema multiforme.
  1. Oral lesions may begin as vesicles or bullae but rapidly become painful superficial erythematous erosions, often with yellowish-white pseudomembrane formation.

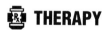

DIAGNOSIS

■ DIFFERENTIAL DIAGNOSIS
- Giant urticaria (lesions less than 24 hours at any one site)
- Vasculitis
- Systemic lupus erythematosus
- Fixed drug eruptions

■ DIAGNOSTIC WORKUP
The diagnosis is usually made on basis of characteristic clinical picture.

THERAPY

■ NONPHARMACOLOGIC
Because the disease is self-resolving, may simply follow course without intervention.

■ MEDICAL
- Symptomatic therapy is initiated, with oral antihistamines for burning or itching.
- Recurrent HSV-associated erythema multiforme may benefit from acyclovir prophylaxis (10 mg/kg/day) for 6 to 12 months.
- No studies support the use of oral steroids.

■ SURGICAL
- Biopsy is rarely needed to confirm the diagnosis.
- No therapeutic surgical procedure is available.

PEARLS & CONSIDERATIONS

■ CLINICAL PEARLS
- Target lesions appear mostly on upper extremities.
- Individual lesions appear fixed at the same skin site for 7 days or more.
  1. Multiforme applies to each lesion.
  2. Lesions do not migrate like they do with urticaria.

■ WEBSITES
- American Academy of Dermatology: www.aad.org
- Society for Pediatric Dermatology: www.spdnet.org

REFERENCES
1. Weston WL: What is erythema multiforme? *Pediatr Ann* 25:106, 1996.
2. Weston WL: Herpes simplex virus-associated erythema multiforme in prepubertal children, *Arch Pediatr Adolesc Med* 151:1014, 1997.
3. Weston WL: Atypical forms of herpes simplex-associated erythema multiforme, *J Am Acad Dermatol* 39:124, 1998.

Author: **Susan Haller Psaila, M.D.**

BASIC INFORMATION

■ DEFINITION

Erythema nodosum is an inflammatory reaction pattern in the skin to several inciting factors; it is the most common type of panniculitis.

ICD-9CM CODE

695.2 Erythema nodosum

■ ETIOLOGY

- Numerous causes exist, including infections, medications, malignant diseases, and a wide group of miscellaneous conditions.
- Streptococcal and respiratory infections are the most common etiologic agents in children.
- In the past, primary tuberculosis was a common cause.
- The cause is unknown in up to 20% of cases.

■ EPIDEMIOLOGY & DEMOGRAPHICS

- The greatest incidence occurs during spring and fall, less commonly during summer.
- It can occur at any age.
- Sex incidence is approximately equal in children.
- Racial and geographic incidences vary, depending on prevalence of diseases that are etiologic factors.

■ HISTORY

- Cutaneous eruption is sometimes associated with low-grade fever, malaise, fatigue, cough, arthralgia, headache, and conjunctivitis.
- Abdominal pain, vomiting, and diarrhea may also appear with the skin findings.

■ PHYSICAL EXAMINATION

- Symmetric, tender, erythematous warm nodules and plaques are present.
- Lesions range in size from 1 to 15 cm and may number from 1 to 10.
- The lesions usually manifest bilaterally, on distal anterior lower extremities.
- More extensive cases can involve the thighs, arms, neck, and rarely, the face.
- Ulceration is not seen, and nodules heal without atrophy or scarring.
- Eruptions last 3 to 6 weeks on average; lesions flatten and become less erythematous during this time.
- Lesions may recur, and some patients may develop chronic and persistent forms.

DIAGNOSIS

■ DIFFERENTIAL DIAGNOSIS

- Common bruises
- Cellulitis/erysipelas
- Deep fungal infections
- Insect bites
- Deep thrombophlebitis
- Angiitis
- Erythema induratum
- Fat-destructive panniculitis

■ DIAGNOSTIC WORKUP

- The diagnosis is usually made on the basis of the characteristic clinical picture.
- If in doubt, bacterial and fungal cultures and skin biopsy may help clarify the diagnosis.

THERAPY

■ NONPHARMACOLOGIC

- The lesions usually regress spontaneously.
- Identification and treatment of underlying causes is necessary.
- Bed rest with leg elevation is useful in patients who are experiencing severe discomfort.

■ MEDICAL

- Nonsteroidal antiinflammatory drugs are helpful when pain, inflammation, or arthralgia is prominent.
- Intralesional corticosteroids often cause rapid involution of lesions.
- Systemic corticosteroids are not indicated, especially if an underlying infectious cause has not been ruled out.

PEARLS & CONSIDERATIONS

■ WEBSITES

- American Academy of Dermatology: www.aad.org
- Society for Pediatric Dermatology: www.spdnet.org

REFERENCES

1. Hurwitz S: *Clinical pediatric dermatology*, ed 2, Philadelphia, 1993, WB Saunders.
2. Labbe L et al: Erythema nodosum in children: a study of 27 patients, *Pediatr Dermatol* 13:447, 1996.
3. Picco P et al: Clinical and biological characteristics of immunopathological disease related erythema nodosum in children, *Scand J Rheumatol* 28:27, 1999.

Author: **Susan Haller Psaila, M.D.**

II

BASIC INFORMATION

■ DEFINITION

Esophageal atresia is a congenital interruption or discontinuity of the esophagus resulting in esophageal obstruction. Tracheoesophageal fistula (TEF) is an abnormal communication (fistula) between the esophagus and trachea. Either atresia or fistula can occur alone (8% and 4%, respectively), but in 86% of patients, both abnormalities are present with an upper esophageal pouch and a fistula from the trachea to the lower esophageal segment.

■ SYNONYMS

- TEF
- Esophageal atresia/tracheoesophageal fistula (EA/TEF)

ICD-9CM CODE

750.3 Congenital esophageal atresia with or without TEF

■ ETIOLOGY

- Abnormal embryogenesis of the esophagus and trachea induced by an unknown factor(s)
- Alteration of the rate and timing of cell proliferation and differentiation during the separation of the esophagus and developing lung bud
- Question environmental teratogens: prolonged maternal exposure to contraceptives, exposure to progesterone and estrogens during pregnancy, infants of diabetic mothers, infants exposed to thalidomide

■ EPIDEMIOLOGY & DEMOGRAPHICS

- The incidence is 1 in 4500 live births.
- Male:female ratio is 1.26:1.
- Chromosomal anomalies (trisomy 13 or 18) occur in 6.6% of patients.
- Polyhydramnios is common.
- Associated anomalies:
  1. Present in 50% to 70% of patients overall
  2. Most common in pure EA and least common in TEF without atresia
  3. VACTERL (**v**ertebral, **a**norectal, **c**ardiac, **t**racheo**e**sophageal, **r**enal, **l**imb) association
  4. Cardiac abnormalities most common (approximately 35%) and account for most deaths
  5. Pure EA associated with the CHARGE syndrome (**c**oloboma, **h**eart defects, **a**tresia choanae, developmental **r**etardation, **g**enital hypoplasia, **e**ar deformities)

■ HISTORY

- Prenatal ultrasound may demonstrate small fetal stomach with polyhydramnios.
- Most infants are symptomatic in the first few hours of life.
- EA results in pooling of oral secretions and/or feedings into a blind upper esophageal pouch, causing excessive drooling, coughing, choking, and regurgitation.
- TEF results in spillage of gastrointestinal (GI) secretions into the trachea, causing cyanosis, coughing, tachypnea, chemical pneumonitis, and wheezing.
- In patients with pure TEF but without EA, symptoms are less evident at birth; they usually have repeated episodes of aspiration and/or pneumonia associated with feeding.

■ PHYSICAL EXAMINATION

- Associated VACTERL abnormalities
  1. Vertebral: meningocele, myelomeningocele
  2. Anorectal: imperforate or anteriorly displaced anus, anal stenosis
  3. Abnormal cardiac examination
  4. Limb abnormalities: absent radius, thumb
- Inability to pass a nasogastric (NG) tube into the stomach
- Stigmata of chromosomal abnormalities: trisomy 13, 18, etc.
- Wheezing or diminished breath sounds

DIAGNOSIS

■ DIFFERENTIAL DIAGNOSIS

- Gastroesophageal reflux (GER)
- Laryngotracheoesophageal cleft
- Tracheomalacia
- Premature (surfactant-deficient) lungs
- Vascular ring

■ DIAGNOSTIC WORKUP

- Plain chest/abdominal radiographs
  1. It is important to exclude congenital heart disease.
  2. Confirm the inability to pass an NG tube into the stomach, and evaluate how far the nasoesophageal tube is able to be passed into the thorax (how close to the carina).
  3. Evaluate the ribs and vertebrae.
  4. Look for a gasless abdomen; the combination of a gasless abdomen and the inability to pass an NG tube into the stomach is diagnostic of pure EA without fistula.
- Echocardiogram
  1. Use to exclude intracardiac abnormalities.

2. Determine which side the aortic arch is on; this finding dictates which side to perform a thoracotomy.
- Ultrasound of spine to exclude tethered cord, occult myelomeningocele, etc.
- Esophagogram to look for a TEF
  1. This study should be done *only* after EA has been excluded (by passage of the NG tube into the stomach).
  2. Study is not necessary if EA has already been demonstrated.

THERAPY
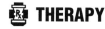

■ NONPHARMACOLOGIC

Minimize the aspiration of GI and salivary secretions by using a nasoesophageal tube to suction secretions and by placing the infant in an upright position.

■ MEDICAL

Administer preoperative broad-spectrum antibiotics.

■ SURGICAL

- The surgical approach is dictated by patient presentation.
  1. Otherwise healthy child with the most common anomaly (EA with distal TEF):
     a. Thoracotomy with division of the fistula and primary end-to-end esophageal reanastomosis
  2. Premature child with respiratory distress syndrome and inability to ventilate: emergent thoracotomy with division of TEF only
     a. No attempt is made to reestablish esophageal continuity.
     b. The resistance to air inflation of the lungs is high; the positive-pressure air will preferentially go down the trachea, across the fistula, and into the stomach. This causes gastric distention with greater risk for aspiration of GI secretions and more difficulty with diaphragm movement.
  3. Placement of gastrostomy tube only; indicated in two general situations:
     a. Palliation for an infant with either complex congenital heart disease or extreme low birth weight (less than 1000 g) who does not have significant respiratory difficulty; the gastrostomy helps prevent the spillover of gastric contents into the trachea during the period required for care of the cardiac lesion and/or prematurity.

b. In a patient with pure EA and without a fistula (gasless abdomen), the distance between the upper and lower esophageal segments is too great to allow for repair in the newborn period. A gastrostomy in this case allows for feeding until the patient is of sufficient size (approximately 20 pounds) to reestablish esophageal continuity using either a colon interposition or a tubular raised portion of stomach to form a neoesophagus.

4. Older infant with TEF and without EA
   a. Neck incision with division and repair of the fistula (thoracotomy not usually necessary)

■ FOLLOW-UP & DISPOSITION

Patient outcome is most influenced by the presence or absence of and the severity of associated anomalies. In most patients with the most common anomaly, oral feedings are begun after a water-soluble contrast study has excluded a leak or stricture at the site of the EA. This study is usually performed from 5 to 10 days postoperatively.

■ PATIENT/FAMILY EDUCATION

- The survival rate is 97% for infants without a major congenital heart disease and birth weight of more than 1500 g.
- The survival rate is 22% for infants who have major congenital heart disease or birth weight of less than 1500 g.

- Possible long-term sequelae of repaired EA and TEF include the following:
  1. GER is very common. This problem often requires antireflux surgery to correct.
  2. Esophageal stricture occurs in 30% to 40% of patients at either the anastomosis or the lower esophageal segment. The cause of this complication may be chronic GER with acid injury to the esophagus or ischemia at the anastomosis.
  3. Recurrent TEF occurs in 3% to 10% of patients.
     a. Presents with recurrent upper respiratory infections, wheezing, pneumonia, choking, or cyanosis with feeds
  4. Tracheomalacia occurs in 10% to 20% of patients.
     a. Difficult to distinguish from GER or recurrent TEF
  5. Esophageal motility problem is almost universal.
     a. Esophageal clearance is delayed.
     b. Clearance may become more of a problem as diet is advanced to more solid foods.

■ REFERRAL INFORMATION

A board-certified pediatric surgeon should manage all infants and children with this anomaly, with the ready availability of pediatric subspecialists, including those from neonatology, anesthesia, urology, neurosurgery, gastroenterology, and cardiology.

⚙ PEARLS & CONSIDERATIONS

■ WEBSITES

- American Academy of Family Physicians: www.aafp.org/afp/990215ap/910.html; an overview of this anomaly along with pictures and references
- EA/TEF: www.eatef.org; the major family support organization
- Family Village: www.familyvillage.wisc.edu/lib_ea-tef.html; family support groups with many helpful links

REFERENCES

1. Dillon PW, Cilley RE: Newborn surgical emergencies: gastrointestinal anomalies, abdominal wall defects, *Pediatr Clin North Am* 40:1289, 1993.
2. Engum SA et al: Analysis of morbidity and mortality in 227 cases of esophageal atresia and/or tracheoesophageal fistula over two decades, *Arch Surg* 130:502, 1995.
3. Foglia RP: Esophageal disease in the pediatric age group, *Chest Surg Clin North Am* 4:785, 1994.
4. Martin LW, Alexander F: Esophageal atresia, *Surg Clin North Am* 65:1099, 1985.
5. Spitz L: Esophageal atresia: past, present, and future, *J Pediatr Surg* 31:19, 1996.
6. Spitz L et al: Oesophageal atresia: at-risk groups for the 1990s, *J Pediatr Surg* 29:723, 1994.

Author: **Brad W. Warner, M.D.**

II

BASIC INFORMATION

DEFINITION

Ewing's sarcoma family of tumors consists of malignancies of neural origin, arising from postganglionic parasympathetic cholinergic neurons. This family of tumors includes Ewing's tumor of bone (87%), extraosseous Ewing's (8%), and peripheral primitive neuroectodermal tumors (PNET) (5%). A PNET of the chest wall is specifically known as an *Askin's tumor*.

ICD-9CM CODE

170.9 Malignant neoplasm of bone and articular cartilage

ETIOLOGY

- No environmental risk factors are identified.
- Reports of Ewing's tumors in patients with congenital abnormalities, constitutional chromosomal abnormalities, or skeletal abnormalities are probably the result of chance.
- Characteristic chromosomal translocation t(11:22) is present in 88% to 95% of Ewing's tumors and produces an aberrant transcription factor.

EPIDEMIOLOGY & DEMOGRAPHICS

- Ewing's sarcoma represents 3% of pediatric cancer.
- There are 200 cases per year in the United States.
- It is the most common malignant bone tumor in children younger than 10 years of age.
- The incidence is 2 to 3 per 1 million per year in whites; it is very rare in African Americans.
- Twenty-seven percent of patients are diagnosed in the first decade of life, 64% in the second decade, and 9% in the third decade.
- The incidence is slightly greater in males than in females.
- Primary sites are as follows:
  1. Central: 47%
     a. Pelvis: 45%
     b. Chest wall: 34%
     c. Spine/paravertebral: 12%
     d. Head/neck: 9%
  2. Extremity: 53%
     a. Distal: 52%
     b. Proximal: 48%

HISTORY

- Pain
- Mass lesion
- Limited range of motion
- Pathologic fracture
- Systemic symptoms, including fever and fatigue
- Respiratory distress caused by chest tumor or pleural effusion

PHYSICAL EXAMINATION

- A mass may be palpable.
- Central axis lesions, such as pelvic primaries, may not be palpable.
- Decreased breath sounds may be heard in patients with Askin's tumor.

DIAGNOSIS

DIFFERENTIAL DIAGNOSIS

- Osteosarcoma
  1. Ewing's sarcoma more likely if central axis or diaphyseal lesion
- Other primary or metastatic malignancy, including rhabdomyosarcoma and other soft tissue sarcomas, lymphoma, and metastatic neuroblastoma
- Infection
- Benign bone tumors

DIAGNOSTIC WORKUP

- Magnetic resonance imaging (MRI) of primary lesion
- Chest radiograph
- Computed tomography (CT) of the chest
- Bilateral bone marrow aspirates and biopsies
- Bone scan
- Biopsy of primary lesion (initial resection usually not possible or recommended)

THERAPY

MEDICAL

- Chemotherapy: The current standard is alternating cycles of vincristine/doxorubicin/cyclophosphamide and ifosfamide/VP-16.
- Other active agents include topotecan.

SURGICAL

Option for surgical removal may be considered if the lesion is resectable without resulting in unacceptable cosmetic or functional impairment.

RADIATION THERAPY

Radiation may be used in place of surgery for unresectable tumors or in addition to surgery if the resection is not complete or if tumor is found too close to the margins of resection.

PROGNOSIS

- The most significant adverse prognostic factor is the presence of metastatic disease. In patients with metastases, 38% have lung nodules, 31% have bone lesions, and 11% have marrow involvement. Of patients with chest wall tumors, 12%

have pleural effusion with or without malignant cells on cytopathologic examination.
- Response to treatment also correlates with survival.
- Current prognosis is as follows:
  1. Between 50% and 70% 5-year survival for localized disease
  2. Less than 30% 5-year survival in patients with metastatic disease

FOLLOW-UP & DISPOSITION

- An MRI/CT scan of the primary lesion, chest radiograph, CT chest scan, and bone scan are generally done every 3 months for 1 year after completion of therapy, then every 4 to 6 months for 2 years, then every year until 10 years off therapy.
- The late effects of chemotherapy may include renal tubular dysfunction, cardiomyopathy, infertility or early menopause, and secondary malignancies, including leukemia and bladder cancer.
- The late effects of radiation depend on the radiation field but may include hypoplasia, leg length discrepancy, hair loss, gonadal failure, and secondary malignancy.

REFERRAL INFORMATION

Patients, including adults younger than 30 years of age, should be referred to pediatric oncologists and treated on formal protocol therapy, if available. Treatment decisions should be made in conjunction with radiation oncologists and surgeons with appropriate oncologic expertise.

PEARLS & CONSIDERATIONS

CLINICAL PEARLS

- Any persistent pain, even after trauma, merits further evaluation, as does pain associated with a mass lesion.
- Because adult oncologists rarely see patients with Ewing's sarcoma, young adults with this disease should be referred to pediatric oncologists.

WEBSITES

- American Cancer Society: www.cancer.org
- National Cancer Institute: www.nci.nih.gov
- OncoLink: University of Pennsylvania Cancer Center: http://oncolink.com

■ SUPPORT GROUPS

Pediatric oncologists can refer patients and parents to local and national organizations for children with cancer and their families. National organizations include the American Cancer Society and Candlelighters.

REFERENCES

1. Buckley JD et al: Epidemiology of osteosarcoma and Ewing's sarcoma in childhood, *Cancer* 83:1440, 1998.
2. Crist WM, Kun LE: Common solid tumors of childhood, *N Engl J Med* 324:461, 1991.
3. Halperin EC et al: Ewing's sarcoma. In Halperin EC et al (eds): *Pediatric radiation oncology,* ed 3, Philadelphia, 1999, Lippincott Williams & Wilkins.
4. Horowitz ME et al: Ewing's sarcoma family of tumors: Ewing's sarcoma of bone and soft tissue and the peripheral primitive neuroectodermal tumors. In Pizzo PA, Poplack DG (eds): *Principles and practice of pediatric oncology,* ed 3, Philadelphia, 1997, JB Lippincott.

Author: **Andrea Hinkle, M.D.**

II

BASIC INFORMATION

■ DEFINITION
Extrahepatic biliary atresia is a fibro-obliterative destructive process involving the extrahepatic biliary tree, which occurs in the first 2 months of life.

■ SYNONYM
Biliary atresia

ICD-9CM CODE
751.61 Extrahepatic biliary atresia

■ ETIOLOGY
- Unknown
- Current hypotheses include the following:
  1. Pathologic interaction between immune response and viral infection (e.g., reovirus, rotavirus)
  2. Malformation syndrome for polysplenia-associated form (less than 20% of cases)

■ EPIDEMIOLOGY & DEMOGRAPHICS
- 1 in 10,000 to 1 in 15,000 live births
- Male = female
- Term infants
- Typically not inherited

■ HISTORY
- Healthy infant
- Persistent jaundice for more than 3 weeks
- Dark urine or pale stools

■ PHYSICAL EXAMINATION
- Healthy infant
- Jaundice
- Typically without apparent associated malformations (more than 80% of cases)
- Hepatomegaly with or without splenomegaly
- Rectal examination that reveals acholic stools

■ MALFORMATIONS ASSOCIATED WITH POLYSPLENIA SYNDROME
- Laterality sequence
  1. Polysplenia
  2. Abdominal situs inversus
  3. Intestinal malrotation
  4. Anomalous portal/hepatic veins (e.g., preduodenal portal vein)
  5. Complex cardiac malformations
- Nonlaterality anomalies
  1. Cardiac (e.g., ventricular septal defect, common atrioventricular canal)
  2. Urinary tract (e.g., solitary kidney, horseshoe kidney)
  3. Gastrointestinal (e.g., Meckel's diverticulum)
  4. Facial (e.g., cleft lip/palate, choanal atresia)

■ DIAGNOSIS

■ DIFFERENTIAL DIAGNOSIS
See Differential Diagnosis in Part I in the section "Jaundice/Hyperbilirubinemia."
- Essential diseases to exclude before surgical repair include the following:
  1. Cystic fibrosis
  2. α_1-Antitrypsin deficiency
  3. Alagille's syndrome

■ DIAGNOSTIC WORKUP
- See Diagnostic Algorithm Part I, Hyperbilirubinemia.
- Diagnostic studies that may suggest extrahepatic biliary atresia include the following:
  1. Liver biopsy (bile duct proliferation, portal expansion, bile duct plugs)
  2. Hepatobiliary excretory scan (e.g., HIDA scan, nonexcretion)
  3. Fasting abdominal ultrasound (absent or hypoplastic gallbladder; *note:* finding of gallbladder or description of common bile duct does not exclude biliary atresia)
- The ultimate diagnosis is made at the time of exploratory laparotomy, with demonstration of destruction of the extrahepatic biliary tree.

■ THERAPY

■ SURGICAL
- Hepatoportoenterostomy (Kasai procedure)
- Potential variants
  1. Gallbladder Kasai
  2. Kasai procedure with ostomy
  3. Kasai procedure with intussusception antireflux valve

■ FOLLOW-UP & DISPOSITION
- Overall results
  1. Complete drainage (postoperative total bilirubin less than 2 mg/dl): Long-term palliation may result in development of biliary cirrhosis over 10 to 20 years.
  2. Incomplete drainage (postoperative total bilirubin 2 to 5 mg/dl): Short-term palliation may result in development of biliary cirrhosis over 2 to 10 years.
  3. Failed procedure (postoperative bilirubin more than 8 mg/dl): Liver failure in 6 to 18 months necessitates immediate liver transplant evaluation.
- Potential postoperative complications include the following:
  1. Cholangitis
  2. Cholestasis
     a. Malabsorption
     b. Pruritus
     c. Xanthoma/xanthelasma
  3. Failure to thrive
  4. Portal hypertension
  5. Synthetic liver failure

■ SPECIAL CONCERNS & POSTOPERATIVE MEDICAL THERAPY
- Cholangitis
  1. Empiric prophylactic antibiotics have not been proven to be beneficial but are used by many.
- Cholestasis
  1. Poor drainage: Empiric ursodeoxycholic acid and steroid boluses have been used.
  2. Malnutrition: Formulas containing medium-chain triglycerides and fat-soluble vitamin supplementation (augmented by d-α-tocopheryl polyethylene glycol 1000 succinate vitamin E) are standard therapy.
  3. Pruritus: Several regimens exist, including ursodeoxycholic acid, rifampin, cholestyramine, and opioid antagonists (antihistamines are commonly used and are relatively ineffective).

■ PATIENT/FAMILY EDUCATION
- Prediagnosis
  1. It is essential to alert parents in well-baby consultation that jaundice persisting beyond 2 weeks of age requires medical follow-up.
  2. The optimal time for surgical treatment is before 60 days of age.
- Postdiagnosis/surgery
  1. The overall prognosis with surgery is good, but a portoenterostomy is typically palliative, with transplantation being the ultimate long-term therapy.
  2. Fever, jaundice, and acholic stools postoperatively can be a sign of cholangitis, which requires immediate therapy.
  3. Hematochezia, hematemesis, or melena requires urgent attention.

■ REFERRAL INFORMATION
- All children with clinically significant direct hyperbilirubinemia should be immediately referred to a pediatric gastroenterologist or a pediatric surgeon for evaluation.
- The following complications should initiate a referral for liver transplant evaluation:
  1. Total bilirubin more than 5 mg/dl 6 months after portoenterostomy
  2. Intractable cholangitis
  3. Failure to thrive
  4. Variceal hemorrhage
  5. Abdominal ascites
  6. Liver synthetic dysfunction

☼ PEARLS & CONSIDERATIONS

■ CLINICAL PEARLS
- Jaundice at birth or jaundice persisting beyond 3 weeks of age requires exclusion of significant liver disease.
- The infant must be NPO (nothing by mouth) for more than 4 hours before abdominal ultrasound.
- Pigmented stools or the finding of a gallbladder on ultrasound does not exclude biliary atresia.
- Always exclude cystic fibrosis, α_1-antitrypsin deficiency, and Alagille's syndrome before performing a portoenterostomy.

■ WEBSITES
- American Gastroenterological Association: www.gastro.org/lliverpg/atresia.htm
- Children's Liver Alliance: www.livertx.org/biliaryatresia.html

■ SUPPORT GROUPS
- American Liver Foundation
- Children's Liver Alliance

REFERENCES

1. Balistreri WF et al: Biliary atresia: current concepts and research directions, *Hepatology* 23:1682, 1996.
2. Chardot C et al: Prognosis of biliary atresia in the era of liver transplantation: French national study from 1986 to 1996, *Hepatology* 30:606, 1999.
3. Davenport M et al: Biliary atresia: the King's College Hospital experience (1974-1995), *J Pediatr Surg* 32:479, 1997.
4. Karrer FM et al: Long term results with the Kasai procedure for biliary atresia, *Arch Surg* 131:493, 1996.
5. McEvoy CF, Suchy FJ: Biliary tract disease in children, *Pediatr Clin North Am* 43:75, 1996.

Author: **Benjamin L. Shneider, M.D.**

II

BASIC INFORMATION

■ DEFINITION
Failure to thrive (FTT) is subnormal growth, regardless of cause, but usually excluding known hormonal or genetic syndromes. Criteria for FTT include low (typically less than the fifth percentile) weight-for-age, weight-for-height, or height-for-age on standard (Centers for Disease Control and Prevention [CDC]) growth charts. Lower-than-expected weight gain for age and current weight and declining growth percentiles also indicate FTT. There is no single agreed-upon criterion. *Nonorganic FTT* typically implies neglect or abuse, but all FTT has an organic component (i.e., malnutrition), and *organic FTT* often has a behavioral component. FTT is a clinical sign, not a specific diagnosis. Uncorrected, FTT may cause long-term cognitive and behavioral impairments.

■ SYNONYMS
- Wasting (below-normal weight-for-height)
- Stunting (below-normal height-for-age)
- Growth delay or growth failure

ICD-9CM CODE
783.4 Failure to thrive

■ ETIOLOGY
One of the following, or more commonly, a combination of the following:
- Inadequate intake: food not available, not offered, or refused, or excessive intake of low-calorie food
  1. These issues may be caused by psychosocial/family stressors, subtle oral-motor deficits, parent-child relationship problems, an acquired food aversion, and neglect or abuse.
  2. These issues occur in approximately 80% of diagnoses.
- Excessive losses: vomiting (e.g., pyloric stenosis, gastroesophageal reflux), chronic diarrhea, malabsorption (e.g., cystic fibrosis, short-gut syndrome, gluten enteropathy)
- Inefficient utilization: hypothyroidism, cyanotic heart disease, genetic syndromes, "psychosocial dwarfism" (rare)
- Increased needs: congenital heart disease, hyperthyroidism, immunodeficiency, other chronic illnesses

■ EPIDEMIOLOGY & DEMOGRAPHICS
- 1% to 2% of hospitalized children
- 5% to 10% of children in poverty
- Age birth to 5 typical
- Males = females

■ HISTORY
- Medical
  1. Prenatal care, infections, exposures, labor and delivery course
  2. Early growth pattern and age of onset of delays
  3. Central nervous system: swallowing difficulty (choking), tactile hypersensitivity
  4. Respiratory: snoring, shortness of breath, chronic cough
  5. Cardiovascular: exercise or feeding intolerance
  6. Gastrointestinal: choking, spitting, vomiting, constipation, greasy or pale stools, excessive gas, distention
  7. Infectious diseases: travel, exposures (e.g., living in shelter), recurrent infections
  8. Allergy: food, environmental reactions, atopy
  9. Family history: genetic diseases, atopy, parental heights and weights
- Nutritional
  1. 24-hour diet recall
  2. Who is responsible for feeding/food preparation?
  3. Formula preparation, juice intake, milk intake
  4. Introduction of solids, timing, any special reaction
  5. Feeding pattern, feeding behaviors, feeding environment (e.g., highchair, TV, others at table, typical events surrounding mealtime)
- Developmental
  1. Milestones, especially gross motor, fine motor, language, self-care, autonomy
  2. Family history of developmental delays
  3. Services in place (e.g., early intervention)
  4. Results of screening questionnaires or tests
- Social/emotional
  1. Family, home constellation, child care (center-based versus family child care)
  2. Financial status, food availability
  3. Separations, trauma (e.g., physical or emotional injury; witness to violence, particularly family violence)
  4. Maternal mental health: depression, substance use, abuse history

■ PHYSICAL EXAMINATION
- Mild FTT may not be apparent, except on growth charts (cheeks often remain chubby even with moderate wasting)
- Signs of moderate to severe malnutrition: decreased energy, thin arms and legs, dry skin, sparse or lanugo hair
- Signs of underlying disorders (often absent): neurologic abnormality, adenoidal facies, dental lesions, heart murmur, clubbing, abdominal distention, surgical scars

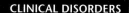

DIAGNOSIS

■ DIAGNOSTIC WORKUP
- Limit screening laboratory tests to a few common ones.
  1. Complete blood count and differential (anemia and decreased lymphocytes as sign of malnutrition, elevated white blood cell count as sign of chronic infection)
  2. Electrolytes (metabolic acidosis as cause or complication)
  3. Urinalysis and culture (chronic infection)
  4. Purified protein derivative (for tuberculosis) and controls (if exposure possible)
  5. Lead (if exposure possible)
- Other investigations as indicated by history (Table 2-7)
- The best index of acute malnutrition is the patient's weight as a percentage of the ideal weight (fiftieth percentile) on the weight-for-height curve. (The "weight-for-height" percentages are shown in Table 2-8.)

THERAPY

- Treat underlying medical diagnoses.
- Intensity of therapy is tied to the severity of undernutrition.
- Level I (primary provider alone)
  1. Nutritional counseling to increase caloric density of feedings (whole milk, cream, added fats and oils; limit of lower-calorie beverages)
  2. Daily multivitamin with zinc and iron
     a. Zinc deficiency results from undernutrition and causes taste bud dysfunction.
  3. Guidance to improve mealtime structure and behaviors: three meals and three snacks, highchair, turn off TV, mild approval for eating, no forced feedings
  4. Close monitoring; if no catch-up, move to level II
- Level II (outpatient team)
  1. Home visits by nutritionist and social worker to assess mealtime interactions and environment and to intervene in patient's environment
  2. Referral for developmental and behavioral intervention (e.g., center- or home-based early intervention program)

TABLE 2-7 Historical Clues

HISTORY	DIAGNOSTIC CONSIDERATION	INVESTIGATION
Spitting, vomiting	Gastroesophageal reflux	Upper gastrointestinal series, pH probe, esophagoscopy
Abdominal distention, cramping, diarrhea	Malabsorption (e.g., cystic fibrosis, celiac disease, lactase deficiency)	D-Xylose test, stool fat, antigliadin titer or biopsy, sweat chloride*
Travel to or from developing country; homeless, overcrowded, or living in shelter	Parasitosis (especially *Giardia*), tuberculosis, inadequate access to cooking facility and refrigeration	Stool O & P, duodenal biopsy, string test, PPD
Snoring, periodic breathing during sleep, restless sleep, noisy or mouth breathing	Adenoid hypertrophy	Lateral neck film (soft tissues and airway)
"Asthma"	Chronic aspiration, cystic fibrosis	Chest film, milk scan, sweat chloride*
Frequent (minor) infections	HIV, other immune deficiency	Serologic tests, immunoglobulins,* PPD with control for anergy*

HIV, Human immunodeficiency virus; *O & P*, stool for ova and parasites; *PPD*, purified protein derivative.
*May be abnormal secondary to malnutrition.

TABLE 2-8 Grading Severity of Failure to Thrive (FTT)

WEIGHT-FOR-HEIGHT PERCENTAGE	GRADE OF UNDERNUTRITION	SEVERITY	LEVEL OF CARE
Ideal			
≥90	0	Pre-FTT or normal	I: Outpatient management by primary physician
≥80 to <90	1	Mild	I or II: Consider adding home visiting, social work
≥70 to <80	2	Moderate	II or III: Consider hospitalization
<70	3	Severe	III: Hospitalize immediately

Adapted from Waterlow.

3. Recruitment of community supports (e.g., parent support groups, respite, parent mental health treatment) as needed
4. Continued close monitoring; if no catch-up, consideration of moving to level III care
- Level III (multidisciplinary in-hospital team or day hospital)
  1. Intensive feeding therapy
  2. Intensive parent support, parent training, and family intervention
  3. Consideration of referral to tertiary care facility with established FTT team

- Move more quickly to higher levels of care depending on child's age and grade of undernutrition (see Table 2-8).

☼ PEARLS & CONSIDERATIONS

■ CLINICAL PEARLS
- The term *failure to thrive* puts parents on the defensive; they tend to see it as their own failure.
- The term *growth deficiency* is less stigmatizing.

- Use a flowchart to track weight and weight gain in grams per day (see Table 2-9) to avoid undertreating.
- Multimodal, coordinated team management works better for established FTT.
- Avoid the temptation to order "shotgun" testing, but aggressively follow up on any hint from the history or physical examination.
- Remember to work simultaneously in four areas: medical, nutritional, developmental, and social.

TABLE 2-9   Expected Weight Gain

AGE	MEDIAN DAILY WEIGHT GAIN (g)	CATCH-UP GROWTH (120% OF AVERAGE g/DAY)	INCREASE LEVEL OF CARE IF NO CATCH-UP BY THIS TIME INTERVAL
0-3 mo	26-31	34	1 wk
≥3-6 mo	17-18	21	2 wk
≥6-9 mo	12-13	15	1 mo
≥9-12 mo	9	11	1 mo
≥1-3 yr	7-9	10	2 mo
≥3-6 yr	5-6	7	3 mo

Adapted from Frank DA et al: *Recommended dietary allowances,* Washington, DC, 1993, National Academy of Sciences, Food and Nutrition Board

REFERENCES
1. Drotar D: Failure to thrive. In Routh D (ed): *Handbook of pediatric psychology,* New York, 1988, Guildford Press.
2. Frank DA, Zeisel SH: Failure to thrive, *Pediatr Clin North Am* 35:1187, 1988.
3. Sills RH: Failure to thrive: the role of clinical and laboratory evaluation, *Am J Dis Child* 139:967, 1978.
4. Kessler D, Dawson P (eds): *Failure to thrive and pediatric undernutrition: a transdisciplinary approach,* Philadelphia, 1999, Paul H Brookes.
5. Waterlow JC: Classification and definition of protein-calorie malnutrition, *Br Med J* 3:566, 1972.

Author: **Robert Needlman, M.D.**

BASIC INFORMATION

DEFINITION

A febrile seizure is one occurring in the presence of fever higher than 38.0° C in a child between the ages of 6 months and 6 years of age. Excluded are patients with a history of afebrile seizures, electrolyte abnormality, or central nervous system (CNS) infection. Simple febrile seizures last less than 15 minutes, are generalized, and if occurring in a series, have a total duration less than 30 minutes. Complex febrile seizures last more than 15 minutes, are focal, or occur in a series with total duration longer than 30 minutes.

SYNONYM

Febrile convulsions

ICD-9CM CODE

780.31 Febrile seizure

ETIOLOGY

Genetic factors play a role in expression.
- Single febrile seizure: polygenic model
- Multiple episodes: dominant with incomplete penetrance

EPIDEMIOLOGY & DEMOGRAPHICS

- Occurs in 2% to 4% of children
- At least 2.5 times incidence in first-degree relatives compared with random population

HISTORY

- Most febrile seizures occur on the first day of illness.
- The seizure is often the presenting symptom.
- Most febrile seizures are of the simple type (90%), with brief bilateral clonic or tonic-clonic movements and no postictal paralysis or prolonged somnolence.

PHYSICAL EXAMINATION

- Examination findings may demonstrate a focus of infection.
- Assess neurologic examination carefully:
  1. Mental status
  2. Meningeal signs
  3. Focal neurologic deficits

DIAGNOSIS

DIFFERENTIAL DIAGNOSIS

- Most important differential diagnosis is meningitis or encephalitis.
- Chills are fine, rhythmic, oscillatory movements about a joint, not clonic in nature.
- Focal febrile seizures may need to be differentiated from seizures caused by CNS mass lesions (e.g., tumor, intracranial bleeding).

DIAGNOSTIC WORKUP

- Routine laboratory studies (including neuroimaging and electroencephalogram [EEG]) are not indicated in most cases of simple febrile seizures.
- Examination of cerebrospinal fluid should be carried out according to the following guidelines:
  1. Lumbar puncture should be strongly considered in any infant younger than 12 months of age because clinical signs of meningitis are not reliable in this age group.
     a. Between 12 and 18 months, lumbar puncture should be considered.
     b. Older than 18 months, lumbar puncture is indicated only when meningeal signs are present or if an adequate neurologic examination cannot be performed.
- If clinically indicated, obtain a complete blood count and blood and urine cultures (to rule out bacteremia and urinary tract infection).
- Complex febrile seizures may warrant further investigation when indicated.
  1. Stat blood glucose, electrolytes, Ca^{2+}, Mg^{2+} if prolonged seizure or postictal somnolence
  2. EEG and/or computed tomography/magnetic resonance imaging scan of the head if a focal seizure or persistent neurologic deficit is detected.

THERAPY

NONPHARMACOLOGIC

Protection of the airway is the most important therapeutic intervention in the seizing child.
- Provide oxygen.
- Position the head.

MEDICAL

- Administer antipyretics, such as acetaminophen 15 mg/kg orally or rectally; ibuprofen 8 to 10 mg/kg orally.
- Any patient with a seizure lasting more than 15 minutes should be treated with midazolam 0.1 mg/kg intravenously or rectally; the dose may be repeated two more times in 5-minute intervals if the seizure persists.
- Administer dilantin 15 to 20 mg/kg intravenously slow load if midazolam is ineffective.
- Administer phenobarbital 15 to 20 mg/kg intravenously slow load for recalcitrant seizures.

FOLLOW-UP & DISPOSITION

- The child should be observed until both the health care provider and parents are satisfied with the child's appearance after the temperature is reduced.
- Follow-up may be needed if blood and urine cultures are obtained.

PATIENT/FAMILY EDUCATION

- For simple febrile seizures, there is no risk of brain injury.
- Most simple febrile seizures do not indicate any underlying brain abnormality.
- Overall, the risk of recurrence of febrile seizures is 30%; future risk is inversely proportional to the age of first episode.
- The incidence of subsequent epilepsy in children having a febrile seizure is increased (1%) compared with the incidence of epilepsy in the general population (0.5%).
- The risks of recurrence of febrile seizures and/or development of subsequent epilepsy are increased in children with a history of developmental delay and/or complex febrile seizures.

PREVENTIVE TREATMENT

- Early administration of antipyretics during febrile illnesses is advocated; however, their efficacy is limited.
- Daily prophylactic use of anticonvulsants has a very limited role.
  1. Modest efficacy (66% reduction in recurrence) must be weighed against adverse effects on behavior and sleep patterns.
  2. Prophylactic anticonvulsant treatment does not appear to reduce the sequelae of prolonged seizures or subsequent development of epilepsy.
  3. The first-line prophylactic anticonvulsant is phenobarbital.
- Rectal administration of diazepam at the time of febrile illness is also a treatment option.

REFERRAL INFORMATION

Consultation with a pediatric neurologist is recommended in the following cases:
- For most cases of complex febrile seizures
- When considering use of prophylactic anticonvulsant for recurrent febrile seizures

☼ PEARLS & CONSIDERATIONS

■ CLINICAL PEARLS

A brief, generalized seizure from which the child recovers quickly to baseline neurologic status is unlikely to be caused by meningitis.

■ WEBSITE

Epilepsy Foundation of America:
www.efa.org/news/fever.html

REFERENCES

1. Fenichel GM: *Clinical pediatric neurology,* ed 2, Philadelphia, 1993, WB Saunders.
2. Oski FA: *Principles and practice of pediatrics,* Philadelphia, 1994, JB Lippincott.
3. Practice parameter: the neurodiagnostic evaluation of the child with a first simple febrile seizure, *Pediatrics* 97: 769, 1996.

Author: **Paul Lehoullier, M.D.**

BASIC INFORMATION

■ **DEFINITION**
Fibromyalgia syndrome is diffuse pain and the presence of tender points (as demonstrated on physical examination) in association with other symptoms (see the following discussion), but in the absence of inflammatory or other disease that could account for the discomfort.

■ **SYNONYMS**
• Juvenile primary fibromyalgia
• Fibrositis
• Fibromyositis

ICD-9CM CODE
729.0 Fibromyalgia syndrome

■ **EPIDEMIOLOGY & DEMOGRAPHICS**
• Fibromyalgia predominantly affects adolescents and older white women.
• Few studies have studied prevalence in children.
  1. One cross-sectional analysis of 338 schoolchildren 9 to 15 years of age yielded a prevalence of 6%.
  2. Others have suggested a lower prevalence of 2%.

■ **HISTORY**
At time of diagnosis, patients typically describe a gradual accumulation of the following:
• Widespread pain (above and below the waist and on both the right and left sides of the body) of the soft tissues, muscles, and tendons
• Fatigue
• Restless and/or nonrestorative sleep
• Headache
• Depressed mood
• Dizziness
• Abdominal pain and irritable bowel-like symptoms
• Dysmenorrhea
• Subjective swelling of hands
• Paresthesias in extremities

■ **PHYSICAL EXAMINATION**
• The only abnormality is the presence of tender points in any of the 18 symmetric and characteristic sites.
• Diagnostic criteria for fibromyalgia in adults stipulate at least 11 of 18 tender points.
  1. In adolescents, fewer points are more usual.
  2. Examination technique calls for palpation with 4 kg of pressure.

 DIAGNOSIS

■ **DIFFERENTIAL DIAGNOSIS**
• Myofascial pain syndrome
• Chronic fatigue syndrome
• Depression
• Thyroid disease
• Hypermobility syndrome
• Somatization disorder

■ **DIAGNOSTIC WORKUP**
• Laboratory studies are normal, including complete blood count with differential, erythrocyte sedimentation rate, and creatine phosphokinase.
• Radiographs are normal.
• Muscle biopsy is without signs of inflammation.

THERAPY

■ **NONPHARMACOLOGIC**
• Initiate a consistent sleep/wake schedule.
• Encourage regular, moderate exercise.
• Explore psychotherapy options.
• Reinstitute a daily routine, school attendance, and so forth.

■ **MEDICAL**
• Consider low-dose tricyclic medication at 1 to 2 hours before bedtime to restore restful sleep.
• Consider a low-dose selective serotonin reuptake inhibitor, particularly in association with significant depression.
• Nonsteroidal antiinflammatory drugs are not usually beneficial but are sometimes useful.

■ **FOLLOW-UP & DISPOSITION**
• Patients require regular contact with providers, and improvement occurs gradually.
• Despite attainment of remission, recurrence of symptoms is common, particularly in times of stress and/or with erratic sleep/wake schedules.

■ **PATIENT/FAMILY EDUCATION**
• It is important to point out that the response to treatment and prognosis for adolescents tends to be better than that for adults.
• Beware of unsubstantiated, nonpeer-reviewed information.
• Involvement of family in the treatment plan is helpful.

■ **PREVENTIVE TREATMENT**
Anticipation of stressful events and/or disruption of sleep/wake schedule as a time to intensify therapy can decrease the severity and duration of disease flare.

■ **REFERRAL INFORMATION**
Referral to a physical therapist, occupational therapist, and/or psychotherapist/counselor may be necessary.

PEARLS & CONSIDERATIONS

■ **CLINICAL PEARLS**
• Adolescents may have only a few tender points.
• Palpation of tender points requires significant pressure (4 kg).
• A consistent sleep/wake schedule (even on weekends) is important.
• Every effort should be made to have the patient attend school.

■ **WEBSITE**
Arthritis Foundation: www.arthritis.org

REFERENCES
1. Ballinger SH, Bowyer SL: Fibromyalgia: the latest great imitator, *Contemp Pediatr* 14:140, 1997.
2. Siegel DM, Janeway D, Baum J: Fibromyalgia syndrome in children and adolescents, clinical features a presentation and status at follow-up, *Pediatrics* 101:377, 1998.
3. Wolfe F et al. The American College of Rheumatology 1990 Criteria for the Classification of Fibromyalgia, *Arthritis Rheum* 33:160, 1990.
Author: **David M. Siegel, M.D., M.P.H.**

II

BASIC INFORMATION

■ DEFINITION

Folliculitis is the superficial or deep inflammation of the hair follicle as a result of infection, physical injury, or chemical injury. Furuncles (or boils) represent deep bacterial folliculitis. They are painful, circumscribed perifollicular abscesses that have a tendency to central necrosis and suppuration. Carbuncles may be considered large, deep-seated abscesses made up of aggregates of interconnected furuncles that drain at multiple points on the cutaneous surface.

■ SYNONYMS

- Sycosis barbae (folliculitis barbae): when in the bearded area
- Bockharts impetigo: superficial folliculitis

ICD-9CM CODES

704.8 Folliculitis
680.9 Furunculosis (deep folliculitis)
680.9 Carbuncle

■ ETIOLOGY

- Superficial infectious folliculitis
  1. Bacterial
     a. Often found to contain normal skin flora
     b. *Staphylococcus aureus*
     c. *Pseudomonas aeruginosa*
     d. Others (rare): *Streptococcus, Proteus,* coliform bacteria
  2. Fungal
     a. *Pityrosporum ovale* (Malassezia)
     b. *Candida albicans* (immunocompromised patients)
  3. Viral
     a. Herpes simplex viruses types 1 and 2
     b. Varicella-zoster virus
- Superficial noninfectious folliculitis
  1. Caused by obstruction of pilosebaceous follicles, resulting in follicular plugging and inflammation (may become secondarily infected)
     a. Steroid acne (actually often caused by *Pityrosporum ovale*)
     b. Occlusive dressings with polyethylene or adhesive
     c. Occupational contact with oils
     d. Occupational or therapeutic contact with tars
     e. Complication of any epilation method (e.g., shaving, waxing, depilatory creams, electrolysis, electric rotating coil devices)
- Deep folliculitis (furunculosis)
  1. *S. aureus*
  2. Gram-negative organisms (rare)
  3. Eosinophilic pustular folliculitis (Ofuji disease) in immunocompromised patients

■ EPIDEMIOLOGY & DEMOGRAPHICS

- Folliculitis, furuncles, and carbuncles occur most commonly on hair-bearing areas of the skin that are subject to friction, perspiration, and maceration.
  1. Particularly face, scalp, back of the neck, axillae, buttocks, and perineum
  2. Other predisposing factors: hyperhidrosis and preexisting dermatitis
  3. Reduced host resistance also a risk factor
     a. Diabetes mellitus
     b. Immunodeficiencies
- The incidence is not known.
  1. Some forms, such as folliculitis barbae, are thought to be extremely common.
  2. Other forms (e.g., after epilation methods) are rare.
- Demodex mites are an extremely common infestation in humans.
  1. Some studies have shown a clear association with histologic and clinical folliculitis.
  2. It is not clear if the Demodex is causative or preferentially selects follicles with inflammation.

■ HISTORY

- *Pseudomonas* folliculitis occurs after exposure to whirlpools, hot tubs, and less commonly, community swimming pools and water slides.
- Cases have been reported after use of contaminated recreational diving suits, synthetic and loofah sponges, and after skin epilation.

■ PHYSICAL EXAMINATION

- The manifestations of infection of the hair follicle vary clinically with the location and depth of follicular involvement.
  1. Superficial folliculitis (Bockharts impetigo) is an infection at the follicular orifice.
     a. Tiny, superficial red papules or dome-shaped, thin-walled yellow pustules
     b. 1 to 2 mm in diameter
     c. Painless but may be pruritic
     d. Occur in crops
     e. Heal in 7 to 10 days
  2. *Pseudomonas* folliculitis is characterized by discrete pruritic papules and erythematous papulopustular lesions.
     a. Usually develop within 1 to 2 days of exposure
     b. Greatest density on areas of the body covered by bathing suits
- Furunculosis appears as a tender, erythematous nodule.
  1. Furunculosis is circumscribed, perifollicular abscesses.

2. The overlying skin becomes thin and tense.
3. The abscess tends to become centrally necrotic, leaving a core of pus.
4. Healing often results in a slightly depressed scar.
- Confluence of two or more adjacent areas of furunculosis produces a tender erythematous tumor called a *carbuncle* that becomes soft and fluctuant after several days.

DIAGNOSIS

■ DIFFERENTIAL DIAGNOSIS

- Fungal infections
- Molluscum contagiosum
- Varicella (chicken pox) or zoster (shingles)
- Scabies
- Insect bites
- Contact dermatitis
- Papular atopic dermatitis
- Miliaria
- Steroid acne
- Pruritic folliculitis of pregnancy
If localized to the face or neck:
- Acne vulgaris
- Pseudofolliculitis barbae (ingrown hair)
  1. A common inflammatory disorder of the pilosebaceous follicles of the beard
  2. Shaved hairs curve inward, with resultant repenetration of the skin
     a. On reentry into the epidermis, the hairs grow in a curved or arcuate path.
     b. This creates an inflammatory foreign body reaction.
- Folliculitis keloidalis nuchae (acne keloidalis nuchae)
  1. Chronic perifollicular inflammation with scar and keloid
  2. Nape of the neck
  3. Seen in males after onset of puberty
- Herpetic sycosis
  1. This is a folliculitis in the beard area caused by herpes simplex.

■ DIAGNOSTIC WORKUP

- History and physical examination are often sufficient to form a diagnosis.
- Gram stain or culture of a lesion is occasionally helpful.

THERAPY

■ NONPHARMACOLOGIC
- The treatment of choice for superficial folliculitis, including *Pseudomonas,* is good personal hygiene, including frequent, thorough handwashing and daily skin cleansing with soap and warm water.
- Avoid offending agents.
- Shave with a clean razor.
- For early lesions in deep folliculitis, use warm compresses to promote drainage.

■ MEDICAL
- Superficial folliculitis
  1. Topical antibiotics, such as mupirocin (Bactroban) or fusidic acid, are helpful.
  2. Topical keratolytics, such as the benzoyl peroxide gels, should be applied twice a day for 4 to 5 days
  3. Systemic antibiotics are rarely required.
  4. For *Pityrosporum* folliculitis, an oral imidazole antifungal drug, such as itraconazole or ketoconazole, should be used.
- Deep folliculitis
  1. If severe, widespread, or persistent, use systemic antibiotics with good antistaphylococcal coverage for 10 days.
  2. If large and fluctuant, incision and drainage are indicated.
- Recurrences of staphylococcal infections: consideration of elimination of possible *S. aureus* carriage in the anterior nares
  1. Apply mupirocin to the anterior nares twice a day for 4 weeks.
  2. Take rifampin orally for 5 days.

■ FOLLOW-UP & DISPOSITION
- Reemphasize proper hygiene and prevention measures at follow-up visits.
- Evaluation for diabetes and immunodeficiencies is not warranted until there are recurrences or concomitant systemic infections.

■ PREVENTION & PATIENT/FAMILY EDUCATION
- Avoid using sponges for bath or shower (use washcloths).
- Avoid sharing razors, towels, and washcloths.
- Ensure proper chlorination of public swimming facilities, hot tubs, spas, and the like.
- Follow the advice of local health departments regarding the avoidance of streams, lakes, and so forth at times of high bacteria counts or chemical residues.

■ REFERRAL INFORMATION
Referral to a dermatologist is recommended if the diagnosis is uncertain, if the condition does not respond to usual therapy, or if you are considering steroid acne or Ofuji disease.

PEARLS & CONSIDERATIONS

■ CLINICAL PEARLS
- *Pityrosporum* (Malassezia) folliculitis is a true entity different from tinea versicolor, even though it is caused by the same organism.
  1. Patients with this form of folliculitis often have concomitant tinea versicolor, seborrheic dermatitis, and acne vulgaris.
  2. The predisposing factors of *Pityrosporum* folliculitis are similar to those of tinea versicolor.
     a. A history of treatment with corticosteroids or antibiotics (e.g. tetracycline)
     b. Diabetes mellitus
     c. Possibly Cushing's syndrome
  3. Many cases of presumed steroid acne actually are *Pityrosporum* folliculitis.
  4. A histopathologic diagnosis is essential for appropriate therapy.
- Patients with Behçets disease often present with papulopustular lesions that are sterile folliculitis or acnelike lesions on an erythematous base, which appear as a papules and in 1 to 2 days become pustular.

REFERENCES
1. Feigin RD, Cherry, JD (eds): *Textbook of pediatric infectious diseases,* ed 4, Philadelphia, 1998, WB Saunders.
2. Hurwitz S: *Clinical pediatric dermatology,* ed 2, Philadelphia, 1993, WB Saunders.
3. Weston WL, Lane AT, Morelli JG: *Color textbook of pediatric dermatology,* ed 2, St Louis, 1996, Mosby.
Author: **Larry Denk, M.D.**

II

BASIC INFORMATION

■ DEFINITION
Bacterial food poisoning is a gastrointestinal illness caused by ingestion of food contaminated with bacteria or bacterial toxins.

ICD-9CM CODE
005.9 Food poisoning

■ ETIOLOGY
Categorized as invasive (inflammatory) or noninvasive (noninflammatory)
- Invasive: *Campylobacter,* enteroinvasive *Escherichia coli* (EIEC), *Salmonella, Shigella, Vibrio parahaemolyticus,* and *Yersinia;* intestinal tissue invaded; fecal leukocytes present
- Noninvasive: *Bacillus cereus, Staphylococcus aureus, Clostridium botulinum, Clostridium perfringens,* enterotoxigenic *E. coli* (ETEC), enterohemorrhagic *E. coli* (EHEC); fecal leukocytes absent

■ EPIDEMIOLOGY & DEMOGRAPHICS
- The incidence in the United States is estimated at 6 to 81 million cases per year.
- Most identifiable cases and deaths are caused by bacteria.
- Peak incidence varies by specific organism.
  1. Summer: *S. aureus, Salmonella, Shigella*
  2. Summer and fall: *C. botulinum, V. parahaemolyticus*
  3. Spring and fall: *Campylobacter jejuni*
  4. Winter: *C. perfringens, Yersinia*

■ HISTORY
- What is the patient's recent travel history?
- What foods were eaten at the suspected meal?
- What was the incubation period of the illness?
- What are the presenting signs and symptoms?

■ PHYSICAL EXAMINATION
- Any combination of gastrointestinal signs and symptoms with or without fever is suspect.
- The cause should be suspected on basis of the incubation period and major symptoms.
- A short incubation period (1 to 16 hours) is the result of ingestion of a preformed toxin and is noninvasive.
  1. *S. aureus:* within 30 minutes to 6 hours, severe abdominal cramps, nausea, vomiting, diar-

rhea, occasionally low-grade fever caused by enterotoxins
  a. Associated with ingestion of contaminated meats, filled pastries, and egg and potato salads
  2. *B. cereus:* two clinical forms: a short incubation (emetic) form characterized by vomiting, abdominal cramps, and 33% with diarrhea, and a long incubation (diarrheal) form characterized by abdominal cramps and watery diarrhea
  a. The illness is usually mild.
  b. Fever is unusual and if present resolves within 12 to 24 hours.
  c. The most likely food is unrefrigerated rice.
  3. *C. perfringens:* severe, crampy, midepigastric pain with watery diarrhea
  a. Fever and vomiting are unlikely.
  b. Symptoms usually resolve in 24 hours.
  c. It is caused by a heat-labile toxin.
  d. Implicated foods include beef, poultry, gravies, and Mexican-style foods.
  e. Outbreaks are related to cooked meat or poultry that is allowed to cool without refrigeration.
- Moderate incubation period (16 to 48 hours): some toxin-mediated, some are invasive
  1. Toxin producers
  a. *C. botulinum:* diarrhea with or before paralysis, severity related to amount of toxin ingested, unusual nerve palsies with descending paralysis; associated with home-canned foods
  b. ETEC: most common cause of traveler's diarrhea; after 1- to 2-day incubation period, abdominal cramps and diarrhea; resolves in 3 or 4 days; associated with contaminated water, salad, or rice
  c. EHEC: severe abdominal cramps, watery diarrhea, bloody diarrhea possible (O157:H7), noninvasive, no fever; complications: hemolytic uremic syndrome (HUS); associated with contaminated beef (especially hamburger), water, salad dressings, and raw milk
  d. *V. cholerae:* varies from a mild to life-threatening illness associated with voluminous, painless diarrhea, nausea, and vomiting; hypovolemic shock possible in 4 to 12 hours if fluid losses exceed intake; recovery within 1 week; associated with ingestion of contami-

nated water or food (especially raw or undercooked shellfish), moist grains, or dried or raw fish
  2. Invasive organisms
  a. *Salmonella:* incubation period of 12 to 48 hours followed by nausea, vomiting, diarrhea, and abdominal cramps typical; fever possible; outbreaks associated with contaminated poultry, beef, pork, eggs, dairy products, vegetables, and fruits
  b. *Shigella:* asymptomatic infection possible, but some with fever, watery diarrhea; may progress to bloody diarrhea and dysentery; usually self-limited, resolving in a few days; with severe illness, complications (e.g., bacteremia, HUS, seizures, colonic perforation) possible; transmission usually person-to-person but can occur via fecal contamination of food or water; associated with contaminated lettuce and egg salads
  c. *C. jejuni:* incubation period of about 24 hours; prodrome of fever, headaches, and myalgias, followed by diarrhea with fever and abdominal pain; diarrhea mild to profuse and bloody; resolves in 1 week; associated with undercooked poultry, unpasteurized milk, drinking from freshwater streams
- Longer incubation period
  1. *Yersinia enterocolitica* and *Y. pseudotuberculosis*
  a. Incubation period is usually 4 to 6 days.
  b. Presents with fever, diarrhea, and abdominal pain lasting 1 to 3 weeks.
  c. Mesenteric adenitis syndrome can mimic acute appendicitis.
  d. It is associated with uncooked pork (chitterlings or raw pork intestines), unpasteurized milk, contaminated water, and tofu.
  e. Stools often contain leukocytes, blood, and mucus.
  2. *Vibrio parahaemolyticus*
  a. Incubation period is 15 hours (range of 4 to 96 hours).
  b. Associated with coastal or cruise ship outbreaks during the summer months.
  c. Symptoms present with explosive, watery diarrhea; nausea; vomiting; abdominal cramps; and headache.
  d. Symptoms resolve in 1 week.
  e. Associated with contaminated seafood that is eaten raw or not thoroughly cooked, such as crab, shrimp, and oysters.

3. EIEC: rare in the United States
   a. Fever and bloody diarrhea
   b. Dysentery possible
4. *Listeria:* incubation period of 2 to 8 weeks
   a. Infection is rare in healthy people; more likely in pregnant women, newborns, and immunocompromised patients.
   b. It presents as fever, flulike illness, and headaches.
   c. Implicated foods are unpasteurized milk, soft cheeses, undercooked poultry, paté, and unwashed raw vegetables.

🔬 DIAGNOSIS

■ DIFFERENTIAL DIAGNOSIS
- Viruses (Norwalk, Rotavirus)
- Parasites *(Entamoeba histolytica, Giardia lamblia)*
- Toxins (ciguatoxins, scombroid toxin, mushrooms)
- Heavy metals, including copper, cadmium, tin, and zinc

■ DIAGNOSTIC WORKUP
- Test stool for fecal leukocytes and blood.
- Cultures should be obtained. (*Note:* Some organisms require special culture requirements, and the laboratory should be notified if the following are suspected: *Yersinia, C. botulinum, Vibrios, E. coli* O157:H7.)
- Examine stool for ova and parasites.
- Examine stool for *Clostridium difficile* toxin if current or recent antibiotic use reported.
- If botulism suspected, send food, serum, and stool for a toxin assay.
- Obtain blood cultures for febrile, toxic patients.

℞ THERAPY

■ NONPHARMACOLOGIC
Supportive therapy and rehydration are the primary therapy.

■ MEDICAL
- No antimicrobial agents needed for noninvasive organisms
  1. *B. cereus, S. aureus, C. perfringens, V. parahaemolyticus, Yersinia,* EHEC, and EIEC
- ETEC
  1. Trimethoprim-sulfamethoxazole (TMP-SMX) for 3 days (10 mg/kg/day TMP component divided every 12 hours)
- *Salmonella*
  1. No antimicrobial treatment is available for gastroenteritis.
  2. Consider antimicrobial therapy in the following patients with an increased risk of invasive disease:
     a. Infants younger than 3 months old
     b. Immunocompromised patients
  3. Consider therapy for invasive disease (e.g., bacteremia, osteomyelitis).
  4. Drug chosen should be based on susceptibilities.
- Shigellosis
  1. Antibiotics (ampicillin or TMP-SMX based on susceptibility testing) shorten duration of disease and eliminate organisms from stool. Duration of treatment is 5 days.
- *Campylobacter*
  1. Erythromycin shortens the duration of illness and prevents relapse. Duration of treatment is 5 to 7 days.

■ FOLLOW-UP & DISPOSITION
- Most infections are self-limited and do not require therapy.
- Serious complications are possible in an immunocompromised host.
- Postinfectious syndromes include the following:
  1. Reiter's syndrome: *Salmonella,* shigellosis, *Campylobacter, Yersinia;* HLA-B27 positive individuals
  2. Guillain-Barré syndrome: *Campylobacter*

■ REFERRAL INFORMATION
Hospitalize if severe illness or complications develop and consider consultation with pediatric infectious disease specialist or pediatric gastroenterologist.

🔆 PEARLS & CONSIDERATIONS

■ CLINICAL PEARLS
- Food poisoning is often underreported and underdiagnosed.
- All cases should be reported to the local health department.

■ WEBSITE
Centers for Disease Control and Prevention: www.cdc.gov

REFERENCES
1. American Academy of Pediatrics: In Peter G (ed): *1997 Red Book: report of the Committee on Infectious Diseases,* ed 24, Ill, 1997, American Academy of Pediatrics.
2. Pavia AT: Foodborne and waterborne disease. In Long SS et al (eds): *Principles and practice of pediatric infectious disease,* New York, 1997, Churchill Livingstone.
Author: **Cynthia Christy, M.D.**

BASIC INFORMATION

■ DEFINITION
Peptic acid disease results in compromise of the gastric (gastritis) and/or duodenal mucosa with diffuse inflammation of the mucosa, which may lead to discrete erosions (superficial lesions), or ulcerations.

■ SYNONYMS
Peptic acid disease includes gastritis, duodenitis, gastric ulcers, duodenal ulcers, and peptic ulcer disease.

ICD-9CM CODES
535.5   Gastritis
535.50 Gastritis without hemorrhage
535.51 Gastritis with hemorrhage
533.9   Peptic ulcer
533.4   Peptic ulcer with hemorrhage
535.60 Duodenitis
535.61 Duodenitis with hemorrhage
531.3   Acute gastric ulcer
531.9   Gastric ulcers

■ ETIOLOGY
- Peptic acid disease (gastritis, duodenitis, ulcers) results from an imbalance between the protective mechanisms and aggressive factors in the upper gastrointestinal (GI) tract.
  1. Protective
     a. Mucous-bicarbonate barrier
     b. Prostaglandins
     c. Growth factors
     d. Cell turnover
     e. Microcirculation
  2. Aggressive
     a. Excess acid
     b. Excess pepsin
     c. Ischemia/hypoxia
     d. Bile acids/drugs/caustic agents/ethanol
     e. Infections (viral, *Helicobacter pylori*)
- Acid is required for development or perpetuation of mucosal damage.
- Traditionally, this condition is classified as primary (no specific cause could be identified) or secondary.
  1. The majority of primary disease is now believed to be related to *H. pylori* infection.
  2. *H. pylori* is a gram-negative spiral-shaped organism that colonizes gastric epithelium and can cause gastritis as well as peptic ulcer disease.
- Causes of secondary gastritis and ulcers include the following:
  1. Physiologic stress (burns, head injury, sepsis, shock, trauma)
  2. Drug-related (nonsteroidal anti-inflammatory drugs [NSAIDs], aspirin, corticosteroids, chemotherapy, ethanol)
  3. Caustic substances
  4. Viral infections (a number of viral agents can compromise the gastric mucosa and result in a postviral gastritis)
  5. Excessive acid production (Zollinger-Ellison syndrome, renal failure, hyperparathyroidism)
  6. Other (eosinophilic gastroenteritis, Crohn's disease, Ménétrier's disease)

■ EPIDEMIOLOGY & DEMOGRAPHICS
- Prevalence in infants and children not well defined.
  1. Peptic acid–related diseases, particularly gastritis, are an important cause of abdominal pain and upper GI symptoms.
- Primary ulcer disease is much less prevalent in infants and young children because of the lower prevalence of *H. pylori.*
- *H. pylori* acquisition increases with age.
  1. Therefore the prevalence of related diseases is higher in adolescents.
- Other factors that increase the prevalence of *H. pylori* are poor socioeconomic environment and living with other household members with *H. pylori* disease.
- *H. pylori* infection has been associated with the development of gastric adenocarcinoma (1% to 2%) and MALT (mucosa-associated lymphoid tissue) lymphomas (rare in children).
- Increased incidence of peptic acid disease is seen in settings that predispose to secondary gastritis/ulcer disease.
  1. Hospitalized patients (particularly in intensive care units)
  2. Children taking certain medications (NSAIDs, steroids, chemotherapy)
  3. Following viral illnesses (postviral gastritis)

■ HISTORY
- Symptoms vary with age.
  1. Infants may present with irritability, vomiting, and failure to thrive.
  2. School-aged children are more likely to present with abdominal pain.
- Characteristics of pain are as follows:
  1. Epigastric (above the umbilicus)
  2. Awakening at night with pain
  3. May be worse with meals
  4. Exacerbated by acidic foods
  5. Relieved with antacids
- Associated symptoms include the following:
  1. Nausea
  2. Vomiting
  3. Early satiety
- A precipitating event may be identified:
  1. Viral illness
  2. Medication
  3. Hospitalization or surgery
- History that may be suggestive of risk factors for *H. pylori* includes the following:
  1. Lower socioeconomic environment
  2. Other household members with *H. pylori* disease

■ PHYSICAL EXAMINATION
- Physical examination may be normal.
- Physical findings suggestive of peptic acid disease include the following:
  1. Epigastric and/or right upper quadrant tenderness
  2. Hemoccult-positive stools
  3. Weight loss if intake has been compromised
  4. Tachycardia or pallor if there has been significant GI blood loss

🔬 DIAGNOSIS

■ DIFFERENTIAL DIAGNOSIS
- Functional abdominal pain
- Esophagitis
- Nonulcer dyspepsia
- Inflammatory bowel disease (IBD)
  1. Crohn's disease involving the upper GI tract
- Hepatobiliary disease
- Pancreatic disease

■ DIAGNOSTIC WORKUP
- Diagnosis can be made with a careful history and physical examination followed by a clinical response to a trial of acid suppression.
  1. Acid suppression is the therapy of choice for any peptic acid–related disorder; therefore differentiating among the different conditions is not necessary to initiate therapy.
- If the diagnosis is unclear or the response to acid suppression is questionable, further evaluation can be pursued.
Laboratory
- Nonspecific
  1. Complete blood count, erythrocyte sedimentation rate to identify iron deficiency anemia and evaluate for IBD
  2. Stool hemoccult
  3. Liver function tests to evaluate for hepatobiliary disease
  4. Amylase, lipase to evaluate for pancreatic disease
- Specific: noninvasive screening for *H. pylori*
  1. Serology: IgG, IgA, *H. pylori* titers
     a. Children have reduced antibody levels; therefore these are not as sensitive or specific in children younger than 7 to 9 years of age.

b. These tests are not reliable for following response to therapy or recurrent disease.

2. Urea breath test (UBT): ^{13}C UBT and ^{14}C UBT

a. Use of the stable isotope (^{13}C) is preferable in children (not validated for children younger than 2 years of age).

b. Currently, the most sensitive and specific noninvasive test and can be used to follow response to therapy and recurrence in adults.

c. This test may not be readily available to pediatricians.

3. Stool antigen

a. Preliminary studies suggest that this may be a sensitive and specific test in both children and adults.

Diagnostic imaging
- Upper GI (UGI) series
  1. UGI is fairly insensitive for superficial mucosal inflammation (gastritis, duodenitis) and for gastric ulcers.
  2. An air-contrast UGI series can identify approximately 90% of duodenal ulcers.
  3. Nonspecific findings include antral spasm and a thickened proximal duodenal fold.
  4. An UGI usually does not contribute to the diagnostic workup of peptic acid disease in children.
- Abdominal ultrasound
  1. Can be used to rule out other causes of abdominal pain (hepatobiliary and pancreatic disease)
- Endoscopy (esophagogastroduodenoscopy [EGD])
  1. This is the most sensitive and specific diagnostic test.
  2. It should be performed if presenting symptoms are severe or empiric therapy fails.
  3. It is preferable to radiographic studies.
  4. This test can identify the location and severity of disease as well as verify the presence of *H. pylori* by histology and/or rapid urease test.
     a. Gastric biopsy tissue is placed in medium containing urea; the presence of *H. pylori* results in a color change in the medium as urea is broken down by the urease produced by the organism.
- Management of a child with suspected gastritis or peptic ulcer disease integrates diagnostic studies with response to therapy (see following discussion)

THERAPY

■ MEDICAL
- History and examination consistent with gastritis/peptic acid disease
  1. Treat with acid suppression (H_2 blocker) and discontinue potential cause (e.g., NSAIDs).
  2. Response: Continue treatment for 6 to 8 weeks.
  3. Partial response: Change to a proton pump inhibitor (PPI) or refer to a gastroenterologist.
  4. No response or a recurrence of symptoms after treatment: Screen for *H. pylori* or refer to a gastroenterologist.
  5. Positive test for *H. pylori*: Provide empiric therapy or refer to a gastroenterologist.
  6. Negative test: Refer to a gastroenterologist for further evaluation (endoscopy).
- Medications available for acid suppression
  1. H_2 blockers block histamine-stimulated acid secretion and are first-line medications for gastritis/peptic acid disease (non–*H. pylori*).
  2. Medications are available in liquid preparations.
  3. Doses are given to a maximum of the adult dose.
     a. Cimetidine 20 to 40 mg/kg/day divided two to four times per day
     b. Ranitidine 1 to 2 mg/kg/dose twice daily (three times daily in infants and toddlers)
     c. Famotidine 0.5 to 1 mg/kg/dose twice daily
  4. PPIs block the gastric proton pump itself and are recommended for severe or refractory disease and for the treatment of *H. pylori*.
     a. Doses are not well established in children.
     b. Medications do not come in liquid preparations, and crushing or chewing the tablets or granules results in inactivation of the medication in the stomach.
     c. Granules from the capsules may be swallowed without chewing.
     d. A liquid suspension can be prepared using bicarbonate to protect from inactivation.
     e. Doses are given to the maximum of the adult dose: omeprazole 0.7 to 3.5 mg/kg/day as a single dose or divided twice daily; dosages for lansoprazole and rabeprazole are not established.
- Therapy for *H. pylori*
  1. Combination therapies for eradication of *H. pylori* include a strong acid suppressor (PPI) and two antibiotics effective against *H. pylori*.

2. Duration of treatment is 10 to 14 days; twice-daily regimen enhances compliance (adult dose).
   a. Omeprazole 1 mg/kg/day divided twice daily (20 mg twice daily), *plus*
   b. Clarithromycin 15 mg/kg/day divided twice daily (500 mg twice daily), *plus*
   c. Amoxicillin 50 mg/kg/day divided twice daily (1 g twice daily), *or*
   d. Metronidazole 20 mg/kg/day divided twice daily (500 mg twice daily)
3. Because compliance and/or tolerance can be an issue, assessing response to therapy with a urea breath test in 4 to 6 weeks is advisable when available.
4. Whether asymptomatic individuals with *H. pylori* should be treated to reduce the long-term risk for gastric cancer is controversial.
5. No association has been found between *H. pylori* and chronic recurrent abdominal pain. These children should not be routinely tested.
- Other medications
  1. Sucralfate: binds to damaged mucosa and provides a protective barrier against peptic acid injury
     a. Four-times-daily dosage schedule can be difficult.
     b. Sucralfate should not be given with meals or other medications.
     c. Use with caution in patients with renal disease.
     d. Dosages in pediatric patients are not well established: 125 to 250 mg/dose four times daily in infants/toddlers; 0.5 to 1 g in older children and adolescents.
  2. Antacids: buffer acid
     a. Provide fairly immediate relief when used as an adjunct to acid suppression
     b. 0.5 ml/kg/dose
  3. Prostaglandins: enhance mucosal protection and can buffer acid
     a. Narrow therapeutic index
     b. Not widely used in children
  4. Bismuth compounds: provide a protective barrier and enhance mucosal protection
     a. Still used in therapeutic regimens for *H. pylori*
     b. Not widely used as primary therapy in children
- General therapeutic measures
  1. Avoid acidic foods if they increase symptoms.
     a. They do not cause irritation but may exacerbate symptoms before mucosa has healed.
  2. Avoid smoking and alcohol (adolescents).

■ REFERRAL INFORMATION
- Patients should be referred to a gastroenterologist based on the pediatrician's comfort level with the acid suppression medications and treatment regimens for *H. pylori*.
  1. *H. pylori* disease is generally less prevalent in pediatric patients than in adults with peptic acid symptoms; referral to a gastroenterologist may precede the diagnostic workup for *H. pylori*.
  2. Patients may be referred following failed response to an empiric trial of acid suppression therapy (H_2 blockers or PPIs) or persistent symptoms after treatment.
- A gastroenterologist should be consulted for any child with severe symptoms, including vomiting suggesting gastric outlet obstruction; hematemesis; or other evidence of significant GI bleeding, severe pain, anorexia, and weight loss.
- Severe pain and peritoneal signs on examination suggesting perforation require emergency evaluation by a surgeon and a gastroenterologist.

■ PATIENT/FAMILY EDUCATION
- Children should complete the 6- to 8-week course of medication.
- Foods that are spicy or acidic do not cause peptic acid disease but may aggravate symptoms before mucosal healing is complete.
- Mental and emotional stress does not cause gastritis or ulcers but may exacerbate symptoms.

☼ PEARLS & CONSIDERATIONS

■ CLINICAL PEARLS
- Medications that suppress acid do not primarily heal the mucosa; they minimize perpetuation of injury by acid and allow the body to repair the damage. It may take a few weeks before a child's symptoms improve significantly, so an empiric trial should not be deemed a failure until the medication has been taken as prescribed for at least 2 weeks.
- Infants and younger children tend to present with complications of peptic ulcer disease.
- The index of suspicion for *H. pylori*–related disease should be higher in children who are from a lower socioeconomic background, live in crowded households, or live in households where other members have *H. pylori*.
- Comfort level with the clinical diagnosis and medications should dictate referral to a gastroenterologist.

REFERENCES
1. Gold BD et al: *Helicobacter pylori* infection in children: recommendations for diagnosis and treatment, *J Pediatr Gastroenterol Nutr* 31:490, 2000.
2. Imrie C, Drumm B: Pathophysiology, epidemiology, diagnosis and treatment of *Helicobacter pylori* disease in childhood, *Int Semin Pediatr Gastroenterol Nutr* 8:10, 1999.
3. Moyer MS: Gastritis and peptic ulcer disease in children, *Int Semin Pediatr Gastroenterol Nutr* 8:1, 1999.

Author: **M. Susan Moyer, M.D.**

BASIC INFORMATION

■ DEFINITION
- Gastroesophageal reflux (GER) describes the effortless retrograde movement of gastric contents into the esophagus and, at times, into the mouth. Gastroesophageal reflux disease (GERD) is any symptom or tissue damage secondary to reflux of gastric contents.
- GERD is a clinical diagnosis that may be objectively confirmed by several diagnostic tests; it may present without the concomitant findings of erosions in the esophagus, just as tissue damage may be identified in the absence of typical symptoms.
- Infantile reflux becomes symptomatic during the first months after birth and resolves by 1 to 2 years of age in at least 80% of patients.
- Adult reflux may develop on a background of infantile reflux in some children, but it often appears anew in children beyond infancy, and it tends to persist, waxing and waning symptomatically.

■ SYNONYMS
- Reflux esophagitis
- GER
- GERD

ICD-9CM CODES
530.81 Esophageal reflux
530.11 Gastroesophageal reflux, gastro-esophageal reflux disease

■ ETIOLOGY
- GERD is a multifactorial disorder, but the key event in the pathogenesis is the movement of acid and/or other noxious substances from the stomach into the esophagus.
- Under normal circumstances, GER is prevented by an antireflux barrier, consisting of the lower esophageal sphincter (LES) and the effect of the crural diaphragm, located at the gastroesophageal junction.
- The increased frequency of reflux in infants younger than 4 months of age suggests developmental immaturity of the LES, which is innervated by the vagus nerve and regulated by a variety of neurotransmitters.
- Transient LES relaxation (TLESR) is an abrupt decrease in pressure across the sphincter, which is part of the reflex that normally permits gas to escape from the stomach and is unrelated to swallowing or peristalsis. In children and adults with GER, the frequency and duration of TLESRs is increased.
- Impaired luminal clearance of gastric acid, secondary to esophageal dysmotility and delayed gastric emptying, is another factor in the pathogenesis of GERD.

- Patients with hiatal hernia can have progressive disruption of the diaphragmatic sphincter, depending on the extent of axial herniation, and thus may experience GER.
- GERD also commonly occurs in patients who have had an esophageal operation (especially repair of esophageal atresia) and in those who are neurologically disabled.

■ EPIDEMIOLOGY & DEMOGRAPHICS
- Mildly symptomatic reflux is extremely common and may be so benign as to be considered virtually normal.
- Twenty percent of otherwise normal infants regurgitate to an extent that their parents consider it a problem.
- Seven percent of infants have severe enough symptoms to come to medical attention; less than 2% of whom require investigation.
- Less than 0.5% of infants have GERD severe enough to warrant fundoplication.
- Very-low-birth-weight infants are more likely to have GERD, and up to 10% have reflux-associated apnea, bradycardia, or bronchopulmonary dysplasia exacerbations.
- Significant reflux disease occurs in 1% to 3% of older children.
- Children with neurologic disease, chronic respiratory disease, increased abdominal pressure or abdominal distention, or vagal dysfunction or injury are at increased risk for GERD.

■ HISTORY
- Infantile regurgitation is the most common and obvious presentation of GERD, but this may not require further investigation if no other symptoms are present.
- When regurgitation is associated with weight loss, irritability, or ill appearance, a thorough evaluation is warranted.
- Infants may present with extraesophageal manifestations, including the following:
  1. Recurrent pneumonia
  2. Wheezing or asthma
  3. Stridor or hoarseness
  4. Apnea
  5. Apparent life-threatening event (ALTE)
  6. Sandifer syndrome (dystonic posturing or arching resulting from reflux)
- Older children may mention the following more common symptoms:
  1. Heartburn or chest pain
  2. Epigastric pain
  3. Bilious taste in the mouth
  4. Dysphagia or odynophagia in more severe cases
- In addition, hoarseness, nocturnal cough, wheezing or asthma, hema-

temesis, or anemia may be attributable to GERD in children.

■ PHYSICAL EXAMINATION
- The physical examination in an infant or child with GERD is often normal.
- Possible physical findings include the following:
  1. Irritability
  2. Ill appearance
  3. Pallor
  4. Weight loss
  5. Posturing and twisting of the head and neck
  6. Stridor or wheezing
  7. Epigastric tenderness

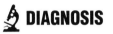 **DIAGNOSIS**

■ DIFFERENTIAL DIAGNOSIS
- Gastrointestinal obstruction: pyloric stenosis, malrotation, intermittent volvulus
- Allergic (eosinophilic) esophagitis or gastroenteritis
- Esophageal or gastroduodenal dysmotility
- Gastritis duodenitis
  1. *Helicobacter pylori*
  2. Nonsteroidal antiinflammatory drug induced
  3. *Giardia*
- Inborn errors of metabolism
- Drug or toxin
  1. Ipecac
  2. Lead poisoning
  3. Vitamin A toxicity
- Nutrient allergies or intolerances
- Neurologic disorders
  1. Arnold-Chiari malformation
  2. Hydrocephalus with shunt dysfunction
  3. Increased intracranial pressure
  4. Pseudoobstruction
- Psychosocial disorders
  1. Cyclic vomiting
  2. Psychogenic vomiting
  3. Bulimia

■ DIAGNOSTIC WORKUP
- Infants and children presenting with uncomplicated regurgitation and/or heartburn may not need a confirmatory diagnostic test.
  1. The positive predictive value of these symptoms is high.
  2. Symptom resolution is often used as a clinical endpoint.
- Guaiac-positive stools are common.
- Patients with atypical or extraesophageal symptoms, as well as individuals not responding to empiric medical therapy, those with frequently recurring symptoms, and those with progressive symptoms, should undergo diagnostic evaluation and may require referral to a gastroenterologist.

II

- The choice of diagnostic test depends on the clinical question.
  1. A contrast study of the upper gastrointestinal tract should be performed in all patients who have chronic regurgitation to eliminate the possibility of anatomic causes of delayed gastric emptying.
     a. It is the most sensitive test for detecting esophageal strictures.
     b. It is useful in evaluating motor function and detecting hiatal hernia.
     c. It is not useful to rule in or out the diagnosis of GER.
  2. The 24-hour pH probe is the most sensitive method for diagnosing GER.
     a. An episode of reflux is defined as a decrease in the intraluminal pH to less than 4.
     b. The frequency of reflux, the overall time of esophageal exposure to acid, and the longest reflux episodes are recorded.
     c. In infants, reflux more than 9% of the time and in older children and adults reflux more than 4% of the time is considered significant.
     d. Prolonged alkaline reflux (pH greater than 7), which is usually caused by bile reflux, can cause symptoms and create significant tissue damage.
  3. Endoscopy with biopsy is the most appropriate test to assess the extent of mucosal damage.
     a. It is useful in the detection of esophagitis, Barrett's esophagus, hiatal hernia, strictures, and antral or duodenal webs.
     b. It allows the opportunity for therapeutic intervention (stricture dilation).
  4. Gastroesophageal scintiscan (radionuclide gastric emptying study) is the best method for calculating the rate of emptying.
     a. Approximately 50% of children with GERD have delayed gastric emptying.
     b. This is especially important when fundoplication is being considered.
  5. Esophageal manometry is rarely used in the diagnosis of GERD; however, it may be used to evaluate peristalsis and to assess the function of the LES when an underlying motility disorder is suspected.

℞ THERAPY

Uncomplicated GERD in infants is usually a self-limiting problem that resolves by 12 to 18 months of age, and only a thorough physical examination and parental reassurance are necessary.

■ NONPHARMACOLOGIC
- The infant should be kept upright as much as possible in the postprandial period.
- High-osmolality formulas should be avoided (osmolality: soy-based < lactose-based < elemental).
  1. Whey-based formulas may empty more rapidly from the stomach but have not been shown to significantly decrease GER.
- Smaller and more frequent feedings may be attempted.
- Thickened feeds may diminish the number of regurgitation episodes.
  1. However, this may lead to occult reflux episodes of long duration.
  2. This may increase the risk of esophageal and pulmonary complications.
- In older children, the following behavioral modifications should be recommended:
  1. Prohibit eating 1 to 3 hours before bedtime.
  2. Elevate the head of the bed.
  3. Avoid known LES relaxants (e.g., caffeine, chocolate, peppermint, garlic) and acidic foods (citrus fruits and tomatoes).
  4. Promote weight loss in obese patients.

■ MEDICAL
- Medical intervention is indicated in patients with GERD who have recurrent episodes or suspected complications.
- In adults, H_2-receptor antagonists (H_2RAs) achieve partial or complete resolution of symptoms in 50% to 70% of patients.
  1. All H_2RAs are equally effective when used in equivalent doses.
- Because of the greater antisecretory effect of proton pump inhibitors (PPIs), the success of this class of agent is superior to H_2RAs in terms of symptom relief and healing.
  1. From 70% to 90% of adult patients report partial or complete resolution of symptoms.
  2. The various PPIs appear to be equally effective when used in equivalent doses.
  3. Safety and dosing of these agents in young children are not well established.

- Prokinetic agents (e.g., metoclopramide, bethanechol, low-dose erythromycin, cisapride) may be useful in children with delayed gastric emptying and GERD.
  1. Cisapride is no longer recommended because of its association with prolonged QT interval and cardiac arrhythmias.
  2. Therapy with erythromycin in very young infants may increase the risk of pyloric stenosis.
  3. Metoclopramide rarely causes tardive dyskinesia and should not be used in patients with underlying seizure disorders.
- In infants and children, combination therapy with acid blockade and prokinetic agents generally yields faster and more satisfying results than either agent alone.
- Therapy is usually continued for 6 to 8 weeks if clinical improvement is noted. If no improvement occurs, further evaluation is necessary.
- The cause of reflux is often not correctable (e.g., motility disturbance, neurologic disease), and multiple courses of treatment are necessary.

■ SURGICAL
Surgery may be considered in the following cases:
- In cases refractory to medical therapy
- In those with severe complications
- In children who face a lifetime of therapy because of recurrent relapses when medications are withdrawn

■ FOLLOW-UP & DISPOSITION
See "Therapy."

■ PATIENT/FAMILY EDUCATION
- Possible complications include esophagitis, esophageal stricture, Barrett's esophagus, recurrent pneumonia, asthma, nocturnal cough, apnea, and possibly ALTEs.
- Infants commonly outgrow the illness, but in older children, the disease is typically one of dysmotility, possibly necessitating long-term or frequent courses of therapy.
- Dietary and behavioral changes may improve the course.

■ REFERRAL INFORMATION
- Patients with recurrent, complicated, or refractory disease should be referred to a gastroenterologist.
- A surgeon may be consulted when complications are severe, medications are ineffective, or the patient does not tolerate or desire long-term medical treatment.
- Neurologists, geneticists, psychiatrists, or toxicologists may be consulted if other causes for recurrent vomiting are being considered.

☼ PEARLS & CONSIDERATIONS

■ CLINICAL PEARLS

- Suspect reflux in patients with refractory asthma or recurrent pneumonia.
- Patients often have a family history of allergy or atopic disease.
- Children with GER often avoid spicy tomato sauces and acidic juices before diagnosis.
- Some patients with reflux complain of a burning sensation in the throat and not in the chest.
- Reflux and constipation often coincide in the same patient.

■ WEBSITES

- Diagnosis Health.com: www.diagnosishealth.com/gerd
- MediConsult: www.mediconsult.com/heartburn

REFERENCES

1. Faubion WA, Zein NN: Gastroesophageal reflux in infants and children, *Mayo Clin Proc* 73:166, 1998.
2. Fennerty MB et al: The diagnosis and treatment of gastroesophageal reflux disease in a managed care environment: suggested disease management guidelines, *Arch Intern Med* 156:477, 1996.
3. Hogan WJ: Spectrum of supraesophageal complications of gastroesophageal reflux disease, *Am J Med* 103:77S, 1997.
4. Orenstein SR: Infantile reflux: different from adult reflux, *Am J Med* 103:114S, 1997.

Authors: **Sujata Chakravarti, M.D., and Elizabeth Mannick, M.D.**

II

BASIC INFORMATION

■ DEFINITION
Giardiasis is a small intestine infection with the Protozoan parasite *Giardia lamblia intestinalis*.

ICD-9CM CODE
007.1 Giardiasis

■ ETIOLOGY
- The life cycle of *Giardia* consists of two stages.
- The cyst is the infectious form.
  1. It is relatively inert and environmentally resistant.
  2. Excystation occurs in the duodenum.
- Two trophozoites (vegetative stage) are produced from each cyst.
  1. The trophozoites replicate in the crypts of the duodenum and upper jejunum.
  2. Mechanical attachment to the surface of the intestine occurs after excystation.
  3. They reproduce asexually by binary fission.
- Some of the trophozoites encyst in the ileum.

■ EPIDEMIOLOGY & DEMOGRAPHICS
- *Giardia* is the most potent human protozoal enteropathogen.
- Prevalence rates vary from 2% to 5% in the industrialized world to 20% to 30% in the developing world.
- High-risk groups for giardiasis include the following:
  1. Infants and young children
  2. Travelers
     a. High attack rates (30% to 40%) occur with travel to certain parts of Russia (e.g., St. Petersburg).
     b. Within the United States, Colorado ski resorts, other mountainous parts of the United States, and national parks have high prevalence areas.
  3. Immunocompromised patients
     a. Agammaglobulinemia or hypogammaglobulinemia states are associated with chronic giardiasis.
     b. It is not a major clinical problem with acquired immunodeficiency syndrome (AIDS).
- *Giardia* isolates from beavers and calves appear to be infective for humans.
- Ingestion of viable cysts can occur by drinking fecally contaminated water.
- Other modes of transmission include direct fecal-oral transmission in situations of overcrowding and poor sanitary standards.
  1. Higher prevalence in day-care centers, mental institutions
  2. Higher prevalence in sexually active male homosexuals
- Humans serve as a major reservoir of infection worldwide.
- Other reservoirs include fresh surface water and wild and domestic animals.

■ HISTORY
- Presents as asymptomatic (carrier), acute diarrhea, or chronic diarrhea
- Asymptomatic infection
  1. This is the most common form of infection.
  2. Infection occurs in both adults and children.
  3. Host factors such as immune and nonimmune defense mechanisms as well as variation in parasite virulence may play a role in preventing disease expression.
- Acute giardiasis
  1. Incubation period of about 1 to 2 weeks
  2. Acute onset with diarrhea (95%)
     a. Stools typically profuse and watery
     b. Usually no associated blood or mucus
  3. Other findings include the following:
     a. Malaise (85%)
     b. Cramping, abdominal pains (75%)
     c. Bloating (70%)
     d. Weight loss (65%)
     e. Nausea (60%)
     f. Marked flatulence (35%)
     g. Vomiting (25%)
     h. Fever (13%)
  4. Untreated: some resolve in 1 to 2 weeks; up to 50% develop chronic giardiasis
- Chronic giardiasis
  1. More profound constitutional symptoms
  2. Headache and malaise
  3. Weight loss
  4. Abdominal bloating
  5. Persistent diarrhea, which can be intermittent in nature
  6. Steatorrhea

■ PHYSICAL EXAMINATION
- May have signs of dehydration
- Failure to thrive
- Weight loss
- Abdominal distention
- Abdominal tenderness
- Perianal erythema
- Stool guaiac usually heme negative
- Edema (protein-losing enteropathy in chronic giardiasis occasionally seen)

■ COMPLICATIONS
- The major complications of giardiasis are nutritional insufficiency and growth impairment.
- Rarely, allergic (food) and immune phenomena such as arthralgia and urticaria have been described.

DIAGNOSIS

■ DIFFERENTIAL DIAGNOSIS
- Other forms of acute diarrhea
  1. Infectious enteritis: viral, bacterial, or other protozoal
  2. Traveler's diarrhea
  3. Allergic reactions
  4. Food poisoning
- Chronic diarrhea
  1. Malabsorption syndromes, including celiac disease
  2. Toddler's diarrhea
  3. Cystic fibrosis
  4. Lactase and other disaccharidase deficiency
  5. Chronic constipation with overflow incontinence
  6. Allergic enterocolitis
  7. Irritable bowel syndrome
  8. Inflammatory bowel disease
  9. Motility disorders
  10. Tuberculosis
  11. AIDS

■ DIAGNOSTIC WORKUP
- The diagnosis of giardiasis can often be made on clinical history and examination.
  1. History of travel to high-risk areas important
     a. Diarrhea usually begins toward the end of the holiday and persists on return.
     b. Traveler's diarrhea occurs early and resolves rapidly.
- Demonstrate *Giardia* cysts or trophozoites in feces or specimens obtained from the small intestine.
  1. Stool microscopy
     a. Motile trophozoites may be seen in wet preparations of fresh stool.
     b. More commonly, cysts are identified after staining the stool with trichrome or iodine.
     c. Examination of a single stool specimen detects up to 70%.
     d. Approximately 85% detection is achieved after examination of three different specimens passed on different days.
  2. Small bowel sampling
     a. Samples of duodenal fluid obtained by aspiration (string test) can be examined for trophozoites.
     b. A small bowel biopsy or impression smear may be examined histologically for trophozoites.
     c. Small bowel biopsy may show partial villus atrophy.
- Immunodiagnosis may be used for diagnosis.
  1. Fecal antigen detection
     a. Enzyme-linked immunosorbent assay
     b. Sensitivities and specificities of 87% to 100%

c. Less commonly used methods: indirect fluorescent antibody test, immunodiffusion
2. Serology
   a. Anti-*Giardia* antibodies in serum not clinically helpful, in general
- Stool is negative for leukocytes.
- Complete blood count may demonstrate macrocytic anemia (folate deficiency).
- Vitamin deficiencies, especially folic acid, are common. Vitamin B_{12} and vitamin A deficiencies are also occasionally reported.

℞ THERAPY

■ MEDICAL
- Three major classes of drugs of proven benefit in the treatment of *Giardia*: nitroimidazole derivatives, acridine dyes such as mepacrine, and the nitrofurans such as furazolidone
- Metronidazole
  1. Dosage: 15 to 20 mg/kg/day for 10 days
  2. Adult dosing: 2 g/day for 3 days or 400 mg three times daily for 7 days
  3. Efficacy: 90%
  4. Side effects:
     a. Nausea, vomiting
     b. Dizziness
     c. Headache
     d. Metallic taste
     e. Rash
     f. Reversible neutropenia
     g. Potential mutagenicity
     h. Disulfiram-like reaction with alcohol
     i. Peripheral neuropathy
- Tinidazole
  1. Dosage: 50 to 75 mg/kg, single dose
  2. Adult dosing: 2 g, single dose
  3. Efficacy: 90%
  4. Side effects: same as for metronidazole

- Mepacrine
  1. Dosage: 2 mg/kg three times daily for 5 to 7 days
  2. Adult dosing: 100 mg three times daily for 7 to 10 days
  3. Efficacy: 90%
  4. During pregnancy: avoid
  5. Side effects:
     a. Nausea, vomiting
     b. Abdominal cramps
     c. Skin discoloration
     d. Toxic psychosis
     e. Hepatitis
     f. Anemia
     g. Psoriasis
     h. Hepatic impairment (in elderly)
- Furazolidone
  1. Dosage: 2 mg/kg three times daily for 7 to 10 days
  2. Adult dosing: 100 mg four times daily for 7 to 10 days
  3. Efficacy: 80%
  4. In glucose-6-phosphate dehydrogenase deficiency: avoid because leads to hemolysis
  5. Side effects: nausea and vomiting

■ PREVENTIVE TREATMENT & PATIENT/FAMILY EDUCATION
- Public health interventions are required to ensure that water supplies are *Giardia* free and that methods are available to monitor the presence of the parasite in drinking water.
- Personal hygiene education is important.
  1. Most filtration devices provide satisfactory decontamination.
  2. Neither chlorine nor iodine-based chemical disinfection results in 100% cyst inactivation, although the latter is superior.
  3. Heating to 70° C for 10 minutes is also a practical alternative.

■ REFERRAL INFORMATION
For confusing cases or those with negative stool ova and parasite, consider pediatric gastroenterology consultation for small bowel biopsy.

⚙ PEARLS & CONSIDERATIONS

■ CLINICAL PEARLS
- Encourage good handwashing technique.
- Consider *Giardia* in workup for failure to thrive, especially in daycare attendees and in those with appetite suppression, with or without history of acute diarrhea.
- Obtain history of swimming in fresh water lakes, creeks, or ponds or of well water ingestion when clinical history is suspicious for *Giardia*.

■ WEBSITES
- Center for Food Safety & Applied Nutrition: http://vm.cfsan.fda.gov/~mow/chap22.html
- Centers for Disease Control and Prevention: www.cdc.gov/ncidod/dpd/parasites/giardiasis/default.htm
- Virtual Hospital: www.vh.org/Patients/IHB/IntMed/Infectious/Giardiasis.html

REFERENCES
1. Brandborg LL: Giardiasis and traveler's diarrhea, *Gastroenterology* 78:1602, 1980.
2. Farthing MJG: Giardiasis, *Gastroenterol Clin* 25:493, 1996.
3. Goka AKJ et al: Diagnosis of giardiasis by specific IgM antibody enzyme-linked immunosorbent assay, *Lancet* 2:184, 1986.
4. Lewis DJM, Freedman AR: *Giardia lamblia* as an intestinal pathogen, *Dig Dis* 10:102, 1992.
5. Pickering LK et al: Occurrence of *Giardia lamblia* in children in day care centers, *J Pediatr* 104:522, 1984.
6. Zaat JOM, Mank TG, Assendelft WJJ: A systematic review on the treatment of giardiasis, *Trop Med Int Health* 2:63, 1997.

Author: **Alka Goyal, M.D.**

II

BASIC INFORMATION

■ DEFINITION
Gingivostomatitis herpes is a viral infection causing characteristic lesions of the gums and mouth.

■ SYNONYMS
- Gingivostomatitis
- Stomatitis

ICD-9CM CODES
054.2 Herpetic gingivostomatitis
528.0 Stomatitis

■ ETIOLOGY
- Gingivostomatitis is usually caused by herpes simplex virus type 1 (HSV-1); less frequently, herpes simplex virus type 2 (HSV-2)
- Incubation period is 2 to 12 days (mean is approximately 4 days).
- Viremia: Outside of the neonate and immunosuppressed host, viremia is unlikely to play a major role. Spread within the host occurs largely via direct cell-to-cell transfer.
- Shedding: Oral shedding after primary infection occurs for up to 23 days (mean of 7 to 10 days).
- Latency: After entry and infection of nerve endings, virions are transported via retrograde axonal transport to the nuclei of sensory ganglia associated with the site of inoculation.
  1. A permanent copy of viral genetic material is inserted into the host's genome.
  2. This allows both recurrence of symptomatic (usually less severe) disease and periodic shedding of virus during asymptomatic intervals.
- Immune response: Antibody production may be detected as early as a few days after infection and functions most critically via its role in antibody-dependent cellular cytotoxicity. Specific cellular immunity is detectable in the second to third week of infection.

■ EPIDEMIOLOGY & DEMOGRAPHICS
- Most children with primary HSV infection are asymptomatic. Of those who are symptomatic, gingivostomatitis is the most common presentation (5% to 26%).
- Distribution is worldwide.
- Humans are the sole reservoir for transmission to other humans.
- No seasonal variation exists.
- Transmission: Direct contact of oral mucosa with infected oral or genital secretions or lesions. Autoinoculation of skin from oral lesions can occur (e.g., Whitlow in the case of nail biting or thumb sucking during an episode of gingivostomatitis).

- Prevalence: Seroprevalence studies may underestimate infection.
  1. Not all individuals with documented HSV infection seroconvert.
  2. Prevalence is influenced by age, geographic location, and socioeconomic status.
  3. Seroconversion occurs at an earlier age in developing countries.
  4. In the United States, serologic evidence of infection is approximately 20% to 30% by 5 years of age and 40% to 80% by early adolescence. The annualized rate of infection among university students is approximately 5% to 10%.

■ HISTORY
- Symptoms present as systemic illness with high fever and malaise (often with extreme discomfort).
  1. Fetor oris
  2. Reluctance to eat or drink
  3. Coryza and/or otalgia also possible
- Exposure to an individual with HSV infection, symptomatic or asymptomatic, is the cause.
- Infection in immunocompromised patients (particularly those with cell-mediated defects) and in neonates may produce disseminated disease requiring systemic therapy.
- Patients with eczema, burns, or otherwise altered integument in contact with herpetic lesions may exhibit severe and even life-threatening symptoms requiring systemic therapy.
- History: There is more than one strain of both HSV-1 and HSV-2.
  1. Past infection with one strain of HSV-1 is not necessarily protective against infection with another strain of HSV-1; the same holds true for HSV-2.
  2. History of infection with HSV-2 in association with new-onset HSV-1, and vice versa, has been associated with attenuation of symptoms.

■ PHYSICAL EXAMINATION
- Fetor oris
- Vesicular lesions on an erythematous base on and around the lips, gingiva, anterior tongue, floor of the mouth, and anterior (hard) palate
  1. Up to 50% of patients may have additional lesions along the anterior pillars or soft palate.
  2. Lesions may extend about the lips and chin, down the neck, or about the nares, even in the immunocompetent child.
- Vesicles
  1. Break down rapidly, often by the time of presentation, appearing as 1- to 3-mm shallow white/gray ulcers on an erythematous base

- Lesions appear that bleed easily and may become covered with a black crust
- Gums generally mildly swollen, erythematous, ulcerated, and friable; often bleeding with contact.
- Cervical, submental, and preauricular nodes often swollen and tender.
- Middle ear effusion possible

DIAGNOSIS

■ DIFFERENTIAL DIAGNOSIS
- Herpangina: This is characterized by small ulcers in the *posterior* pharynx with little or no gingival or buccal involvement. It is often associated with a more acute onset, shorter duration, more mild oral discomfort, and seasonal occurrence.
- Hand-foot-and-mouth (HFM) disease: Although the distribution of oral lesions in HFM is also anterior, the gums and lips are typically uninvolved and the illness is usually more mild.
  1. Peripheral lesions on hands and feet are often bilaterally symmetric (in contrast to HSV gingivostomatitis with concurrent digital autoinoculation) and do not crust.
- Erythema multiforme minor (EM): This is usually distinguished by its accompanying generalized target-like rash.
  1. Although EM may be associated with HSV, it is thought to be a type of allergic response to *recurrent,* rather than primary, HSV infection.
- Stevens-Johnson syndrome: Diffuse mucous membrane lesions are accompanied by generalized integument exfoliation.
- Aphthous stomatitis: Oral lesions are similar but are neither preceded by vesicle formation nor accompanied by fever or systemic symptoms. Extraoral lesions do not occur.
- Mucositis from chemotherapeutic agents: The most recognizable form is marginal or necrotizing gingivitis characterized by a periapical line of erythema, swelling, and tenderness, with "punched-out" craters in the interdental papillae that bleed readily and may become covered with a pseudomembrane. Differentiation may require laboratory identification.
- Impetigo: Extraoral HSV lesions are often confused with impetigo.
  1. The presence of intraoral lesions suggests the need to search for a different diagnosis.
  2. Recurrent "impetigo," especially in the same location on the face, should prompt the diagnosis of HSV.

■ DIAGNOSTIC WORKUP

- Diagnosis usually based on clinical criteria
- Confirmatory tests
  1. Rapid and specific
     a. Fluorescent antibody, enzyme-linked immunosorbent assay, etc.: Commercially available kits report sensitivity and specificity of 90% to 95%. With appropriate reagents, viral typing may also be performed.
     b. Polymerase chain reaction is generally impractical for mucosal lesions because of the presence of inhibitors.
        (1) A scraping from the base of an unroofed vesicle in which the number of viable viral particles is significantly greater than after progression to the ulcerated or crusted stage provides the best material for analysis.
        (2) Despite the significantly lower viral count, a swab from an ulcer crater or crust may still be sufficient in the absence of intact vesicles.
  2. Rapid but nonspecific
     a. Tzanck smear
     b. Giemsa or other tissue stains
     c. Electron microscopy
  3. Less rapid but specific
     a. Tissue culture is the gold standard. HSV grows rapidly with high titer samples positive by 12 to 24 hours and low titer samples by 5 to 7 days (mean of 2 to 3 days).

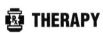

THERAPY

■ NONPHARMACOLOGIC

- Usually supportive
- Oral or intravenous hydration
  1. Cold, nonacidic fluids, slush, and/or popsicles may provide both hydration and symptomatic relief.

■ MEDICAL

- Symptomatic relief of oral lesions
  1. 1:1 solution of diphenhydramine to aluminum and magnesium hydroxide (Benadryl:Maalox) as a swish and swallow (maximum dosage of 5 mg/kg/day of diphenhydramine)
  2. Viscous lidocaine no longer recommended in young children
     a. Potential for methemoglobinemia
     b. Risk of either self-injury from chewing on anesthetized lips/oral mucosa or anxiety because of numbness of the mouth and throat

- Consideration of one of the following agents to prevent secondary bacterial infection:
  1. Chlorhexidine gluconate oral rinse (Peridex), approximately 5 ml in the younger child and 10 ml in the older child as a swish and spit performed after tooth brushing and without subsequent rinsing or oral intake for a 15-minute interval
  2. Gentian violet 0.5% solution painted over mucosal surface two to three times per day
- Antiviral therapy
  1. In otherwise healthy individuals, antiviral therapy generally is not indicated.
  2. Acyclovir is the drug of choice for those with immunocompromised status, underlying inflammatory skin condition, or neonatal disease.
     a. Ensure adequate hydration.
     b. Adjust the dose for renal dysfunction.
  3. Broad-scale use of acyclovir for primary HSV gingivostomatitis is not recommended despite some evidence to suggest a shorter course of illness if acyclovir is begun within 24 hours of onset of illness in children.
     a. Suggested dosing if necessary for primary mucocutaneous infection:
        (1) 15 mg/kg/day or 750 mg/m^2/day intravenously, divided every 8 hours for 7 days
        (2) 1200 mg/m^2/day orally, divided every 8 hours for 7 to 10 days
     b. Any question of accompanying encephalitis
        (1) 30 mg/kg/day or
        (2) 1500 mg/m^2/day divided every 8 hours for 14 to 21 days

■ FOLLOW-UP & DISPOSITION

- Close follow-up is often required to ensure adequate hydration. Dehydration requiring hospitalization is not uncommon (up to 25% of children in some studies).
- Rare but potential complications in children include herpetic epiglottitis, lymphangitis, central nervous system infection, otitis media, and secondary bacterial infection.

■ PATIENT/FAMILY EDUCATION

- Course of illness
  1. Following a prodrome of malaise and fever, evolution of lesions extends over 4 to 5 days, followed by an additional week of resolution, at minimum (approximate 2- to 3-week duration of illness).
  2. Because the epidermis rather than the dermis is typically involved

in the case of extraoral lesions, healing without scarring is the rule.
- Recurrence
  1. The most common manifestation of recurrent oral HSV is herpes labialis (fever blisters or cold sores), which is estimated to occur in 25% to 50% of individuals with primary oral HSV-1 infection.
  2. Recurrences are often triggered by febrile illnesses, local trauma, sun exposure, stress, or menstruation and involve the site of initial inoculation as well as closely contiguous areas.
  3. Most individuals experience a local prodrome (pain, burning, tingling, itching) lasting from 6 hours to several days, followed by the eruption of papules, which progress to vesicles (the most painful stage), and finally ulcers and crusts.
  4. Most recurrences resolve by 5 to 10 days.
  5. Antiviral therapy for recurrent HSV labialis is of little clinical benefit. Little data exist with respect to the development of drug resistance.
- Return to day care or school
  1. Only children with primary HSV gingivostomatitis who do not have control of oral secretions, are biters, or are too ill to comfortably participate in activities should be excluded from group child care.

■ PREVENTIVE TREATMENT

- Individuals with latent infection may shed virus from the site of initial inoculation while both symptomatic and asymptomatic; however, it is prudent to avoid direct contact with lesions or oral secretions during symptomatic periods.
- Sun block may minimize the frequency of recurrences triggered by sunlight.

۞ PEARLS & CONSIDERATIONS

■ CLINICAL PEARLS

- Anecdotal reports suggest excellent symptomatic relief from *Radiacare* (oral rinse containing acemannan hydrogel from *Aloe vera L.*), often used for radiation-induced oral mucositis.
  1. The dose is 5 ml (younger child) to 15 ml (older children and adults) as a swish and spit four times per day.
  2. Increased oral contact time is thought to enhance effectiveness.
  3. The rinse is good tasting and safe if swallowed.

4. To date, no large trials are available for this indication in children.

- HSV-1 is an important cause of acute pharyngitis in the college-age population, accounting for 5% to 24% of cases (double to triple that caused by group A streptococci in this age group). Approximately 10% to 35% of cases are accompanied by at least one herpeslike lesion of the mouth, throat, or lips or have tender or swollen gingiva.

REFERENCES

1. American Academy of Pediatrics: Herpes simplex. In Peter G (ed): *1997 Red Book: report of the Committee on Infectious Diseases,* ed 24, Elk Grove Village, Ill, 1997, American Academy of Pediatrics.

2. Amir J et al: Treatment of herpes simplex gingivostomatitis with acyclovir in children: a randomized double blind placebo controlled study, *Br Med J* 314:1800, 1997.

3. Connelly BL, Stanberry LR: Herpes simplex virus infections in children, *Curr Opin Pediatr* 7:19, 1995.

4. Halperin SA et al: Absence of viremia in primary herpetic gingivostomatitis, *Pediatr Infect Dis J* 2:452, 1983.

5. Kohl S: Herpes simplex virus. In Feign RD, Cherry JD (eds): *Textbook of pediatric infectious diseases,* ed 4, Philadelphia, 1998, WB Saunders.

6. Kuzushima K et al: Clinical manifestations of primary herpes simplex virus type 1 infection in a closed community, *Pediatrics* 87:152, 1991.

7. Kuzushima K et al: Prophylactic oral acyclovir in outbreaks of primary herpes simplex virus type 1 infection in a closed community, *Pediatrics* 89:379, 1992.

8. McMillan JA et al: Pharyngitis associated with herpes simplex virus in college students, *Pediatr Infect Dis J* 12:280, 1993.

9. Schmitt DL et al: Herpes simplex type 1 infections in group daycare, *Pediatr Infect Dis J* 10:729, 1991.

10. Whitley RJ, Kimberlin DW, Roizman B: Herpes simplex viruses, *Clin Infect Dis* 26:541, 1998.

Author: **C. Elizabeth Trefts, M.D.**

BASIC INFORMATION

DEFINITION
Congenital glaucoma is potentially blinding eye damage secondary to increased intraocular pressure occurring in children younger than 2 years of age.

SYNONYMS
- Infantile glaucoma
- Developmental glaucoma
- Buphthalmos: descriptive term meaning "ox eye," referring to the significant enlargement of the eye that can occur from high pressure
- Pediatric glaucoma

ICD-9CM CODE
743.20 Congenital glaucoma

ETIOLOGY
- Although this is a developmental anomaly of the structures of the outflow pathways of the eye, the exact mechanism is not proven.
- Maldevelopment results in decreased aqueous outflow, causing increased intraocular pressure that damages the eye.

EPIDEMIOLOGY & DEMOGRAPHICS
- 1 in 10,000 to 1 in 30,000 live births
- 75% bilateral eye involvement
- 65% of patients male
- 90% sporadic, 10% familial (most autosomal recessive)
- 25% diagnosed by 6 months, 80% by 1 year

HISTORY
- Large eye(s)
- Epiphora (tearing)
- Photophobia
- Eyelid spasm

PHYSICAL EXAMINATION
- Large eye (corneal enlargement more than 12 mm, normal newborn corneal diameter is 10 mm)
- Corneal edema (hazy to dense opacification)
- Blue/gray eye coloring secondary to edema
- Decreased vision

DIAGNOSIS

DIFFERENTIAL DIAGNOSIS
- Nasolacrimal duct obstruction (ipsilateral rhinorrhea is more consistent with glaucoma)
- Conjunctivitis
- Corneal abrasion
- Trauma
- Iritis

DIAGNOSTIC WORKUP
- Referral to an ophthalmologist is advised with any symptoms of tearing, photophobia, or eyelid spasm.
- Refer for an enlarged and/or possibly opacified cornea.
- Diagnosis is made by the ophthalmologist after a complete eye examination, usually done under general anesthesia.

THERAPY

- Medical treatment with pressure-lowering drops is rarely effective (unlike adult glaucoma).
- Surgery is the preferred treatment for congenital glaucoma; a trabeculotomy or goniotomy is performed to relieve outflow obstruction, thereby decreasing intraocular pressure.
- Surgical treatment is associated with success rates of 80% or greater if the disease is recognized promptly.
  1. Glaucoma associated with other ocular or systemic diseases has a lower success rate.

FOLLOW-UP & DISPOSITION
Lifelong follow-up is needed with the ophthalmologist; routine examinations are necessary to monitor intraocular pressure and rule out ocular damage.

PATIENT/FAMILY EDUCATION
Patients should be evaluated by a geneticist because this disease can be hereditary and associated with multisystem genetic disorders.

PREVENTIVE TREATMENT
In the future, genetic testing may be available.

REFERRAL INFORMATION
All patients should be referred to an ophthalmologist immediately.

PEARLS & CONSIDERATIONS

CLINICAL PEARLS
- Tearing thought to be caused by a nasolacrimal obstruction may be glaucoma.
- Large eyes can be glaucomatous eyes.
- Glaucoma usually causes blindness if left untreated.

WEBSITE
www.health.yahoo.com/health/ Diseases and Conditions/Disease Feed Data/Glaucoma/

REFERENCES
1. Brandt JD: Congenital glaucoma. In Yanoff M, Duker JS (eds): *Ophthalmology,* London, 1999, Mosby.
2. Wagner RS: Glaucoma in children, *Pediatr Clin North Am* 40:855, 1993.
Author: **Kristina Lynch-Guyette, M.D.**

II

BASIC INFORMATION

■ DEFINITION

Acute glomerulonephritis (AGN) is kidney disease characterized by proliferation and inflammation of the glomeruli. Clinically, there is sudden onset of hypertension, edema, hematuria, proteinuria, oliguria, and azotemia. The process generally is self-limited.

ICD-9CM CODES

580.9 Acute glomerulonephritis
580.0 Poststreptococcal glomerulonephritis

■ ETIOLOGY

- Most cases are postinfectious, with poststreptococcal glomerulonephritis being the most common. Other infectious agents include the following:
  1. Bacteria *(Streptococcus viridans, Staphylococcus aureus, Klebsiella pneumoniae, Treponema pallidum)*
  2. Viruses (hepatitis B, cytomegalovirus, Epstein-Barr virus, Coxsackie, mumps)
  3. Rickettsiae
  4. Fungi
  5. Parasites
- Acute poststreptococcal glomerulonephritis (APSGN) is the most studied disease type.
  1. The exact pathogenetic mechanism is not completely understood, but it is believed to be an immune complex–mediated process.
  2. APSGN typically occurs 7 to 10 days after a pharyngitic group A β-hemolytic streptococcal infection (often involving strains M type 12, 1, 4, 3, 25, 49) or 14 to 21 days after streptococcal skin infections (strains 49, 55, 2, 57 or 60).
- Not all strains of streptococci lead to nephritis, suggesting that organism characteristics are also important.
- Histologically, AGN is characterized by a diffuse exudative and proliferative glomerulonephritis. Immunofluorescence reveals granular immunoglobulin G (IgG) and C3 deposits along the capillary walls. Electron microscopy reveals subepithelial deposits.

■ EPIDEMIOLOGY & DEMOGRAPHICS

- The actual incidence of APSGN is unknown because many cases are subclinical.
  1. According to one series, the incidence of APSGN (including subclinical cases) is estimated to be about 25% after streptococcal infection.
- APSGN occurs sporadically or in epidemics.
- It is mainly a disease of children, with typical age range between 2 and 8 years.
  1. Fewer than 5% of patients are younger than 2 years old.
- Male:female ratio is approximately 2:1.

■ HISTORY

- Abrupt onset of gross hematuria
- Acute onset of edema and weight gain over several days
- Oliguria
- Pallor
- Pharyngitis 7 to 10 days before or impetigo 14 to 21 days before
- Nonspecific symptoms: headache, malaise, lethargy, anorexia, fever, abdominal pain, weakness
- Poor history of growth: suggests possible underlying chronic illness, which may be acute presentation of chronic glomerulonephritis
- Other illness symptoms include the following:
  1. Concomitant pharyngitis or upper respiratory infection symptoms suggest possible IgA nephropathy.
  2. Preceding illness symptoms suggest another infectious agent besides those caused by streptococcus.
  3. Purpuric rash, abdominal pain, and arthritis suggest Henoch-Schönlein purpura.
  4. Malar rash, arthritis, fever, and malaise suggest systemic lupus erythematosus.
  5. Persistent fever suggests subacute bacterial endocarditis–associated glomerulonephritis.
  6. Persistent fever in patients with ventriculoatrial shunts suggests possible shunt nephritis.
- Family history of renal disease
  1. Associated family history of hearing loss suggests hereditary nephritis—Alport's.

■ PHYSICAL EXAMINATION

- HEENT
  1. Funduscopic examination with atrioventricular nicking or arteriolar narrowing indicates hypertensive changes.
  2. Periorbital edema suggests volume overload.
  3. Erythema and/or exudate of pharynx suggests concomitant infection.
- Cardiac
  1. Hypertension, jugular venous distention, gallop, and tachycardia all indicate volume overload.
  2. New murmur may be secondary to volume overload or suggestive of nephritis associated with subacute bacterial endocarditis.
- Pulmonary
  1. Rales and/or cough may indicate pulmonary edema.
- Abdomen
  1. Distention and ascites suggest fluid overload.
- Extremities
  1. Edema
  2. Joint swelling or erythema
- Skin
  1. Pallor indicates anemia.
  2. Healed skin lesions are suggestive of recent impetigo.
  3. Purpura suggests Henoch-Schönlein purpura.
  4. Malar rash suggests lupus.
- Neurologic
  1. Rarely, seizures and/or coma may occur secondary to hypertensive encephalopathy.
- Growth parameters
  1. Weight and height, if decreased, suggest chronic illness.

DIAGNOSIS

■ DIFFERENTIAL DIAGNOSIS

- Henoch-Schönlein purpura
- Other postinfectious glomerulonephritides
- Subacute bacterial endocarditis–associated nephritis
- Shunt nephritis
- Acute presentation of chronic glomerulonephritis
  1. IgA nephropathy
  2. Membranoproliferative glomerulonephritis (MPGN)
  3. Systemic lupus erythematosus (SLE)
- Rapidly progressive glomerulonephritis

■ DIAGNOSTIC WORKUP

- Diagnosis is generally made on clinical grounds with typical history, physical examination, and evidence of previous streptococcal infection either by culture done at time of infection or by serology.
- Urine studies should be obtained.
  1. Decreased urine volume
  2. Hematuria with or without red blood cell (RBC) casts
  3. Proteinuria—generally trace to 2+; unusual to be nephrotic range
- Chemistries
  1. Blood urea nitrogen and creatinine may be increased.
  2. Electrolyte changes—hyperkalemia, acidosis, and hyperphosphatemia may be present.
- Hematology
  1. Anemia
- Hypocomplementemia (C3) during the acute phase occurs in 90% of patients with APSGN.
  1. Typically normalizes within 6 to 8 weeks.
  2. Failure of C3 to normalize after 6 to 8 weeks raises concern that the diagnosis is MPGN or SLE.

- Elevated ASO titer occurs in 80% of patients.
  1. Rise in titers starts approximately 2 weeks after infection and peaks at approximately 3 to 5 weeks.
  2. Elevation is blunted if the patient is treated with antibiotics early in the course of pharyngitis.
  3. If the initial infection was impetigo, only 30% have an increase in ASO titer.
- Anti-DNase B titer is the most sensitive indicator of prior streptococcal infection.
- See "Patient/Family Education" for the typical course for resolution of oliguria, hypertension, hematuria, proteinuria, and C3.
- Definitive diagnosis is made by renal biopsy, but biopsy is generally not required. Indications for consideration of biopsy include atypical presentation:
  1. Age younger than 2 years or older than 12 years
  2. Presence of nephrotic syndrome
  3. Significant systemic symptoms
  4. Abnormal growth curve
  5. Atypical course—delay in resolution of glomerulonephritis (see "Patient/Family Education" for typical course description).

🗈 THERAPY

■ NONPHARMACOLOGIC
- Predominantly dietary:
  1. Salt restriction
  2. Potassium and phosphate restriction—as indicated by laboratory values
  3. Fluid restriction
  4. If significantly volume overloaded, fluid restriction should equal insensible water losses plus urine output.

■ MEDICAL
- Diuretics can be given.
  1. Used to treat hypertension because hypertension occurs secondary to fluid and salt retention

2. Used to decrease edema
3. Used to improve urine output in oliguric states
- Antihypertensives, in addition to diuretics, may be required to treat hypertension.
- Phosphate binders (e.g., calcium carbonate with meals) should be used for hyperphosphatemia, if present.
- For documented concurrent infection, antibiotics are needed.
- Nephrotic medications should not be used.
- If the patient has severe renal failure, with severe electrolyte abnormalities or uremia, refer to a pediatric nephrologist for consideration of dialysis (required in a few patients).
- Consider hospital admission.
  1. Oliguria, hypertension, renal insufficiency, electrolyte disorders (e.g., hyperkalemia)

■ FOLLOW-UP & DISPOSITION
- Monitor blood pressure, renal function, and urinalysis for presence of blood and protein.
- Frequency of follow-up depends on severity of disease.
  1. Monitoring may be at weekly to monthly intervals (depending on disease severity) for the first 6 months and then at 3- to 6-month intervals until hematuria and proteinuria are resolved for 1 year.
  2. Once hematuria and proteinuria are resolved for 1 year, yearly urinalysis and blood pressure checks are recommended.

■ PATIENT/FAMILY EDUCATION
- Recovery is generally complete for APSGN; however, approximately 1% to 2% may have residual urinalysis abnormalities or hypertension.
- APSGN generally does not occur more than once.
- The typical course is as follows:
  1. Oliguria and azotemia generally resolve within 2 weeks.
  2. Hypertension resolves within 3 weeks.
  3. Gross hematuria resolves within 3 weeks.

4. C3 normalizes by 6 to 8 weeks.
5. Proteinuria generally resolves by 6 months.
6. Hematuria generally resolves by 12 months.

■ REFERRAL INFORMATION
Refer to a pediatric nephrologist if the patient has hypertension, oliguria, renal insufficiency, significant systemic symptoms, atypical course, nephrotic-range proteinuria, severe electrolyte abnormalities, uremia, or persistently low C3.

⚙ PEARLS & CONSIDERATIONS

■ CLINICAL PEARLS
- Presence of RBC casts signifies glomerulonephritis, but the absence does not rule it out.
- The ideal time to examine urine is immediately after the patient voids.
- If gross hematuria is present, it may be easier to detect casts by examining one drop of unspun urine instead of spun urine.
- Treatment with antibiotics at the time of pharyngitis or impetigo does *not* affect the incidence of APSGN. Antibiotic therapy is important to provide prophylaxis against development of future rheumatic heart disease.

REFERENCES
1. Brenner RM, Petersen J: Postinfectious glomerulonephritis, *Nephrol Rounds* 3, 2000.
2. Falk RJ, Jennette JC, Nachman PH: Primary glomerular diseases. In Brenner BM, Rector FC (eds): *Brenner and Rector's the kidney*, ed 6, Philadelphia, 2000, WB Saunders.
3. Jordan SC, Lemire JM: Acute glomerulonephritis: diagnosis and treatment, *Pediatr Clin North Am* 29:857, 1982.
4. Madaio MP, Harrington JT: Current concepts: the diagnosis of acute glomerulonephritis, *N Engl J Med* 309: 1299, 1983.
Author: **Ayesa Mian, M.D.**

BASIC INFORMATION

■ DEFINITION
The nephritic syndrome is characterized by hematuria, proteinuria, oliguria, and volume overload. Acute glomerulonephritis generally has an abrupt onset and is self-limited. Chronic glomerulonephritis may present with an abrupt or insidious onset and does not generally resolve on its own and, indeed, may progress to chronic renal failure. The chronic glomerulonephritides of childhood discussed in this section include membranoproliferative glomerulonephritis (MPGN), Henoch-Schönlein purpura (HSP), IgA nephropathy (IgAN), systemic lupus erythematosus (SLE), and Alport's nephritis.

ICD-9CM CODES
583.9   Glomerulonephritis
287.0   Henoch-Schönlein purpura
583.0   IgAN
710.0   SLE nephritis
759.89 Alport's nephritis

Membranoproliferative Glomerulonephritis
■ SYNONYMS
- Mesangiocapillary glomerulonephritis
- MPGN

■ ETIOLOGY
- Diffuse mesangial proliferation and thickening of capillary walls are seen.
  1. Primary (idiopathic) or secondary (associated with other diseases)
- Idiopathic is the most common type in children and is classified into three subtypes.
  1. MPGN type I
     a. Type I is the most common subtype.
     b. It is an immune complex disease with unknown antigen.
     c. Immune complex formation leads to complement activation via the classical pathway.
     d. Immune complex deposition in glomeruli (mesangium and subendothelial space) is seen.
     e. Immunofluorescence microscopy reveals immunoglobulins and classical complement pathway proteins.
  2. MPGN type II
     a. Type II is considered "dense deposit disease."
     b. Dense ribbonlike deposits are present within the basement membranes of the glomeruli, tubules, and Bowman's capsules; deposits do not appear to contain immunoglobulins.

     c. Complement activation occurs via the alternative pathway.
        (1) C3 nephritic factor is an antibody that binds C3bBb and prevents inactivation of this complex, resulting in continued C3 breakdown because C3bBb normally cleaves C3 into C3a and C3b.
        (2) However, no correlation exists between C3 nephritic factor and disease activity.
     d. Immunofluorescence is positive for C3 but not immunoglobulins.
  3. MPGN type III
     a. Similar to type 1
     b. Deposits in subepithelial space, subendothelial space, and mesangium
     c. Complement activation via alternative pathway
- MPGN can be secondary to other diseases.
  1. Systemic immune complex disease
     a. SLE
     b. HSP
  2. Infections
     a. Subacute bacterial endocarditis
     b. Shunt nephritis
     c. Human immunodeficiency virus (HIV)
  3. Chronic liver disease
     a. Hepatitis B or C
     b. α_1-Antitrypsin deficiency
  4. Other
     a. Lymphoma
     b. Sickle cell disease
     c. Hemolytic uremic syndrome

■ EPIDEMIOLOGY & DEMOGRAPHICS
Occurs in older children and young adolescents (ages 8 to 16 years of age)

■ CLINICAL MANIFESTATIONS
- Presentations
  1. Asymptomatic hematuria and proteinuria detected on routine urinalysis
  2. Acute nephritic picture
  3. Acute nephrotic picture
  4. Rapidly progressive glomerulonephritis: accounts for a few patients
- Symptoms/signs
  1. Preceding respiratory infection in approximately 50% of cases
  2. Gross hematuria in approximately 20%
  3. Nephrotic syndrome in approximately 70%; may have history of edema and weight gain (see the section "Nephrotic Syndrome")
  4. Hypertension in approximately 30%
     a. May have headaches or blurry vision
  5. Asymptomatic hematuria and proteinuria in 20% to 40%
  6. Azotemia in approximately 30%

  7. Secondary forms may be suggested by history of malar rash, purpura, weight loss, arthritis, recurrent infections, cardiac disease, ventriculoatrial shunt, blood transfusion, jaundice

🔬 DIAGNOSIS

■ DIFFERENTIAL DIAGNOSIS
- Acute poststreptococcal glomerulonephritis (APSGN)
  1. C3 returns to normal in 6 to 8 weeks with APSGN but remains low with MPGN.
  2. Proteinuria is mild to moderate with APSGN and mild to nephrotic range with MPGN.
  3. Serum albumin is mildly low with APSGN and moderately to severely low with MPGN.
  4. Hypertension is transient with APSGN and persistent with MPGN.
- IgAN

■ DIAGNOSTIC WORKUP
- Urinalysis with proteinuria and/or hematuria
- Quantitated proteinuria with spot urine protein:creatinine ratio or 24-hour urine for protein
- Hypocomplementemia
  1. C3 low in approximately 75% of cases (types I, II, and III)
  2. C4 often low in type I; normal in type II
- Renal biopsy required to make diagnosis

💊 THERAPY

■ MEDICAL
- Idiopathic MPGN
  1. Treatment with steroids is controversial, but many pediatric nephrologists treat with alternate-day prednisone for a prolonged course (at least 2 years).
  2. Treatments with cytotoxic agents and antiplatelet agents have been tried with variable success.
  3. Other medical interventions include the following:
     a. Antihypertensives if hypertensive
     b. Diuretics with or without albumin if nephrotic and edematous
- Secondary forms of MPGN
  1. Treat the underlying disease.

■ REFERRAL INFORMATION
Patients require referral to a pediatric nephrologist for both diagnosis and management.

■ **FOLLOW-UP & PATIENT/FAMILY EDUCATION**
• If untreated, 50% progress to renal failure within 10 years.
  1. The risk is greater if the patient presents with renal insufficiency, nephrotic syndrome, severe hypertension, a biopsy revealing more than 50% crescents, or marked interstitial fibrosis.
• A retrospective pediatric study suggests better preservation of renal function with alternate-day steroid treatment as compared with no treatment.
• If the patient is nephrotic, need to discuss with parents the potential complications of nephrotic syndrome, such as peritonitis (see "Complications" in the section "Nephrotic Syndrome").
• If steroids are used, review the side effects of steroids (see the section "Nephrotic Syndrome").

 PEARLS & CONSIDERATIONS

■ **CLINICAL PEARLS**
• Patients are often initially diagnosed as APSGN but do not follow the typical course.
  1. C3 remains low for more than 8 weeks.
  2. Nephrotic-range proteinuria is present.

IgA Nephropathy

 BASIC INFORMATION

■ **SYNONYM**
Berger's disease

■ **ETIOLOGY**
• Primary
  1. Pathogenesis is incompletely understood.
  2. Presence of mesangial IgA and C3 deposits suggests that immune complex deposition leads to activation of complement via the alternative pathway and renal injury.
• Secondary (associated with other diseases)
  1. Systemic disease (HSP, SLE, cystic fibrosis, celiac disease, Crohn's disease)
  2. Malignancy (non-Hodgkin's lymphoma)
  3. Infections (*Mycoplasma, Toxoplasma*)
  4. Other (chronic liver disease)

■ **EPIDEMIOLOGY & DEMOGRAPHICS**
• IgAN is the most common glomerulonephritis in the world.

• The male:female ratio is 2:1 to 6:1.
• Lower prevalence exists in African Americans.
• It occurs at all ages but is most common in the second and third decades of life.
• IgAN is uncommon in children younger than 10 years of age.

■ **CLINICAL MANIFESTATIONS**
Variable presentations
• Gross hematuria
  1. May be asymptomatic
  2. May be associated with loin pain
  3. Often associated with upper respiratory infection and typically occurs after 1 to 2 days as compared with 1 to 2 weeks with post-streptococcal glomerulonephritis
  4. Less often associated with other infections (e.g., diarrhea)
  5. Variable intervals between episodes
  6. Microscopic hematuria persists between episodes of gross hematuria
  7. More common presentation in children compared with adults
• Asymptomatic hematuria with or without proteinuria
  1. Hematuria persistent
  2. Acute nephritic syndrome
  3. Nephrotic syndrome
  4. Mixed nephritic-nephrotic syndrome

 DIAGNOSIS

■ **DIFFERENTIAL DIAGNOSIS**
Other glomerulonephritides
• MPGN
• HSP
• APSGN
• Alport's nephritis

■ **DIAGNOSTIC WORKUP**
• No specific laboratory or serologic test is available to diagnose IgAN.
• IgA levels are elevated in the serum of approximately 50% of patients.
• C3 is generally normal with IgA nephropathy but can be low as with APSGN, MPGN, and SLE.
• Quantitated proteinuria with spot urine protein/creatinine or 24-hour collection should be done to rule out nephrotic range proteinuria.
• Renal biopsy is required.

 THERAPY

Possible treatments (e.g., prednisone, fish oil, angiotensin-converting enzyme inhibitors) should be considered by the pediatric nephrologist after reviewing the biopsy.

■ **FOLLOW-UP & PATIENT/FAMILY EDUCATION**
• If the patient is nephrotic, need to discuss with parents the potential complications of nephrotic syndrome, such as peritonitis (see "Complications" in the section "Nephrotic Syndrome").
• If steroids are used, review side effects of steroids.

■ **PROGNOSIS**
• Approximately 25% go into clinical remission if mild disease.
• Approximately 30% develop chronic renal failure.
• Estimated that 1% to 2% develop end-stage renal failure (ESRD) each year from the time of diagnosis.

■ **REFERRAL INFORMATION**
All patients should be followed by a pediatric nephrologist.

Henoch-Schönlein Purpura

 BASIC INFORMATION

■ **DEFINITION**
Systemic vasculitis characterized by palpable purpura, abdominal pain, arthralgias, and nephritis. IgA circulating immune complexes deposit in skin, kidney, and other organs.

■ **ETIOLOGY**
• HSP is an immune complex disease with IgA immune complexes associated with small vessel vasculitis.
• The pathogenesis is unknown.

■ **EPIDEMIOLOGY & DEMOGRAPHICS**
• HSP predominantly affects children, although can occur rarely in adults.
• HSP is rare in children younger than 2 years.
• Peak incidence age is 4 to 5 years.
• HSP often follows an upper respiratory infection.
• Renal disease is more likely to be severe in older children.

■ **CLINICAL MANIFESTATIONS**
• Symptoms may occur in any order.
  1. Skin
    a. Almost all children exhibit skin lesions at some point in the course.
    b. Skin lesions start as erythematous macules; some develop into urticarial papules and then become purpuric.
    c. In younger children, rash may be more urticarial and associated with localized edema.
    d. Rash generally involves extensor surfaces of extremities and buttocks, with symmetric distribution and sparing of trunk.

    e. Recurrent crops of the purpuric rash may occur for 3 months.
2. Joints
    a. Joint involvement occurs in approximately 70% of patients.
    b. Consists of arthralgias and peri-articular edema.
    c. Major joints affected are knees, ankles, elbows, and wrists.
    d. Symptoms are transient and leave no permanent damage.
3. Gastrointestinal (GI) disease
    a. GI involvement occurs in approximately 50% to 70% of patients.
    b. Symptoms include colicky abdominal pain, vomiting, melena, and hematochezia.
    c. Intussusception is a complication.
4. Renal disease
    a. Renal disease is common, with an incidence estimated at 20% to 100%, depending on the series.
    b. Renal disease generally develops within days to weeks after onset.
    c. Involvement may be isolated microscopic hematuria, microscopic hematuria and proteinuria, hypertension, or nephrotic syndrome.
    d. Gross hematuria is not common.
    e. No correlation exists between the severity of extrarenal manifestations and the severity of kidney disease.
    f. Renal disease is a major cause of long-term morbidity.
5. Constitutional symptoms
    a. Fever, malaise, and weakness may be present.

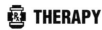 DIAGNOSIS

■ DIFFERENTIAL DIAGNOSIS
- Polyarteritis nodosa
- SLE
- Other vasculitides

■ DIAGNOSTIC WORKUP
- The diagnosis is generally made clinically by the presence of a combination of the aforementioned symptoms.
- Laboratory studies include the following:
  1. Blood urea nitrogen, creatinine, total protein, albumin
  2. Urinalysis
  3. Spot urine protein/creatinine on first morning specimen or 24-hour urine for protein and creatinine
- If atypical rash or course, check antinuclear antibodies (ANA), antineurophilic cytoplasmic antibody, complement levels, complete blood count, and coagulation studies.

- A renal biopsy is generally done if the diagnosis is in question or if associated with nephrotic syndrome.
  1. Shows mesangial IgA deposition
- A skin biopsy reveals leukocytoclastic vasculitis with IgA deposition in vasculature.

THERAPY

■ MEDICAL
- Steroids are beneficial for abdominal pain.
- If no evidence of nephritis is present at the time of diagnosis:
  1. Consider treatment with prednisone (dosage: 1 mg/kg/day for 14 days) as potential prophylaxis for development of nephritis.
  2. Monitor urinalysis (UA) and blood pressure one to three times per week initially, then once a week to once every other week until systemic manifestations resolve and UA normalizes.
  3. If abnormalities are present, quantitate proteinuria and monitor renal function.
  4. Monitor closely for development of nephritis in first 4 months.
- If evidence of nephritis is already present at the time of diagnosis:
  1. Steroids are not proven to be beneficial.
  2. If associated with nephrotic syndrome, renal insufficiency, or hypertension, refer to a pediatric nephrologist for evaluation, follow-up, and consideration of therapy.

■ FOLLOW-UP & PATIENT/FAMILY EDUCATION
- Long-term morbidity is related to renal disease.
- If the patient is nephrotic, need to discuss with parents the potential complications of nephrotic syndrome, such as peritonitis (see "Complications" in the section "Nephrotic Syndrome").

■ PROGNOSIS
- Ninety-five percent of children have complete renal recovery from acute illness.
  1. Most have good long-term renal prognosis, especially if involvement included isolated hematuria or hematuria with mild proteinuria.
  2. Long-term studies show up to 25% have late deterioration, even if full renal recovery initially.
     a. With pregnancy, more than 30% develop hypertension or proteinuria.
- Less than 1% develop ESRD.
  1. Poor prognostic indicators include

acute nephritic presentation, persistent nephrotic syndrome, and more than 50% crescents on renal biopsy.

■ REFERRAL INFORMATION
- Refer to a pediatric nephrologist if the patient has nephritic syndrome, nephrotic syndrome, renal insufficiency, or hypertension.
- Patients with chronic nephritis secondary to HSP should all be followed by a pediatric nephrologist.

Systemic Lupus Erythematosus

■ BASIC INFORMATION

See the section "Systemic Lupus Erythematosus."

■ SYNONYM
Lupus nephritis

■ ETIOLOGY
- SLE is a disease of generalized autoimmunity with an unclear pathogenesis.
- Excess of polyclonal B-cell activation results in production of various antibodies, including autoantibodies.
- Tissue deposition of immune complexes leads to inflammation.

■ EPIDEMIOLOGY & DEMOGRAPHICS
- Incidence and prevalence not well established
- Less common in children
- Increased frequency in Hispanic, Asian, and African Americans
- Female predominance with female:male ratio as follows:
  1. 2:1 in prepubertal children
  2. 4.5:1 in adolescents
  3. 8:1 to 12:1 in adults
  4. 2:1 in patients older than 60 years of age

■ CLINICAL MANIFESTATIONS
- Constitutional symptoms—common initial symptoms
  1. Fever
  2. Weight loss
  3. Malaise
  4. Fatigue
- Oral mucosa
  1. Ulcers
- Skin
  1. Malar rash present in approximately one third of children
  2. Photosensitivity
  3. Discoid rash
- Joint
  1. Swelling
  2. Arthritis
  3. Pain
- Central nervous system
  1. Seizures
  2. Altered mental status or behavior

- Cardiovascular
  1. Hypertension (headaches, visual disturbances)
  2. Pericarditis (chest pain)
- Respiratory
  1. Pleurisy
- GI
  1. Vasculitis (abdominal pain)
- Renal manifestations when SLE nephritis is present*
  1. Proteinuria: approximately 100%
  2. Nephrosis: 45% to 65%
  3. Granular casts: 30%
  4. Red blood cell casts: 10%
  5. Microhematuria: 80%
  6. Gross hematuria: 1% to 2%
  7. Impaired renal function: 40% to 80%
  8. Rapid decline in renal function: 30%
  9. Acute renal failure: 1% to 2%
  10. Hypertension: 15% to 50%
  11. Hyperkalemia: 15%
  12. Tubular abnormalities: 60% to 80%

🔬 DIAGNOSIS

■ DIFFERENTIAL DIAGNOSIS
- HSP
- Other collagen vascular diseases

■ DIAGNOSTIC WORKUP
- American College of Rheumatology Criteria (see the section "Systemic Lupus Erythematosus")
- Diagnosis of SLE renal disease
  1. Renal biopsy to determine class of involvement (World Health Organization [WHO] classification)
     a. Class I: normal
        (1) No evidence of renal disease
        (2) Normal urinalysis
     b. Class II: mesangial hypercellularity
        (1) Mild hematuria with or without proteinuria
        (2) Renal insufficiency (rare)
        (3) Good prognosis
     c. Class III: focal proliferative glomerulonephritis
        (1) Hematuria
        (2) Proteinuria (may be nephrotic)
        (3) Hypertension
        (4) Mild renal insufficiency
     d. Class IV: diffuse proliferative glomerulonephritis
        (1) Hematuria
        (2) Proteinuria (may have nephrotic syndrome)
        (3) Hypertension, renal insufficiency
        (4) Most common and most severe form of nephritis
     e. Class V: membranous nephropathy
        (1) Profound and persistent proteinuria, generally nephrotic
     f. Class VI: advanced sclerosing
- Laboratory tests
  1. ANA
     a. ANA positive in 90% of SLE patients
     b. Anti-dsDNA, anti-C1q, anti-Sm strongly associated with nephritis
     c. Anti Ro/La present at most in low titers in patients with nephritis
     d. If negative ANA and anti-SSA/Ro positive, usually little or no renal disease
  2. Antiphospholipid antibodies
     a. Present in one third of patients with nephritis
     b. Can be associated with renal arterial, venous, and glomerular capillary thrombi
  3. Complement levels
     a. Depressed at presentation in more than 75% of patients, more common in nephritis
     b. C4 and C1q more depressed than C3
  4. Complete blood count: may have leukopenia, hemolytic anemia, and/or thrombocytopenia
  5. Chemistries: blood urea nitrogen, creatinine, total protein, albumin
  6. Urinalysis: quantitate proteinuria with spot urine protein/creatinine or 24-hour collection
- Role of renal biopsy
  1. To confirm diagnosis of SLE nephritis
  2. To determine class of nephritis because class influences prognosis and therapy

℞ THERAPY

■ MEDICAL
- To be recommended by pediatric rheumatologist and/or pediatric nephrologist
- Acute phase: treatment of severe life-threatening disease; goal to get disease under control
  1. High-dose corticosteroids
  2. Pulse solumedrol
  3. Cytotoxic agents—Cytoxan
- Chronic phase: long-term management of chronic disease; goal to minimize side effects and keep disease under control
  1. Steroids
  2. Cytoxan
     a. For severe class III, class IV, and cerebritis
     b. Allows steroid sparing
     c. Side effects: alopecia, nausea, vomiting, hemorrhagic cystitis, infection, sterility, and malignancy
  3. Azathioprine (Imuran)
     a. Effective with nonrenal manifestations
     b. Allows steroid sparing
  4. Mycophenolate mofetil
  5. Cyclosporine
     a. May help decrease proteinuria and help spare steroids
  6. Antimalarials
     a. Hydroxychloroquine
     b. Chloroquine
  7. Nonsteroidal antiinflammatory drugs
     a. Aspirin
     b. Ibuprofen
  8. Therapy is recommended based on type and severity of renal and extrarenal manifestations.

■ FOLLOW-UP & PATIENT/FAMILY EDUCATION
- Patients may require more than one renal biopsy in a lifetime because class of nephritis can change over time.
- If patient is nephrotic, need to discuss with parents the potential complications of nephrotic syndrome.
- Course is variable and depends on renal and extrarenal manifestations.
- Renal prognosis depends on class of nephritis.
  1. Prognosis is improved for class IV; 5-year renal survival has improved from less than 30% to more than 90% with introduction of Cytoxan.
  2. Infection and renal failure are leading causes of death from SLE.

■ REFERRAL INFORMATION
Patients with SLE nephritis should be followed by a pediatric nephrologist and/or pediatric rheumatologist.

⚙ PEARLS & CONSIDERATIONS

■ CLINICAL PEARLS
The course of SLE varies dramatically and is unpredictable.

Alport's Nephritis

 BASIC INFORMATION

■ DEFINITION
Alport's nephritis is a generalized, inherited disorder of basement membranes characterized by hematuria, which progresses over time to include proteinuria and renal insufficiency/failure, sensorineural hearing loss, and ocular abnormalities.

---

*Data from Cameron JS: *J Am Soc Nephrol* 10:413, 1999.

■ ETIOLOGY

Alport's syndrome: Abnormal formation of glomerular basement membrane results from underexpression of the α-3, α-4, or α-5/6 chains of type IV collagen.

■ EPIDEMIOLOGY & DEMOGRAPHICS

- Gene frequency estimated at 1 in 10,000 in the United States.
- Cases have been reported in all ethnic groups.
- X-linked Alport's syndrome (XLAS) accounts for approximately 80% of cases.
  1. Genetic defect is a mutation in COL4A5 (gene coding for α-5/6 chain of type IV collagen).
     a. In 10% to 15% of cases, mutation is a deletion.
     b. In others, mutation is a point mutation.
- Autosomal-recessive cases are also reported, involving mutations in COL4A3 or COL4A4.

■ CLINICAL MANIFESTATIONS

- Affected males with XLAS:
  1. Primary finding is hematuria.
     a. May be persistent and microscopic or intermittent and gross, typically after an upper respiratory infection.
     b. Typically develop hematuria within the first decade of life.
     c. About 70% present before the age of 6 years.
  2. Proteinuria eventually develops in affected males, and the amount progressively increases with increasing age and may reach nephrotic range.
  3. Affected males eventually progress to ESRD, but the rate of progression is variable.
- Heterozygous females with XLAS:
  1. Hematuria
     a. Affected individuals may have intermittent microscopic hematuria.
     b. However, about 10% do not have hematuria.
  2. Proteinuria
     a. May or may not be present
  3. Course generally more benign than that for affected males; may maintain reasonably good renal function even when elderly
  4. Presence of gross hematuria in childhood, nephrotic syndrome, and diffuse glomerular basement thickening suggest progressive nephritis in affected women
- Hypertension also occurs with increasing age.

- Hearing loss is not congenital but is generally detectable by late childhood/early adolescence.
  1. Deafness occurs in approximately 55% of males and 45% of females.
  2. Hearing loss occurs early on, detectable only by audiometry with decreased hearing in the range of 2000 to 8000 Hz.
  3. Hearing loss worsens with time to include other frequencies.
- Ocular anomalies occur in approximately 15% to 30% and include anterior lenticonus.
  1. The presence of anterior lenticonus is generally associated with progression to ESRD before age 30 years.

🔬 DIAGNOSIS

■ DIFFERENTIAL DIAGNOSIS

- IgAN
- MPGN
- Thin basement membrane disease

■ DIAGNOSTIC WORKUP

- Based on the following:
  1. Presence of hematuria with or without proteinuria, hypertension, and renal failure
  2. Associated with familial hematuria and sensorineural hearing loss in patient or affected relative
  3. Progression to ESRD in an affected relative
- Renal biopsy reveals the following:
  1. Absence of α-3, α-4, or α-5 chains of type IV collagen from glomerular basement membrane and distal tubular basement membrane suggests diagnosis of Alport's nephritis.
  2. Variable width of glomerular basement membrane (thick or thin) is seen with basket-weaving and lamellation.
- Linkage analysis is feasible in families with large pedigree where X-linked inheritance is suspected. In such a family, if the mutation has been identified, direct mutational analysis can be done.

💊 THERAPY

- No proven therapy is available to slow progression of the disease.
- Supportive care is instituted once the patient is in renal failure.

■ FOLLOW-UP & PATIENT/FAMILY EDUCATION

- All patients with Alport's nephritis should be followed by a pediatric nephrologist.
- Periodic audiometry and ophthalmology examinations should be conducted.

⟠ PEARLS & CONSIDERATIONS

■ CLINICAL PEARLS

All chronic glomerulonephritides may have an acute presentation.

■ WEBSITES

- Alport's Syndrome Home Page: www. cc.utah.edu/~cla6202/ASHP.htm
- Henoch-Schönlein Pediatric Database: www.icondata.com/health/pedbase
- IgA Nephropathy Foundation Home Page: www.igan.org
- SLE Home Page: www.hamline.edu/~lupus/
- Support group for parents—NephKids: http://cnserver0.nkf.med.ualberta.ca/nephkids
- Website for Children with SLE: www.kidshealth.org/kid/health_problems/life_lupus.html

■ SUPPORT GROUP

NephKids Cyber-Support Group for Parents of Children with Kidney Disease

REFERENCES

1. Andreoli SP: Chronic glomerulonephritis in childhood, *Pediatr Clin North Am* 42:1487, 1995.
2. Appel GB, Radhakrishnan J, D'Agati V: Secondary glomerular disease. In Brenner BM, Rector FC (eds): *Brenner and Rector's the kidney*, ed 6, Philadelphia, 2000, WB Saunders. 1396-1398.
3. Falk RJ, Jennette JC, Nachman PH: Primary glomerular diseases. In Brenner BM, Rector FC (eds): *Brenner and Rector's the kidney*, ed 6, Philadelphia, 2000, WB Saunders.
4. Mollica F, et al: Effectiveness of early prednisone treatment in preventing the development of nephropathy in anaphylactoid purpura, *Eur J Pediatr* 151:40, 1992.

Author: **Ayesa Mian, M.D.**

BASIC INFORMATION

■ DEFINITION
Gonorrhea is an infection of the eye, skin, genital tract, joint, pharynx, or blood caused by the gram-negative diplococcus *Neisseria gonorrhoeae*.

■ SYNONYMS
- Pelvic inflammatory disease (PID)
- Sexually transmitted disease (STD)
- Vaginal infection

ICD-9CM CODES
098.0, 098.40 Gonococcal conjunctivitis
098.19 Pelvic infection
098.15 Cervical infection

■ ETIOLOGY
- STD with *Neisseria gonorrhoeae,* a gram-negative diplococcus
- Infants exposed to an infected mother in the birth canal

■ EPIDEMIOLOGY & DEMOGRAPHICS
- In 1997, 324,901 cases of gonorrhea were reported in the United States.
- Ophthalmia neonatorum occurs in 2% to 5% of live births.
- Adolescent girls and men 20 to 24 years of age have the highest rates of infection.
- The rate for 15- to 19-year-olds is 530 per 100,000.
- PID is an ascending infection of the upper genital tract.
  1. Gonorrhea is responsible for 50% of cases of PID.
  2. Up to one third of untreated cases of gonorrhea infection result in PID.
- Coinfection with *Chlamydia trachomatis* is common.

■ HISTORY
- Newborn
  1. Ophthalmia neonatorum occurs after an incubation of less than 3 days.
     a. Discharge is initially watery, becoming thick and mucopurulent.
     b. Discharge occurs after the incubation period and, if not treated, progresses to corneal involvement in most cases.
     c. Some cases do have a benign limited course.
     d. Disease is often bilateral.
     e. Transmission is the result of exposure to infected cervical exudate during delivery.
     f. There is a history of not receiving ocular prophylaxis in the newborn period.

  2. Scalp abscesses caused by gonorrhea occur after in utero fetal monitoring.
  3. Disseminated infections are rare.
- Prepubertal
  1. Presents as vaginitis
     a. Vaginal discharge
     b. Dysuria, frequency, urgency
  2. Sexual abuse unless proven otherwise
- Adolescents
  1. One third of genital tract infections are asymptomatic.
  2. Urethritis occurs approximately 1 week after exposure.
     a. Dysuria
     b. Mucoid discharge, which becomes purulent
  3. In females, abdominal pain, pelvic pain or fullness, dysuria, and discharge are the common complaints.
  4. Fever, vomiting, and anorexia also occur, especially with more extensive disease.
  5. Extension from genital mucosal infections can lead to less common presentations.
     a. Scrotal pain (epididymitis) may occur.
     b. Right upper quadrant pain, vomiting, and anorexia occur with perihepatitis, Fitzhugh Curtis.
     c. Painful and enlarged lesions (bartholinitis) can be present.
     d. PID presents with mild to severe anorexia, abdominal or pelvic pain, and fever.
  6. Pharyngitis is often asymptomatic but may present with an exudative sore throat.
  7. From 1% to 3% of adolescents who are untreated develop disseminated gonococcal infection.
     a. Presents with septic arthritis or with systemic signs (fever, chills, and polyarthralgias).
     b. Rash with tender skin lesions may be present.

■ PHYSICAL EXAMINATION
- Neonates
  1. Mucopurulent eye discharge
  2. Scalp abscesses
  3. Sepsis (lethargy, apnea, bradycardia, tachypnea, color changes, blood pressure instability or hypotension)
- Prepubertal
  1. Vaginal discharge is associated with sexual abuse.
- Adolescents
  1. Vaginitis (discharge is thick, white-green-yellow) is present in the sexually active teen.
  2. Cervical motion tenderness occurs with discharge.
  3. Urethritis (penile discharge and dysuria) is the most common finding in infected males.

  4. Pustules are seen on erythematous bases; petechiae, papules, and macules on extremities often overlie septic joints.
  5. Tenosynovitis and arthritis are seen, especially of the knee.

DIAGNOSIS

■ DIFFERENTIAL DIAGNOSIS
- Newborn conjunctivitis
  1. Chemical conjunctivitis (silver nitrate prophylaxis)
  2. *Chlamydia* conjunctivitis
  3. Lacrimal duct obstruction
  4. Viral conjunctivitis
- Vaginitis/PID
  1. *Chlamydia*
  2. *Trichomonas*
  3. Herpes simplex virus
  4. Polymicrobial infections

■ DIAGNOSTIC WORKUP
- History and physical examination may narrow the differential diagnosis to bacterial infection or STD.
- Positive culture on selective media (Thayer-Martin-chocolate agar supplemented with antibiotics) is the gold standard.
  1. Culture is definitive.
  2. It should be the basis for diagnosis in the evaluation of the prepubertal child because of legal implications.
- Gram stains of exudate from eyes, endocervix, vagina, male urethra, and skin lesions
  1. Identification of gram-negative intracellular diplococci can be helpful.
- Nonculture methods for identification gaining popularity
  1. DNA probes (polymerase chain reaction and ligase chain reaction)
     a. Urine-based tests (DNA probes) are used to screen for asymptomatic infections (e.g., screening in juvenile detention center settings and in clinic catering to adolescent patients).
     b. Urine-based tests are less invasive and increase compliance (acceptance of testing) in obtaining data.
  2. Enzyme immunoassay tests
- It is important to test for coinfections (e.g., *Chlamydia*, syphilis, human immunodeficiency virus, *Trichomonas*) with any STD.

THERAPY

■ NONPHARMACOLOGIC
Inappropriate even with asymptomatic infection because the risk of spread is high.

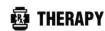

■ MEDICAL

• Uncomplicated sexually transmitted gonococcal infections of the genital tract include two antimicrobials for broad-spectrum coverage.
  1. One of the following:
     a. Cefixime 400 mg orally in a single dose
     b. Ceftriaxone 125 mg intramuscularly in a single dose
     c. Ciprofloxacin 500 mg orally in a single dose
     d. Ofloxacin 400 mg orally in a single dose
  2. And one of the following:
     a. Azithromycin 1 g orally in a single dose
     b. Doxycycline 100 mg orally twice a day for 7 days

■ PATIENT/FAMILY EDUCATION

• Primary prevention
  1. Abstinence
  2. Postponement of sexual involvement
  3. Sexual risk reduction
  4. Condom use
• Secondary prevention
  1. Access to medical care
  2. Partner notification

■ PREVENTIVE TREATMENT

Anticipatory guidance regarding sexual behavior and risk taking needs to be addressed at health care visits.

■ REFERRAL INFORMATION

Positive gonorrhea results need to be reported to the appropriate public health authorities as per individual state laws.

⚙ PEARLS & CONSIDERATIONS

■ CLINICAL PEARLS

In general, antibiotics are used to cover both gonorrhea and *Chlamydia* because coinfection is common, but cultures may not be positive.

■ WEBSITES

• American Medical Association: www.ama-assn.org/
• Centers for Disease Control and Prevention: www.cdc.gov

REFERENCE

1. Peter G, Committee on Infectious Diseases, American Academy of Pediatrics: *1997 Red Book: report of the Committee on Infectious Diseases,* ed 24, American Academy of Pediatrics.

Author: **Maureen Kays, M.D.**

BASIC INFORMATION

■ DEFINITION

Granuloma inguinale is a granulomatous ulcerative disease of the skin and subcutaneous tissues of the genital area. It is rare in the United States.

■ SYNONYM

Donovanosis

ICD-9CM CODE

099.2 Granuloma inguinale

■ ETIOLOGY

An intracellular gram-negative bacterium called *Calymmatobacterium granulomatosis* related most closely to the *Klebsiella* species

■ EPIDEMIOLOGY & DEMOGRAPHICS

- Granuloma inguinale is the major cause of genital ulcers in many tropical regions of the world, including Papua New Guinea, southeast India, eastern South Africa, and the Caribbean.
- The highest incidence occurs in tropical and subtropical areas.
- The incubation period ranges from 8 to 80 days.
- It is transmitted through sexual intercourse with a person with an active infection.
- Young children can become infected by contact with infected secretions.

■ HISTORY

- Any travel to endemic countries
- Any sexual contact with a person with genital ulcer disease

■ PHYSICAL EXAMINATION

- Subcutaneous genital nodules progress to painless ulcers that may bleed.
- There may be single or multiple nodules.
- Involvement of the anal area is seen in 5% to 10% of cases.
- Extragenital lesions (of face, mouth, or liver) occur in approximately 6% of cases.
- Pseudobubo is an inguinal mass that represents subcutaneous extension to the inguinal area and mimics inguinal lymphadenopathy.

DIAGNOSIS

■ DIFFERENTIAL DIAGNOSIS

- In the United States, most young, sexually active patients with genital ulcers have either genital herpes, syphilis, or chancroid (other possibilities include tuberculosis and carcinoma).
- Lymphogranuloma venereum, blastomycosis, and other granulomatous diseases are also part of the differential diagnosis.

■ DIAGNOSTIC WORKUP

- Most cases are diagnosed on the basis of characteristic clinical findings.
- Confirmation of the diagnosis can be made by the following methods:
  1. Histologic examination of punch biopsy specimens taken from the edge of active lesions
  2. Scrapings from the edges of active lesions
  3. A crush preparation made from granulation tissue obtained with a thin scalpel
     a. The crush preparation is made by taking a piece of granulation tissue from a lesion and crushing it between slides. The smear then should be air dried and stained with Wright or Giemsa stain. Donovan bodies are dark-staining, intracellular inclusions seen in large mononuclear cells.

THERAPY

■ MEDICAL

- Administer trimethoprim-sulfamethoxazole or doxycycline for children 8 years or older.
- Treat for a minimum of 3 weeks or until lesions heal.
- Alternative regimens include the following:
  1. Erythromycin (used in pregnant and lactating women)
  2. Ciprofloxacin
  3. Gentamicin 1 mg/kg intravenously every 8 hours (should be considered for resistant cases)
- Evaluate the patient for other sexually transmitted diseases if lesions do not respond within the first few days of therapy.
- Healing begins within 7 days of therapy.

■ FOLLOW-UP & DISPOSITION

- Patients should be followed weekly clinically until signs and symptoms have resolved.
- Healing occurs in 3 to 5 weeks, except in severe cases.

■ PATIENT/FAMILY EDUCATION

- "Safe sex" recommendations should be reviewed.
- Sexual contacts should be examined and treated prophylactically in the following cases:
  1. If they had sexual contact with the patient during the 60 days preceding the onset of symptoms.
  2. If they have clinical signs and symptoms of the disease.
- Relapse occurs frequently. Can occur 6 to 18 months later despite effective initial therapy.

PEARLS & CONSIDERATIONS

■ CLINICAL PEARLS

- Most genital ulcer disease in the United States is caused by herpes, syphilis, or chancroid.
- A secondary bacterial infection may develop in the lesions, or coinfection with another sexually transmitted pathogen can occur.

■ WEBSITE

Centers for Disease Control and Prevention: www.cdc.gov/nchstp/dstd/STD98T06.htm

REFERENCES

1. Centers for Disease Control and Prevention: Granuloma inguinale (donovanosis). In *1998 guidelines for treatment of sexually transmitted diseases*, Atlanta, 1998, Centers for Disease Control and Prevention.
2. Hart GL: Donovanosis, *Clin Infect Dis* 25:24, 1997.
3. Paterson DL: Disseminated donovanosis (granuloma inguinale) causing spinal cord compression: case report and review of donovanosis involving bone, *Clin Infect Dis* 26:379, 1998.

Author: **Cynthia Christy, M.D.**

II

BASIC INFORMATION

■ DEFINITION
Guillain-Barré syndrome is an acute polyradiculoneuropathy that classically presents with ascending paresthesias, weakness, areflexia, and autonomic dysfunction.

■ SYNONYMS
- Acute idiopathic polyneuritis
- Landry's ascending paralysis
- Postinfective polyneuritis
- Kussmaul-Landry paralysis

ICD-9CM CODE
357.0 Guillain-Barré syndrome

■ ETIOLOGY
- Guillain-Barré syndrome appears to be caused by a humoral immuno-pathologic mechanism, based on acute presentation, pathology, and response to immunotherapy.
- Approximately 75% of patients have a history of recent antecedent infection.
- Acute inflammatory demyelinating polyneuropathy (AIDP) variant:
  1. Demyelination of both motor and sensory nerves
  2. Lymphocytic infiltration
  3. Macrophage-mediated demyelination
  4. Most common form in the United States, Western Europe, and Australia
- Acute motor axonal neuropathy (AMAN) variant involves axonal degeneration.
  1. More severe
  2. Higher morbidity and mortality
- Acute motor sensory axonal neuropathy (AMSAN) variant involves both demyelination and axonal degeneration.

■ EPIDEMIOLOGY & DEMOGRAPHICS
- Annual incidence in the developed world is between 1 and 2 cases per 100,000 population.
- The male:female ratio is 1.5:1.
- Guillain-Barré syndrome affects all ages, but bimodal peaks occur in young adults and the elderly.

■ HISTORY
- From 50% to 70% of patients have a nonspecific viral illness in the preceding month.
- Guillain-Barré syndrome most commonly presents with symmetric weakness, paresthesias, and areflexia.
  1. Begins in lower extremities
  2. Progresses cephalad to trunk, upper extremities, bulbar muscles
  3. Weakness may begin in upper extremities and progress caudad
- Weakness may progress to flaccid paralysis.

- Three stages exist:
  1. Progression phase: worsening symptoms for days to weeks
  2. Plateau phase: static symptoms for days to weeks
  3. Recovery: usually begins 2 to 4 weeks after halt of progression; recovery continues for weeks to months, up to 12 months in some cases
- Approximately 40% of patients have sensory complaints.
- Fifty percent of patients have bulbar involvement that may result in oculomotor weakness, dysphagia, facial weakness, and respiratory insufficiency.
- From 15% to 20% of patients progress to respiratory failure requiring mechanical ventilation.
- Patients may have associated severe autonomic dysfunction, including tachyarrhythmias, bradyarrhythmias, and labile blood pressure.
- Bowel and bladder dysfunction is rare.
- Fever is not typical.
- Miller-Fisher variant is characterized by acute external ophthalmoplegia, ataxia, and areflexia.
- Incomplete recovery occurs in up to 28% of patients.

■ PHYSICAL EXAMINATION
- The patient is usually afebrile.
- Examine skin for ticks.
- Examine spine for tenderness.
- Meningismus and papilledema are rare and more compatible with other diagnoses.
- Symmetric motor weakness, usually with distal to proximal progression, is found.
  1. From 5% to 10% of patients may have initial involvement of upper extremities.
- Absent and symmetric deep tendon reflexes are noted in areas of weakness.
  1. Very early in disease, there may be deep tendon reflexes in proximal areas while absent in distal regions.
- Forty-six percent of patients may have some sensory loss, but a sharp sensory level suggests another diagnosis.
- Patients have an ataxic gait out of proportion to weakness.
- Patients may have cranial nerve involvement with facial weakness, oculomotor palsy, and diminished swallowing.
- Autonomic disturbance can be life-threatening.
  1. Tachyarrhythmia
  2. Bradyarrhythmia
  3. Hypertension
  4. Hypotension
- From 10% to 20% of patients will progress to respiratory failure, which

is best monitored by forced vital capacity.

🔬 DIAGNOSIS

■ DIFFERENTIAL DIAGNOSIS
- Acute cerebellar ataxia
  1. Can have associated hypotonia
  2. Cerebrospinal fluid (CSF) protein usually normal and pleocytosis more common
- Spinal cord diseases (e.g., compression myelopathy, transverse myelitis)
  1. Patients usually have distinct spinal level of sensory loss and paresthesias.
  2. Transverse myelitis often presents with back pain and distinct sensory level with paraparesis.
  3. Epidural abscess often presents with fever, back pain, and lower extremity weakness.
- Poliomyelitis
  1. Usually, paralysis is asymmetric, with no sensory deficits.
- Diphtheria
  1. Early signs include palatal paralysis, difficulty swallowing, blurred vision followed by cranial nerve involvement, loss of reflexes, and neuropathy.
- Tick paralysis
  1. Irritability and anorexia are followed by ascending weakness.
  2. Weakness is usually rapidly progressive.
  3. Ticks are commonly located in nuchal or occipital area.
  4. Removal of a tick is diagnostic.
- Porphyria
  1. Attacks usually include abdominal pain, disturbed consciousness, apparent psychosis, seizures, and rapidly progressive peripheral neuropathy.
- Botulism
  1. In children younger than 1 year of age with acute weakness, botulism is most likely.
  2. In infants, constipation may be the first symptom, followed by decreased feeding and ptosis.
  3. In older children, it commonly presents with diplopia, photophobia, and blurred vision, followed by difficulty swallowing and increasing weakness.
- Myasthenia gravis
  1. History of slow progression and episodic weakness with ptosis and/or ophthalmoplegia
  2. Reflexes and sensation normal
- Heavy metal intoxication (e.g., lead, arsenic, mercury, thallium)
  1. Encephalopathy almost always precedes peripheral nerve disease.
  2. With lead intoxication, foot drop may precede encephalopathy.

3. Often, erythema and tremors are seen with mercury poisoning.
- Glue sniffing
- Drug-induced toxic neuropathy
  1. Reported with amitriptyline, dapsone, glutethimide, hydralazine, isoniazid, nitrofurantoin, and vincristine
- Organophosphate poisoning
  1. Usually also have pupillary changes, salivation, and gastrointestinal disturbance
- Lyme disease
  1. In stage 2, patients may have neuropathy, encephalopathy, cranial neuropathy, or peripheral radiculoneuropathy.
  2. History of erythema chronicum migrans is helpful.
- Polymyositis
  1. Onset can be sudden or chronic, with proximal muscle weakness, especially pelvic and shoulder girdles.
  2. Dysphagia and neck weakness are common.
  3. Elevated muscle enzymes are noted.
- Black widow spider bite
  1. Symptoms depend on the number of bites and/or the amount of venom.
  2. Immediate pain, burning, and erythema occur at the site of the bite.
  3. Exquisite abdominal pain with boardlike abdomen may follow in 30 minutes.
  4. Approximately 57% of patients have lower extremity weakness.

■ **DIAGNOSTIC WORKUP**
- CSF examination (the following findings are typical during the second week of disease)
  1. Normal opening pressure
  2. CSF protein elevation
     a. About 50% will have elevation in first week of illness, with increasing CSF protein over ensuing weeks.
     b. Peak protein is between 80 and 200 mg/dl.
  3. CSF cell count
     a. It rarely exceeds 10 lymphocytes/mm^3.
     b. Cell count greater than 50 suggests an alternative diagnosis.
  4. Normal glucose
  5. Cultures with no growth
- Urine for porphyrins

- Complete blood count and erythrocyte sedimentation rate usually normal
- Lyme titer
- Human immunodeficiency virus serology
- Urine heavy metal screen
- Electrodiagnostic studies
  1. Nerve conduction studies show evidence of multifocal demyelination, with possible superimposed axonal degeneration. Typically, conduction block, marked slowing of conduction velocity, prolonged distal latency, and temporal dispersion are seen.
  2. Typical electrophysiologic features may not be apparent until clinical weakness well established.
  3. Electromyography may show abnormal recruitment of motor units.

🧪 **THERAPY**

■ **NONPHARMACOLOGIC**
- Admit the patient to the hospital to monitor respiratory status and autonomic instability and to provide supportive care.
- Provide nutritional support.
- Consult neurology and obtain electrodiagnostic studies.
- Monitor forced vital capacity every 6 hours for signs of impending respiratory failure.
- Monitor the patient's ability to protect the airway (intubation may be necessary if absent/diminished gag reflex is present).
- Monitor skin for decubiti.
- Indications of impending respiratory failure include the following:
  1. Rapidly decreasing vital capacity
  2. Breathlessness/fatigue
  3. Deteriorating arterial blood gases
  4. Dysphagia and shoulder weakness
  5. Rapidly progressive paralysis

■ **MEDICAL**
- For patients with rapidly progressive disease, bulbar paralysis, or impending respiratory distress or for those unable to walk, treatment with plasmapheresis or intravenous immune globulin has been shown to be effective.
- Pain management may be problematic.

■ **SURGICAL**
- Respiratory support, intubation, and ventilation
- Tracheostomy if long-term ventilator support is anticipated

■ **FOLLOW-UP & DISPOSITION**
- Recovery phase may continue for up to 1 year. Most rapid recovery occurs in the first 6 months after recovery begins.
- Approximately 80% of patients have full recovery in 12 months.
- Patients may need symptomatic support and physical therapy.
- Rarely, patients will have relapsing disease and may need repeated immunomodulatory treatment.

■ **REFERRAL INFORMATION**
Refer to pediatric neurologist.

⚙ **PEARLS & CONSIDERATIONS**

■ **CLINICAL PEARLS**
- Fever is not typical.
- Bowel involvement is rare.
- Preceding *Campylobacter jejuni* infection often heralds more severe form of Guillain-Barré syndrome.
- Dysphagia and facial weakness herald respiratory failure.
- In an infant with progressive weakness, think first of botulism.
- Search skin carefully for ticks.

■ **WEBSITE**
Guillain-Barré Syndrome Foundation International: www.webmast.com/gbs/; provides emotional support and assistance to people affected with Guillain-Barré syndrome; fosters research and disseminates information

■ **SUPPORT GROUP**
Consult Guillain-Barré Syndrome Foundation International through their website.

REFERENCES
1. Evans OV, Vedanarayanan V: Guillain-Barré syndrome, *Pediatr Rev* 8:10, 1997.
2. Fulgham JR, Wijdicks EFM: Update on neurologic critical care: Guillain-Barré syndrome, *Crit Care Clin* 13:1, 1997.
Author: **Ellen Gellerstedt, M.D.**

BASIC INFORMATION

■ DEFINITION
Hand, foot, and mouth (HFM) disease is an enteroviral infection characterized by a particular pattern of exanthem (eruption of the skin) and enanthem (eruption of the mucous membranes).

■ SYNONYMS
- HFM syndrome
- Vesicular stomatitis with exanthem
- "Hoof and mouth disease" (popular misconstruction)

ICD-9CM CODE
079.2 Hand, foot, and mouth disease

■ ETIOLOGY
- The major cause is Coxsackie virus A16, followed by Coxsackie virus A5.
- Other agents include Coxsackie virus types A9, A10, B1, B3, B5, and enterovirus 71.
- See the section "Herpangina" for other details on pathophysiology.
- The incubation period is 2 to 10 days.
- Viral shedding from the oropharynx occurs days 3 to 22 after infection, and from stool up to 3 to 4 months after infection.

■ EPIDEMIOLOGY & DEMOGRAPHICS
- In the human host, enteroviruses are well known to demonstrate high rates of subclinical infection.
- In the case of Coxsackie A16, however, the clinical expression rate of the typical syndrome is particularly high.
  1. Children younger than 5 years of age demonstrate the highest clinical expression rates (100%), followed by school-aged children (38%) and adults (11%).
- Although the oral eruption occurs in 90% of all symptomatic cases, the associated exanthem occurs in only 64%, most of whom are children.
- Illness in adults is more easily misidentified.

■ HISTORY
- Sudden onset of fever (38.3° to 41° C) accompanied by anorexia, sore mouth, and malaise is typically reported.
- Fever typically lasts 1 to 2 days and is quickly followed by the appearance of enanthem of 1 to 6 days' duration.
- The exanthem follows 1 to 2 days after the onset of fever and oral eruption, persisting for 2 to 7 days before clearance.

- Illness is generally relatively mild and self-limited, although other manifestations of enteroviral illness may ensue (e.g., meningitis, encephalitis, myocarditis).

■ PHYSICAL EXAMINATION
- Oral lesions chiefly involve the buccal mucosa and tongue but may include the soft and hard palate and gingivae.
  1. They begin as small, 3- to 8-mm erythematous macules, which rapidly progress to vesicles and may coalesce into bullae.
  2. Most typically, they ulcerate before resolution.
- The typical exanthem is peripherally distributed, involving the extremities (hands more often than feet).
  1. Lesions are generally more common on the dorsal and interdigital surfaces.
  2. They often may be found on the palms, soles, and buttocks.
  3. They are small (3 to 7 mm), tender, and consist of mixed papules and vesicles with surrounding erythema.
- Atypical lesions may occur at sites of trauma, such as under rings on fingers, on the medial aspect of the palms (traumatized by frequent writing), on the toes of individuals with tight-fitting shoes, and on the perineum of children in diapers, as well as on the elbows, knees, and shins.

DIAGNOSIS

■ DIFFERENTIAL DIAGNOSIS
- *Herpetic gingivostomatitis:* Patients are generally more ill appearing, typically with higher fever and cervical adenopathy. Except for in concurrent Whitlow, lesions are usually confined to the mouth.
- *Herpangina:* The enanthem resembles HFM disease but is distributed more posteriorly, consistently involving the soft palate and fauces. There are no cutaneous lesions.
- *Varicella:* Patients usually are more ill appearing, demonstrating both more extensive and centrally distributed skin lesions and distinctly less oral involvement. Unlike varicella, the lesions of HFM disease heal by absorption and do not evolve to form pustules and crusts.
- *Aphthous stomatitis:* Oral lesions do not have a vesicular phase and are not typically accompanied by fever or systemic symptoms. There is no exanthem.

■ DIAGNOSTIC WORKUP
- The workup is usually based on clinical findings.
- Confirmation may be obtained via direct culture of oral lesions, skin lesions, or the throat.
- Fluorescent antibody testing of lesions is in the investigational phase.

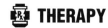

THERAPY

■ NONPHARMACOLOGIC
- Treatment is usually supportive, including hydration.
- Cold, nonacidic fluids, popsicles, and/or slush may provide symptomatic relief.

■ MEDICAL
Patients with humoral immune deficiency may experience more severe disease requiring intravenous immune globulin.

■ FOLLOW-UP & DISPOSITION
Follow-up should be provided as required to ensure adequate hydration and to observe for signs of more severe enteroviral disease.

■ PATIENT/FAMILY EDUCATION
- Control measures include proper handwashing and personal hygiene, especially after diaper changes, etc.
- Children may return to day care/school when oral lesions are unaccompanied by drooling and illness has resolved enough to allow comfortable return to activities.

✷ PEARLS & CONSIDERATIONS

■ CLINICAL PEARLS
- Enterovirus 71 has been identified as the etiologic agent in several fatal outbreaks of HFM disease characterized by progression within 2 to 7 days to refractory shock, pulmonary edema, and encephalomyelitis.
- Randomized trials are under way to evaluate the antiviral agent Placinoral for specific enteroviral infections, including central nervous system disease.
  1. Placinoral is thought to act by preventing the attachment and/or uncoating of viral RNA.
  2. Early results have demonstrated some beneficial effect.
  3. The drug is available on a compassionate-use basis.

REFERENCES

1. Chang LY et al: Fulminant neurogenic pulmonary edema with hand, foot, and mouth disease, *Lancet* 352:367, 1998.
2. Cherry JD: Enteroviruses: coxsackieviruses, echoviruses, and polioviruses. In Feign RD, Cherry JD (eds): *Textbook of pediatric infectious diseases,* ed 4, Philadelphia, 1998, WB Saunders.
3. Lum LCS et al: Fatal enterovirus 71 encephalomyelitis, *J Pediatr* 133:795, 1998.
4. Messner J et al: Accentuated viral exanthems in areas of inflammation, *J Am Acad Dermatol* 40:345, 1999.
5. Modlin JF: Coxsackieviruses, echoviruses, and newer enteroviruses. In Mandel GL, et al (eds): *Principles and practice of infectious diseases,* New York, 1995, Churchill Livingstone.
6. Rotbart HA: Enterovirus infections, *Rep Pediatr Infect Dis* 4:57, 1994.
7. Slavin KA: Hand-foot-and-mouth disease, *Arch Pediatr Adol Med* 152:506, 1998.
8. Thomas I, Janniger CK: Hand, foot, and mouth disease, *Cutis* 52:265, 1993.
9. US Department of Health and Human Services: Deaths among children during an outbreak of hand, foot, and mouth disease: Taiwan, Republic of China, April-July 1998, *MMWR Morb Mortal Wkly Rep* 47:629, 1998.
10. Zaoutis T, Klein JD: Enterovirus infections, *Pediatr Rev* 19:183, 1998.

Author: **C. Elizabeth Trefts, M.D.**

II

BASIC INFORMATION

DEFINITION
Head lice is an arthropod infection of the scalp and neck, most commonly seen in children; it is caused by the head louse.

SYNONYM
Pediculosis capitis

ICD-9CM CODE
132.0 Head lice

ETIOLOGY
- *Pediculosis humanus capitis* is a wingless insect that is an obligate human parasite.
- The parasite requires the vascular environment of the scalp for a blood meal every 4 to 6 hours
- The insect has a three-stage life cycle: egg, nymph, and adult.
  1. Once the egg has hatched, it takes 7 to 10 days to reach the nymph stage.
  2. The nymph takes 2 to 3 weeks to mature into an adult that can continue the fertilization and egg production cycle.
- Transmission occurs via direct contact with an infected person's hair and by sharing combs, hats, and other accessories.
- The adult louse may remain on bedding or upholstery for a brief time.
  1. Viability once removed from the scalp is less than 24 hours.

EPIDEMIOLOGY & DEMOGRAPHICS
- Infection occurs worldwide, with 6 to 12 million persons infected each year in the United States.
- The highest incidence occurs among school-aged children.
  1. The prevalence ranges from 10% to 40%.
- No significant difference exists among race, sex, or socioeconomic status.
  1. Head lice are slightly less common in African Americans.
  2. Adult lice have difficulty attaching to the oval-shaped hair shaft common among African Americans.

HISTORY
- Children usually present for evaluation after an adult (e.g., caregiver, teacher, school nurse, camp counselor) identifies presumed lice or nits on the scalp.
- Other children may be referred for evaluation because of outbreaks in day care or at school.
- A history of pruritus is reported if the infection has been present for a longer time.

PHYSICAL EXAMINATION
- Physical examination is important to verify active infection.
  1. Artifacts, such as dandruff, hair gel, hair spray residue, dirt, or other insects, may be mistaken for lice.
  2. Perform the examination in a well-lit room or in natural sunlight for 3 to 5 minutes.
     a. Lice are sensitive to light and hide in hair strands.
  3. A magnifying aid offers assistance.
- Two main factors to consider on physical examination are as follows:
  1. *What* is seen?
  2. *Where* is it located?
- The adult head louse is grayish white, is 3- to 4-mm long, and favors the front of the scalp.
  1. Adult lice are difficult to locate.
  2. Grayish color may be replaced by red or brown if the insect has just ingested a blood meal.
- Unhatched eggs are small, oval, whitish, and transparent, and they are attached firmly to one side of the hair shaft.
  1. Eggs are laid 1 to 3 mm from the scalp for warmth and moisture.
  2. Eggs can usually be visualized at the nape of the neck and behind the ears.
- Hatched egg shells or nits have the following characteristics:
  1. Easier to visualize
  2. More reflective
  3. Located ½ to ¾ inch from the scalp
- Examination of the scalp may reveal evidence of a secondary bacterial infection.

DIAGNOSIS

DIFFERENTIAL DIAGNOSIS
Ensure appropriate diagnosis and eliminate confusion with benign particles; there is no other differential for scalp infection of this type.

DIAGNOSTIC WORKUP
- Detecting live lice on the head or unhatched, viable eggs near the scalp secures the diagnosis.
- Nits detected farther out on the hair shaft that do not, by definition, contain eggs are not an indication of active infection.
- Samples of presumed lice or eggs may be collected and sent to the Harvard School of Public Health for analysis (see website for more information).

THERAPY

- Treatment should be considered only when active lice or viable eggs are observed.
- Successful therapy usually does not rely on one method but requires an integrated approach with patience and perseverance.

NONPHARMACOLOGIC
- The most important step in effective treatment involves removal of viable eggs from the hair shafts.
  1. This treatment should be used in conjunction with a pediculicide.
  2. This requires patience on the part of the child and the adult because several sessions are often needed.
  3. Several devices have been designed for egg removal.
     a. A fine-toothed comb helps remove the eggs from the hair shafts.
  4. Some people advocate a prerinse of 50% water and 50% vinegar to aid in the removal of the eggs.
     a. No scientific evidence supports this approach.
     b. Additional over-the-counter preparations are available that claim to loosen the egg from the shaft for easy removal.
- Environmental control has centered on careful cleaning of the clothing, bedding, hats, stuffed animals, and upholstery.
  1. Because viability of the louse once removed from the host is less than 24 hours, this is probably not necessary.
  2. No scientific data indicate that fomite control has any effect on reinfestation.
- Occlusive nonpharmacologic methods have recently been recommended for difficult cases.
  1. Petroleum jelly, olive oil, pork fat, or mayonnaise can be placed on the scalp in large quantities and covered overnight with a shower cap.
  2. Presumably, these products occlude the respiratory systems of the lice.
  3. Removal of eggs is critical because unhatched eggs are not affected by the occlusive treatment and will ultimately mature into adult lice.

MEDICAL
- Medical therapies can best be divided into topical pediculicides and oral agents.
  1. The safety of the child is the overriding concern because the infestation presents no risk to the host.

2. Pediculicides, which are neurotoxins, are recommended first.
3. These medications potentially affect mammalian nervous systems.

- Permethrin is a synthetic compound derived from pyrethrin.
  1. It acts on the nerve cell membrane of the parasite, disrupting the sodium channel transport, delaying repolarization, and paralyzing the insect.
  2. Permethrin is available as an over-the-counter 1% crème rinse that remains active on the hair for 2 weeks after the initial application.
  3. Many clinicians recommend reapplication 7 to 10 days later if evidence of continued infection is present.
  4. Permethrin compounds are safe for use in infants older than 2 months of age.
     a. An available over-the-counter preparation is Nix.
     b. A 5% permethrin compound (Elimite) is available by prescription and can be used with a shower cap overnight in cases where resistance is suspected.
- Pyrethrins are natural insecticidal compounds derived from the chrysanthemum flower that also act as a neurotoxin on the adult lice, similar to permethrin.
  1. In combination with piperonyl butoxide, an additive that inhibits the metabolism of pyrethrin, its insecticidal activity reaches 100%, and its ovicidal activity is approximately 70% to 80%. Available over-the-counter preparations include RID, Pronto, A-200, R & C shampoo, and others.
  2. A second application is required in 7 to 10 days to kill any newly hatched nymphs because this agent does not have residual activity.

- Lindane, another pediculicide, exhibits central nervous system toxicity.
  1. It was once available as an over-the-counter product (Kwell).
  2. It is currently available only by prescription because it has been associated with seizures in some patients who used it incorrectly.
  3. The insecticidal and ovicidal activity is less than that seen with permethrin or pyrethrin.
- Ivermectin is an anthelmintic agent structurally similar to the macrolide antibiotics without the antibacterial activity.
  1. A single oral dose of ivermectin, 200 µg/kg, with repeat dosing 10 days later, is effective in eradicating head lice.
- Trimethoprim-sulfamethoxazole has also been shown in one study to eradicate lice infestations.
  1. This medication is less popular among dermatologists than the other options.

■ FOLLOW-UP & DISPOSITION

- Careful reexamination of the scalp for lice or eggs is necessary even after pediculicide application, in conjunction with manual removal techniques.
- Examination by a member of the health care team should be performed before labeling the child as a treatment failure.
- Suspected treatment failures have been reported in increasing frequency and may be the result of the following factors:
  1. Misdiagnosis (misidentification or lack of active infection)
  2. Noncompliance
  3. Resistance by lice to the insecticide
  4. New infestation
  5. Lack of ovicidal or residual properties of the product

☼ PEARLS & CONSIDERATIONS

■ CLINICAL PEARLS

- Louse's saliva ultimately sensitizes people to their bites, thereby exacerbating irritation and increasing the chance of secondary infection.
- When applying topical pediculicides, always apply to dry hair.
  1. Water stimulates lice to temporarily shut down their respiratory systems and the medication becomes ineffective.
- When using the permethrin product, do not use conditioning shampoos or conditioners for 2 to 3 weeks after application.
  1. They interfere with the residual action of the medication.
     a. Prophylactic treatment of all household members is not routinely advised.
  2. Only those with active infection should be treated to help prevent true lice resistance.

■ WEBSITES

- Harvard School of Public Health: www.hsph.harvard.edu/headlice
- HeadLice.org: www.headlice.org/special/mission

REFERENCES

1. Burkhart CG, Burkhart CN, Burkhart KM: An assessment of topical and oral prescription and over the counter treatments for head lice, *J Am Acad Dermatol* 38:979, 1998.
2. Chesney PJ, Burgess IF: Lice: resistance and treatment, *Contemp Pediatr* 15:181, 1998.
3. Schachner LA: Treatment of resistant head lice: alternative therapeutic approaches, *Pediatr Dermatol* 14:409, 1997.

Author: **Kate Tigue, M.D.**

II

BASIC INFORMATION

■ **DEFINITION**
Headache is a symptom. Three clinically defined symptom patterns (migraine, cluster, and tension) include most pediatric recurrent headaches.

■ **SYNONYM**
Cephalalgia

ICD-9CM CODES
346.9   Migraine headache, idiopathic
346.2   Cluster headache
307.81 Tension headache
784.0   NOS headache

■ **ETIOLOGY**
• There are numerous potential causes of pain in the head.
• Migraines are thought by many to relate to a primary abnormality of constriction and dilation of cranial vessels.
• Others believe that abnormal brainstem neuronal activity precedes vascular changes.

■ **EPIDEMIOLOGY & DEMOGRAPHICS**
• Headaches are very common.
• Approximately 40% of 7-year-olds and 75% of 15-year-olds will have experienced recurrent headaches.
• Approximately 5% of school-aged children have migraine headaches.
• The female:male ratio is 3:1 in adults but 1:1 in children.
• Migraine headaches are inherited by a heterogeneous autosomal-dominant pattern with incomplete penetrance.

■ **HISTORY**
• Migraine headache
  1. Age of presentation is usually 7 to 14 years of age.
  2. True migraines occur in approximately 10% of children presenting with recurrent headaches.
  3. Triggers of migraines include the following:
     a. Many foods and chemicals, such as monosodium glutamate (MSG)
     b. Drugs
     c. Environmental factors, such as bright lights or noise
     d. Psychosocial factors, such as emotional stress
  4. Diagnostic criteria of Prensky should be reviewed: must have at least three of the following features:
     a. Hemicranial pain
     b. Throbbing or pulsatile character of the pain
     c. Associated abdominal pain, nausea, or vomiting

  d. Complete relief after rest
  e. Motor, visual, or other sensory aura
  f. Family history of migraine in first-degree relatives
  5. Children may not have typical auras, but prodrome symptoms may include fatigue, irritability, dizziness, tinnitus, personality change, or pallor.
  6. Pain may be unilateral but changes sides.
  7. Duration is generally less in children: 2 to 4 hours compared with 4 to 72 hours in adults.
  8. Migraines rarely awaken patients from sleep.
  9. Children's headaches tend to follow a similar pattern whenever they occur.
• Cluster headache
  1. These headaches present as severe, boring pain behind one eye with facial swelling on that side.
  2. They last approximately 1 hour each and occur in clusters.
  3. Cluster episodes may last for days or weeks.
  4. Not usually found in children younger than 10 years of age.
• Tension headache
  1. Tension headache is also known as *muscle contraction* or *stress headache.*
  2. This type of headache occurs in diverse locations in the head.
  3. No aura is associated with this type of headache.
  4. Nausea or vomiting rarely occurs, usually in the afternoon.
  5. Pain worsens as the day progresses.
  6. Pain is reported as mild to moderate in intensity.
  7. The headache may last 30 minutes to days.
  8. Photophobia may be prominent and therefore hard to distinguish from migraines in children.
• Other types of headache
  1. Other possible causes of headache include the psychosomatic recurrent pain syndromes, similar to chronic recurrent abdominal pain.
  2. These headaches are usually associated with stresses at school or home.
  3. Depression may present as recurrent headache.

■ **PHYSICAL EXAMINATION**
• A complete physical, including thorough neurologic examination and blood pressure, is generally unremarkable in children with recurrent headaches.
• Red flags, findings that are suspicious for another cause, include the following:
  1. Seizure
  2. Trauma

  3. Very specific description of the headache
     a. Pain in a single, specific location that can be pointed at with one finger
     b. Headache that stays in the one spot and is getting worse
  4. A change in gait or personality
  5. Sudden and severe onset with the first episode
  6. Pain with waking up that gets better after arising from bed or that is relieved with vomiting
  7. Pain that is set off by coughing
  8. Presence of an ill contact with meningitis/encephalitis or similar infection
  9. Altered development or mental status
  10. A constant headache that is worse with lying down or with Valsalva maneuver
  11. Fever
  12. Nuchal rigidity
  13. Petechiae
  14. Intense irritability
  15. Bulging fontanel
  16. Altered head circumference
  17. Cushing's triad
      a. Decreased heart rate
      b. Increase respiratory rate
      c. Increased blood pressure
  18. Severe hypertension
  19. Papilledema

 DIAGNOSIS

■ **DIFFERENTIAL DIAGNOSIS**
• Increased intracranial pressure (ICP)
  1. Pseudotumor cerebri
  2. Mass (benign or malignant tumor)
  3. Hydrocephalus
  4. Intracranial bleeding (subdural, epidural, or intracerebral)
• Central nervous system (CNS) infection
  1. Meningitis
  2. Encephalitis
  3. Brain abscess
• Vasculitis
• Arteriovenous malformation
• Aneurysm
• Analgesic abuse
  1. "Analgesic abuse headache" can occur with regular, frequent use of analgesics.
• Depression

■ **DIAGNOSTIC WORKUP**
• Computed tomography (CT) scan or magnetic resonance imaging if elevated ICP is suspected.
• Lumbar puncture if meningitis or encephalitis is a concern.
• A normal CT scan with increased opening pressure on the spinal tap is consistent with pseudotumor cerebri.

℞ THERAPY

■ NONPHARMACOLOGIC
- Reassure the patient that the headache is not caused by a brain tumor or other serious cause.
- Instruct the patient to lie down in a quiet and dark room.
- Biofeedback and other behavioral techniques may be helpful in migraines.
- A simple tension headache is best treated with rest and relaxation.

■ MEDICAL
- Acetaminophen and/or ibuprofen should be given early in the course of a migraine.
- Other medications for migraines include the following:
  1. Promethazine
     a. Initial dose 1 mg/kg orally; repeat at 0.25 to 1 mg/kg every 4 to 6 hours; maximum 25 mg
     b. Contraindications (CIs): use of sedatives, narcotics, asthma
  2. Chlorpromazine
     a. 1 mg/kg intramuscularly for severe attacks
     b. CIs: use of CNS depressants, phenothiazine hypersensitivity, symptoms of Reye's syndrome
  3. Metoclopramide
     a. 0.1 to 0.2 mg/kg orally; maximum 10 mg
     b. CIs: gastrointestinal obstruction, seizure disorder, pheochromocytoma
  4. Dihydroergotamine mesylate
     a. 0.5 to 1 mg intravenously over 3 minutes in children older than 10 years; can repeat in 8 hours
     b. CIs: vascular disease, hypertension, liver or kidney disease, use of vasoconstrictors
  5. Sumatriptan (Imitrex) a selective 5-hydroxytryptamine (5HT)-1-agonist
     a. 6 mg subcutaneously
     b. CIs: vascular or cardiac disease, uncontrolled hypertension, use of monoamine oxidase inhibitors (MAOIs), hemiplegic or basilar migraine, use of an ergot-type medication or other 5HT-agonist, severe liver disease
     c. Expensive
     d. Available forms: subcutaneous, oral, and intranasal
- Acute attacks can be treated with sumatriptan or 100% oxygen.
- Because migraine is a recurrent problem, narcotics and other addictive drugs should be avoided.

■ PREVENTIVE TREATMENT
- A headache diary is useful for trying to identify triggers.
- Detection of and avoidance of triggers can help manage the problem.
- Prophylactic medications may be used when migraines recur with frequency and severity that limit normal functioning.
  1. Propranolol
     a. 1 to 4 mg/kg/day; start at low dosage and increase slowly
     b. CIs: asthma, heart disease
  2. Amitriptyline
     a. 6 to 12 years old: 10 to 30 mg/day divided twice daily
     b. Younger than 12 years: 10 to 50 mg/day divided into three doses
     c. CI: use of MAOIs
  3. Cyproheptadine
     a. Younger than 6 years: 0.125 mg/kg two to three times per day; maximum 12 mg/day
     b. 6 to 14 years old: 4 mg two to three times per day; maximum dose 16 mg/day
     c. CI: use of MAOIs
  4. Riboflavin
     a. 400 mg four times per day
     b. CIs: none
- Medicines used in prevention of cluster headache include the following:
  1. Methysergide
  2. Lithium
  3. Corticosteroids
- Acetaminophen or ibuprofen can be used for tension headaches.
- Management of chronic tension headaches should focus on identifying and avoiding predisposing factors.

■ FOLLOW-UP & DISPOSITION
The patient should be followed until resolution or significant improvement is achieved and as needed for acute recurrences and evaluation of medication side effects.

■ REFERRAL INFORMATION
With difficult-to-manage headaches, referral to a neurologist and/or mental health specialist is recommended.

☼ PEARLS & CONSIDERATIONS

■ CLINICAL PEARLS
- Mnemonic for features of migraines
  Mother (family history)
  Intermittent
  Grinding/throbbing
  Relief with rest
  Aura
  Idiopathic (rule out other causes of headache)
  Nausea/vomiting
  Eyes and ears (photophobia and phonophobia)
  Search for triggers
- All (oral) medications for migraine work better if given earlier in the course. Thus it is important for patients and caregivers to try to recognize sensations that precede an attack.

■ WEBSITE
Contemporary Pediatrics: www.contpeds.com; contains variety of articles on headaches and other topics

REFERENCES
1. Forsyth R, Farrell K: Headache in childhood, *Pediatr Rev* 20:39, 1999.
2. O'Hara J, Koch TK: Heading off headaches, *Contemp Pediatr* 15:97, 1998.
3. Winner PK: Headaches in children, *Postgrad Med* 101:81, 1997.
Author: **C. Andrew Aligne, M.D.**

II

BASIC INFORMATION

■ **DEFINITION**

Complete heart block (CHB) is a brady-cardic rhythm caused by failure of impulse conduction from the atria to the ventricles with complete atrioven-tricular dissociation. The atrial rate is usually higher than the ventricular rate.

■ **SYNONYMS**

- Complete atrioventricular block
- Third-degree atrioventricular block

Unless bradycardia is concurrent, *atrioventricular dissociation* is not an acceptable synonym because this entity may exist with normal rates of at least one pacemaker (e.g., sinus bradycardia with an appropriate junctional rate) and with ventricular tachycardias.

ICD-9CM CODE

746.86 Congenital heart block

■ **ETIOLOGY**

- Congenital due to transplacental immunoglobulin G (IgG) antibody transfer in occult or overt maternal connective tissue disease (especially systemic lupus erythematosus)
- Congenital in the setting of left atrial isomerism (polysplenia) with an atrioventricular septal defect or in patients with levotransposition of the great vessels
- Acquired as a result of damage to the atrioventricular node and bundle of His during surgical repair of congenital and acquired cardiac defects
- Acquired as a result of infections: en-docarditis, myocarditis, diphtheria, Lyme disease
- Acquired in systemic diseases: acute rheumatic fever, myotonic and mus-cular dystrophies, Kearns-Sayre syndrome
- Acquired as a result of tumor infiltra-tion: mesothelioma

■ **EPIDEMIOLOGY & DEMOGRAPHICS**

- Congenital CHB occurs in 1 in 15,000 to 1 in 25,000 births.
- The mortality of congenital CHB in utero is high if hydrops is present.
- The incidence of surgically induced CHB has progressively decreased and is currently quite low (less than 5%), seen most commonly in the setting of complex cardiac malformation repair.
- The incidence of CHB in systemic disease and infection is very low.
- Atrioventricular nodal mesothelio-mas are extremely rare cardiac tumors.

- Congenital CHB caused by fetal exposure to anti-Ro (SSA/Ro) and anti-La (SSB/La) occurs in only 1% to 5% of mothers with collagen vascular disease, but the recur-rence rate for subsequent pregnan-cies is 20%.
- No gender predilection is seen with congenital or acquired CHB.

■ **HISTORY**

- Fetal bradycardia
- Fetal hydrops/intrauterine death
- Fatigue
- Diminished exercise capacity
- Syncope
- Sudden death
- History of associated malformations or history of systemic illnesses (listed under "Etiology")

■ **PHYSICAL EXAMINATION**

- Bradycardia but usually regular rhythm
- Wide pulse pressure
- Low cardiac output
- Manifestations of associated malfor-mations or systemic illnesses (see "Etiology")

🔬 **DIAGNOSIS**

■ **DIFFERENTIAL DIAGNOSIS**

- Sinus bradycardia
- Type II second-degree atrioventricu-lar block

■ **DIAGNOSTIC WORKUP**

- Electrocardiogram/cardiac monitor-ing to determine atrial and ventricu-lar rates
- Echocardiogram to look for structural abnormalities, tumor, and myocar-dial dysfunction
- Holter (ambulatory) monitor to assess
  1. Lowest rate (e.g., during sleep)
  2. Stability of escape pacemakers
  3. Escape ventricular or higher-grade ventricular ectopy
  4. Intermittent atrial capture of the ventricles
- Anti-Ro and anti-La antibodies
  1. Congenital CHB in the absence of structural heart disease likely rep-resents maternal collagen vascular disease (especially systemic lupus erythematosus).
- Exercise test in older patients

℞ **THERAPY**

In general, patients with CHB need to be paced if symptoms, structural heart disease, or rate-related low cardiac output is present.

■ **MEDICAL**

Isoproterenol infusion (0.05 to 0.4 μg/kg/min) to increase the ventricular rate as a bridge to more definitive therapy, but observe for ventricular ectopy

■ **SURGICAL**

Temporary ventricular or, preferably, permanent dual chamber cardiac pace-maker implantation

■ **FOLLOW-UP & DISPOSITION**

- All patients with CHB require follow-up by a pediatric cardiologist.
- All patients with pacemakers require enrollment in a pacemaker clinic with regularly scheduled transtele-phonic assessment and office appointments.

■ **REFERRAL INFORMATION**

All patients with CHB should be referred to a pediatric cardiologist.

⚙ **PEARLS & CONSIDERATIONS**

■ **CLINICAL PEARLS**

- Surgically induced or myocarditis-related CHB may be transient. If re-version to sinus rhythm does not occur in 2 weeks, switch from tempo-rary to permanent pacemaker implantation.
- Immune-mediated congenital CHB is permanent.
- Despite satisfactory pacing, the infant with immune-mediated CHB may succumb to the development of a congestive or dilated immune-related cardiomyopathy during the first 2 years of life.

■ **SUPPORT GROUPS**

Helping Hearts (or a local organiza-tion) or similar related parent groups for patients with congenital or ac-quired heart disease

REFERENCES

1. Buyon JP et al: Autoimmune-associated congenital heart block: de-mographics, mortality, and recurrence rates obtained from a national neona-tal lupus registry, *J Am Coll Cardiol* 31: 1658, 1998.
2. Friedman RA: Congenital A-V block: pace me now or pace me later? *Circula-tion* 92:283, 1995.
3. Schmidt KL et al: Perinatal outcome of fetal complete atrioventricular block: a multicenter experience, *J Am Coll Cardiol* 17:1360, 1991.
4. Weindling SN et al: Duration of com-plete atrioventricular block after congenital heart disease surgery, *Am J Cardiol* 82:525, 1998.

Authors: **J. Peter Harris, M.D., and Chloe G. Alexson, M.D.**

BASIC INFORMATION

■ DEFINITION

Heat-related illness (HRI) covers a spectrum of electrolyte disturbances and temperature elevation encountered in athletes and the general population, often during seasonal heat waves. *Heat cramps* are painful, sustained contractions of leg muscles associated with prolonged exercise, a normal core temperature, sodium depletion, and dehydration. *Heat exhaustion* is a more serious level of dehydration caused by excessive sweating in a hot environment. Core temperatures seen in heat exhaustion are often elevated to 38° to 40° C, with associated orthostasis, syncope, nausea, and vomiting. *Heat stroke* is a life-threatening emergency caused by extreme core temperature elevation (higher than 42° C), with water and sodium loss. Heat stroke may be *exertional* (occurring in otherwise healthy athletes) or *classic* (seen in the elderly and infants).

■ SYNONYM

Sunstroke

ICD-9CM CODES

992.2 Heat cramps
992.5 Heat exhaustion
992.0 Heat stroke

■ ETIOLOGY

- Heat cramps are thought to occur because of inadequate perfusion secondary to dehydration and from sodium depletion.
  1. Both reactions accentuate calcium activity in skeletal muscle.
  2. Cramps occur mainly in hamstring and calf muscles.
- Heat exhaustion is a more severe level of dehydration.
  1. Heat exhaustion is the result of sweating induced by sustained or recurrent exercise.
  2. Plasma volume and sweat production fall as dehydration ensues, further reducing the body's ability to cool.
  3. Elevated core temperature (higher than 40° C) increases the metabolic demand in a setting where the cardiovascular system may not be able to respond proportionately (preload is reduced).
- Heat stroke is severe hypovolemic shock.
  1. Dangerously elevated core temperature (higher than 42°C [107.6° F]) is present.
  2. Diffuse cellular injury occurs from shock (oxygen debt) as well as severe hyperpyrexia.
  3. Lactic acidosis, neuronal injury, and rhabdomyolysis result.
     a. Generalized loss of cellular homeostasis

     b. Impaired calcium metabolism
     c. Poor mitochondrial function
  4. A generalized inflammatory response may develop, leading to coagulopathy (disseminated intravascular coagulation) and pulmonary, renal, and hepatic injury similar to that seen in the sepsis syndrome.
  5. Historically, mortality is estimated to be as high as 50% to 80%.
  6. Recent data suggest that aggressive therapy may lower mortality to 15% to 20%.

■ EPIDEMIOLOGY & DEMOGRAPHICS

- Highly at-risk individuals include infants, victims of diarrheal illness, and elderly persons with underlying medical conditions.
- Events increase during seasonal heat waves.
  1. Those particularly at risk inhabit poor areas of northern American cities.
  2. Tenants in older buildings lacking air conditioning are particularly susceptible.
- Global warming may increase the incidence in the future.
- Infants and child athletes are more prone to climatic heat stress than are adults because of their higher rate of heat transfer from the environment, higher baseline metabolic rates, and lesser ability to sweat.
- Adolescent and child athletes may exercise poor judgment and ignore, or be unaware of, the warning signs of HRI. This may increase their risk of morbidity.
- Accidental deaths occur with infants and children locked in automobiles.
  1. In summer climates, the interior and trunk temperature of automobiles can reach higher than 65° C (150° F) in just 15 minutes.
  2. Cracking open the window does not prevent rapid overheating.

■ HISTORY

- Histories should include a description of and the duration of exercise and environmental conditions to which the patient has been exposed.
- Inquire about chronic illness (i.e., cystic fibrosis) or recent activity (attempted weight loss), which may increase the risk of fluid and electrolyte imbalance.
- Symptoms reported may include the following:
  1. Shaking chills
  2. Headache
  3. Nausea
  4. Excessive sweating
  5. Dry skin (anhydrosis)
  6. Extreme fatigue
  7. Leg cramps
  8. Light-headedness or dizziness

  9. Confusion
  10. Loss of consciousness

■ PHYSICAL EXAMINATION

Potential findings include the following:
- Tachycardia
- Elevated temperature
- Piloerection on chest and arms
- Either excessive perspiration or anhydrosis (dry skin)
- Combativeness, aggressiveness
- Progressive obtundation with loss of consciousness

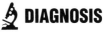 **DIAGNOSIS**

■ DIFFERENTIAL DIAGNOSIS

- In the presence of an appropriate history, the diagnosis is often straightforward.
- HRI should be expected during seasonal heat waves and is often clearly diagnosed in athletes during competitive events.
- The differential diagnosis includes many illnesses that induce fever and mental status changes, including, but not limited to, the following:
  1. Generalized viral illnesses, bacterial sepsis
  2. Encephalitis, meningitis
  3. Head trauma

■ DIAGNOSTIC WORKUP

- Assess the ABCs (airway, breathing, and circulation).
  1. Airway control may be necessary for the most severe heat stroke patients.
  2. Volume status must be determined.
     a. Dehydration is a key component in the pathophysiology of heat stroke.
     b. Tachycardia, followed by hypotension, may occur in decompensated shock.
- Check electrolytes.
  1. Many abnormalities can be found in HRI.
     a. Look for disturbances of sodium and potassium (increased or decreased)
     b. Hypocalcemia
     c. Hyperphosphatemia
- Rhabdomyolysis can be detected by myoglobinuria or elevated serum creatine kinase (CK).
- In severe heat stroke, an arterial blood gas, liver function studies, coagulation assays, CK, and urinary myoglobin should be obtained.
- Initial evaluation of core (rectal temperature) is indicated. If severely elevated, urgent external cooling measures are indicated.

II

THERAPY

■ NONPHARMACOLOGIC

- Heat cramps are treated nonpharmacologically with the following methods:
  1. Rest
  2. Oral rehydration
  3. Local massage
- Symptoms resolve and further evaluation is not indicated.
- Patients should reduce their level of activity and begin a more gradual conditioning regimen.
- In addition to the aforementioned measures, more aggressive treatment should be initiated for heat exhaustion:
  1. Rehydration of 1 to 2 L over several hours for an adolescent or adult should be started.
     a. Oral rehydration is indicated for a fully conscious patient, parental rehydration if decreased mental status is exhibited.
  2. Immediate cooling measures should be initiated.
     a. Move the patient into the shade.
     b. Dry sweat and moisture from the skin (to increase evaporative heat loss).
     c. Further cooling can be achieved by applying ice to sites of superficial great vessels (i.e., neck, axillae, and groin).
  3. Monitor (rectal) temperature closely. *An increasing core temperature despite initial therapy and cooling measures indicates the presence of heat stroke, which is a medical emergency.*

■ MEDICAL

- Heat stroke is a medical emergency necessitating transport to a medical facility. Core temperatures may rise above 42° C, putting the patient at risk for generalized cellular necrosis, imminent cardiovascular collapse, and death.
  1. Begin external cooling with ice application to neck, axillae, and groin. Remove the patient's clothing, cover the patient with a wet sheet, and focus a fan or air conditioning directly on the patient.
  2. Initiate rapid intravenous fluid administration (normal saline 20 ml/kg or 800 ml/m^2) over the first hour.
     a. Give a normal saline bolus (10 ml/kg) as necessary for blood pressure support.
     b. Inotropic support may be necessary.
     c. Urine output should be monitored to assess the ongoing fluid resuscitation (urinary catheter should be placed).
  3. Monitor electrolytes and treat any imbalances accordingly.
  4. Reassess ABCs.
     a. The airway should be protected. Intubation is indicated for the comatose or seizing patient.
     b. Gastric decompression is indicated to prevent vomiting and aspiration.
  5. Treat seizures if they occur.
     a. Benzodiazepines are the usual first-line medical therapy. Diazepam 0.1 to 0.2 mg/kg for children, 2 mg for adults, is given.
  6. Consider treating rigors/shivering with similar benzodiazepine dosing.

■ FOLLOW-UP & DISPOSITION

- Patients should be monitored for 24 to 48 hours for signs of secondary cellular injury after recovery of normothermia and return of normal mental status.
- Delayed complications include neurologic injury, rhabdomyolysis, and hepatic injury.
- Children with heat stroke should be cared for in a pediatric intensive care unit.

■ PREVENTIVE TREATMENT

- Activity level and sports participation should be tailored to climatic conditions. The American Academy of Pediatrics has published generalized exercise guidelines (see website reference).
- Common sense strategies include ensuring adequate hydration with exercise, allowing for acclimatization to a warm environment, and wearing appropriate lightweight clothing.
- During seasonal heat waves, cool baths and visits to air-conditioned public areas (e.g., shopping malls, libraries) should be encouraged.
- Fans alone lose their effectiveness when the ambient temperature exceeds 32° C (90° F).
- Help parents understand the susceptibility of children to HRI and the dangers of leaving children unattended in automobiles.

PEARLS & CONSIDERATIONS

■ CLINICAL PEARLS

Remember that environmentally induced hyperthermia is not altered by the administration of antipyretics (e.g., acetaminophen, ibuprofen).

■ WEBSITE

American Academy of Pediatrics: www.aap.org/policy/098.html; American Academy of Pediatric policy statement on climatic stress and the child athlete

REFERENCES

1. Anonymous: Heat-related mortality: United States, 1997, *MMWR Morb Mortal Wkly Rep* 47:473, 1998.
2. Duthie DJR: Heat-related illness, *Lancet* 352:1329, 1998.
3. Shaffer TE et al: Climatic stress and the exercising child, *Pediatrics* 69:808, 1982.
4. Simon HB: Current concepts: hyperthermia, *N Engl J Med* 329:483, 1993.
5. Squire DL: Heat illness, *Pediatr Clin North Am* 37:1085, 1990.

Author: **William Harmon, M.D.**

BASIC INFORMATION

■ DEFINITION
The classification of Mulliken and Glowacki in 1982 separates hemangioma and vascular malformation. *Hemangiomas* are benign vascular tumors in which a growth phase, marked by endothelial cell proliferation, is followed by involution and fibrosis. Hemangiomas are differentiated from *vascular malformations,* which are hamartomas. Vascular malformations do *not* proliferate or involute; are composed of aberrant but mature endothelial cells, which may be capillary (e.g., port wine stain), lymphatic (i.e., cystic hygroma), venous, arterial, or combined channel anomalies; are always present; and grow with the child.

■ SYNONYMS
- Strawberry hemangioma
- Strawberry mark
- Strawberry birthmark

ICD-9CM CODE
228.00 Hemangioma

■ ETIOLOGY
- Hemangiomas are mostly caused by angiogenesis—new vessels arising from existing vasculature.
- Vasculogenesis, in which new blood vessels are made from endothelial cells, may play a role.
- The rapid increase in size with proliferation of cells followed by cessation of growth and eventual involution is not well understood.

■ EPIDEMIOLOGY & DEMOGRAPHICS
- Hemangiomas are the most common soft tissue tumor of infancy.
- Approximately 5% to 12% of 1-year-olds have hemangiomas.
- They are rarely familial (in less than 10%).
- The female:male ratio is 3:1; vascular malformations occur in equal female:male ratios.
- The incidence is increased in fair-skinned children.
- The incidence is increased in very-low-birth-weight premature infants.
- Fewer than half of hemangiomas are present at birth; most (80%) of the rest develop within the first few weeks.
- Approximately 80% of patients have one, 20% have two, and less than 5% have 3 or more hemangiomas; rarely, disseminated neonatal hemangiomatosis is seen.
- Approximately 60% occur in the head and neck, 25% on the trunk, and 15% on an extremity.

- Approximately 15% deep, and 20% to 25% are combined superficial and deep.
- Neither site, size, depth, presence at birth, diameter of proliferative phase, sex, nor race predicts which hemangiomas will involute completely.
- Approximately 50% resolve by 5 years of age, and 90% resolve by 9 years of age.

■ HISTORY
- The history typically is of little help.
- The typical course is of erythematous growth.
- Hemangioma can be associated with multiple anomalies if numerous hemangiomas are present—PHACE syndrome

    Posterior fossa abnormality
    Hemangiomas
    Arterial anomalies
    Coarctation of the aorta
    Eye abnormalities (cataract, microphthalmia, abnormal retinal vessels)
  1. The female:male ratio is 8:1.
- Hemangiomas of the lumbosacral region are a potential marker for occult spinal malformations.

■ PHYSICAL EXAMINATION
- A pale macule with threadlike telangiectasia may be present in newborns.
- Hemangiomas are bright red, elevated, and slightly compressible as they enlarge, especially if superficial.
- When they lie deeper in the skin, hemangiomas may look like a "bluish" fullness under skin.
- Size can range from a few millimeters to centimeters.
- Patients usually have one or two lesions, but occasionally multiple lesions are present.
- A rapid increase in size occurs over months.
  1. The maximum size is reached at approximately 6 to 8 months in superficial type.
  2. Maximum size not reached until 12 to 14 months in deep hemangiomas.
- Slower involution occurs after 6 to 9 months.
  1. Involution begins with central pallor and fading of bright red color.
  2. Hemangiomas eventually disappear.
     a. From 10% to 40% have residual skin changes.
- Large lesions may leave atrophic, wrinkled skin at the site after resolution.

■ COMPLICATIONS
- Ulceration
  1. Most common complication
  2. May be quite painful
  3. Risk of infection, hemorrhage, and scar formation
- Kasabach-Merritt phenomenon
  1. Associated with consumptive coagulopathy, anemia, and thrombocytopenia
  2. Most common within the first 4 to 5 months of life
  3. Usually occurs in massive, deep hemangioma, which may be a different lesion than a simple hemangioma
  4. May also grow for 2 to 5 years
- Vital structure compromise
  1. Periorbital lesions may lead to amblyopia or astigmatism.
  2. Periauricular lesions may obstruct the external auditory canal.
  3. Airway lesions may present with hoarseness, stridor, and/or "noisy" breathing.
     a. Hemangiomas involving the chin, lips, and mandibular region of the face increase the risk of airway hemangioma.
- Visceral hemangiomas
  1. High morbidity occurs because of high flow with high-output cardiac failure and anemia.
  2. If multiple, especially facial, hemangiomas are present, consider visceral lesions (especially liver).
- Lumbosacral hemangiomas
  1. These are associated with lumbosacral spine abnormalities, in particular tethered cord.
- Large facial hemangiomas
  1. These may be associated with Dandy-Walker syndrome or other posterior fossa abnormalities, such as PHACE syndrome (see information under "History").

🔬 DIAGNOSIS

■ DIFFERENTIAL DIAGNOSIS
- Tumors
- Vascular malformations
- Pyogenic granuloma
- Kaposiform hemangioendothelioma
- Spindle cell hemangioendothelioma
- Infantile hemangiopericytoma

■ DIAGNOSTIC WORKUP
- The diagnosis is usually clinical.
- Larger lesions, especially hepatic or other large congenital lesions, are more difficult to diagnose.
  1. In these lesions, Doppler ultrasonography is useful.
     a. Differentiates from solid tumors

b. Differentiates from arteriovenous malformations and lymph vessel and capillary anomalies
2. Magnetic resonance imaging also differentiates hemangiomas from other vascular malformations and soft tissue tumors.

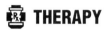

THERAPY

■ NONPHARMACOLOGIC
• Wait and watch approach
• Significant parental emotional support
• More chance of scar with intervention than with waiting for natural involution

■ MEDICAL
• If large or life-threatening
  1. Systemic steroids
     a. Administer 2 to 3 mg/kg/day for weeks to months.
     b. Rapid taper of steroid during proliferative phase may lead to rebound.
     c. Ideal length of therapy is controversial.
  2. Intralesional steroid
     a. 1 to 3 doses
     b. Less than 3 to 5 mg/kg triamcinolone per lesion
  3. Potent topical steroids
     a. Improvement in one series only
     b. Contraindicated in periocular area because of skin atrophy and necrosis with potential occlusion of central retinal artery
  4. Recombinant interferon-alfa
     a. Angiogenesis inhibitor

b. Some success in patients with life threatening lesions who failed corticosteroid therapy
c. Side effects: irritability, neutropenia, liver function test abnormalities, and spastic diplegia
5. Laser systems
   a. Flash lamp-pumped pulsed dye
      (1) Less effective for hemangiomas compared with success in port-wine stains
      (2) Best used in thin superficial malformations (penetrates only 1 mm)
   b. Continuous wave
      (1) Higher risk of scarring
      (2) Operator dependent
6. Bleomycin
   a. When injected into hemangiomas, bleomycin is reported to decrease their size, but general use has not been evaluated.

■ SURGICAL
• The patient may need tracheostomy for subglottic hemangioma.
• Embolization is used for large cutaneous lesions that have not responded to medical therapy.
• Surgical excision may be useful for pedunculated lesions and those that are life-threatening and unresponsive to medical management.
• Surgery is mostly used to repair residual abnormalities after regression of hemangioma.

■ FOLLOW-UP & DISPOSITION
• Follow patients for complete regression.
• Cosmetic surgical repair can be attempted late, if residual skin changes persist.

■ PATIENT/FAMILY EDUCATION
• Stress the benign nature and natural course of involution of these lesions.
• If the lesion ulcerates, bleeds, or suddenly increases in size, parents should seek medical attention.
• If the lesion obstructs a vital structure with its growth, parents should seek medical attention.

■ REFERRAL INFORMATION
Dermatologic referral is warranted if specific therapy is needed.

PEARLS & CONSIDERATIONS

■ CLINICAL PEARLS
• The course of hemangiomas is quite typical; an atypical course suggests a different diagnosis.
• Parents need significant emotional support, especially with hemangiomas that are on the head and neck (and thus easily noticed by others).

■ WEBSITE
HealthLink: www.healthlink.mcw. edu/article/936041445.html

REFERENCES
1. Drolet BA, Esterly NP, Frieden IJ: Hemangiomas in children, *N Engl J Med* 341:173, 1999.
2. Wahrman J, Honig P: Hemangiomas, *Pediatr Rev* 15:266, 1994.
3. Garzon MC, Frieden IJ: Hemangiomas: when to worry, *Pediatr Ann* 29:58, 2000.
4. Dohil MA, Baugh WP, Eichenfield LF: Vascular and pigmented birthmarks, *Pediatr Clin North Am* 47:801, 2000.
Author: **Lynn C. Garfunkel, M.D.**

BASIC INFORMATION

■ DEFINITION

Hemolytic disease with ABO incompatibility is hemolysis of neonatal red blood cells (RBCs) secondary to incompatibility between a type O mother and a type A or B newborn.

■ SYNONYM

ABO isoimmunization

ICD-9CM CODE

773.1 Hemolytic disease due to ABO isoimmunization

■ ETIOLOGY

- In a Type O mother, the naturally occurring maternal immunoglobulin G (IgG) anti-A or anti-B antibodies cross the placenta and attach to fetal and neonatal type A or type B RBCs. The degree of fetal and neonatal hemolysis is usually much milder than that which occurs with RhD hemolytic disease because of the following factors:
  1. Most anti-A and anti-B antibodies are immunoglobulin M (IgM) and do not cross the placenta.
  2. Anti-A and anti-B do not bind complement on the fetal RBC membrane.
  3. A and B antigens are present on many tissues other than RBCs, thus diluting the pool of anti-A and anti-B antibodies available to attach to RBC membranes.
  4. There are relatively few A and B antigen sites on fetal and neonatal RBCs.

■ EPIDEMIOLOGY & DEMOGRAPHICS

- In one large series, 28% of ABO-incompatible babies had a weakly positive direct Coombs' test and only 2% of these required an exchange transfusion.
- The severity of hemolysis does not increase with subsequent pregnancies as it does in RhD hemolytic disease.

■ HISTORY

- Hydrops is very rare.
- Early neonatal jaundice, usually observed during the first 24 hours, may be reported.

■ PHYSICAL EXAMINATION

- Jaundice
- Liver and spleen usually normal in size

DIAGNOSIS

■ DIFFERENTIAL DIAGNOSIS

- Hemolytic disease caused by other RBC antigen-antibody systems, including Rh disease, Kell, Duffy, Kidd, and so on
- Sepsis
- RBC membrane enzyme defects, such as glucose-6-phosphate deficiency (G6PD) and pyruvate kinase deficiency

■ DIAGNOSTIC WORKUP

- Anti-A or anti-B antibodies in cord and neonatal blood
- Positive direct Coombs' test on cord and neonatal blood

- Anemia
- Spherocytes seen on peripheral blood smear

THERAPY

- Phototherapy is administered to control hyperbilirubinemia.
- An exchange transfusion is occasionally required to prevent the bilirubin level from reaching a degree that would put the infant at risk for acute bilirubin encephalopathy (kernicterus on neuropathology).

■ FOLLOW-UP & DISPOSITION

Neonates with significant hemolysis should have serial follow-up hematocrits at 1- to 2-week intervals to identify those infants with a continued slow hemolysis who may require a "top-up" transfusion with packed RBCs.

PEARLS & CONSIDERATIONS

■ CLINICAL PEARLS

The rapidity and degree of hemolysis are difficult to predict. Bilirubin levels must be monitored carefully.

REFERENCE

1. Bowman JM: Immune hemolytic disease. In Nathan DG, Orkin SH, Oski FA (eds): *Nathan and Oski's hematology of infancy and childhood,* vol 2, Philadelphia, 1998, WB Saunders.

Author: **James W. Kendig, M.D.**

II

BASIC INFORMATION

■ DEFINITION
Hemolytic disease of the newborn resulting from Rh incompatibility is hemolysis of fetal and neonatal RhD antigen–positive red blood cells (RBCs) caused by RhD antibodies acquired transplacentally from a sensitized RhD-negative mother.

■ SYNONYM
Erythroblastosis fetalis caused by RhD

ICD-9CM CODE
773.0 Hemolytic disease due to Rh isoimmunization

■ ETIOLOGY
- Fetal RhD-positive RBCs (inherited from the father) cross the placenta of an RhD-negative mother and stimulate the maternal immune system to produce anti-RhD antibodies.
- These maternal immunoglobulin G (IgG) antibodies, in turn, cross the placenta of the current or a future pregnancy to cause hemolysis of the fetal and neonatal RhD-positive RBCs.

■ EPIDEMIOLOGY & DEMOGRAPHICS
- The prevalence of RhD-negative individuals varies by racial and geographic origin.
  1. 15% to 20% in northern Europe
  2. 5% in sub-Saharan Africa
  3. Less than 1% in Asia
- With the introduction in 1968 of RhD immune globulin to prevent the sensitization of RhD-negative mothers, the incidence of this disease has declined exponentially.

■ HISTORY
- The history is variable depending on the degree of maternal sensitization and fetal RBC hemolysis.
- The usual history is that of an RhD-negative mother with climbing serial anti-D antibody titers during the pregnancy.
- With increasing severity of fetal hemolysis, delta O.D. 450 (an index of fetal hemolysis) measurements are elevated on serial samples of amniotic fluid obtained by amniocentesis.
- The newborn infant is anemic and develops progressive hyperbilirubinemia, which may lead to acute bilirubin encephalopathy (kernicterus on neuropathology) if untreated.
- Severe fetal hemolysis may cause hydrops.

■ PHYSICAL EXAMINATION
- The newborn infant may be pale at birth but rapidly develops jaundice.
- The liver and spleen are enlarged because of fetal extramedullary hematopoiesis.
- The newborn infant with hydrops has the following additional symptoms:
  1. Severe subcutaneous edema
  2. Hepatosplenomegaly
  3. May have ascites
  4. May have pleural and pericardial effusions

DIAGNOSIS

■ DIFFERENTIAL DIAGNOSIS
The differential diagnosis includes maternal sensitization with fetal and neonatal hemolysis secondary to other RBC antigen-antibody systems.
- ABO
- Kidd
- Kell
- Duffy
- C/c and E/e alleles of the Rh system

■ PRENATAL DIAGNOSTIC WORKUP
- The RhD-sensitized pregnancy is followed with serial RhD antibody titers and with serial ultrasound examinations (to look for hydrops).
- With climbing antibody titers, amniocentesis should be done to evaluate delta O.D. 450 values of the amniotic fluid.
- With increasing delta O.D. 450 values, cordocentesis should be performed to measure the fetal hematocrit.

■ POSTNATAL DIAGNOSTIC WORKUP
- Samples of umbilical cord blood and neonatal blood are positive for anti-D antibodies.
- Direct antiglobulin test (Coombs' test) is positive.
- The reticulocyte count is elevated.
- Erythroblasts are seen on the blood smear.
- Progressive anemia and hyperbilirubinemia develop.

THERAPY

■ PRENATAL THERAPY
With recent technological developments in the field of fetal-maternal medicine, intravascular fetal transfusions (via cordocentesis) with packed RBCs may be administered to the fetus with severe anemia and early hydrops.

■ DELIVERY ROOM THERAPY
The infant delivered with severe hydrops requires aggressive resuscitation.
- Intubation
- Assisted ventilation
- Administration of packed RBCs
- Prompt thoracentesis and paracentesis if required

■ NEONATAL INTENSIVE CARE UNIT THERAPY
- The infant usually requires one or more double-volume exchange transfusions to prevent the bilirubin from climbing into the toxic range.
- Phototherapy assists in controlling the rate of rise of the bilirubin.

■ FOLLOW-UP & DISPOSITION
- Late anemia may develop because of continued slow hemolysis.
  1. Serial hematocrits should be checked at 1- to 2-week intervals during the first 6 to 8 weeks,
  2. Transfusion with packed RBCs may be needed if symptomatic anemia recurs.
- Late sequelae of neonatal bilirubin toxicity include choreoathetoid cerebral palsy, hearing impairment, and dental dysplasia.

■ PREVENTION OF RhD SENSITIZATION OF THE RhD-NEGATIVE MOTHER
- Antepartum
  1. At 28 weeks' gestation, all RhD-negative mothers should have an RhD antibody screen.
  2. If negative, RhD immunoglobulin (300 μg) is administered intramuscularly.
- Postpartum
  1. If the newborn infant is RhD positive, the mother should receive at least 300 μg of RhD immunoglobulin.
  2. The hospital blood bank should perform a Kleihauer-Betke stain of the maternal blood to evaluate the degree of fetal-to-maternal hemorrhage.
  3. In the case of a large fetal-to-maternal bleed, additional doses of RhD immunoglobulin may be required to prevent maternal sensitization.

■ REFERRAL INFORMATION
Pregnant RhD-sensitized women should be referred to a regional center staffed with specialists in high-risk obstetrics and neonatology.

☼ PEARLS & CONSIDERATION

■ CLINICAL PEARLS

- ABO incompatibility between an RhD-negative mother and an RhD-positive fetus (i.e., mother O negative and fetus A or B positive) helps protect the RhD-negative mother against RhD sensitization.

- Unsensitized RhD-negative pregnant women should receive RhD immunoglobulin after the following events:
  1. Spontaneous and induced abortion
  2. Amniocentesis
  3. An ectopic pregnancy
  4. Abdominal trauma

REFERENCE

1. Bowman JH: Immune hemolytic disease. In Nathan DG, Orkin SH, Oski FA (eds): *Nathan and Oski's hematology of infancy and childhood,* Philadelphia, 1998, WB Saunders.

Author: **James W. Kendig, M.D.**

II

BASIC INFORMATION

■ DEFINITION
Hemolytic uremic syndrome (HUS) is a syndrome of acute renal failure, microangiopathic hemolytic anemia, and thrombocytopenia.

■ SYNONYM
HUS

ICD-9CM CODES
584.9 Acute renal failure
283.11 Hemolytic uremic syndrome

■ ETIOLOGY
There are many causes of HUS. All involve endothelial cell injury of some kind.
- Infectious
  1. *Escherichia coli* O157:H7
     a. *E. coli* O157:H7 is the most common cause of HUS in children, followed by other enterohemorrhagic *E. coli* strains and *Shigella dysenteriae* type 1.
     b. These bacteria cause diarrhea-positive (D+) cases of HUS through the production of shigatoxins (verotoxins).
     c. The secreted toxin is absorbed and binds to a cell surface glycolipid receptor. The complex is internalized and disrupts cellular protein synthesis. In the gastrointestinal (GI) tract, this leads to bloody diarrhea.
     d. Systemically absorbed toxin affects many organs, especially the kidneys, in which there is a very high concentration of the glycolipid receptor on the glomerular endothelium in young children. Damaged endothelium sets off thrombus formation.
  2. *Streptococcus pneumoniae*
     a. Neuraminidase exposes the Thomsen-Friedenreich antigen on cells leading to immune damage.
  3. Human immunodeficiency virus (HIV)
  4. Other infectious agents
- Noninfectious (these are known as atypical or diarrhea-negative [D-] HUS)
  1. Idiopathic
  2. Hereditary: autosomal-dominant and autosomal-recessive forms; complement factor H deficiency
  3. Drugs: cyclosporine, tacrolimus, mitomycin C, oral contraceptives
  4. Pregnancy
  5. Malignant hypertension

■ EPIDEMIOLOGY & DEMOGRAPHICS
Most cases of HUS are secondary to infection with *E. coli* O157:H7.
- D+ HUS is caused by *E. coli* O157:H7:
  1. D+ HUS is the most common cause of acute renal failure in children in North America.
  2. Peak incidence occurs in children younger than 5 years of age.
  3. It occurs sporadically (most cases) and in epidemics.
  4. The disease peaks between June and September.
  5. Most cases result from contaminated beef products, but can also result from person-to-person contact, contaminated fruit, unpasteurized cider and milk, vegetables, and water.

■ HISTORY
- Typical (D+) HUS
  1. Diarrheal prodrome in 90%; bloody in 75%
  2. Abrupt onset of pallor, prostration, hematuria, oliguria, and edema, usually as GI symptoms resolving
  3. Signs and symptoms of renal failure predominate; may have involvement of any organ system
     a. History of offending drugs or affected family members and lack of diarrheal prodrome in atypical forms.

■ PHYSICAL EXAMINATION
Depends on organs involved
- Signs of acute renal failure: hypertension, edema, congestive heart failure, tachycardia
- Hematologic: pallor, bleeding
- Central nervous system (CNS) signs: lethargy, seizures, focal deficits, coma
- GI signs: vary from abdominal tenderness to acute surgical abdomen

DIAGNOSIS

The diagnosis is made by documenting the classic triad of acute renal failure, microangiopathic hemolytic anemia, and thrombocytopenia.

■ DIFFERENTIAL DIAGNOSIS
- Typical (D+) versus atypical (D-) HUS
- Thrombotic thrombocytopenic purpura
- Disseminated intravascular coagulation
- Henoch-Schönlein purpura

■ DIAGNOSTIC WORKUP
- Blood urea nitrogen, creatinine, electrolytes for abnormalities

- Complete blood count, blood smear, platelet count, prothrombin time (PT), partial thromboplastin time (PTT), Coombs' test, reticulocyte count, bilirubin level
  1. Anemia, fragmented red blood cells (RBCs), thrombocytopenia, elevated white blood cell count, reticulocytes elevated, bilirubin elevated
  2. PT, PTT usually normal
  3. Coombs' test negative (except in pneumococcal-related HUS)
- Urinalysis: macroscopic hematuria, proteinuria, pyuria, cellular, granular, hyaline casts
- Stool culture for bacteria (notify laboratory specifically that *E. coli* O157:H7 is being considered); approximately 30% of cultures are positive
- Free fecal shigalike toxin (approximately 50% yield)
- Serologic testing for antibodies to verotoxin producing *E. coli* (VTEC)
- Stool guaiac
- Amylase and lipase if pancreatitis suspected
- Imaging studies of GI tract, CNS, chest, and kidneys as indicated by course and examination
- Kidney biopsy if atypical or a prolonged course

THERAPY

- Therapy of typical (D+) HUS is supportive, with correction of fluid, electrolyte, and acid-base abnormalities. Up to 90% of patients may require dialysis.
- Judicious use of packed RBC and platelet transfusions (symptomatic anemia; bleeding) should be exercised.
- Verotoxin binders are currently undergoing clinical trials.
- Plasmapheresis and plasma exchange are needed for atypical cases, but not for typical (D+) HUS.
- Corticosteroids and intravenous immunoglobulin do not appear to be effective.
- The role of antibiotics in the progression from *E. coli* hemorrhagic colitis to typical (D+) HUS is controversial. They do not appear to help and may lead to more severe disease.
- Antimotility medications are a known risk factor for progression from hemorrhagic colitis to HUS and should be avoided.

■ FOLLOW-UP & DISPOSITION
- Mortality is now less than 5% for typical (D+) HUS but is significantly higher for atypical forms.

- Long-term sequelae include the following:
  1. As many as 40% of patients with typical (D+) HUS have some chronic renal abnormalities after 10 years (proteinuria [18%], hypertension [6%], decreased creatinine clearance [16%], end-stage renal disease [3%]). Up to 47.5% of children with atypical forms of HUS progress to end-stage renal disease.
  2. Proteinuria persisting longer than 1 year from HUS portends a poorer renal prognosis.
  3. Approximately 8% of children with typical (D+) HUS have long-term neurologic sequelae (e.g., retardation, seizures, motor deficit, learning and behavioral problems, blindness).
  4. Recurrence in a kidney transplant is uncommon with typical (D+) HUS. There is a high risk of recurrence in atypical (D-) HUS.

■ PATIENT/FAMILY EDUCATION
- Most patients with typical (D+) HUS recover completely.
- Atypical (D-) HUS can be hereditary.

- Preventive measures should be communicated (see following discussion).

■ PREVENTIVE TREATMENT
- Practice good handwashing technique.
- Cook meats, particularly ground beef, thoroughly (to internal temperature of 155° F [68.3° C]).
- Avoid unpasteurized milk and cider.
- Wash fruits and vegetables well.
- Children with hemorrhagic colitis should not return to day care until two stool cultures for *E. coli* O157:H7 have been negative.

■ REFERRAL INFORMATION
The input of a pediatric nephrologist should be obtained.

✸ PEARLS & CONSIDERATIONS

■ CLINICAL PEARLS
- HUS often occurs abruptly just as the child appears to be improving from a bout of colitis.
- Siblings who develop HUS more than 1 year apart probably have a familial form of HUS.

■ WEBSITE
The Lois Joy Galler Foundation: www.loisjoygaller.org

■ SUPPORT GROUPS
- NEPHKIDS: email discussion group for parents of children with kidney disease. To subscribe, email the message "subscribe nephkids" to majordomo@ualberta.ca
- KidTalk: email list for children with renal disease: http://home.nycap.rr.com/jazzer/kidtalk.html
- Support-Group.com has a chat room on HUS: www.support-group.com/cgi-bin/sg/get_links?hus
- Local chapters of the National Kidney Foundation

REFERENCES
1. Kaplan BS, Meyers KE, Schulman SL: The pathogenesis and treatment of hemolytic uremic syndrome, *J Am Soc Nephrol* 9:1126, 1998.
2. Pickering LK, Obrig TG, Stapleton FB: Hemolytic-uremic syndrome and enterohemorrhagic *Escherichia coli*, *Pediatr Infect Dis J* 13:459, 1994.

Author: **William S. Varade, M.D.**

BASIC INFORMATION

DEFINITION
Hemophilia is a hereditary bleeding disorder that is caused by a deficiency or defect in a blood clotting factor. Rare cases are acquired.

SYNONYMS
- Hemophilia "A": "Classic hemophilia" caused by a factor VIII deficiency/defect.
- Hemophilia "B": "Christmas disease" caused by a factor IX deficiency/defect.

ICD-9CM CODE
286.0 Hemophilia

ETIOLOGY
- Factor VIII or IX deficiency may be qualitative, quantitative, or both.
- Delayed clot formation secondary to reduced thrombin generation.
- Factor VIII is a very large gene (186 kb).
  1. Multiple deletions, mutations, and insertions are described.
  2. Intron 22 mutations (homologous recombination) is a common defect in severe hemophilia A.

EPIDEMIOLOGY & DEMOGRAPHICS
- Hemophilia A and B are X-linked recessive disorders.
- Hemophilia A is the most common, although it is rare in the population of live male births.
  1. Hemophilia A is found in all ethnic groups throughout the world.
  2. All sons of affected males are normal.
  3. All daughters of affected males are obligate carriers.
  4. Sons of carriers have a 50:50 risk of disease (daughters have a 50:50 carrier risk).
- Hemophilia B is clinically identical to hemophilia A.
  1. Hemophilia B occurs in 1 of 30,000 male births; 4:1 ratio of hemophilia A:B.
  2. Factor VIIIa is a cofactor for factor IXa; therefore deficiency of either factor causes decreased factor IX activity. It may be qualitative or quantitative.
  3. Severity patterns, genetic patterns, laboratory features, and differential diagnosis are similar to those of hemophilia A.
  4. Course and prognosis are similar to those seen with hemophilia A (although less inhibitors).
- Other hemophilias include, in order of frequency, deficiencies of factors XI, X, VII, V, and II.
  1. The degree of severity is important in management.
  2. Products are available for some deficiencies; plasma is used for many.

HISTORY & PHYSICAL EXAMINATION
Clinically, patients may have mild, moderate, or severe disease. The clinical features usually correlate with the severity of the factor deficiency. Clinical features are similar in hemophilia A and B.
- Hematomas
  1. These are characteristic of hemophilia (unusual in patients with platelet disorders).
  2. Patients with severe hematomas can have dissection (retropharyngeal/retroperitoneal).
  3. Muscle bleeding can lead to compartment syndromes.
- Hemarthrosis
  1. Approximately 75% of hemophilia bleeding is joint related.
  2. Joints are most commonly affected in the following order: knees, elbows, ankles, shoulders, wrists, and hips.
  3. Patients often have a target joint, resulting in a cycle of inflammation and rebleeding.
  4. If not treated quickly, hemarthrosis can result in chronic pain/joint destruction, and ultimately osteoporosis, bone cysts, and joint space narrowing.
- Pseudotumors
  1. These tumors usually occur within the tendons or bones.
- Hematuria
  1. Hematuria is often seen during the lifetime of a hemophiliac.
  2. Hematuria is usually from the renal pelvis.
  3. Treat with factor replacement. (Prednisone is sometimes used. Avoid Amicar.)
- Neurologic complications
  1. Intracranial bleeding is usually seen with trauma.
  2. Spinal bleeding is rare.
  3. Peripheral nerve compression can be seen secondary to muscle bleeding.
- Mucous membrane bleeding
  1. Epistaxis is common (hemoptysis often structural).
  2. Ulcer disease is common secondary to nonsteroidal antiinflammatory drugs used for arthritis.
- Surgery and procedures
  1. It is common for patients to bleed with surgery. Prevention is key.
  2. Mild bleeding in patients often is discovered postoperatively.
  3. Dental extractions are a common cause of morbidity.
  4. Bleeding may be delayed for hours or days.
  5. Infected wound hematomas may occur.
  6. Perioperative hemophilia needs are based on the type of surgery and the severity of the hemophilia.

DIAGNOSIS

DIFFERENTIAL DIAGNOSIS
- von Willebrand disease (severe)
  1. Usually has a prolonged bleeding time
  2. Different inheritance pattern
- Other hereditary bleeding disorders
  1. Clinically similar with deficiency of factor IX and factor XI
  2. Similar laboratory features: factor XII deficiency (no bleeding)

DIAGNOSTIC WORKUP
- Prolongation of the activated partial thromboplastin time (aPTT) is seen, with normal prothrombin time (PT) and normal bleeding time.
- Patients with mild hemophilia may have a normal aPTT.
- The aPTT corrects with normal plasma (unless inhibitor present).
- Functional factor VIII can be measured with a clotting assay.
  1. Factor VIII:C measures coagulant activity.
- Immunologic factor VIII can be measured with an immunoassay.
  1. Factor VIII: Ag can measure normal and abnormal factor VIII.
- Factor levels expressed in units: 1 unit in 1 ml of plasma if normal (100%).
  1. Severe: less than 1% factor activity; spontaneous bleeding is recognized during infancy.
  2. Moderate: 2% to 5% factor activity; may have spontaneous bleeding, commonly have trauma-related bleeding.
  3. Mild: 6% to 30% factor activity; trauma-related bleeding, surgical bleeding; may go unrecognized until adult years.
  4. Carriers may be symptomatic but if so are usually mild clinically.

THERAPY

NONPHARMACOLOGIC
- General principles are as follows:
  1. Have a sense of urgency.
  2. Avoid acetylsalicylic acid (ASA, aspirin) and antiplatelet drugs (if possible).
  3. Avoid intramuscular injections.
  4. Follow patients in a specialized center.
  5. Trust the patients because they know the disease.
  6. Local measures include pressure, rest, ice, topical thrombin, and sutures.

■ MEDICAL

- General principles
  1. Have clotting factor concentrates available.
  2. Time procedures appropriately for factor coverage (not weekends).
- Factor replacement
  1. Recombinant factor is used; in the future, gene therapy will likely be available.
- Dosing
  1. Based on the following criteria:
     a. Severity of the hemophilia
     b. Severity and site of the bleeding
     c. Size of the patient
  2. Issues to consider include the dosing interval, the desired level, and the treatment duration.
- Other agents/modalities
  1. DDAVP: In patients with mild to moderate hemophilia, factor VIII levels are transiently raised (peak at 30 to 60 minutes), often to a safe level, to control bleeding or prevent procedure-related bleeding. If use of this therapy is anticipated, a DDAVP trial should be performed to assess the patient's response (dose 0.3 µg/kg intravenously).
  2. Recently, intranasal DDAVP (Stimate) has become available.
     a. Different formulation than DDAVP for enuresis and diabetes insipidus
  3. Amicar is an antifibrinolytic drug that is useful with dental work and mucosal bleeding. Hematuria is a contraindication.
  4. Corticosteroids are often useful for hematuria and hemarthrosis.
- Hemophilia B treatment
  1. Basic principles are the same as those for hemophilia A.
  2. Until recently, the only available products were prothrombin complex concentrates, which have potential thrombotic risk with repeat dosing. More highly purified products are now available with minimal contamination of other proteins (monoclonal products). Recently, recombinant factor IX (Benefix) has become available.
  3. Dosing has a *major difference with factor VIII;* only 50% plasma recovery.
     a. There is extravascular binding and a longer half-life.

■ MEDICAL COMPLICATIONS

- Factor VIII inhibitors
  1. Antibodies to factor VIII develop in approximately 15% of patients with hemophilia A.
     a. Usually seen in patients with severe disease and frequent exposure to factor.
     b. Inhibitors tend to run in families and are seen in African Americans more than Caucasians.
     c. Patients may be low-responders or high-responders.
  2. Treatment of inhibitors includes the following:
     a. Factor VIII (high-dose or continuous infusion)
     b. Prothrombin complex concentrates (PCCs)/activated PCCs
     c. Porcine factor VIII (may be cross-reactive)
     d. Recombinant VIIa (recently available)
     e. Immune tolerance regimens
- Hepatitis
  1. Almost all multitransfused patients (pre-1985) have evidence of hepatitis.
     a. Approximately 90% are HBsAb positive, and 10% are HBsAg positive.
     b. The prevalence of hepatitis C is extremely high.
     c. Approximately 50% of patients develop chronic active hepatitis or cirrhosis.
        (1) Some success has been achieved with α-interferon/ribavirin.
        (2) Human immunodeficiency virus (HIV) worsens the natural history of hepatitis C.
- HIV infection
  1. Many early pediatric HIV cases described were hemophiliacs.
  2. Approximately 80% to 90% of severe (older) hemophiliacs are HIV positive.
  3. Most seroconverted between 1978 and 1985.
  4. Essentially no treatment-related conversions have occurred since 1985.
- Other infections
  1. Hepatitis A is associated with rare transfusion-related cases (can vaccinate now).
  2. Parvovirus is also associated with rare transfusion-related cases.
  3. Creutzfeldt-Jakob disease is a theoretical concern, yet no cases have been reported in hemophiliacs.

■ SURGICAL

- Surgical intervention may be needed to evacuate a hematoma.
- Patients occasionally undergo synovectomy.

■ FOLLOW-UP & DISPOSITION

- Home therapy
  1. Infants are usually treated at hemophilia centers.
  2. Parents of young children learn to infuse at home.
  3. Preteens often learn self-infusion.
- Prophylaxis
  1. Commonly used in Europe and is increasing in the United States. Decreases chronic joint damage. Overall may not truly increase cost/use.
  2. Aim for factor level trough of more than 1%.
  3. Can be timed with activities (e.g., Little League)

■ PATIENT/FAMILY EDUCATION

- By the late 1970s, life expectancy approached that of nonhemophiliacs.
  1. Life expectancy for persons born from 1971 to 1980 is 68 years.
  2. Life expectancy for persons born from 1981 to 1990 is 49 years (because of acquired immunodeficiency syndrome epidemic).
- Causes of death are historically bleeding.
  1. Other causes of death and related comorbidities include the following:
     a. The development of inhibitors
     b. Chronic liver disease
     c. Secondary to hepatitis B and/or C
     d. HIV-related complications

■ REFERRAL INFORMATION

A multidisciplinary team should be involved in the care of patients with hemophilia. The team includes medical, nursing, social services, dental, orthopedics, physical therapy, infectious disease, and gastrointestinal personnel, as well as support groups.

✺ PEARLS & CONSIDERATIONS

■ WEBSITES

- The Mary M. Gooley Hemophilia Center, Inc.: www.hemocenter.org
- The National Hemophilia Foundation: www.hemophilia.org
- The World Federation of Hemophilia: www.wfh.org

Author: **Ronald L. Sham, M.D.**

BASIC INFORMATION

DEFINITION
Hemoptysis is expectoration of blood from sputum arising from the oral cavity, larynx, trachea, bronchi, or lungs.

ICD-9CM CODE
786.3 Hemoptysis

ETIOLOGY
- Loss of integrity between pulmonary vasculature and bronchial tree, as in infection, bronchiectasis, or foreign body erosion
- Alveolar hemorrhage syndromes such as hereditary hemorrhagic telangiectasia or arteriovenous malformations (AVMs)
- Pulmonary infarction (e.g., cocaine, pulmonary thromboembolism)
- Vasculitis
- Coagulopathy

EPIDEMIOLOGY & DEMOGRAPHICS
- Acute lower respiratory infection is the most common cause (approximately 40% of cases).
- Bronchiectasis, resulting from cystic fibrosis (CF) or other chronic pulmonary infections, is also common, especially in a referral population.
  1. Approximately 1% to 15% of patients with bronchiectasis develop hemoptysis.
- Congenital heart disease, once a common cause of hemoptysis in pediatric patients, is uncommon now because of the availability of early corrective surgery.

HISTORY
- One must first elucidate that the bleeding is actually coming from the tracheobronchial tree.
- Sputum is usually bright red, rust-colored, or frothy.
- Inquire about constitutional symptoms (e.g., fever, weight loss), choking spells, recent infections or trauma, calf pain, or hematuria.
- Hemoptysis may be preceded by dyspnea, pleuritic pain, or a gurgling noise in the airway.
- With *hematemesis,* the vomited blood may be of coffee-ground consistency, clotted, darkened color, or mixed with food, or it may be preceded by epigastric discomfort or nausea.
- With *epistaxis,* the differentiation may be more difficult, but blood is often spit or vomited, increased in production with the head tilted back, or associated with anterior nasal bleeding.

PHYSICAL EXAMINATION
- First examine the material, checking for food particles, acidity, or clots, all of which are more common in *hematemesis.*
- Pallor may indicate anemia from chronic disease.
- Digital clubbing may indicate chronic suppurative lung disease, pulmonary AVM, or congenital heart disease.
- Other bruises or signs of trauma may support concomitant pulmonary contusion.
- Check for telangiectasias elsewhere on the body.
- A missing tooth may support a foreign body aspiration.
- Localized pulmonary examination findings include consolidation, wheezes (foreign body, endobronchial lesions), unequal breath sounds, pleural rubs (pneumonia, collagen vascular disease, pulmonary embolism), and bruits (AVM).

🔬 DIAGNOSIS

Made primarily from history, with supportive features from physical examination

DIFFERENTIAL DIAGNOSIS
- Acute infection of the lower respiratory tract
  1. Pneumonia: bacterial, viral, tuberculosis, fungal (especially aspergillosis), or parasitic
  2. Tracheobronchitis
- Bronchiectasis, especially in patients with CF and ciliary dyskinesia
- Foreign body aspiration
- Lung abscess
- Pulmonary AVM
- Hereditary hemorrhagic telangiectasia (Osler-Weber-Rendu syndrome)
- Trauma (iatrogenic, penetrating, blunt)
- Alveolar hemorrhage syndrome (may be idiopathic or associated with systemic lupus erythematosus, Goodpasture's syndrome, Henoch-Schönlein purpura, or Wegener's granulomatosis)
- Congenital heart disease
- Primary pulmonary hemosiderosis: may be associated with cow's milk protein allergy (Heiner syndrome)
- Pulmonary thromboembolism
- Tumor (uncommon as a cause overall, but a common feature in bronchial carcinoid syndrome)
- Coagulopathy
- Drugs (aspirin [ASA], propylthiouracil, cocaine)
- Unexplained hemoptysis: following workup is imperative

DIAGNOSTIC WORKUP
- The pH of expectorated material is alkaline; in hemotemesis, the pH is acidic.
- Laboratory tests include the following:
  1. Complete blood count assessment for anemia with chronic disease or elevated white blood cell counts with acute infectious process
  2. Erythrocyte sedimentation rate to look for collagen vascular disease
  3. Prothrombin time (PT)/partial thromboplastin time (PTT) for vitamin K deficiency or liver disease
  4. Sputum Gram stain and culture for bacteria, fungi, and mycobacteria
  5. Urine analysis to assess hematuria
  6. Blood urea nitrogen and creatinine
- Specialized testing should be performed as needed.
  1. Tuberculosis and/or aspergillus skin testing
  2. Immunoglobulin E
  3. Sweat chloride test for CF
  4. Milk precipitins (Heiner syndrome)
  5. Antiglomerular basement membrane antibodies (Goodpasture's syndrome)
  6. Antinuclear antibodies (systemic lupus erythematosus)
  7. Antineutrophil cytoplasmic antibody (Wegener's granulomatosis)
  8. Consideration of renal biopsy if signs of renal involvement
- Imaging includes the following:
  1. Chest radiograph (one third are normal)
     a. AVM
     b. Bronchiectasis
     c. Infiltrates
     d. Adenopathy
        (1) Most foreign bodies are radiolucent; therefore consider expiratory-inspiratory films to check for ball-valve obstruction.
  2. ^{99}Technetium-tagged red blood cell scan can identify the site of bleeding in approximately 50% of cases.
  3. Chest computed tomography (CT) scan is the procedure of choice to further define pulmonary parenchymal disease.
     a. Magnetic resonance imaging is more useful for vascular structures.
     b. Ventilation-perfusion (V/Q) scan or spiral chest CT scan should be obtained to evaluate for pulmonary embolus.
- Selective bronchoscopy may be needed in the following cases:
  1. Laboratory workup complete and cause not defined
  2. Continued bleeding

- Bronchiole alveolar lavage with or without biopsy may be needed.
- Removal of foreign bodies may be necessary.

THERAPY

■ NONPHARMACOLOGIC
In most cases, hemoptysis is self-limited and not a sign of more serious disease.

■ MEDICAL
- In massive hemoptysis, remember airway, breathing, and circulation (ABCs of resuscitation).
  1. Mechanical ventilation with frequent suctioning may be necessary to maintain airway patency.
- Once the airway is protected, a diagnostic/therapeutic rigid bronchoscopy (for concomitant mechanical ventilation) can be performed.
  1. Clotted material is removed.
  2. Iced saline or topical epinephrine can be instilled to control bleeding.
- If this does not control the bleeding, balloon tamponade may be attempted.
- If this fails, the patient should be sent for selective bronchial arteriography followed by embolization of the suspected vessel(s).
  1. Gelfoam, Ivalon, or bucrylate may be used.

2. Bronchial artery embolization is contraindicated if a spinal artery arises from the suspected bronchial artery.
   a. In this case, the bronchial artery is cannulated.
   b. Embolization material is injected.
- Up to 90% of bleeding can be controlled with the previous measures.

■ SURGICAL
- Surgical intervention is necessary only for failed medical treatment.
- Laser therapy may be an option in the future.
  1. Approximately 70% of patients have minor and 20% have major recurrences.
- Surgical therapy with resection of the affected segment is indicated for severe recurrences.

■ PATIENT/FAMILY EDUCATION
- Most cases of hemoptysis are self-limited.
- For most cases, safe and effective therapeutic options are available.
- In more complex cases, a pulmonologist can often dictate the most effective strategy for the workup.

■ REFERRAL INFORMATION
Any patient with persistent, severe, or recurrent hemoptysis should be considered for referral to a pulmonologist.

PEARLS & CONSIDERATIONS

■ CLINICAL PEARLS
- The first objective is to firmly confirm that one is dealing with hemoptysis rather than epistaxis or hematemesis.
- Infections of the respiratory tree account for nearly half of the cases overall, whereas foreign body aspiration is a common cause in toddlers.
- Malignancy is a rare cause.

■ WEBSITES
- American College of Rheumatology: www.rheumatology.org
- American Lung Association: www.lungusa.org
- Cystic Fibrosis Foundation: www.cff.org

REFERENCES
1. Fabian MC, Smitheringale A: Hemoptysis in children: the hospital for sick children experience, *J Otolaryngol* 25: 44, 1996.
2. Nelson WE et al: *Nelson textbook of pediatrics,* ed 15, Philadelphia, 1999, WB Saunders.
3. Pianosi P, Al-sadoon H: Hemoptysis in children, *Pediatr Rev* 17:344, 1996.
Author: **Steven Joyce, M.D.**

II

BASIC INFORMATION

■ DEFINITION
Intracranial hemorrhage refers to bleeding that occurs inside the skull but not necessarily within the brain (intracerebral). It is classified by location. Epidural blood is situated between the skull and the dura, subdural blood is situated between the dura and the underlying brain, and subarachnoid blood is beneath the arachnoid and separated from the brain by the pia. Subdural bleeding is further classified by the time interval between injury and the onset of symptoms. They are acute (up to 24 hours), subacute (1 to 10 days), or chronic (more than 10 days).

■ SYNONYMS
- Epidural hematoma, epidural hemorrhage, or epidural bleed
- Subdural hematoma, subdural hemorrhage, or subdural bleed
- Intracranial hemorrhage, intracranial hematoma, or intracranial bleed

ICD-9CM CODES
431 Intracerebral hemorrhage
432 Nontraumatic extradural hemorrhage
432.1 Nontraumatic subdural hemorrhage
432.9 Nonspecified nontraumatic intracranial hemorrhage
767 Subdural and cerebral hemorrhage due to birth trauma
852 Subarachnoid, subdural, and extradural hemorrhage following injury
853 Other and unspecified intracranial hemorrhage following injury
Both 852 and 853 can be modified with a fourth digit (.1) to signify an association with an open intracranial wound and require a fifth digit modifier to signify the association with loss of consciousness.

■ ETIOLOGY
- Most cases of intracranial bleeding in newborn and pediatric populations result from trauma.
- Subdural hematomas in newborns result from birth trauma caused by cephalopelvic disproportion, abnormal presentation, precipitant deliveries, and the use of mechanical devices during delivery.
- Trauma resulting from automobile accidents is the usual mechanism of injury resulting in intracranial bleeding.
- Inflicted injury caused by abuse or assault may also cause intracranial bleeding.

- Primary hematologic conditions (e.g., hemophilia, idiopathic thrombocytopenic purpura) can be associated with spontaneous intracranial bleeding. Most cases of bleeding in these patients also occur as a result of trauma.

■ EPIDEMIOLOGY & DEMOGRAPHICS
- Trauma is the leading cause of death and disability among American children, and brain injury is the leading cause of death from trauma.
- The major causes of pediatric brain injury (and traumatic intracranial bleeding) are falls, motor vehicle crashes, and recreational activities.
- As with all types of trauma, males have approximately twice the rate of brain injuries compared with females.
- Rates of injury are fairly stable throughout childhood but increase dramatically at age 15 years.
- The more severe the head injury, the more likely there is to be associated intracranial bleeding.
  1. Approximately 70% of epidural hemorrhages and about 30% of subdural hemorrhages are associated with skull fracture.
- The following is true among children younger than 2 years of age:
  1. Approximately 25% of head injuries requiring hospital admission are caused by abuse.
  2. Subdural hemorrhages in young children more commonly result from child abuse than from unintentional injury.
  3. Intracranial bleeding is caused by blunt trauma and shaking injury with secondary damage to the bridging cortical veins.
- Approximately 20% of subdural hemorrhages are bilateral.
- Epidural hematomas usually occur in older children with blunt unintentional trauma to the temporal lateral aspect of the skull.
- Most epidural hemorrhages are unilateral.
- Epidural hematomas are less common than subdural hematomas.
- Retinal hemorrhages rarely occur in unintentional brain injury. Their presence usually implies that the child is the victim of shaken-impact syndrome.
- Most falls resulting in brain injury and intracranial bleeding are falls from heights of more than 10 feet.
  1. Epidural hematomas can occur in infants from falls of less than 4 feet (especially in the presence of a skull fracture) because of their high center of gravity and tendency to land head first.

- The risk of bleeding complications in patients with coagulopathy is directly related to the severity of the condition (e.g., critically low factor level or platelet count less than $5000/mm^3$).
  1. The location of bleeding is consistent with the mechanism of injury.
  2. Rarely, such bleeding occurs as a spontaneous event.

■ HISTORY
- Because most instances of intracranial bleeding are associated with trauma, a history of trauma should always be sought.
- Precise details should be elicited, including the following:
  1. Time, location, and description of how the injury occurred
  2. Whether there was loss of consciousness
  3. The duration of loss of consciousness
  4. Whether there were any posttraumatic neurologic changes, such as focal neurologic signs, seizures, or a lucent period before the onset of confusion or coma
- Explanations that are not consistent with the severity of the injury or the developmental level of the child should be investigated further.
- Important aspects of the child's medical history include the following:
  1. Concurrent illnesses associated with falls or increased bleeding, such as epilepsy, poor judgment or impulsive behavior, and a personal or family history of coagulopathy
  2. Baseline level of neurodevelopmental functioning
  3. Immunization status (especially tetanus)
  4. Current medications (especially aspirin and ibuprofen) and allergies
  5. Time of last meal
  6. Potential airway foreign bodies at the time of the injury
- Health care providers should be aware of the presentation of intracranial bleeding associated with birth trauma.
  1. Newborns may present with seizures after 48 hours of age.
  2. Subarachnoid and subdural hemorrhages are the most commonly seen types of bleeding.
  3. A history of cephalopelvic disproportion, abnormal presentation, precipitous delivery, or the use of mechanical devices may be elicited.
  4. Significant intracranial bleeding may be found in the absence of external signs of trauma.

■ PHYSICAL EXAMINATION

- Physical assessment should begin with the familiar "ABCDE" mnemonic—airway, breathing, circulation, disability, and exposure.
  1. Airway instability can be both a cause and an effect of head injury.
  2. Monitoring vital signs is critical for initial assessment and ongoing care.
  3. Recognition and control of shock is important for adequate central nervous system (CNS) perfusion.
  4. Hypovolemic shock is rare in isolated head injury; if shock occurs, look for other sources of blood loss.
- Initial neurologic examination should focus on the level of consciousness, the presence of abnormal neurologic signs, and size and reactivity of the pupils.
  1. Level of consciousness is the best indicator of insufficient perfusion oxygenation of the brain.
  2. Pupil changes can indicate a herniation syndrome.
- Carefully examine the fundi for papilledema and retinal hemorrhages.
  1. Abnormalities of ocular gaze suggest orbital fracture or impending herniation.
- The head should be examined carefully, looking for the following:
  1. Lacerations and contusions of the scalp
  2. Tenderness to palpation or indentations of the skull
  3. Tension of the anterior fontanel in the infant
  4. Basilar skull fracture, which is suggested by the following:
     a. Periorbital hemorrhage (raccoon eyes)
     b. Ecchymosis behind the ears (Battle's sign)
     c. Bleeding from the nose or ears and cerebrospinal fluid (CSF) rhinorrhea or otorrhea (glucose positive)
- The most important feature of the examination of children with a head injury is serial and frequent reassessment.
  1. Use a reliable, easily reproducible system with good interrater reliability, such as the Glasgow Coma Scale with its pediatric modification (PGCS)—a grading system of consciousness based on three parameters (eye opening, verbal response, and best motor response) (see Part III, Emergency Medicine, Boxes 3-3 and 3-4).
  2. Initial results serve as a baseline against which subsequent results should be compared.
  3. Deteriorations demand reevaluation and may require therapeutic intervention.

🔬 DIAGNOSIS

■ DIFFERENTIAL DIAGNOSIS

- With a known history of significant trauma or minor trauma in a patient at high risk for intracranial bleeding, diagnostic evaluation is done to determine the extent and nature of the injuries and to determine the potential need for emergent neurosurgical intervention.
- Children who present with physical findings that are inconsistent with the history given should be evaluated for other sites of traumatic injury. Abuse should be considered.
- Newborns with intracranial bleeding associated with birth trauma may present with the following:
  1. Seizures
  2. Apnea
  3. Vomiting
  4. Irritability
  5. External signs of trauma: may or may not be present
- Differential diagnosis in infant with altered mental status includes the following:
  1. Apparent life-threatening event (ALTE) (see the section "Sudden Infant Death Syndrome")
  2. Shaken baby syndrome
  3. CNS infection
  4. Seizure
  5. Poisoning
  6. Inborn error of metabolism
  7. Hypoglycemia, hyponatremia
  8. Stroke
- Differential diagnosis in older children with altered mental status if trauma or history for trauma not obvious includes the following:
  1. Meningitis
  2. Encephalitis, encephalopathy
  3. Seizure disorder
  4. Ingestion
  5. Intoxication
  6. Drug exposure, overdose
  7. Metabolic abnormality (inborn error of metabolism, hypoglycemia, hyponatremia)
  8. Stroke
  9. Tumor
  10. Vitamin A intoxication

■ DIAGNOSTIC WORKUP

- Computed tomography (CT) scan is the test of choice for patients with a head injury who are suspected of having intracranial bleeding.
- CT scan of the head should be performed for patients with any of the following:
  1. A history of or findings on examination that suggest an underlying bleeding problem
  2. Posttraumatic loss of consciousness, seizures, amnesia, disorientation, or other mental status change

  3. Hemiparesis, anisocoria, ocular palsy, or other focal neurologic signs
  4. Severe head injury with a PGCS score of 8 or less
  5. Presence of a penetrating skull injury or a palpably depressed skull fracture
  6. An unexplained decline in the PGCS of 2 points or more
  7. Signs or symptoms of elevated intracranial pressure (ICP)
  8. Retinal hemorrhages
  9. Unconscious patients in need of emergent chest or abdominal surgery
- Contrast is not required; significant intracranial blood is quite evident without contrast.
- CT images of the head may miss some linear, stellate, and basilar skull fractures.
- Significant findings on CT scan include the following:
  1. Cerebral hyperemia is evident as an increased density with blurring of the gray-white margins.
  2. Cerebral hyperemia with increased ICP appears as obliteration of the cisterns and ventricles (early sign) and shift of the midline structures.
  3. Fresh blood is seen as an area of increased density (whiter) than surrounding tissue.
  4. Epidural hemorrhages are lens-shaped areas of increased signal located in the temporal-parietal regions. They are usually unilateral and are commonly associated with a skull fracture.
  5. Acute subdural hematomas are crescent-shaped areas of increased density that spread diffusely along the inner table of the skull. They are usually frontal in location.
- Magnetic resonance imaging (MRI) is usually not needed in the acute situation.
  1. MRI is more sensitive in detecting hypothalamic and brainstem infarcts and nonhemorrhagic intracranial lesions and in distinguishing acute on top of more chronic bleeding. It can also be used in subsequent evaluations of the child with persistent signs or symptoms.
  2. Availability of MRI and the challenge of sedation and monitoring make MRI less practical than CT scan for the acutely injured patient.
- Ultrasonography can be helpful in newborns and young infants with open fontanelles.
- Radiologic evaluation should not be undertaken until the patient is stabilized.
  1. Because epidural hematomas result from arterial bleeding that

can progress rapidly, some patients with hemiparesis, signs of herniation, and respiratory failure may require neurosurgical intervention before the diagnosis can be confirmed with CT.

- Although most cases of epidural bleeding and some cases of subdural bleeding are associated with a skull fracture, normal skull films do not exclude the possibility of intracranial bleeding.
- Subdural hemorrhages are a classic feature of the shaken baby syndrome. In these injuries, subdural hemorrhages occasionally may be bilateral and located posteriorly in the interhemispheric fissure.
- Most newborns with intracranial hemorrhages associated with birth trauma are asymptomatic. These bleeds are most commonly small subarachnoid collections that require no intervention.

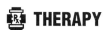 **THERAPY**

■ **NONPHARMACOLOGIC**
- Initial management should be directed at correcting life-threatening problems and preventing secondary brain injury.
- The frequency of pupil examination, level of consciousness checks, and repeated neurologic examination should be dictated by the patient's acuity in conjunction with neurosurgical consultation.
- Attention to the airway, respirations, and circulation take immediate precedence over the management of the head injury.
  1. Clear and secure the patient's airway while maintaining neck stability.
  2. Place the patient on a cardiorespiratory monitor.
  3. Provide supplemental oxygen.
  4. Ensure ventilation.
     a. If needed, orotracheal (not nasal) intubation using a rapid-sequence intubation technique to minimize elevations of ICP
  5. Control bleeding and treat shock to maintain cerebral perfusion pressure.
- If herniation is imminent, hyperventilation is indicated.
- Elevate the head of the bed of all head-injured patients.

■ **MEDICAL**
- Pharmacologic agents have limited usefulness in the emergency management of pediatric head trauma.
- Lidocaine (1 to 1.5 mg/kg intravenously) can be given to suppress the cough reflex before intubation.
- Rapid-sequence induction with Pavulon, atropine, succinylcholine,

and thiopental is needed for intubation to protect the airway and minimize elevations of ICP.
- Osmotic agents such as mannitol may rarely be necessary to decrease ICP but are never used prophylactically and are begun only if fluid resuscitation has been ensured. Furosemide is often used as an adjunct to mannitol therapy.
- Hypotonic fluids should be avoided and fluid status reevaluated frequently given the potential for inappropriate antidiuretic hormone release.
- Prophylactic use of anticonvulsants is unwarranted. Phenytoin (10 to 20 mg/kg slow intravenous infusion) is the most commonly used anticonvulsant for the treatment of acute, traumatic seizures.

■ **SURGICAL**
- Neurosurgical consultation is indicated for patients with severe head injury with loss of consciousness, depressed skull fractures, linear skull fractures that cross the middle meningeal artery groove, or basal skull fractures, and is indicated if imaging studies reveal acute bleeding that has a mass effect or the potential for one.
- Epidural and acute subdural hemorrhages are managed with emergent surgical drainage and support.
- In the young infant with open sutures, subdural taps can be performed for diagnostic and therapeutic purposes, but they generally are not used to evacuate acute bleeds.
- A burr hole approach to the hematoma may be required emergently.
- Depressed skull fractures are often associated with brain laceration and may require intraoperative hemostasis and elevation of the depressed fragment.
  1. In the absence of an intracerebral bleed, many pediatric depressed fractures are managed conservatively.
  2. The potential for the subsequent development of a seizure focus should be considered.
- A unique fracture of infants and young children is the "growing" or diastatic fracture. Such fractures occur in young children experiencing rapid brain growth and result from a skull fracture with a dural tear.
  1. In the postinjury period, rapid growth of the brain is associated with extrusion of the brain or a CSF cyst (leptomeningeal cyst) through the dural defect, preventing fusion of the fracture margins.
  2. It presents clinically as an enlarging skull defect following head injury.

3. This complication is treated neurosurgically.
- Most subarachnoid and small intracerebral hemorrhages do not require surgical drainage and are managed conservatively.

■ **PATIENT/FAMILY EDUCATION & PROGNOSIS**
- The prognosis for head injury is worse with associated intracranial bleeding.
- Many individuals have significantly reduced scores on neuropsychologic tests.
- About 15% of these children will subsequently develop epilepsy.
- The outcome for children with severe head injury is in general better than that for adults with the same severity score. Note, however, that children with epidural and subdural hemorrhage are a special subgroup with a poorer prognosis.
- All families whose children sustain major head injury experience major stress and require early intervention with social and rehabilitation services.

■ **PREVENTIVE TREATMENT**
- Most significant pediatric head trauma is caused by accidental injuries related to accidents involving motor vehicles or recreational vehicles and falls.
- Primary prevention of such accidental injuries through education and the use of restraints and safety equipment is strongly encouraged.
- Early recognition of infants and children at risk for or being victimized as a result of child abuse is crucial.
  1. Many children who subsequently become victims of serious abuse with significant head trauma have been previously identified as being at risk.
  2. Vigilant follow-up of such families is required.

■ **REFERRAL INFORMATION**
- Children with serious head trauma associated with intracranial bleeding require hospitalization and monitoring in an intensive care setting.
- Neurosurgical consultation and operative intervention are indicated for children with epidural and acute subdural hemorrhages and for children with depressed skull fractures associated with cerebral laceration.
- Consultation with a neurologist may be needed for the child with seizures or CNS disability resulting from the head injury.
- Involvement of social services and rehabilitative services is almost always needed for children and families who have experienced severe head injury.

☼ PEARLS & CONSIDERATIONS

■ CLINICAL PEARLS

- Most intracranial hemorrhages in pediatric patients are caused by moderate or severe head injury resulting from accidental or intentional injury.
- Epidural hematomas are seen with a history of a direct traumatic blow, usually across the middle meningeal artery groove.
  1. There is generally a lucid period followed by headache with a change in mental status associated with pupillary changes and hemiparesis.
  2. CT demonstrates a lens-shaped epidural collection of arterial and venous blood with mass effect.
  3. Treatment consists of emergent surgical drainage and supportive care.
- Subdural hematomas are more common than epidural hematomas in pediatric patients. They result from venous bleeding of the bridging veins that cross the dura and are a classic feature of shaken baby syndrome.
  1. These are usually associated with a slower time course than epidural bleeding.
  2. Generally, they present with symptoms of elevated ICP, and retinal hemorrhages may be found on physical examination.
  3. CT shows a crescent-shaped collection of blood that spreads diffusely along the inner table of the skull.
  4. Acute bleeding usually requires emergent surgical drainage and carries a poorer prognosis than epidural bleeding because of the underlying brain injury. Most chronic cases of bleeding are managed conservatively without surgery.
- A high index of suspicion for the possibility of intentional injury should be considered if the history contains discrepancies or is inconsistent with the extent of the observed trauma.

■ WEBSITES
- National Resource Center for Traumatic Brain Injury: www.neuro. pmr.vcu.edu
- Virtual Hospital: www.vh.org/ Patients/IHB/Neuro/BrainInjury/ 00TableOfContents.html; information for patients and families

REFERENCES

1. American Board of Pediatrics: Closed head injury: guides for record review, *Pediatr Rev* suppl:1, 1993.
2. Dolan M: Head trauma. In Barkin RM (ed): *Pediatric emergency medicine: concepts and clinical practice*, St Louis, 1992, Mosby.
3. Kaufman BA, Dacey RG: Acute care management of closed head injury in childhood, *Pediatr Ann* 23:18, 1994.
4. Raphaely RC et al: Management of severe pediatric head trauma, *Pediatr Clin North Am* 27:715, 1980.
5. Rivara FP: Epidemiology and prevention of pediatric traumatic brain injury, *Pediatr Ann* 23:12, 1994.
6. Rossman NP et al: Acute head trauma in infancy and childhood: clinical and radiologic aspects, *Pediatr Clin North Am* 26:707, 1979.

Author: **Lynn R. Campbell, M.D.**

II

BASIC INFORMATION

■ DEFINITION
Henoch-Schönlein purpura (HSP) is a systemic vasculitis with palpable purpura, colicky abdominal pain, arthritis, and nephritis.

■ SYNONYMS
- Anaphylactoid purpura
- Purpura rheumatica
- Hypersensitivity vasculitis
- HSP

ICD-9CM CODE
287.0 Henoch-Schönlein purpura
Others depending on findings and organ involvement

■ ETIOLOGY
Deposition of immunoglobulin A (IgA)-containing immune complexes in small blood vessel walls leading to a leukocytoclastic vasculitis

■ EPIDEMIOLOGY & DEMOGRAPHICS
- Peak is at age 4 to 5 years but can occur at any age.
- Males and females are affected equally.
- Incidence is more common in winter and spring.
- HSP is often preceded by upper respiratory infection; rarely associated with drug or food ingestion.

■ HISTORY
- Red, papular rash that becomes purpuric on the lower extremities and buttocks; less extensive on upper extremities
- Swelling of scalp, periorbital area, hands, and feet seen in infants in absence of renal disease
- Colicky abdominal pain (more than 50%)
- Gastrointestinal bleeding (bloody stools, hematemesis)
- Arthralgias and arthritis (in up to 75%; ankles and knees more often than hands)
- Macroscopic hematuria
- Hemoptysis (rare, although 95% have subclinical lung involvement)
- Neurologic involvement (rare; headache, mental status changes, seizures, focal neurologic deficits, mononeuropathies, polyradiculoneuropathies)

■ PHYSICAL EXAMINATION
- Symmetric, palpable, petechial rash on buttocks and extensor surfaces of the extremities occurring in crops; becomes purpuric; may be macular, papular, urticarial, or bullous
- Edema of scalp, hands, and feet in infants
- Abdominal tenderness

- Arthritis, particularly of knees and ankles more than elbows and hands
- Hypertension
- Testicular swelling (approximately 10% of males)

DIAGNOSIS

Typical rash in the absence of thrombocytopenia

■ DIFFERENTIAL DIAGNOSIS
- Acute hemorrhagic edema of childhood
- Systemic lupus erythematosus
- Drug reaction
- Erythema multiforme
- Urticaria
- Cryoglobulinemia
- Testicular torsion
- Juvenile rheumatoid arthritis
- Intussusception
- Acute surgical abdomen

■ DIAGNOSTIC WORKUP
- Prothrombin time (PT), partial thromboplastin time (PTT), and platelet count are usually normal.
- Stool guaiac is often positive.
- Skin biopsy (in questionable cases) shows leukocytoclastic vasculitis with IgA and C3 deposition.
- Blood urea nitrogen (BUN), creatinine, electrolytes, and albumin may be abnormal if there is significant renal involvement.
- Urinalysis may show hematuria (up to 90% of patients), proteinuria, leukocytes, and casts with renal involvement.
- Serum IgA level is elevated in 50% of cases.
- Abdominal ultrasound may show intussusception (most are ileoileal in HSP, with average age 6 years).
  1. Kidneys may show "medical renal disease," a descriptive term that indicates abnormal appearance of the kidneys on ultrasound but is nonspecific regarding cause.
- Kidney biopsy is indicated if renal insufficiency and/or nephrotic range proteinuria are present.
  1. May show a proliferative, crescentic, necrotizing glomerulonephritis with IgA and C3 deposition

THERAPY

■ MEDICAL
- Nonsteroidal antiinflammatory agents can be prescribed for arthritis.
  1. Use with caution in the presence of renal disease or gastrointestinal (GI) bleeding.
- Corticosteroids may hasten the re-

covery of abdominal pain and painful edema.
- Corticosteroids are *not* indicated for established mild renal involvement.
  1. Use of corticosteroids is controversial for the *prevention* of renal disease.
- Antihypertensives are given for elevated blood pressure.
- High dosages of pulse steroids and/or cytotoxic agents, and perhaps plasmapheresis, are used for rapidly progressive glomerulonephritis, crescentic glomerulonephritis, and nephrotic syndrome.

■ SURGICAL
If severe GI involvement exists, intussusception, bowel infarction, or bowel ulceration with GI bleeding can be present and should be treated as needed.

■ FOLLOW-UP & DISPOSITION
- The patient may have a relapsing course with recurrent bouts of rash and arthritis.
  1. Generally becomes milder over time with eventual resolution
- Renal involvement generally occurs within 3 months of the onset of rash.
  1. Need to follow serial urinalyses even if rash, arthralgias, and abdominal pain are improving.
  2. The incidence of renal involvement in HSP has been reported to be 20% to 100% depending on the definition used. A true estimate is difficult to determine.
- Renal involvement is the most significant complication, with 2% to 5% progressing to chronic renal failure.
  1. Renal insufficiency, heavy proteinuria with or without nephrotic syndrome, and significant hypertension are poor prognostic indicators.
- Deterioration of renal function has occurred even with apparent resolution of renal involvement and 20 years after onset.
  1. Patients must be monitored long term with blood pressure and urinalyses.
    a. If these are abnormal, BUN and creatinine should also be evaluated.

■ PATIENT/FAMILY EDUCATION
- The patient may have recurrent bouts of rash and arthralgias, but these generally become less frequent and milder with time.
- Most cases resolve completely without sequelae.
- Renal involvement is the most serious complication and may occur even as other symptoms are resolving. Even so, most renal findings resolve without sequelae.

■ PREVENTIVE TREATMENT
- None known
  1. Corticosteroids have been suggested to prevent renal involvement in early HSP, but this is controversial.

■ REFERRAL INFORMATION
- Patients with significant renal involvement should be referred to a pediatric nephrologist.
- Pediatric gastroenterology or surgery referral may be indicated for severe GI findings.
- In questionable cases, referral to a dermatologist for skin biopsy may be indicated.

☼ PEARLS & CONSIDERATIONS

■ CLINICAL PEARLS
Patients who are older at presentation are more likely to have severe renal involvement and a poorer prognosis.

■ SUPPORT GROUPS
For those with renal involvement:
- NEPHKIDS is an email discussion group for parents of children with kidney disease. To subscribe, email the message "subscribe nephkids" to majordomo@ualberta.ca.
- KidTalk is an email list for children with renal disease: http://home.nycap.rr.com/jazzer/kidtalk.html.
- Local chapters of the National Kidney Foundation can provide information and support.

REFERENCES
1. Alon U, Warady BA, Hellerstein S: The kidney in systemic disease: part II—autoimmune and vascular disorders, *Adv Pediatr* 40:325, 1993.
2. Choong CK, Beasley SW: Intra-abdominal manifestations of Henoch-Schönlein purpura, *J Paediatr Child Health* 34:405, 1998.
3. Goldstein AR et al: Long-term follow-up of childhood Henoch-Schönlein nephritis, *Lancet* 339:280, 1992.
4. Szer IS: Henoch-Schönlein purpura: when and how to treat, *J Rheumatol* 23:1661, 1996.
Author: **William S. Varade, M.D.**

II

BASIC INFORMATION

■ DEFINITION
Hepatitis A virus (HAV) infects hepatocytes and produces a clinical spectrum of disease ranging from asymptomatic infection to acute, fulminant hepatitis.

■ SYNONYM
Infectious hepatitis

ICD-9CM CODE
070.0 Hepatitis A

■ ETIOLOGY
- HAV is a 27-nm, icosahedral, nonenveloped, single-stranded RNA virus belonging to the family hepatovirus of the genus Picornaviridae that resembles enteroviruses in its transmission and replication.
- HAV infects exclusively human and primate hepatocytes with minimally cytopathic properties but induces a host immune response resulting in its characteristic disease.
- Transmission is primarily by a fecal-oral mode, with an attack rate as high as 90%.
- Fecal-oral route is by either person-to-person contact or ingestion of contaminated water or food (e.g., undercooked shellfish).
- HAV exists at the highest concentrations in stool and bile. It can rarely be transmitted by transfusion of blood but is not believed to be transmissible by saliva, urine, or semen.
- Infection can occur perinatally if the mother is incubating HAV, but the outcome is almost universally benign.

■ EPIDEMIOLOGY & DEMOGRAPHICS
- Overall seroprevalence of HAV in the United States is approximately 38%, with 11% by the age of 5 and almost three fourths of adults past their fifth decade.
- HAV accounted for almost 43% of all acute hepatitis reported in the United States in 1999.
- The incidence in the United States is quoted at 9.1 per 100,000, but this is likely grossly underreported because of mild or asymptomatic illness.
- In underdeveloped countries, antibody can be found in virtually 100% of adults.
- In order of importance, risk factors in U.S. surveillance were found to be (1) contact with an infected individual (26%), (2) exposure to a day-care facility (14%), (3) intravenous drug use (11%), (4) recent travel (4%), or (5) as part of suspected water or food outbreak (3%).
- Forty-two percent of cases are

without known risk factors, but half of these cases notably contained a child younger than 6 years of age in the household.

■ HISTORY
- The average incubation period is 28 days, with a range of 15 to 50 days.
- In children younger than 6 years of age, 70% are asymptomatic, whereas adolescents and adults have symptoms more than 70% of the time.
- Prodromal symptoms include fatigue, anorexia, nausea, vomiting, and abdominal pain.
- After the prodrome, less than 5% of children (compared with 30% of adolescents and adults) develop the characteristic symptoms of jaundice, pruritus, dark urine, and so forth.
- Only a small percentage of symptomatic children are hospitalized, with a case fatality of approximately 0.1% compared with 1.8% in adults older than age 50.

■ PHYSICAL EXAMINATION
- Eighty-five percent of symptomatic patients have mild hepatomegaly and liver tenderness.
- Both posterior cervical lymphadenopathy and splenomegaly occur in 15% of cases.
- Less than 5% of symptomatic children are icteric. When present, jaundice generally clears within 2 weeks.
- Complications include complete hepatic failure, which is rare.

🔬 DIAGNOSIS

■ DIFFERENTIAL DIAGNOSIS
- See "Differential Diagnosis" and diagnostic algorithms for jaundice/hyperbilirubinemia.
- In particular, hepatitis E, which is virtually nonexistent within the United States, resembles HAV in transmission, course, and prognosis, with the exception of its greater association with complications during pregnancy and fetal loss.

■ DIAGNOSTIC WORKUP
- In week 2 through the initial week of jaundice, HAV can be cultured in stool; however, this method is impractical for standard workups.
- In week 2, serum aminotransferases (aspartate aminotransferase [AST] and alanine aminotransferase [ALT]) begin to rise, often peaking in weeks 3 through 6 at levels higher than 500, and usually normalizing by week 8.
- Aminotransferases are closely followed by elevation of the bilirubin level.
- Immunoglobulin M (IgM)-specific antibody is detectable 25 to 30 days

after infection and persists at a detectable level for 2 to 3 months.
- Immunoglobulin G (IgG)-specific antibody is detectable within 40 days of infection and persists at elevated levels indefinitely.
- Liver biopsy is seldom warranted.

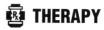 **THERAPY**

■ NONPHARMACOLOGIC
HAV is generally self-limited, and recovery within 4 to 6 weeks is typical. Therapy is generally supportive and includes good nutrition and avoidance of further liver trauma (i.e., hepatotoxic drugs).

■ MEDICAL
For the rare patient with dramatic cholestasis, a short course of prednisolone can mitigate both the disease process and its associated symptoms.

■ SURGICAL
Fulminant HAV is a rare event, but when it does occur, it most often strikes patients younger than 10 or older than 40. When acute liver failure does occur, transplant options should be promptly considered.

■ FOLLOW-UP & DISPOSITION
Chronic HAV does not exist, and infection confers lifelong immunity.

■ PATIENT/FAMILY EDUCATION
Sexual and household contacts of patients with acute HAV infection should receive 0.02 ml/kg immunoglobulin within 2 weeks of exposure.

■ PREVENTIVE TREATMENT
- Prevention includes attention to good hygiene and avoidance of contaminated water and food sources.
  1. Strict handwashing is especially important in day-care and institutional settings.
  2. Special precautions should be taken with regard to water sources and food preparation when visiting endemic areas. (Eighty-four percent of U.S. travel-related cases involved excursions to Mexico.)
- Pooled human immune serum immunoglobulin (ISIG) has existed for more than half a century and can be used prophylactically before an exposure (i.e., travel) or within 2 weeks of exposure (i.e., HAV-positive household contact).
  1. Serious adverse events associated with administration of ISIG are extremely rare.
  2. There are no reported cases of hepatitis B, hepatitis C, or human immunodeficiency virus transmission with administration of ISIG.

3. When administered within 2 weeks of HAV exposure, ISIG is more than 85% effective in preventing HAV infection.

4. When administered before exposure, ISIG prevents HAV infection in up to 95% of patients and confers immunity for 3 to 5 months.

• Two HAV vaccines are widely available: HAVRIX (SmithKline Beecham) and VAQTA (Merck & Co.); they cost approximately $60 per dose.

1. Both are inactivated vaccines and are fairly free of adverse effects other than local irritation (20% to 50%) and fever (5%).

2. A first dose of HAV vaccine is effective within 1 month but should be followed by a second dose in 6 to 12 months if further HAV exposure is predicted.

3. Vaccination efficacy is believed to be 95% or greater, and by kinetic models of antibody decline, it confers immunity for at least 20 years.

4. HAV vaccine is recommended for people traveling to endemic areas, intravenous drug users, male homosexuals, people with occupational exposures, and people with chronic liver disease.

■ REFERRAL INFORMATION

Consider referral to a gastroenterologist or hepatologist if patients present with an extended or fulminant course of HAV.

☼ PEARLS & CONSIDERATIONS

■ CLINICAL PEARLS

• The Centers for Disease Control and Prevention (CDC) has recently changed its recommendations (as of October 1999) to include immunization of children living in areas with more than 20 cases of HAV per 100,000 persons and to consider immunization at more than 10 cases per 100,000 persons.

• From 6% to 12% of those with HAV develop a relapsing form. Although these patients have multiple bouts between remissions, they do not develop chronic disease.

• Although rarer than in hepatitis B and C, extrahepatic symptoms in HAV exist and include evanescent rash, arthralgias, vasculitis, and glomerulonephritis.

■ WEBSITES

• CDC: http://cdc.gov/ncidod/diseases/hepatitis; updated guidelines
• Hepatitis Central: http://hepatitis-central.com/hcv/maintoc.html; information and resources

■ SUPPORT GROUPS

Connections to local support groups can be made through the American Liver Foundation: http://sadieo.ucf.edu/alf/alffinal/

REFERENCES

1. Duff P: Hepatitis in pregnancy, *Semin Perinatol* 22:277, 1998.
2. Feldman M: *Siesenger & Fordtran's gastrointestinal and liver disease,* ed 6, Philadelphia, 1998, WB Saunders.
3. Kane M: Hepatitis viruses and the neonate, *Clin Perinatol* 24:181, 1997.
4. Prevention of HAV through active or passive immunization, *MMWR Morb Mortal Wkly Rep* 48(RR-12):1, 1999.
5. Sokal E: Viral hepatitis throughout infancy to adulthood *Acta Gastroenterologica Belgica* LXI:170, 1998.
Author: **Jason Emmick, M.D.**

BASIC INFORMATION

■ DEFINITION
Hepatitis B virus (HBV) is a highly infectious DNA virus that primarily causes acute liver disease but that also leads to chronic disease in many patients. Hepatitis D virus (HDV) is a passenger virus requiring the presence of HBV and may occur as a simultaneous coinfection or as a superinfection in an HBV carrier.

ICD-9CM CODES
070.30 HBV, acute
070.32 HBV, chronic
070.52 HDV

■ ETIOLOGY
- HBV is a partially double-stranded DNA virus from the family of Hepadnaviridae.
- HBV contains three primary structural antigens: surface (HBsAg), core (HBcAg), and e-antigen (HBeAg).
- HBV can be transmitted via infected blood, semen, vaginal secretions, and saliva.
- Nonserous secretions (i.e., breast milk) contain minimal to no HBV particles.
- In industrial countries, infection most often results from sexual activity (26%), intravenous drug use (23%), and occupational exposure (3%), and more rarely from perinatal or household contact, hemodialysis, and surgery.
- No clear risk factor is identified in one fourth of HBV infections.
- Perinatal transmission occurs in as little as 10% of cases when the mother has only HBsAg, but it occurs as often as 90% when she is also seropositive for HBeAg.
- HDV is a small passenger virus that uses excess HBsAg to coat an inner core of single-stranded, circular RNA.

■ EPIDEMIOLOGY
- Worldwide, HBV ranks as the ninth cause of mortality, with an estimated 400 million carriers by the year 2001.
- In the United States, 300,000 people are infected each year, resulting in 17,000 hospitalizations and 5000 annual deaths from its various complications.
- In all pregnancies, 0.1% to 0.2% of mothers have acute HBV, and 0.5% to 1.5% have chronic disease.
- Although children represent only 1% to 3% of the reported HBV cases in the United States, they constitute as much as 30% of the chronic cases.
- Superinfection with HDV in a patient who is seropositive for HBeAg is a major risk factor for chronic liver disease.

- Of those with chronic HBV, 15% to 30% develop cirrhosis. with a small subset of this group developing hepatocellular carcinoma (HCC).

■ HISTORY
- Neonatal and early childhood HBV infections are often asymptomatic.
  1. Up to 90% of children younger than 1 year of age, but only a few older children and adults (10% to 15%), develop chronic HBV.
  2. Early childhood carriers of HBV generally spend 10 to 20 years in an immunotolerant state during which silent and active replication of HBV occurs.
- Acute HBV results in fulminant hepatitis and death in less than 1% of patients.
- Most older children and adults acquire protective levels of antibody, experience complete resolution of symptoms, and go on to have lifelong immunity.
- Symptomatic children develop malaise and anorexia about 6 weeks after exposure.
- Jaundice develops in one fourth of all infected children and peaks in weeks 8 to 12.

■ PHYSICAL EXAMINATION
- Liver tenderness, hepatomegaly, splenomegaly, and lymphadenopathy are common.
- Jaundice may be present.
- More often than in hepatitis A virus (HAV) or hepatitis C virus (HCV) infections, there is skin and joint involvement.
  1. Arthritis of interphalangeal-metacarpal joints
  2. Urticaria/angioedema
- A small subset of patients develop polyarteritis nodosa, glomerulonephritis, leukocytoclastic vasculitis, Raynaud's phenomenon, or Guillain-Barré syndrome.

DIAGNOSIS

■ DIFFERENTIAL DIAGNOSIS
See "Differential Diagnosis" and diagnostic algorithms for jaundice/hyperbilirubinemia.

■ DIAGNOSTIC WORKUP
- In acute HBV, aminotransferases begin to rise by 8 weeks after exposure, peak at 10 to 12 weeks, and normalize around months 5 to 6.
  1. Alanine aminotransferase (ALT) tends to be greater than aspartate aminotransferase (AST), and both generally peak at more than 500 IU/L.
  2. Both rise soon after the presence of HBeAg, HBsAg, and HBV DNA.

- They are soon followed by more modest elevations in bilirubin (5 to10 mg/dl).
- Acute HBV is demonstrated by detection of surface antigen (HBsAg) and immunoglobulin M (IgM) antibody to the core antigen.
- HBV DNA by polymerase chain reaction is a highly sensitive and direct measure of infectivity.
- The presence of HBeAg is indicative of high HBV levels of inoculum or viral replication.
- Antibody to HBsAg confers protective immunity and is found in those immunized for HBV or who have cleared the infection.
- Patients with chronic HBV maintain HBsAg along with IgG antibody to the core antigen.
- In chronic HBV, AST/ALT often remain modestly elevated (50 to 200 IU/L).
- HDV can be detected by IgM to HDV, and its presence should be sought in flares of chronic HBV and in particularly fulminant cases of HBV.

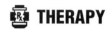

THERAPY

■ NONPHARMACOLOGIC
For both HBV and HDV, treatment is limited to supportive care and avoidance of further liver trauma (i.e., hepatotoxic drugs and alcohol).

■ MEDICAL
- Treatment is indicated for children with active viral replication and elevated liver function tests
- As in adults, pooled data have demonstrated that treatment with interferon results in loss of HBV DNA and HBeAg 20% to 58% of the time, compared with 8% to 17% in controls.
- Successful interferon treatment results in histologic and clinical improvements.
- There appears to be no role for "steroid priming" for either children or adults.
- Use of nucleoside analogs (i.e., lamivudine and famciclovir) is still experimental in children but is likely to emerge as a key component of chemotherapeutic combination therapy.

■ SURGICAL
Transplantation should be considered early in the course of impending liver failure.

■ FOLLOW-UP & DISPOSITION
- HCC secondary to HBV has been reported in childhood but most often occurs later as an adult.
  1. HCC more often occurs in cirrhotic patients (90%).
  2. HCC risk is up to 390-fold greater in patients with chronic HBV.

■ PATIENT/FAMILY EDUCATION
- Condoms reduce, but do not prevent, the spread of HBV to sexual partners.
- Seronegative household members or sexual partners of HBV-infected individuals should receive immunoprophylaxis with HBV immunoglobulin (HBIG), followed by the HBV immunization series.

■ PREVENTIVE TREATMENT
- Most industrialized nations now routinely screen all pregnant mothers for HBV and vaccinate all children in early life.
- Newborns of HBV-positive mothers should receive HBIG and begin the HBV vaccine series within 12 hours of life.
- Two similar recombinant HBV vaccines are available.
  1. Both contain an inactivated portion of surface antigen in a yeast vector.
  2. The vaccine series consists of three doses given at month 0, 1, and 6.

3. The vaccine confers protection in 95% of healthy recipients and may last a lifetime.
4. Vaccination carries no risk of transmission and no absolute contraindications except severe hypersensitivity to yeast or other vaccine components.
5. Severe reactions are rare; the vaccine costs about $30 per pediatric dosing.
- HBIG should be given to seronegative patients who have been exposed to HBV. It is approximately 90% effective in preventing HBV in exposed neonates.
- There is no cure for HDV, and strategies rely on treatment and prevention of HBV.

■ REFERRAL INFORMATION
Consider referral to a gastroenterologist or hepatologist for all patients with chronic or complicated courses of HBV/HDV.

☼ PEARLS & CONSIDERATIONS

■ CLINICAL PEARLS
- Vaccine effectiveness is not altered by simultaneous administration of HBIG but is compromised by gluteal rather than deltoid injection.
- Cesarean section delivery does not reduce the transmission rate of HBV to neonates.
- A small percentage of patients in the United States have viral mutations with no detectable HBeAg (but can be picked up by HBV DNA) and tend to have more virulent disease.

■ WEBSITES & SUPPORT GROUPS
See the section "Hepatitis A."

REFERENCES
1. Arnot R: The evolving efforts to control HBV, *Pediatr Infect Dis J* 17: S26, 1998.
2. Duff P: Hepatitis in pregnancy, *Semin Perinatol* 22:277, 1998.
3. Feldman M: *Siesenger & Fordtran's gastrointestinal and liver disease,* ed 6, Philadelphia, 1998, WB Saunders.
4. Kane M: Hepatitis viruses and the neonate, *Clin Perinatol* 24:181, 1997.
5. Lee W: Hepatitis B virus infection, *N Engl J Med* 337:1733, 1997.
6. Nelson W: *Nelson textbook of pediatrics,* ed 15, Philadelphia, 1996, WB Saunders.
7. Sokal E: Viral hepatitis throughout infancy to adulthood, *Acta Gastroenterologica Belgica* LXI:170, 1998.
8. Vajro PL: Interferon: a meta-analysis of published studies in pediatric chronic HBV, *Acta Gastrenterologica Belgica* 61:219, 1998.
Author: **Jason Emmick, M.D.**

II

BASIC INFORMATION

■ DEFINITION
Hepatitis C virus (HCV) is an RNA virus that is generally asymptomatic in its first 20 years but most often leads to chronic liver disease.

■ SYNONYM
Non-A/non-B hepatitis

ICD-9CM CODES
070.51 HCV, acute
070.54 HCV, chronic

■ ETIOLOGY
- HCV is a single-stranded, enveloped RNA virus from the Flaviviridae family.
- The principle risk factors for acquisition of HCV are intravenous drug use (60%), transfusions, and sexual intercourse (less than 20%), with a minor role played by perinatal transmission.
- In one study, two thirds of intravenous drug users tested seropositive for HCV.
- Although HCV accounts for up to 90% of hepatitis resulting from transfusion, the blood supply has been relatively free of this entity since July 1992.
- Reported vertical transmission rates range widely from only 3% up to 44%, being more common in immunocompromised mothers and those with high HCV titers.
- Sexual transmission appears to be rare among monogamous partners but increased in more sexually promiscuous settings.
- Although low levels of HCV are found in breast milk of HCV-infected mothers, this has not yet been proven to be a route of transmission.
- About 10% of HCV-infected individuals have no clear risk factor.

■ EPIDEMIOLOGY & DEMOGRAPHICS
- Worldwide, it is estimated that 170 million people have chronic HCV.
- In the United States, it is estimated that 4 million people have HCV, with the full peak of infection not expected to crest for another 10 to 20 years.
- Males and people ages 20 to 39 years are at highest risk for HCV infection.
- It is estimated that 1% to 3% of the present obstetric population is seropositive for HCV.
- A recent examination of 55 children who contracted hepatitis C in Japan when they received a transfusion related to either malignancy or cardiac surgery demonstrated the following findings:
  1. Approximately 60% to 80% of the children progressed to chronic HCV.
  2. Alanine aminotransferase (ALT) levels varied widely from 100 to 1000 for 1 to 6 years after infection before falling to near-normal levels.
  3. Children had lower levels of necroinflammation and fibrosis than would be expected in adult counterparts.

■ HISTORY
- Only about 20% of patients report initial vague symptoms of fatigue, anorexia, nausea, malaise, and abdominal discomfort after the 40- to 90-day incubation period.
- Eighty-five percent of HCV-infected individuals progress to chronic liver disease.
  1. Risk factors for poor prognosis include alcohol intake, age older than 40, male gender, and necroinflammatory findings on liver biopsy.
- Progression of HCV is insidious in children, and most are asymptomatic at 20 years of age or older.
- Of those with chronic HCV, 20% progress to cirrhosis after 20 to 50 years, with as many as 1% to 4% of these patients developing hepatocellular carcinoma (HCC) per year.

■ PHYSICAL EXAMINATION
- Jaundice is occasionally seen in acute infection but, when seen with chronic HCV, generally represents hepatic decompensation.
- HCV is well known for extrahepatic disease and may manifest itself in a wide variety of ways:
  1. Necrotizing skin lesions
  2. Arthritis
  3. Hepatosplenomegaly
  4. Purpura

DIAGNOSIS

■ DIFFERENTIAL DIAGNOSIS
See "Differential Diagnosis" and diagnostic algorithms for jaundice/hyperbilirubemia.

■ DIAGNOSTIC WORKUP
- Initially, enzyme immunoassay (EIA) is used, with positive results confirmed by recombinant immunoblot assay (RIBA) or HCV RNA by polymerase chain reaction (PCR).
  1. EIA has a sensitivity that approaches 97%, but it may not be accurate in the first 6 months after exposure.
  2. EIA cannot distinguish among acute, chronic, and resolved HCV infections.
  3. RIBA assays for four HCV antigens.
  4. A RIBA that is positive for two or more antigens is confirmatory for HCV infection.
  5. A RIBA with only one antigen detected is considered indeterminant.
- The ALT is most often used to follow liver disease but may often fluctuate or even be normal despite ongoing hepatic damage.
- HCV RNA uses PCR amplification and exists in qualitative and quantitative forms.
  1. Qualitative HCV RNA is the more sensitive test and can detect the virus as soon as 2 weeks after exposure.
  2. Quantitative HCV RNA can be used to judge prognosis and treatment response.
- Genotype testing exists in several versions and can help predict prognosis and treatment response (i.e., the common U.S. genotype 1 is the least responsive).
- Liver biopsy is a valuable tool in determining patients who are likely to progress to cirrhosis: those with marked necroinflammation, septal fibrosis, or partial nodularity.
- Hepatitis C patients are at high risk for developing the following:
  1. Essential mixed cryoglobulinemia
  2. Porphyria cutanea tarda
  3. Leukocytoclastic vasculitis
  4. Keratoconjunctivitis
  5. Arthritis
  6. Glomerulonephritis
  7. Thyroiditis
  8. Pulmonary fibrosis

THERAPY

■ NONPHARMACOLOGIC
Strict emphasis is placed on avoiding additional liver insults (i.e., alcohol and hepatotoxic drugs) as well as preventing and/or immunizing against the other viral hepatites.

■ MEDICAL
- In general, treatment criteria for adults and children older than 2 years of age are elevated transaminases, abnormal liver histology, and positive HCV RNA titers.
- Typical treatment regimens consist of 3 million units of interferon given three times per week for 6 months.
  1. Treatment leads to 15% to 25% sustained (more than 6 months) response.

2. Positive prognostic factors include young age, HCV genotypes other than type 1, short duration of disease, low HCV RNA levels, and absence of cirrhosis.
3. Higher dosages and longer courses of interferon may increase the response rate and duration.
4. Interferon often results in flulike symptoms shortly after administration.
5. Later complications include bone marrow suppression, fatigue, severe depression, alopecia, interstitial pulmonary fibrosis, and autoimmune disorders.

- Concomitant use of ribavirin may increase the interferon response, but it is not commonly in use for children.

■ SURGICAL

- HCV-related liver disease now rates as the single most common reason for liver transplantation in the United States.
  1. Recurrence of HCV occurs in as many as 95% of the transplant cases.
  2. The risk of HCV in previously naive hosts is more than 25% during liver transplantation.
  3. Although the risk is lower in the pediatric population, extrahepatic reservoir and immunosuppressive therapy contribute to the high HCV rates seen.

■ FOLLOW-UP & DISPOSITION

- Periodic measurement of ALT as a rough marker of disease activity is recommended.
- Periodic ultrasound and α-fetoprotein levels should be performed as a screening test for HCC in longstanding HCV infection.

■ PATIENT/FAMILY EDUCATION

- HCV-infected persons should be cautioned against sharing razors and toothbrushes with household members or having unprotected sexual activity.
- Strict avoidance of alcohol should be adamantly encouraged because its use is the single strongest risk factor for progression to end-stage liver disease.

■ PREVENTIVE TREATMENT

- Prevention mainly relies on avoidance of previously mentioned risk factors.
- Immune globulins are ineffective, and the promise of an HCV vaccine is distant.

■ REFERRAL INFORMATION

Consider referral to a gastroenterologist or hepatologist for all patients with chronic or complicated courses of HCV.

⟨⟩ PEARLS & CONSIDERATIONS

■ CLINICAL PEARLS

Occasionally, a single HCV DNA can be negative despite HCV infection, and ALT can be normal despite ongoing necroinflammation.

■ WEBSITES & SUPPORT GROUPS

See the section "Hepatitis A."

REFERENCES

1. Duff P: Hepatitis in pregnancy, *Semin Perinatol* 22:277, 1998.
2. Feldman M: *Siesenger & Fordtran's gastrointestinal and liver disease,* ed 6, Philadelphia, 1998, WB Saunders.
3. Hoshiyama A: Clinical and histologic features of chronic HCV infection after blood transfusion in Japanese children, *Pediatrics* 105:62, 2000.
4. Kane M: Hepatitis viruses and the neonate, *Clin Perinatol* 24:181, 1997.
5. Moyer M: HCV infection, *Adv Pediatr Infect Dis* 14:109, 1999.
6. Recommendations for prevention and control of HCV infection and HCV-related chronic disease, *MMWR* 47 (RR-19):1, 1998.
7. Sokal E: Viral hepatitis throughout infancy to adulthood, *Acta Gastroenterologica Belgica* LXI:170, 1998.
8. Zignego A: Extrahepatic manifestations of HCV infection: facts and controversies, *J Hepatol* 31:369, 1999.

Author: **Jason Emmick, M.D.**

II

BASIC INFORMATION

■ DEFINITION
An abdominal wall hernia is protrusion of a viscus through an opening in the wall of the abdominal cavity. The hernial orifice is the defect in the innermost aponeurotic layer of the abdomen, and the hernial sac is an outpouching of peritoneum.

■ TYPES
- Umbilical hernia
- Epigastric hernia
- Spigelian hernia
- Lumbar hernia
- Parastomal hernia
- Incisional hernia

■ SYNONYMS
- Rupture
- Mass
- Bulge

ICD-9CM CODES
533.1   Umbilical
553.29 Epigastric
553.29 Spigelian
553.8   Lumbar
569.69 Parastomal
553.21 Incisional

■ ETIOLOGY
- Umbilical hernias result from a failure of complete obliteration of the site where fetal umbilical vessels join the placenta during gestation.
  1. In teens and adults, obesity, multiple pregnancies, and ascites may be precursors.
- Epigastric hernias, which are located between the xiphoid process and the umbilicus, result from congenital fascial defects arising at the site of penetration of the fascia by blood vessels or from tears in the linea alba induced by coughing, straining, or abdominal distension.
  1. Epigastric hernias are differentiated from diastasis recti, which is a broad attenuation but not a defect in the linea alba.
- Spigelian hernias occur along the subumbilical portion of Spieghel's semilunar line and through Spieghel's fascia, which is an intrinsically weak area of the abdominal wall from segmental banding of the internal oblique and transversus abdominis muscles at the lateral border of the rectus sheath.
- Lumbar hernias of congenital origin result from a diffuse muscle deficiency of the musculofascial layers and occur in the following areas:
  1. Inferior lumbar triangle of Petit bounded by the latissimus dorsi, the external oblique muscle, and the iliac crest

  2. Superior lumbar triangle of Grynfeltt-Lesshaft bounded by the twelfth rib, the internal oblique muscle, and the sacrospinalis muscle
- Parastomal hernias usually occur lateral to the ostomy when the stoma emerges through the attenuated semilunar line rather than the rectus sheath.
- Incisional hernias are caused by wound infection, obesity, and poor suture closure technique.
  1. Closure suture should be nonabsorbable, continuous, and four times the length of the incision.

■ EPIDEMIOLOGY & DEMOGRAPHICS
- Umbilical hernias are seen in 1 of every 6 children.
  1. They are 6 to 10 times more common in African-American than Caucasian children.
  2. These hernias are more often seen with low birth weight.
  3. They are more common with trisomy 13, 18, and 21.
  4. They are more common with hypothyroidism, mucopolysaccharidoses, and Beckwith-Weidemann syndrome.
- Epigastric hernias are common hernias in children and are usually small and multiple.
  1. Preperitoneal fat protrudes through small defects in the midline fascia.
  2. If located immediately above the umbilicus, they are called *supraumbilical hernias* and may contain bowel.
- Spigelian hernias are rarely seen in childhood.
- Lumbar hernias are among the rarest of abdominal wall hernias and may be congenital, posttraumatic, or postoperative. Congenital lumbar hernias are associated with rib and vertebral anomalies, leading to the designation of lumbocostovertebral syndrome.
- Parastomal and incisional hernias occur with incidences below 5% and are most often related to technical error at operation.

■ HISTORY
- Umbilical hernias spontaneously close in most children by 3 years of age. Spontaneous closure is unlikely after 4 years of age and with defects larger than 1.5 cm in internal diameter. Umbilical hernias in children rarely incarcerate.
- Epigastric hernias are often asymptomatic bulges in the midline but may present with pain and tenderness associated with a palpable, usually irreducible, mass in the subcutaneum.

- Spigelian hernias may present with a mass or bulge in either lower quadrant of the abdomen. Pain may be a presenting symptom.
- Lumbar hernias protrude with crying. Congenital lumbar hernias may be apparent in neonates. A history of trauma also may be elicited (i.e., flank incision after nephrectomy).
- Parastomal hernias rarely are painful but may interfere with irrigations of an ostomy or adherence of stomal appliances.
- Incisional hernias have a propensity to enlarge.
  1. They are often difficult to repair.
  2. They may entrap underlying omentum or bowel, causing pain or obstruction.

■ PHYSICAL EXAMINATION
- Umbilical hernias protrude when the child strains or cries and spontaneously reduce when the child is supine and at rest.
  1. Fascial rings smaller than 1 cm in children younger than 3 years of age usually close spontaneously.
  2. Proboscus-like hernias with redundant skin may be referred for surgical repair early for social, cosmetic, or skin integrity concerns.
- Epigastric hernias present as palpable protrusions in the midline from the xiphoid to the umbilicus.
  1. They are readily apparent when the child holds his or her arms above the head and performs a Valsalva maneuver.
  2. Most are irreducible and produce discomfort out of proportion to their size.
- Spigelian hernias are difficult to diagnose because they are interparietal and are contained by the aponeurosis of the external oblique.
  1. They may appear as intermittent masses in the lower abdomen, lateral to the edge of the rectus abdominus muscle
  2. They are accentuated by crying or straining.
- Lumbar hernias present as flank swellings that protrude with crying.
  1. Most are easily reducible on examination.
- Parastomal hernias are more common with colostomies than with ileostomies and are located lateral to the ostomy.
- Incisional hernias underlie visible scars and are palpable defects in the fascia that protrude with increased intraabdominal pressure.
  1. Overlying skin is atrophic and devoid of subcutaneous fat.

🔬 DIAGNOSIS

■ DIFFERENTIAL DIAGNOSIS
- Lipoma
- Hematoma
- Soft tissue neoplasm

■ DIAGNOSTIC WORKUP
- Umbilical hernias are recognized on physical examination.
  1. The diameter of the fascial defect and not the length of protrusion is prognostically significant.
  2. The incarceration rate is 1 per 1500 hernias in childhood.
- Epigastric hernias are accentuated on physical examination by the Valsalva maneuver and by having the child raise his or her arms above the head.
  1. Protuberance is seen midline, above the level of the umbilicus.
- Spigelian hernias, unless large, are difficult to diagnose on physical examination.
  1. Ultrasound and computed tomography (CT) may reveal hernias that are too small to detect clinically.
- Lumbar hernias may be apparent on physical examination, but CT may define the precise anatomy of the defect.
- Parastomal and incisional hernias after surgery are accentuated on physical examination by maneuvers that increase intraabdominal pressure.

℞ THERAPY

■ NONPHARMACOLOGIC
Umbilical hernias less than 1 cm in diameter will likely close spontaneously.

■ SURGICAL
- Surgical repair of umbilical hernias is indicated in many instances, such as the following:
  1. If they persist beyond 4 to 5 years of age, surgery should be performed.
  2. Defects larger than 1.5 cm in diameter may be repaired earlier.
  3. Proboscus-like defects may be repaired as early as 1 to 2 years of age.
  4. Other absolute indications for surgical repair include incarceration, strangulation, perforation, and evisceration, all of which are rare events in children.
- Epigastric hernias should be repaired operatively even in the absence of symptoms because they are predisposed to gradual enlargement and are more difficult to repair in adults.
  1. Hernias should be marked at skin level before induction of anesthesia because they are extremely difficult to palpate once relaxation has occurred.
- Spigelian hernias should be surgically repaired to prevent incarceration and strangulation. They should be marked before anesthesia.
- Lumbar hernias in children may allow primary closure, but prosthetic mesh is occasionally required to accomplish closure of large defects or recurrences.
- Parastomal hernias may be repaired at the time of stomal closure by moving the stoma to a new location or by implanting prosthetic mesh about the stoma.
- Incisional hernias in children usually can be primarily closed 6 to 8 months after the initial operation to allow underlying intraabdominal adhesions to mature. Defects in excess of 5 cm often require insertion of a permanent synthetic mesh.

■ FOLLOW-UP & DISPOSITION
In the absence of wound infection, chronic disease states, connective tissue disorders, or malnutrition, recurrence rates after operative repair of abdominal wall hernias in children are negligible.

■ PATIENT/FAMILY EDUCATION
- The most difficult task in dealing with children with umbilical hernias is convincing the family that observation only is successful in most cases.
- After surgical repair of any abdominal wall hernia, children should avoid excessive physical activity and contact sports for 4 weeks.

■ REFERRAL INFORMATION
Children with abdominal wall hernias should be referred to a pediatric surgeon. Operative repair is generally an outpatient procedure under general anesthesia.

⚙ PEARLS & CONSIDERATIONS

■ WEBSITES
- American Medical Association: www.ama-assn.org/insight/h_focus/men_hlth/hernia/hernia.htm#top
- Hernia information: www.hernia.org
- YourHealth.com: www.yourhealth.com

REFERENCES
1. Kapur P, Caty MG, Glick PL: Pediatric hernias and hydroceles, *Pediatr Clin North Am* 45:773, 1998.
2. Oldham KT, Colombani PM, Foglia RP: *Surgery of infants and children: scientific principles and practice*, Philadelphia, 1997, Lippincott-Raven.
3. Wantz G (moderator): *Incisional hernia: the problem and the cure*, Symposium, *J Am Coll Surg* 188:429, 1999.
Authors: **Walter Pegoli, Jr., M.D., and George T. Drugas, M.D.**

II

BASIC INFORMATION

DEFINITION
Hernias arising above the abdominal crural crease are *inguinal,* and those arising below the crease are *femoral.* Indirect inguinal hernias pass obliquely or indirectly toward and into the scrotum, in which case they are called *scrotal hernias.* Direct inguinal hernias protrude directly outward and forward through the floor of the inguinal canal. Femoral hernias are protrusions of peritoneum through a defect on the medial side of the femoral sheath.

SYNONYM
Inguinal bulge or rupture

ICD-9CM CODES
550.90 Inguinal hernia
553.00 Femoral hernia
550.10 Incarcerated hernia
603.9 Hydrocele

ETIOLOGY
- Failure of the processus vaginalis to close accounts for nearly all inguino-scrotal abnormalities seen in infancy and childhood.
- Direct hernias result from congenital or acquired muscular insufficiencies of the floor of the inguinal canal.
- For women, the increased diameter of the true pelvis, as compared with that of men, proportionately widens the femoral canal, which predisposes women to femoral herniation.
- Femoral hernias are extremely rare, with a 2:1 female:male ratio.

EPIDEMIOLOGY & DEMOGRAPHICS
- Inguinal hernia
  1. The incidence of inguinal hernias in children ranges from 0.8% to 4.4%, highest in infancy.
  2. Approximately one third of children with hernias are younger than 6 months old at operation.
  3. The incidence of inguinal hernia is highest in premature infants, ranging from 16% to 25% of all premature infants.
  4. Males are affected approximately six times more often than females.
  5. Right-sided hernias are predominant.
     a. 60% occur on the right
     b. 30% on the left
     c. 10% bilateral
  6. Approximately 11.5% of patients have a positive family history of inguinal hernia.

- Femoral hernia
  1. Femoral hernias account for less than 1% of all groin hernias in children.

HISTORY
- Inguinal or scrotal bulge, which may come and go
  1. Accentuated with increased intraabdominal pressure (cough, strain, Valsalva)
- Perinatal factors that increase risk of hernias
  1. Prematurity
  2. Mechanical ventilation
  3. Bronchopulmonary dysplasia

PHYSICAL EXAMINATION
- A mass that is visible above the inguinal ligament, possibly extending to the ipsilateral scrotum, is a classic finding in patients with inguinal hernia.
- "Silk glove sign" (thickening "smoothness" of the spermatic cord) is a useful finding in patients in whom an inguinal hernia is suspected clinically but is not evident.
- Inguinal hernias may be associated with undescended testis.
- Noncommunicating hydroceles (peritesticular fluid collections) do not change in size or decompress with manual compression.
  1. They have a high incidence of spontaneous resolution by 1 year of age.
- Femoral hernias are located medial to the femoral vessels and do not extend into the scrotum.
  1. From 15% to 20% are incarcerated at initial presentation.

DIAGNOSIS

- Made on physical examination
- Ultrasound (duplex) if differential includes torsion of testis and/or appendix testis

DIFFERENTIAL DIAGNOSIS
- Testicular torsion
- Inguinal or femoral lymphadenitis
- Torsion of appendix testis
- Lipoma of the spermatic cord
- Hydrocele of the spermatic cord

THERAPY

- Femoral and inguinal hernias do not spontaneously resolve and should be surgically repaired because of the high risk of incarceration.

- In patients younger than 1 year old with an unilateral inguinal hernia, contralateral exploration is indicated because of the high risk of bilaterality.
- Most patients can undergo ambulatory hernia repair.
- Femoral hernias should be repaired to prevent incarceration and strangulation.

FOLLOW-UP & DISPOSITION
- Several complications that are associated with herniorrhaphy require long-term follow-up.
  1. Iatrogenic undescended testis (trapped testicle)
  2. Injury to vas deferens (sterility if bilateral)
  3. Testicular atrophy
- Repeated evaluation of the scrotal content over time is necessary to evaluate for possible postoperative complications.

PATIENT/FAMILY EDUCATION
- Patients and/or their families should be informed of the association of infertility and herniorrhaphy in men (secondary to injury to the vas deferens or testicular atrophy).
- Repair of an indirect inguinal hernia in childhood does not preclude the development of a direct inguinal hernia in adulthood.

REFERRAL INFORMATION
Children with inguinal and femoral hernias should be referred to a pediatric surgeon for definitive surgical correction.

PEARLS & CONSIDERATIONS

CLINICAL PEARLS
To reduce an incarcerated hernia, place the child in a warm dark room, use warm hands and adequate sedation, and apply constant pressure at the apex of the sac.

WEBSITE
Hernia information: www.hernia.org

REFERENCE
1. Lloyd DA, Rintala RJ: Inguinal hernia and hydrocele. In O'Neill JA, Rowe MI, Grosfeld J (eds): *Pediatric surgery,* ed 5, vol 2, St Louis, 1998, Mosby.

Authors: **Walter Pegoli, Jr., M.D., and George T. Drugas, M.D.**

BASIC INFORMATION

DEFINITION

Although some authors consider herpangina to be a specific, febrile, enteroviral illness characterized by a typical enanthem, others restrict the term to the oropharyngeal eruption itself, which can also occur in conjunction with other clinical constellations caused by enterovirus, including encephalitis, meningitis, myocarditis, and so forth.

SYNONYMS

- Mouth ulcers
- Coxsackie mouth ulcers
- Stomatitis

ICD-9CM CODE

074.0 Herpangina

ETIOLOGY

- Herpangina is most commonly caused by the Coxsackie viruses of group A (1-10, 16, 22).
- Other agents include Coxsackie virus B (1-5), echovirus (6, 9, 11, 16-17, 22, 25), and herpes simplex.
- Incubation period is 2 to 10 days.
- The nasopharynx is the site of inoculation.
  1. Although most of the inoculum is swallowed, some viral replication occurs in the pharynx, followed by spread to the upper respiratory lymphatics.
  2. Acid stability permits survival of the virus past the stomach, with subsequent passage through intestinal lining cells to Peyer's patches, where primary replication occurs.
- Minor viremia follows the replication of virus in Peyer's patches, resulting in subsequent seeding of numerous organ systems.
  1. At this time, the oral lesions typical of herpangina appear.
  2. Other sites may also be seeded at this time, including the central nervous system, heart, lungs, and liver.
  3. Replication in these sites produces a second, major viremia.
- Minor and major viremia commonly correlate with the biphasic appearance of fever and symptoms often characteristic of enteroviral infection.
- Virus may be cultured from the oropharynx during days number 10 to 22 after infection and from stool for up to 2 to 4 months.
- The immune response is humoral.

EPIDEMIOLOGY & DEMOGRAPHICS

- Humans are considered the only natural hosts. Other animals may acquire infection, most likely from direct contact with humans or human excreta.
- Shellfish may support a source of enteroviral storage during cold-weather intervals.
- In temperate climates, attack rates peak in summer and fall, although sporadic cases may occur throughout the year. Prevalence is yearlong in tropical climates.
- Transmission is person-to-person by the fecal-oral and possibly oral-oral routes.
  1. Flies (from which enteroviruses have been recovered) and swimming/wading pools have also been implicated as a means of spread.
  2. Vertical transmission of enteroviruses from mother to infant in the peripartum period has been documented.
- Children are considered the main susceptible cohort.
  1. Spread in the community is most likely to be from child to child, and then within family groups.
- Enteroviral infections in the neonate are generally more severe than in older persons.

HISTORY

- Onset is usually abrupt, with fever preceded only occasionally by a short (few-hour) prodrome of listlessness and anorexia.
- Temperature varies widely from normal to 41° C, with the higher temperatures occurring in younger children.
- Drooling, sore throat, coryza, head and/or backache, myalgia, vomiting, and/or diarrhea are common.
- In most instances, the classic oropharyngeal lesions are present from the onset of fever or shortly thereafter.
- Although occasionally associated with other forms of more severe enteroviral infection, such as aseptic meningitis, most instances of herpangina are mild, without complication.

PHYSICAL EXAMINATION

- Patients are generally only mildly ill appearing.
- Characteristic lesions begin as moderately painful, punctate macules but rapidly progress through papular, vesicular, and then ulcerative stages. They are most commonly seen as discrete ulcers on an erythematous base.
- Ulcerative lesions are initially small (1 to 2 mm) but may enlarge to 3 to 4 mm over a few days. The erythematous base varies in diameter up to 10 mm.
- Lesions average 5 in number but range from 2 to 14 and are most commonly located on the anterior tonsillar pillars. They may also be found on the uvula, soft palate, tonsils, pharyngeal wall, posterior buccal mucosa, and rarely, the dorsum or tip of the tongue.
- Beyond the discrete lesions, the rest of the pharynx varies from normal to erythematous.

DIAGNOSIS

DIFFERENTIAL DIAGNOSIS

- *Herpetic gingivostomatitis:* Lesions are typically larger and predominantly more anteriorly located. Involvement of the gingivae and lymphadenopathy, which are common in herpetic gingivostomatitis (HGS), are not seen in herpangina. Patients with HGS are generally more ill appearing and have higher fevers.
- *Hand, foot, and mouth disease:* Oral lesions are typically more anterior, with cutaneous lesions on the hands, feet, and often also the buttocks.
- *Aphthous stomatitis:* Oral lesions are often larger and more anterior. They are not typically accompanied by fever or systemic symptoms.

DIAGNOSTIC WORKUP

- The diagnostic workup is usually clinical.
- Confirmation, when necessary, can be obtained via a direct culture of oral lesions or throat.

THERAPY

NONPHARMACOLOGIC

- Treatment is usually supportive, including hydration. Cold, nonacidic fluids, popsicles, and/or slush may provide symptomatic relief as well.
- Observation for manifestations of more severe enteroviral illness is necessary.

FOLLOW-UP & DISPOSITION

As required to ensure adequate hydration or to reassess in the event of complication

PATIENT/FAMILY EDUCATION

- The illness is self-limited, lasting 3 to 7 days.
- Control measures include handwashing and personal hygiene, especially after diaper changes.

- Children may return to day care/school when mouth lesions are unaccompanied by drooling and illness has resolved enough to allow comfortable return to activities.

❂ PEARLS & CONSIDERATIONS

■ CLINICAL PEARLS

Acute lymphonodular pharyngitis is a variant of the syndrome associated with Coxsackie A10 infection.
- The lesions, which are found in the same distribution as herpangina, are small, firm, white nodules packed with lymphocytes.
- Unlike the lesions of herpangina, which progress to vesicles before ultimate ulceration, lymphonodular lesions simply recede.
- There is little difference in clinical course, however, and thus no reason for separating the two entities.

REFERENCES

1. Cherry JD: Enteroviruses: coxsackieviruses, echoviruses, and polioviruses. In Feigin RD, Cherry JD (eds): *Textbook of pediatric infectious diseases,* ed 4, Philadelphia, 1998, WB Saunders.
2. Cherry JD: Herpangina. In Feigin RD, Cherry JD (eds): *Textbook of pediatric infectious diseases,* ed 4, Philadelphia, 1998, WB Saunders.
3. Modlin JF: Coxsackieviruses, echoviruses, and newer enteroviruses. In Mandel GL et al (eds): *Principles and practice of infectious diseases,* New York, 1995, Churchill Livingstone.
4. Rotbart HA: Enterovirus infections, *Rep Pediatr Infect Dis* 4:57, 1994.
5. Zaoutis T, Klein JD: Enterovirus infections, *Pediatr Rev* 19:183, 1998.

Author: **C. Elizabeth Trefts, M.D.**

BASIC INFORMATION

■ DEFINITION
Herpes simplex type 1 (HSV1) and herpes simplex type 2 (HSV2) cause a range of cutaneous, mucocutaneous, central nervous system (CNS), and disseminated infections. Primary infections are defined as initial HSV2 infections in individuals who have not previously been infected with HSV1 and vice versa. Once infected, herpes viral infections can reactivate from latent infection in regional sensory nerves.

■ SYNONYMS
Herpetic infections are generally described by their location.
* Oral herpes
  1. Recurrent oral herpes lesions are commonly called *cold sores* or *fever blisters.*
* Genital herpes
* Herpetic gingivostomatitis
* Herpetic pharyngitis
* Herpetic whitlow
* Herpetic conjunctivitis
* Herpetic keratoconjunctivitis
* Herpes meningoencephalitis

ICD-9CM CODES
054.9   Herpes
054.10 Genital herpes
054.2   Herpetic gingivostomatitis
054.79 Herpetic pharyngitis
054.6   Herpetic whitlow
054.43 Herpetic conjunctivitis
054.43 Herpetic keratoconjunctivitis
054.3   Herpes meningoencephalitis

■ ETIOLOGY
* HSV1 and HSV2 enter the host by direct skin or mucous membrane contact with the virus.
* HSV1 usually causes infections above the waist.
* HSV2 usually causes infections below the waist.
* In individuals beyond the newborn age, HSV typically causes an asymptomatic or localized initial infection at the site of inoculation and then enters regional sensory nerves, where it establishes latent infection.
* When HSV subsequently reactivates, it may cause asymptomatic shedding or recurrent lesions.

■ EPIDEMIOLOGY & DEMOGRAPHICS
* HSV1 and HSV2 infections are extremely common; the seroprevalence depends on the population studied.
* In many parts of the world, most individuals acquire HSV1 infection during childhood.
* Recently, in the United States, HSV1 infection has become less common in childhood.

* The prevalence of HSV2 infection has increased in the United States.
  1. Twenty percent of the adult population in this country is infected with HSV2.

■ HISTORY
* In most cases of HSV infections, there are no symptoms and the individual is unaware of the infection.
* Individuals with primary mucocutaneous or cutaneous herpes infections may complain of a painful rash at the site and manifest other constitutional symptoms, such as fever and malaise (see also "Herpetic Gingivostomatitis").
  1. Children with herpetic gingivostomatitis have painful oral ulcers.
     a. Fever and malaise
     b. Decreased oral intake
     c. Drooling
* Those with symptomatic recurrent infections may recognize a prodrome of pain or dysthesias in the area.
* Infants with perinatal herpes infections may have a history of delivery after prolonged rupture of membranes.
  1. Rarely is there a history of maternal genital herpes or oral herpes contact.
  2. These infants may develop meningoencephalitis, disseminated disease, or disease localized to the skin, eye, and mouth.
  3. These infants may have symptoms attributable to pneumonitis or sepsis syndrome.
* Beyond the newborn period, disseminated HSV infection is rare but may occur in immunocompromised patients.
* Patients with HSV meningoencephalitis may have fever, altered mental status, and/or focal or generalized seizures.

■ PHYSICAL EXAMINATION
* Localized vesicular rash is characteristic of symptomatic infections but often is absent in cases of disseminated or CNS herpes infections.
* Vesicles may rupture, drain, and crust, giving the impression of purulence.
* Mucous membrane lesions may evolve into ulcers.
* Distribution of gingivostomatitis typically includes the lips, anterior oral cavity, gingiva, buccal mucosa, and tongue, and may involve the posterior palate and pharynx.
* Patients with disseminated HSV infections may have tachypnea, respiratory distress, or hemodynamic instability.
* Patients with HSV meningoencephalitis may have nuchal rigidity and/or focal neurologic signs.

⚗ DIAGNOSIS

■ DIFFERENTIAL DIAGNOSIS
* Localized cutaneous or mucocutaneous infections may be confused with impetigo, varicella-zoster virus infections, candidiasis, or noninfectious dermatitis.
* Genital HSV infections may be confused with other sexually transmitted infections, including chancroid and syphilis.
* Gingivostomatitis may be confused with enterovirus infections (herpangina) or aphthous stomatitis.
* Perinatal herpes infection may be confused with bacterial sepsis, cutaneous staphylococcal infection, enterovirus infection, or congenital cytomegalovirus infection.
* Herpetic meningoencephalitis or meningitis may be confused with aseptic meningitis or meningoencephalitis of other causes, bacterial meningitis, or subarachnoid hemorrhage.

■ DIAGNOSTIC WORKUP
* HSV can be identified in skin or mucous membrane lesions by virus isolation in tissue culture or fluorescent antigen detection.
* Except in cases of HSV2 meningitis associated with primary genital infections, HSV is generally not isolated from cerebrospinal fluid (CSF) in tissue culture.
  1. Polymerase chain reaction is a sensitive method to detect HSV in CSF.
  2. HSV meningoencephalitis causes CSF pleocytosis, often predominantly lymphocytes, red blood cells, and elevated CSF protein.
  3. Electroencephalogram typically shows focal spike and wave abnormalities. A characteristic finding of paroxysmal lateralizing epileptiform discharges is described.
* Magnetic resonance imaging (MRI) can also help in the diagnosis of HSV meningoencephalitis.
  1. MRI detects lesions in the limbic system a few days before computed tomography (CT) scan.
* Disseminated infections, including perinatal infections, may be associated with the following:
  1. Pneumonitis apparent on chest radiograph
  2. Hepatitis detected by measuring liver function tests
  3. Disseminated intravascular coagulation detected by clotting studies
* Serology can detect individuals who are at risk for primary disease.
  1. Commercially available tests cannot differentiate between antibodies to HSV1 and HSV2.

II

⊞ THERAPY

- Primary or moderately severe cutaneous or mucocutaneous infections
  1. Oral acyclovir 20 mg/kg/dose every 8 hours or 400 mg three times daily, or
  2. Oral valacyclovir 1000 mg twice a day for 5 days, or
  3. Oral famciclovir 250 mg every 8 hours for 5 days for primary genital infections
     a. 125 mg twice a day for 5 days for recurrent episodes
  4. Topical acyclovir: limited benefit for cutaneous lesions
- Severe infections, including perinatal HSV infection and HSV meningoencephalitis
  1. Intravenous acyclovir 10 to 20 mg/kg/dose every 8 hours
- Resistance to acyclovir: occurs in some immunocompromised patients
  1. These infections may respond to foscarnet.
- Suppression of frequent HSV recurrences: oral acyclovir 5 mg/kg/dose every 8 hours
- Ophthalmologic HSV infections: treated with systemic and topical antivirals, usually in consultation with an ophthalmologist

■ FOLLOW-UP & DISPOSITION

- Patients with uncomplicated cutaneous or mucocutaneous herpes infections do not require additional follow-up.
- Patients who experience frequent recurrences require regular follow-up to assess the need for and the effectiveness of suppressive therapy.
- Patients with severe herpes infections, including perinatal HSV infections, meningoencephalitis, and keratoconjunctivitis, require close monitoring to assess the effectiveness of therapy and to evaluate for the development of complications or side effects from antiviral therapy.
- Patients with CSF or ophthalmologic infection require subsequent evaluation for the residual effects of infection.
- Recurrent episodes during infancy require evaluation and are generally treated with intravenous acyclovir.

■ PATIENT/FAMILY EDUCATION

- Young infants are particularly vulnerable to HSV infection.
  1. Limit contact with people with oral lesions.

2. When contact between an infant and an individual with active HSV lesions is unavoidable, the person should cover the lesion and wash his or her hands carefully before handling the infant.
3. Infants at risk of developing perinatal HSV infection or who have had perinatal infection should be evaluated if rash, fever, or lethargy occurs.
- Patients may feel stigmatized and require reassurance to alleviate feelings of guilt and embarrassment.
  1. HSV is transmitted by physical contact with infected skin or mucous membranes.
  2. Asymptomatic infections and asymptomatic shedding are common, and people may transmit the virus without realizing that they are infected.
- Immunocompromised patients and young infants should not come in contact with children with gingivostomatitis because they transmit HSV in their oral secretions.
- Individuals with genital HSV infections should always use condoms because the virus may be transmitted at times when no symptoms are apparent.

■ PREVENTIVE TREATMENT

- Frequent recurrences as well as virus shedding may be suppressed with antiviral therapy.
- Regular and correct condom use will decrease, but not prevent completely, the transmission of genital herpes.
- Individuals, such as intensive care unit nurses and respiratory therapists, who have occupational exposures to oral or genital secretions should wear gloves to prevent herpetic whitlow.
  1. Gloves should be worn for contact with herpetic lesions.
- Transmission of HSV to infants of mothers with active genital lesions during labor may be decreased by delivering the infant by cesarean section before or as soon as possible after rupture of membranes (4 hours or less).

■ REFERRAL INFORMATION

- Infants and other individuals with severe HSV infection should be referred to a specialist in infectious diseases.

- Patients with ophthalmic HSV infection or facial lesions in the area of the eye should be referred to an ophthalmologist.
- Patients with HSV meningoencephalitis or radiculomyelopathy should be refered to a neurologist.

☼ PEARLS & CONSIDERATIONS

■ CLINICAL PEARLS

- HSV should be considered in the differential diagnosis of infections that fail to respond to antibiotics and are associated with negative bacterial cultures.
- Although HSV lesions often appear somewhat purulent, they rarely become superinfected.
- A young child with suspicious genital lesions requires a thorough evaluation and a high index of suspicion for child sexual abuse.

■ SUPPORT GROUPS

- American Social Health Association Resource Center, P.O. Box 13287, Research Triangle Park, NC 27709, 919-361-8400
- National Herpes Hotline, 919-361-8488
- CDC National STD Hotline, 800-227-8922

REFERENCES

1. Brown ZA et al: The acquisition of herpes simplex during pregnancy: its frequency and impact on pregnancy outcome, *N Engl J Med* 337:509, 1997.
2. Fleming DT et al: Herpes simplex virus type 2 in the United States, 1976 to 1994, *N Engl J Med* 337:1105, 1997.
3. Prober CG et al: The management of pregnancies complicated by genital infections with herpes simplex virus, *Clin Infect Dis* 15:1031, 1992.
4. Whitley R et al: A controlled trial comparing vidarabine with Acyclovir in neonatal herpes simplex virus infection, *N Engl J Med* 324:444, 1991.
5. Whitley R et al: Predictors of morbidity and mortality in neonates with herpes simplex virus infections, *N Engl J Med* 324:450, 1991.

Author: **Paula Annunziato, M.D.**

BASIC INFORMATION

■ DEFINITION
Chickenpox is the primary infection caused by the varicella-zoster virus. Zoster is caused by reactivation of the latent varicella-zoster virus.

■ SYNONYMS
• Chickenpox is varicella.
• Zoster is herpes zoster or shingles.

ICD-9CM CODES
052.9 Chickenpox
053.9 Zoster

■ ETIOLOGY
• Both chickenpox and zoster are caused by the varicella-zoster virus, which is a member of the herpesvirus family.
• Chickenpox results from primary infection.
• Zoster results from reactivation of the latent virus in the sensory ganglia.

■ EPIDEMIOLOGY & DEMOGRAPHICS
• In temperate climates, most individuals develop chickenpox during childhood.
• Fifteen percent of otherwise healthy people subsequently develop zoster.
  1. Zoster is more common in older individuals but can occur in younger patients.
  2. Immunocompromised individuals are more likely than the general population to develop zoster.
• Patients from tropical climates may not develop chickenpox during childhood and may be at risk for primary infection during adulthood.

■ HISTORY
Chickenpox
• Fever
• Malaise
• Pruritic rash starting on the head and face and spreading to other parts of the body
• Exposure to varicella-zoster virus 10 days to 3 weeks before the onset of illness
Zoster
• Painful, localized rash that reflects the distribution of one to three dermatomes
• Generally does not cross the midline

■ PHYSICAL EXAMINATION
Chickenpox
• Chickenpox is characterized by a generalized rash consisting of papules, pustules, vesicles, and crusted lesions.
  1. In mild cases, fewer than 50 lesions develop.
  2. In severe cases, more than 500 lesions develop.

• Patients may have fever, cough, or abdominal pain.
• Moderate to severe cough or abdominal pain may indicate disseminated disease with varicella hepatitis or pneumonia.
Zoster
• Zoster is characterized by a papular to vesicular rash limited to one to three dermatomes.
• Involvement of more than three dermatomes indicates disseminated zoster.
• In a variant of zoster, zoster sine herpetica, no rash is evident.

DIAGNOSIS

■ DIFFERENTIAL DIAGNOSIS
• Herpes simplex virus infection
• Impetigo
• Staphylococcal or streptococcal skin infection
• Arthropod bites
• Allergic skin reaction

■ DIAGNOSTIC WORKUP
• The diagnosis is often made on the basis of history and physical examination findings alone.
• Tzanck prep, direct fluorescent antigen detection, or virus isolation from a skin lesion can also be diagnostic.
• Serologic testing can identify whether a person is at risk of developing chickenpox but is not helpful in making the diagnosis of chickenpox or zoster.
• Patients with evidence of complications, such as bacterial skin superinfection, pneumonia, or hepatitis, need appropriate diagnostic testing, such as culture of purulent skin lesions, chest radiograph, and liver function testing.

THERAPY

■ NONPHARMACOLOGIC
Chickenpox
• Keep the child comfortable.
• Administer cool or warm baths with oatmeal (Aveeno).
• Apply calamine lotion for pruritus.
Zoster
• Apply cool compresses to the area of pain.
• Keep the affected area clean.

■ MEDICAL
Chickenpox
• Antipyretics (acetaminophen) are given.
• Oral acyclovir, if used, is given in doses of 20 mg/kg/dose four times daily

(maximum dose, 3200 mg/day) for 5 days.
  1. This therapy decreases the duration of illness by 1 to 2 days in uncomplicated cases if instituted in the first 24 hours of rash.
  2. Antiviral therapy may lessen the incidence of complications in adolescents, adults, and pregnant women and is recommended for these groups.
• Immunocompromised individuals who develop chickenpox are generally treated with intravenous acyclovir at dosages of 1500 mg/m^2/day divided every 8 hours.
• Severe cases of chickenpox, including those complicated by pneumonia or sepsis syndrome, require therapy with intravenous acyclovir.
Zoster
• Antiviral therapy is usually not recommended for otherwise healthy children with zoster.
• Immunocompromised children who develop zoster are usually treated with intravenous acyclovir (see previous section).
• Adults with zoster may be treated with oral acyclovir 800 mg five times a day for 7 days, famciclovir 500 mg three times a day for 7 days, or val-acyclovir 1000 mg three times a day for 7 days.
• The addition of systemic steroids to the treatment of zoster may have some benefit on zoster-associated pain and subsequent postherpetic neuralgia, but this therapy is controversial.

■ FOLLOW-UP & DISPOSITION
Chickenpox
• Uncomplicated cases in children generally resolve in 5 to 7 days and do not require additional follow-up.
• Adolescents and adults are at greater risk of complications and may warrant closer follow-up.
• Cases in immunocompromised patients require close follow-up and should be referred to an infectious diseases specialist.
• Potential complications include bacterial superinfection, including cellulitis, necrotizing fasciitis, and toxic shock syndrome; pneumonia; varicella pneumonitis; hepatitis; post-varicella ataxia; and skin scarring.
• Complications such as cellulitis require systemic antimicrobial treatment and close follow-up because of the high incidence of group A streptococcal superinfection.
  1. May lead to toxic shock syndrome
  2. May lead to sepsis syndrome
  3. May lead to necrotizing fasciitis
• Patients who develop sepsis syndrome, cellulitis, pneumonia, hepatitis, or encephalitis should be hospitalized for therapy and observation.

- Referral to a neurologist may be warranted for cases of postvaricella ataxia.

Zoster
- Uncomplicated cases in those younger than 50 years of age resolve in 2 to 3 weeks and do not require additional follow-up.
- Patients with zoster involving the third branch of the facial nerve may develop keratoconjunctivitis and require urgent referral to an ophthalmologist.
- Immunocompromised patients with zoster should be followed closely in consultation with an infectious diseases specialist.
- Potential complications include bacterial superinfections, skin scarring, and disseminated zoster, which may lead to pneumonitis, hepatitis, or encephalitis. Facial zoster may cause infections of the eye or facial nerve palsy. Long-term sequelae in older individuals include postherpetic neuralgia and muscle weakness.
- Patients who experience pain more than 1 month after zoster have postherpetic neuralgia, a chronic pain syndrome that may be refractory to conventional pain management.
  1. This complication occurs more often in those older than 50 years of age at the time of zoster infection.
  2. Patients with postherpetic neuralgia may benefit from referral to a neurologist or a pain management specialist.
  3. Other sequelae that warrant referral to a neurologist include muscle weakness and atrophy.

■ PATIENT/FAMILY EDUCATION
Chickenpox
- Acetaminophen is given for fever.
- Antiitch creams and lotions, such as calamine lotion, and Aveeno oatmeal baths may be helpful.
- Avoid aspirin because of the association with Reye's syndrome.
- Avoid nonsteroidal antiinflammatory drugs (e.g., ibuprofen) because of a possible association with invasive group A streptococcal superinfection.
- Chickenpox is highly contagious; more than 90% of susceptible individuals develop the infection after household exposure.

- Patients should seek advice if they develop high fever, painful redness around one or more skin lesions, lethargy, moderate to severe cough, or moderate or severe abdominal pain.

Zoster
- Treatment with lotions or creams containing capsaicin may help alleviate zoster-associated pain.
- Varicella-susceptible people who are in contact with patients with zoster may develop chickenpox.
- Patients should seek advice if the rash extends beyond the area of three dermatomes or involves the skin around the eye or if the patient develops high fever, moderate to severe cough, moderate to severe abdominal pain, or weakness.

■ PREVENTIVE TREATMENT
- The live attenuated varicella vaccine is recommended for immunocompetent individuals older than 1 year of age who have not had chickenpox previously.
  1. One dose is administered to those younger than 12 years of age.
  2. Two doses are administered to those older than 12 years of age.
- Varicella-zoster immune globulin prevents or ameliorates the symptoms of chickenpox if administered within 72 hours of exposure and is recommended for susceptible patients who are at risk for severe infection.
  1. Newborns whose mothers developed chickenpox in the period between 5 days before delivery and 2 days after delivery
  2. Premature infants less than 28 weeks' gestation or birth weight less than 1000 g
  3. Immunocompromised patients
- There are currently no means of preventing zoster.

■ REFERRAL INFORMATION
Referral to specialists in infectious diseases, ophthalmology, neurology, pain management, or physical rehabilitation may be appropriate, as mentioned previously.

☼ PEARLS & CONSIDERATIONS

■ CLINICAL PEARLS
- Children who develop chickenpox during the first year of life are more likely to develop zoster at a young age.
- Zoster in an infant or young child who has no known history of chickenpox may result from congenital infection, and the mother should be asked if she had chickenpox during pregnancy.
- Women who develop chickenpox during pregnancy are at high risk for complications such as pneumonia and death, and they should be treated with appropriate antiviral therapy.
- The risk of mother-to-infant transmission during pregnancy is estimated to be less than 2%, and the congenitally infected infant may manifest a spectrum of signs or symptoms ranging from asymptomatic infection to the full congenital varicella syndrome.
- Current data concerning the use of acyclovir during pregnancy can be obtained by calling the Acyclovir in Pregnancy Registry at 800-722-9292, extension 39437.

■ WEBSITES
- Centers for Disease Control and Prevention: www.cdc.gov/ncidod/srp/varicella.htm
- VZV Research Foundation: www.vzvfoundation.org

REFERENCES
1. Gershon AA: Varicella zoster virus. In Feigin RD, Cherry JD (eds): *Textbook of pediatric infectious diseases,* ed 4, Philadelphia, 1998, WB Saunders.
2. McCrary ML, Severson J, Tyring SK: Varicella zoster virus, *J Am Acad Dermatol* 41:1, 1999.
3. Wharton M: The epidemiology of varicella-zoster virus infections, *Infect Dis Clin North Am* 10:571, 1996.
4. White CJ: Clinical trials of varicella vaccine in healthy children, *Infect Dis Clin North Am* 10:595, 1996.
5. Whitley RJ, Gnann JW: Acyclovir: a decade later, *N Engl J Med* 327:782, 1992.
Author: **Paula Annunziato, M.D.**

BASIC INFORMATION

DEFINITION
Hirschsprung's disease is a genetic disorder characterized by congenital absence of ganglion cells in the colon extending proximally to a variable distance from the internal anal sphincter (rectum).

SYNONYMS
- Colonic aganglionosis
- Congenital megacolon

ICD-9CM CODE
751.3 Hirschsprung's disease

ETIOLOGY
- Approximately 80% of cases are caused by genetic mutations that are autosomal dominant with incomplete penetrance.
  1. Of current interest are mutations in the RET proto-oncogene and the endothelin 3 genes.
- Genetic defect or mutation causes failure of neural crest cells to migrate caudad along the vagus and enter the bowel wall, with a resulting absence of ganglion cells for variable distances in the colon starting at the internal anal sphincter in the rectum.
- The ganglion cells in the myenteric plexus of Auerbach and the submucosal plexus of Meissner are part of the enteric nervous system. Their absence interrupts the expression of the parasympathetic nerves, inhibiting relaxation of the affected muscles.
  1. Affected bowel remains contracted.
  2. There is loss of peristalsis.
  3. There is loss of the rectosphincteric reflex. A bolus of stool in the rectum does not result in relaxation of the internal anal sphincter.

EPIDEMIOLOGY & DEMOGRAPHICS
- The incidence is 1 per 5000 live births.
- No racial predilection is seen.
- The male:female ratio is as follows:
  1. Rectosigmoid disease: 4:1
  2. Total colonic aganglionosis: 2:1
- Family history may be positive.
  1. Approximately 6% to 8% of patients have a positive family history.
  2. About 21% in patients with total colonic aganglionosis have a positive family history.
  3. The risk of Hirschsprung's disease in siblings of an affected child is 4% and increases as the length of affected bowel increases.

- Increased prevalence of other disorders is seen.
  1. Multiple endocrine neoplasia types IIa and IIb
  2. Trisomy 21 (4% to 13%)
  3. Waardenburg's syndrome
  4. Smith-Lemli-Opitz syndrome
  5. Ondine's curse
  6. Von Recklinghausen's syndrome
  7. Type D brachydactyly
- Only 4% to 8% of patients with Hirschsprung's disease are premature.
- Age at diagnosis varies, but most are diagnosed in the first month of life.
  1. Younger than 1 month: 41% to 64%
  2. From 1 month to 1 year: 21% to 35%
  3. Older than 1 year: 15% to 26%
- Various lengths of the colon can be involved.
  1. Rectosigmoid (75%)
  2. Variable lengths beyond the rectosigmoid (10% to 15%)
  3. Entire colon (8%)
  4. Short segment and ultrashort segment (less than 5 cm) Hirschsprung's disease also described
  5. Small and large bowel (less than 1%)
- Mortality rate is 2.4% to 6%.
  1. Mortality may be related to other underlying disorders.
  2. Mortality is higher in the presence of enterocolitis.

HISTORY
- Constipation (difficulty passing a bowel movement) since birth
- Presentation in the newborn period
  1. Vomiting (most common clinical feature)
  2. Abdominal distention
  3. Constipation
  4. Failure to pass meconium within 48 hours of birth
  5. General symptoms of bowel obstruction
  6. Evidence of sepsis in the presence of enterocolitis
- Presentation in older infants and children
  1. Constipation (most common clinical feature)
  2. Abdominal distention
  3. Vomiting
  4. History of problems with stooling since birth
  5. Absence of significant encopresis
  6. Poor weight gain

PHYSICAL EXAMINATION
- Rectal examination
  1. Increased rectal tone on digital examination
  2. Explosive bowel movement after digital examination
  3. No stool in rectal vault
- Abdominal distention

- Signs of enterocolitis: fever, explosive stools (with or without gross blood), significant abdominal distention, and in severe cases, hypovolemic shock
- Failure to thrive (older children with underlying chronic enterocolitis)

DIAGNOSIS

DIFFERENTIAL DIAGNOSIS
- Infants
  1. Atresia (anal, colonic, jejunoileal)
  2. Meconium plug syndrome or ileus, small left colon syndrome
  3. Microcolon
  4. Hypothyroidism
  5. Anal stenosis
  6. Congenital pseudoobstruction
  7. Neuronal dysplasia
  8. Incarcerated hernia (inguinal or internal)
  9. Gastrointestinal tract duplications
  10. External obstruction (ovarian, mesenteric cysts)
  11. Sepsis with ileus (in severely ill infants)
- Older children
  1. Functional constipation
  2. Pseudoobstruction, primary or secondary
  3. Anterior displacement of the anus

DIAGNOSTIC WORKUP
- Early diagnosis is important.
- Plain abdominal radiograph (kidney, ureter, and bladder) may suggest the diagnosis of Hirschsprung's disease.
  1. Distended bowel loops with an abrupt cut-off below the pelvic brim
  2. Relatively airless rectum (unless a digital rectal examination has been performed or the infant has received an enema or suppository)
  3. In infants with enterocolitis, grossly distended loops of bowel with bowel wall thickening and, in some cases, evidence of perforation
- Barium enema (unprepped):
  1. The infant or child should not receive a bowel prep before the study because it could modify the findings.
  2. Findings suggestive of Hirschsprung's disease include the following:
     a. Radiographically apparent transition zone between the narrow aganglionic bowel and the dilated unaffected bowel
     b. Rectal diameter narrower than the sigmoid colon
     c. Delayed evacuation of barium at 24 hours (least reliable finding)

3. Barium enema is diagnostic in approximately 80% of patients with Hirschsprung's disease.
4. In total colonic aganglionosis, there is no transition zone.
5. Barium enema is less diagnostic in patients with short or ultrashort segment disease.

- Rectal biopsy:
  1. Rectal biopsy is required for definitive diagnosis.
  2. The specimen can be obtained by suction or punch rectal biopsy.
     a. Suction rectal biopsy is the initial procedure of choice.
     b. This can be done at the bedside without sedation.
  3. Biopsy is performed by both surgeons and pediatric gastroenterologists.
  4. Findings on the biopsy that support the diagnosis include the following:
     a. Absence of ganglion cells
     b. Positive acetylcholinesterase stain
        (1) Staining with acetylcholinesterase allows identification of hypertrophied nerves.
  5. Complications of the suction rectal biopsy are rare and include perforation (less than 1%) and an inadequate specimen (a biopsy with insufficient submucosa or taken too low in the rectum).
  6. It may be difficult to diagnose short or ultrashort segment Hirschsprung's disease.
  7. Occasionally, a full-thickness surgical biopsy is required to make the diagnosis if an adequate specimen cannot be obtained.

- Anorectal manometry:
  1. Anorectal manometry measures the reaction of the internal anal sphincter (aganglionic in all cases of Hirschsprung's disease) to balloon distention in the rectum.
  2. Normally, the sphincter will relax when the balloon is inflated.
  3. In Hirschsprung's disease, the internal anal sphincter does not relax or the tone actually increases.
  4. Positive predictive value is approximately 90%, and there are few false-negative test results.
  5. This is a more reliable screening test than barium enema but requires expertise in anorectal manometry.
  6. This test is particularly reliable for short and ultrashort segment Hirschsprung's disease.

- Selection of diagnostic tests is as follows:
  1. Highly suspicious: rectal biopsy
  2. Suspicious: barium enema before rectal biopsy

3. Suspicious but barium enema is nondiagnostic: manometry or rectal biopsy
4. Suspicious of short or ultrashort segment disease and both barium enema and rectal biopsy are nondiagnostic: manometry

THERAPY

■ MEDICAL
- Medical management is reserved for stabilizing the infant before surgery.
  1. Restore fluid and electrolyte balance.
  2. Perform adequate evacuation of the colon with saline enemas.
  3. Provide broad-spectrum antibiotics if enterocolitis is expected.

■ SURGICAL
- Operative intervention is the definitive treatment.
- Remove affected bowel and place normally innervated bowel at the anus. There are three established surgical procedures:
  1. Duhamel (side-to-side rectal colonic anastomosis)
  2. Soave (endorectal pull-through)
  3. Swenson (coloanal anastomosis)
- Traditionally, a diverting colostomy was created at a level in which the presence of ganglion cells was verified histologically. The definitive procedure was performed at a later time.
- All three procedures can now be performed as a single stage, and even newer techniques include the laparoscopically assisted approach.
- Staged repairs are still recommended in some patients:
  1. Ill patients and those who require emergent fecal diversion
  2. Those with massive gastrointestinal dilation who require defunctionalization to shrink the bowel before the definitive procedure
- A more limited procedure may be used for patients with ultrashort segment Hirschsprung's disease.
  1. Anorectal myectomy: A full-thickness, 2- to 3-cm-long strip is cut through the internal anal sphincter.

■ FOLLOW-UP & DISPOSITION
- Approximately 65% to 85% of patients eventually achieve good results with normal bowel habits, no soiling, and infrequent constipation.
- About 5% to 10% have severe constipation or incontinence.
- Approximately 25% of patients require reoperation for stenosis, prolapse, obstruction, abscess drainage, sphincterotomy, or surgical revision.

- Children with neurologic compromise and those with trisomy 21 tend to have more problems with constipation and/or incontinence.
- Postoperative enterocolitis may occur in up to 25% of patients.
- Enterocolitis is the most significant complication, preoperatively and postoperatively, of Hirschsprung's disease.
  1. Overall incidence varies from 20% to 60%.
  2. Until recently, enterocolitis was the major cause of mortality.
  3. It usually presents with the clinical triad of explosive watery diarrhea, abdominal distention, and fever.
  4. Treatment includes the following:
     a. Immediate intravenous hydration (hypovolemic shock)
     b. Frequent rectal irrigation with warm saline enemas
     c. Intravenous antibiotics, including metronidazole
  5. Postoperatively, mechanical factors (anastomotic stricture or leak, intestinal obstruction) contribute to an increased risk of developing enterocolitis.

■ REFERRAL INFORMATION
- Refer to a gastroenterologist or pediatric surgeon for definitive diagnosis (rectal biopsy) if Hirschsprung's disease is suspected by history and physical examination.
- If the clinical diagnosis is equivocal, a barium enema can be performed before referral.
- If the barium enema supports the diagnosis, the patient should be referred directly to the surgeon.
- An infant or child who develops clinical symptoms of enterocolitis postoperatively should be stabilized if necessary (fluid resuscitation, intravenous antibiotics) and immediately referred to the surgeon.

■ PATIENT/FAMILY EDUCATION
- Genetic counseling: There is an increased incidence of Hirschsprung's disease in subsequent children, which is 4% on average and increases with the length of colon involved.
- Postoperatively, parents should be able to recognize the symptoms and signs of enterocolitis and contact their pediatrician or surgeon immediately.

PEARLS & CONSIDERATIONS

■ CLINICAL PEARLS
- Consider Hirschsprung's disease in any infant or child who does not pass meconium in the first 48 hours of life or who is constipated from birth.

- Consider Hirschsprung's disease in an older child who has a history of longstanding constipation not associated with encopresis and who cannot have a bowel movement without a laxative.
- Consider Hirschsprung's disease with increased tone, empty rectal vault, and explosive evacuation of stool after a digital rectal examination.
- The clinical triad of explosive watery stools, abdominal distention, and fever in a child with Hirschsprung's disease requires immediate intervention with intravenous fluids, antibiotics, and rectal irrigation.

■ RESOURCES FOR PARENTS

American Pseudo-obstruction and Hirschsprung's Disease Society (APHS): phone: 978-685-4477; website: aphs@tiac.net

REFERENCES

1. Fortuna RS et al: Critical analysis of the operative treatment of Hirschsprung's disease, *Arch Dis Surg* 131: 520, 1996.
2. Nowicki MJ, Bishop PR: Organic causes of constipation in infants and children, *Pediatr Ann* 28:293, 1999.
3. Pearl RH et al: The approach to common abdominal diagnoses in infants and children, *Pediatr Clin North Am* 45:1287, 1998.
4. Puri P, Ohshiro K, Wester TL: Hirschsprung's disease: a search for etiology, *Semin Pediatr Surg* 7:140, 1998.

Author: **M. Susan Moyer, M.D.**

II

BASIC INFORMATION

■ **DEFINITION**

The histiocytoses are a group of disorders characterized by infiltration and proliferation of cells of either monocyte-macrophage or dendritic lineage.

■ **CLASSIFICATION & SYNONYMS**
- Class I histiocytoses
  1. Langerhans' cell histiocytosis (LCH), Histiocytosis X
     a. Eosinophilic granuloma (bone lesions alone)
     b. Hand-Schüller-Christian disease (bone lesions, diabetes insipidus, exophthalmos)
     c. Letterer-Siwe disease (disseminated disease)
- Class II histiocytoses
  1. Primary hemophagocytic lympho-histiocytosis (HLH)
     a. Infection-associated hemophagocytic syndrome (IAHS), virus-associated hemophagocytic syndrome (VAHS)
     b. Familial erythrophagocytic lymphohistiocytosis (FEL)
     c. Sporadic hemophagocytic lymphohistiocytosis
  2. Other class II histiocytoses
     a. Sinus histiocytosis with massive lymphadenopathy (SHML), Rosai-Dorfman disease
     b. Histiocytic necrotizing lymphadenitis, Kikuchi's disease
     c. Juvenile xanthogranuloma
     d. Self-healing reticulohistiocytosis
- Class III histiocytoses
  1. Malignant histiocytosis, histiocytic medullary reticulosis
  2. Acute monocytic leukemia (M5 AML)
  3. Histiocytic lymphoma
  4. Histiocytic sarcoma

ICD-9CM CODES
202.3 Malignant histiocytosis
202.5 Histiocytosis X, acute
206.0 Acute monocytic leukemia
277.8 Histiocytosis X, chronic
289.9 Erythrophagocytosis

■ **ETIOLOGY**
- Class I histiocytoses
  1. This is a reactive disorder characterized by a proliferation of Langerhans cells, perhaps secondary to a defect in immunoregulation.
  2. Although generally not considered a neoplasm, recent studies demonstrate that lesional cells are clonal in origin.
- Class II histiocytoses
  1. This is a nonmalignant accumulation of mononuclear phagocytic cells (non-Langerhans cells)

throughout the reticuloendothelial system.
  2. HLH may be secondary to an inappropriate response to various infectious or noninfectious stimuli.
  3. A defect in humoral or cellular immunity is postulated in HLH.
  4. Increased levels of various cytokines and of activated T cells are observed in HLH.
  5. Low natural killer cell activity is described in FEL.
  6. SHML is a nonmalignant, locally invasive disorder of unknown origin.
- Class III histiocytoses
  1. This group includes malignant histiocytic disorders such as acute monocytic leukemia and the rare neoplasms of true histiocytes, malignant histiocytosis, and histiocytic lymphoma.
  2. Each of these disorders arises from the clonal proliferation of malignant cells of monocyte-macrophage lineage.

■ **EPIDEMIOLOGY & DEMOGRAPHICS**
- Class I histiocytoses
  1. Peak age is between 1 and 4 years.
  2. Male:female ratio is 2:1.
- Class II histiocytoses
  1. Most children are diagnosed before 3 months of age.
  2. The familial form of the disorder has an autosomal recessive pattern of inheritance.
  3. SHML occurs primarily during the first two decades, and the male:female ratio is 1:1.
- Class III histiocytoses
  1. Malignant histiocytosis (MH) is reported in all decades of life.
  2. MH is rare and accounts for less than 1% of non-Hodgkin's lymphoma (NHL).

■ **HISTORY**
- Class I histiocytoses
  1. Symptoms reflect the extent of disease.
  2. With solitary bone lesions, there may be mild discomfort at affected sites.
  3. Pulmonary eosinophilic granuloma may present as a mild respiratory illness of sudden onset.
     a. Cough
     b. Fast breathing and shortness of breath
  4. When central nervous system (CNS) involvement is present, signs and symptoms include the following:
     a. Subtle neurologic findings
     b. Seizures
     c. Pituitary dysfunction
        (1) Growth failure
        (2) Increased thirst

        (3) Polyuria
        (4) Polydipsia
  5. With disseminated histiocytosis, recurrent fevers are common.
  6. A rash resembling seborrheic dermatitis or "cradle cap" may be present.
  7. Disseminated LCH is more common in children younger than age 2.
- Class II histiocytoses
  1. Symptoms of HLH are nonspecific.
     a. Irritability
     b. Anorexia
     c. Fever
     d. Diarrhea
     e. Vomiting
     f. Pallor
  2. The diagnosis of FEL requires a family history of HLH.
  3. A wide range of viral, bacterial, fungal, mycobacterial, rickettsial, and parasitic diseases have been associated with hemophagocytic syndromes.
  4. Patients with SHML generally present with systemic symptoms.
     a. Fever
     b. Massive lymphadenopathy, typically cervical
- Class III histiocytoses
  1. Symptoms are nonspecific.
     a. Fever
     b. Weakness
     c. Weight loss
     d. Abdominal pain

■ **PHYSICAL EXAMINATION**
- Class I histiocytoses
  1. Lytic bone lesions may be found anywhere but are especially common in the cranial region.
     a. Physical examination findings may include tenderness at the site of bone lesions.
     b. The most common sites of bone lesions are the skull, pelvis, femur, orbit, ribs, humerus, mandible, tibia, vertebrae, and clavicle.
     c. Exophthalmos, otitis media, and dental anomalies, including early loss of deciduous teeth, may be observed.
  2. A skin rash resembling seborrheic dermatitis may be present. The rash typically consists of crops of scaling, crusted, yellow-brown macules and papules.
  3. Thrombocytopenia arising from splenomegaly or bone marrow infiltration may give rise to mucosal bleeding or may render skin rashes hemorrhagic.
  4. Bone marrow infiltration may lead to signs of anemia.
     a. Pallor
     b. Increased heart rate
     c. Heart murmur

5. Mucosal ulcers involving the mouth, perianal region, or gastrointestinal tract may be present.
6. Signs of multisystem disease include the following:
   a. Fever
   b. Irritability
   c. Wasting and growth failure
   d. Lymphadenopathy
   e. Hepatosplenomegaly
   f. Increased respiratory rate and shortness of breath
   g. Cough
- Class II histiocytoses
  1. In HLH, signs of multisystem disease include the following:
     a. Pallor
     b. Tachycardia
     c. Heart murmur
     d. Petechiae
     e. Tachypnea
     f. Cough
     g. Seizures
     h. Disorientation
     i. Nystagmus
  2. Hepatosplenomegaly and enlarged lymph nodes are common in HLH.
  3. Erythematous or purpuric maculopapular rash, jaundice, and edema may also be present in HLH.
  4. SHML is associated with massive lymph node enlargement and may be locally destructive.
- Class III histiocytoses
  1. Signs of histiocytic malignancies are nonspecific.
     a. Fever
     b. Pallor
     c. Heart murmur
     d. Weight loss
     e. Hepatosplenomegaly
     f. Jaundice
     g. Generalized lymphadenopathy
  2. Skin lesions include the following:
     a. Raised nodules
     b. Subcutaneous infiltrates

🔬 DIAGNOSIS

■ DIFFERENTIAL DIAGNOSIS
- Class I histiocytoses
  1. The diagnosis of LCH is based on pathologic examination of lesions from involved tissues.
  2. A presumptive diagnosis may be based on light microscopy identification of granulomatous lesions and cells consistent with LCH.
  3. Positive stains for two of the following: ATPase, S-100, α-D-mannosidase, or peanut lectin provide additional support for the diagnosis.
  4. Definitive diagnosis requires immunohistochemistry staining for CD1a (OKT6) and/or electron microscopy for Birbeck granules.

5. The differential diagnosis for skin lesions includes the following:
   a. Diaper rash
   b. Scabies
   c. Atopic dermatitis
   d. Seborrhea
6. Both benign and malignant disorders may present as lytic bone lesions.
   a. Bone cysts
   b. Giant cell tumors
   c. Osteosarcoma
   d. Ewing's sarcoma
   e. Metastatic neuroblastoma
   f. Malignant fibrous histiocytoma
   g. Primary lymphoma of the bone
   h. Bone marrow involvement should raise the possibility of leukemia.
- Class II histiocytoses
  1. Diagnostic criteria for HLH include the following:
     a. Fever higher than 38.5° C for 7 days
     b. Splenomegaly (larger than 3 cm)
     c. Cytopenia affecting at least two lineages (hemoglobin lower than 9 g/dl, platelets lower than 100,000/μl, or absolute neutrophil count less than 1000/μl)
     d. Laboratory evidence of either hypertriglyceridemia (more than 2.0 nmol/L) or hypofibrinogenemia (less than 150 mg/dl)
     e. Histopathologic evidence of hemophagocytosis in the bone marrow, spleen, or lymph nodes
  2. Other abnormal findings in HLH may include increased transaminases, hyponatremia, hyperferritinemia, and cerebrospinal fluid (CSF) pleocytosis; however, these findings are not required for diagnosis.
  3. A family history of HLH is required to make the diagnosis of FEL.
  4. SHML and the other class II histiocytoses are generally diagnosed by biopsy.
  5. The differential diagnosis of HLH is that of a generalized multisystem disease:
     a. Sepsis/infection
     b. Lymphoid malignancies
     c. The possibility of an underlying immune deficiency should be considered.
- Class III histiocytoses
  1. MH is diagnosed by histologic examination of involved tissue, usually a lymph node or bone marrow biopsy. Cells are at a stage of differentiation between that of the fixed tissue histiocyte and the monocyte/monoblast.

2. Acute monocytic leukemia (M5) is primarily diagnosed by bone marrow biopsy.
3. True histiocytic lymphoma is a localized neoplasm, in contrast to MH, which is systemic and involves the entire reticuloendothelial system.
4. Pathologically, a histiocytic lineage is suggested by the antigen CD68 and special stains with the enzymes lysozyme and nonspecific esterase.
5. MH and true histiocytic lymphoma are rare.
6. The differential diagnosis of leukemia includes the following:
   a. Juvenile rheumatoid arthritis
   b. Infectious mononucleosis
   c. Immune thrombocytopenia purpura
   d. Aplastic anemia
   e. Leukemoid reactions
   f. Common pediatric malignancies
      (1) Neuroblastoma
      (2) Ewing's sarcoma
      (3) Rhabdomyosarcoma
      (4) Hodgkin's lymphoma
      (5) NHL

■ DIAGNOSTIC WORKUP
- Class I histiocytoses
  1. Complete blood count (CBC), liver function tests, coagulation studies
  2. Chest radiograph to look for pulmonary involvement and skeletal survey to look for bone lesions
  3. Tissue from involved lesion(s) to confirm the diagnosis
  4. Urine osmolality to look for evidence of diabetes insipidus
  5. Additional tests such as bone marrow aspiration, head computed tomography scan, biopsy of involved organs, or endocrinologic evaluations: may be indicated for some patients
- Class II histiocytoses
  1. A detailed family history looking for HLH and parental consanguinity is needed.
  2. Biopsy of bone marrow, lymph node, spleen, liver, or lungs is necessary to establish the diagnosis and to demonstrate the presence of hemophagocytosis.
  3. CBC, triglycerides, and fibrinogen are required.
  4. Increased circulating soluble interleukin-2 receptors, increased ferritin, CSF pleocytosis (mononuclear cells), and increased transaminases may provide supportive evidence for the diagnosis.
  5. A thorough search for associated infections, including, but not limited to, viruses such as Epstein-Barr virus, cytomegalovirus, and

adenovirus, should be made in all patients with a diagnosis suggestive of HLH.

6. In HLH, consider performing additional tests to exclude the possibility of an underlying immune disorder.

- Class III histiocytoses
  1. Imaging studies of the chest and brain define the extent of disease and are important for staging the malignancies.
  2. Bone marrow and lymph node biopsies establish the pathologic diagnosis.
  3. CSF examination for staging and to exclude CNS involvement by malignancy.
  4. CBC and liver function tests may help define the extent of disease but do not establish the diagnosis, which requires a pathologic tissue.

℞ THERAPY

- Class I histiocytoses
  1. The clinical course of LCH depends on the extent of disease (organ involvement) and the age of the child. Children younger than 2 years of age have a higher mortality rate.
  2. The treatment approach to LCH is not universally agreed upon, but given the disease's propensity for spontaneous remission, many experts advise the use of less intensive therapies directed at preventing the progression of lesions while minimizing systemic toxicity.
  3. Patients with localized disease of the skin, bone, or lymph node have an excellent prognosis. Therapeutic options may include observation, intralesional steroids, and curettage.
  4. For patients with multiple organ involvement, organ dysfunction, or progressive lesions after treatment with less intensive therapy, combination chemotherapy and/or systemic steroids may be indicated.

5. Low-dose radiation therapy may be effective but carries the risk of secondary malignancy.
6. The mortality rate is approximately 10%.

- Class II histiocytoses
  1. When indicated, specific antibacterial or antiviral therapy may be of benefit in IAHS or VAHS.
     a. IAHS may resolve in those patients who recover from their acute infection.
  2. For patients with FEL, the clinical course may be one of rapid deterioration with an average life expectancy as short as 6 weeks.
     a. Treatment regimens for FEL may include corticosteroids, chemotherapeutic agents, or cyclosporine, but responses may be of limited duration.
  3. Bone marrow transplant may offer the best hope for long-term survival.

- Class III histiocytoses
  1. Malignant histiocytosis is an aggressive neoplasm, and multiagent chemotherapy is required.
  2. Prolonged disease-free survival with current chemotherapy regimens approaches 50%.
  3. Bone marrow transplantation is a therapeutic option.

■ REFERRAL INFORMATION

Although most histiocytic disorders of childhood are not true malignancies, a pediatric hematology-oncology specialist generally follows children with one of these disorders.

☼ PEARLS & CONSIDERATIONS

■ CLINICAL PEARLS
- The lytic bone lesion is the clinical hallmark of LCH.
- Seborrheic dermatitis is often present on the scalps of infants with LCH; biopsy and appropriate electron microscopy or histopathologic studies are diagnostic.
- The age of onset is the major clinical feature distinguishing HLH from the malignant histiocytosis.

- The chemotherapeutic agent etoposide should be used with caution in patients with LCH or HLH because of concerns of an increased risk of secondary malignancy.
- Acute monocytic leukemia (M5 AML) may have an increased risk of fatal hemorrhage.

■ WEBSITE
The Histiocytosis Association of America: www.histio.org/us/

REFERENCES

1. Henter J-I, Elinder G, Ost A: Diagnostic guidelines for hemophagocytic lymphohistiocytosis, *Semin Oncol* 18: 29, 1991.
2. Imashuku S: Differential diagnosis of hemophagocytic syndrome: underlying disorders and selection of the most effective treatment, *Int J Hematol* 66:135, 1997.
3. Janka G et al: Infection- and malignancy-associated hemophagocytic syndromes: secondary hemophagocytic lymphohistiocytosis, *Hematol Oncol Clin North Am* 12:435, 1998.
4. Ladisch S, Jaffe ES: The histiocytoses. In Pizzo PA, Poplack DG (eds): *Principles and practice of pediatric oncology,* ed 3, Philadelphia, 1997, Lippincott-Raven.
5. Lanzkowsky P: *Manual of pediatric hematology and oncology,* ed 2, New York, 1995, Churchill Livingstone.
6. Malone M: The histiocytoses of childhood, *Histopathology* 19:105, 1991.
7. Stéphan JL: Histiocytoses, *Eur J Pediatr* 154:600, 1995.
8. Sullivan JL, Woda BA: Lymphohistiocytic disorders. In Nathan DG, Orkin SH (eds): *Nathan and Oski's hematology of infancy and childhood,* ed 5, Philadelphia, 1998, WB Saunders.
9. Writing Group of the Histiocyte Society: Histiocytosis syndromes in children, *Lancet* 1:208, 1987.

Author: **Charles B. Foster, M.D.**

BASIC INFORMATION

■ DEFINITION
Histoplasmosis is an endemic mycosis with multiple clinical patterns caused by the fungus *Histoplasma capsulatum* variety *capsulatum*.

■ SYNONYMS
- Ohio valley disease
- Cave disease
- Darling's disease
- Reticuloendotheliosis
- Reticuloendothelial cytomycosis

ICD-9CM CODES
115.00 American histoplasmosis
115.05 With pneumonia

■ ETIOLOGY
- *H. capsulatum* is a thermally dimorphic fungus.
- In cultures at temperatures below 35° C and on natural substrates (soil), it grows as a white to brownish fungus.
- The yeast form is found within cells of the reticuloendothelial system and in culture when grown at 37° C.

■ EPIDEMIOLOGY & DEMOGRAPHICS
- Histoplasmosis is worldwide in distribution, but in the United States, the endemic areas are the Ohio-Mississippi-Missouri, the St. Lawrence, and the Rio Grande River valleys.
- Up to 80% of adults in endemic areas are skin test positive.
- The primary reservoir is soil contaminated with bird or bat droppings.
- No human-to-human or animal-to-human transmission has been documented.

■ CLASSIFICATION
- Asymptomatic disease (normal host, mild exposure)
- Pulmonary disease
  1. Acute (normal host with heavy exposure) mild, moderate, severe forms
  2. Mediastinal adenopathy with or without obstructive (esophagus, tracheobronchial) symptoms
  3. Mediastinal fibrosis—rare
     a. Most cases occur in persons between the ages of 20 and 40 years.
     b. Uncommon in children
  4. Chronic disease with cavitation
     a. Occurs in patients with underlying structural lung disease, such as emphysema
     b. Uncommon in children
- Pericarditis, usually an immunologic reaction rather than fungal invasion
- Primary cutaneous infection
- Disseminated, progressive infection

(infants, acquired immunodeficiency syndrome, immunocompromised)
1. Acute (infants or immunocompromised individuals), subacute (only one third in pediatric age group), and chronic (adults)
2. Central nervous system involvement (usually meningitis) in 10% to 30% of patients
- Presumed ocular histoplasmosis; not clear if *H. capsulatum* truly is a cause of choroiditis in patients without disseminated disease

■ HISTORY
- Exposure to chicken houses, bird roosts, attics, caves, old buildings, or travel to endemic areas may be reported.
- Most patients (more than 95% of normal hosts with mild exposure) are asymptomatic.
- Fever, chills, headache, myalgia, anorexia, cough, and chest pain characterize acute pulmonary histoplasmosis, a flulike illness.
- With acute disseminated disease, patients are severely ill with fever and often have gastrointestinal symptoms.
  1. Cough may develop.

■ PHYSICAL EXAMINATION
- Fever
- Tachypnea, dyspnea with moderate to severe disease
- Signs of airway obstruction—stridor, supraclavicular retractions, wheezing, poor air exchange
- Hepatosplenomegaly and erythema nodosum possible
- Pericardial rub
- Clubbing

DIAGNOSIS

■ DIFFERENTIAL DIAGNOSIS
- Endemic mycoses (blastomycosis, coccidiodomycosis)
- Influenza
- Tuberculosis
- Sarcoidosis
- Q fever
- Leukemia (in differential for acute, disseminated infection)
- Addison's disease

■ DIAGNOSTIC WORKUP
- Chest radiograph
  1. About 75% of patients with mild acute pulmonary disease have a normal radiograph.
  2. Twenty-five percent with mild disease show small infiltrates.
  3. Heavy pulmonary inoculation may lead to a diffuse reticulo-nodular pattern or a miliary pattern.

- Culture
  1. Culture is positive in 85% (blood, bone marrow, urine, or respiratory cultures) of patients with disseminated infection.
  2. With diffuse interstitial or miliary pulmonary infiltrates, cultures of sputum, alveolar lavage specimens, or lung tissue are positive in up to 70% of cases.
  3. Approximately 50% of patients with meningitis have positive cerebrospinal fluid cultures.
- Antigen
  1. Detected in the urine of 90% of patients with disseminated infection and 75% with diffuse acute pulmonary disease
- Serology
  1. High levels of antibodies develop within 6 weeks of exposure in most patients and decline to low or undetectable levels over a 2- to 5-year period.
  2. Serology is positive in approximately 90% of patients with symptomatic histoplasmosis.
- Histoplasmin skin test
  1. Skin test reactivity persists for years after recovery from histoplasmosis.
  2. Background positivity rates of 50% to 80% in endemic areas severely limit its diagnostic value.

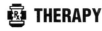

THERAPY

■ NONPHARMACOLOGIC
Supportive therapy is all that is needed for most patients with acute pulmonary histoplasmosis (mildly ill).

■ MEDICAL
- Amphotericin B (0.5 to 1.0 mg/kg/day intravenously) is given for central nervous system (CNS) infections or severe infections.
  1. Total dose of 30 to 35 mg/kg; most patients without CNS disease can be changed to itraconazole after 1 to 2 weeks of amphotericin B
- Itraconazole is given for moderately ill patients or after initial treatment with amphotericin B.
  1. Pediatric dosage is 5 mg/kg once daily.
- Corticosteroids in addition to antifungal therapy may be helpful for patients with obstructive pulmonary disease or adult respiratory distress syndrome.

■ SURGICAL
May be indicated in select patients with obstruction of thoracic structures caused by enlarged mediastinal nodes

II

■ FOLLOW-UP & DISPOSITION

- If antifungal therapy is indicated, treatment should be continued until clinical findings of histoplasmosis have resolved.
- Antigen levels can be used to follow therapy and should be normal before stopping antifungal agents.
- For acute pulmonary disease, 1 to 3 months of therapy may be sufficient, but longer courses of 6 to 12 months may be needed with granulomatous mediastinitis.
- For disseminated disease, antifungal therapy should probably be given for 12 months.

■ PATIENT/FAMILY EDUCATION

Most patients with acute pulmonary disease improve in a few weeks, but some are fatigued for several months.

■ PREVENTIVE TREATMENT

- Immunocompromised patients should avoid activities known to be associated with increased risk of exposure, such as cleaning chicken coops, disturbing soil beneath bird-roosting sites, and exploring caves.
- Patients infected with human immunodeficiency virus who complete initial therapy should receive lifelong suppressive therapy with itraconazole to prevent disseminated disease or recurrence.

■ REFERRAL INFORMATION

Infectious disease consultation should be obtained for patients with moderate to severe disease or immunocompromised patients.

۞ PEARLS & CONSIDERATIONS

■ CLINICAL PEARLS

- Infants are at risk for acute disseminated disease and may present with a pancytopenia and be confused with acute leukemia.
- The highest yield for culture and fungal stain in disseminated disease is the bone marrow.
- Adrenal function should be measured in patients with disseminated histoplasmosis with hypotension, hyponatremia, or a poor response to therapy because Addison's disease develops in 10% to 20%.

■ WEBSITES

For patients
- Association of State and Territorial Directors of Health Promotion and Public Health Education: www.astdhpphe.org/infect/histo.html
- Centers for Disease Control and Prevention: www.cdc.gov/ncidod/dbmd/diseaseinfo/histoplasmosis_g.htm

For physicians
- Centers for Disease Control and Prevention: www.cdc.gov/ncidod/dbmd/diseaseinfo/histoplasmosis_t.htm
- Indiana University–Purdue University Indianapolis: www.iupui.edu/histodgn
- International Association of Physicians in AIDS Care: www.iapac.org/clinmgt/diseases/fungal/histo.html

REFERENCES

1. Bradsher RW: Histoplasmosis and blastomycosis, *Clin Infect Dis* 22(suppl 2): S102, 1996.
2. Centers for Disease Control and Prevention: 1997 USPHS/IDSA guidelines for the prevention of opportunistic infections in persons infected with human immunodeficiency virus, *MMWR Morb Mortal Wkly Rep* 46 (RR-12):20, 1997.
3. Wheat J: Histoplasmosis: experience during outbreaks in Indianapolis and review of the literature, *Medicine* 76: 339, 1997.
4. Wiedermann BL: Histoplasmosis. In Feigin RD, Cherry JD (eds): *Textbook of pediatric infectious diseases*, ed 4, Philadelphia, 1998, WB Saunders.

Author: **Robert R. Wittler, M.D.**

BASIC INFORMATION

DEFINITION

A hordeolum is an acute infection of one of the eyelid glands. It is essentially an abscess because pus forms within the lumen of the infected gland. When it affects the meibomian (posterior) glands, it is relatively large and is known as an *internal hordeolum.* The smaller and more superficial *external hordeolum* (sty) is an infection of the anterior glands of Moll or Zeis.

SYNONYM

Sty or stye

ICD-9CM CODES

373.1 Hordeolum
373.11 External hordeolum
373.12 Internal hordeolum

ETIOLOGY

- Approximately 75% to 95% of cases of hordeolum are caused by *Staphylococcus aureus.*
- Occasional cases are caused by *Streptococcus pneumoniae,* other streptococci, gram-negative enteric organisms, or mixed bacterial flora.

EPIDEMIOLOGY & DEMOGRAPHICS

- The incidence and prevalence are unknown.
- No gender predilection exists.
- It may occur at any age, although it is rare in the neonatal period.

HISTORY

- Abrupt onset of pain, erythema, and swelling of the eyelid is reported.
- The intensity of pain is directly proportional to the amount of eyelid swelling.

PHYSICAL EXAMINATION

- A localized, tender mass in the eyelid, typically 5 to 10 mm in diameter, is observed.
- There may be preauricular adenopathy.
- It may be associated with blepharitis.
- An internal hordeolum may point toward the conjunctival side of the lid and may cause conjunctival inflammation.
- An external hordeolum always points to the skin surface of the lid margin and may spontaneously drain.

DIAGNOSIS

DIFFERENTIAL DIAGNOSIS

- Chalazion (chronic lipogranuloma caused by retention of secretions of a meibomian gland)
- Eyelid cellulitis (preseptal cellulitis)
- Eyelid abscess
- Allergy or contact dermatitis with tarsal conjunctival edema
- Herpes simplex infection involving the periocular area
- Dacryocystitis (infection of the lacrimal sac)
- Molluscum contagiosum of the eyelid
- Pyogenic granuloma
- Acute dacryoadenitis (inflammation of the lacrimal gland)
- Chronic diseases
  1. Diseases such as tuberculosis, sarcoid, Hodgkin's disease, lymphatic leukemia, lymphosarcoma, and mononucleosis may produce lacrimal gland swelling with a palpable mass in the upper outer portion of the orbit.
- Kaposi's sarcoma of the ocular adnexa
  1. This may mimic hordeolum and has been reported as the initial presenting sign of acquired immunodeficiency syndrome.
  2. Papillomas of the conjunctiva caused by papillomavirus
  3. Malignancy
  4. The eyelids are subject to the usual tumors of the skin and pilosebaceous structures, including basal cell carcinoma and sebaceous carcinoma (meibomian gland carcinoma).

DIAGNOSTIC WORKUP

- Generally, none is necessary.
- If incision and drainage are performed, specimens should be sent for bacterial culture.

THERAPY

NONPHARMACOLOGIC

Both internal and external hordeolum usually spontaneously resolve or respond to warm compresses applied for 10 to 15 minutes, several times per day.

MEDICAL

- An antibacterial ophthalmic ointment instilled into the conjunctival sac and on the eyelids is indicated only if concomitant conjunctivitis or blepharitis is present.
- A systemic antistaphylococcal antibiotic is usually necessary only if early eyelid cellulitis is suspected, but it could also be considered in a patient with difficult recurrences.

SURGICAL

Incision and drainage are rarely needed.

FOLLOW-UP & DISPOSITION

Follow up in 1 week to be sure that resolution is complete.

PATIENT/FAMILY EDUCATION

Advise patients and parents to not attempt squeezing the lesion.

PREVENTIVE TREATMENT

Good personal hygiene, with frequent face (including eyelids) and handwashing, is helpful.

REFERRAL INFORMATION

Referral to an ophthalmologist is necessary if visual acuity or ocular movement is affected, if the diagnosis is in doubt, or if surgical drainage is necessary.

PEARLS & CONSIDERATIONS

CLINICAL PEARLS

- Seborrheic, allergic, or staphylococcal blepharitis may coexist with a hordeolum.
- Disorders of the lacrimal gland are rare in children; however, acute dacryoadenitis is included in the differential diagnosis and may occur with viral infections, most often mumps.

REFERENCES

1. Feigin RD, Cherry JD: *Textbook of pediatric infectious diseases,* ed 4, Philadelphia, 1998, WB Saunders.
2. Nelson LB: *Harley's pediatric ophthalmology,* ed 4, Philadelphia, 1998, WB Saunders.
Author: **Larry Denk, M.D.**

II

BASIC INFORMATION

■ DEFINITION
Human granulocytic ehrlichiosis (HGE) is an acute, febrile, nonspecific illness occurring through the bite of ixodes ticks, which can result in hospitalization and/or death, particularly in the elderly.

ICD-9CM CODE
288.0 HGE

■ ETIOLOGY
- "Agent of HGE" is a still unnamed *Ehrlichia* species related to *E. phagocytophilia* and *E. equi*.
- Genus *Ehrlichia* consists of small, gram-negative, obligate intracellular organisms within the rickettsial family.
- Organisms form microcolonies of elementary bodies (morulae), which rupture into the circulation to infect other leukocytes.

■ EPIDEMIOLOGY & DEMOGRAPHICS
- This disease is transmitted by a tick vector—*Ixodes scapularis* (dammini), the principal vector in the northeastern and southeastern United States.
- Peak incidence is from May to July but occurs year-round.
- The incubation period is 1 to 3 weeks after a tick bite or exposure.
- Approximately 75% of cases occur in the upper midwestern and northeastern United States.
- Most cases are sporadic.
- Perinatal transmission has been documented.

■ HISTORY
- The patient may report history of tick bite or potential tick exposure.
- Abrupt onset of fever (often higher than 39° C), accompanied by headache, malaise, and myalgia, are reported.
- Nausea, vomiting, and anorexia are common.
- Less common are diarrhea, cough, and abdominal pain.

■ PHYSICAL EXAMINATION
- Fever
- Rash
  1. Occurs in approximately one third of patients.
  2. It is pleomorphic, variable in appearance, and commonly involves the trunk, but spares the hands and feet.
  3. Occurs several days to 1 week after onset and is short-lived (several days).
  4. More common in children.
- Central nervous system—photophobia, lethargy, confusion

■ COMPLICATIONS
- Adult respiratory distress syndrome
- Acute renal failure
- Secondary and opportunistic infection (herpes, disseminated candidiasis, and yeast pneumonitis)
- Disseminated intravascular coagulation
- Seizure
- Encephalopathy
- Coma

DIAGNOSIS

■ DIFFERENTIAL DIAGNOSIS
Extensive and varies according to organ systems most affected
- Other tickborne diseases: Rocky Mountain spotted fever, babesiosis, Lyme disease
- Human monocytic ehrlichiosis
- Viral hepatitis
- Epstein-Barr virus
- Tularemia
- Murine typhus
- Leptospirosis
- Gastroenteritis

■ DIAGNOSTIC WORKUP
- Complete blood count (CBC)
  1. Leukopenia and thrombocytopenia (70% to 80%)
  2. Mild anemia (50%)
- Mildly elevated erythrocyte sedimentation rate and lactic dehydrogenase
- Elevated hepatic transaminases
- Cerebral spinal fluid: lymphocytic or neutrophilic pleocytosis
- Blood smears: examination of peripheral blood smears for morulae insensitive
- Fourfold increase or decrease in antibody titer between acute and convalescent sera, obtained 2 to 4 weeks apart
  1. Antibody titers are obtained via indirect immunofluorescent antibody detection using *E. equi* antigen.
- Polymerase chain reaction: sensitive and facilitates early confirmation of acute illness, but is not yet widely available for clinical purposes

THERAPY

■ NONPHARMACOLOGIC
Supportive care and adequate hydration should be maintained.

■ MEDICAL
- Very little is known to be helpful.
- Doxycycline is the drug of choice.
  1. 4 mg/kg/day in two divided doses (maximum, 100 mg)
  2. Continue for 3 days after defervescence, with a 5- to 7-day minimum duration of therapy.
- Chloramphenicol has been used in children younger than 9 years of age. Risks and benefits must be weighed against those of doxycycline.
- Rifampin has been used in pregnancy.
- Parenteral nutrition may be necessary.
- Pain management should be initiated as needed.

■ FOLLOW-UP & DISPOSITION
- Repeat CBC to make sure values are normalizing.
  1. Leukopenia and thrombocytopenia reach nadir at the end of the first week.
- Obtain convalescent antibody titers approximately 4 weeks after acute illness.

■ PATIENT/FAMILY EDUCATION
- The mean duration of illness is 3 weeks; recovery without sequelae usually occurs.
- Inform parents of strategies for preventing tick bites.

■ PREVENTIVE TREATMENT
- Prevention is directed primarily at minimizing the risk of tick bites.
- Preventive clothing includes long pants tucked into socks, long sleeves, and shoes (not sandals).
- Insect repellents:
  1. N-N-diethyl-m-Tolamide (DEET): 10% or less concentration for children; avoid hands and face.
  2. Permethrin is available as a repellent for shoes and clothes.
     a. Should not be applied to skin
     b. Very effective against ticks
- Perform a postexposure inspection in high-risk areas.

PEARLS & CONSIDERATIONS

■ CLINICAL PEARLS
- Tick removal: Disinfect area, grasp with forceps as close to skin as possible, and pull straight out, then disinfect the skin again.
- Tick should be saved for county health department for appropriate identification.

■ CONSIDERATIONS
Very little is known about this disease in children; most information is based on adult patients who required hospitalization.

■ WEBSITE

For parents, information about tick prevention

• Encyclopedia.com: www. encyclopedia.com/articles/ 06292.html

REFERENCES

1. American Academy of Pediatrics: Human granulocytic/ehrlichiosis. In Pickering LK (ed): *2000 Red Book: report of the Committee on Infectious Diseases,* ed 25, Elk Grove Village, Ill, 2000, American Academy of Pediatrics.

2. Fritz CL, Glaser CA: Ehrlichiosis, *Infect Dis Clin North Am* 12:123, 1998.

3. Horowitz HW et al: Perinatal transmission of the agent of human granulocytic ehrlichiosis, *N Engl J Med* 339: 375, 1998.

4. Jacobs RF, Schutze GE: Ehrlichiosis in children, *J Pediatr* 131:184, 1997.

Author: **Kristen Smith Danielson, M.D.**

II

BASIC INFORMATION

■ DEFINITION

Primary infection with human herpesvirus-6 (HHV-6) causes an acute, self-limited, undifferentiated febrile illness that persists for 3 to 6 days. Although all children acquire infection with HHV-6 in infancy or early childhood, only a few develop roseola during infection with HHV-6. Roseola is a clinical syndrome consisting of an acute, nonspecific febrile illness that persists for 3 to 6 days, followed by the appearance of a characteristic rash on defervescence caused by HHV-6 and human herpesvirus-7 (HHV-7).

■ SYNONYMS
- Exanthem subitum
- Pseudorubella
- Exanthem criticum
- Sixth disease
- Three-day fever
- Rose rash of infants

ICD-9CM CODE
057.8 Other specified viral exanthemata—roseola infantum

■ ETIOLOGY
Most cases of roseola infantum are caused by primary infection with HHV-6. A few cases are caused by infection with HHV-7.

■ EPIDEMIOLOGY & DEMOGRAPHICS
- HHV-6 causes ubiquitous human infection among widely distributed populations throughout the world.
- The peak age of acquisition of primary HHV-6 infection is 6 to 9 months, with 66% of infants having evidence of prior infection by 12 months of age.
- More than 95% of children acquire HHV-6 infection before 24 months of age.
- Primary infection with HHV-6 is recognized year-round in an equal number of males and females.
- Thirty percent of children develop clinically recognized roseola infantum during infancy or early childhood, with only rare cases identified before 3 months or after 4 years of age.

■ HISTORY
- Abrupt onset of high fever for 3 to 6 days is the hallmark of primary infection with HHV-6 (87% of children with temperatures higher than 39° C) and roseola.

- Nonspecific symptoms of illness, including malaise, irritability, nasal congestion, and gastrointestinal complaints, are common.

■ PHYSICAL EXAMINATION
- Children generally appear nontoxic (8% with initial diagnosis of sepsis).
- Inflamed tympanic membranes (62%) and high fever (mean temperature of 39.6° C) are the most consistent physical findings in primary HHV-6 infection.
- Febrile seizures are the most common complication of primary HHV-6 infection (13%).
- Rash occurs in approximately 20% of children with primary HHV-6 infection.
- Inflamed tympanic membranes, mild palpebral erythema, occipital lymphadenopathy, mild injection of the pharynx and tonsils, small ulcerative or erythematous lesions on the uvula and/or soft palate, and a bulging fontanelle are most commonly described in roseola.
- Rash on defervescence is the clinical hallmark of roseola.
- The rash is made up of discrete, 2- to 5-mm erythematous, blanching macules or maculopapules that are most prominent on the neck and trunk but can spread to the extremities and face.

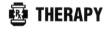

DIAGNOSIS

■ DIFFERENTIAL DIAGNOSIS
The syndrome of roseola infantum is diagnosed clinically based on the appropriate history of fever followed by rash in a generally well-appearing infant. Primary infection with HHV-6 can be accurately diagnosed by isolation of the virus from blood coupled with seroconversion (only available through research laboratories)

■ DIAGNOSTIC WORKUP
Primary HHV-6 infection is not distinguished by any specific general laboratory finding.

THERAPY

■ NONPHARMACOLOGIC
No specific therapy is available for either roseola or primary HHV-6 infection.

■ MEDICAL
Symptomatic treatment of fever is often recommended.

■ FOLLOW-UP & DISPOSITION
- The prognoses for both roseola and primary HHV-6 infection are usually excellent, with full recovery the general rule.
- Long-term sequelae are rare and tend to be caused by central nervous system involvement.

■ PATIENT/FAMILY EDUCATION
- All children acquire infection with HHV-6 in infancy or in early childhood, making it one of the most common childhood illnesses.
- HHV-6 is probably spread from person to person by saliva because the viral DNA is commonly present in the saliva of normal adults and children.
- No means are available to prevent infection with HHV-6.
- Limited information suggests that febrile seizures accompanying primary HHV-6 infection are less likely to recur than febrile seizures resulting from other causes.

■ PREVENTIVE TREATMENT
No means are presently available to prevent infection with HHV-6.

■ REFERRAL INFORMATION
Most children with roseola can be cared for by their pediatrician. Referral to a neurologist for the management of seizures is generally not necessary.

PEARLS & CONSIDERATIONS

■ WEBSITES
- Canadian Pediatric Society general information: www.cps.ca/english/carekids/infections/Roseola.htm
- Canadian Pediatric Society statement: www.cps.ca/english/statements.ID/id90-09.htm

REFERENCES
1. Barone SR, Kaplan MH, Krilov LR: Human herpesvirus-6 infection in children with first febrile seizures, *J Pediatr* 127:95, 1995.
2. Braun DK, Dominguez G, Pellett PE: Human herpesvirus 6, *Clin Micro Rev* 10:521,1997.
3. Caserta MT, Hall CB: Human herpesvirus-6, *Ann Rev Med* 44:377, 1993.

4. Cherry JD: Roseola infantum (exanthem subitum). In Feigin RD, Cherry JD (eds): *The textbook of pediatric infectious diseases,* ed 4, Philadelphia, 1998, WB Saunders.

5. Hall CB, Caserta MT: Human herpesvirus 6 and 7. In Mandell GL, Wilfert CM (eds): *Atlas of infectious diseases,* vol XI, Philadelphia, 1999, WB Saunders.

6. Hall CB et al: Human herpesvirus-6 infection in children, *N Engl J Med* 331:432, 1994.

7. Jee SH et al: Risk of recurrent seizures after a primary human herpesvirus 6-induced febrile seizure, *Pediatr Infect Dis J* 17:43, 1998.

Author: **Mary T. Caserta, M.D.**

BASIC INFORMATION

■ DEFINITION
Hydrocephalus is increased volume of cerebrospinal fluid (CSF) within the cerebral ventricles that typically is associated with increased intracranial pressure (ICP).

■ SYNONYMS
• Water on the brain
• Ventriculomegaly

ICD-9CM CODES
742.3 Congenital
331.3 Acquired communicating
331.4 Acquired obstructive
741.0 Spina bifida with hydrocephalus

■ ETIOLOGY
• Imbalance between the production and absorption of CSF
• Communicating
  1. Obstruction of the subarachnoid space (posthemorrhagic, postinfectious)
  2. Developmental failure of arachnoid villi
  3. Excessive CSF production (choroid plexus tumor)
  4. Associated with Chiari malformation (neural tube defect)
• Obstructive
  1. Aqueductal stenosis
  2. Mass lesions (neoplasm, cyst, hematoma, aneurysm)
  3. Acquired obstruction (hemorrhage, infection)
  4. Obstruction of fourth ventricle (Dandy Walker malformation, arachnoiditis)
  5. May develop with achondroplasia or Hurler's disease (mucopolysaccharidosis)

■ EPIDEMIOLOGY & DEMOGRAPHICS
• Birth prevalence is 10 in 1000 in preterm infants, and 1 in 1000 in term infants.
• X-linked hydrocephalus occurs.
• In general, most congenital cases are multifactorial, with a recurrence risk of 4%.

■ HISTORY
• If congenital, a family history of hydrocephalus or neural tube defect may be found.
• Signs of acute increased intracranial pressure include the following:
  1. Headache, vomiting, lethargy, irritability, high-pitched cry
  2. Change in vision
  3. Seizures
• Signs of chronic increased ICP include the following:
  1. Learning disabilities (difficulties with attention, information processing, memory)

  2. Discrepancy between verbal and performance scales on IQ score
  3. Change in personality or performance in school
  4. Precocious puberty

■ PHYSICAL EXAMINATION
• Progressive enlargement of head circumference
• Strabismus or paralysis of upward gaze (setting sun sign, Perinaud's phenomenon)
• Spasticity of lower extremities
• Bulging fontanelle, spreading of sutures in infancy
• Papilledema

🔬 DIAGNOSIS

■ DIFFERENTIAL DIAGNOSIS
• Large head may be caused by the following:
  1. Subdural hematoma
  2. Degenerative diseases (Tay-Sachs disease, Canavan disease, metachromatic leukodystrophy, Alexander disease)
  3. Skeletal disorders (achondroplasia, Russell-Silver syndrome, mucopolysaccharidosis)
  4. Meningeal infiltration (neuroblastoma, histiocytosis)
• Cerebral atrophy may lead to large ventricles (hydrocephalus ex vacuo) but small head size.
• Hydranencephaly is characterized by complete absence of cerebrum supplied by the anterior and middle cerebral arteries.

■ DIAGNOSTIC WORKUP
• Obtain serial measurements of head circumference.
• Neuroimaging can be done (e.g., ultrasound, computed tomography [CT] scan or magnetic resonance imaging) scan of the head to look for ventricular size and structural abnormalities.
• ICP may be determined through a ventricular tap or lumbar puncture (if not contraindicated).
• Radionuclide studies can be used to determine ventricular and spinal perfusion.
• Neuroimaging plus shunt series are used to evaluate for ventricular shunt dysfunction.

🔲 THERAPY

■ NONPHARMACOLOGIC
• Appropriate referral is needed for educational evaluation, stimulation, and therapies (e.g., Early Intervention Program).

• Braces (e.g., ankle-foot orthosis) can be applied if spasticity is present.
• Repeated lumbar or ventricular punctures (taps) have been used to treat hydrocephalus secondary to intracranial hemorrhage.

■ MEDICAL
• The combination of acetazolamide (Diamox) plus furosemide (Lasix) is effective in *transiently* reducing ICP and has been used to treat hydrocephalus secondary to intracranial hemorrhage or to temporize when surgical shunt placement is not possible.
• Oral medications such as diazepam (Valium), Lioresal (Baclofen), and tizanidine (Zanaflex); injections with botulinum toxin (Botox); intrathecal baclofen; and selective dorsal rhizotomy may help decrease spasticity.

■ SURGICAL
• Ventricular-peritoneal shunts are used for most forms of hydrocephalus.
  1. Some newer valves have adjustable pressures.
  2. If the peritoneal cavity is not available, the distal end may be placed in the pleural space.
  3. Ventricular-atrial shunts are no longer used because of the risk of pulmonary microemboli and shunt-related nephritis.
• Endoscopic third ventriculostomy is extremely useful to treat obstructive hydrocephalus.

■ FOLLOW-UP & DISPOSITION
• Routine clinical monitoring, including monitoring of pubertal development, is advised.
• Routine head CT scans should be obtained to evaluate ventricular size.
• Close communication should be maintained with the school or Early Intervention Program.

■ PATIENT/FAMILY EDUCATION
• Inform the family and child of signs and symptoms of increased ICP (ventricular shunt failure).
• Help families and educators develop realistic expectations for the child.

■ PREVENTIVE TREATMENT
• All women of child-bearing age should receive 0.4 mg of folic acid daily periconceptionally to decrease the occurrence of neural tube defects.
• Prenatal surgery to shunt hydrocephalus has thus far not been successful; however, continuing attempts are being made to improve the procedure.

■ REFERRAL INFORMATION

- All children should be referred to a neurosurgeon for treatment and follow-up.
- All children 0 to 3 years of age who have significant hydrocephalus should be referred to an Early Intervention Program.
- All children older than 3 years of age who have neural tube defects should be referred to their school district's Committee on Special Education or Committee on Preschool Special Education.

☼ PEARLS & CONSIDERATIONS

■ CLINICAL PEARLS

- The signs and symptoms of ventricular shunt malfunction may be subtle. Consider a CT scan of the head plus shunt series.
- Papilledema is a late sign of increased ICP.
  1. If it is present, it is useful.
  2. If it is absent, it is not useful.

- Determining how a ventricular shunt valve empties and fills is not reliable in deciding whether a shunt has failed.
- Tapping a malfunctioning shunt with a 25-gauge butterfly needle may save the life of a child whose shunt is obstructed.
- In a child who has meningomyelocele with hydrocephalus, ventricular shunt failure may cause signs of Chiari malformation or tethered spinal cord.

■ WEBSITES

- Hydrocephalus Association: http://neurosurgery.mgh.harvard.edu/ha/
- Hydrocephalus Center: www.patientcenters.com/hydrocephalus/
- Hydrocephalus Foundation, Inc: www/hydrocephalus.org/

■ SUPPORT GROUP

Hydrocephalus online discussion group, HYCEPH-L: listserv@listserv/utoronto.ca

REFERENCES

1. Boaz JC, Edwards-Brown MK: Hydrocephalus in children: neurosurgical and neuroimaging concerns, *Neuroimaging Clin North Am* 9:73, 1999.
2. Dias MS, Li V: Pediatric neurosurgical disease, *Pediatr Clin North Am* 45:1539, 1998.
3. Drake JM et al: Randomized trial of cerebrospinal fluid shunt valve design in pediatric hydrocephalus, *Neurosurgery* 43:294, 1998.
4. du Plessis AJ: Posthemorrhagic hydrocephalus and brain injury in the preterm infant: dilemmas in diagnosis and management, *Semin Pediatr Neurol* 5:161, 1998.
5. Tuli S, Alshail E, Drake J: Third ventriculostomy versus cerebrospinal fluid shunt as a first procedure in pediatric hydrocephalus, *Pediatr Neurosurg* 30:11, 1999.

Author: **Gregory S. Liptak, M.D.**

II

BASIC INFORMATION

■ **DEFINITION**
Hydronephrosis (HN) is a descriptive term indicating an enlarged renal pelvis, usually found by radiologic study.

■ **SYNONYMS**
• Pelvocaliectasis
• Nephrohydrosis
• Caliectasis

ICD-9CM CODE
591 Hydronephrosis

■ **ETIOLOGY**
• Obstruction
  1. Bilateral HN with hydroureter suspicious for posterior urethral valves
  2. Unilateral HN without hydroureter suspicious for ureteropelvic junction (UPJ) obstruction
  3. Unilateral HN with hydroureter suspicious of ureterovesical junction obstruction (megaureter)
• Vesicoureteral reflux
• High urine output
• Associated with a syndrome such as prune-belly syndrome

■ **EPIDEMIOLOGY & DEMOGRAPHICS**
• The prevalence in the general population is unknown.
• Frequency found on antenatal ultrasound is 1 in 200 to 1 in 700.

■ **HISTORY**
• Eighty percent of infants with antenatal HN are asymptomatic at birth.
• Abdominal pain is present.
• Hematuria occurs after minor trauma.
• Urinary tract infection may be present.
• Failure to thrive may occur.

■ **PHYSICAL EXAMINATION**
• Asymptomatic palpable mass in newborn
• Hypertension

🔬 **DIAGNOSIS**

■ **DIFFERENTIAL DIAGNOSIS**
• Multicystic dysplastic kidney (MCDK)
• Extrarenal pelvis (normal variant)
• Peripelvic cyst

■ **DIAGNOSTIC WORKUP**
• Renal ultrasound to confirm the presence and laterality of HN and to evaluate the renal parenchyma and bladder
• Voiding cystourethrogram (VCUG) to identify vesicoureteral reflux, bladder function, and urethral anatomy
• Diuretic renal scan to assess for obstruction
  1. Nuclear scintigraphy with technetium-labeled DPTA (^{99m}Tc-diethlenetriamenpentaacetic acid) is the study of choice.
  2. Water-loading and/or a diuretic study are needed to diagnose the obstruction.
  3. These studies also provide information on the differential function of kidneys.
  4. A standard intravenous pyelogram is not adequate to detect the obstruction.
  5. MCDK demonstrates no function in an abnormal kidney.
• For infants with a history of antenatal HN:
  1. Renal ultrasound should be performed within the first few days of birth.
  2. If normal, ultrasound should be repeated in 7 to 10 days because of risk of false-negative result.
  3. VCUG can be performed at any time within the first month of life.
  4. Diuretic renal scan should be done after 2 weeks of age because of physiologically low glomerular filtration rate (GFR) in immediate postnatal period.
• For children with confirmed HN:
  1. These children need to have their blood urea nitrogen (BUN), creatinine, and electrolytes measured.
  2. BUN and creatinine provide an estimate of the GFR.
  3. Abnormalities in potassium and bicarbonate may indicate subtle renal dysfunction.
• Urinalysis
  1. A urinalysis should be done on first-morning urine to evaluate concentrating ability (specific gravity 1.020 or higher) and to assess for the presence of proteinuria, which would be suspicious for parenchymal scarring.

💊 **THERAPY**

Therapy depends on the cause.

■ **MEDICAL**
Newborns with a history of antenatal HN should receive antibiotics to suppress urinary tract infection until the cause of HN is determined.
  2. Amoxicillin 10 to 15 mg/kg/day
  3. Cefazolin 20 to 30 mg/kg/day

■ **SURGICAL**
• Surgical correction depends on the cause of HN.
• Bilateral HN with hydroureter implies bladder outlet obstruction and requires urgent surgical relief of obstruction. Bladder catheterization may provide temporary drainage.
• Surgical repair of unilateral HN caused by a UPJ obstruction may be deferred if no impairment of renal function is observed.

■ **FOLLOW-UP & DISPOSITION**
• The immediate postoperative course of children with obstruction may be complicated by polyuria caused by postobstruction diuresis.
• Most obstructed kidneys have some return of function.
• Maximal return of function occurs within the first 12 to 24 months.
• Long-term follow-up of renal function is required in all children with obstruction because of the risk of delayed renal deterioration.
• Children with HN secondary to vesicoureteral reflux require yearly VCUG and antibiotic prophylaxis until resolution of reflux.

■ **PATIENT/FAMILY EDUCATION**
Although up to 1% of newborns have a prenatal diagnosis of HN, only 20% to 70% of those with this antenatal diagnosis of HN are found to have significant urinary pathology.

■ **REFERRAL INFORMATION**
All children with HN should be referred to a pediatric nephrologist or urologist for evaluation.

☼ **PEARLS & CONSIDERATIONS**

■ **WEBSITES**
For parents and physicians, information on neonatal HN:
• Digital Urology Journal: Neonatal Hydronephrosis: www.duj.com/hydronephrosis.html
• University of Michigan Health System Section of Urology: www.um-urology.com/clinic/pediatric/hydroneph.html

■ SUPPORT GROUP

Nephkids is an Internet-based support group for parents with children with kidney disease; it is moderated by a pediatric nephrologist and supported by the National Kidney Foundation. Information on enrolling is available at http://cnserver0.nkf.med.ualberta.ca/nephkids.

REFERENCES

1. Blachar A et al: Clinical outcome and follow-up of prenatal hydronephrosis, *Pediatr Nephrol* 8:30, 1994.
2. Dudley JA et al: Clinical relevance and implications of antenatal hydronephrosis, *Arch Dis Child* 76:F31, 1997.
3. Elder JS: Antenatal hydronephrosis: fetal and neonatal management, *Pediatr Clin North Am* 44:1299, 1997.
4. Kass EJ, Bloom D: Anomalies of the upper urinary tract. In Edelmann CM Jr (ed): *Pediatric kidney disease,* ed 2, Boston, 1992, Little, Brown.

Author: **Melissa Gregory, M.D.**

BASIC INFORMATION

■ DEFINITION
Hypercholesterolemia is elevation above specified levels of total and/or low-density lipoprotein (LDL) cholesterol. This is important because it is one of several risk factors associated with atherosclerosis and coronary artery disease (CAD). Screening for elevated lipids, although recommended by the American Academy of Pediatrics (AAP) for children in high-risk families, is still controversial.

■ SYNONYM
Hyperlipidemia

■ ICD-9CM CODE
272.0 Hypercholesterolemia

■ ETIOLOGY
- Defects in apolipoproteins or lipoprotein receptors lead to elevations in cholesterol and/or triglycerides (TG).
- Lipoproteins transport lipids in blood. They consist of the following:
  1. Free and esterified cholesterol
  2. TG
  3. Phospholipids
  4. Apo or apolipoproteins
     a. Stabilize lipid complex
     b. Factors for plasma enzymes
     c. Interact with receptors for lipid uptake
     d. Chylomicrons: intestinally synthesized lipoprotein
     e. Liver apoproteins: primarily involved with atherosclerosis
        (1) Very-low-density lipoprotein (VLDL); practically speaking equivalent to TG ÷ 5
        (2) LDL
        (3) High-density lipoprotein (HDL)
- Blood lipid abnormalities increase risk for CAD.
  1. LDL increase, increases risk of CAD.
  2. HDL increase, decreases risk of CAD.
- Lifestyle susceptibility for CAD also includes the following:
  1. Diet high in cholesterol and fat
  2. Sedentary life routines
  3. Tobacco exposure
  4. Obesity

■ EPIDEMIOLOGY & DEMOGRAPHICS
- Approximately 7% of 10- to 15-year-olds have coronary vessel lesions.
- About 14% of 15- to 20-year-olds have coronary vessel lesions.
- About 21% of 20- to 25-year-olds have coronary vessel atherosclerosis.
- White males have higher levels than nonwhite males.
- Females, especially in adolescence and young adulthood, have elevated levels.

■ HISTORY
- Patients may have the following:
  1. Family history of premature heart disease
  2. Low level of physical activity
  3. Obesity
- Determine personality type.
- Obtain diet details: milk and dairy, types of meat and fats.
- Most patients with atherosclerosis are asymptomatic.
- Look for symptoms of diseases that secondarily cause hyperlipidemia.
  1. Hypothyroid, diabetes mellitus, Cushing's syndrome
  2. Renal disease
  3. Drug use and abuse (glucocorticosteroids, oral contraceptives, seizure medications, Retin-A, anabolic steroids, alcohol)

■ PHYSICAL EXAMINATION
- Growth (weight)
- Blood pressure
- Evidence of lipid deposition
  1. Xanthomas: yellow, orange, non-painful, palpable, lesions commonly found on the elbow, knees, or Achilles tendon
  2. Corneal arcus
- Goiter
- Hepatomegaly
- Signs of nephrosis (hypertension, edema)

⚬ DIAGNOSIS

■ DIFFERENTIAL DIAGNOSIS
- Familial hypercholesterolemia
  1. Autosomal dominant (AD) inheritance pattern
  2. Homozygotes 1 per 1,000,000 births
  3. LDL receptor defect or absence
  4. Type II electrophoretic pattern
  5. Severe coronary atherosclerosis beginning at 10 years of age
  6. Aortic valve disease common; tendon xanthomas seen
  7. Heterozygotes for disease develop atherosclerotic heart disease at age 30
- Familial combined hyperlipidemia
  1. AD, most common familial lipid abnormality
  2. One to two percent in adult population
  3. Approximately 10% of population with premature atherosclerosis
  4. Increased hepatic production of LDL or VLDL or both or decreased clearance of TG-rich particles
  5. Type IIa pattern if cholesterol alone elevated
  6. Type IV pattern if TG alone elevated
  7. Type IIb pattern if TG and cholesterol elevated
- Hyperapo-β-lipoproteinemia
  1. Elevated LDL
  2. Increased risk of CAD
  3. Variant of familial combined hyperlipidemia
- E protein defects
  1. VLDL particles are elevated.
  2. Characteristic type III (or broad β) pattern is seen.
  3. Alone, patients with this abnormality do well, but this condition is often associated with elevated TG or cholesterol, which is associated with early CAD
  4. Also, if associated with other acquired problems, such as obesity, the risk of CAD increases.
- Secondary causes
  1. Medication
     a. Steroids
     b. Anticonvulsants
     c. Oral contraceptives
     d. Isotretinoin
     e. Thiazides
  2. Endocrine
     a. Diabetes mellitus
     b. Hypothyroidism
     c. Hyperaldosteronism/hyperreninemia
  3. Renal
     a. Nephrosis
     b. Renal failure
  4. Liver
     a. Obstructive liver disease
     b. Hepatitis
  5. Storage disease
     a. Gaucher disease
     b. von Gierke's disease
  6. Other
     a. Acute intermittent porphyria
     b. Anorexia
     c. Systemic lupus erythematosus
     d. Obesity
  7. Drugs of abuse
     a. Alcoholism
     b. Anabolic steroid misuse

■ DIAGNOSTIC WORKUP
- Total cholesterol (T cholesterol) = LDL cholesterol + HDL cholesterol; where HDL cholesterol = TG ÷ 5 (for TG less than 400 mg/dl)
  1. Average T cholesterol in children 2 to 18 years of age: approximately 150 mg/dl
  2. Average LDL cholesterol: approximately 100 mg/dl
- Normal cholesterol, however, not known
- Acceptable cholesterol
  1. T cholesterol: less than 170 mg/dl
  2. LDL cholesterol: less than 110 mg/dl
- Borderline (75th to 95th percentile) cholesterol values
  1. T cholesterol: 170 to 199 mg/dl
  2. LDL cholesterol: 110 to 129 mg/dl

- High cholesterol (above the 95th percentile)
  1. T cholesterol: greater than 200 mg/dl
  2. LDL cholesterol: greater than 130 mg/dl
- LDL cholesterol receptor deficiency
  1. T cholesterol: 240 mg/dl and often greater than 300 mg/dl
- Screening
  1. Screening for symptoms of secondary causes of hyperlipidemia should occur for all children with elevated cholesterol levels (e.g., thyroid-stimulating hormone, blood sugar, cortisol, renal function, liver function) (see "Differential Diagnosis")

℞ THERAPY

■ NONPHARMACOLOGIC
- Diet mainstay of therapy
- Must provide adequate calories for growth and development
- Calories maintained by increasing carbohydrate
- Step 1 diet (only for children older than 2 years of age)
  1. 30% of total calories as fat, less than 10% saturated fat
  2. Less than 300 mg/day cholesterol
- Step 2 diet (for children older than 2 years of age)
  1. 30% of calories as fat, but less than 7% saturated fats
  2. Limit of cholesterol to less than 200 mg/day

■ MEDICAL
- Reserved for the following cases:
  1. Children older than 10 years of age, and
  2. Children who failed dietary manipulation for 6 to 12 months
- Drug therapy is indicated if the preceding two parameters are met and:
  1. Greater than 190 mg/dl LDL cholesterol, or
  2. Greater than 160 mg/dl LDL cholesterol and family history of premature heart disease, or
  3. Greater than 160 mg/dl LDL cholesterol and multiple associated risk factors
- The desired effect of medications is lower T cholesterol and LDL cholesterol by 15%.
- Current medications for children include the following:
  1. Bile acid sequestrants (resins)
     a. Usually need to supplement with vitamin D and folic acid
     b. Cholestyramine
        (1) Dosage: 8 to 10 g/day (low dosage)
        (2) First-line medication for children
        (3) Unpalatable

        (4) Side effects: nausea and bloating
     c. Colestipol
        (1) Dosage: 10 g/day
  2. Hydroxymethylglutaryl coenzyme A (HMG-CoA) reductase inhibitors ("statins")
     a. Inhibit rate-limiting step in cholesterol synthesis and secondarily stimulate synthesis and activity of LDL cholesterol, which enhances cholesterol clearance
     b. Long-term studies not available in children
     c. Not approved for use in children
     d. Potential use in those with significantly elevated levels and/or significant risks or premature disease in close family members
  3. Fibric acid derivatives (fibrates)
     a. Reduce TG, increase HDL cholesterol, have variable effect on LDL cholesterol
     b. Little data in children; not currently recommended
  4. Nicotinic acid
     a. Limited use in children
     b. Major tolerability and adverse effects
     c. Side effects: skin flushing, glucose intolerance, elevated liver enzymes
     d. Not currently recommended

■ COMPLEMENTARY & ALTERNATIVE THERAPIES
- Fish oil (omega-3 fatty acid)
  1. There is questionable evidence of generalizable effectiveness.
  2. Short-term use in children with renal disease showed decreased TG level.

■ PATIENT/FAMILY EDUCATION
- It is unusual for atherosclerotic heart disease to be the result of one specific cause.
- Causes include the following:
  1. Age: increases with increasing age
  2. Weight: increases with increasing weight
  3. Sex: higher risk of CAD later in life for males
  4. Family history of premature heart disease
  5. Cigarette smoking
  6. Diabetes mellitus
  7. Low level of exercise
  8. Dietary intake high in fat and total calories

■ FOLLOW-UP & PREVENTIVE TREATMENT
- Direct proof that intervention and treatment decrease the risk of CAD is not available.
- Evidence suggests that early awareness and appropriate care will decrease risks later in life.

☼ PEARLS & CONSIDERATIONS

■ CLINICAL PEARLS
- Never make the diagnosis of hyperlipidemia on the basis of total cholesterol alone.
- Approximately 10% to 15% of children with elevated T cholesterol have normal LDL cholesterol and elevated HDL cholesterol.
- Other risk factors for CAD include the following:
  1. Cigarette smoking: Discourage.
  2. High blood pressure: Identify and treat.
  3. Obesity: Avoid or reduce.
  4. Regular aerobic exercise: Encourage.
  5. Diabetes mellitus: Diagnose and treat.

■ WEBSITE
American Heart Association: www.americanheart.org/Heart_and_stroke_A-Z_Guide/cholscr.html

■ SUPPORT GROUPS
Local diet and weight control groups

REFERENCES

1. American Academy of Pediatrics, Committee on Nutrition: Cholesterol in childhood, *Pediatrics* 101:141, 1998.
2. Canter CF: A pediatrician primer of lipid metabolism and its relationship to coronary heart disease, *Pediatr Ann* 21:217, 1992.
3. Newman TB, Garber AM: Cholesterol screening in children and adolescents, *Pediatrics* 105:637, 2000.
4. Newman TB et al: Problems with the report of expert panel on blood cholesterol levels in children and adolescents, *Arch Pediatr Adolesc Med* 149:241, 1995.
5. Shamir R, Fisher EA: Dietary therapy for children with hypercholesterolemia, *Am Fam Physician* 61:675, 2000.
6. Skinivasan SR, Berensen GS: Serum lipids and lipoproteins in children, *Pediatr Ann* 21:220, 1992.
7. Snetselaar L, Lauer R: Diet and heart disease, *Semin Pediatr Gastroenterol Nutr* 2:6, 1991.
8. Starc TJ, Deckelman RJ: Diet and heart disease, *Semin Pediatr Gastroenterol Nutr* 2:4, 1991.
9. Starc TJ, Deckelman RJ: Evaluation of hypercholesteremia in children, *Pediatr Rev* 17:94, 1996.
10. Tonstad S: Role of lipid-lowering pharmacotherapy in children, *Paediatr Drugs* 2:12, 2000.

Author: **Lynn C. Garfunkel, M.D.**

II

BASIC INFORMATION

■ DEFINITION
Hyperkalemia is present when the serum potassium level is greater than 5.5 mEq/L (nl = 3.5 to 5.5 mEq/L)

ICD-9CM CODE
276.7 Hyperkalemia

■ ETIOLOGY
- Spurious hyperkalemia
  1. Caused by hemolysis during blood sampling
  2. Caused by blood sampling distal to potassium infusion (e.g., blood drawn from a central line's distal port, when total parenteral nutrition solution is infusing into a proximal port)
  3. Thrombocytosis (more than 500,000 platelets/mm^3), leukocytosis (more than 50,000/mm^3): potassium release during the clotting process (serum) but not in plasma (in vivo)
- Acidemia
- Hyperosmolality
- Diabetic ketoacidosis
- Renal failure (acute or chronic)
- Salt-losing congenital adrenal hyperplasia (21-hydroxylase deficiency)
- Adrenal insufficiency
- Hypoaldosteronism
- Rhabdomyolysis
- Crush injuries and burns
- Tumor lysis syndrome
- Intravascular hemolysis
- Transfusion with old (hemolyzed) blood
- Excessive intake (e.g., salt substitutes, potassium-containing antibiotics)
- Drug induced
  1. Succinylcholine (hyperkalemia peaks after 5 minutes)
  2. Potassium-sparing diuretics (e.g., spironolactone, amiloride)
  3. Angiotensin-converting enzyme inhibitors (e.g., captopril, enalapril)
  4. β-Blockers
  5. Heparin
  6. Digoxin toxicity
- Malignant hyperthermia

■ EPIDEMIOLOGY & DEMOGRAPHICS
- Spurious values are the most common and are caused by blood sampling techniques (heelsticks/fingersticks, tourniquets).
- The epidemiology and demographics of true hyperkalemia are associated with the conditions causing it.

■ HISTORY
- Medication and dietary history (especially a combination of spironolactone, captopril/enalapril, other diuretics, and potassium chloride supplement)

- Urine output: evidence of oliguria (renal failure), polyuria (diabetes, renal failure)
- Pink, red, or dark urine (myoglobinuria, hemoglobinuria, glomerulonephritis)
- Fatigue or weakness (adrenal insufficiency, hyperkalemic familial periodic paralysis, renal failure)

■ PHYSICAL EXAMINATION
- Usually, no direct physical examination findings are apparent, except those related to the underlying disease process (e.g., tachypnea may suggest a compensatory respiratory alkalosis induced by an underlying metabolic acidosis).
- Cardiac arrhythmias may be present.
- Muscle weakness or ascending paralysis may occur with high levels and/or with the syndrome of hyperkalemic periodic paralysis.

DIAGNOSIS

- Standard laboratory test of serum potassium
  1. Whole blood potassium is lower than serum potassium.
- Supportive
  1. Electrocardiogram (ECG): Progression of findings often correlates with increasing potassium levels.
     a. Peaked T waves (precordial leads)
     b. Decreased amplitude of R wave
     c. Widened QRS
     d. Prolonged PR interval
     e. Absent P wave
     f. Sine wave (potassium greater than 8.0)
  2. Ventricular arrhythmias may occur at any point, and progression of findings may occur extremely rapidly (minutes).
  3. A normal ECG does not rule out hyperkalemia.
     a. Only 20% of patients with hyperkalemia have a peaked T wave.

THERAPY

- If potassium is higher than 6.0 mEq/L, maintain a continuous cardiac monitor.
- Prepare for management of ventricular arrhythmias.
- If potassium is lower than 6.5 mEq/L:
  1. Discontinue all exogenous potassium.
  2. Administer sodium polystyrene sulfonate (Kayexalate).
     a. 1 to 2 g/kg orally, nasogastrically, or rectally in 20% sorbitol every 6 hours
     b. Monitor for sodium overload

  3. Consider furosemide (0.5 to 1.0 mg/kg intravenously).
  4. Consider albuterol nebulization (2.5 mg in 3.0 ml saline); its β-agonist effect will drive potassium intracellularly.
  5. Monitor potassium levels hourly.
- If potassium is higher than 6.5 mEq/L or lower than 6.5 mEq/L and likely to rise rapidly (renal failure/tissue necrosis):
  1. Discontinue potassium, give Kayexalate, and consider furosemide as previously mentioned.
  2. Administer intravenous 10% calcium gluconate 100 mg/kg (1 ml/kg) up to 20 ml, over 10 minutes monitoring for bradycardia and hypotension.
     a. Will stabilize myocardial cell membranes immediately
     b. May repeat in 1 hour; follow calcium level
  3. If a central line or well-functioning peripheral intravenous line is in place, may use 10% calcium chloride 20 mg/kg (0.2 ml/kg) up to 5 ml (500 mg) instead.
     a. Infiltration causes severe tissue necrosis.
  4. Sodium bicarbonate (NaHCO$_3$) 1 to 2 mEq/kg intravenous bolus over 5 to 15 minutes can be used to shift potassium intracellularly by inducing alkalemia.
     a. This dose may repeat every 1 to 4 hours as necessary.
     b. Follow pH.
  5. Administer a glucose and insulin infusion: 1 g/kg glucose with 0.3 unit insulin/g glucose mixed together and administered over 2 hours.
  6. Monitor potassium levels hourly until potassium is lower than 6.0; if no response, prepare for dialysis to remove potassium from body.

■ FOLLOW-UP & DISPOSITION
- Determine the cause of hyperkalemia.
- Monitor potassium if the cause is not amenable to therapy or continued risks exist.
  1. Usually, if the underlying disease can be treated, hyperkalemia resolves.

■ PATIENT/FAMILY EDUCATION
Educate the patient (and family) about medication side effects when appropriate.

■ REFERRAL INFORMATION
- Hospital admission and possible intensive care unit referral for the following conditions:
  1. Potassium greater than 6.0 mEq/L and risk factors present
  2. Potassium greater than 6.5 mEq/L and not responsive to initial treatments

- Endocrinology/metabolic or nephrology referral may be needed.

☼ PEARLS & CONSIDERATIONS

■ CLINICAL PEARLS
- Whenever hyperkalemia is suspected to be caused by the technique only, either a repeat (STAT) venous specimen should be drawn without a tourniquet or an arterial puncture performed with free-flowing blood. Do not assume a spurious value until a clear reason is determined.

- Administration of potassium supplements to a patient with an intestinal ileus or poor intestinal motility may result in acute hyperkalemia when ileus or dysmotility resolves because of the sudden absorption of the previously administered, unabsorbed, accumulated potassium.

REFERENCES

1. Brem AS: Disorders of potassium homeostasis, *Pediatr Clin North Am* 37: 419, 1990.
2. Cronan KM, Norman ME: Renal and electrolyte emergencies. In Fleisher GR, Ludwig SL (eds): *Textbook of pediatric emergency medicine*, ed 3, Baltimore, 1993, Williams & Wilkins.
3. Kemper MJ, Harps E, Muller-Wiefel DE: Hyperkalemia: therapeutic options in acute and chronic renal failure, *Clin Nephrol* 46:67, 1996.
4. Wood EG, Lynch RE: Fluids and electrolyte balance. In Fuhrman BP, Zimmerman JJ (eds): *Pediatric critical care*, ed 2, St Louis, 1998, Mosby.

Author: **Elise van der Jagt, M.D.**

II

BASIC INFORMATION

■ **DEFINITION**

Hypernatremia is present when the serum sodium concentration is higher than 150 mEq/L; normal is 135 to 145 mEq/L.

■ **SYNONYM**

- None
  1. *Hypertonicity* is not a synonym for, but rather a result of, hypernatremia. Other substances besides sodium may cause hypertonicity, the increased amount of solute in the extracellular space as compared with the intracellular space (e.g., mannitol, glucose).

ICD-9CM CODE
276.0 Hypernatremia

■ **ETIOLOGY**

- Increased sodium intake
  1. Oral route: improperly made-up formula, boiled skim milk, accidental poisoning, rarely breastmilk
  2. Intravenous: intravenous fluids containing excess sodium or sodium bicarbonate
  3. Salt water near-drowning
- Decreased fluid intake
  1. Water
  2. Formula or breastmilk
- Increased water loss compared with sodium loss
  1. Diarrhea: infectious, malabsorptive, sorbitol induced
  2. Diabetes insipidus (DI): central or nephrogenic
  3. Renal tubular dysfunction secondary to obstructive uropathy or renal dysplasia
  4. Diuretics, mannitol, glucose, lithium, cyclophosphamide, cisplatin
  5. Increased respiratory or dermal water (insensible) losses

■ **EPIDEMIOLOGY & DEMOGRAPHICS**

- Hypernatremia is most commonly associated with dehydration secondary to gastroenteritis.
  1. About 10% of infants with dehydration from gastroenteritis have hypernatremia.
- The mortality of acute hypernatremia is 8% to 45%.
  1. Estimates are based on older literature.
  2. Current practices may lead to better results.
- In chronic hypernatremia, 10% mortality is reported.
  1. Morbidity is high among survivors.
- Hypernatremia is often associated with hypocalcemia and hyperglycemia.

- It has been associated with breastfed infants in the first several weeks of life.
  1. Usually first infant
  2. Older women
  3. Middle and upper socioeconomic class
  4. Well educated

■ **HISTORY**

- Diarrhea, nausea, and/or vomiting
- Thirsty unless gastritis
- Type and quantity of fluid intake (high salt content?)
- Breastfed infant in first 2 to 3 weeks of life
- Amount of urine output
  1. If high, consider central or nephrogenic DI, salt poisoning, excess diuresis from diuretics, hyperglycemia, or osmolar agents.
  2. If low, consider dehydration from poor intake or excess diarrheal or skin losses.
- Weight loss/gain
- Neurologic symptoms: irritability, high-pitched cry, seizures, coma
- Medications: furosemide, thiazides, mannitol, sorbitol, sodium bicarbonate, intravenous fluid sodium content

■ **PHYSICAL EXAMINATION**

- Weight (compare with a previous weight if known)
- Temperature: fever caused by infection or dehydration
  1. Fever increases insensible water loss.
  2. For every degree centigrade, fluid requirements increase by 10% to 12%.
- General/neurologic: obtunded, lethargic, irritable, high-pitched cry, seizures
- State of hydration: cardiovascular examination
  1. Fluid deficit: tachycardia, decreased pulses, decreased capillary refill, decreased distal extremity temperature, decreased skin turgor, decreased blood pressure, dry mucous membranes
  2. Fluid overload: edema, puffy eyelids, moist mucous membranes, hypertension
- Skin turgor: relatively well preserved compared with hyponatremic and isonatremic dehydration
  1. Velvety skin
  2. Doughy abdomen
- Anterior fontanelle: sunken, flat, or depressed; may be bulging if sagittal sinus thrombosis or bleed
- Respiratory rate: tachypnea (fever, acidosis, hyperventilation from increased intracranial pressure from intracranial bleeding)

 DIAGNOSIS

■ **DIFFERENTIAL DIAGNOSIS**
See "Etiology."

■ **DIAGNOSTIC WORKUP**

- Serum sodium should be obtained.
- Urine output should be determined.
  1. Low urine output suggests dehydration.
  2. Normal to high urine output suggests DI, renal tubular dysfunction, or salt poisoning.
- The cause of hypernatremia is refined by obtaining additional laboratory testing.
  1. Blood urea nitrogen (BUN), creatinine, chloride, potassium, bicarbonate, glucose
  2. Urine specific gravity, pH, sodium, osmolality, potassium, chloride
     a. High urine sodium (more than 40 mEq/L)
        (1) Sodium and/or volume overload
        (2) Renal tubular dysfunction or renal failure
        (3) Cerebral salt wasting
        (4) Diuretic use (furosemide, thiazides)
     b. Low urine sodium (less than 10 mEq/L) with low urine osmolality (less than 100 mOsm/L) and/or low urine specific gravity (less than 1.003)
        (1) DI
        (2) Inadequate circulating blood volume with secondary aldosterone secretion
        (3) Primary hyperaldosteronism or use of spironolactone
  3. Fractional excretion of sodium:
     $(U_{Na} \div P_{Na}) \times (P_{Cr} \div U_{Cr}) \times 100\%$
     a. Fractional excretion of sodium less than 1% suggests a prerenal cause, such as dehydration, or an absolute deficit sodium.
     b. Fractional excretion of sodium more than 2% suggests renal disease (serum sodium usually low or normal, however).

 THERAPY

■ **NONPHARMACOLOGIC**

- Observe for neurologic deterioration suggestive of cerebral edema and increased intracranial pressure (anterior fontanelle, Glasgow Coma Scale score).
- Provide assistance with breastfeeding, including lactation aids.

■ MEDICAL

- Hypernatremia caused by water loss
  1. If signs of circulatory failure are present, restore intravascular volume rapidly with 20 ml/kg intravenous normal saline.
  2. Then slowly replace water deficit so that serum sodium falls 10 to 12 mEq/24 hr.
  3. Use D_5 ¼ normal saline with potassium chloride (as appropriate) at rates that result in replacement of deficit over the predicted number of days it takes to decrease sodium back to normal while providing maintenance fluids.
     a. This should take at least 48 hours and may be up to 4 to 5 days depending how hypernatremic the child was.
     b. It is critical that fluid be given no faster than over 48 hours because sodium may drop too fast otherwise.
  4. Although D_5 ¼ normal saline with potassium chloride (combination of replacement and maintenance fluid) is hypotonic compared with serum, slow replacement results in a slow decrease in serum sodium with decreased risk of cerebral edema.
  5. If caused by central DI, administer either of the following:
     a. DDAVP (desmopressin acetate) intranasally at 5 to 40 µg every 8 to 24 hours as needed or intravenously at 0.5 to 4 µg/dose every 8 to 24 hours as needed
     b. Aqueous vasopressin 50 mU/kg/hr continuous intravenous drip, increase as necessary to 150 to 300 mU/kg/hr while monitoring urine output, urine specific gravity, and osmolality
     c. Aim for urine output of 1 ml/kg/hr and urine specific gravity of 1.010 or higher.

- Hypernatremia caused by excess intake or decreased excretion
  1. Discontinue all sodium intake and provide hyponatremic fluids for maintenance.
  2. Furosemide helps promote natriuresis and may be considered.
  3. Allow sodium to decrease at a rate of 10 to 12 mEq/24 hr.
  4. In the case of oliguric renal failure, dialysis should be considered.

■ FOLLOW-UP & DISPOSITION

- Monitor serum sodium every 4 hours initially to ensure slow (10 to 12 mEq/24 hr) decrease.
- Monitor neurologic examinations every 2 hours until stable for 24 hours, then at longer intervals.
- Ongoing neurologic and developmental assessments by primary care provider are necessary.

■ PATIENT/FAMILY EDUCATION

- Instruct parents regarding the proper mixing of formulas.
- Provide instruction on the sodium content of various fluids (e.g., Gatorade).
- Explain normal urine output, the signs of dehydration, and the symptoms of DI (e.g., polyuria, polydipsia).
- Ensure that proper administration of intranasal DDAVP is given if central DI is present.

■ PREVENTIVE TREATMENT

- Proper intake of fluids, including formula and breastmilk
- Proper use of medications
- Proper identification of signs of dehydration

■ REFERRAL INFORMATION

May need to consider intensive care unit for the following conditions:
- Sodium higher than 160 mEq/L

- 10% dehydration and/or evidence of circulatory compromise
- Neurologic signs and/or symptoms with need for hourly neurologic monitoring
- Newly diagnosed central DI
- Need for multiple blood draws for laboratory tests; may require arterial line
- Other electrolyte abnormalities, along with significant hypernatremia

☼ PEARLS & CONSIDERATIONS

■ CLINICAL PEARLS

- Meticulous fluid calculations are essential, especially for deficits.
- If serum sodium is dropping too fast when correcting, either decrease the rate of fluid administration (probably overestimated deficit) or increase sodium in the fluids.
- In DI, the degree of hypernatremia does not correlate well with the BUN; often, the BUN is minimally elevated, even though the patient is free water depleted and sodium is high.
- Aqueous vasopressin is easier to regulate than intranasal or intravenous bolus desmopressin.

REFERENCES

1. Conley SB: Hypernatremia, *Pediatr Clin North Am* 37:365, 1990.
2. Cronan KM, Norman ME: Renal and electrolyte emergencies. In Fleisher GR, Ludwig SL (eds): *Textbook of pediatric emergency medicine*, ed 3, Baltimore, 1993, Williams & Wilkins.
3. Wood EG, Lynch RE: Fluids and electrolyte balance. In Fuhrman BP, Zimmerman JJ (eds): *Pediatric critical care*, ed 2, St Louis, 1998, Mosby.
Author: **Elise van der Jagt, M.D.**

II

BASIC INFORMATION

■ DEFINITION

- *Normal blood pressure* is systolic and diastolic blood pressure less than the 90th percentile for age and sex. High-normal refers to blood pressures in the 90th to 95th percentiles.
- *Hypertension* (HTN) is an average systolic or diastolic blood pressure greater than or equal to the 95th percentile for age and sex measured on at least three separate occasions (see Tables 2-10 and 2-11).
- *Secondary hypertension* refers to those cases in which an identifiable cause exists (see "Etiology"), whereas in *essential* (or *primary*) *hypertension*, no underlying disorder is identified.
- Hypertension guidelines are as follows:
  1. Neonates at age 7 days: Significant hypertension is systolic blood pressure above 100 mm Hg; serious hypertension is systolic blood pressure above 110 mm Hg.
  2. Neonates from age 8 to 30 days: Significant hypertension is systolic blood pressure above 110 mm Hg; serious hypertension is systolic blood pressure above 120 mm Hg.
  3. Refer to Tables 2-10 and 2-11 for blood pressure values of children aged 1 to 17 years.

■ SYNONYM

High blood pressure

ICD-9CM CODES

401.9	Unspecified
401	Essential HTN
401.1	Benign
401.0	Malignant
403	Hypertensive renal disease
402	Hypertensive heart disease
405	Secondary HTN
405.01	Renovascular

■ ETIOLOGY

- The likelihood of finding a secondary cause of HTN in childhood is directly related to the degree of the

---

TABLE 2-10 Blood Pressure Levels for the 90th and 95th Percentiles of Blood Pressure for Boys Aged 1 to 17 Years by Percentiles of Height

AGE (yr)	BLOOD PRESSURE PERCENTILE*	SYSTOLIC BLOOD PRESSURE BY PERCENTILE OF HEIGHT, mm Hg†							DIASTOLIC BLOOD PRESSURE BY PERCENTILE OF HEIGHT, mm Hg†						
		5%	10%	25%	50%	75%	90%	95%	5%	10%	25%	50%	75%	90%	95%
1	90th	94	95	97	98	100	102	102	50	51	52	53	54	54	55
	95th	98	99	101	102	104	106	106	55	55	56	57	58	59	59
2	90th	98	99	100	102	104	105	106	55	55	56	57	58	59	59
	95th	101	102	104	106	108	109	110	59	59	60	61	62	63	63
3	90th	100	101	103	105	107	108	109	59	59	60	61	62	63	63
	95th	104	105	107	109	111	112	113	63	63	64	65	66	67	67
4	90th	102	103	105	107	109	110	111	62	62	63	64	65	66	66
	95th	106	107	109	111	113	114	115	66	67	67	68	69	70	71
5	90th	104	105	106	108	110	112	112	65	65	66	67	68	69	69
	95th	108	109	110	112	114	115	116	69	70	70	71	72	73	74
6	90th	105	106	108	110	111	113	114	67	68	69	70	70	71	72
	95th	109	110	112	114	115	117	117	72	72	73	74	75	76	76
7	90th	106	107	109	111	113	114	115	69	70	71	72	72	73	74
	95th	110	111	113	115	116	118	119	74	74	75	76	77	78	78
8	90th	107	108	110	112	114	115	116	71	71	72	73	74	75	75
	95th	111	112	114	116	118	119	120	75	76	76	77	78	79	80
9	90th	109	110	112	113	115	117	117	72	73	73	74	75	76	77
	95th	113	114	116	117	119	121	121	76	77	78	79	80	80	81

From National High Blood Pressure Education Program Working Group on Hypertension Control in Children & Adolescents: Update on Task Force Report on High Blood Pressure, *Pediatrics* 98:649, 1996.
*Blood pressure hypercentile was determined by a single measurement.
†Height percentile was determined by standard growth curves.

blood pressure elevation and inversely related to the age of the child.
- The most common causes of hypertension vary by age group.
  1. Newborn: renal artery thrombosis, renal artery stenosis, renal vein thrombosis, congenital renal abnormalities, and coarctation of the aorta
  2. Infant: coarctation of the aorta, renovascular disease, and renal parenchymal disease
  3. Age 1 to 6 years: renal parenchymal disease, renovascular disease, and coarctation of the aorta
  4. Age 6 to 12 years: renal parenchymal disease, renovascular disease,

essential hypertension, and coarctation of the aorta
  5. Age 12 to 18 years: essential hypertension, iatrogenic, and renal parenchymal disease

■ **EPIDEMIOLOGY & DEMOGRAPHICS**
- By definition, 5% of children have blood pressure high enough to be considered hypertensive.
- Although blood pressure has been shown to be higher in African-American children compared with Caucasian children, the differences have not been believed to be clinically relevant and the current reference standards for children do not

distinguish between racial or ethnic groups.
- There appears to be a familial genetic influence on development because children from families with HTN tend to have higher blood pressure than children from normotensive families.

■ **HISTORY**
- Neonatal history (especially umbilical artery catheterization)
- Medical history: renal disease (glomerulonephritis, polycystic kidneys, Henoch-Schönlein purpura), systemic lupus erythematosus, urinary tract infections, renal trauma, diabetes mellitus, cardiac surgery

TABLE 2-10 **Blood Pressure Levels for the 90th and 95th Percentiles of Blood Pressure for Boys Aged 1 to 17 Years by Percentiles of Height—cont'd**

AGE (yr)	BLOOD PRESSURE PERCENTILE*	SYSTOLIC BLOOD PRESSURE BY PERCENTILE OF HEIGHT, mm Hg†							DIASTOLIC BLOOD PRESSURE BY PERCENTILE OF HEIGHT, mm Hg†						
		5%	10%	25%	50%	75%	90%	95%	5%	10%	25%	50%	75%	90%	95%
10	90th	110	112	113	115	117	118	119	73	74	74	75	76	77	78
	95th	114	115	117	119	121	122	123	77	78	79	80	80	81	82
11	90th	112	113	115	117	119	120	121	74	74	75	76	77	78	78
	95th	116	117	119	121	123	124	125	78	79	79	80	81	82	83
12	90th	115	116	117	119	121	123	123	75	75	76	77	78	78	79
	95th	119	120	121	123	125	126	127	79	79	80	81	82	83	83
13	90th	117	118	120	122	124	125	126	75	76	76	77	78	79	80
	95th	121	122	124	126	128	129	130	79	80	81	82	83	83	84
14	90th	120	121	123	125	126	128	128	76	76	77	78	79	80	80
	95th	124	125	127	128	130	132	132	80	81	81	82	83	84	85
15	90th	123	124	125	127	129	131	131	77	77	78	79	80	81	81
	95th	127	128	129	131	133	134	135	81	82	83	83	84	85	86
16	90th	125	126	128	130	132	133	134	79	79	80	81	82	82	83
	95th	129	130	132	134	136	137	138	83	83	84	85	86	87	87
17	90th	128	129	131	133	134	136	136	81	81	82	83	84	85	85
	95th	132	133	135	136	138	140	140	85	85	86	87	88	89	89

TABLE 2-11 **Blood Pressure Levels for the 90th and 95th Percentiles of Blood Pressure for Girls Aged 1 to 17 Years by Percentiles of Height**

AGE (yr)	BLOOD PRESSURE PERCENTILE*	SYSTOLIC BLOOD PRESSURE BY PERCENTILE OF HEIGHT, mm Hg†							DIASTOLIC BLOOD PRESSURE BY PERCENTILE OF HEIGHT, mm Hg†						
		5%	10%	25%	50%	75%	90%	95%	5%	10%	25%	50%	75%	90%	95%
1	90th	97	98	99	100	102	103	104	53	53	53	54	55	56	56
	95th	101	102	103	104	105	107	107	57	57	57	58	59	60	60
2	90th	99	99	100	102	103	104	105	57	57	58	58	59	60	61
	95th	102	103	104	105	107	108	109	61	61	62	62	63	64	65
3	90th	100	100	102	103	104	105	106	61	61	61	62	63	63	64
	95th	104	104	105	107	108	109	110	65	65	65	66	67	67	68
4	90th	101	102	103	104	106	107	108	63	63	64	65	65	66	67
	95th	105	106	107	108	109	111	111	67	67	68	69	69	70	71
5	90th	103	103	104	106	107	108	109	65	66	66	67	68	68	69
	95th	107	107	108	110	111	112	113	69	70	70	71	72	72	73
6	90th	104	105	106	107	109	110	111	67	67	68	69	69	70	71
	95th	108	109	110	111	112	114	114	71	71	72	73	73	74	75
7	90th	106	107	108	109	110	112	112	69	69	69	70	71	72	72
	95th	110	110	112	113	114	115	116	73	73	73	74	75	76	76
8	90th	108	109	110	111	112	113	114	70	70	71	71	72	73	74
	95th	112	112	113	115	116	117	118	74	74	75	75	76	77	78
9	90th	110	110	112	113	114	115	116	71	72	72	73	74	74	75
	95th	114	114	115	117	118	119	120	75	76	76	77	78	78	79

From National High Blood Pressure Education Program Working Group on Hypertension Control in Children & Adolescents: Update on Task Force Report on High Blood Pressure, *Pediatrics* 98:649, 1996.
*Blood pressure percentile was determined by a single measurement.
†Height percentile was determined by standard growth curves.

- Family history: hypertension, athero-sclerosis, preeclampsia, toxemia, renal disease, tumors (risk for essential hypertension and inherited renal/endocrine diseases)
- Review of systems: abdominal pain, dysuria, hematuria, frequency, nocturia, enuresis (may suggest underlying renal disease or infection); joint pains and/or swelling, facial or peripheral edema (nephritis); weight loss, failure to gain weight, flushing, sweating, fevers, palpitations (pheochromocytoma); muscle cramps, weakness, constipation (hypokalemia and hyperaldosteronism); age of menarche, sexual development (hydroxylase defi-ciency); ingestion of prescription, over-the-counter, or illicit drugs

■ **PHYSICAL EXAMINATION**
- General: pallor, facial or pretibial edema (renal disease)
- Café-au-lait spots, neurofibromas (Von Recklinghausen's disease)
- Moon face, hirsutism, buffalo hump, truncal obesity, striae (Cushing's syndrome)
- Webbing of neck, low hairline, wide-spaced nipples (Turner syndrome)
- Elfin facies, poor growth, retardation (Williams syndrome)
- Thyroid enlargement or nodules (hyperthyroid or hypothyroid)
- Cardiovascular
  1. Murmur, absent or delayed femoral pulses, low leg blood pressure relative to arm blood pressure (aortic coarctation)
  2. Heart size, tachycardia, hepatomegaly, tachypnea (heart failure)
  3. Bruits over great vessels (arteritis or arteriopathy)
- Abdomen
  1. Epigastric bruit (renovascular disease or arteritis)
  2. Unilateral or bilateral masses (Wilms' tumor, neuroblastoma, pheochromocytoma, polycystic kidneys)
- Neurologic: hypertensive funduscopic changes, Bell's palsy, neurologic deficits (chronic and/or severe acute hypertension).

TABLE 2-11 **Blood Pressure Levels for the 90th and 95th Percentiles of Blood Pressure for Girls Aged 1 to 17 Years by Percentiles of Height—cont'd**

AGE (yr)	BLOOD PRESSURE PERCENTILE*	SYSTOLIC BLOOD PRESSURE BY PERCENTILE OF HEIGHT, mm Hg†							DIASTOLIC BLOOD PRESSURE BY PERCENTILE OF HEIGHT, mm Hg†						
		5%	10%	25%	50%	75%	90%	95%	5%	10%	25%	50%	75%	90%	95%
10	90th	112	112	114	115	116	117	118	73	73	73	74	75	76	76
	95th	116	116	117	119	120	121	122	77	77	77	78	79	80	80
11	90th	114	114	116	117	118	119	120	74	74	75	75	76	77	77
	95th	118	118	119	121	122	123	124	78	78	79	79	80	81	81
12	90th	116	116	118	119	120	121	122	75	75	76	76	77	78	78
	95th	120	120	121	123	124	125	126	79	79	80	80	81	82	82
13	90th	118	118	119	121	122	123	124	76	76	77	78	78	79	80
	95th	121	122	123	125	126	127	128	80	80	81	82	82	83	84
14	90th	119	120	121	122	124	125	126	77	77	78	79	79	80	81
	95th	123	124	125	126	128	129	130	81	81	82	83	83	84	85
15	90th	121	121	122	124	125	126	127	78	78	79	79	80	81	82
	95th	124	125	126	128	129	130	131	82	82	83	83	84	85	86
16	90th	122	122	123	125	126	127	128	79	79	79	80	81	82	82
	95th	125	126	127	128	130	131	132	83	83	83	84	85	86	86
17	90th	122	123	124	125	126	128	128	79	79	79	80	81	82	82
	95th	126	126	127	129	130	131	132	83	83	83	84	85	86	86

DIAGNOSIS

■ DIAGNOSTIC WORKUP
- Initial evaluation
  1. Complete blood count
  2. Serum electrolytes, blood urea nitrogen, creatinine, calcium, uric acid
  3. Urinalysis and urine culture
  4. Plasma renin activity
  5. Lipid panel
  6. Renal ultrasound
- Suspicious of secondary hypertension or persistent elevation
  1. Echocardiography (check left ventricular wall thickness)
  2. Renal scan with angiotensin-converting enzyme (ACE) inhibitor
  3. Urine catecholamines
  4. Plasma and urinary steroids
  5. Renal artery imaging or renal vein renin sampling

THERAPY

The goals of therapy are to achieve a reduction in blood pressure below the 95th percentile and to prevent the occurrence of long-term sequelae.

■ NONPHARMACOLOGIC
The following therapies should be advocated for high-normal blood pressures and as a complement to pharmacologic interventions:
- Weight reduction
- Exercise
- Dietary interventions, such as sodium restriction and heart-healthy diet, to decrease fat intake
- Smoking cessation
- Alcohol and drug avoidance

■ MEDICAL
- See Table 2-12 for medications used in chronic hypertension therapy, which include the following:
  1. Diuretics
  2. β-Blockers
  3. ACE inhibitors
  4. Calcium channel blockers
- The aforementioned drugs may be used alone or in combination.
- Pharmacologic therapy should be directed at the underlying cause of HTN when possible.
  1. Those who benefit from salt restriction may do well with dietary

TABLE 2-12 Treatment of Chronic Hypertension in Children

DRUG	DOSAGE	COMMENTS
Diuretics		
Hydrochlorothiazide	20-30 mg/kg/day PO ÷ every 12 hr	Monitor for ↓ K, ↑ glu, ↑ uric acid
Chlorothiazide	2-3 mg/kg/day PO ÷ every 12 hr	Monitor for ↓ K, ↑ glu, ↑ uric acid
Chlorthalidone	Dose not established in pediatrics	Longer acting than thiazides
Furosemide	2-3 mg/kg/day PO ÷ every 6-12 hr	Monitor for ↓ K, ↑ glu, ↑ uric acid, loop diuretic, hypercalciuria
Ethacrynic acid	2-3 mg/kg/day PO ÷ every 6-12 hr	Monitor for ↓ K, ↑ glu, ↑ uric acid, loop diuretic
Bumetanide	0.02-0.3 mg/kg/day PO ÷ every 6-12 hr	Monitor for ↓ K, ↑ glu, ↑ uric acid, loop diuretic
Spironolactone	1-3 mg/kg/day PO ÷ every 6-12 hr	Aldosterone antagonist
Triamterene	2-3 mg/kg/day PO ÷ every 6-12 hr	Distal tubule blocker of Na:K exchange
Acetazolamide	5 mg/kg/day PO	Carbonic anhydrase inhibitor not useful in patients with hypertension
Vasodilators		
Hydralazine	0.75-3.0 mg/kg/day PO ÷ every 6-8 hr	↑ Heart rate, headache, lupuslike syndrome (rare in pediatrics)
Minoxidil	0.05-1.0 mg/kg/day PO ÷ every 12 hr	Salt and water retention, hirsutism
Prazosin	0.05-0.5 mg/kg/day PO ÷ every 8-12 hr	Give first dose with patient supine
Calcium Channel Antagonist		
Nifedipine (extended release)	0.25-3 mg/kg/day PO ÷ every 12-24 hr	↑ Heart rate, flushing, headache, dizziness
β-Adrenergic Antagonist		
Propranolol	0.5-6.0 mg/kg/day PO ÷ every 6-12 hr	Avoid in patients with asthma or CHF, ↓ glu
Atenolol	1-2 mg/kg/day PO ÷ every 12-24 hr	↓ Bronchospasm and bradycardia
Labetalol	1-3 mg/kg/day PO ÷ every 6-12 hr	α- and β-blockade
α-Adrenergic Antagonist		
Clonidine	0.05-0.6 mg/kg/day PO ÷ every 6-12 hr	Initial drowsiness, rebound HTN with abrupt discontinuation
Angiotensin-Converting Enzyme (ACE) Inhibitors		
Captopril	0.02-2.0 mg/kg/day PO ÷ every 12 hr (infants) 0.5-6.0 mg/kg/day PO ÷ every 8 hr (children)	↑ K, ↓ platelets, neutropenia, cough, caution in renal artery stenosis, ↓ GFR
Enalapril	0.15-? mg/kg/day PO ÷ every 12-24 hr	↓ GFR, ↑ K, ↓ platelets, ↓ WBC count

From Bartosh SM, Aronson AJ: *Pediatr Clin North Am* 46:235, 1999.
↓, Decreased; ↑, increased; *CHF*, congestive heart failure; *GFR*, glomerular filtration rate; *glu*, glucose level; *HTN*, hypertension; *K*, potassium level; *Na*, sodium; *PO*, by mouth; *WBC*, white blood cell.

TABLE 2-13   Antihypertensive Drug Therapy for Hypertensive Emergencies in Children

DRUG	DOSAGE
Nifedipine	0.25-0.5 mg/kg PO prn; may be repeated two times if no response
Sodium nitroprusside	0.5-1 μg/kg/min IV initially; may be increased stepwise to 8 μg/kg/min maximum
Labetalol	0.2-1 mg/kg/dose IV; may be increased incrementally to 1 mg/kg/dose until response achieved; 0.25-2 mg/kg/hr maintenance, either bolus or IV infusion
Esmolol	500-600 μg/kg IV load dose over 1-2 min then 200 μg/kg/min; may be increased by 50-100 μg/kg every 5-10 min to maximum of 1000 μg/kg
Diazoxide	1-5 mg/kg/dose IV bolus up to maximum of 150 mg/dose
Hydralazine	0.2-0.4 mg/kg IV prn; may be repeated two times if no response
Minoxidil	0.1-0.2 mg/kg oral

From National High Blood Pressure Education Program Working Group on Hypertension Control in Children & Adolescents: Update on Task Force Report on High Blood Pressure, *Pediatrics* 98:649, 1996.
IV, Intravenous; *PO*, by mouth; *prn*, as needed.

interventions and a thiazide diuretic.
2. Patients with high renin hypertension, as in renovascular disease, often benefit from ACE inhibitors.
- Emergency therapy is indicated for children with extreme elevation of blood pressure.
  1. Extreme hypertension is a blood pressure greater than 1.3 to 1.5 times the 95th percentile.
  2. See Table 2-13 for medications used in hypertensive emergencies.
- Immediate therapy is also indicated for those with evidence of end-organ damage.
  1. Heart failure
  2. Malignant renal changes
  3. Funduscopic changes
  4. Symptoms consistent with encephalopathy

■ **FOLLOW-UP & DISPOSITION**
Monitor blood pressure often until correction of underlying disorder is achieved or lifelong.

■ **PATIENT/FAMILY EDUCATION**
Explain the long-term sequela and reasons to treat even though no current symptoms are present.

■ **PREVENTIVE TREATMENT**
Early diagnosis of high-normal blood pressures with implementation of non-pharmacologic measures may decrease the onset of hypertension in those at risk (i.e., positive family history).

■ **REFERRAL INFORMATION**
Referral to a cardiologist, nephrologist, or endocrinologist may be considered if a specific disorder is suspected. Surgical specialists may also be needed depending on the underlying cause.

⚙ **PEARLS & CONSIDERATIONS**

■ **CLINICAL PEARLS**
- Cuff size is important.
  1. Cuff bladder width should be at least 40% of the circumference of the arm measured midway between the olecranon and acromion.
  2. Cuff bladder length should cover 80% to 100% of the arm.
- Systolic blood pressure is determined by the onset of the tapping Korotkoff sounds.
- Diastolic blood pressure has recently been established as the fifth Korotkoff sound (disappearance of sounds) in children of all ages.
- Approximately 60% to 80% of secondary hypertension in childhood is caused by renal parenchymal disease.
- Essential hypertension is rare in children 10 years or younger.

- Because of the teratogenic risk with fetal exposure during second and third trimester, ACE inhibitors should be used with extreme caution in sexually active adolescent females.

■ **WEBSITE**
For physicians and families of those with hypertension:
- P\S\L Group: www.pslgroup.com/hypertension.htm

REFERENCES
1. Bartosh SM, Aronson AJ: Childhood hypertension: an update on etiology, diagnosis and treatment, *Pediatr Clin North Am* 46:235, 1999.
2. Hohn AR: Diagnosis and management of hypertension in childhood, *Pediatr Ann* 6:105, 1997.
3. National High Blood Pressure Education Program, Working Group on Hypertension Control in Children and Adolescents: Update on the 1987 Task Force Report on High Blood Pressure in Children and Adolescents: A Working Group Report from the National High Blood Pressure Education Program, *Pediatrics* 98:649, 1996.
4. Sinaiko AR: Hypertension in children, *N Engl J Med* 335:1968, 1996.
Author: **Marc A. Raslich, M.D.**

BASIC INFORMATION

■ **DEFINITION**

Hyperthyroidism is a clinical condition typified by manifestation of an elevated T_4 and/or T_3 level, usually caused by Graves disease.

■ **SYNONYM**

Thyrotoxicosis

ICD-9CM CODES

242.00 Graves disease without thyroid storm
242.90 Thyrotoxicosis without mention of goiter

■ **ETIOLOGY**

• Graves disease is caused by production of immunoglobulin G (IgG) thyroid-stimulating immunoglobulins (TSI).
  1. These antibodies bind to the thyroid-stimulating hormone (TSH) receptors on the thyroid gland and stimulate production of thyroid hormones and thyroid growth.
• Hyperthyroidism can also occasionally be caused by the presence of a hyperfunctioning thyroid nodule (adenoma).

■ **EPIDEMIOLOGY & DEMOGRAPHICS**

• Graves disease is six times more prevalent in females than in males.
• There is an increased incidence at puberty and in families with a history of autoimmune thyroid disease (Graves or Hashimoto thyroiditis).

■ **HISTORY**

• General
  1. Weight loss (less commonly weight gain occurs)
  2. Increased urination and thirst
  3. Heat intolerance
• Endocrine
  1. Goiter possible
  2. Menstrual disturbances (decreased flow)
• Nervous system complaints
  1. Sleep disturbance: difficulty falling asleep and/or difficulty staying asleep
  2. Difficulty concentrating
  3. Emotional lability
  4. Decline in school performance
  5. Fatigability
  6. Tremor or worsening of handwriting
• Cardiovascular
  1. Palpitations or perception of tachycardia
• Gastrointestinal
  1. Increased appetite
  2. Loose stools

■ **PHYSICAL EXAMINATION**

• General
  1. Markedly "fidgety"
  2. Weight loss
• Endocrine
  1. Diffusely enlarged thyroid gland without palpable nodules
• Nervous system
  1. Fine motor tremors
  2. Tongue fasciculations
  3. Proximal muscle weakness
  4. Hyperreflexia
• Cardiovascular
  1. Increased pulse pressure
  2. Tachycardia
  3. Hyperactive precordium
  4. High-output flow murmur
• Skin
  1. Warm skin
  2. Sweaty palms
  3. Absence of acne in adolescents
• Eyes
  1. Exophthalmos (less common in children than adults, only one third of children)

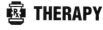 **DIAGNOSIS**

■ **DIFFERENTIAL DIAGNOSIS**

• Hyperthyroidism is often confused with nonthyroid conditions involving the central nervous system, including the following:
  1. Attention deficit/hyperactivity disorder, behavioral problems
  2. Psychiatric conditions
  3. Stimulant use
• Hyperthyroidism also may be confused with cardiovascular conditions.
  1. Tachycardia (from anemia)
  2. Arrhythmia
• Differential diagnosis for hyperthyroid state includes the following:
  1. Hyperfunctioning nodule
  2. Exogenous thyroxine ingestion
  3. "Hashitoxicosis": early hyperthyroid phase of Hashimoto's thyroiditis

■ **DIAGNOSTIC WORKUP**

• Diagnosis often obvious from history and physical examination, especially if diffusely enlarged thyroid is evident, obviating need for any further evaluation beyond simple thyroid function tests
• Thyroid function tests
  1. TSH should be suppressed below the normal range in all forms of hyperthyroidism (except for extremely rare cases of TSH-secreting adenoma).
  2. Free T_4 should be elevated.
     a. Total T_4 is not necessary if free T_4 is measured, but it should also be elevated.
  3. T_3 is not routinely needed.
     a. May be helpful in diagnosis if

TSH is suppressed with normal free T_4 (adenomas and some Graves disease, primarily with T_3 toxicosis)
  4. Thyroid-stimulating antibodies (TSI) are present.
     a. Levels are elevated but do not need to be measured if the diagnosis is evident from the history and physical examination.
• Radioiodine uptake and imaging generally not needed
  1. Helpful in identifying a hyperfunctioning nodule *or*
  2. Helpful in differentiating "Hashitoxicosis" (low uptake) from Graves disease (high uptake)

THERAPY

■ **MEDICAL**

• Methimazole (Tapazole) or propylthiouracil (PTU) is the usual first-line therapy in children and adolescents.
  1. Initial dosing in adolescents is typically methimazole 10 mg three times daily or PTU 100 mg three times daily (half this amount for preadolescent children).
  2. Repeat free T_4 level should be obtained in 4 to 6 weeks; if free T_4 is dropping into the normal range, the dosage can be gradually reduced, often to once daily if using methimazole.
• Propranolol, starting at 10 mg three times daily, can be used in selected severely affected patients to help control symptoms while awaiting the therapeutic effects of medication or radioiodine.
• Radioiodine therapy with ^{131}I is usually considered second-line therapy in adolescents.
  1. Used primarily in context of adverse reaction to medical therapy (neutropenia), failure to control hyperthyroidism on medication, or patient preference for definitive therapy
  2. Associated with a high risk of permanent hypothyroidism requiring lifelong thyroid replacement

■ **SURGICAL**

• Partial thyroidectomy as treatment for Graves disease has fallen out of favor behind medical management and radioiodine because of the small but finite risk of surgical complications, including hypoparathyroidism and recurrent laryngeal nerve damage.
• However, surgery is still the treatment of choice for pregnant patients, for those who require immediate de-

finitive therapy, and if radioiodine therapy is not possible (e.g., iodine allergy) after failure of medical management.

- Excision of a hyperfunctioning nodule is the treatment of choice, is curative, and is not associated with complications of thyroidectomy (as outlined previously).

■ FOLLOW-UP & DISPOSITION

- For patients treated with PTU or methimazole, the key to management is consistent regular thyroid function testing with subsequent appropriate adjustments of medication.
- Once thyroid values are stabilized, thyroid function tests every 3 to 4 months is usually adequate.
- Trial off of medication can be considered after a couple of years if the dosage of medication is low (i.e., 5 to 7.5 mg of methimazole daily), there have been no recent relapses of free T_4 into the hyperthyroid range, and the thyroid gland is small.

■ PATIENT/FAMILY EDUCATION

- It is imperative that patients and family understand that neutropenia, a rare, reversible adverse effect of methimazole or PTU, can be life-threatening if it goes unrecognized.
  1. Perioral lesions or fevers should be evaluated immediately with a complete blood count with differential.
- Significant changes in clinical status

between regular visits should be reported to the physician as soon as they are noted and followed-up with repeat thyroid function tests.

■ REFERRAL INFORMATION

- Many pediatricians prefer to refer all patients with hyperthyroidism to a pediatric endocrinologist for management and education.
- For children with hyperthyroidism that does not readily come under control who are receiving medical management, those with adverse effects to therapy, or those being considered for radioiodine or surgery, referral should be strongly considered.

☼ PEARLS & CONSIDERATIONS

■ CLINICAL PEARLS

- TSH may not be a reliable indicator of the hyperthyroid state early after beginning therapy because of the lag in pituitary recovery.
- The duration of Graves disease in children is much longer than in adults and may take years to remit.
  1. If the euthyroid state is maintained for 1 year or longer off medications, there is a good chance that long-term remission from Graves disease will be achieved.
- Neonatal Graves disease, caused by

the transplacental passage of maternal stimulating antibodies, is rare but life-threatening and should receive immediate attention.

■ WEBSITES

- National Graves' Disease Foundation: www.ngdf.org
- Thyroid Foundation of America: www.allthyroid.org

■ SUPPORT GROUPS

Visit www.ngdf.org/groups.htm for listing of local support groups.

REFERENCES

1. American Association of Clinical Endocrinologists: Practice standard for adults with hyperthyroidism, available at: www.aace.com/clinguideindex.htm
2. Foley TP: Disorders of the thyroid in children. In Sperling MA (ed): *Pediatric endocrinology,* Philadelphia, 1996, WB Saunders.
3. Rivkees SA, Sklar C, Freemark M: Clinical review 99: the management of Grave's disease in children, with special emphasis on radioiodine treatment, *J Clin Endocrinol Metab* 83:3786, 1998.
4. Segni M et al: Special features of Grave's disease in early childhood, *Thyroid* 9:871, 1999.
5. Zimmerman D, Lteif AN: Thyrotoxicosis in children, *Endocrinol Metab Clin North Am* 27:109, 1998.

Author: **Craig Orlowski, M.D.**

II

BASIC INFORMATION

■ DEFINITION
Hypertrophic cardiomyopathy is excessive hypertrophy and specific abnormalities of cardiac muscle, such as myofiber disarray or glycogen deposits, resulting in cardiac dysfunction.

■ SYNONYMS
- Hypertrophic obstructive cardiomyopathy (HOCM/HCM)
- Asymmetric septal hypertrophy (ASH)
- Idiopathic hypertrophic subaortic stenosis (IHSS)
- Concentric left ventricular hypertrophy or hypertrophic nonobstructive cardiomyopathy

ICD-9CM CODES
425.1 Obstructive
425.4 Nonobstructive

■ ETIOLOGY
- Numerous and diverse
- Idiopathic—no cause identified
- Primary myocardial
  1. Familial: actin, myosin, troponin abnormalities seen within families
     a. Autosomal, X-linked, and spontaneous mutations identified
  2. Diseases related to energy creation or utilization
     a. Fatty acid transport defects resulting in deposition of storage products within myocytes
     b. Carnitine deficiency
     c. Abnormal glucose utilization
        (1) Hyperinsulinemia and infants of diabetic mothers both may develop hypertrophic cardiomyopathy.
     d. Mitochondrial dysfunction
- Secondary myocardial
  1. Endocrine: hypothyroidism, infant of a diabetic mother, tyrosinemia
  2. Neuromuscular: Friedreich's ataxia
  3. Drugs: glucocorticosteroid
  4. Other: Noonan syndrome, multiple lentigines

■ EPIDEMIOLOGY & DEMOGRAPHICS
- The true incidence and prevalence in infants and children is not known.
- A large database is currently being developed for North America.

■ HISTORY
- May present as sudden death and be found only by autopsy
- Often found on evaluation of a new murmur
- Syncope, particularly on exertion
- Neurologic or seizure disorder

- Chest pain, particularly on exertion
- Incidental finding of enlarged heart on chest radiograph
- Strong family history of sudden death or heart disease
- Rarely, symptoms of congestive heart failure (shortness of breath, dyspnea, orthopnea)

■ PHYSICAL EXAMINATION
- Look for characteristic features of syndromes, such as Noonan syndrome, or coarse facial features of storage diseases.
- Muscle weakness and organomegaly may support the diagnosis of neuromuscular or storage diseases.
- Retinal lesions (seen in Kearn-Sayre syndrome) should prompt an evaluation for mitochondrial dystrophy.
- Cardiac examination may be remarkable for displaced and/or hyperdynamic point of maximum impulse, brisk carotid upstroke.
- Murmurs are characteristically as follows:
  1. Systolic ejection in nature
  2. Usually located at the base
  3. Increased with Valsalva maneuver
  4. No ejection clicks as might be heard with valvar stenosis

DIAGNOSIS

■ DIFFERENTIAL DIAGNOSIS
- Dilated cardiomyopathy
- Structural heart disease
- Valvar stenosis
- Athletic heart—an accentuated left ventricular hypertrophy in response to vigorous athletic activity

■ DIAGNOSTIC WORKUP
- Chest radiograph
  1. May show enlarged cardiac silhouette, but usually normal
  2. Rarely, pulmonary venous congestion
- Electrocardiogram
  1. Nonspecific ST-T wave changes, in particular, inversion of the T waves and ST-segment depression
  2. Severe left ventricular hypertrophy and/or right ventricular hypertrophy dependent on the affected chamber
  3. Axis deviation to support the vector of ventricular hypertrophy
  4. Often interventricular conduction delay
  5. High-grade arrhythmia: ventricular ectopia
- Echocardiogram
  1. This is the most accurate, rapid, and widely used technique for initial evaluation and monitoring of left ventricular anatomy, outflow tract obstruction, and function.

  2. Classically, there is asymptomatic septal left ventricular hypertrophy with hyperdynamic function.
  3. Hypertrophy may occur anywhere within the ventricle, and there may be concentric left ventricular hypertrophy.
  4. There may be near obliteration of the left ventricular cavity in systole.
  5. There may systolic anterior motion of the mitral valve.
  6. There may be left and/or right ventricular outflow tract obstruction, depending on the site of ventricular hypertrophy.
- Exercise stress test to evaluate for ischemic changes and to assess the outflow tract gradient during exertion
- Blood tests
  1. Complete blood count with differential, if an infant
     a. Male infants with low white blood cell count, urine amino acid abnormalities, and any form of cardiomyopathy may have the lethal mitochondrial dystrophy known as Barth syndrome.
  2. Blood chemistry looking for chronic acidosis
  3. Urine amino acids
  4. Serum organic acids
  5. Thyroid studies
  6. Carnitine
  7. Troponin I or T if suspicious of ischemic changes
- Genetic evaluation and skeletal muscle biopsy if indicated
- Neurologic evaluation if syndrome suspected

THERAPY

■ NONPHARMACOLOGIC
- Restrict from weight-lifting.
- May need to restrict vigorous (competitive) activity as well.
  1. Dependent on family history, personal history, and clinical manifestations
- Do not allow dehydration.

■ MEDICAL
- Avoid inotropes (no digoxin).
- β-Blockade or calcium channel blockers may be used.

■ SURGICAL
- Pacemaker implantation may reduce the outflow tract gradient by regulating the diastolic time interval.
- An automated cardiac defibrillator may be necessary if a history of ventricular tachycardia or fibrillation is present.
- Surgical myomectomy may be required.

- Cardiac transplantation is considered when other therapy has failed.

■ FOLLOW-UP & DISPOSITION

- The natural history of cardiomyopathy is not well known and may be quite variable.
- Long-term follow-up with a cardiologist is necessary.
- Patients who undergo cardiac transplantation are followed closely for the remainder of their lives.

■ PATIENT/FAMILY EDUCATION

- Explain the associated family history of cardiac disease and sudden death.
- Infants and children with dysmorphology or genetic syndromes should undergo cardiac evaluation.
- Infants and children with known neuromuscular disease should be followed by a cardiologist.

■ REFERRAL INFORMATION

Regular follow-up with a cardiologist is necessary.

☼ PEARLS & CONSIDERATIONS

■ CLINICAL PEARLS

- A new-onset systolic murmur at the midleft sternal border requires further investigation.
- Screening electrocardiograms with left ventricular hypertrophy, particularly in the presence of a murmur, should be evaluated by a pediatric cardiologist.
- Patients with a strong family history of sudden death should be evaluated by a pediatric cardiologist.
- Patients with syncope or chest pain on exertion require further evaluation.

■ WEBSITE

Nicholas Institute of Sports Medicine and Athletic Trauma: www.nismat. org/card_cor/abnormal.html

REFERENCES

1. Colan SD et al: Cardiomyopathies. In Fyler DC (ed): *Nadas' pediatric cardiology*, Philadelphia, 1992, Mosby.
2. Wynne JE, Braunwald E: The cardiomyopathies and myocarditides. In Braunwald E (ed): *Heart disease*, Philadelphia, 1997, WB Saunders.
3. Maron BJ: Hypertrophic cardiomyopathy. In Emmanouilides GC et al (eds): *Heart disease in infants, children, and adolescents: including the fetus and young adult*, Baltimore, 1995, Williams & Wilkins.

Author: **Michelle A. Grenier, M.D.**

II

BASIC INFORMATION

■ DEFINITION
Hypocalcemia is present when the total serum calcium concentration is less than 7.0 mg/dl and the ionized calcium is less than 3.5 mg/dl (depending on the particular ion-selective electrode used).

ICD-9CM CODE
275.41 Hypocalcemia

■ ETIOLOGY
- Early-onset hypocalcemia (during the first 3 days of life)
  1. Prematurity: multifactorial from abrupt discontinuation of maternofetal calcium transfer, inappropriate parathyroid hormone (PTH) response, high calcitonin, resistance to 1,25-dihydroxyvitamin D in very low-birth-weight infants, and decreased calcium intake
  2. Infants of insulin-dependent diabetic mothers (IDMs): maternal magnesium deficiency, hypoparathyroidism, and high calcitonin
  3. Birth asphyxia: increased endogenous phosphate load, high calcitonin, decreased calcium intake, and bicarbonate (alkali) therapy (see the section on "Tetany")
  4. Hypoparathyroidism secondary to maternal hyperparathyroidism
  5. Gestational exposure to anticonvulsants: may be related to the accelerated metabolism of 25-hydroxyvitamin D
- Late-onset hypocalcemia (usually at the end of the first week of life)
  1. Term infants fed a cow milk–derived formula or other high-phosphate diet (e.g., cereals) with immaturity of renal tubular phosphate excretion
  2. Hypoparathyroidism: primary or secondary
  3. Hypomagnesemia
  4. Intestinal calcium malabsorption
  5. Phototherapy: may relate to melatonin disturbance
  6. Maternal factors: decreased vitamin D intake or sunlight exposure
  7. Exchange transfusion with citrate-containing blood

■ EPIDEMIOLOGY & DEMOGRAPHICS
- About 30% to 90% of preterm infants develop hypocalcemia. Less mature infants have a greater probability of developing hypocalcemia.
- About 20% to 50% of IDMs develop hypocalcemia.
- About 30% of newborns who have an Apgar score below 7 at 1 minute of age may develop hypocalcemia.

■ HISTORY
- Nonspecific signs include apnea, seizures, jitteriness, increased extensor tone, clonus, hyperreflexia, and stridor (laryngospasm).
- Asymptomatic or clinically mild signs are present in preterm infants with early-onset hypocalcemia.
- High-pitched cry, Chvostek sign, and Trousseau sign are useful in older infants but are of little diagnostic value in the first few days of life.

⚗ DIAGNOSIS

The diagnosis is made based on serum total or ionized calcium level.

■ DIAGNOSTIC WORKUP
- Monitor serum calcium levels in infants at risk for developing hypocalcemia.
  1. Preterm infants less than 1500 g: at 12, 24, 48 hours of life
  2. Sick or stressed infants: at 12, 24, 48 hours of life and then as indicated
- Measure serum calcium, ionized calcium, phosphorus, and magnesium.
  1. Elevated serum phosphorus suggests phosphorus loading, renal insufficiency, or hypoparathyroidism.
  2. Magnesium level of 1 mg/dl or less strongly suggests primary hypomagnesemia.
- Assess albumin, PTH as needed, rarely 25-hydroxyvitamin D, and 1,25-dihydroxyvitamin D and renal function.
- An electrocardiographic QTc interval longer than 0.4 second (because of prolonged systole) is an indicator of hypocalcemia and may help in monitoring therapy.
- Examine the chest roentgenogram for thymic silhouette if DiGeorge syndrome is suspected.

℞ THERAPY

■ NONPHARMACOLOGIC
- Early-onset hypocalcemia
  1. Hypocalcemic preterm infants who have no clinical signs and are not ill from any other cause may not require specific treatment.
  2. This condition often resolves spontaneously by day 3.

■ MEDICAL
- Calcium preparations: calcium gluconate 10% solution (elemental calcium content 9 mg/ml) for intravenous use or oral use; calcium supplementation at dosages of 30 to 75 mg elemental calcium/kg/day (in four to six divided doses), titrated to the response of patient
- Early-onset hypocalcemia
  1. Ill infants or infants with severe hypocalcemia (serum calcium less than 6 mg/dl, ionized calcium less than 3 mg/dl) is usually treated.
- Late-onset hypocalcemia
  1. In phosphorus-induced hypocalcemia, a low-phosphorus formula (or human milk) and oral calcium supplementation, to increase calcium and decrease phosphorus absorption, are indicated.
  2. Hypoparathyroidism requires therapy with vitamin D or one of its metabolites: 1,25-dihydroxyvitamin D (or 1 α-hydroxyvitamin D_3, a synthetic analog)
- Treatment of hypocalcemic seizures, apnea, or tetany (serum calcium level is usually less than 5.0 to 6.0 mg/d)
  1. Emergency calcium therapy: 1 to 2 ml of calcium gluconate 10% per kg by intravenous infusion over 10 minutes
     a. Monitor heart rate and the infusion site to avoid cardiac arrhythmia and skin necrosis: Calcium infusion should be temporally stopped if bradycardia occurs.
     b. Repeat the dose in 10 minutes if no clinical response occurs.
  2. Maintenance calcium therapy
     a. Following the initial dose, maintenance calcium should be given parenterally or orally: 75 mg/kg/day for the first day, half the dose next day, half again, and discontinue.
     b. The duration of supplemental calcium therapy varies with the cause of hypocalcemia: 2 to 3 days for early hypocalcemia and possibly for lifetime for hypocalcemia caused by hypoparathyroidism or malabsorption.
- Symptomatic hypocalcemia unresponsive to calcium therapy: may be caused by hypomagnesemia
  1. Magnesium sulfate 50% solution (500 mg or 4 mEq/ml); 0.1 to 0.2 ml (50 to 100 mg)/kg, intravenously (infuse slowly over 10 minutes) or intramuscularly (may cause local tissue necrosis). Repeat dose every 6 to 12 hours. Obtain serum magnesium before each dose.

■ FOLLOW-UP & DISPOSITION
- In most cases, early neonatal hypocalcemia resolves within the first week of life.

- Prolonged hypocalcemia should prompt the physician to investigate other, more permanent causes.
- Regular follow-up monitoring of serum calcium concentration and appropriate monitoring of underlying disease (e.g., PTH concentration) are necessary to watch for recurrence of hypocalcemia.

■ PREVENTIVE TREATMENT
- Early neonatal hypocalcemia can be prevented in neonates at risk by oral and parenteral calcium supplementation (75 mg elemental calcium/kg/day).
- Maintenance of normal maternal vitamin D status may secondarily prevent late hypocalcemia in some infants.

- Treatment should be used to prevent hypocalcemia for high-risk newborns who exhibit cardiovascular compromise and require cardiotonic drugs or blood pressure support.
  1. Use a continuous calcium infusion by central catheter to maintain a total calcium higher than 8.0 mg/dl and an ionized calcium level higher than 4.0 mg/dl.
  2. Commonly used dosages range from 20 to 75 mg/kg/day.
- The most effective prevention of neonatal hypocalcemia includes prevention of prematurity and birth asphyxia, judicious use of bicarbonate therapy, and minimization of the occurrence of respiratory alkalosis from excessive mechanical ventilation.

☼ PEARLS & CONSIDERATIONS

■ CLINICAL PEARLS
If neonatal hypocalcemia accompanies hypomagnesemia, hypocalcemia may not be corrected unless hypomagnesemia is first rectified.

REFERENCES
1. Itani O, Tsang RC: Calcium, phosphorus, and magnesium in the newborn: pathophysiology and management. In Hay WW (ed): *Neonatal nutrition and metabolism,* St Louis, 1991, Mosby.
2. Demarini S, Mimouni FB, Tsang RC: Disorders of calcium, phosphorus and magnesium metabolism. In Fanaroff AA, Martin RJ (eds): *Neonatal-perinatal medicine: diseases of the fetus and infant,* St Louis, 1998, Mosby.
Authors: **Reginald Tsang, M.D., M.B.B.C., and Ran Namgung, M.D., Ph.D.**

BASIC INFORMATION

■ **DEFINITION**
Hypokalemia is present when the serum potassium level is less than 3.5 mEq/L (normal is 3.5 to 5.5 mEq/L).

ICD-9CM CODE
276.8 Hypokalemia

■ **ETIOLOGY**
- Decreased intake: anorexia nervosa, high-carbohydrate diet
- Increased renal and/or urinary losses
  1. Diuretics (furosemide, thiazides), gentamicin, amphotericin, carbenicillin, corticosteroids
  2. Hyperaldosteronism, adrenal adenomas, renin-producing tumors, Cushing's syndrome, licorice ingestion
  3. Renovascular disease
  4. Renal tubular acidosis, Fanconi's syndrome, chronic cystic renal disease, Bartter's syndrome
  5. Osmotic diuresis from glycosuria
  6. Hypomagnesemia, hypochloremia
- Increased gastrointestinal losses
  1. Diarrhea and/or malabsorption
  2. Vomiting or nasogastric suction
  3. Laxative abuse
  4. Ileostomy
- Redistribution of potassium from extracellular or intravascular space to intracellular space
  1. Endogenous catecholamines, β-agonists, including inhaled medications (e.g., albuterol)
  2. Alkalemia
  3. Increased insulin levels

■ **EPIDEMIOLOGY & DEMOGRAPHICS**
- The most common cause of hypokalemia is diuretic use.
- The epidemiology and demographics of hypokalemia are associated with the conditions causing it.

■ **HISTORY**
- Medication and dietary history
- Fatigue or weakness (hypokalemic familial periodic paralysis, hypomagnesemia)
- Diarrhea
- Vomiting or ileus
- Nasogastric suction

■ **PHYSICAL EXAMINATION**
- Cardiac arrhythmias: premature ventricular and/or atrial contractions, heart block ventricular tachycardia, ventricular fibrillation
- Decreased cardiac output and perfusion occur with severe hypokalemia
- Decreased bowel sounds from intestinal ileus
- Mental apathy
- Muscle weakness

- Ascending paralysis may occur with the syndrome of hypokalemic periodic paralysis.

DIAGNOSIS

■ **DIFFERENTIAL DIAGNOSIS**
- For muscle weakness, see Hypotonia algorithm.
- For congestive heart failure and arrhythmia, see the section "Congestive Heart Failure."
- For hypokalemia, see "Etiology."

■ **DIAGNOSTIC WORKUP**
- Serum potassium
  1. Whole blood potassium is lower than serum potassium.
- Electrocardiogram: flattened and/or inverted T wave, U wave, ST-segment depression, atrial and ventricular arrhythmias
- Urine potassium
  1. Low suggests total body potassium depletion.
  2. High suggests renal potassium wasting.

THERAPY

- Urgency of treatment depends on the level of serum potassium, the rate of potassium loss, the number of risk factors present for cardiac arrhythmias and/or neurologic abnormalities, and the presence of physical signs and symptoms secondary to hypokalemia.
  1. The presence of signs or symptoms suggests that immediate and aggressive treatment is necessary.
     a. Cardiac arrhythmias
     b. Muscle weakness (lower extremities, then upper extremities and respiratory muscles)
  2. The absence of symptoms but a high number of risk factors suggests that rapid treatment is required.
     a. Risk factors
        (1) Use of potassium-depleting diuretics, especially furosemide; even one dose will result in significant kaliuresis within 1 hour of administration
        (2) Ongoing significant gastrointestinal losses
        (3) Association with other electrolyte abnormalities (hypomagnesemia, hypophosphatemia, hypocalcemia, hypochloremia)
        (4) Intrinsic cardiac conduction abnormalities, such as prolonged QT syndrome

        (5) Myocarditis
        (6) Cardiomyopathy (especially dilated)
        (7) Within the first few days after cardiac surgery, especially if cardiopulmonary bypass and/or ventriculotomy
        (8) Digoxin
        (9) Known history of hypokalemic periodic paralysis
  3. The absence of both symptoms and risk factors suggests that correction may be done less emergently.
- If risk factors (especially cardiac) are present and serum potassium is less than 3.0 mEq/L (less than 3.5 if immediately preoperative or postoperative for cardiac surgery)
  1. Place patient on a cardiac monitor.
  2. Increase concentration of potassium in maintenance fluids to 40 mEq/L (peripherally) and up to 100 mEq/L centrally.
  3. Immediately administer 1 mEq/kg potassium chloride enterally.
     a. 40 mEq per dose maximum
     b. Enteral route preferable
        (1) Fewer potential arrhythmogenic side effects occur.
        (2) Absorption is almost as rapid (within 1 hour) as giving potassium intravenously over 1 hour.
  4. If enteral route is not appropriate (ileus, emesis), may administer 0.5 mEq/kg up to maximum of 20 mEq potassium chloride intravenously over 1 hour.
     a. Peripherally, use a concentration of less than 40 mEq/L (to avoid the potential for serious infiltration and injury).
     b. On rare occasions, when risk factors are present, in the absence of a central line but with an extremely well-functioning intravenous line, higher concentrations may have to be used because of volume considerations.
     c. Centrally, may use up to a concentration of 100 mEq/L (0.1 mEq/ml) potassium chloride.
     d. Check potassium level 1 hour after infusion is complete or 2 hours after enteral administration and repeat as necessary until potassium is within 3.0 to 3.5 mEq/L.
  5. Hold diuretics until potassium is corrected to greater than 3.0 mEq/L
  6. Avoid alkalemia.
  7. Correct other electrolyte abnormalities, especially magnesium and chloride.

- If no risk factors or signs and symptoms are present and serum potassium is higher than 3.0 mEq/L, use oral medications and a high-potassium diet.
  1. Medications: Various preparations are available in either liquid, tablet, or capsule formulations.
     a. The starting dose in a low-risk situation is 1 to 2 mEq/kg/24 hr divided twice per day up to 10 to 20 mEq twice per day as an adult.
  2. Consider potassium-sparing diuretics (spironolactone, amiloride) if required.
  3. Dietary intake should include potassium-rich foods (e.g., prune juice, tomato juice, orange juice, grape juice, bananas—1 mEq potassium/inch).

■ FOLLOW-UP & DISPOSITION

Follow-up with frequent serum potassium levels is imperative until the patient is stable, especially if the underlying cause is not resolved.

■ PATIENT/FAMILY EDUCATION

- Educate the patient (and family) about the importance of compliance with oral potassium preparations, especially if taking multiple diuretics.
- Educate the patient (and family) about potassium-rich foods (may require nutrition consultation).

■ REFERRAL INFORMATION

May consider endocrinology, metabolic, and/or renal consultations based on the underlying cause

☼ PEARLS & CONSIDERATIONS

■ CLINICAL PEARLS

- Administration of potassium supplements in a patient with an intestinal ileus or poor intestinal motility may result in acute hyperkalemia (caused by sudden absorption of the previously administered, accumulated potassium) at the time of ileus/dysmotility resolution.
- If potassium chloride infiltrates a peripheral vein, hyaluronidase should be infiltrated into the area to minimize tissue injury.
- Because a significant risk of arrhythmias exists, a cardiac monitor should always be used while infusing a potassium bolus into a central vein or catheter. Serial boluses should not be administered in rapid succession without measuring a serum potassium level in between.
- If serum chloride is low, potassium will be difficult to replete. Replete chloride aggressively along with potassium supplementation. Arginine chloride may need to be used.

REFERENCES

1. Brem AS: Disorders of potassium homeostasis, *Pediatr Clin North Am* 37: 419, 1990.
2. Cronan KM, Norman ME: Renal and electrolyte emergencies. In Fleisher GR, Ludwig SL (eds): *Textbook of pediatric emergency medicine*, ed 3, Baltimore, 1993, Williams & Wilkins.
3. Wood EG, Lynch RE: Fluids and electrolyte balance. In Fuhrman BP, Zimmerman JJ (eds): *Pediatric critical care*, ed 2, St Louis, 1998, Mosby.

Author: **Elise van der Jagt, M.D.**

II

BASIC INFORMATION

■ DEFINITION
Hyponatremia is present when the serum sodium concentration is less than 130 mEq/L.

■ SYNONYMS
Hyponatremia is not synonymous with *hypotonic* or *hyposmolar*. Patients with hyponatremia may be isotonic, hypotonic, or hypertonic depending on other solutes in the extracellular space that cannot traverse the cell membrane.

ICD-9CM CODE
276.1 Hyponatremia

■ ETIOLOGY
- Sodium loss
  1. Gastrointestinal
     a. Secretory and nonsecretory diarrhea
     b. Ileostomy
  2. Renal disease
     a. Tubular dysfunction
     b. Postobstructive uropathy
     c. Polyuric renal failure, chronic renal disease
     d. Heavy metal poisoning
  3. Hypoadrenalism with salt wasting
     a. Congenital adrenal hyperplasia
     b. Addison's disease
     c. Hypoaldosteronism
  4. Cerebral salt wasting
  5. Diabetic ketoacidosis, hyperglycemia with secondary urinary losses
  6. Excessive skin losses
     a. Cystic fibrosis
     b. Heat exhaustion
  7. Third-space losses
     a. Peritonitis
     b. Burn edema
     c. Postsurgery
  8. Diuretics
     a. Furosemide
     b. Thiazides
- Increased intravascular and/or total body water
  1. Excessive oral or intravenous (IV) administration of hyponatremic fluids
     a. Inappropriate formula mixing
     b. Psychogenic
     c. Forced water intoxication
  2. Syndrome of inappropriate antidiuretic hormone secretion (SIADH)
  3. Hyperglycemia
     a. Osmolar substance attracts water and thus results in hyponatremia (dilutional effect).
     b. Once the hyperglycemia overrides the renal threshold, glycosuria with water loss and eventual total body water depletion occurs.
  4. Severe pulmonary disease
     a. Asthma
     b. Pneumonia
     c. Bronchiolitis

  5. Congestive heart failure
  6. Oliguric renal failure
  7. Liver failure
  8. Medications (DDAVP [desmopressin acetate], mannitol administration)
  9. Hypothyroidism
- Inadequate intake (dietary salt restriction)
- Artificially low
  1. High blood lipid content
  2. High blood protein content

■ EPIDEMIOLOGY & DEMOGRAPHICS
- Hyponatremia is most commonly associated with dehydration secondary to gastroenteritis, especially Rotavirus.
- In hospitalized patients, it is often related to the following conditions:
  1. Excess antidiuretic hormone (ADH) secretion secondary to surgery, pain, and mechanical ventilation
  2. Diuretic therapy
  3. Third-space losses

■ HISTORY
- Diarrhea
- Nausea and/or vomiting
  1. Central nervous system disease
  2. Gastroenteritis
  3. Adrenal
  4. Renal disease
- Type and quantity of fluid intake (low salt content?)
- Amount of urine output
  1. High urine output in the face of hyponatremia suggests physiologic correcting of fluid overload with associated:
     a. Dilutional hyponatremia
     b. Salt wasting from renal, adrenal, or cerebral disease
     c. Diuretic therapy
- Weight loss/gain
- Neurologic symptoms
  1. Headache
  2. Altered sensorium
  3. Lethargy or coma
  4. Seizures
- Muscle weakness and cramps
- Medications (e.g., furosemide, thiazides)

■ PHYSICAL EXAMINATION
- State of hydration
  1. Fluid deficit: tachycardia, decreased pulses, decreased capillary refill, decreased distal extremity temperature, decreased skin turgor, decreased blood pressure, dry mucous membranes
  2. Fluid overload: edema, puffy eyelids, moist mucous membranes, hypertension
- Weight (compare with a previous weight if known)
- Anterior fontanelle: sunken, flat, or bulging
- Respiratory rate: tachypnea (seen

with fever, acidosis, congestive heart failure, fluid overload, respiratory disease)
- Fever: infection
- Neurologic: obtunded, lethargic, hyperreflexia or hyporeflexia, muscle weakness, seizures

DIAGNOSIS

■ DIFFERENTIAL DIAGNOSIS
See "Etiology."

■ DIAGNOSTIC WORKUP
- Serum sodium is obtained.
- The cause of hyponatremia is refined by obtaining additional laboratory examinations.
- Blood urea nitrogen (BUN), creatinine, chloride, potassium, bicarbonate, and glucose are measured.
- Urine specific gravity, pH, sodium, potassium, and creatinine are obtained.
  1. High urine sodium (more than 20 mEq/L) suggests the following:
     a. Volume overload
     b. Adrenal insufficiency
     c. Renal tubular dysfunction/ renal failure
     d. Cerebral salt wasting
     e. Increased ADH, SIADH
     f. Diuretic use (e.g., furosemide, thiazides)
  2. Low urine sodium (less than 10 mEq/L) suggests the following:
     a. Inadequate circulating blood volume with secondary aldosterone secretion
     b. Absolute sodium deficit from lack of intake or excess gastrointestinal and/or skin losses
     c. Primary hyperaldosteronism
     d. Spironolactone
- Fractional excretion of sodium: $(U_{Na} \div P_{Na}) \times (P_{Cr} \div U_{Cr}) \times 100\%$
  1. Fractional excretion of sodium less than 1% suggests a prerenal cause or absolute deficit of sodium.
  2. Fractional excretion of sodium more than 2% suggests renal disease.

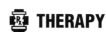

THERAPY

■ MEDICAL
- If seizures or coma is present and sodium is less than 125 mEq/L, give 3% saline.
  1. Calculate mEq sodium to give (125 - serum sodium) × (weight in kg) × 0.6
  2. Give over 4 hours.
- If hyponatremic from water overload, restrict water and give furosemide (water greater than sodium loss)

- If renal failure, may require dialysis and/or oral sorbitol administration to induce diarrhea.
- If dehydrated and sodium is 120 to 130 mEq/L without neurologic deficits, make up deficit fluids in 24 hours (one half in first 8 hours and remainder in next 16 hours) using normal saline to replace the sodium deficit and maintenance sodium requirements.
- If sodium is less than 120 mEq/L and has decreased over longer than 48 hours, correct sodium no faster than 10 to 12 mEq/24 hr.
- If sodium is less than 120 mEq/L and has decreased over less than 48 hours, may correct more rapidly.
- Monitor for neurologic deterioration if sodium is less than 125 mEq/L and has occurred acutely over 48 hours.

■ FOLLOW-UP & DISPOSITION
- Neurologic intensive monitoring is not required when sodium is higher than 125 mEq/L.
- The cause must be determined so that hyponatremia does not recur.

■ PATIENT/FAMILY EDUCATION
- Proper formula mixing
- Side effects of diuretics
- Information about underlying illness or disease process

■ PREVENTIVE TREATMENT
- Careful evaluation of fluid balance—intake and output
- Careful monitoring of urine output for patients at risk for SIADH
- Proper IV and oral fluid administration (containing sufficient sodium)

■ REFERRAL INFORMATION
Hospitalization and potential intensive care setting may be needed for the following:
- Serum sodium less than 125 mEq/L
- Hyponatremia associated with any neurologic symptoms
- Hyponatremia and renal failure
- Hyponatremia and more than 10% dehydration
- Hyponatremia and any disease that requires frequent monitoring of cardiovascular, neurologic, renal, or respiratory systems

☼ PEARLS & CONSDERATIONS

■ CLINICAL PEARLS
Urine sodium, specific gravity, osmolality, and serum BUN and osmolality provide the critical information for making an etiologic diagnosis.

REFERENCES
1. Berry PL, Belsha CW: Hyponatremia, *Pediatr Clin North Am* 37:35, 1990.
2. Cronan KM, Norman ME: Renal and electrolyte emergencies. In Fleisher GR, Ludwig SL (eds): *Textbook of pediatric emergency medicine*, ed 3, Baltimore, 1993, Williams & Wilkins.
3. Gruskin AB, Sarnaik A: Hyponatremia: pathophysiology and treatment—a pediatric perspective, *Pediatr Nephrol* 6:280, 1992.
4. Wood EG, Lynch RE: Fluids and electrolyte balance. In Fuhrman BP, Zimmerman JJ (eds): *Pediatric critical care*, ed 2, St Louis, 1998, Mosby.
Author: **Elise van der Jagt, M.D.**

II

BASIC INFORMATION

DEFINITIONS
- *Hypothermia* is a reduction of core body temperature to 35° C (89° F) or lower. Hypothermia may be divided into mild (core temperature 32° to 35° C), moderate (28° to 32° C), and severe (less than 28° C).
- *Frostbite* is the actual freezing of tissue and may be divided into superficial and deep forms.

SYNONYMS
Cold injury (a general term encompassing hypothermia, frostbite, frostnip, immersion foot [trench foot], chilblains [pernio])

ICD-9CM CODES
991.0 Frostbite of the face
991.1 Frostbite of the hand
991.2 Frostbite of the foot
991.3 Frostbite of the other/unspecified
991.4 Immersion foot
991.5 Chilblains
991.6 Hypothermia
991.8 Other specified effects of reduced temperature
991.9 Other unspecified effects of reduced temperature

ETIOLOGY
- Hypothermia and frostbite are the result of exposure to conditions resulting in excessive heat loss. This may be a body of water, such as with near-drowning.
- Hypothermia may also be the result of abnormal control of body temperature, seen in such conditions as sepsis, hypothyroidism, hypopituitarism, and hypoadrenalism.
- Infants are at relatively higher risk for hypothermia, as are those with an immature or inappropriate behavioral response to the cold.
- Hypothermia and frostbite may be the result of inflicted injury (child abuse), such as punishment by cold exposure, or neglect.

EPIDEMIOLOGY & DEMOGRAPHICS
- Hypothermia and frostbite are often associated with outdoor activities.
- They may complicate an injury, especially multiple trauma and near-drowning.
- The homeless are at increased risk, as are those with mental illness or intoxication.
- Frostbite is more common in males, probably reflecting behavioral rather than biologic differences.

HISTORY
- Usually obvious: exposure to cold environment
Hypothermia
- The diagnosis of hypothermia may be missed, especially in association with other injury, such as multiple trauma.
- More subtle complaints include dizziness, confusion or poor judgment, mood changes, or irritability.
- Hypothermia may present with unresponsiveness, coma, or cardiac arrest of unknown origin.
Frostbite
- Initial complaints of frostbite include a feeling of cold and thickness, usually in an extremity, which then becomes associated with numbness. At this point, the injury is termed *frostnip;* rewarming causes tingling in the affected area and prevents permanent injury.
- Frostnip progresses to frostbite if the area is not rewarmed. As sensation diminishes, numbness and cold are replaced with a feeling of clumsiness or absence of the limb.

PHYSICAL EXAMINATION
Hypothermia
- Accurate temperature recording may be problematic because many thermometers do not accurately record low body temperatures.
  1. Ideally, use a rectal thermometer designed for a wide range of temperatures, the end of which should not be buried in cold stool.
  2. Bladder or esophageal temperature probes may also be used.
- Bradycardia or other dysrhythmias are common in moderate to severe hypothermia.
- Bradypnea may be appropriate because metabolic demands are diminished.
- Coma and apparent lifelessness, including absent cardiac activity and respiratory effort, may be present in severe hypothermia.
- At 34° to 35° C, vigorous shivering is seen. Shivering ceases below 30° to 32° C, as glycogen stores are depleted (may occur earlier in small children).
- Central nervous system changes, such as amnesia and dysarthria, develop as core temperature falls below 33° C. These progress to ataxia, apathy, and stupor as temperature continues to fall.
Frostbite
- Superficial injury: waxy, edematous skin, may be erythematous, with firm white plaques and decreased sensation. Clear blisters form, which reach the distal portion of the affected extremity.

- Deep injury: absent sensation and hemorrhagic blister formation occur.

DIAGNOSIS

DIFFERENTIAL DIAGNOSIS
- *Immersion foot* (trench foot) is the result of prolonged exposure to cold, wet conditions. Its course and treatment are generally similar to those of frostbite.
- *Chilblains* (pernio) are localized skin changes, such as erythema, cyanosis, plaques, and nodules, as a result of chronic cold exposure. Treatment is supportive.

DIAGNOSTIC WORKUP
- Frostbite and mild hypothermia do not require diagnostic testing.
Moderate to severe hypothermia
- Arterial blood gas reflects overall acid-base and respiratory status.
- Rapid glucose determination: Hypoglycemia may precipitate or complicate hypothermia.
- Check complete blood count with platelet count.
- Prothrombin time/partial thromboplastin time and fibrinogen level may reveal disseminated intravascular coagulation. Low fibrinogen is associated with poorer outcomes.
- Electrolyte panel: Serum potassium higher than 10 mEq/L predicts a poor outcome.
- Electrocardiogram (ECG) and continuous cardiorespiratory monitoring are important:
  1. ECG may show a characteristic J or "Osborne" wave, a positive deflection immediately following the R wave.
  2. Dysrhythmias are commonly seen in severely hypothermic patients.
  3. Atrial dysrhythmias are often benign.
  4. Asystole or ventricular fibrillation may be present.
- Consider a toxicology screen, cervical spine imaging, and a chest radiograph.

THERAPY

- Treatment of hypothermia takes priority over treatment of frostbite!
- Carefully remove cold, wet clothing; wet skin should be carefully dried.
Hypothermia
- Although the patient may appear lifeless, resuscitative efforts, including cardiopulmonary resuscitation (CPR), should generally be continued until the temperature is at least 30° to 32° C.

- Severely hypothermic patients should be handled gently because even minor jostling may precipitate dysrhythmias.
- Obtunded or unresponsive patients should undergo gentle endotracheal intubation.
- Asystole or ventricular fibrillation should be treated with CPR.
  1. Defibrillation of the hypothermic patient is often ineffective but may be attempted.
- Intravenous (IV) drugs are generally ineffective at temperatures below 30° C.
  1. Bretylium is probably the most effective drug for treatment of ventricular fibrillation in hypothermia.
     a. The dose is not well tested.
     b. The usual recommendation is 5 mg/kg by rapid infusion.
     c. If no response, a second dose of 10 mg/kg may be given.
- Mild hypothermia requires external rewarming.
  1. Passive rewarming: Provide a warm environment and insulated blankets.
  2. Active rewarming: Initiate truncal application of warm packs or warmed blankets.
  3. Avoid thermal injury to damaged skin.
- Moderate hypothermia requires core rewarming.
  1. Warmed (42° to 44° C) IV fluids are given to replace cold-induced diuresis and third-spacing.
  2. Warm (40° to 42° C), humidified oxygen is provided.
  3. Consider warm peritoneal, gastric, bladder, rectal, and/or thoracic lavage.
- Severe hypothermia requires cardiopulmonary bypass with extracorporeal rewarming, as well as warmed oxygen and IV fluids.
- Hypoglycemia should be treated with IV glucose.

- If sepsis is suspected, broad-spectrum antibiotics should be administered.
- Endocrine insufficiency may require hormonal supplementation.

Frostbite
- Rubbing or application of snow should be avoided.
- Do not use hair dryers or heaters.
- Rapidly rewarm by immersion of extremity in warm (38° to 43° C) water bath, usually for 20 to 30 minutes, longer if fully frozen. This therapy should be delayed until core body temperature is at least 32° C.
- Clear blisters should be debrided, but hemorrhagic blisters should be left intact.
- Tetanus immunization status should be updated if necessary.
- Wound infection is common; consider administration of broad-spectrum antibiotics.
- Intense pain on rewarming is common; analgesia will be needed.
- Amputation should be delayed until devitalized tissue is clearly demarcated.

■ **FOLLOW-UP & DISPOSITION**
- Patients with moderate-severe hypothermia or deep frostbite may be best managed at a pediatric referral center with critical care, burn unit, and surgical support.
- Frostbite may affect growth plates, leading to bone growth abnormalities, requiring orthopedic referral. Sensory changes, including increased sensitivity to cold, may be lifelong.

■ **PREVENTIVE TREATMENT**
- Appropriate clothing should be worn, and drugs and alcohol should be avoided when cold exposure is anticipated.
- Eyes, testicles, and nipples should be protected to prevent frostbite of these sensitive areas.

☼ PEARLS & CONSIDERATIONS

■ **CLINICAL PEARLS**
- "No one is dead until he or she is warm and dead."
- External active rewarming should be applied to the trunk only, avoiding extremities.
- External rewarming of the moderately to severely hypothermic patient may make matters *worse*.
- *Avoid* gradual rewarming of frostbitten extremities because further tissue damage may result. Partial thawing followed by refreezing is even worse.
- When giving warmed (42° to 44° C) IV fluids, avoid lactate, which is poorly metabolized by the hypothermic liver.
  1. Normal saline or D_5NS is preferred.
  2. To warm, place a 1-L bag in the microwave for 1 to 2 minutes on "high" setting and mix thoroughly.

■ **WEBSITES**
- Hypothermia: Islandnet.com: www.islandnet.com/sarbc/hypo.html
- For parents: KidsHealth: www.kidshealth.org/parent/firstaid/frostbite.html

REFERENCES
1. Decker W: Hypothermia. In Adler J (ed): *Emedicine: emergency medicine,* Boston, 1998, Boston Medical Publishing, www.emedicine.com/emerg/topic279.html.
2. Hofstrand HJ: Accidental hypothermia and frostbite. In Barkin RM (ed): *Pediatric emergency medicine: concepts and clinical practice,* ed 2, St Louis, 1997, Mosby.
3. Mechem CC: Frostbite. In Adler J (ed): *Emedicine: emergency medicine,* Boston, 1998, Boston Medical Publishing, www.emedicine.com/emerg/topic279.html.
Author: **Gregory P. Conners, M.D., M.P.H.**

BASIC INFORMATION

■ DEFINITION

Hypothyroidism is an abnormally low level of circulating thyroid hormones (T_4 and T_3) resulting in clinical manifestations of hypometabolism.

■ SYNONYMS

- Congenital
  1. Cretinism
     a. Old term used to describe clinical constellation of mental and physical developmental delays resulting from untreated congenital hypothyroidism
- Acquired hypothyroidism (immune mediated)
  1. Hashimoto thyroiditis
  2. Autoimmune thyroiditis
  3. Chronic lymphocytic thyroiditis

ICD-9CM CODES

243   Congenital hypothyroidism
245.2 Hashimoto thyroiditis

■ ETIOLOGY

- Congenital
  1. Thyroid gland dysgenesis occurs sporadically. The cause is unknown; it is sometimes associated with an ectopic gland.
  2. Fifteen percent have a hormonogenesis defect inherited in an autosomal recessive pattern.
- Acquired
  1. Hashimoto thyroiditis is a T-cell autoimmune-mediated destruction of the thyroid gland.
  2. Other nonautoimmune forms of hypothyroidism include the following:
     a. Exposure to neck irradiation
     b. Neck surgery
     c. Low dietary iodine
     d. Excessive intake of goitrogens (Brassica family of vegetables)
     e. Antithyroid medications (propylthiouracil [PTU], methimazole)

■ EPIDEMIOLOGY & DEMOGRAPHICS

- Congenital: 1 in 4,000 births, usually sporadic except in dyshormonogenesis
- Autoimmune: 1.2% in U.S. teenagers, with peak incidence in early to mid puberty
- Female:male ratio: 2:1 in adolescence (compared to 10:1 in adults)

■ HISTORY

- Symptoms of clinical hypothyroidism include the following:
  1. Poor energy level
  2. Constipation
  3. Cold intolerance
  4. Weight gain
  5. Reduced appetite
  6. Paleness
- Thyroid enlargement may be noted, especially in Hashimoto thyroiditis.
- In infants:
  1. Delayed development and poor growth if untreated
  2. Hypothyroid infants often described as "good babies" because of reduced crying

■ PHYSICAL EXAMINATION

- Signs of clinical hypothyroidism
  1. Infants
     a. Poor linear growth
     b. Poor weight gain
     c. Relative bradycardia
     d. Large anterior and posterior fontanelles
     e. Large tongue
     f. Hoarse cry
     g. Umbilical hernia
     h. Facial puffiness
     i. Jaundice (unconjugated hyperbilirubinemia)
     j. Feeding difficulties
  2. Newborn period: signs may be subtle or absent
  3. Children and adolescents
     a. Poor linear growth
     b. Bradycardia
     c. Excessive weight gain (rarely extreme)
     d. Dry skin
     e. Paleness
     f. Lethargy
     g. Slow relaxation phase of deep tendon reflexes (test at Achilles)
- Thyroid examination
  1. Congenital
     a. Usually no thyroid tissue palpable
     b. Goiter in 15% with dyshormonogenesis
  2. Hashimoto
     a. Goiter with cobblestone surface (bosselation)
     b. May have no palpable tissue if late in process
     c. Initially, gland may be smooth and soft but later becomes firm or hard

DIAGNOSIS

■ DIFFERENTIAL DIAGNOSIS

- Primary (thyroid underactivity)
  1. Acquired
     a. Hashimoto thyroiditis (chronic lymphocytic thyroiditis)
     b. Iodine deficiency
     c. Iatrogenic radiation-induced hypothyroidism
     d. Surgical removal
  2. Congenital
     a. Transient hypothyroidism from transplacental passage of maternal blocking antibodies (maternal autoimmune thyroid disease)
     b. Transient from maternal use of antithyroid medications (PTU or methimazole)

■ DIAGNOSTIC WORKUP

- Thyroid function tests in both congenital and acquired forms include the following:
  1. Thyroid-stimulating hormone (TSH) alone is generally sufficient for screening for primary (thyroid) hypothyroidism and should be elevated, often markedly.
  2. Free (or total) T_4 should also be measured if a secondary (pituitary) or tertiary (hypothalamic) pathologic condition is suspected or possible.
     a. TSH will be low in secondary or tertiary hypothyroid states.
     b. Therefore it is not useful as a sole test in this situation.
  3. Antithyroid antibodies (antithyroglobulin and antimicrosomal [antiperoxidase]) are helpful in confirming the autoimmune nature of thyroiditis in acquired hypothyroidism.
- Newborn screening programs using dried blood spots collected at 24 to 48 hours of age are now routine in almost all industrialized countries.
  1. In the United States, the primary screen most commonly measures TSH values in all infants.
  2. Infants with TSH above a certain cut-off value then have total T_4 measured.
  3. These programs, initiated in the 1970s, have dramatically reduced the incidence of mental retardation associated with unrecognized congenital hypothyroidism because hypothyroid infants were rarely diagnosed clinically before several months of age.
- Thyroid scan (^{99m}Technetium or 123-Iodine) or, alternatively, ultrasound in congenital hypothyroidism, is used to detect ectopic gland.
  1. This is not needed in all babies because treatment will be instituted based on thyroid function test results.
- Ultrasound is generally not needed in acquired hypothyroidism from Hashimoto thyroiditis, but it is often obtained in patients presenting with goiter.
  1. In this case, ultrasound may be read as "multinodular goiter" corresponding to intrathyroidal lymphoid follicles typical of a gland with Hashimoto's thyroiditis.

℞ THERAPY

■ NONPHARMACOLOGIC
None, except for dietary iodine supplementation in areas where endemic goiters occur as a result of nutritional iodine deficiency

■ MEDICAL
- Synthetic L-thyroxine (e.g., Synthroid, Levoxyl) is dosed at 75 to 100 $\mu g/m^2$/day for children and adolescents.
  1. The initial dose in congenital hypothyroidism is L-thyroxine 10 to 15 $\mu g/kg$/day.
- T_3, or triiodothyronine (e.g., Cytomel), is used only in special circumstances.
- Desiccated thyroid preparations are antiquated.
  1. There is no good clinical evidence that combinations of T_4 and T_3, as found in desiccated preparations, are superior to T_4 alone.

■ FOLLOW-UP & DISPOSITION
- Congenital hypothyroidism requires very close follow-up with frequent thyroid function testing.
  1. The American Academy of Pediatrics and the American Thyroid Association recommend repeat T_4 and TSH levels on the following schedule:
     a. 2 and 4 weeks after initiation of therapy
     b. Every 1 to 2 months during the first year of life
     c. Every 2 to 3 months from age 1 year to 3 years
     d. Then every 3 to 12 months until growth is completed
     e. After 2 to 3 years of age, a trial off therapy can be tried for infants believed to have had transient hypothyroidism
- Acquired hypothyroidism can usually be managed adequately by remeasuring TSH and free T_4 at 4 to 6 weeks after initiation of therapy (and after dose changes), and then every 6 months during the growing years, or every 12 months in older adolescents.

■ PATIENT/FAMILY EDUCATION
- Thyroid replacement should ideally be taken on an empty stomach and not be taken with iron or soy products.
- Missed doses can be made up by doubling the dose the next day.
- Any change in clinical status in a patient receiving replacement therapy suggestive of hypothyroidism or hyperthyroidism should prompt communication with the physician and repeat thyroid function tests.

■ PREVENTIVE TREATMENT
- Iodine supplementation (usually in salt) effectively prevents hypothyroidism resulting from iodine deficiency in persons living in iodine-deficient areas.
- In families with multiple first-degree relatives with autoimmune thyroid disease, screening with TSH and anti-thyroid antibodies may identify affected children early in course of disease.

■ REFERRAL INFORMATION
- All patients with severe congenital hypothyroidism should be managed, if possible, by a pediatric endocrinologist in the first several years of life because of the possibility of developmental problems if not treated optimally.
- Uncomplicated cases of Hashimoto's thyroiditis can generally be treated in the primary care setting by physicians familiar with thyroid replacement therapy.

☼ PEARLS & CONSIDERATIONS

■ CLINICAL PEARLS
- Soy formula can significantly impede thyroid hormone absorption and should be avoided.

- Newborn infants who have a sibling with congenital hypothyroidism should not have thyroid function tests drawn in the first 24 hours of life, despite common parental desire.
  1. The postnatal surge in TSH immediately after birth complicates interpretation of thyroid function tests at this age.
- Because of the wide range of normal free or total T_4 values and the sensitivity of TSH to small changes in thyroid hormone levels, an individual with an elevated TSH can be hypothyroid despite normal population range thyroid hormone levels.

■ WEBSITES
- The MAGIC Foundation: www.magicfoundation.org/congthyr.html; good resource for parents regarding congenital hypothyroidism
- Thyroid Disease Manager: www.thyroidmanager.org/Chapter15/15-4.htm; outstanding site with exhaustive up-to-date online textbook on all aspects of thyroid disease
- Thyroid Foundation of America: www.allthyroid.org; good general link for patient and physician
- The Thyroid Society: www.the-thyroid-society.org/med_letter2.html; short article for parents

REFERENCES
1. Brown R, Larsen PR: Thyroid gland development and disease in infancy and childhood. In DeGroot LJ, Hennemann G (eds): *The thyroid and its diseases*, 1999. Online text www.thyroidmanager.org/Chapter15/15-frame.htm.
2. Fisher DA: Hypothyroidism, *Pediatr Rev* 15:227, 1994.
3. Foley TP Jr: Disorders of the thyroid in children. In Sperling MA (ed): *Pediatric endocrinology*, Philadelphia, 1996, WB Saunders.
4. Rapaport R: Congenital hypothyroidism: expanding the spectrum, *J Pediatr* 136:10, 2000.
Author: **Craig Orlowski, M.D.**

BASIC INFORMATION

■ DEFINITION
Thrombocytopenia is caused by antibody-mediated destruction of platelets. Children typically present with signs and symptoms of mucocutaneous bleeding. Immune thrombocytopenic purpura (ITP) can be acute (resolves within 6 months) or chronic (persists longer than 6 months).

■ SYNONYMS
- Idiopathic thrombocytopenic purpura
- Autoimmune thrombocytopenic purpura
- Werlhof's disease

ICD-9CM CODE
287.3 Immune thrombocytopenic purpura

■ ETIOLOGY
- Antibody-mediated destruction of platelets occurs.
- Antibody-coated platelets are removed by the reticuloendothelial system, especially the spleen.
- Acute ITP is associated with a recent viral illness in two thirds of cases.
  1. Acute ITP can be caused by specific viral infections, such as Epstein-Barr virus (EBV), human immunodeficiency virus (HIV), or varicella.
- Many children with chronic ITP have autoantibody to platelet antigens, such as glycoprotein (GP) IIbIIIa or GP IbIX, and thus have true autoimmune disease.
- ITP is associated with other autoimmune disorders, such as lupus, Evans' syndrome, and antiphospholipid antibody syndrome.
- ITP may be caused by certain medications: carbamazepine, valproate, quinidine, heparin.
- ITP is also associated with recent vaccinations (e.g., MMR, DPT)

■ EPIDEMIOLOGY & DEMOGRAPHICS
- The peak age of acute ITP is 2 to 4 years, but it can occur at any age.
- The annual incidence is 4 to 8 per 100,000 population.
- The male:female ratio is 1:1 in childhood and 1:3 in adolescence.
- A slight increase occurs in winter and spring.
- Most cases in children (80% to 90%) resolve within 6 to 12 months.
- Chronic ITP is more common in children older than 10 years (especially girls) and younger than 1 year of age.

■ HISTORY
- A relatively short history (days to weeks) of easy bruising and/or petechiae is reported in a child who is otherwise healthy.
- Minimal or no trauma is associated with bruises.
- Less commonly, children present with epistaxis, prolonged menses, hematuria, or gastrointestinal bleeding.
- Two thirds of children have a history of an antecedent viral illness in the month before presentation.
- No other systemic or constitutional illnesses are present.

■ PHYSICAL EXAMINATION
- General: well-appearing child, normal vital signs
- Skin
  1. Bruises (large and small)
  2. Sometimes palpable hematomas
  3. Petechiae
- Mucus membranes: palatal petechiae, subconjunctival or retinal hemorrhage
- No lymphadenopathy or hepatosplenomegaly

DIAGNOSIS

■ DIFFERENTIAL DIAGNOSIS
- For the underlying cause of ITP, see "Etiology."
  1. Autoimmune: systemic lupus erythematosus (SLE), antiphospholipid antibody syndrome, Evans' syndrome
  2. Infection: HIV, EBV, varicella
  3. Medications: carbamazepine, quinidine, valproate, heparin
- Other causes of thrombocytopenia include the following:
  1. Bone marrow disorders: thrombocytopenia-absent radii syndrome, aplastic anemias, leukemias, Wiskott-Aldrich disease
  2. Platelet disorders: type IIB von Willebrand disease, Bernard-Soulier syndrome, giant platelet syndromes
  3. Neonatal thrombocytopenia, alloimmune thrombocytopenia
  4. Medications: sulfonamides
  5. Other: hemolytic uremic syndrome, disseminated intravascular coagulation, thrombotic thrombocytopenic purpura, Kasabach-Merritt syndrome (cavernous hemangioma)
- Other causes of bleeding include von Willebrand disease, nonsteroidal antiinflammatory drugs (NSAIDs), trauma, abuse, hemophilias, and liver disease.

■ DIAGNOSTIC WORKUP
- Made on the basis of the history, physical examination, and limited laboratory studies: a well-appearing child with a brief history of bruising, petechiae, and/or bleeding who has an isolated profound thrombocytopenia and no other hematologic or other laboratory abnormalities
- Complete blood count, differential, platelet count, reticulocyte count
- Prothrombin time, activated partial thromboplastin time
- Peripheral blood smear to look at platelet size and number, red blood cell and white blood cell morphology
- Erythrocyte sedimentation rate
- Tests of liver and renal function, urinalysis
- Optional: Coombs' test, antinuclear antibodies, IgG, IgA, IgM
- Bone marrow aspirate (optional): recommended in the thrombocytopenic child who has anemia and/or leukopenia, the child who has hepatosplenomegaly, or a child with presumed ITP who will be treated with glucocorticoids

THERAPY

- The decision to treat and what to treat with is based primarily on the extent of bleeding and the platelet count.
- The child's desired level of activity and family concerns and wishes should be considered.

■ NONPHARMACOLOGIC
- Observation: Because there is a high rate of spontaneous recovery (50% to 75% within 1 month of diagnosis), selected children with minimal signs of bleeding and platelet counts higher than 10,000/mm^3 can be observed.
  1. Children should not be given NSAIDs.
  2. They should not participate in contact sports or activities that put them at risk of head trauma.

■ MEDICAL
- Treatment is indicated for any patient with active bleeding, extensive bruising or petechiae, or a very low platelet count (e.g., less than 10,000/mm^3).
- Treatment of asymptomatic patients with low (less than 20,000/mm^3) platelet counts is controversial.
- Prednisone is given at 2 mg/kg/day divided twice a day orally.
  1. In general, a bone marrow aspirate is done first.
     a. This is done to ensure that no leukemia is present.
     b. Prednisone partially treats and could mask an early diagnosis of leukemia.
  2. Taper over 1 to 4 weeks to maintain the platelet count in a safe range (20,000 to 50,000) with no evidence of bleeding.

3. Toxicity for short-term use includes mood changes, increased appetite, weight gain, hypertension, and diabetes.
- Anti-D antibody (WinRho) is dosed at 50 μg/kg and given intravenously over 3 to 5 minutes.
  1. This treatment is effective only in Rh-positive children.
  2. The platelet count rises in a few days and drops again in 2 to 3 weeks.
  3. Toxicity includes anemia, chills, and headache.
- Intravenous gamma globulin (IVIG) is dosed at 1 g/kg and given intravenously over 6 to 12 hours.
  1. This treatment is most effective in quickly raising the platelet count (24 to 72 hours).
  2. Treatment usually requires admission to the hospital.
  3. The platelet count remains elevated for 3 to 4 weeks.
  4. More than 50% of children develop headaches, vomiting, and fever.
  5. Allergic reaction and blood product–associated infections are two risks.

■ SURGICAL
- Splenectomy is reserved for children older than 5 years of age with severe ITP refractory to, or only transiently responsive to, medical therapies beyond 12 months.
  1. ITP permanently resolves in 70% to 80% of children after splenectomy.
  2. The risks of splenectomy include surgical and anesthesia complications and postsplenectomy sepsis.

■ FOLLOW-UP & DISPOSITION
- The aforementioned therapies do not cure ITP, but they are effective in temporarily controlling it.

- ITP resolves within 1 month of diagnosis in 50% of children, within 6 months in 75%, and within 12 months in 90%.
- The likelihood of life-threatening hemorrhage, such as a central nervous system hemorrhage, is less than 1%.
- Patients should be followed closely by their pediatrician and pediatric hematologist/oncologist until the platelet count is consistently within the normal range.
  1. Decisions regarding ongoing therapy depend on the extent of bleeding, the platelet count, and the child's desired level of activity.
  2. Children with ongoing thrombocytopenia should be periodically reevaluated for autoimmune diseases such as SLE, Evans' syndrome, or the antiphospholipid antibody syndrome.

■ PATIENT/FAMILY EDUCATION
- ITP is a self-limited disease with a low likelihood of recurrence.
- ITP is not cancer or leukemia and is not associated with and does not lead to cancer.
- Children with ITP must avoid activities that put them at risk of head trauma and should not take medications that increase their risk of bleeding, especially NSAIDs.
- In most instances, children with ITP can continue to attend school or day care.

■ REFERRAL INFORMATION
Children with thrombocytopenia should be referred to a pediatric hematologist/oncologist.

✪ PEARLS & CONSIDERATIONS

■ CLINICAL PEARLS
- Platelets are large on the peripheral blood film of children with ITP.
- Children with ITP may have bruises in unusual places (e.g., inner thighs, axillae).
- Splenomegaly and lymphadenopathy are *not* seen in ITP and suggest another illness.

■ WEBSITES
- National Institute of Diabetes & Digestive & Kidney Diseases: www.niddk.nih.gov/health/hematol/pubs/itp/itp.htm
- UltraNet Communications, Inc.: www.ultranet.com/itpsoc/

■ SUPPORT GROUPS
The ITP Society, Contact a Family (www.cafamily.org.uk)

REFERENCES
1. Beardsley DS, Nathan DG: Platelet abnormalities in infancy and childhood. In Nathan DG, Orkin SH (eds): *Nathan and Oski's hematology of infancy and childhood,* ed 5, Philadelphia, 1998, WB Saunders.
2. George J et al: Idiopathic thrombocytopenic purpura: a practice guideline developed by explicit methods for the American Society of Hematology, *J Am Soc Hematol* 88:3, 1996.
3. Medeiros D, Buchanan G: Current controversies in the management of idiopathic thrombocytopenic purpura during childhood, *Pediatr Clin North Am* 43:757, 1996.
4. Murphy S, Nepo A, Sills R: Thrombocytopenia, *Pediatr Rev* 20:64, 1999.
Authors: **Matthew Richardson, M.D., and David N. Korones, M.D.**

BASIC INFORMATION

■ DEFINITION
Impetigo is a highly contagious superficial skin infection largely affecting infants and children.

ICD-9CM CODE
684 Impetigo

■ ETIOLOGY
- The upper epidermis is invaded by pathogenic *Staphylococcus aureus* or group A streptococcus *(Streptococcus pyogenes)*
- Microscopic breaks (such as trauma from scratching) in the epidermal barrier increase the risk of infection.

■ EPIDEMIOLOGY & DEMOGRAPHICS
- Colonization of the skin with the pathogens precedes clinical lesions by several days to months.
- Penicillinase-producing staphylococci represent an increasing proportion of impetigo in children in the United States.
- A high transmission rate is enhanced by crowded conditions and low socioeconomic environments.

■ HISTORY
- The patient may report a history of recent trauma to the skin, such as insect bite, varicella, eczema, or a superficial abrasion.
- Constitutional symptoms (e.g., fever) are unusual.

■ PHYSICAL EXAMINATION
- Impetigo begins as small vesicles that easily unroof, progressing to a "honey-crusted" appearance with serous drainage on an erythematous base.
- The face and extremities are the most common sites of involvement.
- *Bullous impetigo* refers to lesions that have transparent, fragile, flaccid bullae or an outer rim of desquamation where bullae have ruptured.

🔬 DIAGNOSIS

■ DIFFERENTIAL DIAGNOSIS
- Nummular dermatitis
- Herpes simplex infections
- Contact dermatitis
- Kerion

■ DIAGNOSTIC WORKUP
- The workup is based on clinical findings.
- Routine culture of the lesions is not indicated. Cultures may be obtained on those lesions that do not respond to standard therapy.

💊 THERAPY

■ MEDICAL
- Antimicrobial should cover both *S. aureus* and group A streptococcus.
- Uncomplicated, localized impetigo may be treated topically.
  1. Bacitracin or mupirocin ointment three times a day for 7 to 10 days
- Widespread impetigo is usually treated systemically.
  1. Dicloxacillin 15 to 50 mg/kg/day (four times per day) or cephalexin 40 mg/kg/day divided (two to four times per day) for 5 to 10 days
  2. Alternative: erythromycin; however, many resistant staphylococcal strains exist

■ FOLLOW-UP & DISPOSITION
Extensive cases should be reevaluated at the end of therapy to determine response to therapy.

■ PATIENT/FAMILY EDUCATION
- Good handwashing is important to prevent spreading.
- Children may return to school or day care after a minimum of 24 hours of appropriate therapy.

⚙ PEARLS & CONSIDERATIONS

■ CLINICAL PEARLS
- Bullous impetigo is almost always caused by *S. aureus* and mediated by production of an epidermolytic toxin, so systemic therapy is preferred.
- Nephritogenic strains of streptococci can cause impetigo.
  1. Antimicrobial therapy in these cases does not prevent development of poststreptococcal glomerulonephritis.

■ WEBSITE
- Encyclopedia.com: www. encyclopedia.com/articles/ 06292.html
  1. "Beating Impetigo" for parents
  2. "What Is Impetigo?"

REFERENCES
1. American Academy of Pediatrics: Group A streptococcal infections. In Pickering LK (ed): *2000 Red Book: report of the Committee on Infectious Diseases,* ed 25, Elk Grove Village, Ill, 2000, American Academy of Pediatrics.
2. American Academy of Pediatrics: Staphylococcal infections. In Pickering LK (ed): *2000 Red Book: report of the Committee on Infectious Diseases,* ed 25, Elk Grove Village, Ill, 2000, American Academy of Pediatrics.
3. Jain A, Daum RS: Staphylococcal infection in children: part 1, *Pediatr Rev* 20: 183, 1999.
4. Weston WL, Lane AT, Morelli JG: *Color textbook of pediatric dermatology,* ed 2, St Louis, 1996, Mosby.
Author: **Kristen Smith Danielson, M.D.**

BASIC INFORMATION

■ DEFINITION

- Inflammatory bowel disease (IBD) includes chronic, idiopathic inflammatory disorders of the gastrointestinal (GI) tract. IBD is generally divided into ulcerative colitis (UC) and Crohn's disease (CD), although overlap does exist.
- UC is inflammation that is restricted to the colon and that almost universally begins in the rectum, extending variable distances proximally without any "skip" areas. Inflammation is limited to the mucosa.
- CD is inflammation that can involve any part of the GI tract from the mouth to the anus. Inflammation is transmural.

■ SYNONYMS

- CD
  1. Ileocolitis
  2. Terminal ileitis
  3. Granulomatous enterocolitis
- UC
  1. Ulcerative proctitis (limited to the rectum)
  2. Pancolitis (involving the entire colon)

ICD-9CM CODES

555.9 Crohn's disease
556.9 Ulcerative colitis

■ ETIOLOGY

- Although the pathogenesis of IBD is still unknown, there is a genetic predisposition involving dysregulation of the immune response to an environmental trigger.
  1. Either an appropriate immunologic response to an exogenous trigger that is not subsequently downregulated or an inappropriate mucosal immune response to normal luminal (endogenous) stimuli
- Genetics may also play a role.
  1. Most likely, several genes are involved.
  2. Current interest has focused on loci on chromosomes 12 and 16.
  3. There are several different types of CD and UC that may be related to different underlying gene defects.
  4. There is an association with class II alleles of the HLA complex, which is different for UC and CD.
- The precise mechanisms of immune dysregulation leading to the chronic intestinal inflammation have not been elucidated.
- There are a number of different proposed triggers, both endogenous and exogenous.
  1. Infections
  2. Food antigens
  3. Medications that effect mucosal barrier: nonsteroidal antiinflammatory drugs (NSAIDs)
  4. Normal bacterial flora
- Despite some similarities, UC and CD appear to be different diseases.
  1. In UC, mucosal inflammation involves only the colon and almost universally begins in the rectum. The inflammation can involve varying distances from just the rectum to the entire colon.
  2. In CD, transmural inflammation can involve any part of the GI tract from mouth to anus.
     a. Most common site of involvement is the terminal ileum (TI) and cecum/right colon.
     b. There is a higher incidence of upper GI tract involvement in children than in adults.
     c. CD can be limited to the colon, and in these cases, it may be difficult to differentiate from UC (indeterminate colitis).
     d. The transmural inflammation in CD contributes to some of the complications of the disease.
        (1) Fistulas
        (2) Abscesses
        (3) Small bowel obstruction
        (4) Intestinal perforation

■ EPIDEMIOLOGY & DEMOGRAPHICS

- Incidence/prevalence of IBD
  1. In the United States, the prevalence of IBD is estimated to be approximately 100 cases per 100,000 population, and the annual incidence is 2 and 6 cases per 100,000 for UC and CD, respectively.
  2. There is an increased incidence in the following:
     a. Jewish population
     b. Developed countries and northern climates
  3. Incidence is low in Hispanics and African Americans.
- Age
  1. IBD can present at any age, although most have onset of symptoms between the ages of 15 and 40 years (peak between 15 and 25 years).
  2. Approximately 25% of new cases of IBD are diagnosed in individuals younger than 20 years of age.
  3. IBD has been diagnosed in infants and children younger than 5 years of age, although this is uncommon.
- Gender
  1. The male:female ratio is 1:1.
- Morbidity/mortality
  1. Although these diseases can be associated with significant morbidity, longevity is not significantly decreased.
- Genetic factors
  1. Positive family history is the greatest risk factor.
  2. Approximately 10% to 25% of patients have a first-degree relative with IBD.
  3. There is usually concordance for the same type of IBD within sibships.
- Environmental factors
  1. Smoking exacerbates CD but ameliorates UC.
  2. Increased incidence of IBD in developed countries and in northern climates regardless of race or ethnicity suggests an environmental contribution.
  3. Early life events, including frequent infections, have been associated with the development of IBD.
- Cancer risk
  1. Patients with IBD are at increased risk for GI malignancies.
  2. In UC, the risk of developing adenocarcinoma begins to increase about 10 years after diagnosis.
     a. Patients with pancolitis are at particular risk.
     b. Surveillance colonoscopy is recommended after 7 to 10 years' disease duration.
  3. Patients with Crohn's colitis also appear to be at an increased risk for colorectal cancer.
     a. There is also an increased frequency of intestinal lymphomas in CD.

■ HISTORY

- Family history may be positive for IBD.
- Symptoms vary by disease type and region of bowel involved.
- In CD:
  1. Abdominal pain
     a. Epigastric (upper GI tract involvement)
     b. Right lower quadrant (terminal ileum/cecum involvement)
     c. Crampy, lower abdominal, relieved by bowel movement (colonic involvement)
  2. Diarrhea
  3. Hematochezia
  4. Fatigue
  5. Anorexia, weight loss
  6. Nausea, vomiting
  7. Systemic symptoms
     a. Fever, arthralgias, night sweats
- In UC:
  1. Abdominal pain
     a. Often crampy and relieved by passing a stool
     b. Pain with defecation
  2. Diarrhea
     a. May be associated with urgency and tenesmus
  3. Hematochezia
  4. Fatigue
  5. Anorexia, weight loss
  6. Systemic symptoms
     a. Fever, arthralgias, night sweats

■ PHYSICAL EXAMINATION
- Physical findings vary by disease type and region of bowel involved.
- In CD:
  1. Growth delay, short stature
  2. Weight loss
  3. Right lower quadrant tenderness, mass
  4. Perianal disease
     a. Fissures, skin tags, fistulas
  5. Clubbing
  6. Mouth ulcers
  7. Enterocutaneous fistulae
  8. Hemoccult-positive stool
- In UC:
  1. Weight loss
  2. Abdominal tenderness: diffuse, left lower quadrant
  3. Hemoccult-positive stool
- Both CD and UC may present with extraintestinal signs.
  1. Arthritis
  2. Episcleritis, uveitis
  3. Erythema nodosum, pyoderma gangrenosum

🔬 DIAGNOSIS

■ DIFFERENTIAL DIAGNOSIS
The differential diagnosis will vary with the presenting signs and symptoms and with the age of the patient.
- Abdominal pain without diarrhea
  1. CD
  2. Functional abdominal pain
  3. Irritable bowel syndrome (IBS)
  4. Peptic acid disease
  5. Urinary tract disease (younger children)
  6. Hepatobiliary disease
  7. Pancreatitis (uncommon in children)
- Growth delay
  1. CD
  2. Celiac disease
  3. Endocrinopathy
- Anorexia, weight loss
  1. CD
  2. Anorexia nervosa
- Nonbloody diarrhea
  1. CD or UC
  2. Infection
     a. Bacterial
     b. Parasite
  3. IBS
  4. Celiac disease
  5. Lactose intolerance
  6. Postenteritis enteropathy (younger children)
- Bloody diarrhea
  1. CD or UC
  2. Infection
     a. Bacterial
     b. Parasites
  3. Henoch-Schönlein purpura
  4. Hemolytic uremic syndrome
  5. Ischemic colitis
  6. Allergic colitis (infants, toddlers)

- Rectal bleeding without diarrhea
  1. Proctitis (UC or CD)
  2. Fissure, hemorrhoids
  3. Polyp
  4. Allergic proctitis (infants, toddlers)
  5. Meckel's diverticulum
  6. Solitary rectal ulcer
- Children: can present with extraintestinal manifestations; therefore IBD should be considered in the differential diagnosis of the following:
  1. Arthritis, arthralgias, ankylosing spondylitis
  2. Erythema nodosa, pyoderma gangrenosum
  3. Episcleritis, uveitis
  4. Cholelithiasis, nephrolithiasis (particularly CD)
  5. Primary sclerosing cholangitis (particularly UC)

■ DIAGNOSTIC WORKUP
- Laboratory tests
  1. Stool studies
     a. Culture: *Salmonella, Shigella, Campylobacter, Yersinia*
     b. *Escherichia coli* O157:H7
     c. *Clostridium difficile* toxin (can complicate IBD without antibiotic exposure)
  2. Complete blood count, erythrocyte sedimentation rate, iron studies, albumin
- Diagnostic imaging
  1. Upper GI series with small bowel follow-through (UGI/SBFT)
     a. Diagnostic for small intestinal inflammation
  2. Tagged white blood cell (WBC) scan
     a. Infusion of technetium-labeled WBCs
     b. Identifies sites of small and large bowel inflammation
     c. May help differentiate a fixed stricture from an actively inflamed segment of bowel
     d. Has not yet taken the place of UGI/SBFT as initial diagnostic test for small bowel inflammation
- Endoscopic (tissue diagnosis)
  1. Upper endoscopy (esophagogastroduodenoscopy)
     a. Particularly important for diagnosis of CD in patients with upper GI tract symptoms and evidence of inflammation on UGI
  2. Colonoscopy
     a. Provides tissue diagnosis in most cases of UC and CD involving the colon
        (1) UC: Endoscopically, there is continuous mucosal inflammation. Biopsies show inflammation restricted to the mucosa with crypt abscesses, mucus depletion, and crypt architec-

tural distortion. No inflammation is noted in the TI
        (2) CD: Endoscopically, there may be "skip" areas of inflammation or inflammation restricted to the TI. Biopsies show transmural inflammation, "skip" lesions of inflammation within a single sample, and architectural distortion. Granulomas are pathognomonic for CD but are not always seen.
- In most patients, diagnosis made with the combination of an UGI/SBFT and colonoscopy
  1. Suspicious of CD: start with UGI/SBFT followed by colonoscopy
  2. Suspicious of colitis (CD or UC): start with colonoscopy followed by UGI/SBFT to complete evaluation for small bowel involvement
- Child with nonsevere symptoms
  1. The workup, including stool studies, laboratory tests, and an UGI/SBFT, can be initiated by the pediatrician.

💊 THERAPY

■ NONPHARMACOLOGIC
- Nutritional
  1. Compromised nutrition in IBD; related to several factors
     a. Increased demand
     b. Decreased intake
     c. Malabsorption (in CD)
  2. UC
     a. Nutrition is important but does not serve a therapeutic role.
  3. CD
     a. Nutritional therapy has been shown to have a therapeutic and steroid-sparing effect.
     b. This is usually given in the form of nutritional supplements of semielemental or elemental formulas.
        (1) May need to be administered by nasogastric tube as a continuous overnight infusion

■ MEDICAL
- Steroids
  1. Treatment of moderate to severe disease (both CD and UC) still requires steroids.
  2. The dosage is 1 to 2 mg/kg/day for 3 to 4 weeks, or until symptoms subside.
  3. This is not acceptable maintenance therapy.
  4. Many long-term side effects, including compromised growth velocity and osteopenia, have been reported.

- Aminosalicylate preparations
  1. Oral Azulfidine and the newer 5-ASA (5-aminosalicylate) preparations, including the following:
     a. Asacol, Pentasa, Dipentum
     b. Also come as enemas and suppositories for topical treatment of distal colitis
     c. Side effects: diarrhea and abdominal pain and, in rare cases, a colitis indistinguishable from the underlying disease; nephritis has been reported
  2. Released in the distal small bowel and colon and provide a topical antiinflammatory effect
  3. Used for maintenance therapy in colitis (both UC and CD) and for CD involving the distal small bowel
- Immunosuppressants
  1. 6-Mercaptopurine (6-MP), azathioprine
     a. Used in both CD and UC not controlled by 5-ASA preparations
     b. More commonly used in CD (involving small bowel), in which 5-ASA preparations are less effective
     c. Has steroid-sparing effect and is currently used when patients experience a relapse soon after or during attempts to taper steroids
     d. Side effects: marrow suppression, increased risk of infection, hepatotoxicity, GI symptoms, and pancreatitis
  2. Methotrexate
     a. Has been useful in some patients who do not respond to 6-MP or azathioprine
  3. Cyclosporine (CSA), FK-506 (tacrolimus, Prograf)
     a. These medications have been used in the setting of severe or fulminant colitis in an attempt to avoid colectomy and are currently under investigation for refractory perianal CD.
- Antibiotics
  1. Most commonly used antibiotics: metronidazole and ciprofloxacin
  2. Alter (decrease) small bowel enteric organisms
  3. May ameliorate a flare and avoid use of steroids
  4. Not usually used as first-line maintenance therapy
  5. Used for perianal disease and fistulas in CD
- Infliximab (Remicade)
  1. One of the newer immunobiologics that targets the inflammatory cascade
  2. Chimeric antibodies to tumor necrosis factor-α, one of the cytokines responsible for inducing inflammation, given as an intravenous infusion
  3. Currently approved for treating CD: refractory and fistulizing disease
- Treatment of fulminant colitis/toxic megacolon
  1. Intravenous steroids, broad-spectrum antibiotics, nothing by mouth, total parenteral nutrition
  2. If no improvement in approximately 5 days, intravenous CSA, FK-506, or colectomy
     a. CSA/FK-506 can successfully salvage the colon, but most of these patients will eventually undergo colectomy in the next 1 to 2 years.
  3. Colectomy for complications (e.g., hemorrhage, perforation) or intractable disease unresponsive to intravenous steroids or CSA/FK-506.

■ **SURGICAL**
- CD
  1. Approximately 60% to 75% of patients with CD will eventually require surgery.
  2. Surgery is not curative. In most patients, inflammation recurs, usually at or near the site of anastomosis.
  3. Surgery is indicated for the following:
     a. Complications of CD
        (1) Hemorrhage
        (2) Toxic megacolon, fulminant colitis (not responsive to medical therapy)
        (3) Perforation
        (4) Stricture (resection or stricturoplasty)
     b. Intractable, localized disease
- UC
  1. Approximately 25% to 40% of patients will eventually require surgery.
  2. Colectomy cures UC. Currently, the standard procedure is a proctocolectomy with ileoanal pouch anastomosis.
     a. The colon and rectum are removed, leaving the anal muscles. Any residual rectal mucosa is stripped, and a neorectum or pouch is created from the ileum, which is then anastomosed to the anus (ileoanal pouch anastomosis).
     b. Most common complication is pouchitis (i.e., inflammation in the pouch), which usually responds to antibiotics such as metronidazole or ciprofloxacin.
     c. Approximately 8% to 10% of pouches "fail," requiring permanent ileostomy.
  3. Surgery is indicated for the following:
     a. Intractable hemorrhage
     b. Toxic megacolon, fulminant colitis (not responsive to medical therapy)

     c. Perforation (usually associated with toxic megacolon)
     d. Dysplasia, carcinoma
  4. Outcomes are favorably affected by the surgeon's experience.
  5. Although colectomy cures UC, this is often a difficult decision for patients and families.

■ **REFERRAL INFORMATION**
- Any child with suspected IBD should be referred to a gastroenterologist. Referral to a pediatric gastroenterologist is preferred for infants and children and should also be considered for adolescents younger than 14 to 16 years of age.
- Depending on the severity of the symptoms, referral can be made after screening tests.

■ **PATIENT/FAMILY EDUCATION**
- Parents and patients (depending on their age) should be as knowledgeable about the disease as possible, including medications, side effects, and complications of IBD.
- Educational materials are available through the Crohn's and Colitis Foundation of America (see "Website & Support Group").
- Parents and patients should be encouraged to discuss with their physicians information and potential "treatments" they obtain on Internet sites that are not associated with responsible organizations and in books not published by recognized authorities.
- It is important for patients and families to maintain a relationship with their primary care provider as well as their gastroenterologist.

☼ **PEARLS & CONSIDERATIONS**

■ **CLINICAL PEARLS**
- IBD should be considered in any child who presents with any of the following:
  1. Chronic abdominal pain
  2. Growth delay or compromised weight gain
     a. If a child does not grow between yearly well-child visits, consider CD.
  3. Chronic diarrhea with or without blood
  4. Rectal bleeding
  5. Family history of IBD
  6. Unexplained anemia in an older child or adolescent
- Children may present with extraintestinal manifestations and minimal or no GI symptoms.
- IBD is associated with significant morbidity but does not significantly affect longevity.

- These are chronic disorders requiring ongoing medical therapy and, in many patients, surgical intervention as well. There is often a significant emotional and psychosocial impact on both the patient and the family. Early counseling and support should be provided and encouraged.

■WEBSITE & SUPPORT GROUP

- Crohn's and Colitis Foundation of America (CCFA), 386 Park Avenue South, New York, NY 10016-8804; phone: 212-685-3440; 800-932-2423; fax: 212-779-4098; email: info@ccfa.org; website: www.ccfa.org

REFERENCES

1. Baldassano RN, Piccoli DA: Inflammatory bowel disease in pediatric and adolescent patients, *Gastroenterol Clin North Am* 28:445, 1999.
2. Winesett M: Inflammatory bowel disease in children and adolescents, *Pediatr Ann* 26:227, 1997.

Author: **M. Susan Moyer, M.D.**

BASIC INFORMATION

■ DEFINITION
Influenza is an acute, febrile, respiratory illness caused by infection with influenza virus.

■ SYNONYMS
- Flu
- Influenza-like illness (ILI)

ICD-9CM CODE
487.1 Influenza

■ ETIOLOGY
- Respiratory tract infection with influenza virus (an orthomyxovirus) type A or B
- Influenza A: multiple subtypes designated by hemagglutinin (H) and neuraminidase (N) (e.g., H1N1 or H3N2)
- Influenza B: single subtype
- Influenza C: minor cause of the common cold

■ EPIDEMIOLOGY & DEMOGRAPHICS
- Yearly winter outbreaks from November to April are associated with minor antigenic changes in H or N (antigenic drift).
- Sporadic worldwide severe outbreaks (pandemics) are associated with major antigenic changes in H or N (antigenic shift).
- Approximately 20 million cases occur per year in the United States, with 20,000 to 40,000 excess deaths, mostly in adults.
- Children with heart disease; chronic pulmonary disorders, including asthma; diabetes; renal failure; and immunosuppression are at higher risk for influenza complications.

■ HISTORY
- The presentation is nonspecific.
- Typical features are high fever (more than 102° F), sudden onset, myalgias, malaise, and cough.
- The usual course is 7 to 10 days.

■ PHYSICAL EXAMINATION
- Fever, irritability, lethargy, and pharyngeal erythema without exudate are common.
- Rash is rare.

■ COMPLICATIONS
- Pneumonia, bronchitis, sinusitis, otitis media, and exacerbations of chronic bronchitis or asthma can occur.
- Rare manifestations include encephalitis, myocarditis, and Reye's syndrome.

DIAGNOSIS

■ DIFFERENTIAL DIAGNOSIS
- Must be differentiated from other common acute febrile illnesses
  1. Streptococcal pharyngitis (suggested by presence of exudate)
  2. Bacterial pneumonia (suggested by productive cough, consolidation)
  3. Rhinoviral cold (usually with less fever, more rhinorrhea)

■ DIAGNOSTIC WORKUP
- Viral culture is more than 90% sensitive and 100% specific.
- Optimal specimens are nasal or nasopharyngeal swabs; virus can also be detected in sputum, throat swabs.
- Time to positive culture is 5 to 7 days; shell vial technique can shorten to 24 to 48 hours.
- Rapid antigen detection tests are available in several formats.
  1. Directigen (detects flu A only)
  2. BioStar
  3. Zymtec
- All have levels of sensitivity of between 60% and 90% compared with culture, depending on age group (children are better) and study. Results are available within 30 minutes.
- Polymerase chain reaction: Complexity has generally relegated it to a research tool, but when performed properly, it is highly sensitive and specific.
- Other diagnostic tests are dictated by clinical presentation, such as chest radiograph to rule out pneumonia, throat cultures if group A streptococcus is suspected, and so forth.

THERAPY

■ NONPHARMACOLOGIC
- Fluids
- Bed rest

■ MEDICAL
- Symptomatic
  1. Antipyretics and pain relief (*Note:* Aspirin is contraindicated because of possible Reye's syndrome; nonsteroidal antiinflammatory drugs are acceptable)
- Antiviral
  1. Most studies show reductions in the duration of illness in adults if administered within 48 hours of the onset of symptoms; much less information is available regarding the treatment of children.
- Two classes of drugs available:
  1. M2 inhibitors
  2. Neuraminidase inhibitors

- M2 inhibitors
  1. Amantadine
  2. Rimantadine
     a. Rimantadine is active against influenza A but not influenza B.
     b. It is effective for therapy of influenza A in adults.
     c. Only amantadine is licensed for therapy in children in the United States.
     d. Central nervous system (CNS) and gastrointestinal side effects may occur; CNS effects are especially limiting for amantadine.
- Neuraminidase inhibitors
  1. Zanamivir (Relenza) (inhaled)
  2. Oseltamivir (Tamiflu) (oral)
     a. Active against both influenza A and influenza B viruses
     b. Effective for therapy of influenza in adults.

■ PREVENTIVE TREATMENT
- Annual administration of influenza vaccine is the most effective means available to control influenza.
- Inactivated vaccine dosage is as follows:
  1. Two doses are administered 1 month apart in children 8 years old or younger who have not been previously vaccinated.
  2. All others receive one dose.
  3. Dose is 0.5 ml containing approximately 15 μg of each hemagglutinin (trivalent vaccine, H1, H3, B) intramuscularly.
  4. Children 3 and younger receive 0.25 ml.
- Live attenuated vaccine is effective in children, but not yet licensed as of 2000.

■ REFERRAL INFORMATION
Children who develop Reye's syndrome should be referred to appropriate specialists.

PEARLS & CONSIDERATIONS

■ WEBSITE
Centers for Disease Control and Prevention: www.cdc.gov/ncidod/diseases/flu/fluvirus.htm

REFERENCES
1. Nicholson KG: Human influenza. In Nicholson KG, Webster RG, Hay AJ (eds): *Textbook of influenza,* Oxford, 1998, Blackwell.
2. Treanor JJ: Influenza virus. In Mandell GL, Bennett JE, Dolin R (eds): *Principles and practice of infectious diseases,* New York, 1999, Churchill Livingstone.
Author: **John Treanor, M.D.**

BASIC INFORMATION

■ DEFINITION
The venom from any insect sting causes a reaction that ranges from local inflammation to life-threatening anaphylaxis.

ICD-9CM CODE
989.5 Venomous insect

■ ETIOLOGY
- The Hymenoptera are stinging insects whose venom results in anaphylactic fatalities more often than that of any other animal.
- They are divided into the following three groups:
  1. *Vespids:* wasp, hornet, yellow jacket (individuals can sting multiple times)
  2. *Apids:* bumblebee, honeybee, Africanized "killer" bees (individuals can sting only once)
  3. *Fire ants:* red or black (individual and often groups of ants sting multiple times in a semicircular arc) (see Table 2-14)

■ OTHER CLINICAL FINDINGS
- Systemic reactions are anaphylactic and manifest themselves as airway edema, wheezing, urticaria, and/or hypotension.
- A serum sickness–like illness can occur 1 to 2 weeks after an insect sting.
  1. It is characterized by fever, aches, a *painful urticarial* rash, and angioedema.

DIAGNOSIS

- The diagnosis of an insect sting is made on the basis of the history and examination.
- In combination with vital sign monitoring, the history and examination help determine the severity of a reaction.

THERAPY

■ NONPHARMACOLOGIC
- Remove the stinger without touching the venom sac.
- Apply an ice pack.

■ MEDICAL
- Antihistamine: Diphenhydramine is administered at 1 to 2 mg/kg orally, intravenously, or intramuscularly (maximum, 50 mg)
- Analgesia: Acetaminophen 15 mg/kg orally every 4 hours as needed (maximum, 1000 mg) may be given.
- Corticosteroid use, topical or systemic, is of unproven benefit for insect stings.
  1. Therapy for serum sickness, however, consists of several days of corticosteroids and antihistamines.

■ FOLLOW-UP & DISPOSITION
- Twenty percent of patients with systemic reactions experience symptoms of late-phase anaphylaxis that occurs several hours after the first symptoms appear.
- To detect this late-phase reaction, patients who have systemic reactions to stings should have vital sign monitoring for a minimum of 6 hours.

■ PATIENT/FAMILY EDUCATION
- See "Preventive Treatment."
- Alert patients to the signs and symptoms of anaphylaxis.
- Instruct patients on the use of an emergency epinephrine kit.

■ PREVENTIVE TREATMENT
- Avoid stinging insects through the following methods:
  1. Do not wear bright colors.
  2. Avoid garbage bins.
  3. Be aware of areas of nests (e.g., house vines, under awnings).
  4. Avoid perfumes, scented soap, and hair sprays.
  5. Do not walk or play outside in bare feet.
- Use insect repellent.
- Desensitization by immunotherapy may be of benefit to some hypersensitive individuals.

■ REFERRAL INFORMATION
Patients with severe reactions may need to be referred to an allergist for desensitization.

PEARLS & CONSIDERATIONS

■ CLINICAL PEARLS
- A mild reaction in a patient does not preclude a systemic one with later stings.
- Be wary of the late-phase reaction of anaphylaxis.

■ WEBSITES
- Allergy, Asthma & Immunology Online: http://allergy.mcg.edu/alk/insect.html
- Centers for Disease Control and Prevention: www.cdc.gov/niosh/nasd/docs3/me97005.html

REFERENCES
1. Jerrard DA: ED management of insect stings, *Am J Emerg Med* 14:429, 1995.
2. Kemp ED: Bites and stings of the arthropod kind: treating reactions that can range from annoying to menacing, *Postgrad Med* 103:88, 1998.
3. Litoritz TL et al: 1997 Annual Report of the American Association of Poison Control Centers Toxic Exposure Surveillance System, *Am J Emerg Med* 16:443, 1998.

Author: **Robert J. Freishtat, M.D.**

TABLE 2-14 Etiology, Demographics, History, and Physical Examination of Insect Stings

ETIOLOGY	DEMOGRAPHICS	HISTORY	PHYSICAL EXAMINATION
Yellow jacket	Most common sting; found in most areas of the United States	Often hang around garbage; attack in a group if nest is disturbed; painful sting	Usually only one sting, but can be more than 10 stings if a nest is disturbed; wheal and flare
Hornet/wasp	Most areas of the United States	Attack in a group if a nest is disturbed; painful sting	One to five stings; wheal and flare
Africanized "killer" honeybee	South Central and Southwestern United States	Often pursue victims; painful sting	One to hundreds of stings; wheal and flare
Fire ant	South Central and Southwestern United States	Painful sting	Papular becoming pustular lesions in a semicircular arc

BASIC INFORMATION

■ DEFINITION
Intussusception is present when a portion of the alimentary canal telescopes into the distal segment.

ICD-9CM CODE
560.0 Intussusception

■ ETIOLOGY
- Approximately 90% are idiopathic; the probable lead point is an inflamed Peyer's patch adjacent to the ileum.
- Ten percent have an associated lead point: Meckel's diverticulum, intramural hematomas caused by Henoch-Schönlein purpura, intestinal wall tumors, meconium ileus equivalent caused by cystic fibrosis, appendiceal stump, intestinal polyp, or ileal duplication
- An associated lead point is more common with increasing age.
- Seventy-five percent of patients older than age 5 years had an associated lead point.

■ EPIDEMIOLOGY & DEMOGRAPHICS
- The incidence is 0.9 to 4 in 1000 live births.
- Ninety percent are ileocolic.
- Intussusception is the most common cause of intestinal obstruction in children between 3 months and 6 years of age; it rarely occurs outside this range.
- About 60% of cases occur by age 2 years.
- The male:female ratio is 2:1 to 4:1.

■ HISTORY
- Sudden onset of severe, paroxysmal, colicky pain in a previously well child is observed. Between attacks, the child may appear normal.
- Approximately 70% to 80% present with emesis that initially is nonbilious.
- Stools may be loose, and symptoms may be confused with diarrhea.
- Younger children may present with an altered, apathetic mental state, and not complain of pain.
- Fever may be present.

■ PHYSICAL EXAMINATION
- From 50% to 70% of children have a palpable, sausage-shaped mass, most often in the right upper quadrant.
- Stools often have occult blood. Stool containing visible mucus and blood (currant-jelly stool) is a late and inconsistent finding.
- Younger children often present with an apathetic, limp appearance.

🔬 DIAGNOSIS

■ DIFFERENTIAL DIAGNOSIS
- Gastroenteritis tends to have less severe and less regular episodes of pain; however, many children with intussusception do not have apparent pain, and distinguishing from gastroenteritis may be difficult.
- Meckel's diverticulum has painless rectal bleeding.

■ DIAGNOSTIC WORKUP
- Blood and urine tests are noncontributory.
- Plain abdominal radiographs may show signs of obstruction (dilated loops of small intestine) or even a mass; 10% to 30% are normal.
- Ultrasonography is reported to have high sensitivity and specificity.
- Barium enema is diagnostic; however, reduction during the procedure, but before visualization, can occur.

℞ THERAPY

■ NONPHARMACOLOGIC
- Treat dehydration and electrolyte disturbances.
- About 80% can be hydrostatically reduced with a barium enema.

■ MEDICAL
Peritonitis requires appropriate antibiotics.

■ SURGICAL
Signs of intestinal perforation or peritonitis are contraindications to barium enema; surgical reduction is required.

■ FOLLOW-UP & DISPOSITION
About 10% recur after barium enema reduction and require admission to observe for relapse of abdominal pain and vomiting.

■ PATIENT/FAMILY EDUCATION
1% mortality

■ REFERRAL INFORMATION
A pediatric surgeon should be alerted when a child is to undergo a barium enema.

REFERENCES
1. Bhistkul DM et al: Clinical application of ultrasonography in the diagnosis of intussusception, *J Pediatr* 121:182, 1992.
2. Bruce J et al: Intussusception: evolution of current management, *J Pediatr Gastro Nutr* 6:663, 1987.
3. Losek JD: Intussusception: don't miss the diagnosis! *Pediatr Emerg Care* 9:46, 1993.
4. Rachmel A et al: Apathy as an early manifestation of intussusception, *Am J Dis Child* 137:701, 1983.
Author: **James R. Campbell, M.D.**

II

BASIC INFORMATION

■ DEFINITION
Iron is an essential element to human metabolism. Free iron that is not confined to storage proteins or bound to protein carriers can have toxic effects by presenting an oxidative stress to various cellular processes that may lead to free radical formation. Free elemental iron can be overingested in the form of many readily available preparations, including pediatric and adult multivitamins. Iron overingestion can lead to profound systemic toxicity, including shock and organ failure.

■ ICD-9CM CODE
964.0 Iron poisoning

■ ETIOLOGY
- Iron overingestion produces gastrointestinal (GI) disturbance from a direct corrosive effect on mucosa.
- Systemic toxicity derives from widespread disruption of intracellular metabolic processes.

■ EPIDEMIOLOGY & DEMOGRAPHICS
- In recent years, iron overingestion has accounted for an average of 2% of all toxic exposures in pediatric patients.
- Exposures to iron-containing substances average approximately 22,000 per year. Formulations include the following:
  1. Adult iron preparations:
     a. 60 to 90 mg elemental iron per dose
  2. Pediatric iron preparations: 12 to 18 mg elemental iron per dose

Standard Conversions for Common Iron Compounds

Ferrous gluconate	12% elemental iron
Ferrous sulfate	20% elemental iron
Ferrous chloride	28% elemental iron
Ferrous fumarate	33% elemental iron

- Most victims are 6 years of age or younger.

■ HISTORY
- A history of ingestion can often be obtained. The examiner should inquire specifically about the following factors:
  1. Time of ingestion
  2. Exact preparation ingested
     a. Have witness read directly from container or bring container to health care facility.
  3. Quantity of preparation ingested
     a. More than 20 mg/kg is potentially toxic.
     b. The exact amount that correlates with symptoms of toxicity is difficult to specify.
  4. Where preparation was stored
  5. Degree of supervision at time of ingestion
  6. History of prior ingestions
- Iron toxicity should be considered when evaluating any patient with acute onset of abdominal discomfort, nausea, vomiting, diarrhea, and even upper GI bleeding.

■ SIGNS & SYMPTOMS
- Signs and symptoms usually develop within 6 hours of ingestion.
  1. If the patient remains asymptomatic during the 6-hour period after ingestion, subsequent development of clinical toxicity is unusual.
- Clinical stage classification does not necessarily correlate with measured serum iron levels because systemic toxicity generally derives from iron's *intracellular* effects.
  1. *Stage I:* In the first 6 hours, signs and symptoms of direct irritation of the proximal GI tract usually dominate the clinical picture and include abdominal pain, nausea, vomiting, and/or hematemesis, and diarrhea.
     a. Hypotension and frank hypovolemic shock from acute GI losses can occur early in the clinical course.
     b. Consumptive coagulopathy can also develop at this stage.
  2. *Stage II:* After 6 to 12 hours, many patients enter a quiescent phase marked by apparent improvement or even normalization of physiologic status.
  3. *Stage III:* Patients can relapse into marked metabolic derangement from effects of absorbed iron. At this point, there may be dysregulation (by free serum iron) of the coagulation cascade, third-spacing of fluid from GI injury, capillary leak syndrome, ongoing metabolic acidosis with elevated anion gap, cardiac failure from negative inotropic effect, and myocarditis referable to iron-induced myocardial damage. Acute hepatic failure is also possible at this stage and is heralded by elevation of serum transaminases, lactate dehydrogenase and bilirubin. Central nervous system failure can also be seen at this stage.
  4. *Stage IV:* Scarring and stricture formation of the proximal GI tract can occasionally develop up to 4 weeks after the acute ingestion.

DIAGNOSIS

■ DIFFERENTIAL DIAGNOSIS
- Septic shock should be considered in any patient who presents with hypotension, especially in the setting of coagulopathy.
  1. Hypotension can also be a major feature of other toxic exposures, such as antihypertensives, tricyclic antidepressants, and salicylates.
- The GI symptoms seen in stage I iron toxicity may be seen in ingestion of salicylates and nonsteroidal antiinflammatory drugs.
- Stage III toxicity with hepatic involvement may resemble the clinical effects of acetaminophen or mushroom toxicity.

■ DIAGNOSTIC WORKUP
- Serum iron level should be determined 4 to 6 hours after ingestion.
  1. Serum iron levels in excess of 300 µg/dl (normal, 50 to 150 µg/dl) are often associated with clinical symptoms.
  2. Levels in excess of 500 µg/dl are nearly always associated with clinical toxicity.
- Clinical findings consistent with any stage of iron intoxication should be addressed promptly, even if the measured serum iron level is lower than expected.
- Serum iron levels should be repeated at 8- to 12-hour intervals in symptomatic patients.
- Abdominal radiographs should be obtained early to screen for the presence of visible radiopaque iron pills. Absence of radiopaque material on abdominal radiograph should be interpreted with caution because material in the stomach that has already dissolved may not be radiographically apparent.
- Other laboratory studies that are useful early on include arterial blood gas; complete blood count; and serum electrolytes, including glucose, blood urea nitrogen, and creatinine.
  1. Serum transaminases and liver function tests, including coagulation studies, are helpful in the setting of ongoing clinical toxicity.
  2. Some sources suggest that white blood cell elevation higher than 15,000/mm^3 and serum blood glucose higher than 150 mg/dl are helpful in predicting a clinically significant ingestion.
     a. Clinical correlation with these values is inconsistent.
  3. Serum total iron-binding capacity is *not* useful in the management of acute iron toxicity.

℞ THERAPY

- Maintain airway, assist with ventilation if necessary, and support intravascular volume.
  1. In patients with evidence of shock, intravascular volume should be aggressively repleted with intravenous crystalloid or blood, as appropriate.
  2. Serial reevaluation of intravascular volume status is critical, especially if there is ongoing metabolic acidosis.
- In the alert and stable patient with intact airway reflexes, initial decontamination should begin by administering syrup of ipecac if evaluating a patient within 2 hours of ingestion.
  1. Administer 10 ml orally for patients 6 to 12 months of age, 15 ml for those 1 to 12 years old, 30 ml for patients older than 12 years of age.
  2. Ipecac is most effective if administered within 30 minutes of ingestion.
  3. Gastric lavage (with appropriate airway protection) with normal saline should also be considered, especially for intentional ingestions, evidence of pill fragments in stomach on radiography, and when the amount of elemental iron ingested is greater than 20 mg/kg.
     a. Large tablet size and viscous consistency of iron preparations makes recovery of gastric contents difficult.
     b. Lavage with bicarbonate or phosphate-containing solutions, or with enterally administered deferoxamine, is not recommended.
  4. In the setting of significant iron ingestion, GI decontamination is probably best achieved by whole bowel irrigation with a polyethylene glycol solution (GoLYTELY) administered by nasogastric tube at a rate of 250 to 500 ml/hr.
     a. If a sizable tablet mass is suspected or identified radiographically, endoscopy or surgical gastrotomy may be indicated to remove it.
  5. *Activated charcoal is not useful in the setting of isolated iron ingestion because it does not adsorb iron.*
- Chelation therapy should be administered to symptomatic patients with 4- to 6-hour serum iron levels greater than 300 mg/dl and in all patients with 4- to 6-hour levels in excess of 500 mg/dl. The agent of choice for chelation in acute iron toxicity is deferoxamine, a ferric iron chelator with intracellular activity.
  1. Deferoxamine should be given by continuous intravenous infusion at 10 to 15 mg/kg/hr. The intramuscular route of administration is not recommended.
     a. Rapid infusion of deferoxamine may be associated with significant side effects, including a shocklike state with hypotension and oliguria. The rate of administration should be slowed and intravascular volume supported, as needed, to control any side effects of therapy.
  2. The duration of chelation therapy should be guided mainly by the patient's clinical status because serum iron measurement may be inaccurate in the setting of deferoxamine administration.
  3. Chelation should continue until all physiologic disturbances have resolved and laboratory values and imaging studies are normal. Deferoxamine can be given safely to a pregnant patient.
- Throughout the clinical course of the iron-intoxicated patient, one should assess frequently for signs of electrolyte derangement and shock so that aggressive fluid resuscitation can proceed in a timely fashion.
  1. Renal failure may ensue as a result of shock and hypoperfusion or from nephrotoxicity of deferoxamine-iron complex.
  2. Hemodialysis may be useful to assist clearance of the chelated iron complex.

■ FOLLOW-UP & DISPOSITION
- All patients with intentional ingestions should receive an evaluation by psychiatry once they are clinically stable.
- In cases of accidental ingestion, social work consultation is often helpful to assess the degree of supervision in the home.

■ PATIENT/FAMILY EDUCATION
- Parents should be educated about the potential toxicity of iron-containing compounds in the home, including multivitamin preparations. These and other medications should be kept locked and out of the reach of children, even if they are packaged with childproof caps.
- Families should be provided with the phone number of the nearest regional poison center.

■ PREVENTIVE TREATMENT
- The danger of accidental poisoning in the home should be discussed routinely at pediatric health supervision visits, beginning at the 6-month visit.
  1. If syrup of ipecac is provided to the family, parents should be instructed not to administer it unless under the guidance of the regional poison center.
  2. Parents should be instructed to "childproof" the home, including locking vitamin preparations and all other medicines out of the reach of children.
  3. Parents should be provided with the phone number of the regional poison center. They should be instructed to call immediately when they suspect that an inappropriate ingestion may have occurred.

■ REFERRAL INFORMATION
- In general, all patients suspected of having a potentially toxic exposure should be stabilized acutely and referred to the nearest tertiary care center with experience in managing critically ill children.
- The nearest regional poison center should be consulted in all cases of intentional or accidental toxic ingestion.

✷ PEARLS & CONSIDERATIONS

■ CLINICAL PEARLS
- In general, syrup of ipecac should be administered under the guidance of the regional poison center.
  1. Ipecac contains plant alkaloids and causes vomiting (generally within 30 minutes) by direct irritation of gastric mucosa and by stimulation of the central medullary chemotactic trigger zone.
  2. Its effect can be promoted by giving water afterward.
     a. 15 ml/kg in patients 6 months to 1 year, 50 to 240 ml in patients 1 to 12 years of age, 240 to 300 ml in patients older than 12 years of age
  3. The effects of ipecac-induced emesis in achieving gastric decontamination are variable (19% to 62%).
  4. Administration of a single dose of ipecac can result in protracted emesis for several hours.
- Infusion of deferoxamine is typically associated with a change of urine color to orange-red or pink, "vin rose," but efficacy of chelation therapy should not be judged according to whether or not the color change has occurred.
  1. Even in patients with markedly toxic serum iron levels, urine color change may not be observed, especially if the patient is in some degree of hypovolemic or distributive shock.

■ **WEBSITES**
- POISINEX System: www. micromedex.com/products/ pd-poisindex.htm
- TOXNET: http://toxnet.nlm.nih/gov

REFERENCES

1. McGuigan M: Acute iron poisoning, *Pediatr Ann* 25:33, 1996.
2. Mills KC, Curry SC: Acute iron poisoning, *Emerg Med Clin North Am* 12:397, 1994.
3. Nolan RJ: Poisoning. In Hoekelman RA et al (eds): *Primary pediatric care,* ed 3, St Louis, 1997, Mosby.
4. Olson K (ed): *Poisoning and drug overdose,* Englewood Cliffs, NJ, 1994, Appleton & Lange.
5. Perry H, Shannon M: Emergency department gastrointestinal decontamination, *Pediatr Ann* 25:19, 1996.

Author: **Kathleen M. Ventre, M.D.**

BASIC INFORMATION

■ DEFINITION
Irritable bowel syndrome (IBS) is a series of chronic, nonspecific gastrointestinal (GI) symptoms for which no organic cause can be found. The symptoms include abdominal pain with alterations in bowel habits.

■ SYNONYMS
- Irritable colon
- Spastic colon
- Functional GI disorders
- IBS

ICD-9CM CODES
564.1 Irritable colon
536.9 Unspecified functional disorder of the stomach

■ ETIOLOGY
- The cause is unknown.
- The pathophysiology is poorly understood, but there is evidence of the following:
  1. GI dysmotility: inconsistent abnormal small bowel and colonic motility patterns
  2. Abnormalities in sensation: visceral hyperalgesia
  3. Stress and psychologic disturbances

■ EPIDEMIOLOGY & DEMOGRAPHICS
- This condition is a common cause of school absenteeism and utilization of medical care resources in children and adolescents.
  1. It is the most common digestive disease encountered by adult gastroenterologists.
- In community-based studies, abdominal pain occurred weekly in 13% to 17% of middle and high school students.
  1. Six percent of middle school students and 14% of high school students could be classified as having IBS.
  2. In referral specialty clinics, two thirds of children with chronic abdominal pain have symptoms compatible with IBS.
- The relationship between recurrent abdominal pain (RAP) and IBS has not been clearly defined.
  1. Approximately 30% to 50% of patients with RAP continue with pain and may develop IBS that persists into adulthood.
  2. Females with RAP seemed to be at greater risk.
- For adults, the number seeking medical advice may be a small portion of those with IBS.
  1. Other factors are likely to influence the decision to obtain medical advice.

2. The same is probably true in children.

■ HISTORY
Different symptoms may predominate.
- Abdominal pain (recurrent, colicky, periumbilical), particularly in children 5 years and older
  1. Abdominal pain varies in intensity.
  2. Pain may be epigastric or in the right or left side.
  3. Pain may be severe enough to interfere with daily activities.
  4. A bowel movement may relieve pain.
  5. Food ingestion may worsen pain.
- Abnormal bowel movements
  1. In older children, IBS follows a pattern similar to that seen in adults: either constipation, diarrhea, or diarrhea alternating with constipation.
  2. There may be a sensation of difficult or incomplete evacuation.
- Symptoms of upper GI dysfunction: heartburn, nausea, vomiting, bloating
- Autonomic symptoms: pallor, fatigue, headache, dizziness, palpitations, low-grade fever, nausea, vomiting
- Anxiety and depression scores higher for patients with IBS

■ PHYSICAL EXAMINATION
- Normal growth and development
- Normal abdominal examination
  1. Occasionally, mild abdominal distention
  2. Occasionally, periumbilical or generalized tenderness
- Normal physical examination otherwise
  1. Malnutrition, mass lesions, organomegaly, jaundice, ascites, perianal disease, costovertebral pain, skin problems, joint swelling, neuropathy, or guaiac-positive stool are *not* compatible with the diagnosis of IBS.

DIAGNOSIS

- The diagnosis is made on clinical grounds.
- No strict definition in children is available. The "Rome" criteria established for adults include the following:
  1. First, at least 3 months of continuous or recurrent abdominal pain or discomfort relieved by defecation, or associated with a change in the frequency or consistency of stool
  2. Second, two or more of the following at least 25% of the time:
     a. Altered stool frequency

     b. Altered stool form (hard, loose, or watery)
     c. Altered stool passage (straining or urgency, feeling of incomplete evacuation)
     d. Passage of mucus
     e. Bloating or abdominal distention

■ DIFFERENTIAL DIAGNOSIS
- GI infections (particularly *Giardiasis*)
- Inflammatory bowel disease (IBD)
- Lactose intolerance
- *Helicobacter pylori* infections
- Food intolerances or allergies
- Malabsorption
- Gallstones
- Pancreatitis
- Urinary tract infection
- Gynecologic abnormalities (e.g., pelvic inflammatory disease)
- Toxin (lead)
- Constipation
- Unlikely in child who is ill appearing or has progressive symptoms, weight loss, symptoms at night, bleeding, evidence of malabsorption, fever, bilious vomiting, an abnormal physical examination, or a positive family history (e.g., peptic ulcer disease, IBD, gallstones)
- Although recurrent abdominal pain is common, identifiable organic disease found only in a minority

■ DIAGNOSTIC WORKUP
- Screening tests that may be considered for all patients:
  1. Complete blood cell count with differential and reticulocytes
  2. Erythrocyte sedimentation rate
  3. Total protein and albumin
  4. *H. pylori* titer (of questionable use with or without evidence of gastritis or ulcer)
  5. Liver function tests
  6. Pancreatic amylase and lipase
  7. Serum electrolytes
  8. Blood urea nitrogen and creatinine
  9. Urinalysis and urine culture
  10. Stool guaiac
  11. Stool for ova and parasites
- Additional tests (should be performed only if indicated by the history, findings on physical examination, or screening laboratory tests):
  1. Lactose breath test
  2. Blood screening for inflammatory bowel disease (perinuclear antineutrophil cytoplasmic antibodies [p-ANCA] and anti–saccharomyces cerevisia antibodies [ASCA])
  3. Abdominal ultrasound (if possible during acute attack)
  4. Upper GI series with small bowel follow-through
  5. Barium enema
  6. Intravenous pyelogram

II

7. Abdominal computed tomography scan
8. Esophagogastroduodenoscopy
9. Colonoscopy
10. Electroencephalography
11. Functional gallbladder imagining (nuclear medicine with gallbladder emptying)
12. Laparoscopy
13. Other (e.g., porphyrins, lead)

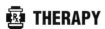 **THERAPY**

■ **NONPHARMACOLOGIC**
Recommended in all patients
• Reassurance, education, and emotional support are critical.
• Nutrition:
  1. Dietary fiber
  2. Elimination of potentially exacerbating foods (consider lactose-free diet)

■ **MEDICAL**
• Initial therapy
  1. Suppression of gastric acid: Use of H_2 blockers (ranitidine, cimetidine, famotidine) or proton pump inhibitors (omeprazole and lansoprazole) may be beneficial, particularly if there is a component of dyspepsia.
  2. Prokinetics may be useful in patients with dyspepsia and constipation.
  3. Loperamide is effective in patients with diarrhea.
• If nonpharmacologic and medical interventions fail:
  1. Antispasmodics and anticholinergics (dicyclomine, hyoscyamine) or calcium channel blockers (diltiazem, peppermint oil, pinaverium) can be tried.
     a. Although placebo-controlled studies in adults have had mixed results, these agents may be effective in children with severe and debilitating symptoms.

2. Antidepressants and anxiolytics have central and peripheral effects.
   a. Effective in patients with visceral hyperalgesia
      (1) Most of the experience has been with tricyclic antidepressants (e.g., amitriptyline, trazodone, desipramine) and benzodiazepines.
3. Psychotherapy and biofeedback may be useful.
4. A multidisciplinary approach is often necessary.

■ **FOLLOW-UP & DISPOSITION**
• Close follow-up should be maintained with frequent visits and physician availability.
• Avoid school absence.

■ **PATIENT/FAMILY EDUCATION**
• Even though the symptoms are functional in nature, they are real.
• The diagnosis of IBS needs to be a positive diagnosis, not one of exclusion.
• Reassurance is important.
  1. There is a low likelihood of finding an organic cause.
  2. There is no physical danger to the child.
• It is important not to let the symptoms become the disease.
• IBS symptoms are associated with high levels of disability and health service use.

■ **PREVENTIVE TREATMENT**
Early intervention is important in children with RAP.

■ **REFERRAL INFORMATION**
• Patients with a poor response to nonpharmacologic and initial medical interventions may need to be evaluated by a gastroenterologist.
• If patients with IBS have a high degree of disability, they may require a multidisciplinary approach.

PEARLS & CONSIDERATIONS

■ **CLINICAL PEARLS**
• Abdominal pain in children younger than 4 years of age needs to be investigated thoroughly.
• IBS should be a main and positive diagnosis.
• Unnecessary diagnostic tests and referrals may only reinforce an already problematic symptom.
• Visits to a physician are related to parental perceptions of the severity of the symptoms.
• Treatment should start with simple interventions.

■ **WEBSITES**
• American Academy of Family Physicians: www.aafp.org/patientinfo/bowel.html
• International Foundation for Functional Gastrointestinal Disorders: www.iffgd.org
• National Institute of Diabetes & Digestive & Kidney Diseases: www.niddk.nih.gov/health/digest/summary/ibskids/index.htm
• National Institute of Diabetes & Digestive & Kidney Diseases: www.niddk.nih.gov/health/digest/pubs/irrbowel/irrbo

REFERENCES

1. Hyams JS et al: Characterization of symptoms in children with recurrent abdominal pain: resemblance with irritable bowel syndrome, *J Pediatr Gastroenterol Nutr* 20:209, 1995.
2. Hyams JS et al: Abdominal pain and irritable bowel syndrome in adolescents: a community-based study, *J Pediatr* 129:220, 1996.
3. Hyman PE, Fleisher DR: Pediatric functional gastrointestinal disorders, *J Pediatr Gastroenterol Nutr* 25:S11, 1997.
4. Thompson WG et al: Functional bowel disease and functional abdominal pain, *Gastroenterol Int* 5:75, 1992.
5. Walker LS et al: Recurrent abdominal pain: a potential precursor of irritable bowel syndrome in adolescents and young adults, *J Pediatr* 132:1010, 1998.
Author: **Samuel Nurko, M.D.**

BASIC INFORMATION

■ DEFINITION

Juvenile ankylosing spondylitis (JAS) is a chronic arthropathy, which includes chronic inflammation of the sacroiliac joints (SIJs), spine, peripheral joints, and enthesis (tendon insertion to bone). It is the prototype of the spondyloarthropathies. These enthesitis-related arthritides share a common link with inflammation in the ligament, tendon, and fascia insertion sites on the bone, as well as the synovium, uveal tract, and gastrointestinal tract. The class I HLA-B27 gene allele is present in a large majority of these patients.

■ SYNONYMS

- Marie-Strumpell disease
- Juvenile spondyloarthropathy (JSpA)
- JAS

ICD-9CM CODE

720.00 Ankylosing spondylitis (juvenile is same ICD-9CM code as adult)

■ ETIOLOGY

- The cause is unknown.
- There is a strong genetic predisposition with associated HLA-B27.
- Suspected antigenic stimulation is suggested by bacterial infections, such as *Salmonella, Shigella, Yersinia,* and *Campylobacter,* which trigger reactive arthritis in the HLA-B27 host.
- How the antigen or what peptides provoke the inflammatory response with the HLA-B27 molecules are not understood.

■ EPIDEMIOLOGY & DEMOGRAPHICS

- Older studies indicate a male:female ratio of 4.5:1 to 6:1; more recent data suggest a 2:1 to 3:1 ratio.
- There is a strong link with HLA-B27 (75% to 90%).
- Prevalence is approximately 1.6 per 100,000; total JSpA is approximately 20 per 100,000.
  1. Prevalence may be higher, but slow progression makes diagnosis difficult during childhood and adolescence.
- The mean age of onset is beyond 10 years of age.

■ HISTORY

- Usually, JAS occurs in an older boy who presents with pain and stiffness in the lower extremity joint(s), especially the feet (tarsal disease), knees, and hip. Upper extremity involvement is uncommon.
- Inflammation in entheses is common: plantar fascia, Achilles tendon insertion, tibial tubercle.
- Lumbar or sacroiliac pain and stiffness occur early in disease in 13% to 24% of patients.
- Fever, lymphadenopathy, and uveitis (acute) may be present early in disease.

■ PHYSICAL EXAMINATION

- Signs of inflammation with swelling or loss of motion with pain in lower extremity joints, especially the feet, knees, ankles, and subtalar joints, may be noted. Hips may be involved early in disease.
- Tenderness and swelling of entheses may be seen. Inspect the Achilles tendon with insertion site on calcaneus. Palpate over plantar fascia, tibial tubercles, greater trochanters, and ischial tuberosities.
- Pain in sacroiliac joint is noted with provocative compression.
  1. Simultaneous, bilateral compression of the hips by the examiner may elicit pain in the SIJ.
  2. In the Patrick test, the patient lies supine and the examiner flexes, abducts, and externally rotates the patient's test leg so that the foot of the test leg is on top of the opposite knee.
     a. The examiner slowly lowers the test leg toward the examining table.
     b. A positive test result occurs when the test leg remains above the opposite leg. In a negative test, the leg will be able to come down to the level of the opposite leg and thigh.
     c. A positive result of the Patrick test may indicate hip disease, iliopsoas spasm, or sacroiliac abnormality.
  3. Gaenslen's sign is demonstrated by having the patient in a supine position, with the knee flexed and the hip on the chest; the other thigh is extended over the edge of the table.
     a. Pain in the hip that is flexed (contralateral to the extended hip) may have pathology.
- Limited lumbar flexion and reduced chest expansion are uncommon early in disease.
- Examine carefully for evidence of acute iritis, psoriasis, nail changes (pitting or onycholysis), oral mucosal lesions, perianal fissure/fistula (Crohn's disease), right lower quadrant mass, or aortic insufficiency.

DIAGNOSIS

■ DIFFERENTIAL DIAGNOSIS

- Juvenile rheumatoid arthritis (JRA) versus JAS:
  1. Tarsal, enthesis, and lower extremity joint inflammation predict JAS.
  2. Presence of SIJ involvement strongly suggests JAS.
- Arthritis associated with psoriasis, Reiter's disease, and inflammatory bowel disease (IBD) must be considered.

■ DIAGNOSTIC WORKUP

- Antinuclear antibodies and rheumatoid factor are usually negative.
- Up to 90% to 95% of patients are HLA-B27 positive.
- Radiographs are not usually abnormal early in disease.
  1. Radionucleotide scan, computed tomography, or magnetic resonance imaging (MRI) of SIJs may be helpful if suspected involvement needs to be confirmed.
  2. MRI is a superb modality to identify disease of the synovium and tenosynovium in selected cases.
- Complete blood count (CBC) with differential, erythrocyte sedimentation rate (ESR), urinalysis, and renal and liver chemistries are necessary to follow the patient and monitor for medication toxicities and systemic complications.

THERAPY

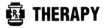

■ NONPHARMACOLOGIC

- Physical therapy is essential: range of motion, strengthening, flexibility, postural exercises, heat/whirlpool.
- Swimming is an avocational sport and is strongly encouraged.
- Orthotics are recommended for foot and enthesis pain relief and support.

■ MEDICAL

- Nonsteroidal antiinflammatory drugs (NSAIDs)
  1. Especially indomethacin 1 to 3 mg/kg/day divided into three to four doses; slow-release product (75 mg total dose) lasts 12 hours in larger patients
  2. Tolmetin sodium 20 to 30 mg/kg/day divided into three doses
  3. Naproxen 10 to 20 mg/kg/day divided into two doses
- Second-line drugs
  1. Sulfasalazine (not only for IBD) up to 50 mg/kg/day
  2. Methotrexate 10 mg/m²/wk orally or subcutaneously; higher dosages may be tolerated later if initial low dosage is not effective
- Intraarticular corticosteroid injections
  1. Triamcinolone hexacetonide 1 mg/kg per joint (up to 40 mg per joint)
  2. Avoid tendon insertion injection—may weaken the tendon, potential for rupture

■ SURGICAL
Late total joint arthroplasty may be necessary, especially hip replacement.

■ FOLLOW-UP & DISPOSITION
- Carefully follow the range of motion of the peripheral joints and lumbar flexion.
- Monitor for loss of lumbar flexion; chest expansion; cervical flexion, extension, and rotation; and postural alterations; this should be done every 3 to 6 months.
- Radiographic reevaluation is done as necessary but may not reveal bone or joint space changes for several years.
- Monitor CBC with differential, blood urea nitrogen, creatinine, ALT, albumin, and ESR.
- Frequently encourage physiotherapy, an often-neglected component of therapy.
- Complications include cartilage and bone erosion, sacroiliac and spinal ankylosis with severe loss of motion, aortic insufficiency, atlantoaxial subluxation, IgA nephropathy, and cauda equina syndrome.

■ PATIENT/FAMILY EDUCATION
- Educate about slow progression.
- Educate about importance of exercise.
- Advise regarding the development of acute, painful red eye (acute iritis), which requires prompt ophthalmologic evaluation.
- Advise regarding diarrhea, blood in stools, and weight loss because clinical IBD develops in some of these patients.
- Advise regarding the development of dyspepsia or epigastric pain secondary to NSAIDs.

■ PREVENTIVE TREATMENT
Physiotherapy is essential to prevent the loss of axial and peripheral joint motion.

■ REFERRAL INFORMATION
A pediatric rheumatologist can be invaluable in helping to establish a diagnosis, follow the patient, and provide an interdisciplinary team for physical management.

⚙ PEARLS & CONSIDERATIONS

■ CLINICAL PEARLS
- Watch for psoriasis, IBD, and uveitis.
- Older boys with pauciarticular-onset JRA may evolve into JAS; prospectively follow for axial involvement.
- Enthesitis in an older boy with signs of inflammation may have early JAS, although repetitive activity (overuse) syndromes are more common.

■ WEBSITES
- KickAS.org: www.kickas.org
- Spondylitis Association of America: www.spondylitis.org

■ SUPPORT GROUPS
- National Ankylosing Spondylitis Foundation
- Local arthritis foundations—usually have support groups
- American Juvenile Arthritis Organization (AJAO)—provides educational and support resources

REFERENCES
1. Burgos-Vargas R, Pacheco-Tena C, Vásquez-Mellado J: Juvenile-onset spondyloarthropathies, *Rheum Dis Clin North Am* 23:569, 1997.
2. Burgos-Vargas R, Vásquez-Mellado J: The early clinical recognition of juvenile-onset ankylosing spondylitis and its differentiation from juvenile rheumatoid arthritis, *Arthritis Rheum* 38:835, 1995.
3. Cabral DA, Malleson PN, Petty RE: Spondyloarthropathies of childhood, *Pediatr Clin North Am* 42:1051, 1995.
4. Calin A, Elswood J: The natural history of juvenile-onset ankylosing spondylitis: a 24-year retrospective case-control study, *Br J Rheum* 27:91, 1998.
Author: **Murray Passo, M.D.**

BASIC INFORMATION

■ DEFINITION
Diagnostic criteria for chronic arthritis in children stipulate the following:
- Age of onset younger than 16 years
- Arthritis: swelling or effusion, or presence of two or more of the following:
  1. Limitation of range of motion
  2. Tenderness or pain on motion
  3. Increased heat in one or more joints
- Duration of disease 1½ months or longer

Based on disease characteristics in the first 6 months after onset, juvenile arthritis is classified as follows:
- Pauciarticular: less than five inflamed joints
- Polyarticular: five or more inflamed joints
- Systemic onset: arthritis with characteristic quotidian fever pattern

Criteria established by the European League Against Rheumatism (EULAR) add the following:
- Juvenile rheumatoid arthritis: five or more joints, rheumatoid factor positive
- Juvenile ankylosing spondylitis
- Juvenile psoriatic arthritis

■ SYNONYMS
- Juvenile chronic arthritis
- Juvenile rheumatoid arthritis
- Idiopathic arthritides of childhood
- Still's disease (usually refers only to systemic onset)

ICD-9CM CODES
714.30 Juvenile rheumatoid arthritis
714.32 Pauciarticular
714.33 Polyarticular
714.31 Systemic onset
720.01 Juvenile ankylosing spondylitis
713.31 Juvenile psoriatic arthritis with psoriasis
713.32 Juvenile psoriatic arthritis without psoriasis

■ ETIOLOGY
Not known

■ EPIDEMIOLOGY & DEMOGRAPHICS
- The incidence is 9.2 to 19.6 cases per 100,000 children.
- Prevalence is 69.1 to 196.3 per 100,000 children.
- The female:male ratio is 3:1 for pauciarticular and 5:1 to 6:1 if uveitis is present, 2.8:1 for polyarticular, and 1:1 for systemic onset.
- The peak age of onset is 1 to 3 years overall, less skewed toward younger children in polyarticular and systemic onset.

■ HISTORY
- Pauciarticular: minimal constitutional symptoms, involved joint(s) often not significantly painful
- Polyarticular: mild to moderate constitutional symptoms, more pain and stiffness
- Systemic onset: prominent constitutional symptoms, patient quite ill and debilitated, especially when febrile

■ PHYSICAL EXAMINATION
- Pauciarticular
  1. Usual absence of fever, knee most commonly affected
  2. Swelling
  3. Warmth
  4. Mild to moderate tenderness
  5. Limitation of range of motion
  6. Uveitis/iridocyclitis, especially in presence of antinuclear antibody (ANA)
- Polyarticular
  1. Mildly febrile
  2. Fatigue
  3. Weight loss
  4. Small and large joints
  5. Symmetric, especially in presence of positive rheumatoid factor (RF)
- Systemic onset: daily spiking fever to higher than 39° C, usually in afternoon or early evening
  1. Irritable
  2. Fatigued
  3. Weight loss
  4. Pale pink, macular, evanescent rash
  5. Lymphadenopathy
  6. Hepatosplenomegaly
  7. Arthritis tends to be polyarticular but may not develop until weeks after onset of systemic features

DIAGNOSIS

■ DIFFERENTIAL DIAGNOSIS
- Infectious arthritis
- Postinfectious arthritis
- Hematologic disorders
- Hemophilic arthropathy
- Neoplasm
- Familial Mediterranean fever
- Sarcoidosis
- Other connective tissue disorders
- Vasculitis
- Inflammatory bowel disease
- Pigmented villonodular synovitis

■ DIAGNOSTIC WORKUP
- Complete blood count with differential and platelet count: leukocytosis, anemia, and thrombocytosis most prominent in systemic onset, least likely in pauciarticular
- Erythrocyte sedimentation rate, C-reactive protein: markedly elevated in systemic onset, moderately elevated in polyarticular, mild to moderate elevation in pauciarticular
- ANA: present in subset of pauciarticular, marker for increased risk of uveitis
- RF: present only in small subset of patients with polyarticular disease
- Liver function tests: elevated in systemic onset
- HLA-B27: present in juvenile ankylosing spondylitis
- Joint radiographs
  1. Erosions appear after persistent disease, especially in polyarticular disease.
  2. Sacroiliitis is seen in ankylosing spondylitis.
  3. Cervical spine films most commonly show fusion, except in RF positive.

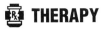

THERAPY

■ NONPHARMACOLOGIC
- Physical therapy (PT)
- Occupational therapy (OT), including heat, ultrasound, and splinting
- Psychotherapy and counseling

■ MEDICAL
- Nonsteroidal antiinflammatory drugs (NSAIDs)
- Disease-modifying antirheumatic drugs, especially methotrexate
- Systemic corticosteroids; intraarticular corticosteroids
- Tumor necrosis factor-α antagonists (etanercept); other immunosuppressants

■ SURGICAL
- Joint replacements (should be performed at as old an age as possible to optimize long bone growth and decrease the number of surgical revisions)
- Tendon-release procedures

■ FOLLOW-UP & DISPOSITION
- Patients require multidisciplinary care with aggressive PT and OT.
- Medications may need to be manipulated depending on the degree of disease activity.
- Surgical consultation is necessary in long-term and persistent cases.

■ PATIENT/FAMILY EDUCATION
- Patients follow very different disease courses; pauciarticular tends to be least problematic.
- The adjustment to a chronic, disabling disease can be challenging.
- Nonmedical therapy is as important as medical.

II

■ **PREVENTIVE TREATMENT OR TESTS**
- Screening slit-lamp examinations for patients at high risk of uveitis
- Monitoring for gastric erosion/ulcer disease in patients on NSAIDs and/or corticosteroids
- Osteoporosis prevention strategies for patients receiving long-term corticosteroids

■ **REFERRAL INFORMATION**
OT, PT, orthopedic surgery, psychology social work, and ophthalmology

PEARLS & CONSIDERATIONS

■ **CLINICAL PEARLS**
- There are no absolutely confirmatory laboratory tests. It is a clinical diagnosis.

- Uveitis occurrence does not relate to the level of joint inflammation.
- Peripheral, large joint arthritis typically precedes any spine involvement in juvenile ankylosing spondylitis.
- Folic acid supplementation for patients receiving methotrexate can decrease side effects.

■ **WEBSITE**
Arthritis Foundation: www.arthritis.org

■ **SUPPORT GROUP**
American Juvenile Arthritis Organization, 1330 W. Peachtree St., Atlanta, GA 30309, 404-872-7100.

REFERENCES

1. Cassidy JT et al: A study of classification criteria for a diagnosis of juvenile rheumatoid arthritis, *Arthritis Rheum* 29:274, 1986.
2. Fink CW: Proposal for the development of classification criteria for idiopathic arthritides of childhood, *J Rheumatol* 22:1566, 1995.
3. Siegel DM: Drug treatment of juvenile arthritis: accepted therapeutic options, *Drugs Today* 34:327, 1998.
4. Siegel DM, Baum J: Juvenile arthritis, *Primary Care* 20:883, 1993.
5. Woo P, Wedderburn LR: Juvenile chronic arthritis, *Lancet* 351:969, 1998.

Author: **David M. Siegel, M.D., M.P.H.**

BASIC INFORMATION

DEFINITION
Kawasaki disease (KD) is an acute multisystemic vasculitis of unknown etiology and is a leading cause of acquired heart disease in children.

SYNONYMS
- Mucocutaneous lymph node syndrome
- Kawasaki syndrome

ICD-9CM CODE
446.1 Kawasaki disease

ETIOLOGY
Unknown but likely to be infectious with immunoregulatory derangements

EPIDEMIOLOGY & DEMOGRAPHICS
- KD usually occurs in children 6 months to 5 years of age.
- It is rare in patients younger than 3 months or older than 8 years of age.
- The U.S. annual attack rate is 6 to 9 per 100,000 children younger than 5 years.
- The male:female ratio is 1.5:1.
- KD occurs year-round but is more common in the winter and spring.
- Geographic and temporal clustering does occur.
- Person-to-person transmission is not documented; it is rare in siblings.
- Recurrence is reported in less than 2% of patients.
- Coronary artery ectasia (dilation) or aneurysms develop in 15% to 25% of untreated children.
- Risk factors for coronary artery abnormalities include the following:
  1. No treatment with intravenous gamma globulin (IVIG)
  2. Male gender
  3. Age younger than 1 year
  4. Long duration of fever (more than 10 days) or biphasic febrile course
  5. Persistent high elevation of acute-phase reactants
  6. High absolute band count
  7. Hemoglobin lower than 10 mg/dl, low platelet count, low albumin
- Coronary dilation occurs as early as 7 days after onset and peaks at 3 to 4 weeks.
- Previously, death occurred in 2 to 3 per 1000 untreated patients as a result of an acute myocardial infarction.
- Highest risk of death, persistence of aneurysms, and late sequelae are most common in patients with giant coronary aneurysms (larger than 8 mm internal diameter).
- Fifty percent of aneurysms regress in 1 to 2 years; the remainder either persist or develop stenosis at the mouth or outlet of the aneurysm.

HISTORY
- Diagnostic criteria are as follows:
  1. Fever, usually high and spiking, of at least 5 days' duration and four or more of the five principal clinical features:
     a. Bilateral nonexudative bulbar conjunctivitis
     b. Red edematous cracked lips, strawberry tongue, pharyngeal erythema
     c. Polymorphous exanthema with perineal accentuation
     d. Palmar and solar erythema with tender induration of the hands and feet and subsequent desquamation 1 to 3 weeks after onset, beginning in the periungual areas
     e. Cervical adenopathy (one or more nodes with a diameter larger than 1.5 cm)—the least common finding, present in 50%
  2. Other diseases with similar findings must be excluded.
- Other findings include extreme irritability, headache, vomiting, abdominal pain, diarrhea, and arthralgia or arthritis.
- Rarely, hearing loss or testicular swelling occurs.

PHYSICAL EXAMINATION
- See "History" for diagnostic criteria.
- Tachycardia greater than expected from fever, gallop rhythm, cardiogenic shock from acute myocarditis, or later myocardial infarction occurs.
- Nuchal rigidity caused by aseptic meningitis may be found.
- Audible mitral regurgitation is present in 1% of patients.

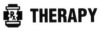 **DIAGNOSIS**

DIFFERENTIAL DIAGNOSIS
- Measles
- Scarlet fever
- Drug reactions
- Stevens-Johnson syndrome
- Other febrile viral exanthemas
- Rocky Mountain spotted fever
- Staphylococcal scalded skin syndrome
- Juvenile arthritis
- Leptospirosis
- Mercury poisoning

DIAGNOSTIC WORKUP
- See "History."
- Elevated acute-phase reactants are seen: erythrocyte sedimentation rate, C-reactive protein (CRP), α_1-antitrypsin, platelet count.

- The following are common:
  1. Neutrophilia with immature forms
  2. Anemia
- The following may be seen:
  1. Hypoalbuminemia
  2. Proteinuria
  3. Sterile pyuria
  4. Cerebrospinal fluid mononuclear pleocytosis
  5. Elevated serum transaminases
- Subclinical pericardial effusions are seen in 30% of patients on echocardiography.
- Gallbladder hydrops are noted on abdominal ultrasound.
- Thrombocytosis peaks at 10 to 14 days.
- Abnormal lipid metabolism (low high-density lipoprotein, high triglycerides) may persist for years.
- These laboratory findings may be helpful if some of the principal findings are not present (early or atypical KD).

THERAPY

MEDICAL
- IVIG is administered at a dose of 2 g/kg over 12 hours.
- IVIG may be repeated with recrudescent or persistent fever (10% of patients).
- Intravenous methylprednisolone has been used in patients who are resistant to IVIG.
- Aspirin is dosed at 80 mg/kg/day orally until the patient is afebrile.
- Aspirin is then dosed at 3 to 5 mg/kg/day for at least 8 weeks.
- Cardiology evaluation, including echocardiograms 2 and 8 weeks after the onset of KD, is necessary.
- If no coronary artery abnormalities are seen at 2 and 8 weeks, aspirin can be discontinued; otherwise, aspirin should continue indefinitely.
- If giant coronary artery aneurysms (larger than 8 mm diameter) are present, warfarin is usually added for satisfactory anticoagulation.
- Administer varicella and influenza vaccines to patients taking aspirin long term.

SURGICAL
- Coronary artery bypass grafts (revascularization) for reversible ischemia caused by coronary artery stenosis if:
  1. The myocardium is viable.
  2. No distal stenoses are present.
- Coronary angioplasty has not been shown to be effective for stenotic lesions.

■ FOLLOW-UP & DISPOSITION
- All patients with KD should initially be evaluated by a pediatric cardiologist with repeat echocardiography at 2 and 8 weeks after onset to detect coronary artery abnormalities.
- Patients with coronary abnormalities require long-term follow-up, with activity restrictions and serial diagnostic testing based on the severity of their coronary lesions.
- Patients with aortic or mitral regurgitation require infective endocarditis prophylaxis.

■ PATIENT/FAMILY EDUCATION
- If coronary artery abnormalities are present, parents should learn basic cardiopulmonary resuscitation.
- The patient's cardiologist should be notified immediately if syncope or acute exercise intolerance develops.
- Whether KD is a risk factor for premature atherosclerotic coronary disease is unknown; nevertheless, a cardiac-healthy lifestyle should be emphasized for patients who have had KD.

■ REFERRAL INFORMATION
- All patients with suspected acute KD should be seen by a pediatric cardiologist and have a baseline echocardiogram.
- Patients with a past history suggestive of KD but no cardiovascular evaluation should be seen by a pediatric cardiologist.

☼ PEARLS & CONSIDERATIONS

■ CLINICAL PEARLS
- The constellation of marked persistent irritability, refusal to bear weight, and confluent perineal erythema may be helpful if KD is in an early stage or is atypical.
- Approximately 90% of patients treated with IVIG are afebrile within 48 hours.

- Despite appropriate therapy, 4% of patients with KD develop coronary aneurysms (giant in 1%).
- Consider obtaining an echocardiogram for unexplained fever in an infant, child, or adolescent lasting 1 week or more.

REFERENCES
1. Akagi T et al: Outcome of coronary artery aneurysms after Kawasaki disease, *J Pediatr* 121:689, 1992.
2. Beiser AS et al: A predictive instrument for coronary artery aneurysms in Kawasaki disease, *Am J Cardiol* 81:1116, 1998.
3. Dajani AS et al: Diagnosis and therapy of Kawasaki disease in children, *Circulation* 87:1776, 1993.
4. Dajani AS et al: Guidelines for long-term management of patients with Kawasaki disease, *Circulation* 89:916, 1994.

Author: **J. Peter Harris, M.D.**

BASIC INFORMATION

■ DEFINITION

A characteristic phenotype in the presence of a 47,XXY chromosome pattern syndrome constitutes Klinefelter syndrome.

■ ICD-9CM CODE

758.7 Klinefelter syndrome

■ ETIOLOGY

- Eighty percent of males with two or more X chromosomes have a 47,XXY genotype.
  1. Males with other sex chromosome abnormalities, such as 48,XXXY; 48,XXYY; or other numerical or structural X chromosome aberrations, generally have a more abnormal phenotype.
  2. In general, the higher the number of X chromosomes, the higher the number of abnormalities.
- Klinefelter syndrome is usually secondary to aberrant segregation of sex chromosomes in meiosis; maternal or paternal errors appear equally likely in most cases.
- The phenotype appears associated with genes mapping to the long arm of the X chromosome.
- Males who are mosaic for a 47,XXY cell line and a normal 46,XY cell line may have a variable phenotype (from normal to Klinefelter syndrome) and a higher likelihood of fertility.

■ EPIDEMIOLOGY & DEMOGRAPHICS

- The incidence of 47,XXY karyotype is 1:500 to 1:1000 male live births.
- Approximately half of 47,XXY conceptions are lost prenatally.

■ HISTORY

- Early literature describes an increased incidence of childhood behavior problems, learning difficulties, and intelligence quotients 10 to 15 points below siblings in boys with Klinefelter syndrome.
  1. Verbal fluency appeared to be most affected.
  2. The typical presentation was a male who came to medical attention in the school years because of behavior or learning problems in conjunction with the characteristic body habitus.
  3. These older reports appear to demonstrate an ascertainment bias.
     a. Only boys who manifested the behavior or learning problems were likely to come to medical attention before puberty.

- Diagnosis of a 47,XXY karyotype is not unusual in infertility clinics or during an evaluation for small testicles in otherwise apparently normal postpubertal males.
- In males diagnosed prenatally with a 47,XXY karyotype, most appear to perform relatively normally in childhood.
- An undefined percentage of boys with a 47,XXY genotype actually manifest the phenotype of Klinefelter syndrome as defined by Dr. Klinefelter's original report.
- The most commonly reported developmental abnormality is delayed expressive speech.
- Postpubertally, males with a 47,XXY karyotype generally have some degree of decreased testosterone production.
  1. Hypergonadotropic hypogonadism
  2. May produce adequate testosterone for virilization at puberty, and may come to medical attention later for small testicles or infertility
- Most affected males appear to have normal sexual function.
  1. Some require exogenous testosterone supplementation to sustain this function.
- Nearly all affected males are infertile; however, a few men with a 47,XXY karyotype have successfully fathered normal children via intracytoplasmic sperm injection (ICSI). (In this procedure, sperm are harvested and injected directly into the oocyte in vitro.)

■ PHYSICAL EXAMINATION

- Normal to tall stature
- Thin body habitus with relatively long legs
- Normal male external genitalia, with small testicles (especially postpubertally)
- Significant incidence of the following:
  1. Gynecomastia
  2. Elbow dysplasia
  3. Intention tremor
- Occasional incidence of the following:
  1. Cryptorchidism or hypospadias
  2. Scoliosis
  3. Diabetes mellitus
  4. Bronchitis
  5. Ataxia
  6. Skin breakdown over lower legs
  7. Germ cell tumors
- Mental deficiency, growth deficiency, and more severe elbow abnormalities in males with more than two X chromosomes (e.g., 48,XXXY)

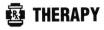 **DIAGNOSIS**

■ DIFFERENTIAL DIAGNOSIS

- Other chromosome abnormalities
- Fragile X syndrome
- Primary endocrine abnormalities
- Marfan's syndrome
- Homocystinuria

■ DIAGNOSTIC WORKUP

- Chromosome karyotype is 47,XXY.
- Buccal smears are no longer recommended because they are unlikely to detect mosaicism, structurally abnormal X chromosomes, or autosomal karyotypic abnormalities.

THERAPY

■ NONPHARMACOLOGIC

- Referral to a developmental and/or behavioral specialist is helpful if behavior or learning problems are present.
- The child may need special educational services for learning difficulties.

■ MEDICAL

- Testosterone therapy is typically needed at adolescence.
  1. The requirement for testosterone supplementation in adulthood is controversial.
  2. Many men report enhanced well-being on supplementation.

■ FOLLOW-UP & DISPOSITION

- Routine pediatric follow-up is needed, with special attention to developmental and behavioral issues in early childhood and virilization, sexual function, and self-esteem in adolescence.
- A slightly increased risk exists for germinal tumors.

■ PATIENT/FAMILY EDUCATION

- A relatively normal childhood can be expected if the child is diagnosed prenatally.
- Behavior and/or learning issues, when present, may require special evaluation and school placement.
- Sexual intercourse is normal, although some men receive testosterone supplementation.
- Infertility may be amenable to sperm manipulation (ICSI) in some men.

■ REFERRAL INFORMATION

- The patient and family should be referred for genetic counseling.
- Affected boys should undergo endocrine evaluation at adolescence.
- Referral for psychological therapy may be necessary if issues of poor

self-esteem, depression, and so forth are apparent

⚙ PEARLS & CONSIDERATIONS

■ CLINICAL PEARLS

Some individuals recommend that the eponym *Klinefelter syndrome* be reserved for the percentage of males who actually exhibit the characteristic phenotype. Thus those diagnosed prenatally or for other reasons who do not experience significant difficulties with growth or performance should be referred to as having "47,XXY karyotype" and not "Klinefelter syndrome."

■ WEBSITES

- Genetic.org: www.genetic.org/ks/
- Klinefelter Syndrome Support Group: http://klinefeltersyndrome.org/index.html
- National Institutes of Health: www.nih.gov/health/chip/nichd/kleinfelter/

■ SUPPORT GROUPS

- *The Even Exchange,* the newsletter of Klinefelter Syndrome and Associates, provides useful information for parents and adult patients. Write to Klinefelter Syndrome and Associates, *The Even Exchange,* P.O. Box 119, Roseville, CA 95678-0119.
- *Klinefelter Syndrome, The X-tra Special Boy,* and *For Boys Only* are publications available from the Genetics Clinic, Crippled Children's Division, Oregon Health Sciences University.

REFERENCES

1. Jones K-L: *Smith's recognizable patterns of human malformations,* Philadelphia, 1997, WB Saunders.
2. Klinefelter HF, Reifenstein EC, Albright F: Syndrome characterized by gynecomastia, aspermatogenesis, without aleydigism and increased excretion of follicle stimulating hormone, *J Clin Endocrinol* 2:615, 1942.
3. Robinson A et al: Sex chromosome aneuploidy: the Denver prospective study, *Birth Defects* (original article series) 26:59, 1990.
4. Willard HF: The sex chromosomes and X chromosome inactivation. In Scriver CR et al (eds): *The metabolic and molecular bases of inherited disease,* New York, 1995, McGraw-Hill.

Author: **Georgianne L. Arnold, M.D.**

BASIC INFORMATION

■ DEFINITIONS & SYNONYMS

Knee pain is acute or chronic pain in or around the knee caused by one of multiple bone, tendon/ligament, muscle, or meniscal abnormalities. Common knee problems discussed here include the following:

- Patellofemoral pain syndrome (PFPS; formerly called *chondromalacia patella*), patellofemoral dysplasia, patellofemoral dysfunction, patellar tracking abnormalities, runner's knee, and peripatellar pain syndrome: referred to variably in orthopedic and sports medicine literature and refer to anterior knee pain from irritation within the patellofemoral joint
- Patellar subluxation and dislocation (PS/D): dislocation of the patella, usually laterally, from femoral articulation, thought by some to be a subset of patellofemoral dysfunction
- Osteochondritis dissecans (OCD): subchondral necrosis of bone involving overlying articular cartilage, usually of femoral condyles, but also patella
- Osgood-Schlatter disease (OGSD): tibial tuberosity apophysitis (see specific section, also)
- Sinding-Larsen-Johansson syndrome (SLJ): traction apophysitis of the patella in a growing child that causes secondary ossification center
- Jumper's knee: patellar tendon apophysitis
- Fractures
  1. Patella fracture
  2. Fracture of tibial physis/tibial spine avulsion
  3. Fracture of femur physis
- Ligament injuries
  1. Anterior cruciate ligament (ACL): strain or rupture of the ligament that goes from the medial aspect of lateral femoral condyle to the central anteromedial tibial plateau
  2. Lateral collateral ligament (LCL): injury of the ligament that extends from the lateral distal femoral epiphysis to the proximal tibial epiphysis
  3. Medial collateral ligament (MCL): injury of the ligament that extends medially from the distal femoral to the proximal tibial epiphysis
  4. Posterior cruciate ligament (PCL): injury of the ligament that extends from the lateral portion of medial femoral condyle to the posterior lateral central tibial plateau
- Meniscal tears/injuries: tear of disc-shaped medial or lateral cartilages that lie between the femoral condyles and the tibial plateau

ICD-9CM CODES

719.46 Knee pain
717.7 Chondromalacia patella
836.3 Patellar dislocation
732.7 OCD
732.4 OGSD, SLJ, patella fracture
727.2 Jumper's knee
821.0 Femur fracture
823.80 Tibia fracture
844.0 Lateral collateral ligament sprain
844.1 Medial collateral ligament sprain
844.2 Acute anterior cruciate ligament sprain
717.83 Old tear anterior cruciate ligament
717.84 Old tear posterior cruciate ligament
836.2 Meniscal tear

■ ETIOLOGY

- The knee is a hinge joint with bony, ligamentous, muscle, and menisci involvement.
  1. Bones involved in the knee
     a. Femur: physis (growth plate) in close proximity to the knee joint
        (1) The distal femoral physis is the most active growth plate in body.
        (2) Medial and lateral condyles articulate with the tibial plateau.
        (3) Condyles are connected by the trochlear groove.
        (4) The anterior portion of the condyles and trochlear groove articulates with the patella.
        (5) Fusion occurs at approximately 15 years of age in girls (range, 12 to 17 years).
        (6) Fusion occurs at approximately 17 years of age in boys (range, 15 to 20 years).
     b. Tibia: proximal growth plate in close proximity to the knee joint
        (1) The physis is responsible for significant growth.
        (2) Flattened tibial plateau articulates with the femoral condyles.
     c. Patella: initially cartilaginous, with ossification beginning as early as 2 to 3 years of age
        (1) The patella is attached within the distal quadriceps.
        (2) It normally tracks parallel to the long axis of the lower extremity, moving caudad with flexion and cephalad with extension.
        (3) It articulates with the intertrochlear groove and femoral condyles.

  2. Ligaments (help stabilize joint): static restraints
     a. ACL and PCL
        (1) The ACL is the most commonly injured ligament.
        (2) The ACL and PCL are the major restraints to anterior and posterior tibial translation.
     b. MCL and LCL
        (1) LCL protects against excessive varus stress.
        (2) MCL protects against valgus stress.
  3. Secondary stabilizing elements
     a. The medial and lateral menisci protect against mechanical loading (shock absorbers).
        (1) Centrally avascular
     b. The joint capsule and tendon sheaths protect against medial and lateral stresses.
        (1) Medial retinaculum
        (2) Lateral retinaculum, iliotibial band
     c. Large tendons and muscles lend dynamic stability to the knee.
        (1) Quadriceps group, anteriorly, laterally, medially—vastus medialis portion medially and vastus lateralis portion laterally
        (2) Hamstrings, posteriorly with medial and lateral heads—biceps femoris laterally and semitendinous medially
        (3) Popliteus muscles, laterally
        (4) Sortorius, medially
        (5) Gastrocnemius posteriorly (lateral and medial heads)
- PFPS
  1. PFPS is the malalignment or abnormal tracking of patella in intercondylar groove.
  2. Tight lateral or weak medial muscles around knee may lead to or exacerbate tracking abnormalities.
  3. Patella may subluxate or dislocate.
     a. These result from abnormal bone and ligament restraints holding patella in place.
     b. Laxity of ligaments, as in trisomy 21 and other neuromuscular disorders, increases risk of patellar subluxations.
- OCD
  1. Separation of an osteochondral fragment
  2. Trauma and ischemia of bone in those with a genetic predisposition
  3. More common in growing children
- OGSD
  1. Incomplete separation of a fragment of cartilaginous or chondro-osseous tuberosity of tibia

2. Often with patella tendon disruption
3. Caused by chronic, repetitive (overuse) trauma of the maturing proximal tibial growth plate
4. Lesions: are microfractures of the tubercle
- SLJ and patellar tendonitis (jumper's knee)
  1. SLJ is traction apophysitis with secondary ossification of the patella.
  2. Repetitive knee flexion activity (e.g., jumping, kicking), an overuse syndrome, leads to microavulsions of the patellar tendon or stress fracture of the patella (SLJ).
- Patella fractures
  1. These fractures result from a direct blow.
  2. Avulsion force proximal or distal to the patella may cause a sleeve fracture.
- Distal femur fractures
  1. High-velocity trauma is the usual cause in a prepubertal child.
  2. Hyperextension with torsion occurs.
  3. Type 2 fractures traverse the growth plate.
- Proximal tibia/tibial spine avulsion fractures
  1. These fractures result from forceful hyperextension or a direct blow to the lower femur.
  2. Avulsion of tibial spine may occur, for example, from bicycle injuries.
  3. In adults, the ACL may tear, but the same stress in a child causes cancellous bone at the ligament attachment to avulse.
- Meniscal tears
  1. These tears result from a twisting motion with the knee flexed and foot planted.
  2. The meniscus splits because of firm attachments to the rotating femur and fixed tibia.

■ **EPIDEMIOLOGY & DEMOGRAPHICS**
- Approximately 10% to 12% of patients presenting with muscular skeletal pain have knee pain.
- Knee injuries account for 30% to 40% of sports medicine injuries in the pediatric and adolescent populations.
- Hypermobility or hypermobile joint increases the risk of injury.
- PFPS:
  1. Pubertal girls most commonly affected
  2. Chondromalacia patella, used only for arthroscopically diagnosed lesion
  3. Wasting of medial quadriceps common
  4. Increased Q angle, but may not play a role in pathogenesis

- OCD:
  1. Lateral portion medial femoral condyle most common location (85%)
  2. Three to four times more common in boys
  3. Late adolescence, early childhood
- OGSD:
  1. Most common form of apophysitis in teens
  2. Typically affects 12- to 14-year-old boys and 10- to 11-year-old girls
  3. Clearly related to growth spurt in adolescents and level of activity
  4. Bilateral in 20% to 30% of patients
  5. Chronic, repetitive trauma to proximal tibial growth plate
  6. Self-limited, but bony prominence may persist
- SLJ and jumper's knee:
  1. Jumping, kicking sport
  2. Self-limited
- Tibial fractures:
  1. Avulsion fracture of the tibial eminence more common in child than ACL disruption
  2. Proximal tibial physis fractures rare
- Distal femur fractures:
  1. Accounts for less than 1% of all fractures
  2. More common in adolescent than prepubertal children
  3. Type 1: uncommon obstetric injury to newborn
  4. Type 2: most common fracture pattern of distal femur
  5. Types 3 and 4: most serious because usually involves the growth plate and 40% of growth is accounted for by the length of the femur
- Ligament injuries:
  1. Less common in preadolescent
     a. Growth plate weaker than ligament; therefore fractures more common
  2. ACL and MCL most commonly injured knee ligaments
  3. Graded for severity
     a. 1: minor fiber dysfunction
     b. 2: moderate, partial fiber disruption
     c. 3: severe injury, complete ligament disruption
- Meniscal tears:
  1. Rare among prepubertal children
  2. More common with high-impact sports

■ **HISTORY**
- Pain
  1. Nonspecific diffuse anterior knee pain with PFPS or occasionally medial to or behind (under) the patella
  2. Specifically over the lower patella in SLJ
- PFPS
  1. Difficulty descending and climbing stairs or squatting

2. Positive theater sign (inability to sit comfortably with knees flexed for several hours)
3. Aching after strenuous activity
4. Swelling, sensation of giving way, and sense of locking vague and less reliable
- Patella subluxation and dislocation
  1. Insidious onset, often bilateral
  2. Poorly localized, all around knee anteriorly and occasionally medially
  3. Acute pain and dramatic when patella dislocates
- Osteochondritis dissecans (OCD)
  1. Knee pain usually activity related, although nonspecific
  2. Often bilateral, but symptoms may be unilateral
  3. Popping, locking, catching, "unstable" feeling
  4. Occasionally intermittent knee swelling reported
- OGSD
  1. Insidious onset of pain
  2. Well-localized pain just below the patella, anteriorly over the proximal tibia
  3. Seen especially with jumping, climbing stairs, kneeling, or squatting
  4. Pain intermittent in some cases
- Patellar fractures
  1. Direct blow to the patella
  2. Acute onset of pain
  3. Swelling
- Tibial fractures
  1. Bicycling or high-impact sport
- Femoral fractures
  1. High-velocity trauma
- Ligament injuries
  1. ACL
     a. Hyperextension or sudden deceleration or valgus and rotational force with foot planted
     b. Pop heard in some cases
     c. Fall to ground and unable to walk without assistance
  2. LCL
     a. Varus force to the knee or hyperextension injury
     b. Pain and tenderness
     c. Swelling within hours if complete rupture
  3. MCL
     a. Valgus or external rotation force to knee with foot planted
- Meniscal tears
  1. Pain
  2. Clicking
  3. Locking
  4. Specific event often recalled by teen

■ **PHYSICAL EXAMINATION**
- General examination
  1. Assess stance and posture.
  2. Evaluate range of motion.
  3. Test ligament stability.
  4. For anterior knee pain, pay attention to the patellofemoral joint.

- PFPS
  1. The patella should face forward while standing upright and while sitting with knees flexed 90 degrees.
  2. Positive apprehension: Passive lateral and medial patellar movement makes the patient uncomfortable.
  3. Positive apprehension with stress: This is pathognomonic for patella instability and tracking malalignment.
     a. Pain and contraction of quadriceps when the patella is gently moved laterally while the patient is supine with leg flexed to less than 30 degrees
  4. Abnormal Q angle:
     a. Angle formed at the center of the patella by the line of pull of the quadriceps tendon and patella tendon
     b. Measured from the central patella to the anterior superior iliac spine proximally and tibial tuberosity distally
     c. Normal: 15 degrees or less in women and less than 10 degrees in men
     d. More than 15 degrees abnormal and increases risk of lateral patellar subluxation
     e. Increased in patients with trisomy 21 and other neuromuscular disorders
- OCD
  1. The examination is often normal.
  2. Firm palpation of femoral condyle in 90 degrees of flexion may elicit pain.
  3. Effusion is sometimes present.
  4. Decreased range of motion may be present.
- OGSD
  1. Tendon prominence of the knee just below the joint is noted.
  2. Pain is increased with resisted extension.
  3. Quadriceps atrophy may be noted.
- SLJ
  1. Point tenderness at the inferior portion of the patella
  2. Tight but weak quadriceps
- Patella fractures
  1. Point tenderness on palpation of patella
  2. Swelling
  3. Decreased range of motion, especially extension
- Tibial spine fractures
  1. Large effusion (hemarthrosis)
- Distal femoral fractures
  1. Acute pain
  2. Swelling, grossly deformed
  3. Circumferential tenderness
- Ligament injuries
  1. ACL
     a. Large effusion within hours

  b. Lachman test
     (1) With patient supine, the hip and knee are flexed 20 to 30 degrees.
     (2) Stabilize the femur and move the tibia anteriorly from the femur.
     (3) The test is positive, indicating an ACL tear, if the anterior translation of the tibia on the femur occurs with a soft endpoint.
  c. Anterior drawer test
     (1) With the patient sitting with the knee flexed 90 degrees, anteriorly displace the tibia from the femur, or the patient may be supine with the hip flexed 45 degrees and the knee flexed 90 degrees.
     (2) The examiner may stabilize the foot by sitting on it.
     (3) The examiner wraps his or her fingers around the calf near the hamstring insertion with the thumbs on either side of the patella along the tibial plateau.
     (4) Significant anterior translation occurs after an ACL tear.
  2. LCL
     a. Local tenderness
     b. Effusion
     c. Limited range of motion
  3. MCL
     a. Local swelling
     b. Pain along MCL course in extension and slight flexion
     c. Laxity with valgus stress
- Meniscal tears
  1. Joint (femoral-tibial) line tenderness
  2. Decreased range of motion
  3. Occasional effusion of knee
  4. Positive McMurray test
     a. This test is nonspecific.
     b. Place fingers along the joint line on a flexed (greater than 120 degrees) knee, then internally (and/or externally) rotate the tibia, while bringing the knee joint to full extension.
     c. A painful pop in the lateral or medial joint line will be elicited.

🔬 DIAGNOSIS

■ DIFFERENTIAL DIAGNOSIS

In addition to excluding the aforementioned common pain syndromes and injuries from each other, consider the following:
- Osteomyelitis
- Tumor
- Slipped capital femoral epiphysis (SCFE)

- Legg-Calvé-Perthes
- Synovitis, bursitis
- Arthritis
  1. Inflammatory (e.g., juvenile arthritis, rheumatic fever)
  2. Infectious (e.g., staphylococcal, salmonellal infections)

■ DIAGNOSTIC WORKUP

- X-ray examination
  1. Anteroposterior (AP) and lateral views
     a. AP best to evaluate distal femoral physis, proximal tibial physis, and patella
        (1) Bipartite patella is an incidental finding; it may become symptomatic after acute trauma.
     b. Lateral for patella position and tibial tubercle
  2. Notch or tunnel view
     a. AP with knee flexed 20 degrees
     b. Notch between distal femoral condyles visualized
     c. Used for diagnosis of osteochondritis dissecans
  3. Sunrise or sulcus view
     a. Shows relationship between the patella and distal femur
     b. Tangential radiograph with knee flexed approximately 45 degrees
     c. Lack of congruence of the patella femoral joint seen with patella subluxation
  4. Standing AP (of entire lower extremity)
     a. To assess angular or torsional malalignment
     b. Femoral anteversion and genu valgum best evaluated
  5. Oblique and stress views and comparison views to evaluate specific types of trauma
  6. In patella subluxation/dislocation:
     a. Look for osteochondral fracture fragments.
  7. In patellar fracture:
     a. May look like small or insignificant bone fragment
     b. Often includes significant radiolucent cartilage being pulled from bone
  8. With ligament injuries, consider radiographic studies
     a. Rule out fractures
     b. May need stress x-ray study under fluoroscopy to visualize nonossified disruptions
  9. In tibial fractures:
     a. Small ossified portion may lead to deceptively normal x-ray examination
- Magnetic resonance imaging
  1. Evaluation of soft tissues not visualized on plain radiography
  2. Controversial still because of both poor sensitivity and specifically and high cost compared with examination and arthroscopy

- Evaluation of knee effusions
  1. Acute associated with trauma
     a. Usually hemarthrosis
     b. Often indication for further orthopedic workup
  2. Chronic
     a. Associated with tumor, infection, rheumatologic or metabolic abnormalities
     b. Clarity, color, viscosity
     c. Cell count
     d. Gram stain and cultures

■ **THERAPY**
- PFPS
  1. Nonpharmacologic
     a. Curtail activities that include weight bearing with flexed knee
     b. Muscle-stretching exercise for quadriceps, hip adductors, and hamstrings
     c. Muscle strengthening, especially quadriceps group (including vastus medialis) and hamstrings
     d. Activity modification with gradual resumption when pain free
     e. Ice before and after activities
  2. Medical
     a. Nonsteroidal antiinflammatory drugs (NSAIDs) for pain
     b. Orthotic support
        (1) May provide symptomatic support
        (2) No evidence that improves patella tracking
- Patella subluxation/dislocation
  1. Nonpharmacologic
     a. Immediate reduction and immobilization with knee extended for 3 to 6 weeks
     b. Nonsurgical rehabilitation and strengthening as for PFPS
  2. Medical
     a. NSAIDs for pain
  3. Surgical
     a. Results not uniformly successful, especially if increased Q angle or flat lateral femoral condyle
- OCD
  1. Treatment goal: to produce a stable and normally functioning articular surface
  2. Nonpharmacologic
     a. Activity modification if nondisplaced lesion
     b. Immobilization so that lesion may heal anatomically before growth plate closure occurs
     c. Non–weight bearing may be necessary
  3. Medical
     a. Pain medications often warranted
     b. No specific medications to resolve fragments

  4. Surgical
     a. If not healed after 3 to 6 months of nonsurgical treatment
     b. Displaced fragments: usually need to be excised
     c. Commonly done arthroscopically
- OGSD
  1. Nonpharmacologic
     a. Rest, activity modification (e.g., restrict sports)
     b. Ice
     c. Quadriceps stretching and strengthening
  2. Medical
     a. NSAIDs useful
     b. Immobilization on rare occasions
     c. Knee pad with cutout to reduce pressure on tuberosity may help
  3. Surgical
     a. Rarely needed
     b. Removal of painful, nonunited ossicle after skeletal maturation
- SLJ and jumper's knee
  1. Nonpharmacologic
     a. Restricted activity: may be necessary temporarily
     b. Quadriceps stretching and strengthening
     c. Cross-training
  2. Medical
     a. NSAIDs
  3. Surgical
     a. Immobilization not usually necessary
- Patella fractures
  1. Nonpharmacologic
     a. Long leg cast or extension knee splint
     b. 4 to 6 weeks usual
     c. Extension knee splint to allow for gradual range-of-motion exercises as pain abates
  2. Medical
     a. Pain medication
  3. Surgical
     a. Displaced, transverse fractures: require surgery (open reduction and internal fixation)
- Distal femur fractures
  1. Surgical
     a. Usually closed reduction and cast immobilization for type 2 fractures
     b. Types 3 and 4 demand anatomic realignment of both the growth plate and articular surface to minimize sequela (growth plate dysfunction)
- Tibial fractures
  1. Medical
     a. Minimally displaced fractures: require nonsurgical immobilization
  2. Surgical
     a. Open reduction and fixation required in displaced fractures

- Ligament injuries
  1. Nonpharmacologic
     a. Grade 1
        (1) Immobilization and restricted activity
        (2) Protected motion in brace
        (3) Several weeks maximum
     b. Grade 2
        (1) Immobilization for longer
        (2) Rehabilitation before returning to activities
  2. Medical
     a. NSAIDs for pain
     b. Compression
     c. Cryotherapy
  3. Surgical
     a. Grade 3
        (1) Surgical repair usually necessary
- Meniscal tears
  1. Nonpharmacologic
     a. Small, peripheral tears: heal without specific therapy
  2. Medical
     a. NSAIDs for acute pain
  3. Surgical
     a. Repair if unstable tear
     b. Removal of fragments, especially medial central, because avascular and poor healing
     c. Meniscectomy; not preferred because poor long-term results

■ **FOLLOW-UP & DISPOSITION**
- For many patients with PFPS, a long-term exercise program will be needed.
- For patients with proximal femoral or distal tibial fractures, long-term growth assessment is needed.
- For ligament injuries:
  1. Return to sports when the following have occurred:
     a. Normal strength
     b. Range of motion comfortably
     c. Nontender
     d. No complaints with sport

■ **PATIENT/FAMILY EDUCATION**
- Most patients with PFPS respond to a nonsurgical approach.
- Recurrence of dislocation occurs in up to 85% of inadequately treated patients.
- SLJ and OSGD are usually self-limited.
- The prognosis in OCD is poor in adults.

■ **PREVENTIVE TREATMENT**
- For many pediatric knee problems, adequate stretch and strengthening with a decrease in repetitive trauma (overuse) will allay problems.
- For asymptomatic OCD, limit activities until lesion heals and treat symptomatic lesions to prevent degenerative arthritis.

■ REFERRAL INFORMATION
- Referral to a sports medicine or occupational therapist for rehabilitation or exercise training
- Referral to an orthopedic surgeon if the diagnosis is unclear, for acute trauma necessitating surgery, and for unresolving pain

☼ PEARLS & CONSIDERATIONS

■ CLINICAL PEARLS
- The most common cause of subacute and chronic knee pain in girls is PFPS.
  1. Special attention to vastus medialis strengthening is important.
- Neoplasm near the knee may present with sports-related trauma.

- Infectious, metabolic, and inflammatory diseases of knee, femur, or tibia may present with knee pain or effusion.
- Proximal tibia and distal femur fractures may be missed early on x-ray examination.
- All children presenting with knee pain should also be evaluated for ipsilateral hip disorders, which can present with knee pain.
  1. SCFE
  2. Transient toxic synovitis
  3. Legg-Calvé-Perthes

■ WEBSITES
- American Academy of Family Physicians: www.aafp.org/afp/991101ap/99110lb.html; PFPS exercises
- Familydoc.com: www.familydoc.com; parent site

REFERENCES
1. Davids JR: Pediatric knee: clinical assessment to common disorders, *Pediatr Clin North Am* 43:1067, 1996.
2. Eilert RE: Adolescent anterior knee pain, *Instructional Course Lectures* 42:473, 1993.
3. Johnson RP: Anterior knee pain in adolescents and young adults, *Curr Opin Rheumatol* 9:159, 1997.
4. Ruffin MT IV, Kiningham RB: Anterior knee pain: the challenge of patellofemoral syndrome, *Am Fam Physician* 47:185, 1993.
5. Smith AD, Tao SS: Knee injuries in young athletes, *Clin Sports Med* 4:629, 1995.
6. Roach JW: Knee disorders and injuries in adolescents, *Adolesc Med* 9:589, 1998.

Author: **Lynn C. Garfunkel, M.D.**

II

BASIC INFORMATION

DEFINITION
Labyrinthitis is a viral or bacterial infection of the inner ear that causes dizziness and reduced or distorted hearing. Closely related is vestibular neuritis, which is caused by a viral infection of one of the two vestibular nerves. The imbalance of information about head positioning is interpreted by the brain to be movement, resulting in the sensation of vertigo. Symptoms include dizziness, vertigo, disequilibrium or imbalance, and nausea.

SYNONYMS
- Vertigo
- Neuronitis
- Inner ear infection

ICD-9CM CODE
386.30 Labyrinthitis

ETIOLOGY
- Viruses (or occasionally bacteria) can enter the inner ear and inflame the labyrinth system or directly affect the vestibular nerve.
  1. Viruses causing labyrinthitis or vestibular neuritis include influenza, herpes, hepatitis, polio, Epstein-Barr virus, measles, rubella, and mumps.
- Chronic, untreated middle ear infections can create a serous labyrinthitis secondary to inflammation.
- Bacteria from the middle ear can spread locally, leading to suppurative labyrinthitis.

EPIDEMIOLOGY & DEMOGRAPHICS
- Five percent of all dizziness is caused by labyrinthitis or vestibular neuritis.
- It occurs equally in all age groups.
- Females are slightly more susceptible than males at a ratio of 1.5:1.

HISTORY
- The early stages may be mild.
- Disequilibrium is present.
- Nausea is common.
- Symptoms are often precipitated by sudden movements or a sudden turn of the head.

PHYSICAL EXAMINATION
- The middle ear may show signs of infection or serous fluid.
- Nystagmus (usually horizontal) may be present at rest or when provoked by head turning.
- Meningeal signs should be evaluated carefully to distinguish from meningitis.
- Labyrinthitis may induce vertigo with a sudden change in head position (e.g., sitting to supine).

DIAGNOSIS

DIFFERENTIAL DIAGNOSIS
- Many drugs can cause dizziness:
  1. Alcohol
  2. Tobacco
  3. Caffeine
  4. Illicit drugs
     a. Cocaine
     b. Amphetamines
     c. Glue sniffing
- Closed head injury
- Hypertension
- Ear trauma
- Allergies
- Anxiety
- Neurologic disease
  1. Central nervous system (CNS) tumor, such as acoustic schwannoma
  2. CNS infection, such as bacterial or viral meningitis
- Headache/migraine
- Ménière's disease

DIAGNOSTIC WORKUP
- Initially, a history and physical examination are all that are necessary.
- If symptoms persist beyond 1 month, recur, or become debilitating, an audiogram and an electronystagmography (ENG) may help distinguish from Ménière's disease and migraine.
  1. An audiogram shows reduced hearing in labyrinthitis.
  2. The ENG characteristically shows reduced responses to motion of one ear.
- A magnetic resonance imaging scan can detect evidence of stroke, tumor, or vestibular nerve impingement but is usually normal in labyrinthitis.

THERAPY

NONPHARMACOLOGIC
Lying still with eyes closed may help reduce the severity of vertigo.

MEDICAL
- Acute episodes are treated symptomatically with medications to reduce nausea and/or dizziness.
  1. Antiemetics
     a. Meclizine
     b. Promethazine
     c. Prochlorperazine
  2. Anxiolytics
     a. Lorazepam
     b. Diazepam
- For protracted nausea and vomiting, hospitalization may be required for intravenous rehydration.

SURGICAL
- Surgical treatment is reserved for those cases caused by mastoiditis, tumor, or vestibular nerve impingement.
- Vestibular nerve ablation is rarely necessary.

FOLLOW-UP & DISPOSITION
- Patients should be monitored to ensure adequate hydration.
- Formal hearing testing should be performed at the end of symptoms to detect subtle hearing deficits that may persist.

PATIENT/FAMILY EDUCATION
- It may take 3 weeks to recover from labyrinthitis. Recovery involves a combination of the following:
  1. Resolution of viral infection
  2. Compensation by the brain for persistent vestibular imbalance
- Some patients experience intermittent symptoms for months, especially associated with sudden head movements.
- Minor sensitivity to head motion can persist for years and may reduce the ability to perform certain activities and sports, such as racquetball, volleyball, or aerobics.

REFERRAL INFORMATION
- Most people recover without a referral to a neurologist or otolaryngologist.
- For those whose symptoms persist or who exhibit concerning neurologic findings, a referral to a specialist who is familiar with vestibular disorders should be made.

PEARLS & CONSIDERATIONS

CLINICAL PEARLS
- About 5% of all dizziness is caused by vestibular neuritis or labyrinthitis.
- Children as young as 1 year of age can experience vertigo, which may mimic seizure activity.
- Any neurologic finding besides nystagmus suggests conditions other than labyrinthitis.

WEBSITE
The Vestibular Disorders Association (VEDA): www.vestibular.org; includes support groups, children's educational sites, and reference books

REFERENCES
1. Lorenzo NY: Labyrinthitis. In Adler J et al: emedicine.com (electronic book on emergency medicine).
2. McDonald DL: Dizziness and vertigo. In Hoekelman RA et al: *Primary pediatric care*, ed 3, St Louis, 1997, Mosby.
Author: **Neil Herendeen, M.D.**

BASIC INFORMATION

■ DEFINITION
Lacrimal duct obstruction is blockage of the nasolacrimal duct drainage system leading to increased eye tearing and potential infection.

■ SYNONYMS
- Nasolacrimal duct obstruction
- Dacryostenosis
- Dacryocystitis (infection of obstructed duct)
- Blocked tear duct

ICD-9CM CODES
375.56 Dacryostenosis
743.65 Congenital dacryostenosis
375.32 Dacryocystitis, acute and subacute
375.42 Chronic dacryocystitis

■ ETIOLOGY
- Congenital
  1. Obstruction of the nasolacrimal duct (the bony canal that carries tears into the nose) prevents drainage of tears produced by the lacrimal gland and promotes mucus build-up within the lacrimal sac.
  2. Obstruction occurs during development of the lacrimal system and typically involves the distal portion of the duct.
  3. Obstruction may represent failure of canalization of the epithelial cells that form the duct, resulting in a thin membrane that occludes the lumen.
- Acquired
  1. Far less common in children and adolescents than in adults
  2. May result from trauma, infection, sinus disease, nasal polyps, tumor, sarcoid, Wegener's granulomatosis, or other granulomatous disease

■ EPIDEMIOLOGY & DEMOGRAPHICS
- The nasolacrimal duct system is not fully patent in as many as 73% of term infants.
- Obstruction resolves spontaneously or remains asymptomatic in all but approximately 6% of patients.

■ HISTORY
- Intermittent and recurrent tearing and mucoid discharge is produced from one or both eyes, usually without conjunctival injection.
- Symptoms usually begin within days to weeks after birth and are often variable and cyclical.

- Associated conjunctival injection and infection may occur and, in rare cases, progress to dacryocystitis.
  1. Mucopurulent discharge with tender swelling of the nasolacrimal sac
  2. Swelling noted along the medial canthus and lower lid
- More than 90% of cases of lacrimal duct obstruction resolve spontaneously in the first 9 to 12 months of life.

■ PHYSICAL EXAMINATION
- Assess for conjunctival injection.
- Assess for erythema or swelling of lacrimal sac and surrounding periorbital tissues.
- Digital pressure of the nasolacrimal sac can be diagnostic as well as therapeutic.
  1. If obstructed, pressure may cause tears and mucus to be released from the puncta.
  2. This may help relieve the distal obstruction.

🔬 **DIAGNOSIS**

■ DIFFERENTIAL DIAGNOSIS
- In a newborn with obstruction and associated infection, other causes of conjunctivitis (*Neisseria gonorrhoeae, Chlamydia,* nonspecific, or allergic) or keratitis need to be considered.
- Congenital glaucoma can present with excessive tearing and light sensitivity, but associated signs include increased intraocular pressure, an enlarged, hazy cornea, and occasionally, lid spasm.
- In an older infant with tearing, consider a foreign body or corneal abrasion.
- Other disorders of the lacrimal drainage system can present with similar symptoms.
  1. Atresia of the lacrimal puncta: increased tearing but milder and without mucoid discharge
  2. Congenital mucocele (dacryocystocele) of the lacrimal sac
     a. Rare; bluish subcutaneous swelling in the medial canthal area
     b. Results from a nonpatent lacrimal sac with both proximal and distal obstruction
     c. Prone to infection and may progress to cellulitis
- In cases of dacryocystitis, assess closely for signs of periorbital or orbital cellulitis.

■ DIAGNOSTIC WORKUP
Consider culture of the eye discharge in cases with associated conjunctivitis or dacryocystitis.

💊 **THERAPY**

Directed toward avoiding infection and minimizing additional obstruction of the sac with discharge and debris

■ NONPHARMACOLOGIC
- Application of warm compresses to the eye to cleanse away discharge and debris
- Massage of nasolacrimal sac
  1. Digital compressing of the nasolacrimal sac results in increased hydrostatic pressure within the canal.
  2. This pressure may force the duct to open (see "Patient/Family Education").

■ MEDICAL
- For mild or low-grade infection accompanying obstruction, use topical antibiotics (ointment preferred over drops) combined with nasolacrimal sac massage.
- If infection is more severe or with accompanying dacryocystitis, take a culture of the discharge and begin treatment with systemic antistaphylococcal antibiotics (oral or intravenous).
  1. Close monitoring is critical.
  2. Orbital cellulitis is a possible complication.

■ SURGICAL
- For cases that do not resolve spontaneously by 1 year of age, referral to a pediatric ophthalmologist is indicated for probing and irrigation of the nasolacrimal duct.
- Additional surgical options include nasolacrimal duct intubation with silastic tubing and pediatric balloon dacryoplasty.

■ FOLLOW-UP & DISPOSITION
See "Therapy."

■ PATIENT/FAMILY EDUCATION
- Parents should be instructed to massage the nasolacrimal sac three to four times daily.
  1. Appropriate massage technique should be performed in the medial canthal area and not down the nasal bone, where the duct is interosseous and not affected by compression.
  2. The initial motion should milk any discharge from the sac upward, followed by firm downward pressure on the nasolacrimal sac.

- Parents should call their child's physician to report signs of infection such as conjunctival injection or periorbital erythema and swelling.

■ PREVENTIVE TREATMENT
See nonpharmacologic therapy described previously to minimize secondary infection.

■ REFERRAL INFORMATION
Infants who do not experience spontaneous resolution by 1 year of age should be referred to a pediatric ophthalmologist.

☼ PEARLS & CONSIDERATIONS

■ CLINICAL PEARLS
- Congenital nasolacrimal duct obstruction is the most common abnormality of the entire lacrimal system in children.
- It presents with recurrent tearing and eye discharge in the early newborn period without conjunctival injection or photophobia.
- Digital massage can be therapeutic in relieving the distal congenital duct obstruction.

REFERENCES
1. Lavrich JB, Nelson LB: Disorders of the lacrimal system apparatus, *Pediatr Clin North Am* 40:767, 1993.
2. Ogawa GSH, Gonnering RS: Congenital nasolacrimal duct obstruction, *J Pediatr* 119:12, 1991.
Author: **Laura Jean Shipley, M.D.**

BASIC INFORMATION

■ DEFINITION
Lactose intolerance is the inability to digest the milk sugar lactose, resulting in a constellation of clinical symptoms following the ingestion of milk products.

■ SYNONYMS
- Lactose malabsorption
- Lactase deficiency
- Hypolactasia

ICD-9CM CODE
271.3 Intestinal lactase deficiency and lactose malabsorption

■ ETIOLOGY
- Lactose malabsorption is caused by a deficiency of the intestinal brush border enzyme lactase.
  1. Lactase breaks down lactose into the monosaccharides glucose and galactose.
  2. Unlike disaccharides, the monosaccharides are absorbed by the small intestine.
- Undigested, and therefore unabsorbable, lactose passes through the intestine, drawing water into the lumen.
- Colonic bacteria ferment lactose, producing gas and volatile fatty acids.
- Congenital alactasia is extremely rare.
- Primary acquired deficiency results from decreasing enzyme activity in the small intestine with age/maturity (postweaning).
- Secondary lactase deficiency results from disease processes that cause injury to the small bowel lining (e.g., celiac disease, Crohn's disease, giardiasis, rotavirus infection, cow's milk or soy protein sensitivity, radiation).
- Transient lactase deficiency occurs in premature infants.
  1. Developmental lactose intolerance
     a. At 26 to 34 weeks' gestation, lactase levels are 30% of term infants' levels.
     b. At 35 to 38 weeks' gestation, lactase levels are 70% of term infants' levels.

■ EPIDEMIOLOGY & DEMOGRAPHICS
- Primary acquired lactase deficiency is more common in some populations.
  1. Up to 70% to 100% prevalence in Asian, African, Eskimo, Native Americans
  2. Less than 20% prevalence in Scandinavians, Anglo-Saxons
- Primary lactose intolerance develops after lactase levels decrease, usually between 3 and 5 years of age. Symptoms may present at any age.

- Secondary lactose intolerance occurs during and often after its causal illness.

■ HISTORY
- Flatulence
- Abdominal pain
- Bloating
- Loose stools (develop within hours after milk ingestion)
- Symptom severity, timing after milk ingestion, and amount of lactose required to elicit them vary depending on the following:
  1. Intestinal lactase levels
  2. Lactose dose and presenting vehicle
  3. Gastric emptying and intestinal transit time
  4. Intestinal secretion in response to osmotic challenge
  5. Bacterial flora

■ PHYSICAL EXAMINATION
- Tympanitic or distended abdomen
- Hyperactive bowel sounds
- Weight loss or poor weight gain (rare)

DIAGNOSIS

■ DIFFERENTIAL DIAGNOSIS
- Cow's milk protein sensitivity
- Giardiasis
- Constipation with encopresis
- Irritable bowel syndrome/recurrent abdominal pain
- Other diseases causing small bowel mucosal injury

■ DIAGNOSTIC WORKUP
- Breath hydrogen test
  1. This test measures exhaled hydrogen gas produced in the colon by bacterial fermentation of undigested lactose.
  2. Serial measurements are obtained after ingestion of a 2-g/kg lactose load.
     a. Abnormal peak demonstrated within 1 to 2 hours indicates lactose malabsorption.
     b. Associated with symptoms indicates lactose intolerance.
- Serum lactose tolerance test
  1. Serial blood glucose levels are drawn after oral lactose ingestion.
  2. Patients with lactase deficiency will not have a normal elevation of blood glucose levels after oral ingestion of lactose.
- Direct assay of enzyme activity (can be obtained from intestinal biopsy)
- Stool pH
  1. Acid stool (pH less than 5) indicative of carbohydrate malabsorption

2. Not specific for lactose malabsorption
3. May be helpful in infants and toddlers

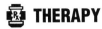

THERAPY

■ NONPHARMACOLOGIC
- A lactose-free or low-lactose diet should be initiated.
  1. Strict elimination is recommended for 2 to 3 weeks to demonstrate complete resolution of symptoms.
  2. Liberalize slowly depending on the symptoms.
- Some patients tolerate digested or fermented milk products such as yogurt, cultured buttermilk, and curds.
- Hidden sources of lactose may be found in baked goods, margarine, lunch meats, salad dressings, candy, and medications.

■ MEDICAL
- Lactase supplements may be taken with milk products.
- Milk containing hydrolyzed lactose is available (Lactaid).
- Calcium supplements are necessary if few dairy products are tolerated.

■ REFERRAL INFORMATION
- Patients should be referred to a pediatric gastroenterologist if an underlying intestinal illness is suspected (e.g., associated weight loss) or if symptoms do not resolve with strict elimination of lactose.
- Consider referral to nutritionist for parental education and advice about diet, especially if caloric intake is a concern.

PEARLS & CONSIDERATIONS

■ WEBSITE
National Digestive Diseases Information Clearinghouse: www.niddk.nih.gov/TOOLS/MAIL_nddic.html

REFERENCES
1. Barnard J: Gastrointestinal disorders due to cow's milk consumption, *Pediatr Ann* 26:244, 1997.
2. Shaw AD, Davies GJ: Lactose intolerance: problems in diagnosis and treatment, *J Clin Gastroenterol* 28:208, 1999.
3. Vesa TH, Marteau P, Korpela R: Lactose intolerance, *Am J Coll Nutr* 19(suppl):165S, 2000.
Author: **Colston McEvoy, M.D.**

BASIC INFORMATION

■ DEFINITION
Lead poisoning is the potential impairment caused by lead ingestion. Lead poisoning is usually silent—no overt symptoms are noted; however, lead affects nearly every organ in the body. The developing central nervous system of the young child is particularly likely to be affected. Common manifestations are a reduction in neurocognitive potential and behavioral disorders. Very high blood lead levels (70 µg/dl or greater) can result in encephalopathy, coma, and death.

■ SYNONYM
Lead toxicity

■ ICD-9CM CODE
984.9 Lead poisoning

■ ETIOLOGY
- Lead-based paint
- Lead-containing dust, soil, water, cosmetics, ceramics, and home remedies
- Lead solder
- Occupational exposure (pottery making, glass production, battery manufacture or recycling, work in lead smelters or incinerators, iron working, pipe fitting, plumbing, demolition work, remodeling, chemical manufacturing, and work on firing ranges)
- Airborne exposure near industrial point sources
- Often found in association with iron deficiency anemia

■ EPIDEMIOLOGY & DEMOGRAPHICS
- Children are primarily susceptible to the toxic effects of lead.
- Lead poisoning occurs in all population groups.
- The highest prevalence is found in poor, African-American children 5 years of age or younger living in older inner-city housing.

■ HISTORY
- Pica
- Exposure to old, peeling paint, lead-containing dust, or other lead sources
  1. Paint used before 1950 had a high content of lead.
- Hyperactivity
- Anemia
- Low dietary intake of iron and/or calcium

■ PHYSICAL EXAMINATION
Usually noncontributory

DIAGNOSIS

■ DIFFERENTIAL DIAGNOSIS
The diagnosis is based on laboratory testing, with nothing else in the differential diagnosis.

■ DIAGNOSTIC WORKUP
- The workup depends on venous lead assay.
- Erythrocyte protoporphyrin levels can help differentiate children with acute and chronic lead exposure.
- Long-bone radiographs may show the presence of "lead lines" in cases of chronic lead exposure.

THERAPY

■ NONPHARMACOLOGIC
- A dietary history and iron studies should be obtained for any child with venous lead levels of 15 µg/dl or higher.
- The adequacy of iron and calcium in the diet should be ensured.
- Environmental home inspection should occur expeditiously for any child whose venous lead level is 20 µg/dl or higher.
- It is always extremely important to get the child out of the environment in which the lead source is found.

■ MEDICAL
- A lead challenge test with a single intramuscular dose of $CaNa_2EDTA$ should be considered for children with blood lead levels of 35 to 44 µg/dl. If the challenge test is positive (excreted urinary lead/$CaNa_2EDTA$ administered 0.6 or higher), the child should undergo a full course of lead chelation.
- Children with a venous lead level of 45 µg/dl or higher or a positive $CaNa_2EDTA$ challenge test should be chelated with either a 5-day parenteral course of 1000 mg/M^2/day of $CaNa_2EDTA$ or a 19-day oral course of 2,3 DMSA (Succimer, Chemet).
  1. Home chelation should never be performed in a hazardous home environment.
- A venous lead level of 70 µg/dl or higher is considered a medical emergency. Children with a venous lead level of 70 µg/dl or higher should receive a 5-day parenteral course of 1500 mg/M^2/day of $CaNa_2EDTA$, as well as 75 mg/M^2 of intramuscular dimercaprol (BAL) every 4 hours for 3 days.

■ FOLLOW-UP & DISPOSITION
- Children completing chelation should not return to a home environment where lead hazards remain.
- Children with elevated venous lead levels (10 µg/dl or higher) should undergo frequent follow-up blood lead testing. Children with higher blood lead levels should undergo more frequent follow-up testing.
- Developmental follow-up is important for children with significantly elevated blood lead levels.

■ PATIENT/FAMILY EDUCATION
- Minimize environmental exposure to lead through the following steps:
  1. Wet-mop uncarpeted floors and wet-wipe window sills often.
  2. Wash children's hands often.
  3. Limit children's exposure to peeling or chipping paint; avoid children's presence in homes where renovations are occurring.
- Maintain an adequate dietary intake of iron and calcium for affected children.

■ PREVENTIVE TREATMENT OR TESTS
Children who are at risk for significant lead exposure by history or who are younger than 36 months of age and either live in areas where 12% or more of children have blood lead levels of 10 µg/dl or higher or where 27% or more of housing was built before 1950 should have blood lead testing.

■ REFERRAL INFORMATION
Referral to the city or county health department should be undertaken whenever a child with a venous lead level of 20 µg/dl or higher is identified.

PEARLS & CONSIDERATIONS

■ CLINICAL PEARLS
- "Lead is toxic wherever it is found, and it is found everywhere."
- Lead poisoning rarely has obvious clinical manifestations. Diagnosis requires screening.

■ WEBSITES & INFORMATION SERVICES
- Alliance to End Childhood Lead Poisoning, 227 Massachusetts Avenue NE, Suite 200, Washington, DC 20002, 202-543-1147, www.aeclp.org
- Centers for Disease Control and Prevention Childhood Lead Poisoning Prevention Program: www.cdc.gov/nced/programs/lead/lead.htm
- Housing and Urban Development Office of Hazard Control: www.hed.gov/lea/leahome.html

- Lead Poisoning Prevention Outreach Program, National Safety Council, Environmental Health Center, 1025 Connecticut Avenue NW, Suite 1200, Washington, DC 20036, 202-974-2476, nsc.org/ehc/lead.htm
- The National Center for Lead Safe Housing: 10227 Wincopin Circle, Suite 205, Columbia, MD 21044, 410-992-0712, www.leadsafehousing.org
- National Lead Information Center (part of the National Safety Council), Environmental Protection Agency, Office of Pollution Prevention and Toxics, 800-424-LEAD, www.epa.gov/lead/nlic.htm

■ SUPPORT GROUP

United Parents Against Lead (UPAL), P.O. Box 24773, Richmond, VA 23224, 804-714-0798, www.home.earthlink.net/~shabazzaupal

REFERENCES

1. Centers for Disease Control and Prevention: *Preventing lead poisoning in young children: a statement by the Centers for Disease Control,* Atlanta, 1991, Department of Health and Human Services.
2. Centers for Disease Control and Prevention: *Screening young children for lead poisoning: guidance for state and local public health officials,* Atlanta, 1997, Department of Health and Human Services.
3. National Academy of Sciences: *Measuring lead exposure in infants, children, and other sensitive populations,* Washington, DC, 1993, National Academy Press.

Authors: **Stanley J. Schaffer, M.D., M.S., and James R. Campbell, M.D., M.P.H.**

BASIC INFORMATION

■ DEFINITION

Left ventricular outflow tract (LVOT) obstruction is an anatomic obstruction to left ventricular outflow at any level, including subvalvular, valvular, supravalvular, and intraaortic, as in coarctation of the aorta. The most severe form is hypoplastic left ventricle syndrome with aortic valve atresia.

■ SYNONYMS

- Aortic stenosis (AS)
- Coarctation of the aorta
- "Coarct"

ICD-9CM CODES

746.3   Aortic valve stenosis
746.81 Subvalve aortic stenosis
747.22 Supravalve aortic stenosis
747.1   Coarctation of the aorta
746.7   Hypoplastic left heart syndrome

■ ETIOLOGY

- Strong genetic determinants of LVOT obstruction
  1. Abnormal in utero flow patterns
  2. Aortic valve annulus may be hypoplastic
- Abnormal in utero valve formation
- Frequent associated anomalies
  1. Ventricular septal defect
  2. Mitral valve abnormalities

■ EPIDEMIOLOGY & DEMOGRAPHICS

- The incidence of congenital heart disease is 1%.
  1. Approximately 10% of these have LVOT obstruction.
  2. The incidence of bicuspid aortic valve is unknown.
- No racial, ethnic, or gender differences exist.
- No known environmental associations have been found.
- Supravalvar AS is associated with Williams syndrome.

■ HISTORY

- Murmur may be heard at birth in severe obstruction.
- Severe obstruction presents in the neonate as congestive heart failure.
  1. Poor feeding
  2. Poor growth
  3. Lethargy
  4. Rapid respiratory rate
  5. Cardiovascular collapse
- In older children, uncommon symptoms include the following:
  1. Chest pain
  2. Syncope
  3. Near-syncope on exertion
- Manifestations of congestive heart failure in an older child may include the following:
  1. Edema (usually facial)
  2. Shortness of breath

3. Dyspnea on exertion
4. Orthopnea
- Congestive heart failure may appear as late as adulthood.
- Coarctation of aorta in the neonate may occur.
  1. May present in the neonatal period as sudden cardiovascular collapse at 7 to 10 days when ductus arteriosus closes
- Coarctation in later infancy and childhood is possible.
  1. Usually identified by diminished or absent femoral pulses, relative (but not necessarily absolute) upper extremity hypertension.
  2. Symptoms uncommon but can include the following:
     a. Headaches
     b. Nose bleeds
     c. Leg pain, particularly in association with exercise

■ PHYSICAL EXAMINATION

- Aortic valve stenosis (AS): usually progressive
  1. A narrow pulse pressure is detected.
  2. A systolic ejection murmur is present in the midleft sternal border to aortic area.
  3. The murmur increases in intensity as obstruction increases in severity.
  4. If turbulence is severe enough, a palpable thrill is felt over murmur, supraclavicular notch.
  5. An ejection click is audible unless the valve is very dysplastic.
  6. An associated decrescendo, hollow, tambour diastolic murmur of aortic valve regurgitation may be present.
- Subaortic stenosis: usually progressive, often rapidly
  1. Murmur is better localized to midleft sternal border or midsternum.
  2. No ejection click is heard.
  3. The patient may have an associated diastolic murmur of aortic valve insufficiency.
- Supravalve AS
  1. May be part of Williams syndrome: Typical Williams syndrome features include "elfin" facies, mental retardation, "cocktail personality," and small, pointed, and irregular teeth.
  2. An ejection systolic murmur and a possible thrill in the aortic area to carotid arteries may be present.
  3. No ejection click is heard.
  4. The aortic closure sound may be accentuated.
  5. Peripheral pulmonary artery stenosis is present in Williams syndrome.
  6. The right arm blood pressure may be higher than the left arm pressure, even without arch obstruction.

- Coarctation of aorta in the neonate
  1. May have no pulses if cardiac function poor or palpable right arm pulse only
  2. Congestive heart failure
  3. Pallor/grayness
  4. No characteristic murmur but may have murmur in pulmonic area
- Coarctation in later infancy and childhood
  1. Well developed, well nourished
  2. Arm pulses more vigorous than leg pulses; leg pulses may be delayed
     a. Blood pressure measured in the arm exceeds the blood pressure measured in the leg.
     b. Normal leg blood pressure should exceed arm pressure by at least 10 mm Hg.
     c. Palpable collateral vessels are felt in the neck and the parascapular area.
     d. No characteristic murmur is present but may have a bruit in the back over the area of coarctation.
     e. May have murmurs of associated defects: aortic valve stenosis, mitral valve regurgitation, ventricular septal defect

DIAGNOSIS

■ DIAGNOSTIC WORKUP

- Aortic valve stenosis
  1. Electrocardiogram
     a. Normal to left ventricular hypertrophy and ischemia
  2. Chest roentgenogram
     a. Normal to prominent ascending aorta (poststenotic dilation)
     b. Enlarged left ventricle
  3. Echocardiogram
     a. Valve structure: number and equality of leaflets
     b. Left ventricular hypertrophy, dilation, function
     c. Gradient across valve
     d. Diameter of aortic and pulmonic annuli (for surgical correction)
  4. Cardiac catheterization and angiography
     a. Direct measurement of transvalve gradient
     b. Left ventricular function
     c. Associated anomalies
- Subaortic stenosis: usually progressive, often rapidly
  1. Electrocardiogram
     a. Same as valve stenosis
  2. Chest roentgenogram
     a. Same as aortic valve stenosis except no poststenotic dilation
  3. Echocardiogram
     a. Define location of obstruction.

b. Define type (e.g., ridge versus muscular).
c. Estimate gradient.
d. Evaluate left ventricular hypertrophy, dilation, and function.
e. Define associated defects.
- Supravalve AS
  1. Electrocardiogram
     a. Same as aortic valve stenosis
  2. Chest roentgenogram
     a. Same as valve stenosis
     b. No poststenotic dilation, although ascending aorta may be prominent
  3. Echocardiogram
     a. Locate obstruction.
     b. Estimate gradient.
     c. Evaluate left ventricular hypertrophy, dilation, function.
     d. Define associated defects.
     e. Cardiac catheterization and angiocardiography: anatomic evaluation of aorta, area of obstruction as part of evaluation for surgical repair
- Coarctation of aorta in the neonate
  1. Electrocardiogram
     a. Not diagnostic; may have increased or decreased left ventricular forces
     b. Usually right ventricular hypertrophy
  2. Chest roentgenogram
     a. Cardiomegaly
     b. Increased pulmonary arterial flow
     c. Pulmonary venous congestion
  3. Echocardiogram
     a. Poor myocardial function
     b. Visible coarctation; may be difficult to identify
     c. Associated defects
  4. Cardiac catheterization and angiocardiography
     a. Not usually indicated
- Coarctation in later infancy and childhood
  1. Electrocardiogram
     a. Usually normal, although may have left ventricular hypertrophy
  2. Chest roentgenogram
     a. Usually normal but may show left ventricular hypertrophy
  3. Echocardiography
     a. This test confirms coarctation and provides localization.
     b. Estimate gradient across coarctation.
     c. Evaluate associated defects.
     d. Evaluate left ventricular hypertrophy, dilation, and function.
  4. Catheterization and angiography
     a. Not always indicated
     b. Give specific delineation of coarctation, associated defects
     c. Evaluate pulmonary hypertension
     d. Left ventricular function

℞ THERAPY

■ NONPHARMACOLOGIC
- Aortic valve stenosis
  1. Follow if not severe: gradient less than 50 mm Hg, no symptoms, normal electrocardiogram

■ MEDICAL
- Aortic valve stenosis
  1. Infants with cardiovascular collapse
     a. Administer prostaglandin to improve systemic cardiac output.
     b. Add conventional agents for congestive heart failure and decreased cardiac output.
- Subvalve AS
  1. Subacute bacterial endocarditis prophylaxis
  2. Treatment of congestive heart failure if necessary
- Neonatal coarctation
  1. Administer prostaglandin to reopen ductus to improve systemic circulation and renal blood flow.
  2. Provide general supportive measures and treatment for congestive heart failure and poor systemic output.

■ SURGICAL
- Aortic valve stenosis
  1. If severe gradient (more than 50 mm Hg), electrocardiographic change, congestive heart failure, or left ventricular dysfunction:
     a. Relieve obstruction by balloon valvuloplasty.
     b. Surgical valvotomy may be needed.
  2. Aortic valve replacement (Ross procedure substituting pulmonic valve for abnormal aortic valve, prosthetic valve, or tissue valve)
     a. Not usually required for first procedure.
     b. Some institutions are now beginning with Ross procedure.
- Subvalve AS
  1. Surgical resection must remove all traces of abnormal tissue to prevent recurrence.
  2. Obstruction by muscle, mitral valve, and so forth may not be surgically approachable.
- Supravalve AS
  1. Surgical repair technically difficult
  2. Depends on left ventricular function and aortic anatomy more than on the specific gradient
- Neonatal coarctation
  1. Surgical resection (or bypass) when stable
  2. May require repeat relief of obstruction in later childhood by balloon dilation or repeat surgery

- Coarctation in later infancy or childhood
  1. Relief of aortic obstruction by balloon angioplasty or surgical resection/bypass
  2. Usually in the preschool period

■ FOLLOW-UP & DISPOSITION
- Although surgical approaches are available for most types of LVOT obstruction, in general, these are palliative rather than curative and repeated surgery is often needed.
- All of these patients deserve lifelong surveillance and follow-up for recurrences after surgery.
- Appropriate protection against bacterial endocarditis is necessary at times of possible bacteremia.
- Patients with coarctation need long-term follow-up for restenosis, aneurysm formation, systemic hypertension, and development of aortic valve stenosis.

■ PATIENT/FAMILY EDUCATION
- Patients and parents need to understand fully the concept of infective endocarditis prophylaxis.
- Patients and parents need to understand that surgical approaches to LVOT obstruction are palliative and not curative.
- Patients and parents need to understand that although small children may not need activity restriction, older children and those with more severe disease may be limited in sports participation.
- Patients and parents need to understand that isometric exercise imposes a significant extra workload on the heart and that such sports as weightlifting, wrestling, and rope climbing may not be permitted.

■ REFERRAL INFORMATION
All patients with suspected LVOT obstruction should be referred to a cardiologist for diagnosis and, if surgery is indicated, a cardiothoracic surgeon.

☼ PEARLS & CONSIDERATIONS

■ CLINICAL PEARLS
- This condition may be minor to severe or lethal.
- Isometric exercise increases left ventricular work by increasing systemic vascular resistance.
- Think of AS or coarctation of the aorta in an infant with cardiovascular collapse because there may be no physical findings to suggest it.
- A family tree may include people with any degree of LVOT obstructive disease.

- Children with LVOT obstruction should be encouraged in early childhood to develop an interest in nonsustained, noncompetitive sports, such as bowling, swimming, and archery, and should have the opportunity to be exposed to music and the arts, allowing them to develop their own leisure time activities that do not depend on hard physical work.
- An ejection click implies a thin mobile valve.

- A normal electrocardiogram does not necessarily mean a mild degree of obstruction.
- LVOT obstruction is usually a progressive disease, particularly when the valve or the immediate subvalve and supravalve areas are involved.
- Surgical approaches to LVOT obstruction are palliative, not curative, and repeat surgery may be necessary.

■ WEBSITES
- For patients: American Heart Association: www.americanheart.org/children
- For patients and physicians: www.mdconsult.com

REFERENCE
1. Park MK: *Pediatric cardiology for practitioner,* St Louis, 1996, Mosby.
Author: **Chloe Alexson, M.D.**

BASIC INFORMATION

■ DEFINITION
Legg-Calvé-Perthes disease (LCPD) is an idiopathic avascular necrosis of the femoral head that may be either partial or total.

■ SYNONYMS
- Legg-Perthes disease
- Perthes disease
- Osteochondrosis, hip

■ ICD-9CM CODE
732.1 Legg-Calvé-Perthes disease

■ ETIOLOGY
- The cause is unknown.
- Theories have focused on a compromise of blood flow to the femoral head.
  1. Intraosseous venous hypertension and venous congestion
  2. Arterial occlusion
  3. Disorders of coagulation (thrombophilia and hyperfibrinolysis, i.e., factor V Leiden, protein C and S deficiencies, anticardiolipin antibodies)
  4. Probably multifactorial

■ EPIDEMIOLOGY & DEMOGRAPHICS
- The incidence varies from 1:1200 to 1:12,500.
- The male:female ratio is 4:1.
- LCPD generally occurs at 4 to 8 years of age (range, 2 to 13 years).
- LCPD is more common in Caucasians and Asians; it is rare in African Americans and Native Americans.
- LCPD may be associated with low birth weight, abnormal birth position, increased parental age, lower socioeconomic status, urban setting, psychologic profiles suggestive of attention deficit hyperactivity disorder, and exposure to passive smoke.
- A delayed bone age may be seen.
- Short stature for age may be noted.

■ HISTORY
- A painless limp that is exacerbated by activity is reported.
- Pain, if present, is located in the groin, anterior thigh, or knee.
  1. *Note:* Pain in the knee of any growing child should prompt a thorough examination of the hip. Hip pathology often presents as pain in the knee.

■ PHYSICAL EXAMINATION
- Antalgic limp
- Limitation of abduction and internal rotation
- Disuse thigh atrophy (may also have atrophy of the buttock and calf)
- Leg length discrepancy
- Hip flexion contracture

- Bilateral involvement in approximately 10%

DIAGNOSIS

■ DIFFERENTIAL DIAGNOSIS
Before radiologic evaluation:
- Transient synovitis
- Synovitis of any cause
  1. Juvenile arthritis
  2. Early septic arthritis
  3. Osteomyelitis

■ DIFFERENTIAL DIAGNOSIS
After radiologic evaluation, usually obvious:
- Bilateral symmetric involvement; consider the following:
  1. Hypothyroidism
  2. Skeletal dysplasia (multiple epiphyseal dysplasia)
- Bilateral involvement also may occur in other systemic disorders:
  1. Renal disease
  2. Steroid medication use
  3. Sickle cell disease

■ DIAGNOSTIC WORKUP
- Laboratory results:
  1. Generally normal complete blood count and erythrocyte sedimentation rate
  2. May show thrombophilia or hyperfibrinolysis
- Plain radiographs reveal various stages of the disease.
  1. Normal
  2. Cessation of growth (decreased size of ossific center)
  3. Subchondral fracture or lucency (crescent sign)
  4. Fragmentation
  5. Reossification
  6. Healed
- A bone scan may be helpful early, before bony changes occur.
  1. Decreased uptake is noted in the involved femoral head.
- Magnetic resonance imaging may be useful before radiographic changes or during the course of the disease.
  1. Ascertain shape of the femoral head.
  2. Image for congruency of joint.
  3. Look for presence of osteochondritis dissecans.

THERAPY

- The prognosis depends primarily on the age of the child and the extent of femoral head involvement.
- The presence of subluxation or extrusion, the duration of the disease process, premature closure of the growth plate, and limited range of motion also may affect outcome.
- Children younger than 6 years of age tend to have less severe disease.

- No treatment has been reported to speed healing of the femoral head.
- Treatment is indicated for pain, limitation of motion, and those with severe disease and poor prognosis.
- The goals of treatment are restoring a normal range of motion and obtaining as round a femoral head as possible by containing the femoral head within the acetabulum.

■ NONPHARMACOLOGIC
- Limitation of activities
- Crutches
- Physical therapy
- Traction
- Petrie casts
- Abduction bracing

■ MEDICAL
Nonsteroidal medication for hip joint irritability and pain

■ SURGICAL
- Adductor tenotomy and/or medial release to help restore motion
- Innominate osteotomy
- Proximal femoral osteotomy
- Arthroscopy or arthrotomy to remove symptomatic osteochondritis dissecans of the femoral head

■ FOLLOW-UP & DISPOSITION
- Follow-up should take place until skeletal maturity to monitor the hip as well as limb length.
- Long-term follow-up suggests that osteoarthritis will develop in the fifth decade.

■ REFERRAL INFORMATION
- Pediatric orthopedic surgeons should be involved in the assessment and care of children with persistent, unexplained limp or pain in the hip, thigh, or knee.
- An abnormal radiograph should prompt referral to a pediatric orthopedist.

REFERENCES
1. Gruppo R et al: Legg-Calvé-Perthes disease in three siblings, 2 heterozygous and one homozygous for the factor V Leiden mutation, *J Pediatr* 132:885, 1998.
2. Herring JA: Current concepts review: the treatment of Legg-Calvé-Perthes disease—a critical review of the literature, *J Bone Joint Surg* 76A:448, 1994.
3. Koop S, Quanbeck D: Three common causes of childhood hip pain, *Pediatr Clin North Am* 43:1053, 1996.
4. Roy DR: Current concepts in Perthes disease, *Pediatr Ann* 28:748, 1999.
5. Thompson GH: Legg-Calvé-Perthes disease. In Pizzutillo PD (ed): *Pediatric orthopaedics in primary practice*, New York, 1997, McGraw-Hill.
Author: **Dennis R. Roy, M.D.**

II

BASIC INFORMATION

■ DEFINITION
Acute lymphoblastic leukemia (ALL) is a malignant transformation and proliferation of a lymphoid progenitor cell.

■ SYNONYMS
- ALL
- Acute lymphocytic leukemia
- Acute lymphatic leukemia

ICD-9CM CODE
204.00 Acute lymphoblastic leukemia

■ ETIOLOGY
- The cause is unknown.
- Most patients have a chromosomal abnormality in the leukemic blast; it is unclear how the genetic change occurs.
- Genetic factors play a role—increased incidence is associated with certain constitutional abnormalities (Down syndrome, neurofibromatosis), identical twins, and familial cases.
- Environmental exposures—ionizing radiation and alkylating agents—may play a role.

■ EPIDEMIOLOGY & DEMOGRAPHICS
- ALL is the most common cancer in the pediatric age group; comprising 25% of all pediatric cancers.
- The incidence is 3:100,000 to 4:100,000 children.
- The peak incidence is 2 to 5 years of age.
- A higher incidence occurs in males and Caucasians.

■ HISTORY
- Symptom duration of days to weeks
- Unexplained fever
- Easy or excessive bruising or other unusual bleeding
- Bone pain, limp
- Anorexia, fatigue

■ PHYSICAL EXAMINATION
- Ill appearance
- Weight loss
- Pallor
- Lymphadenopathy—nontender, firm nodes; disseminated
- Splenomegaly and/or hepatomegaly
- Petechiae, purpura

DIAGNOSIS

■ DIFFERENTIAL DIAGNOSIS
- Infections: infectious mononucleosis (Epstein-Barr virus), cytomegalovirus, pertussis (associated with lymphocytosis)
- Hematologic disorders: idiopathic thrombocytopenic purpura, aplastic anemia
- Malignancy: neuroblastoma, non-Hodgkin's lymphoma
- Nonmalignant disorders: juvenile rheumatoid arthritis

■ DIAGNOSTIC WORKUP
- Complete blood count (CBC): Half of pediatric patients present with a white blood cell (WBC) count of lower than 10,000/mm^3. Need to look at CBC results for evidence of more than one cell line affected (i.e., neutropenia (absolute neutrophil count less than 1000), anemia, and/or thrombocytopenia).
- Review the blood smear for blasts.
- Definitive diagnosis can be made only by bone marrow aspiration.
  1. More than 25% blasts in marrow are required for a diagnosis of leukemia.
  2. Most patients have complete replacement by blasts.
- Multiple biologic studies are performed on marrow blasts for confirmation of the diagnosis and stratification for treatment purposes and prognosis.
  1. Immunophenotyping of surface antigens by flow cytometry
  2. Chromosome analysis (cytogenetics)
  3. Other research tools
- Chemistries: electrolytes, blood urea nitrogen, creatinine, uric acid, liver function tests
- Spinal tap to evaluate cerebrospinal fluid for blasts
- Chest radiograph to assess for significant mediastinal lymphadenopathy

THERAPY

- Because of the intensity of current treatment regimens, most pediatric patients have a central venous access device placed at diagnosis to facilitate treatment.
- Treatment is divided into various phases:
  1. Induction: Goal is to produce remission during the initial 4 to 5 weeks of therapy.
     a. Drugs: vincristine, prednisone, L-asparaginase with or without anthracycline, intrathecal methotrexate
  2. Consolidation: Therapy is directed at the central nervous system (CNS).
     a. Intrathecal methotrexate weekly (for prophylaxis), or
     b. Cranial radiation if CNS leukemia is present
     c. Continued systemic chemotherapy
  3. Intensification: Multiple drugs are administered in an intensive schedule to intensify remission.
  4. Maintenance: Mostly consists of outpatient therapy with monthly visits to a clinic.
     a. Oral 6-mercaptopurine and methotrexate
     b. Monthly pulses of vincristine and/or steroids
     c. Intrathecal therapy every 12 weeks
- The duration of treatment is 2 years for girls and 3 years for boys.
- Most children are (and should be) treated on national cooperative group study protocols (Children's Cancer Group, Pediatric Oncology Group; soon to be Children's Oncology Group).
- A large proportion of adolescents are not included in studies.
  1. Evidence suggests that the outcome is improved when patients are treated on pediatric protocols.

■ SUPPORTIVE TREATMENTS
- Prophylaxis for *Pneumocystis pneumoniae*—trimethoprim-sulfamethoxazole or pentamidine
- Prompt evaluation for fever or other signs of infection (varicella), especially with low absolute neutrophil count
- Transfusions, nutritional support as needed

■ PROGNOSIS
- Seventy percent of patients with ALL are cured.
- "Good-risk" patients (initial WBC count less than 50,000/mm^3, age 1 to 10 years) have an 85% to 90% cure rate.
- "High-risk" patients (older than 10 years; WBC count greater than 50,000/mm^3) have a 65% to 70% cure rate.
- Most relapses occur while on therapy.
  1. A 20% risk of relapse exists after treatment is complete.

■ FOLLOW-UP & DISPOSITION
After therapy, patients need to be followed intermittently for relapse and late effects secondary to treatment.

■ PATIENT/FAMILY EDUCATION
- Parents need to understand that childhood cancer is different than adult cancer and that patients are CURED.
- Parents need to be educated about the side effects of chemotherapy and the signs and symptoms for which they need to contact the medical team.
- School-related issues include repeated absences and learning difficulties secondary to CNS therapy

(especially in patients younger than 6 years of age).

■ REFERRAL INFORMATION

With few exceptions, children and adolescents should be managed primarily by pediatric hematologists-oncologists at medical centers participating in cooperative group trials and with appropriate support staff. Patients are usually followed primarily by the oncology team until their treatment is complete.

☼ PEARLS & CONSIDERATIONS

■ CLINICAL PEARLS
- Leukemia should always be considered in the differential of unexplained fever, bruising, or bone pain.
- When a CBC is obtained, remember to look for evidence of more than one cell line being abnormal.
  1. Increases suspicion of bone marrow abnormality
- Abnormality of more than one lymphoid organ on examination (nodes, spleen, liver) raises suspicion of ALL.

■ WEBSITES
- American Cancer Society: www.cancer.org
- Friends Network: www.cancerfunletter.com; interactive site for kids
- National Cancer Institute: www.nci.nih.gov
- National Childhood Cancer Foundation (Children's Cancer Group): www.nccf.org

■ SUPPORT GROUPS
- Leukemia Society of America, 600 Third Ave., New York, NY 10016, 212-573-8484
- Candlelighters Childhood Cancer Foundation, Inc., 7910 Woodmont Ave., Suite 460, Bethesda, MD 20814, 800-366-2223 or 301-657-8401

REFERENCES

1. Friebert SE, Shurin SB: ALL: diagnosis and outlook, *Contemp Pediatr* 15(2): 118 and 15:39, 1998.
2. Greaves M: A natural history for pediatric acute leukemia, *Blood* 82:1043, 1993.
3. Margolin JF, Poplack DG: Acute lymphoblastic leukemia. In *Principles and practice of pediatric oncology,* ed 3, Philadelphia, 1997, Lippincott-Raven.
4. Pui C-H: Childhood leukemias, review article, *N Engl J Med* 332:1618, 1995.

Author: **Cynthia A. DeLaat, M.D.**

II

BASIC INFORMATION

DEFINITION
Acute myelogenous leukemia (AML) is a malignant transformation and proliferation of any myeloid progenitor cell.

SYNONYMS
- AML
- Acute nonlymphocytic leukemia

ICD-9CM CODE
205.00 Acute myelogenous leukemia

ETIOLOGY
- The cause is unknown.
- Specific genetic abnormalities are present in the leukemia cell, but it is unknown how they arise; myelodysplasia often converts to AML.
- Children with genetic conditions (Down syndrome, Fanconi's anemia) have an increased risk of AML.
- Environmental exposures, such as ionizing radiation, benzene, epipodophyllotoxins, and alkylating agents, are associated with AML.

EPIDEMIOLOGY & DEMOGRAPHICS
- AML constitutes 25% of cases of leukemia in pediatrics.
- No age, sex, or ethnic predisposition exists.
- Most cases of congenital leukemia are AML.

HISTORY
- Unexplained fever, serious infection/sepsis
- Pallor, fatigue, weight loss
- Bruising or bleeding
- Bone pain
- Persistent respiratory or gastrointestinal symptoms

PHYSICAL EXAMINATION
- Cutaneous or mucosal hemorrhage
- Lymphadenopathy
- Hepatosplenomegaly, lymphadenopathy
- Gingival hypertrophy
- Leukemia cutis (bluish skin nodules), especially in the neonate
- Retinal hemorrhage or cotton wool spots on funduscopic examination

DIAGNOSIS

DIFFERENTIAL DIAGNOSIS
- Hematologic disorders: aplastic anemia, idiopathic thrombocytopenic purpura
- Infection: sepsis, disseminated intravascular coagulation (DIC), osteomyelitis

DIAGNOSTIC WORKUP
- Complete blood count: Most patients have significant anemia and thrombocytopenia.
  1. Immature white blood cells (WBCs) (promyelocytes, myelocytes) are reported on the differential.
  2. Twenty percent of patients can present with hyperleukocytosis with a WBC count greater than $100,000/mm^3$.
- Review the blood smear for blasts, nucleated red blood cells.
- Bone marrow aspiration is necessary to make the diagnosis of AML.
  1. More than 25% of myeloblasts is diagnostic.
- Multiple biologic tests are performed on leukemic cells for confirmation of diagnosis and stratification for treatment and prognosis.
  1. Morphology: Seven different subtypes of AML exist (myeloblastic [M0, M1], monocytic, erythroblastic, megakaryocytic, promyelocytic, myelomonocytic). All subtypes are treated the same way except for promyelocytic leukemia.
  2. Immunophenotyping is performed.
  3. Chromosomal analysis is done.
- Coagulation tests include prothrombin time (PT), partial thromboplastin time (PTT), fibrinogen, D-dimer to screen for DIC.
- Blood chemistries include electrolytes, blood urea nitrogen, creatinine, transaminases, and bilirubin.
- Spinal tap is done to evaluate cerebrospinal fluid for involvement by leukemia.

THERAPY

- Treatment for AML entails intensive chemotherapy.
  1. Marrow must be put into a state of aplasia to induce remission.
  2. This results in prolonged periods of pancytopenia and hospitalization.
  3. Side effects such as severe mucositis, liver damage, bleeding complications, and bacterial and fungal infections are common.
     a. These patients require aggressive supportive care.
     b. All patients require a central venous access line.
- The main chemotherapeutic agents for treatment of AML are cytosine arabinoside and anthracyclines.
  1. Several courses of intensive chemotherapy are given to prevent relapse.
  2. The cure rate for AML is about 40%.

- Allogeneic bone marrow transplant is performed in first remission.
  1. This is recommended for patients with AML who have a matched donor in the family.
  2. The cure rate following transplantation is 50% to 70%.

FOLLOW-UP & DISPOSITION
- The risk of relapse is about 50%; therefore patients need to be monitored closely for signs and symptoms of recurrence of leukemia.
- Survivors need to be followed for late-occurring side effects:
  1. Cardiac dysfunction from anthracyclines
  2. Second cancers
  3. Fertility problems

PATIENT/FAMILY EDUCATION
- AML requires aggressive treatment, with many serious side effects and prolonged hospitalizations.
- Family members will be tested at diagnosis to identify compatible bone marrow donors.
- Even with successful completion of treatment, a significant risk of relapse exists.

REFERRAL INFORMATION
Patients with AML need to be treated by a pediatric hematology-oncology team at a medical center experienced in using intensive therapeutic protocols.

PEARLS & CONSIDERATIONS

CLINICAL PEARLS
- Persistent fever of unknown origin, persistent infections, or other chronic signs and symptoms of illness should raise suspicion of AML.
- Patients presenting with AML can be seriously ill secondary to infection or very high WBC count and should be referred promptly for care.
- Patients with Down syndrome have an increased risk of leukemia, especially after transient myeloproliferative syndrome as a neonate.

WEBSITES
- American Cancer Society: www.cancer.org
- Friends Network: www.cancerfunletter.com; interactive site for kids
- National Cancer Institute: www.nci.nih.gov
- National Childhood Cancer Foundation (Children's Cancer Group): www.nccf.org

■ SUPPORT GROUPS

- Leukemia Society of America, 600 Third Ave., New York, NY 10016, 212-573-8484
- Candlelighters Childhood Cancer Foundation, Inc., 7910 Woodmont Ave., Suite 460, Bethesda, MD 20814, 800-366-2223 or 301-657-8401

REFERENCES

1. Golub TR, Weinstein HJ, Grier HE: Acute myelogenous leukemia. In *Principles and practice of pediatric oncology,* ed 3, Philadelphia, 1997, Lippincott-Raven.
2. Greaves M: A natural history for pediatric acute leukemia, *Blood* 82:1043, 1993.
3. Pui C-H: Childhood leukemias, review article, *N Engl J Med* 332:1618, 1995.

Author: **Cynthia A. DeLaat, M.D.**

II

BASIC INFORMATION

■ DEFINITION

Infection caused by *Listeria monocytogenes* is an important zoonosis that is uncommon in the general population. It is predominantly responsible for food poisoning and gastroenteritis; however, in some risk groups (i.e., neonates, pregnant women, and immunocompromised hosts), infection results in life-threatening meningoencephalitis or bacteremia.

■ SYNONYMS

• Listeriosis
• Granulomatosis infantiseptica

ICD-9CM CODES

027.0 *L. monocytogenes*
771.2 Granulomatosis infantiseptica
005.8 Other bacterial food poisoning

■ ETIOLOGY

• *L. monocytogenes:* gram-positive, rod-shaped, facultative anaerobic bacterium
• The only one of six *Listeria* species pathogenic for humans

■ EPIDEMIOLOGY & DEMOGRAPHICS

• *L. monocytogenes* is widespread in nature.
  1. Found commonly in soil, decaying vegetation, and sewage
  2. Also found in the fecal flora of many mammals, including 5% of healthy adults
• Modes of transmission include the following:
  1. Foodborne is the most predominant method.
  2. Vertical transmission to a fetus is possible, but it is not otherwise transmitted from human to human.
• Risk groups are as follows:
  1. Pregnant women
  2. Infants younger than 1 month of age
  3. Patients with malignancy, organ transplantation, or human immunodeficiency virus–induced immunosuppression
  4. Iron overload (transfusion, hemochromatosis)
  5. Adults older than 50 years of age
• The most common foods associated with transmission are "ready-to-eat" foods such as milk, soft cheeses, pâté, delicatessen meats, raw meat, raw vegetables; unreheated hot-dogs and turkey franks; and undercooked poultry.

■ PREDOMINANT CLINICAL SYNDROMES

• Infection in pregnancy
  1. Febrile bacteremia, generally occurring in the third trimester, can result.
  2. The condition may be self-limited but can persist or cause chorioamnionitis.
  3. Premature labor is common.
  4. A 25% risk of stillbirth and neonatal death exists.
• Neonatal infection
  1. Disseminated in utero form, *granulomatosis infantiseptica*
     a. Uncommon but fatal
     b. Widespread microabscesses, especially in the liver and spleen; hepatic, splenic, and cutaneous granulomas present at birth (cutaneous lesions papular or pustular, 1 to 3 mm in size, erythematous base)
  2. More commonly, neonatal infection that mimics group B streptococcal disease
     a. Early-onset sepsis and bacteremia occurring shortly after birth in premature infants
     b. Late-onset meningitis occurring at about 2 weeks of age
• Systemic infection in immunocompromised children and adults
  1. Most commonly pyogenic meningitis has been described.
     a. Somewhat atypical features for bacterial meningitis are seen.
     b. Nuchal rigidity is less common.
     c. Fluctuating mental status is more common.
     d. Blood cultures are more likely positive than cerebrospinal fluid (CSF) cultures.
     e. CSF Gram stains may not show organisms.
  2. Less commonly, brainstem encephalitis (rhomboencephalitis) has been described in adults but not in infants.
     a. Brain abscesses and cerebritis occur at all ages.
  3. Other focal sites of infection are rare.
  4. Systemic infection also occurs in not otherwise immunocompromised older adults.
  5. The incubation period is about 21 days.
• Acute gastroenteritis
  1. Unusual but reported in point-source outbreaks
     a. Accompanied by fever, abdominal pain
     b. Incubation period of about 1 day

■ HISTORY

• Patients often have ingested foods associated with transmission in the preceding month.

• Many patients presenting with bacteremia, central nervous system (CNS) infection, or infection during pregnancy have experienced gastroenteritis in the preceding month.

■ PHYSICAL EXAMINATION

No unique features are seen beyond those discussed under "Clinical Syndromes."

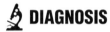

DIAGNOSIS

■ DIFFERENTIAL DIAGNOSIS

• Neonatal sepsis or meningitis
• Atypical meningitis
• Parenchymal brain infection in immunosuppressed patients
• Febrile illnesses in third-trimester pregnant women
• Foodborne outbreaks of febrile gastroenteritis that are not found to be caused by a more common etiology

■ DIAGNOSTIC WORKUP

• Bacterial cultures of blood, CSF, and stool are obtained.
• For CNS disease, magnetic resonance imaging is superior to computed tomography scan in demonstrating early cerebritis or brainstem involvement.

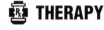

THERAPY

■ MEDICAL

• Although no controlled clinical trials are available, in vitro data, animal model data, and clinical experience suggest that the therapy of choice is the combination of ampicillin plus gentamicin.
• For penicillin-allergic patients, trimethoprim-sulfamethoxazole can be given.
• Cephalosporins are *not* active against *L. monocytogenes.*

■ PREVENTIVE TREATMENT & EDUCATION

• The Centers for Disease Control and Prevention (CDC) recommendations for consumer prevention of listeriosis are as follows:
  1. For all persons
     a. Thoroughly cook raw food from animal sources (e.g., beef, pork, poultry).
     b. Thoroughly wash raw vegetables.
     c. Keep uncooked meats separate from other foods.
     d. Avoid raw or unpasteurized milk.
     e. Wash hands, knives, and cutting boards after handling uncooked meat.

2. For persons at high risk (i.e., immunocompromised hosts, pregnant women, elderly persons)
   a. Avoid soft cheeses (e.g., Mexican-style, Feta, Brie, Camembert, blue-veined cheese, but *not* hard cheeses, cream cheese, cottage cheese, or yogurt); pasteurization may not be fully effective against intracellular *Listeria.*
   b. Reheat leftover foods and "ready-to-eat" preprocessed meats (e.g., hot-dogs) until steaming hot before eating.
   c. Consider avoiding cold cuts and delicatessen foods, although the risk is relatively low.

PEARLS & CONSIDERATIONS

■ CLINICAL PEARLS

- Unlike group B streptococcal infections, recurrent maternal disease in humans is not documented and antibiotics are not indicated for future pregnancies.
- Isolation of "diphtheroids" from blood or CSF should alert the clinician to consider misdiagnosed *L. monocytogenes.*
- *L. monocytogenes* causes monocytosis in the blood of rabbits but not humans; human CSF pleocytosis is most often polymorphonuclear.

■ WEBSITE

Centers for Disease Control and Prevention: www.cdc.gov/health/diseases.htm

REFERENCES

1. Bortolussi R, Kennedy WA: Listeriosis. In Feigin RD, Cherry JD (eds): *Textbook of pediatric infectious diseases,* ed 4, Philadelphia, 1998, WB Saunders.
2. Lorber B: Listeriosis, *Clin Infect Dis* 24:1, 1997.
3. Lorber B: *Listeria monocytogenes.* In Mandell GL, Bennett JE, Dolin R (eds): *Mandell, Douglas, and Bennett's principles and practice of infectious diseases,* ed 5, Philadelphia, 2000, Churchill Livingstone.
4. Tappero JW et al: Reduction in the incidence of human listeriosis in the United States: effectiveness of prevention efforts? *JAMA* 273:1118, 1995.

Author: **Geoffrey A. Weinberg, M.D.**

II

BASIC INFORMATION

■ **DEFINITION**

Lyme disease (LD) is the most common tickborne illness in the United States.

ICD-9CM CODE

088.81 Lyme disease

■ **ETIOLOGY**

LD is caused by infection with the spirochete *Borrelia burgdorferi.*

■ **EPIDEMIOLOGY & DEMOGRAPHICS**

• Cases peak in summer and fall.
• Infestation occurs in rural, heavily wooded areas near the vector.
• More than 90% of cases are concentrated in the Northeast, the upper Midwest, and northern California.
• In the Northeast and upper north-central regions of the United States, *Ixodes scapularis* (the black-legged tick, previously known as *Ixodes dammini*) is the main vector for *B. burgdorferi.*
• *Ixodes pacificus* (the Western black-legged tick) is the primary vector in the Pacific coast states.
• Children and adolescents account for 33% to 50% of reported cases.
• The incidence peaks at ages 5 to 14 years and 30 to 49 years.
• Seventy-five percent of reported children presented with their initial symptoms in the summer months (June, July, and August).
• Boys seem to be at higher risk for infection than girls.
• The mean age of affected children is 9.9 years.

■ **HISTORY**

• Tick bite
• Travel to endemic area
• Arthritis, neurologic disorder, cardiac problems, typical rash of erythema migrans (EM)

■ **PHYSICAL EXAMINATION**

• Stage 1 occurs within days to weeks of when an infected tick inoculates the human host with *B. burgdorferi,* and between 60% and 80% of children develop the characteristic cutaneous finding of EM.
• EM begins as a red papule or macule, usually in the groin, axilla, or thigh, and steadily and rapidly (over 24 to 48 hours) expands to a round or oval lesion (at least 5 cm in diameter) with an erythematous periphery and central clearing.
• Symptoms associated with the rash are reminiscent of a viral syndrome

and can include fever, arthralgia, myalgia, chills, headache, malaise, and fatigue, as well as physical signs composed of lymphadenopathy, hepatosplenomegaly, and less commonly nonexudative pharyngitis, nonproductive cough, and orchitis.
• Stage 2 occurs 3 to 4 weeks after infection. Dissemination of the spirochete occurs, and half of patients manifest secondary skin lesions, which are also annular with central clearing but removed from the original point of inoculation and generally smaller than the primary lesion.
  1. This second stage of the illness is similar to other spirochetal infections (e.g., syphilis), in which these early disease manifestations resolve even without antibiotic therapy.
  2. Other complications seen in the early disseminated stage of the illness involve multiple organs systems, including the following:
     a. Ophthalmologic
        (1) Optic neuritis, keratitis, conjunctivitis, uveitis, choroiditis
     b. Cardiac (4% to 8% of patients)
        (1) Most commonly see complete heart block
        (2) Can include myoperi-carditis
     c. Neurologic (15% to 20% of patients)
        (1) Meningitis, subtle signs of encephalitis (including somnolence, poor memory, and mood change)
        (2) Peripheral neuritis: asymmetric with motor, sensory or mixed manifestations
        (3) Commonly presenting as paralysis of the seventh or facial nerve (Bell's palsy)
        (4) Other: pancreatitis
  3. Serum antibody to *B. burgdorferi* develops during this phase
• Late phase of LD is characterized by more persistent findings and occurs within months to years after the initial infection.
  1. Two thirds of untreated patients have episodic oligoarthritis lasting approximately 1 week, especially involving the knee but also reported in the elbow, wrist, hip, shoulder, and ankle.
  2. Late-stage neurologic disease is less common than arthritis but can persist much longer.
  3. Transplacental passage of *B. burgdorferi* does occur, and case reports of prematurity, syndactyly, rash, cortical blindness, developmental delay, and intrauterine fetal death are present in the literature.

■ **DIAGNOSIS**

• The diagnosis of LD is made primarily by clinical criteria secondarily supported by serologic data.
  1. Isolation of *B. burgdorferi* from a clinical specimen
  2. Diagnostic levels of immunoglobulin M (IgM) or immunoglobulin G (IgG) antibody response to the spirochete in serum or cerebrospinal fluid (CSF)
  3. Significant change in IgM or IgG antibody response to *B. burgdorferi* in paired acute and convalescent serum samples
• IgM antibody becomes detectable in 2 to 4 weeks and peaks between 3 and 6 weeks after the onset of infection.
• The secondary IgG response corresponds to the development of early arthritic symptoms, occurs at 4 to 6 weeks after the onset (later than the IgM response), and can be detectable for years afterward.

■ **DIFFERENTIAL DIAGNOSIS**

• Pauciarticular juvenile arthritis
• Aseptic meningitis
• Multiple sclerosis
• Septic arthritis
• Acute rheumatic fever
• Fibromyalgia syndrome
• Bell's palsy
• Peripheral neuropathy

■ **DIAGNOSTIC WORKUP**

• Serologic testing for LD focuses on these antibody responses using three assays:
  1. Indirect immunofluorescence assay
  2. Enzyme-linked immunosorbent assay
  3. Immunoblotting or the Western Blot assay
• Ongoing work toward a standardized methodology for identification of *B. burgdorferi* antigen using polymerase chain reaction technology for amplification of minute quantities of DNA in serum or urine specimens has resulted in increasing test availability.
• None of these antibody assays are appropriate for screening patients who do not demonstrate a consistent clinical picture, even in hyperendemic areas.

℞ THERAPY

■ MEDICAL

- Antibiotics are effective in most cases of LD, although few controlled trials have been done in children or adults.
- Oral therapy with amoxicillin (for those younger than 9 years) or doxycycline (for those 9 years or older) for 10 to 30 days is indicated for the early manifestations of LD such as EM.
- Equivalent efficacy for the treatment of early LD has been demonstrated for other oral agents such as cefuroxime, amoxicillin/probenecid, and azithromycin in adults.
- Parenteral regimens for 2 to 3 weeks are preferred therapy for late manifestations such as persistent arthritis, severe carditis, meningitis, or encephalitis.
- Ceftriaxone is probably the therapy of choice because of its long half-life and penetration into the CSF in concentrations consistently higher than the MIC_{90} of *B. burgdorferi.*
- Treatment failure can occur with any of the recommended regimens, and re-treatment may (rarely) be necessary.

■ PREVENTIVE TREATMENT

- Prevention of LD involves avoidance of tick exposure in endemic areas.

- Tick repellents, such as DEET (*N,N*-diethylmetatoluamide) for the exposed skin of adults or permethrins for clothing, should be used sparingly.
- Appropriate light-colored clothing, with long sleeves and long pants, is recommended.
- Tick "patrols" or intense scrutiny of the body after potential exposures should be conducted.
  1. Embedded ticks must be removed with tweezers, being careful not to squeeze the body and promote mixing of the tick and human blood.
  2. Studies of antibiotic prophylaxis after a tick bite have shown no definite advantage.
     a. Antibiotic prophylaxis after a tick bite even in an endemic area is not indicated.
- The ultimate strategy in LD prevention is effective vaccination for humans.
  1. On December 22, 1998, the U.S. Food and Drug Administration approved LYMErix (Smith Kline Beecham Biologicals) for individuals 15 years of age and older.
  2. Immunization efficacy (after three doses at 0, 1, and 12 months) is 76% to 92%.
  3. Boosters every 1 to 3 years may be necessary.

  4. Consider immunization in patients who are 15 years old or older and who are at high risk for exposure.

☼ PEARLS & CONSIDERATIONS

■ CLINICAL PEARLS

- LD is a multisystem spirochetal disease with numerous clinical presentations.
- Think of it in case of rash and arthritis in a child from an endemic area with a history of tick bite.

■ WEBSITE

Centers for Disease Control and Prevention: www.cdc.gov

REFERENCES

1. American Academy of Pediatrics: Lyme disease *(Borrelia burgdorferi).* In Pickering LK (ed): *2000 Red Book: report of the Committee on Infectious Diseases,* ed 25, Elk Grove Village, Ill, 2000, American Academy of Pediatrics.
2. Siegel DM: Lyme disease. In Hoekelman RA et al (eds): *Primary pediatric care,* ed 4, St Louis, 2000, Mosby.
3. Steere AC: Lyme disease, *N Engl J Med* 345:115, 2001.

Author: **Cynthia Christy, M.D.**

II

BASIC INFORMATION

DEFINITIONS

- Lymphangitis is an inflammation or infection of the lymphatic system
- Lymphedema is an excess amount of lymph in soft tissue, resulting from primary or secondary lymphatic insufficiency
- Cystic hygroma is a congenital malformation of the lymphatic system, resulting in multiloculated, cystic masses

SYNONYMS

- Lymphedema, primary
  1. Milroy's disease
  2. Meige's disease (lymphedema praecox)
  3. Lymphedema tarda
- Cystic hygroma
  1. Lymphangioma

ICD-9CM CODES

457.2 Lymphangitis
457.1 Lymphedema
228.1 Cystic hygroma
759.89 and 759.90 Congenital anomaly

ETIOLOGY

- Lymphangitis
  1. Radiation
  2. Tumor
  3. Obstruction
- Lymphedema, primary
  1. Several different forms based on age of presentation: congenital lymphedema in infancy, lymphedema praecox in childhood and adolescence, lymphedema tarda in later life
  2. A few cases have a positive family history with autosomal dominant inheritance: Milroy's and Meige's disease
  3. Several different pathologic forms exist, including agenesis, hypoplasia, and obstructive.
  4. Obstruction can be proximal or distal.
  5. A rarer hyperplastic type can be seen and occasionally is associated with megalymphatics.
- Lymphedema, secondary
  1. Acquired secondary to a variety of causes: bacterial lymphangitis (usually streptococci), tumor, filariasis, radiation, surgery, trauma, tuberculosis, dermatitis, parenteral drug use, and rheumatoid arthritis.
  2. Edema associated with abnormalities of the heart, liver, and kidney are not true lymphedema because the lymphatic system is normal in those conditions.

- Cystic hygroma
  1. Congenital failure of the embryologic lymphatic system to establish drainage into the venous system
  2. Results in the formation of multiloculated, cystic lymphatic malformations

EPIDEMIOLOGY & DEMOGRAPHICS

- Lymphangitis
  1. The most common cause of lymphangitis worldwide is *filaria* infection, but bacterial infection (streptococci) is more common in North America.
  2. Infections are often seen as a result of chronic obstruction or malformation.
- Lymphedema, primary
  1. Occurs in 1 per 10,000 people younger than 20 years of age.
  2. A female preponderance exists.
     a. One third are caused by agenesis, hypoplasia, or obstruction of the distal system.
     b. One half are caused by proximal obstruction.
  3. A few patients have a positive family history.
  4. Primary lymphedema is associated with Turner syndrome, Noonan syndrome, yellow nail syndrome, intestinal lymphangiectasia, lymphangiomyomatosis, and arteriovenous malformation.
- Lymphedema, secondary
  1. More common than primary lymphedema.
  2. Increased incidence exists in India and Southeast Asia.
  3. Tumor is an uncommon cause in children.
- Cystic hygroma
  1. Incidence of 1 per 12,000
  2. Predilection for the head and neck but may involve axilla, limbs, trunk, and mediastinum
  3. Approximately 50% to 65% present at birth

HISTORY

- Lymphangitis
  1. Redness and pain of an extremity
  2. Occasionally, fever and systemic symptoms
  3. Travel history
- Lymphedema, primary
  1. Unilateral or bilateral swelling of extremity
  2. May present at birth/infancy, adolescence, or after age 35
  3. May have family history
- Lymphedema, secondary
  1. Unilateral or bilateral swelling of an extremity
  2. Medical history of recurrent infections, cancer, radiation

- Cystic hygroma
  1. Painless mass involving the neck, axilla, head
  2. Stridor and/or cough secondary to airway compression
  3. Dysphagia because of tongue or neck involvement
  4. Sometimes history of fever, redness, pain

PHYSICAL EXAMINATION

- Lymphangitis
  1. Painful, tender erythematous extremity (often lower) with red "streaking" is present.
  2. The extremity may be diffusely swollen, especially when associated with lymphedema.
  3. Fever and local adenopathy may develop.
  4. Cystic hygroma can present as an infected mass.
- Lymphedema
  1. Diffuse swelling and pitting of the extremity (often lower) are seen.
  2. Occasionally, lymphedema is associated with infection.
  3. In secondary forms, surgical or radiation changes to an extremity might be noted.
- Cystic hygroma
  1. Small or large cystic mass involving the neck, axilla, and tongue is seen.
  2. Masses are usually nontender, soft, mobile, and not erythematous (although can get infected).
  3. The mass may transilluminate.
  4. Stridor and respiratory compromise may be noted.

🔬 DIAGNOSIS

DIFFERENTIAL DIAGNOSIS

- Lymphangitis
  1. Superficial thrombophlebitis
  2. Reflex sympathetic dystrophy
  3. Cellulitis
- Lymphedema
  1. Congestive heart failure
  2. Nephrotic syndrome
  3. Deep vein thrombosis (DVT)
  4. Cirrhosis
  5. Hypoalbuminemic states
  6. Myxedema
  7. Reflex sympathetic dystrophy
  8. Pelvic mass or tumor
- Cystic hygroma
  1. Hemangioma
  2. Branchial cleft cyst
  3. Thyroglossal duct cyst
  4. Dermoid or epidermoid cyst
  5. Ranula
  6. Cervical lymphadenitis
  7. Mediastinal mass

■ **DIAGNOSTIC WORKUP**
- Lymphangitis: The history and physical examination (fever, adenopathy, swelling) may be enough to make a diagnosis.
  1. Leukocytosis may be found on complete blood count.
  2. An ultrasound or phlebogram is sometimes necessary to rule out DVT.
- Lymphedema
  1. The diagnosis is generally based on history and physical examination to rule out nonlymphatic causes of edema.
  2. Occasionally, an ultrasound and/or phlebogram can help differentiate from DVT.
  3. Computed tomography (CT) may be needed to assess a focal (pelvic) mass.
  4. Rarely, a lymphangiogram, lymphoscintigram, or CT scan can be used to define abnormal lymphatics.
- Cystic hygroma
  1. History and physical examination are important.
  2. Ultrasound can help in the assessment.
  3. CT can be used to evaluate the extent of complicated masses.
  4. Occasionally, needle aspiration is used for culture and/or pathology to ensure that no infection or tumor is present.
  5. Consider genetic testing or workup for Turner or Noonan syndrome.

▣ **THERAPY**

Lymphangitis
■ **NONPHARMACOLOGIC**
Elevation and local compresses

■ **MEDICAL**
Antibiotics, especially antistreptococcal antibiotics

■ **SURGICAL**
- Occasionally surgical intervention (incision and drainage of abscess)
- For lymphangitis associated with chronic lymphedema, see following Lymphedema discussion.

Lymphedema
■ **NONPHARMACOLOGIC**
- Elevation, compression stockings or devices
- Continued exercise, skin hygiene
- Salt restriction

■ **MEDICAL**
- Diuretics
- Antibiotics/antifungals if infection coexistent
- Treatment of cause in secondary cases (e.g., malignancy)

■ **SURGICAL**
Surgery (drainage procedures, limb reduction, grafting) is mostly palliative.

Cystic Hygroma
■ **MEDICAL**
- No known medical therapies are available.
- Repeated aspiration and radiation treatment in an attempt to shrink or involute, and injection with sclerosing agents have all been tried with little success.

■ **SURGICAL**
- Surgical removal of abnormal lymphatic structures can be attempted.
- Occasionally, immediate aspiration to relieve an airway obstruction is necessary.

■ **FOLLOW-UP & DISPOSITION**
- Lymphangitis
  1. This is a recurrent problem for many individuals, especially if an underlying lymphatic vessel obstruction or abnormality is present.
  2. Antibiotic treatment is effective.
  3. A recurring problem can lead to secondary obstruction (or increased obstruction).
- Lymphedema
  1. This is a chronic problem with progressive increase within the first year of diagnosis, but progression is rare after that.
  2. Approximately 15% require surgical intervention.
- Cystic hygroma
  1. Close follow-up and removal are necessary.
  2. Regression is rare.

■ **PATIENT/FAMILY EDUCATION**
- Lymphangitis
  1. Good skin hygiene
  2. Prompt attention to infection
- Lymphedema
  1. Dietary education
  2. Exercise and compression stockings
  3. Prompt attention to infection
- Cystic hygroma
  1. Parents should be educated about the complications (i.e., acute change in size, hemorrhage, infection, and respiratory compromise).

■ **PREVENTIVE TREATMENT**
Cystic hygroma can sometimes be detected on fetal ultrasound.

※ **PEARLS & CONSIDERATIONS**

■ **CLINICAL PEARLS**
- Cystic hygroma often involves the left side of the neck and is usually not subtle or confused with other things in the differential diagnosis.
- Nonlymphatic causes of edema are far more common and should always be ruled out.

■ **WEBSITES, SUPPORT GROUPS, & RESOURCES**
- Cystic Hygroma Online Support Group: members.tripod.com/ ~chsupport
- Cystic Hygroma-Parent's Place Message Board: rainforest. parentsplace.com/dialog/get
- Lymphedema Foundation: www. lymphedemafoundation.org
- Lymphedema International Network: www.lymphedema.com
- Lymphedema Products: home. earthlink.net
- Lymphedema Support Group: super.sonic.net/LSG/
- National Lymphedema Network: www.lymphnet.org

REFERENCES
1. Brown R, Azizkhan R: Pediatric head and neck lesions, *Pediatr Clin North Am* 45:889, 1998.
2. Cooke JP, Rooke TW: Lymphedema. In Loscalzo J et al (eds): *Vascular medicine*, Boston, 1992, Little, Brown.
3. Harel L et al: Lymphedema praecox seen as isolated unilateral arm involvement: case report and review of the literature, *J Pediatr* 130:492, 1997.
4. Lewis JM, Wald ER: Lymphedema praecox, *J Pediatr* 104:641, 1984.
5. Ninh T, Ninh T: Cystic hygroma in children: a report of 126 cases, *J Pediatr Surg* 9:191, 1974.

Author: **Steven Scofield, M.D.**

II

BASIC INFORMATION

■ DEFINITION

Hodgkin's lymphoma is characterized by the presence of Reed-Sternberg (RS) cells or variants in a background of nonneoplastic cells. RS cells are large cells with abundant cytoplasm and multiple nuclei or multilobed nuclei. They are not pathognomonic, however, and can be found in other disorders. The normal counterpart of the RS cell remains undefined, although a clone of B lymphocyte origin may be most common.

■ SYNONYM

Malignant lymphoma

ICD-9CM CODE

201.9 Hodgkin's disease

■ ETIOLOGY

- Increased incidence in family members: twofold to fivefold increase in siblings, ninefold increase in same-sex siblings, and ninety-ninefold increase in monozygotic twins.
- Increased incidence in patients with evidence of Epstein-Barr virus (EBV), although approximately half of patients with Hodgkin's disease (HD) have no evidence of EBV. EBV-associated antigens are found to a variable degree in HD subtypes as follows:
  1. Mixed cellularity: 32% to 96%
  2. Nodular sclerosing: 10% to 50%
  3. Lymphocyte predominant: 10%
- Anti-EBV titers are elevated before diagnosis of HD.
- A complex deficiency of cellular immunity exists in HD patients.
- There may be an increased incidence in immunocompromised patients, including patients with human immunodeficiency virus/acquired immunodeficiency syndrome, organ transplant patients, and patients with congenital immunodeficiency syndromes.
- HD is rarely seen as a secondary malignancy, in contrast to non-Hodgkin's lymphoma.

■ EPIDEMIOLOGY & DEMOGRAPHICS

- HD accounts for 6% of pediatric cancers.
- Approximately 10% to 15% of cases are diagnosed in children younger than 16 years of age.
- Two age peaks (in developed countries) occur in early adulthood (age 15 to 40) and late adulthood (age older than 55).
- The incidence in males is greater

than in females, particularly in younger children. The male:female ratio in younger children is as follows:
  1. 3:1 to 4:1 in children younger than 10 years of age
  2. 1:1 to 3:1 in older children
- Mediastinal disease is present in 76% of adolescents, 33% of 1- to 10-year-olds.

■ HISTORY

- Enlarged lymph nodes, usually painless and most commonly located in the cervical or supraclavicular region
- Coughing or shortness of breath
- Fever
- Night sweats (drenching, requires changing night clothes and/or sheets)
- Weight loss
- Fatigue
- Abdominal pain, noted in older patients, especially after consuming alcohol
- Pruritus

■ PHYSICAL EXAMINATION

- Enlarged lymph nodes, generally firm and immobile, are present. Ninety percent of patients present with a pattern that suggests contiguous lymphatic spread.
- Decreased breath sounds can be heard if large mediastinal mass is present.
- Superior vena cava syndrome is observed if a large mediastinal mass is present.

⚗ DIAGNOSIS

■ DIFFERENTIAL DIAGNOSIS

- Non-Hodgkin's lymphoma
- Leukemia, particularly T-cell acute lymphoblastic leukemia
- Metastatic disease from other tumor (e.g., neuroblastoma, rhabdomyosarcoma)
- Infection, including viral (e.g., EBV or cytomegalovirus), atypical mycobacterium, cat-scratch disease
- Normal thymus

■ DIAGNOSTIC WORKUP

- Biopsy of enlarged node (excisional or open biopsy recommended)
- Chest radiograph
- Computed tomography (CT) scan of the neck, chest, abdomen, and pelvis
  1. Approximately 50% of patients with normal chest radiographs have chest CT abnormalities.
- Gallium scan to determine presence and extent of gallium avid disease
- Lymphangiography rarely used, especially in children

- Bone marrow aspirates and biopsies in patients with high-risk disease to evaluate for metastatic disease
- Laboratory evaluation
  1. Includes complete blood count, renal and liver function tests as baseline.
  2. Elevated liver enzymes may indicate liver involvement.
- Erythrocyte sedimentation rate (ESR)
  1. Often elevated and may be followed to monitor disease response and recurrence

■ PATHOLOGY

- Frequency of RS cell in pathology specimen is variable. Reactive infiltrate likely results from cytokine release by RS cell.
- Four subtypes exist (first three are considered classical Hodgkin's disease):
  1. Nodular sclerosing
     a. Distinctive because of collagenous bands that divide the lymph node into nodules.
     b. Approximately 70% to 77% of adolescents and 40% to 44% of children younger than 10 years of age are diagnosed with this subtype.
  2. Mixed cellularity
     a. Approximately 11% of adolescents and 33% of children younger than 10 years have this subtype.
     b. This subtype is associated with advanced disease, extranodal extension, and B symptoms.
  3. Lymphocyte depleted
     a. Rare in children; often advanced at diagnosis; poor prognosis
  4. Lymphocyte predominant
     a. More common in males and young children than in adults (33% of cases are in children younger than 15 years of age)
     b. Clinically localized disease, commonly involving one lymph node region with sparing of mediastinum

■ STAGING

- I—One lymph node is involved and may have local extension to adjacent tissue.
- II—Two or more lymph node areas on same side of diaphragm are involved, and local extension to adjacent tissues may occur.
- III—Involved lymph nodes are seen on both sides of the diaphragm and may have extended to adjacent tissue or to the spleen.
- IV—Disease spread to one or more organs outside the lymphatic system, including liver, bone marrow, lungs, occurs.

- Approximately 60% of children are stage I/II; stage IV is less common in children younger than 10 years.
  1. A—asymptomatic, no B symptoms
  2. B—presence of one or more of the following symptoms (occur in approximately one third of patients)
     a. Weight loss, defined as 10% loss over preceding 6 months without known cause
     b. Fever higher than 38° C for 3 days
     c. Night sweats

■ PATHOLOGIC STAGING
- Laparotomy is performed to examine organs, biopsy liver and lymph nodes, and remove the spleen.
- Indications for pathologic staging vary, depending on risk of abdominal disease and potential use of combined modality therapy versus radiation therapy alone.

THERAPY

- Therapy is generally determined on an individual basis in consultation with pediatric oncologists and radiation therapists. Therapy decisions are based on age, stage, pathology, and skeletal maturity. Multiple effective regimens exist using chemotherapy, radiation therapy, or both modalities.
- The current strategy usually uses combination chemotherapy with reduced-dose radiation therapy in high-stage disease or skeletally immature patients.
- Patients who have completed their growth may be candidates for radiation therapy alone.
- There are multiple active chemotherapy regimens. The mechlorethamine (nitrogen mustard), Oncovin (vincristine), prednisone, procarbazine (MOPP) regimen is currently rarely used because of a high incidence of infertility, especially in males, and the risk of secondary leukemia. Current regimens may include doxorubicin, bleomycin, vinblastine, dacarbazine, cyclophosphamide, VP-16, vincristine, and prednisone.
- Radiation therapy may be involved field or extended field. The dose depends on whether it is used as single modality or combined with chemotherapy.

■ PROGNOSIS
- Survival is excellent for all stages of disease, with most recent studies demonstrating 93% 5-year survival and 86% to 92% 10-year survival for

children and adolescents younger than 16 years and 84% 5-year survival for adults.
- High-stage, more than four sites of involvement, large mediastinal adenopathy (LMA, defined as mass exceeding one third the transverse diameter of the chest on posteroanterior chest radiograph), and B symptoms, particularly fever and weight loss, are poor prognostic factors.
- Unlike many other malignancies, salvage rates or cures after relapse are significant. Intensive therapy, such as autologous bone marrow or stem cell transplant, may be required.

■ FOLLOW-UP & DISPOSITION
- The schedule of radiologic monitoring depends on the site and stage of disease. CT scan of initial disease sites and/or chest radiograph may be followed every 3 to 6 months for 3 to 5 years, then yearly until 10 years from therapy. CT scans of the chest, abdomen, and pelvis may also be periodically performed.
- Gallium scan and ESR may be repeated on the same schedule if abnormal at diagnosis.
- Long-term toxicities of chemotherapy may include cardiomyopathy, pulmonary fibrosis, infertility, or early menopause, and secondary malignancies include leukemia and bladder cancer.
- Long-term toxicities of radiation therapy may include hypothyroidism, hypoplasia, coronary artery and valvular disease, and salivary dysfunction, and secondary malignancies include breast, thyroid, and skin cancer. The risk of breast cancer is particularly significant for females receiving radiation during early adolescence. Annual screening mammograms starting 10 years from diagnosis are recommended.

■ PATIENT/FAMILY EDUCATION
- HD is curable using a variety of chemotherapy and radiation therapy regimens. Parents and patients should ask to be fully informed about treatment options and potential risks and benefits. This is important for many reasons, including the following:
  1. The potential long-term toxicities of therapy are considerable. An important component of choosing the appropriate treatment involves finding the right balance between maximizing the likelihood of cure and minimizing the risk of late effects. This balance may differ for different patients.
  2. Selecting the appropriate treatment plan for an individual patient is not straightforward.

Parents and patients may receive different opinions from different physicians. By ensuring they are informed about the risks and benefits of different treatment plans, they can fully participate in decisions regarding therapy.

■ REFERRAL INFORMATION
- Patients should be referred to pediatric oncologists and radiation therapists with experience treating pediatric patients.
- Although medical oncologists have experience treating patients with HD, the medical, psychosocial, and long-term needs of children and adolescents are best met by a team of pediatric specialists.

✷ PEARLS & CONSIDERATIONS

■ CLINICAL PEARLS
- Chest radiographs should be obtained before the surgical procedure because patients may have significant mediastinal adenopathy that may compromise their airway.
- Children and adolescents who have had splenectomies should take prophylactic penicillin and have booster immunizations as appropriate.

■ WEBSITES
- American Cancer Society: www.cancer.org
- National Cancer Institute: www.nci.gov
- OncoLink: University of Pennsylvania Cancer Center: www.oncolink.com

■ SUPPORT GROUPS
- Pediatric oncologists can refer patients and parents to local or national support organizations for children with cancer and their families.
- National organizations include American Cancer Society and Candlelighters.

REFERENCES
1. Jaffe ES (ed): Hodgkin's lymphoma, *Semin Hematol* 36:217, 1999.
2. Halperin EC et al: Hodgkin's disease. In Halperin EC et al (eds): *Pediatric radiation oncology*, ed 3, Philadelphia, 1999, Lippincott Williams & Wilkins.
3. Hudson MM, Donaldson SS: Hodgkin's disease. In Pizzo PA, Poplack DG (eds): *Principles and practice of pediatric oncology*, ed 3, Philadelphia, 1997, JB Lippincott.
Author: **Andrea Hinkle, M.D.**

BASIC INFORMATION

■ DEFINITION

Non-Hodgkin's lymphoma (NHL) represents a heterogeneous group of malignant neoplasms arising from the transformation of cells of lymphocytic or histiocytic origin, which most often appear in lymph nodes or other lymphoid tissue (tonsils, thymus, or Peyer's patches). Heterogeneous by histology, site of origin, and clinical manifestations, NHL often involves the bone marrow and the central nervous system.

■ SYNONYMS

- Malignant lymphoma
- Reticuloendothelial neoplasm
- Specific subtypes
  1. Burkitt's
  2. Non-Burkitt's or small, non-cleaved cell
  3. Lymphoblastic
  4. Large cell or anaplastic
  5. True histiocytic
- Former terms: lymphoreticular neoplasm, giant follicular lymphoma, lymphosarcoma, reticulum cell sarcoma

ICD-9CM CODES

202.8   Non-Hodgkin's lymphoma
200.1-200.8 Specific subtypes

■ ETIOLOGY

- The cause is unknown in most cases; rare cases of familial NHL have been reported.
- A small proportion of cases are seen in association with diseases that are known to carry an increased risk.
  1. Congenital immunodeficiency syndromes
     a. Wiskott-Aldrich syndrome
     b. Ataxia-telangiectasia
     c. X-linked lymphoproliferative syndrome
     d. Severe combined immunodeficiency syndrome
  2. Acquired immunodeficiency states
     a. Acquired immunodeficiency syndrome (AIDS)
     b. Immunosuppressive therapy: postorgan or postmarrow transplantation, high-dose glucocorticosteroids, androgen steroid abuse
- Epstein-Barr virus (EBV) infection is associated with African-type Burkitt's lymphoma or NHL occurring in patients with an underlying immunodeficiency.
- Specific biologic subtypes are associated with distinctive gene translocations, but their role in the pathogenesis of the disease is not known.

■ EPIDEMIOLOGY & DEMOGRAPHICS

- In the United States, approximately 800 children and adolescents younger than 20 years of age are diagnosed with NHL each year.
- A higher incidence is seen in males and Caucasians versus African Americans.
- Peak age is 5 to 15 years.
  1. Burkitt's and non-Burkitt's small, noncleaved cell tumors predominate among 5- to 14-year-olds.
  2. Diffuse large cell lymphomas are most common among 15- to 19-year-olds.
- Prevalence of primary site varies.
  1. Abdominal: 35%
  2. Mediastinal: 26%
  3. Peripheral nodal: 14%
  4. Head and neck region: 13%
  5. Skin, orbit, thyroid, bone, kidney, breast, or gonads: 10%
- Average time from onset of symptoms to diagnosis is 2 to 6 weeks.
- The 5-year survival rate is 72% for those younger than 20 years of age.

■ HISTORY

- The history depends on the anatomic site(s) and extent of involvement.
- Common systemic symptoms include fever, malaise, anorexia, and mild weight loss.
- Abdominal pain and change in bowel habits may occur.
- Airway compression with shortness of breath, cough, and/or wheeze may occur.
- Superior vena cava syndrome with facial edema, headache, and altered mental status has been reported.
- Painless masses (lymph node enlargement) may be noted.
- When primary occurs in head and neck:
  1. Neck masses or jaw enlargement or swelling
  2. Tonsillar enlargement
  3. Congestion, nasal obstruction
  4. Signs of cranial nerve palsy
     a. Double vision
     b. Facial droop
  5. Eye bulging
  6. Soft tissue swelling

■ PHYSICAL EXAMINATION

- Soft tissue swelling or mass
- Organomegaly
- Firm, rubbery hard, nontender enlarged nodes
- Wheeze, dyspnea, stridor (may be heard on pulmonary examination)
- Cervical adenopathy
- Jaw swelling
- Unilateral tonsillar enlargement
- Nasal obstruction
- Signs of cranial nerve palsy
  1. Asymmetric extraocular movement
  2. Facial asymmetry or droop

DIAGNOSIS

■ DIFFERENTIAL DIAGNOSIS

- Benign
  1. EBV or cytomegalovirus mononucleosis
  2. Cat-scratch disease
  3. Histiocytosis
- Malignant
  1. Hodgkin's disease
  2. Leukemia
  3. Rhabdomyosarcoma
  4. Neuroblastoma
  5. Ewing's sarcoma

■ DIAGNOSTIC WORKUP

- For confirmation of the diagnosis to subtype and stage disease
  1. The final diagnosis is based on histology, cytochemistry, cytogenetics, immunophenotype, and molecular studies of the lymph node biopsy (or marrow biopsy when positive).
  2. Biopsy should be done at a center with the capacity to perform all necessary analyses on tissue sample.
- Complete blood count and differential
  1. If counts are abnormal, suspect marrow involvement and do a marrow aspirate.
- Blood chemistries
  1. Elevated urate, calcium, phosphate, or creatinine suggests tumor lysis syndrome.
  2. Lactate dehydrogenase and uric acid are usually elevated.
- Chest roentgenogram to look for mediastinal mass, adenopathy, effusions, and degree of airway compression
- Computed tomography scan of involved areas (neck, chest, abdomen, and pelvis as indicated)
- Bone marrow aspirate and biopsy
  1. When positive, these test can be used to establish the diagnosis without performing a lymph node biopsy.
  2. Marrow involvement (stage 4 lymphoma) is defined as less than 25% blasts.
  3. If there is greater than 25% blasts or blasts circulating in the peripheral blood, leukemia is the diagnosis.
- Spinal fluid
- Pleural or peritoneal fluid analysis when applicable
- Gallium scan
  1. Lymphomas are gallium avid, and this will identify occult/metastatic disease.
- Magnetic resonance imaging may be helpful if bony or paraspinal involvement suspected

- *Urgent* medical situations (cord compression, mediastinal mass with respiratory distress, superior vena cava syndrome, cranial nerve palsy, hyperuricemia, or renal failure from tumor lysis syndrome)
  1. Minimum investigations should be performed based on presenting history and examination so that emergent treatment such as radiation therapy or steroids can be instituted without delay.

🔬 THERAPY

■ MEDICAL
- Initial management often requires treatment of complications arising from the following:
  1. Space-occupying nature of the tumor
  2. Tumor lysis syndrome, the metabolic complications of onset of chemotherapy or the tumor itself, characterized by hyperuricemia, hypocalcemia, hyperphosphatemia, and renal insufficiency
- Multiagent chemotherapy is the mainstay of treatment.
  1. Treatment is based on the stage of disease and the histologic subtype.
  2. Commonly used chemotherapy agents include vincristine, corticosteroids, methotrexate, mercaptopurine, and intrathecal chemotherapy.
  3. Other agents may include anthracycline, cyclophosphamide, and cytosine arabinoside.
  4. Length of treatment varies with the stage and subtype of NHL, from 6 weeks (localized except lymphoblastic) to 1 to 2 years (lymphoblastic and any advanced-stage disease).

- Radiation may be used emergently to treat complications arising from space-occupying lesions (mediastinal mass, hydronephrosis, or spinal cord compression).

■ SURGICAL
Surgery has no role except for biopsy.

■ FOLLOW-UP & DISPOSITION
- Periodic imaging of affected organs is performed during therapy and at regular intervals for 3 to 4 years from diagnosis to monitor for evidence of recurrence.
- Regular medical evaluation with history, examination, and laboratory tests as appropriate should continue yearly for 20 years or more.
  1. Monitor late effects of chemotherapy.
  2. Monitor for secondary malignancies.

■ REFERRAL INFORMATION
All patients should be referred to a pediatric cancer center for diagnosis, management, and follow-up as soon as the diagnosis of NHL or other malignancy is suspected.

☼ PEARLS & CONSIDERATIONS

■ CLINICAL PEARLS
- The presence of a mediastinal mass with respiratory symptoms is an emergency.
  1. The patient should be kept in a sitting position.
  2. Use of general anesthesia avoided. Once an airway is stabilized, immediately refer to a pediatric cancer center.

- An abdominal primary lesion is the most common cause of intussusception in children older than 6 years of age.

■ WEBSITES
For physicians and families:
- CancerNet: http://cancernet.nci.nih.gov/pdq.html
- OncoLink: http://oncolink.upenn.edu/disease/
- Pediatric Oncology Group: www.pog.ufl.edu

■ SUPPORT GROUPS
- National Candlelighters Association can be reached at 800-366-2223 or through their website at www.candle.org.
- National Children's Cancer Society can be reached at 800-5-FAMILY.
- Many cities and state regions have support groups and summer camp programs for patients, parents, siblings, and friends.
- Local cancer centers are aware of local support groups and resources available for each stage of treatment.

REFERENCES
1. Percy CL et al: Lymphomas and reticuloendothelial neoplasms. In Ries LAG et al (eds): *Cancer incidence and survival among children and adolescents,* US SEER Program 1975-1995, Bethesda, Md, 1999, National Cancer Institute, NIH Pub No. 99-4649.
2. Shad A, Magrath I: Malignant non-Hodgkin's lymphomas in children. In Pizzo PA, Poplack DG (eds): *Principles and practice of pediatric oncology,* Philadelphia, 1997, Lippincott-Raven.
Author: **Barbara Asselin, M.D.**

II

BASIC INFORMATION

■ **DEFINITION**
Malaria is a febrile disease caused by intracellular protozoa of the genus *Plasmodium.*

■ **SYNONYM**
Malaria, foul air

ICD-9CM CODE
084.6 Malaria

■ **ETIOLOGY**
- Four species cause disease in humans: *P. falciparum, P. malariae, P. ovale,* and *P. vivax.*
- Malaria is most commonly acquired from the bite of an infected female Anopheles mosquito.
- Sporozoites travel from the blood to the liver, where infection is amplified and merozoites are released into the blood.
- Rupture of infected red blood cells is responsible for periodic fever.
- Some parasites develop gametes taken up by mosquitoes to produce sporozoites.
- Infection also results from inoculation of infected blood through transfusion, contaminated needles, or across the placenta.

■ **EPIDEMIOLOGY & DEMOGRAPHICS**
- Malaria is endemic in tropical areas; most U.S. cases are imported.
- *P. falciparum* and *P. vivax* are the most common species.
- Because of persistent hepatic infection, relapses are found with *P. vivax* and *P. ovale.*
- Widespread drug resistance has important implications for prevention and treatment.

■ **HISTORY**
- Cyclical febrile paroxysms are typical.
- Fevers may be irregular *(P. falciparum)* or at periodic intervals (every 48 hours for *P. vivax* or *P. ovale*) or every 72 hours *(P. malariae).*
- Paroxysm begins with chill, followed by high fever. There may be systemic symptoms, including malaise, headache, seizures, vomiting, and diarrhea. The sweating stage is characterized by fatigue and resolution of fever.
- Patients often appear well between paroxysms.

■ **PHYSICAL EXAMINATION**
- In addition to fever, tachycardia and hypotension may be present.
- Hepatosplenomegaly is common.
- Central nervous system findings (i.e., confusion, seizures, coma) are common in children.

DIAGNOSIS

■ **DIFFERENTIAL DIAGNOSIS**
Symptoms may be suggestive of numerous infectious diseases, including influenza, typhoid fever, tuberculosis, meningoencephalitis, and endocarditis.

■ **DIAGNOSTIC WORKUP**
- A microscopic examination of the blood should be done to look for parasites; in hyperendemic areas, low-level parasitemia may not be the cause of the presenting illness.
- Thick blood smears concentrate red blood cells; multiple smears may be necessary to find the parasite.
- Thin blood smears are needed for species identification and determination of the parasite load.
- Determination if *P. falciparum* is present is critical because of the potential severity of disease.
- *P. falciparum* is suggested by parasitemia in more than 2% of red blood cells, multiple parasites in a single erythrocyte, and banana-shaped gametocytes.
- Antigen assays and polymerase chain reaction are used in selected settings.

THERAPY

■ **MEDICAL**
- Drug choice depends on the *Plasmodium* species, drug resistance patterns, and severity of illness.
- Chloroquine is the main drug used, except for resistant *P. falciparum.*
- Primaquine phosphate is used to prevent relapses with *P. vivax* and *P. ovale.* Screening for glucose-6-phosphate dehydrogenase (G6PD) deficiency is necessary because of associated hemolytic anemia with this drug.
- For current drug recommendations and dosages, refer to the current *Red Book: Report of the Committee on Infectious Diseases and Centers for Disease Control* (CDC) publications.
- Intravenous therapy may be necessary in very ill patients.
- Exchange transfusion has been used with parasitemia greater than 10%.

■ **FOLLOW-UP & DISPOSITION**
Follow-up blood smears in patients with *P. falciparum*

■ **PATIENT/FAMILY EDUCATION**
- Travelers to endemic areas should obtain advice from health care providers familiar with travel medicine.
- In some situations (i.e., pregnancy, very young children, sensitivity to drugs), usual chemoprophylaxis

cannot be used and travel should be avoided.
- Patients should limit the amount of exposed skin and use DEET (N,N-diethylmetatoluamide)-containing repellent.
- Instructions for DEET repellents should be followed carefully.
- Patients should avoid outside activity from dusk until dawn and use protective measures when sleeping.

■ **PREVENTIVE TREATMENT**
- No current vaccine is effective against malaria.
- For current drug recommendations and dosages, refer to the current *Red Book: Report of the Committee on Infectious Disease and Center for Disease Control* (CDC) publications.
- Medications should be stored in childproof containers, out of children's reach.
- For small children, special drug formulations are necessary and can be prepared at a full-service pharmacy.

■ **REFERRAL INFORMATION**
- Patients should be seen by a health care provider 6 to 8 weeks before travel.
- Referral to an infectious disease specialist or travel clinic may be recommended.

PEARLS & CONSIDERATIONS

■ **WEBSITES & HOTLINES**
- CDC: www.cdc.gov/travel
- CDC Fax Information Service: 888-232-3299
- CDC Malaria Hotline: 770-488-7788

REFERENCES
1. American Academy of Pediatrics: Malaria. In Pickering LK (ed): *2000 Red Book: report of the Committee on Infectious Diseases,* ed 25, Elk Grove Village, Ill, 2000, American Academy of Pediatrics.
2. Centers for Disease Control and Prevention: *Health information for international travel 1999-2000,* Atlanta, 1999, Department of Health and Human Services.
3. Krogstad DJ: Plasmodium species (malaria). In Mandel GL, Bennett JE, Dolin R (eds): *Mandell, Douglas and Bennett's principles and practices of infectious diseases,* ed 5, Philadelphia, 2000, Churchill Livingstone.
4. Strickland GT: Malaria. In Strickland GT (ed): *Hunter's tropical medicine and emerging infectious diseases,* ed 8, Philadelphia, 2000, WB Saunders.
Author: **Carol McCarthy, M.D.**

BASIC INFORMATION

■ DEFINITION
A wide variety of marine creatures are capable of human envenomation. Fortunately, the organisms that are by far the most common cause of marine envenomation in the United States have relatively benign venom.

ICD-9CM CODE
989.5 Marine sting

■ ETIOLOGY
- The venom of certain marine animals is of medical significance in the United States because of their relatively common rate of occurrence.
  1. These are members of the phylum *Cnidaria,* which include the following:
     a. Jellyfish
     b. Atlantic Portuguese man-of-war
     c. Sea nettles
     d. Several species of coral
- All have a similar means of envenomation, the nematocyst, which is an injection device for venom.
  1. Tentacles carry nematocysts along their length.
  2. Even after detachment from the animal, the nematocysts can remain active in water for weeks.

■ EPIDEMIOLOGY & DEMOGRAPHICS
- Marine envenomations typically occur in the warmer waters of the south but can happen anywhere in the United States.
- In 1997, The American Association of Poison Control Centers received 2800 reports of marine envenomation.
- Envenomations by more exotic creatures have been noted to occur in tropical fish tanks.

■ HISTORY
- Many victims of marine envenomation are beachgoers who are stung while bathing along the shore.
- Other victims may be unsuspecting divers who touch these creatures.
- Envenomations typically seen in the United States are immediately painful along a line consistent with a tentacle.

■ PHYSICAL EXAMINATION
- Toxicity is dose related.
- Wheals and vesicles are seen in a linear arrangement.

- Varying degrees of urticaria are present.
- Occasionally, systemic symptoms occur, typically respiratory distress.

DIAGNOSIS

The diagnosis of a marine sting is made based on history and physical examination alone.

THERAPY

- Initial management of airway, breathing, and circulation (ABCs), if necessary, should be begun.
- The remainder of therapy is directed at minimizing further envenomation and managing pain.

■ NONPHARMACOLOGIC
Therapy aims to deactivate any remaining nematocysts and venom.
- Rinse with saltwater.
- Remove remaining tentacles with forceps.
- Apply vinegar topically for 30 minutes, which inactivates most venoms.
- Apply shaving cream and shave the affected area with a razor to remove any remains.

■ MEDICAL
- Topical anesthesia may be applied.
  1. Apply eutectic mixture of local anesthetics (EMLA) to small areas under occlusive dressing for 60 minutes.
- Systemic analgesia with narcotics is occasionally necessary.
  1. Morphine 0.1 to 0.2 mg/kg intravenously (IV), intramuscularly (IM), or subcutaneously (SC) (maximum dose, 15 mg) or 0.2 to 0.5 mg/kg orally (maximum dose, 30 mg) every 4 hours as needed
  2. Codeine 0.5 to 1 mg/kg IM, orally (PO), or SC (maximum dose, 60 mg) every 4 hours as needed
  3. Acetaminophen 15 mg/kg PO or rectally every 4 hours as needed
- Systemic antihistamines may be used.
  1. Diphenhydramine 1 to 2 mg/kg IV, IM, or PO (maximum dose, 50 mg) every 6 hours as needed

- Steroid therapy remains controversial.
- The only marine envenomation for which there is an antivenom is *C. fleckeri.*

■ FOLLOW-UP & DISPOSITION
- Most patients can continue symptomatic therapy at home.
- Local discomfort and rash should resolve by 1 to 2 weeks in most cases.

■ REFERRAL INFORMATION
- Envenomation by the box jellyfish (*C. fleckeri*), which is found near Northern Australia, and severe envenomation by the Portuguese man-of-war (*Physalia physalis*) can be life-threatening.
  1. These stings require immediate care in a facility that is capable of airway and cardiac management.
  2. The regional poison control center can be helpful in the management of the sting.

PEARLS & CONSIDERATIONS

■ CLINICAL PEARLS
Local symptomatic treatment is the mainstay of therapy for most marine stings.

■ WEBSITES
- Beach-Net.com (for parents): www.beach-net.com/oceanjfishstings.html
- Women and Children's Hospital (for physicians): www.wch.sa.gov.au/paedm/clintox/cslavh_marine.html

REFERENCES
1. Fenner PJ: Dangers in the ocean: the traveler and marine envenomation. I. Jellyfish, *J Trav Med* 5:135, 1998.
2. Tintanalli JE, Ruiz E, Krome RL: *Emergency medicine: a comprehensive study guide,* ed 4, New York, 1996, McGraw-Hill.
3. Litovitz TL et al: 1997 Annual Report of the American Association of Poison Control Centers Toxic Exposure Surveillance System, *Am J Emerg Med* 16: 443, 1998.
Author: **Robert Freishtat, M.D.**

BASIC INFORMATION

■ DEFINITION
Infant mastitis/breast abscess is breast inflammation, often with abscess formation in the first 2 months of life.

ICD-9CM CODES
771.5 Neonatal infective mastitis
778.7 Neonatal noninfective mastitis

■ ETIOLOGY
- Physiologic breast enlargement secondary to in utero maternal estrogen exposure
- Presence of potentially pathogenic bacteria on mucous membranes and skin
- Virtually all cases caused by *Staphylococcus aureus*
  1. Rare cases are associated with gram-negative organisms (*Salmonella* and *Escherichia coli*), group B streptococcus, and anaerobes.

■ EPIDEMIOLOGY & DEMOGRAPHICS
- The overall incidence is low (the highest incidence was seen in the 1940s to 1950s during the staphylococcal epidemics in hospital nurseries).
- This condition occurs only in term infants because premature infants lack full mammary development.
- Mastitis occurs at age 2 to 8 weeks of life and usually peaks in the third week.
- The female:male ratio is 2:1.
- Bilateral breast involvement is rare.

■ HISTORY
- Increased swelling and redness of the breast is noted.
- Discharge from the affected nipple may be reported.
- Signs of systemic illness are absent.

■ PHYSICAL EXAMINATION
- Fever present in 25% of patients
- Variable irritability

- Breast tenderness on palpation
- Marked erythema and induration of affected breast
- Breast fluctuance and warmth variably present
- Other skin findings possible and include:
  1. More extensive cellulitis beyond the mammary area
  2. Pustular or bullous rash elsewhere

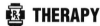

DIAGNOSIS

■ DIFFERENTIAL DIAGNOSIS
The diagnosis is both clinical and microbiologic, with the differential diagnosis mainly centering on the etiologic organism.

■ DIAGNOSTIC WORKUP
- Gram stain and culture (aerobic and anaerobic) of the purulent material must be obtained using one of the following methods:
  1. Gentle manipulation of the nipple
  2. Needle aspiration of the abscess
  3. Surgical incision and drainage of the abscess
- Blood cultures are usually negative.
- Urine and cerebrospinal fluid cultures are not indicated unless clinical evidence of sepsis is present.

THERAPY

■ MEDICAL
- Initial parenteral antimicrobial coverage should be directed at the organism observed on Gram stain.
  1. Generally, a β-lactamase–resistant penicillin is used.
  2. Aminoglycoside is an appropriate choice.
- Once the organism and sensitivities are microbiologically determined, antibiotic coverage can be narrowed.

- The total length of therapy depends on the overall clinical response but usually need not extend beyond 10 to 14 days.

■ SURGICAL
- Prompt incision and drainage is indicated for all abscesses that have not spontaneously drained.
- Incision and drainage is essentially curative.
- An experienced surgeon should perform the surgery to minimize mammary tissue destruction.

■ FOLLOW-UP & DISPOSITION
- Close clinical follow-up is necessary, especially when oral antimicrobial agents are being used.
- Long-term follow-up may reveal evidence of decreased breast tissue compared with the contralateral side once pubertal development is complete.

PEARLS & CONSIDERATIONS

■ CLINICAL PEARLS
- More than two thirds of all breast abscesses in females are found in nursing mothers (2 to 8 weeks postpartum) and not in neonates.
- All infants with mastitis/abscess caused by *Salmonella* have signs and symptoms of gastroenteritis.
- A bacterial throat or nasopharyngeal culture may be useful because it may accurately reflect colonization with *S. aureus*.

REFERENCES
1. Rudoy RC, Nelson JD: Breast abscess during the neonatal period, *Am J Dis Child* 129:1031, 1975.
2. Walsh M, McIntosh K: Neonatal mastitis, *Clin Pediatr* 25:395, 1986.
Author: **Kate Tigue, M.D.**

BASIC INFORMATION

■ **DEFINITION**
Mastoiditis is an acute or subacute infection of the mastoid air cells.

ICD-9CM CODE
383.00 Mastoiditis (acute or subacute)

■ **ETIOLOGY**
• Acute mastoiditis (symptoms less than 1 month in duration)
  1. *Streptococcus pneumoniae*
  2. *Streptococcus pyogenes*
  3. *Staphylococcus aureus*
• Chronic mastoiditis differs in etiologic profile (symptoms 1 month or longer in duration)
  1. *S. aureus*
  2. Gram-negative bacilli (*Pseudomonas aeruginosa*)
  3. Anaerobes (*Peptococcus, Actinomyces,* and *Bacteroides melaninogenicus* most common)
  4. *Mycobacteria* (uncommon in the United States)

■ **EPIDEMIOLOGY & DEMOGRAPHICS**
• Inflammation of mastoid air cells is common in association with acute otitis media.
• Mastoiditis is a natural extension of otitis given the continuity of the mucoperiosteal lining from mastoid to middle ear; about one third of cases occur with a first episode of otitis media.
• Mastoiditis is uncommon in the antibiotic era.
  1. In the preantibiotic era, 25 of 1000 deaths at Los Angeles County Hospital from 1928 to 1933 were attributed to complications of acute otitis media.
  2. In the postantibiotic era, 0.25% of deaths were attributed to complications of acute otitis media.

■ **HISTORY**
• Acute
  1. Fever
  2. Otalgia
  3. Retroauricular swelling and pain with downward and outward deviation of the auricle
  4. Otorrhea or a bulging, immobile, opaque tympanic membrane
  5. If treated with antibiotics, will have a history of either initial improvement then relapse with fever, pain, and swelling, or no response to antibiotics
• Chronic
  1. Longstanding otitis media—usually months to years
  2. With or without fever
  3. Persistent or intermittent ear drainage

  4. Hearing loss
  5. Persistent ear pain
• Complications
  1. Subperiosteal abscess
  2. Bezold abscess (dissection of pus into deep neck structures)
  3. Cerebellar abscess
  4. Epidural abscess
  5. Subdural abscess
  6. Empyema
  7. Labyrinthitis
  8. Venous sinus thrombosis
  9. Bacteremia
  10. Temporal bone osteomyelitis
  11. Conductive hearing loss
  12. Septic emboli
  13. Facial nerve palsy
  14. Meningitis
  15. Otitic hydrocephalus (intracranial hypertension secondary to lateral sinus obstruction)

■ **PHYSICAL EXAMINATION**
• Acute
  1. Fever
  2. Abnormal tympanic membrane
  3. Mastoid tenderness, swelling, and erythema
  4. Downward and outward displacement of auricle
  5. Fluctuance if pus disrupts the bone and forms a subperiosteal abscess.
     a. In infants, fluctuance is above the ear, pushing the pinna inferiorly and out.
     b. In children, fluctuance is posterior to the ear, pushing the pinna superiorly and out.
• Chronic
  1. With or without fever
  2. With or without postauricular swelling
  3. Mucopurulent drainage from perforated tympanic membrane
  4. Hearing loss

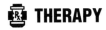 **DIAGNOSIS**

■ **DIFFERENTIAL DIAGNOSIS**
• Posterior auricular lymphadenopathy
• Mumps
• Histiocytosis
• Leukemia
• Lymphoma
• Bone cysts
• Mastoid tumors

■ **DIAGNOSTIC WORKUP**
Consider further workup in all cases of otitis media that are not responsive to antibiotics and in all cases of suppurative intracranial processes with no known focus.
• Tympanocentesis
  1. Gram stain and culture

• Computed tomography (CT) scan of the temporal bone for confirmation of clinical impression
  1. Nonspecific clouding of mastoid cells
     a. Serous otitis media can cause cloudy mastoids on CT scan.
  2. Necrosis and coalescence of bony septa
  3. Bony destruction
  4. Hypoaeration
• Lumbar puncture when meningeal signs are present
• Immunologic evaluation in cases in which other recurrent infections have occurred

■ **THERAPY**

■ **MEDICAL**
• The team approach of primary care physician and otolaryngologist recommended
• Tympanocentesis for diagnosis and treatment
  1. Tympanostomy tubes
  2. Myringotomy
• Antibiotics tailored to Gram stain and known etiologic agents
  1. In acute mastoiditis: ceftriaxone, cefotaxime, or clindamycin (in penicillin-allergic patient)
  2. If central nervous system involvement is suspected: vancomycin to cover resistant pneumococci or staphylococci
  3. In chronic mastoiditis: no treatment until surgical cultures obtained
  4. Examples of empiric therapy regimens for chronic mastoiditis
     a. Ticarcillin/clavulanate, piperacillin/tazobactam, ceftazidime, or imipenem may be used.
  5. Therapy then tailored depending on culture results
     a. Length of therapy is similar to treatment of osteomyelitis.
     b. Intravenous therapy is given until a clinical response is achieved and then may be changed to oral therapy.
  6. Change to oral therapy appropriate only if adequate oral absorption can be maintained, the etiologic organism has been identified, and an appropriate oral agent for treatment is available
  7. Duration of therapy: minimum of 3 weeks

■ **SURGICAL**
Surgical intervention is indicated for therapeutic drainage and/or debridement if any of the following are present:
• Fluctuance

II

- CT scan indicative of bony involvement
- Complications of mastoiditis (see previous section, "History")
- Failure of medical therapy within 48 hours

■ **FOLLOW-UP & DISPOSITION**
- Evaluation of hearing loss
- Careful evaluation for response to therapy and complications
- Primary prevention
  1. Early and complete treatment of otitis media

■ **REFERRAL INFORMATION**
Appropriate consultation with oto-laryngologists, surgeons, and neurosurgeons for specific complications and pediatric infectious disease specialists is recommended.

⚡ **PEARLS & CONSIDERATIONS**

Rare, but not extinct

REFERENCES
1. American Academy of Pediatrics: Mastoiditis. In Peter G (ed): *1997 Red Book: report of the Committee on Infectious Diseases,* ed 24, Elk Grove Village, Ill, 1997, American Academy of Pediatrics.
2. Lewis K, Newman A, Cherry J: Mastoiditis. In Feigin RD, Cherry JD (eds): *Textbook of pediatric infectious diseases,* ed 4, Philadelphia, 1998, WB Saunders.
Author: **Maureen Kays, M.D.**

BASIC INFORMATION

■ DEFINITION
Measles is an acute viral illness characterized by fever, cough, coryza, conjunctivitis, and a characteristic exanthem and enanthem.

ICD-9CM CODE
055.9 Measles

■ ETIOLOGY
Measles virus is an RNA virus of one serotype, classified as *Morbillivirus* in the *Paramyxovirus* family.

■ EPIDEMIOLOGY & DEMOGRAPHICS
- Measles is transmitted by direct contact with infectious droplets and less commonly by airborne spread.
- Peak incidence in temperate areas is winter and spring.
- In the prevaccine era, 400,000 cases were reported in the United States each year. Measles was epidemic and occurred in biennial cycles in urban areas.
- The highest attack rates were in children ages 5 to 9 years old.
- Encephalitis occurs in approximately 1 in 2000 reported cases.
- Death occurs in 1 of every 3000 cases. Mortality is highest in infants and adults.
- Vaccination efforts have reduced the incidence of measles by 99%.

■ HISTORY
- The incubation period is 10 ± 2 days.
- A 3-day prodrome of upper airway tract symptoms with fever is seen.
- Malaise, fever, coryza, conjunctivitis, and cough follow, with increasing severity over the next 2 to 4 days.
- Maximum temperature is 39.5° C (103° F).
- Conjunctivitis is associated with tearing and photophobia.
- Exanthem appears 2 weeks after exposure:
  1. At peak of fever and respiratory symptoms
  2. Appears first on head, behind ears, and spreads centrifugally to the feet
  3. Becomes confluent by the third day
  4. Fades following the reverse course of its appearance; desquamation possible
- Modified illness occurs in the partially immune individual:
  1. Same sequence, yet milder
  2. Most commonly occurs after immune globulin is given to an exposed susceptible host
  3. Also occurs in infected unimmunized infants modified by transplacentally acquired maternal antibody

- Atypical illness occurs in some immunized patients exposed to wild-type virus.
  1. Seen primarily in the 1970s in young adults who received killed measles vaccine
  2. Similar incubation period
  3. Sudden high fever in prodrome, headache, abdominal pain, and myalgia
  4. Rash first seen distally with spread upward
  5. Rash may be vesicular
  6. Respiratory distress with pneumonia
  7. Atypical measles: not contagious
- Complications of measles include pneumonia and secondary bacterial infection, which are the leading causes of death.
  1. Otitis media is the most common complication.
  2. Cardiac involvement: Clinically significant myocarditis and pericarditis occur rarely.
  3. Encephalitis may occur during the rash.
  4. Black measles (a confluent hemorrhagic rash) is a severe, often fatal, complication, but it is rarely seen.
  5. Subacute sclerosing panencephalitis is a rare degenerative central nervous system disease caused by persistent infection.

■ PHYSICAL EXAMINATION
- Prodrome lasts approximately 3 days.
  1. Fever, coryza, rhinitis, and conjunctival injection predominate.
  2. Koplik spots are the pathognomonic enanthem.
     a. White spots (about 1 mm in size) appear on a bright red background on the buccal mucosa and increase in number to coalesce on most of the buccal and lower labial mucosa.
- The exanthem stage typically begins on the fourteenth day after exposure, at the peak of the respiratory symptoms.
  1. Fever peaks then begins to clear after the third or fourth day.
  2. Koplik spots disappear over the next 3 days.
  3. Exanthem starts behind the ears and along the hairline.
  4. By the third day, the rash involves face and spreads to lower extremities sequentially from head to toe (centrifugally).
  5. Maculopapular erythematous discrete lesions appear, which progress to a confluent rash.
  6. Appearance of lesions can be vesicular on an erythematous base.
  7. On day 3 or 4, the rash fades to a copper color and fine desquamation occurs.
     a. Fever breaks on day 3 or 4,

with resolution of respiratory symptoms.
     b. Pharyngitis and generalized lymphadenopathy are often present.

DIAGNOSIS

- Exclude illnesses whose main signs include an exanthematous rash.
  1. Infectious mononucleosis and drug eruptions are the most confusing alternative diagnoses.
- Exposure and immunization history are helpful in limiting the differential diagnosis.
- The presence of Koplik spots is pathognomonic.
- Specific diagnosis is made by the following:
  1. Viral isolation
  2. Detection of measles antigen in exfoliated cells and tissues by fluorescent antibody
  3. Neutralizing antibody titer rise in sequential serum samples
  4. Specific measles immunoglobulin M (IgM) antibody (false-positive IgM ELISA results may occur)

THERAPY

- No specific antiviral treatment is available.
- Symptomatic treatment of fever, maintenance of hydration, and antitussive therapy should be provided.
- Vitamin A (single dose of 200,000 IU orally) (100,000 IU for children 6 to 12 months of age) repeated the following day and at 4 weeks in clinically deficient children should be administered to all infected children who live in areas of known vitamin A deficiency.
- Any infected child with any of the following risk factors should be considered for vitamin A supplementation:
  1. Hospitalized 6-month-old to 2-year-old with measles
  2. Immunodeficiency (human immunodeficiency virus [HIV], immunosuppressive therapy, congenital immunodeficiencies)
  3. Clinical evidence of vitamin A deficiency (by ophthalmologic criteria)
  4. Impaired intestinal absorption (short gut syndrome, cystic fibrosis, biliary obstruction)
  5. Moderate to severe malnutrition (including eating disorders)
  6. Recent immigration from areas where measles mortality rates are 1% or greater

TABLE 2-15   Recommendations for Administration of Live Measles Virus Vaccine

CATEGORY	RECOMMENDATIONS
Unvaccinated, no history of measles (12-15 mo)	A two-dose schedule (with MMR) is recommended if born after 1956. The first dose is recommended at 12-15 mo; the second is recommended at 4-6 yr.
Children 12 mo in area of recurrent measles transmission	Vaccinate; a second dose is indicated at 4-6 yr (at school entry).
Children 6-11 mo in epidemic situations	Vaccinate (with monovalent measles vaccine or, if not available, MMR); revaccination (with MMR) at 12-15 mo is necessary, and a third dose is indicated at 4-6 yr.
Children 11-12 ys who have received one dose of measles vaccine at 12 mo	Revaccinate (1 dose).
Students in college and other post–high school institutions who have received one dose of measles vaccine at 12 mo	Revaccinate (1 dose).
History of vaccination before first birthday	Consider susceptible and vaccinate (2 doses).

MMR, Measles-mumps-rubella.

■ **PATIENT/FAMILY EDUCATION**

Immunization results in serologic evidence of immunity in 99% of those receiving two doses, at least 1 month apart starting at older than 12 months of age.

■ **PRIMARY PREVENTION**
• See Table 2-15
• Live measles virus vaccine
  1. Attenuated
  2. Monovalent or in combination (measles-rubella, measles-mumps-rubella [MMR])
  3. Produces mild, noncommunicable infection
  4. Development of antibodies in 95% of susceptible children
  5. Durable protection
  6. First dose by 15 months of age, on or after first birthday
  7. A second dose given by 12 years, preferably given between 4 and 6 years
  8. Consider susceptible if born after 1957 and without documentation of vaccination, physician-diagnosed illness, or titers confirming infection
  9. In outbreaks: interval between vaccinations should be at least 1 month
• Adverse events
  1. Fever in 5% to 15% occurs in 7 to 12 days after receiving the vaccine.
  2. Transient rashes appear in 5% of vaccine recipients.
  3. Transient thrombocytopenia can occur.
  4. Rare hypersensitivity reactions are usually minor and consist of urticaria or wheal and flare at the site of injection.
    a. Children with egg allergies are at low risk for anaphylactic reactions; skin testing is not predictive of reactions to MMR vaccine.
    b. Reactions are attributed to small amounts of neomycin or gelatin in the vaccine.
• Precautions
  1. Minor illnesses with fever are not a contraindication.
  2. Children with anaphylactic reactions to eggs, neomycin, or gelatin should be evaluated by an allergist before receiving the measles vaccine and may require skin testing and desensitization before receiving measles vaccine.
  3. The risk of thrombocytopenia is increased in children with history of thrombocytopenia.
    a. The benefit versus risk of vaccine and illness need to be considered.
• Recent administration of immune globulin
  1. May interfere with the serologic response to measles vaccine, and measles immunization should be delayed as detailed in Table 2-16.
• Immunodeficient hosts
  1. Live virus should not be given to severely immunodeficient children.
  2. An interval of 3 months should be observed from cessation of any immunosuppressive therapy and vaccination.
  3. High-dose corticosteroids necessitates an interval of 1 month.
  4. HIV infection is not a contraindication unless the child is severely immunocompromised (low CD4 T lymphocyte counts).
  5. Pregnant women should not receive the vaccine.
• Secondary prevention: see Table 2-17
• Measles vaccine
  1. If given within 72 hours of exposure, may provide some protection against measles
• Immune globulin
  1. Immune globulin can be given to susceptible children within 6 days of exposure to prevent or modify infection.
  2. The usual dose is 0.25 ml/kg intramuscularly.
  3. Immunocompromised children should receive 0.5 ml/kg intramuscularly.
  4. Maximum dose is 15 ml.
• Indications for immune globulin
  1. Susceptible household contacts
  2. Infants younger than 12 months
  3. Pregnant women
  4. Immunocompromised hosts
  5. HIV-infected children regardless of immunization status, unless patient is receiving intravenous immune globulin at regular intervals, whose last dose was within 3 weeks of exposure

■ **REFERRAL INFORMATION**
• Consultation with a pediatric infectious disease specialist may be warranted in complicated cases and exposures.
• Report all cases of measles to the local health department and Infection Control Committee in hospitalized patients.

TABLE 2-16   Recommendations for Time Interval for Administration of Measles Vaccine Following Administration of Immune Globulin

HISTORY OF RECEIVING IMMUNOGLOBULIN FOR:	INTERVAL (MO) BEFORE VACCINATION
Tetanus (as TIG)	3
Hepatitis A prophylaxis (as IG) Contact prophylaxis	3
International travel	3
Hepatitis B prophylaxis (as HBIG)	3
Rabies prophylaxis (as RIG)	4
Measles prophylaxis (as IG): standard host	5
Immunocompromised host	6
Varicella prophylaxis (as VZIG)	5
Blood transfusion Washed RBCs	0
RBCs, adenine-saline added	3
Packed RBCs	5
Whole blood	6
Plasma or platelet products	7
Replacement (or therapy) of immune deficiencies (as IVIG)	8
ITP (as IVIG)	8
RSV-IVIG	9
ITP	10
ITP or Kawasaki disease	11

HBIG, Hepatitis B immune globulin; *IG,* immune globulin; *ITP,* immune thrombocytopenic purpura; *IVIG,* intravenous immune globulin; *RBCs,* red blood cells; *RIG,* rabies immune globulin; *RSV,* respiratory syncytial virus; *TIG,* tetanus immune globulin; *VZIG,* varicella-zoster immune globulin.

TABLE 2-17   Recommendations for Control of Measles Outbreaks

SETTING	CONTROL MEASURES
Outbreaks in preschool-age children	Age for vaccination should be lowered to 6 mo in outbreak area if cases occur in children younger than 1 yr.*
Outbreaks in institutions: child care centers, K-12 grades, colleges, and other institutions	All students, their siblings, and school personnel born after 1956 who do not have documentation of immunity to measles† should be immunized.
Outbreaks in medical facilities	Revaccination of all medical workers born after 1956 who have direct patient contact and who do not have proof of immunity to measles.† Vaccination may also be considered for workers born before 1957. Susceptible personnel who have been exposed should be relieved from direct patient contact from the fifth to the 21st day after exposure (regardless of whether they received measles vaccine or immune globulin) or, if they become ill, for 4 days after the rash develops.

*Children initially vaccinated before their first birthdays should be revaccinated at 12 to 15 months of age. A third dose should be administered at 4 to 6 years of age.
†Proof consists of documentation of physician-diagnosed measles disease, serologic evidence of immunity to measles, or documentation of receipt of two doses of measles vaccine on or after the first birthday.

✷ PEARLS & CONSIDERATIONS

■ **WEBSITES**
- Centers for Disease Control and Prevention (CDC): www.cdc.gov/
- *Morbidity and Mortality Weekly Report* (MMWR): www2.cdc.gov/mmwr

REFERENCES

1. American Academy of Pediatrics: Measles. In Pickering LK (ed): *2000 Red Book: report of the Committee on Infectious Diseases,* ed 25, Elk Grove Village, Ill, 2000, American Academy of Pediatrics.
2. The Centers for Disease Control and Prevention: Measles in the United States—1999, *MMWR Morb Mortal Wkly Rep* 49:557, 2000.
3. Cherry J: Measles virus. In Feigin RD, Cherry JD (eds): *Textbook of pediatric infectious diseases,* ed 4, Philadelphia, 1998, WB Saunders.

Author: **Maureen Kays, M.D.**

BASIC INFORMATION

■ **DEFINITION**

- *Meckel's diverticulum* is an ileal out-pouching that occurs from the incomplete atresia of the vitelline duct (also known as the *omphalomesenteric duct* [OMD]) in the embryo. It may contain ileal mucosa or ectopic mucosa of gastric, pancreatic, or jejunal/colonic origin. Partial or incomplete attenuation of the OMD can also lead to persistent fistula formation to the umbilicus, umbilical cysts in which the distal duct only remains intact, or fibrous bands. These bands course from the Meckel's diverticulum to the base of the mesentery and may act as sites for internal herniation of the small intestine or intestinal obstruction.
- *Meckel's diverticulitis* is an inflammation of the Meckel's diverticulum. This results from obstruction at the base leading to infection within the blind-ending diverticulum (similar mechanism to appendicitis).

ICD-9CM CODES

751.0   Meckel's diverticulum
751.0   Omphalomesenteric duct
759.89 Umbilical cyst

■ **ETIOLOGY**

- The causes of persistence and incomplete atresia of the OMD are unknown.
- Complications arising from a Meckel's diverticulum occur secondary to the presence of this diverticulum.
  1. Bleeding is precipitated by ulceration of the ileal mucosa at a site next to the ectopic gastric mucosa.
     a. The ulcer may be within the main ileal lumen or within the diverticulum.
  2. Intussusception is caused by the Meckel's diverticulum acting as a lead point.
- Persistence of a portion of the embryonic fistula tract (intraumbilical fistula, umbilical cyst) may lead to mucoid or meconium drainage from the umbilicus.
- Residual OMD bands may cause obstruction.

■ **EPIDEMIOLOGY & DEMOGRAPHICS**

- Meckel's diverticulum occurs in approximately 2% of the population.
- Males represent 75% of symptomatic patients.
- Approximately 60% of diverticula present in childhood, 50% by the third year of life.
- The typical diverticulum is approximately 2 inches in length and arises within the terminal 2 feet of the ileum.

- There are two primary types of ectopic mucosa seen: gastric and pancreatic.
- The two most common complications are bleeding and obstruction of the diverticulum or the small intestine.
- The type of presentation depends on the patient's age.
  1. Hemorrhage is the most common complication (40%) and occurs more commonly in younger infants.
  2. Older patients present more commonly with symptoms of inflammation.

■ **HISTORY & PHYSICAL EXAMINATION**

- Rectal hemorrhage is typically "currant jelly" in appearance, of significant volume, and often without stool.
- Bleeding may be accompanied by mild cramps, but other significant gastrointestinal symptoms are rare.
- Mere guaiac-positive stools are rare.
- When obstruction of the diverticular base occurs, leading to diverticulitis, symptoms are indistinguishable from those of appendicitis.
  1. Nausea, anorexia, fever, and/or abdominal pain may occur.
  2. There may be a palpable, central suprapubic mass.
  3. Most are recognized when patients undergo laparotomy for presumed appendicitis.
     a. When a normal appendix is identified, further exploration leads to the diagnosis.
- Intussusception from a Meckel's lead point is clinically indistinguishable from other types of intussusception.
  1. However, with Meckel's, there is a much larger risk for recurrence if the diverticulum is not appreciated (and corrected).
- Obstruction may also be caused by internal herniation or volvulus around an OMD band.
- Fistulas to the umbilicus through an OMD present with drainage at the base of the umbilicus.
  1. Drainage may be of enteric secretions if the OMD is completely patent.
  2. A periumbilical rash and inflammation surrounding the umbilicus may occur.
  3. Incomplete patency (i.e., fibrosed at the intestinal end) may lead to mucoid drainage at the umbilicus.
- Other umbilical anomalies (e.g., cysts) may also present as a mass or an infection under the umbilicus.
- Persistence of umbilical "granulation tissue" in the newborn should provoke further investigation.

🔬 **DIAGNOSIS**

■ **DIFFERENTIAL DIAGNOSIS**

- The differential diagnosis depends on the anomaly and presentation.
- Intestinal obstruction and diverticulitis present as an acute abdomen and have a definitive diagnosis made, in most cases, at the time of laparotomy.
- The differential diagnosis of mildly symptomatic or asymptomatic rectal bleeding includes the following:
  1. Rectal fissure, trauma
  2. Juvenile polyp or polyposis syndrome
  3. Ulcerative colitis
  4. Foreign body
  5. Vascular malformation
  6. Coagulopathy

■ **DIAGNOSTIC WORKUP**

- ^{99m}Tc sodium pertechnetate scanning assists in the identification of a Meckel's if there is ectopic gastric mucosa in the diverticulum.
  1. When visualized, this is a helpful procedure.
  2. Unfortunately, false-negative studies approach 40%, even with enhancement using H_2 blockers or pentagastrin.
- Barium studies and computed tomography (CT) are rarely helpful.
- Laparoscopy is both diagnostic and therapeutic and has become the primary mode of diagnosis and treatment for suspected Meckel's bleeding when the diagnosis is not secured.
- In patients with persistent drainage from the umbilicus, a direct sinogram with water-soluble contrast will often disclose the tract and any communication with the intestinal tract.
- Ultrasound or CT will help identify cysts and sinus tract remnants.
  1. These can be identified (and corrected) during operative exploration of the umbilicus in patients undergoing umbilical hernia repair.

℞ **THERAPY**

■ **SURGICAL**

- Patients with symptomatic Meckel's diverticulum should undergo operative removal of the diverticulum and correction of other coincident complications.
- When resection is undertaken for bleeding, care to excise all ectopic mucosa and the diverticulum is necessary.
  1. In the face of active bleeding, resection of the ulcer is curative.

2. In the case of intussusception, the diverticulum is resected along a healthy margin after reduction.
3. Inflamed diverticulum should be excised.

- OMD bands should be excised in all cases; any intestinal obstruction is also relieved.
- The use of diagnostic and resection techniques during laparoscopy has simplified the risk of exploration in the case of undiagnosed rectal bleeding in the young child.
  1. This procedure has replaced more complex imaging and angiography, simplifying and expediting management.

☼ PEARLS & CONSIDERATIONS

■ CLINICAL PEARLS

- The "Rule of Twos" indicates the following:
  1. 2 years old
  2. 2 feet from the terminal ileum
  3. 2 inches long
  4. 2 types of ectopic mucosa: gastric, pancreatic
  5. 2 major complications: bleeding, obstruction
  6. 2 primary routes for diagnosis: Meckel's scan, laparoscopy
- In cases of undiagnosed intractable abdominal pain, consider Meckel's diverticulum: intermittent intussusception, recurrent inflammation, ectopic ulceration.
- Intractable granulation tissue at the umbilicus may represent ectopic tissue from an incompletely patent OMD.

REFERENCES

1. Brown RL, Azizkhan RG: Gastrointestinal bleeding in infants and children: Meckel's diverticulum and intestinal duplication, *Semin Pediatr Surg* 8:202, 1999 (review).
2. Connolly LP et al: Meckel's diverticulum: demonstration of heterotopic gastric mucosa with technetium-99m-pertechnetate SPECT, *J Nucl Med* 39: 1458, 1998.
3. Lee KH et al: Laparoscopy for definitive diagnosis and treatment of gastrointestinal bleeding of obscure origin in children, *J Pediatr Surg* 35:1291, 2000.
4. Martin JP, Connor PD, Charles K: Meckel's diverticulum, *Am Fam Physician* 61:1037, 2000 (review).
5. Peeker R, Hjalmas K: Ileoileal intussusception with a leading Meckel's diverticulum, *Am Fam Physician* 58:659, 1998.
6. Snyder CL: Meckel's diverticulum. In Ashcraft KW et al (eds): *Pediatric surgery*, ed 3, Philadelphia, 2000, WB Saunders.
7. Swaniker F, Soldes O, Hirschl RB: The utility of technetium 99m pertechnetate scintigraphy in the evaluation of patients with Meckel's diverticulum, *J Pediatr Surg* 34:760, 1999.

Author: **Frederick Ryckman, M.D.**

BASIC INFORMATION

■ **DEFINITION**

Bacterial meningitis is inflammation of the meninges, the membranes covering the brain and spinal cord, as a result of bacterial infection.

■ **SYNONYM**

Leptomeningitis

ICD-9CM CODES

320.9 Bacterial meningitis, not otherwise specified
320.1 Gram positive
320.82 Gram negative
320.81 Anaerobic

■ **ETIOLOGY**

- Most cases of bacterial meningitis arise hematogenously.
- Occasional cases result from the spread from contiguous foci of infection or meningeal defects of congenital or traumatic origin.
- Microbiologic etiology depends on the patient's age.
  1. Younger than 1 to 2 months of age
     a. Group B streptococcus: 52%
     b. *Escherichia coli* and other gram-negative enteric bacilli: 27%
     c. *Listeria monocytogenes:* 6%
     d. Anaerobes: 3%
     e. Other gram-positive organisms (enterococci, pneumococci, staphylococci): 7%
     f. Other gram-negative organisms (*Haemophilus influenzae, Neisseria meningitidis, Pseudomonas* species): 5%
  2. Older than 2 to 3 months of age
     a. *Streptococcus pneumoniae*
     b. N. meningitidis
     c. Together, account for 95% of cases
     d. Occasionally: *H. influenzae, Salmonella* species, *L. monocytogenes,* Group B streptococcus, anaerobes

■ **EPIDEMIOLOGY & DEMOGRAPHICS**

- Depends on the causative agent
- Pneumococcal meningitis
  1. There are 83 stereotypes, but 9 cause most invasive disease.
  2. The organism is a frequent inhabitant of the upper respiratory tract.
  3. Meningitis most commonly occurs in the very young (younger than 8 months of age) and after head injury.
  4. Higher incidence is found in African Americans than in whites.
  5. The incidence of antibiotic resistance to penicillin and even third-generation cephalosporins is increasing.

- Meningococcal meningitis
  1. There are nine serogroups; the most invasive disease in the United States is caused by group B (younger children) or group C (older children) meningococci.
  2. Two percent to fifteen percent of healthy persons (particularly adults) harbor the organism in the nasopharynx.
  3. The endemic attack rate for invasive disease is 1 to 3 cases per 100,000 population per year.
  4. Meningitis most often occurs in children younger than age 5 years, with peak attack rate at 6 to 12 months of age; another peak occurs in adolescence.
  5. The secondary attack rate in household and other close contacts (e.g., day-care contacts) of an index case is approximately 1000-fold greater than the endemic attack rate.
- Group B streptococcal meningitis
  1. There are seven major serotypes, but meningitis is usually caused by serotype III organisms.
  2. Meningitis can be a manifestation of either early-onset (younger than 5 to 7 days of age) or late-onset (older than 7 days of age) infection.
     a. Early-onset infection results from vertical transmission of the organism from mother to infant shortly before or during delivery.
     b. Five percent to thirty-five percent of pregnant women in the United States are colonized rectally, vaginally, or both.
     c. In the absence of maternal chemoprophylaxis, 40% to 70% of colonized women transmit the organism to their infants, and 1 to 4 infants per 1000 live births develop invasive disease (pneumonia, bacteremia, and/or meningitis).
     d. There is usually a history of maternal obstetric complications (prematurity, prolonged rupture of membranes, chorioamnionitis, intrapartum fever, group B streptococcal bacteriuria).
  3. Late-onset infection usually occurs at 3 to 4 weeks of age (range, 1 week to 8 months).
     a. It may result from vertical transmission of the organism from mother to infant at the time of delivery, but with delayed hematogenous dissemination.
     b. It more likely results from horizontal transmission of the organism from nursery personnel, caregivers at home, and others to the infant.
     c. The disease usually presents as bacteremia, meningitis, or focal infections (septic arthritis, osteomyelitis, cellulitis).

■ **HISTORY**

- Fever: may or may not be present in the neonate; virtually always present in nonneonates; variable height
- Vomiting
- Headache
- Altered mental status: most helpful symptoms in infants are either excessive lethargy or irritability
- Poor feeding
- Apnea, respiratory distress in neonates

■ **PHYSICAL EXAMINATION**

- Meningeal signs (signs of meningeal irritation): nuchal rigidity, positive Kernig's sign (leg is flexed 90 degrees at hip; knee cannot be extended beyond 135 degrees), positive Brudzinski's sign (legs are flexed involuntarily when neck is flexed); usually present in older children but may not be present (or be present late in course) in infants younger than 1 year of age
- Bulging fontanelle: in infants
- Rash (petechiae and/or purpura): may or may not be present in meningococcal infection
- Shock: manifested by diminished peripheral perfusion (capillary refill longer than 2 seconds), decreased urine output, depressed mental status, late hypotension
- Papilledema: very rare; when present, look for brain abscess, venous sinus thrombosis, subdural fluid collection
- Seizures: occur in approximately 20%; those occurring before or during the first 2 to 4 days of hospitalization and that are not difficult to control are not associated with a poor neurologic prognosis
- Focal neurologic signs: occur in 14% to 24%; are associated with a poorer neurologic prognosis
- Cranial nerve palsies: involvement of those controlling extraocular movements (III, IV, VI) is usually transient; VIII nerve involvement (cochlear or vestibular) is often permanent
- Other signs of increased intracranial pressure (ICP): marked depression of consciousness; hypertension; bradycardia; irregular respirations; dilated, sluggishly reactive pupils; decorticate or decerebrate posturing (These signs are uncommon but may occur.)

II

DIAGNOSIS

■ DIFFERENTIAL DIAGNOSIS
- Other forms of meningitis (viral, tuberculous, fungal, parasitic/protozoal)
- Encephalitis
- Brain abscess
- Subdural empyema
- Head injury
- Intoxications
- Brain tumors

■ DIAGNOSTIC WORKUP
- A lumbar puncture (LP) to collect cerebrospinal fluid (CSF) is the principal diagnostic test.
  1. LP is generally safe, although there is a risk of cerebral herniation in patients with significantly elevated ICP.
  2. LP should be deferred in patients with significant depression of consciousness (no response to pain), hypertension, bradycardia, decorticate or decerebrate posturing, irregular respirations, or pupillary dilation/sluggish reaction to light.
     a. Treat presumptively for meningitis and lower ICP until deemed safe to perform an LP.
- CSF should be collected for the following:
  1. Cell count: white blood cell (WBC) count usually greater than 1000/mm^3 (normal, less than 10/mm^3); may be less if early infection or fulminant disease
  2. Differential: usually see a predominance of polymorphonuclear leukocytes
  3. Glucose: usually moderately to severely depressed (less than 60% of the blood sugar)
  4. Protein: usually elevated
  5. Gram stain: usually positive, unless the patient has very early infection, has been pretreated with antibiotics, or has *L. monocytogenes* infection
  6. Culture: CSF should be inoculated onto sheep's blood agar, onto chocolate agar, and into nutrient broth; culture usually positive, although if the patient has been pretreated with antibiotics, it may be negative
  7. Latex agglutination: may be used to detect antigens of *S. pneumoniae*, *H. influenzae* type b, *N. meningitidis*, and group B streptococcus in the CSF
     a. Sensitivity proportional to the amount of antigen present
     b. Useful in patients who have been pretreated with antibiotics, which might render CSF Gram stain and culture falsely negative, but need not be performed in every patient with suspected bacterial meningitis
- Use CSF analysis to differentiate among the various types of meningitis
  1. Viral meningitis
     a. CSF cell count is usually 50 to 500/mm^3, although occasionally higher.
     b. There may be polymorphonuclear WBC predominance early, but a shift to mononuclear WBC predominance usually occurs within 12 to 24 hours.
     c. Glucose is usually normal or only mildly depressed; protein is usually modestly elevated.
     d. Gram stain, latex agglutination, and bacterial cultures are negative.
     e. Viral cultures and viral polymerase chain reaction (PCR) may be positive.
  2. Tuberculous meningitis
     a. CSF cell count is usually 50 to 500/mm^3.
     b. There is polymorphonuclear WBC predominance early, but a shift to mononuclear WBC predominance usually occurs later.
     c. Glucose is usually moderately low (15 to 35 mg/dl), lower than what is usually observed in viral meningitis but not as low as in many cases of bacterial meningitis.
- Obtain blood cultures.
  1. Positive in 60% to 90% of patients with hematogenously acquired bacterial meningitis
  2. Highest yield if obtained early in the clinical course
- If skin lesions are present:
  1. Gram stain of skin lesions can assist in the diagnosis of meningococcal infection.
- Computed tomography (CT) scan of the head is primarily useful in assessing for complications of meningitis (hydrocephalus, subdural effusions, infarcts), but it is not helpful in establishing the diagnosis of meningitis.

THERAPY

■ SUPPORTIVE CARE
- Admit to the pediatric intensive care unit (PICU) or neonatal intensive care unit (NICU) initially for close observation.
- Monitor vital signs, peripheral perfusion, urine output, and mental status for signs of shock. Treat shock initially with isotonic fluids (crystalloids usually, occasionally colloids); vasopressors may be needed later.
- Initiate fluid therapy.
  1. Correct dehydration and shock, but do not overhydrate.
  2. Monitor for evidence of the syndrome of inappropriate secretion of antidiuretic hormone (SIADH), which is manifested by hyponatremia, hyposmolality, possible oliguria, and high urinary sodium excretion.
     a. Restrict fluids if SIADH develops.
  3. Perform frequent neurologic evaluations for the first 2 to 3 days after the onset of therapy.
  4. Observe for seizures: If they develop and are not caused by a metabolic derangement (hypoglycemia, hyponatremia, hypocalcemia), treat with phenytoin or fosphenytoin (either is preferred in children older than 1 month because they do not depress mental status) or phenobarbital, with or without a benzodiazepine (for rapid seizure control).
- Monitor head circumference of infants daily. A rapid increase suggests development of hydrocephalus or large subdural effusions.
- Observe for evidence of marked elevation of ICP. Treat suspected markedly increased ICP with mannitol (with or without furosemide) and possible hyperventilation (latter is useful only for acute management of impending herniation).
- Monitor for evidence of disseminated intravascular coagulation (DIC). Treat DIC with fresh frozen plasma, cryoprecipitate, and platelets as needed.

■ ANTIBIOTIC THERAPY
- Therapy should always be given parenterally.
- Empiric therapy is as follows:
  1. Younger than 1 month of age: ampicillin plus cefotaxime
     a. Consider also the addition of vancomycin if CSF Gram stain shows gram-positive diplococci characteristic of pneumococci or if CSF bacterial antigen testing supports a diagnosis of pneumococcal meningitis.
  2. Between 1 month and 3 months of age: ampicillin plus cefotaxime plus vancomycin
  3. Older than 3 months of age: cefotaxime plus vancomycin
     a. Vancomycin may be eliminated if CSF Gram stain shows gram-negative diplococci characteristic of *N. meningitidis* or if CSF bacterial antigen testing supports a diagnosis of meningococcal meningitis.

- Therapy for specific pathogens
  1. Group B streptococcus: penicillin G or ampicillin plus gentamicin
     a. This combination is synergistic against most isolates of the organism and should be used initially.
     b. Once a satisfactory clinical and microbiologic response has been achieved, penicillin G can be given alone.
     c. Therapy is usually continued for a minimum of 14 days.
  2. Gram-negative enteric bacilli/Enterobacteriaceae: cefotaxime with or without an aminoglycoside
     a. Meropenem is an alternative agent if the organism is resistant to third-generation cephalosporins.
     b. Therapy is usually continued for a minimum of 21 days.
  3. *S. pneumoniae:* vancomycin plus cefotaxime or ceftriaxone
     a. There is an increasing prevalence of strains demonstrating intermediate or high resistance to penicillin (some of which are also resistant to third-generation cephalosporins); therefore this combination should be used for initial therapy pending susceptibilities.
     b. If the organism is found to be sensitive to penicillin by a reliable methodology (e.g., the E test), penicillin alone can then be used.
     c. If the organism is resistant to penicillin but sensitive to cefotaxime or ceftriaxone, either of these cephalosporins can be used.
     d. If the organism is resistant to penicillin and to the third-generation cephalosporins, vancomycin should be continued with cefotaxime or ceftriaxone.
     e. The addition or substitution of rifampin for vancomycin can be considered in some circumstances after consultation with a specialist in infectious diseases.
     f. Therapy is continued for a minimum of 10 to 14 days.
  4. *N. meningitidis:* penicillin or a third-generation cephalosporin (cefotaxime or ceftriaxone)
     a. Therapy is continued for a minimum of 7 days.
- Antiinflammatory therapy
  1. Dexamethasone
     a. Efficacy of this agent, when given shortly before or at the time of administration of the first dose of parenteral antibiotic therapy, was established

to reduce the frequency of hearing loss and/or neurologic sequelae in patients with *H. influenzae* type b meningitis.
     b. Similar efficacy has not been firmly established in children with meningitis caused by other organisms.
     c. Its use can be considered in patients 6 weeks of age or older who have pneumococcal or meningococcal meningitis.
     d. The recommended dosage is either 0.6 mg/kg/day in four divided doses for 2 days or 0.8 mg/kg/day in two divided doses for 2 days.

■ SURGICAL
- One indication for surgery is hydrocephalus requiring ventriculoperitoneal shunt insertion.
- Large, symptomatic subdural effusions may also require surgical drainage.

■ FOLLOW-UP & DISPOSITION
- The mortality rate for bacterial meningitis is 1% to 5% (15% to 30% in neonates). Morbidity depends on several factors (e.g., age of the patient, duration of the illness before initiating effective therapy, the specific pathogen, bacterial inoculum, host defense defects).
- Overall, up to 50% of patients sustain neurologic sequelae.
- Follow-up is directed at monitoring for the rare (less than 1%) occurrence of relapse of infection after a course of antibiotic therapy and monitoring for neurologic sequelae, including hearing loss, motor abnormalities, language disorders/delay, seizures, hydrocephalus, and mental retardation.
  1. Screening for hearing loss using audiometry or, in the young child, brainstem auditory-evoked potentials, is usually done at the completion of the course of parenteral antibiotic therapy.
  2. Careful assessment of the child's neurodevelopment is essential.
  3. Consultation with a child neurologist may be indicated in select cases.

■ PATIENT/FAMILY EDUCATION
- Parents should be educated about the mortality rate and the overall frequency of neurologic sequelae (up to 50%) after bacterial meningitis.
- The types of possible neurologic sequelae can be discussed.
- Parents should be aware that their child's hearing will be evaluated before hospital discharge and that close neurodevelopmental follow-up will be needed.

- The small risk of relapse of infection (less than 1%) should also be discussed.

■ PREVENTIVE TREATMENT
- The widespread use of the conjugate *H. influenzae* type b vaccines has largely eliminated this organism as a cause of bacterial meningitis.
- Although a nonconjugate pneumococcal vaccine has been available for many years, it is not reliably immunogenic in the children who would benefit the most from it (those younger than 2 years of age).
  1. A heptavalent conjugate pneumococcal vaccine became available for young children in the year 2000. It contains seven serotypes (4, 6B, 9V, 14, 18C, 19F, 23F). The routine schedule is for doses at 2, 4, 6, and 12 to 15 months.
- A quadrivalent meningococcal vaccine against groups A, C, Y, and W-135 *N. meningitidis* is available but is not reliably immunogenic in children younger than 18 to 24 months of age.
  1. Routine immunization of children with this vaccine is not currently recommended.
  2. Immunization is recommended for children older than age 2 years in high-risk groups (e.g., those with functional or anatomic asplenia, terminal complement component deficiencies) or as an adjunct to chemoprophylaxis to control outbreaks of disease caused by one of the serogroups contained in the vaccine.
- Chemoprophylaxis of household and other close contacts (day-care contacts, nursery school contacts, and those having contact with the index patient's oral secretions through sharing of foods or beverages or kissing during the 7 days before onset of disease in the index case) of patients with invasive *N. meningitidis* infections is usually effective in preventing secondary cases. Available effective chemoprophylactic agents include rifampin, ceftriaxone, and ciprofloxacin.

■ REFERRAL INFORMATION
- Most patients with bacterial meningitis should be referred to a center containing a PICU or NICU.
  1. Subspecialty consultation with a pediatric infectious disease specialist, neonatologist, child neurologist, and a pediatric neurosurgeon should be available.
- Therapy should be begun promptly at the hospital to which the patient first presents for care.

PEARLS & CONSIDERATIONS

■ CLINICAL PEARLS

- Physicians caring for children must maintain a high level of vigilance to detect the child who has bacterial meningitis. The most common clinical manifestations are fever, vomiting, headache, and altered mental status (excessive irritability or lethargy).
- The diagnosis is established through performance of an LP to collect CSF for analysis.
- Parenteral antibiotic therapy should be promptly administered.

■ WEBSITES

- Centers for Disease Control and Prevention: www.cdc.gov/ncidod/dbmd/diseaseinfo/meningitis_g.htm
- The Meningitis Foundation of America: www.musa.org/welcome/htm

■ SUPPORT GROUP

The Meningitis Foundation of America has information on its website that can be of considerable assistance to patients who have had meningitis or families who have had a family member with meningitis. Stories of patients who survived or died from bacterial meningitis are located at this site.

REFERENCES

1. Committee on Infectious Diseases, American Academy of Pediatrics: Therapy for children with invasive pneumococcal infections, *Pediatrics* 97:289, 1997.
2. Committee on Infectious Diseases, American Academy of Pediatrics: Policy statement: recommendations for the prevention of pneumococcal infections, including the use of pneumococcal conjugate vaccine (Prevnar), pneumococcal polysaccharide vaccine, and antibiotic prophylaxis (RE9960), *Pediatrics* 106:362, 2000.
3. Feigin RD, Pearlman E: Bacterial meningitis beyond the neonatal period. In Feigin RD, Cherry JD (eds): *Textbook of pediatric infectious diseases*, vol 1, ed 4, Philadelphia, 1998, WB Saunders.
4. Feigin RD, McCracken GH, Klein JO: Diagnosis and management of meningitis, *Pediatr Infect Dis J* 11:785, 1992.
5. McCracken GH: Current management of bacterial meningitis in infants and children, *Pediatr Infect Dis J* 11:169, 1992.

Author: **Robert A. Broughton, M.D.**

BASIC INFORMATION

■ DEFINITION
Viral meningitis is an inflammation of the meninges caused by many different viruses.

■ SYNONYM
Aseptic meningitis

ICD-9CM CODE
047.9 Unspecified viral meningitis

■ ETIOLOGY
- Enteroviruses (EV) account for 85% to 95% of cases for which an etiologic is agent identified.
  1. Most common are Coxsackie B5 and Echoviruses 4, 5, 9, and 11
- Five percent are caused by Arboviruses (occur in summer and fall).
  1. St. Louis encephalitis virus most common vector-transmitted cause of aseptic meningitis
     a. It is seen throughout the United States.
     b. Aseptic meningitis accounts for 15% of all symptomatic cases of St. Louis encephalitis.
- Aseptic meningitis is the most common neurologic presentation of mumps infection.
  1. It occurs in winter and spring.
  2. Cerebrospinal fluid (CSF) pleocytosis occurs in more than 50% of patient with mumps.
  3. Except for parotitis, the clinical manifestations differ little from EV cases; encephalitis may also occur.
  4. Neurologic involvement is three times more common in males than in females.
- Many other viruses may cause meningitis, including the following:
  1. Herpes simplex type 2 (see the section "Herpes Simplex Virus Infections")
  2. Human herpesvirus type 6
  3. Human immunodeficiency virus type 1 (HIV-1)
  4. Adenovirus
  5. Varicella-zoster virus
  6. Epstein-Barr virus
  7. Lymphocytic choriomeningitis
     a. Transmitted by rodents
     b. Clinical manifestations in only 15% of those infected
     c. Remainder asymptomatic or mildly ill
  8. Encephalomyocarditis virus
  9. Cytomegalovirus
  10. Rhinoviruses
  11. Measles
  12. Rubella
  13. Influenza types a and b
  14. Parainfluenza
  15. Parvovirus B19
  16. Rotavirus
  17. Coronavirus
  18. Variola

■ EPIDEMIOLOGY & DEMOGRAPHICS
- EV
  1. This is most common in infants younger than 1 year of age.
  2. In temperate climates, most cases occur in summer and fall; cases occur year round in tropical and subtropical climates.
  3. Spread is from person to person, fecal/oral, respiratory droplets.
  4. Incubation period is 4 to 6 days.
  5. Fewer than 1 per 1000 infected persons develop meningitis.
- Other agents
  1. Arboviruses
     a. Usually accompanying brain involvement (meningoencephalitis) unless caused by St. Louis and California viral infections (see the section "Encephalitis")
  2. Mumps
     a. Usually accompanied by brain involvement
  3. Most infections with measles, rubella, and variola viruses that involve the central nervous system (CNS) are encephalitic

■ HISTORY
- Fever
- Headache (usually retro-orbital or frontal)
- Photophobia
- Anorexia, nausea, vomiting, abdominal pain, diarrhea
- Meticulous history of exposures in past 2 to 3 weeks
  1. Travel
  2. Insects
  3. Pets (especially horses)
  4. Medications
  5. Injections
  6. Other exposures
- Seizures: occur occasionally, may occur because of high fever alone

■ PHYSICAL EXAMINATION
- Meningeal signs
  1. Nuchal rigidity
  2. Positive Kernig's and Brudzinski's signs
     a. Kernig's: When the leg is flexed 90 degrees at the hip, the knee cannot be extended beyond 135 degrees.
     b. Brudzinski's: The legs are flexed involuntarily when the neck is flexed.
     c. These signs are usually present in older children.
     d. They may not be present in infants younger than 1 year of age.
- Young infants: fever, irritability, and lethargy most commonly
- Bulging fontanelle
- Exanthem, enanthem
- Occasionally myalgia
- Muscle weakness (rare)

■ DIAGNOSIS

■ DIFFERENTIAL DIAGNOSIS
- Other forms of meningitis: may present identically to cases caused by viruses
  1. Bacterial: including certain bacteria that do not readily stain or grow in standard culture systems (i.e., *Mycoplasma*)
  2. Fungal
  3. Tuberculosis
  4. Parasitic/protozoal
- Parameningeal infections (e.g., pneumonia, vertebral osteomyelitis)
- Malignancy
  1. Leukemia
  2. Brain tumor
- Immune diseases
  1. Behçet's syndrome
  2. Systemic lupus erythematosus
  3. Sarcoidosis
- Miscellaneous
  1. Kawasaki disease
  2. Heavy metal poisoning
  3. Intrathecal injections
  4. Foreign bodies
  5. Antimicrobial agents or other drugs
     a. Trimethoprim-sulfamethoxazole
     b. Nonsteroidal antiinflammatory drugs
     c. Chemotherapy
  6. Epidermoid (dermoid or other cysts)

■ DIAGNOSTIC WORKUP
- Lumbar puncture to collect CSF for the following:
  1. Cell count: white blood cell (WBC) count usually 50 to 500/mm^3; may be up to 1000/mm^3
  2. Differential: may be a polymorphonuclear WBC predominance early, but shift to mononuclear predominance usually occurs within 12 to 24 hours
  3. CSF glucose: usually normal or mildly depressed
  4. CSF protein: usually normal to mildly elevated
  5. Gram stain: negative for bacteria
  6. Culture: for bacteria
- CSF, blood, rectal, and nasopharyngeal swabs should be collected for viral cultures.
- Paired serum specimens (day 0 and days 10 to 21) can be collected for antibody titer rises if cultures no growth for viruses and bacteria.
- History and clinical findings may require additional culture for mycobacteria, fungal, or protozoal infection.
- Atypical cells may require examination of cytopathology to exclude tumor.
- Enterovirus and herpes simplex virus infections can be confirmed by polymerase chain reaction (PCR): At

II

least 65% to 70% of culture-negative CSF in patients with aseptic meningitis are enterovirus positive by PCR.

- Identification of specific viral pathogen is possible in as many as 55% to 70% of cases when consistent diagnostic methods applied.

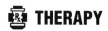 **THERAPY**

■ NONPHARMACOLOGIC
- Supportive care
  1. Fluids
  2. Analgesics
     a. Avoid aspirin because of associated risk of Reye's syndrome.
  3. Need for hospital admission based on possibility of treatable bacterial disease, toxicity, and need for hydration and pain control
  4. Observe for seizures (rare)

■ MEDICAL
- No specific antibiotic therapy is available for enteroviral disease (some efficacy of intravenous gamma-globulin in agammaglobulinemic patients).
- Acyclovir is available to treat meningitis caused by herpes simplex virus.
- Antibiotics may be started empirically while awaiting results of bacterial cultures (see the section "Bacterial Meningitis").
  1. Antibiotics should be given parenterally.
  2. Antibiotics may be used depending on the clinical scenario, for example:
     a. Toxic patient
     b. CSF with a higher WBC count
     c. A young patient with an unclear clinical picture

■ FOLLOW-UP & DISPOSITION
- Prognosis depends on the cause.
  1. Enteroviral meningitis: most children recover completely
     a. Ten percent have CNS complications, including focal seizures, weakness, and/or obtundation or coma.
        (1) Infants in first few months of life may have increased risk of problems with language and development.
        (2) These infants need formal developmental evaluation at age 3 to 6 years of age.
  2. Herpes simplex meningitis (see the section "Herpes Simplex Virus Infection")

■ PATIENT/FAMILY EDUCATION
- Parents should be educated about its good prognosis in general (this is etiology specific and most true with the EV).
- Possible low risk of neurologic sequelae can be discussed.
- Parents should be aware that the child's hearing and neurodevelopmental status should be monitored.

■ PREVENTIVE TREATMENT
- Handwashing: thorough and frequently
- Child care centers
  1. Wash objects and surfaces with a diluted bleach solution.
     a. 1 cup chlorine-containing household bleach in 1 gallon water

■ REFERRAL INFORMATION
- Most patients with viral meningitis can be treated by their primary care provider.
- Subspecialty consultation may be needed in complicated cases.
  1. Pediatric infectious disease
  2. Neurology

PEARLS & CONSIDERATIONS

■ CLINICAL PEARLS
- The common presenting signs of fever, vomiting, headache, and irritability need attention to exclude meningitis, especially in the young infant.
- The diagnosis is established by lumbar puncture to collect CSF for cell counts and culture.
- Parenteral antibiotics are not needed to treat viral meningitis but may be used empirically if bacterial meningitis cannot be reasonably excluded from the differential diagnosis.

■ WEBSITES
- AOL Government Guide: www. governmentguide.com
- Centers for Disease Control and Prevention: www.cdc.gov/ viralmeningitis
- Meningitis Foundation of America: www.musa.org

■ SUPPORT GROUP
The Meningitis Foundation of America has a large amount of information on its website that can be of considerable assistance to patients who have had meningitis or families who have had a family member with meningitis.

REFERENCE
1. Cherry JD: Aseptic meningitis and viral meningitis. In Feigin RD, Cherry JD (eds): *Textbook of pediatric infectious diseases,* vol 1, ed 4, Philadelphia, 1998, WB Saunders.
Authors: **Cynthia Christy, M.D., and H. Reid Mattison, M.D.**

BASIC INFORMATION

■ DEFINITION

Meningococcemia is bacteremia and sepsis syndrome with fever, petechiae and purpura, and hemodynamic instability caused by the organism *Neisseria meningitidis,* a Gram-negative intracellular diplococci.

■ SYNONYMS

- Meningococcal septicemia
- Purpura fulminans
- Waterhouse-Friderichsen syndrome

ICD-9CM CODES

036.2   Meningococcemia
V03.89 Meningococcal vaccine

■ ETIOLOGY

- *N. meningitidis* is acquired in the nasopharynx.
- Asymptomatic colonization occurs.
- Bloodstream invasion occurs when complex interactions involving organism attachment factors, cofactors such as other infective agents, often respiratory viruses, and host immune status are in concert.
- Lipopolysaccharide endotoxin mediates cytokine release from activated monocytes, macrophages, and endothelial cells.
- Cytokines such as tumor necrosis factor, interleukins 1 and 6, and gamma-interferon result in hypotension, myocardial depression, and increased vascular permeability.
- Direct capillary leakage, endothelial tissue damage, and end-organ damage result in necrosis of skin, digits, and mucosal surfaces, as well as adrenal hemorrhage (Waterhouse-Friderichsen syndrome).
- *N. meningitidis* has an outer polysaccharide capsule that serves to identify different serotypes; A, B, C, W135, and Y account for invasive disease.
- Almost all isolates in the United States are still susceptible to penicillin; other parts of the world may have increasing penicillin resistance.
- U.S. isolates are often resistant to sulfonamides but rarely resistant to rifampin.
- *N. meningitidis* can also cause meningitis, septic arthritis, pericarditis, pneumonia, and conjunctivitis.
- Chronic meningococcemia is an uncommon presentation of periodic fever without shock or sepsis syndrome, often accompanied by recurrent petechiae and splenomegaly, and may mimic Henoch-Schönlein purpura.

■ EPIDEMIOLOGY & DEMOGRAPHICS

- Transmission occurs from person to person by the respiratory route via pharyngeal secretions.
- Approximately 60% to 90% of cases occur in children.
- Overcrowding, such as in day cares, barracks, and household contacts, is a risk factor for spread.
- Most people exposed become carriers and do not develop disease; however, they are the major source of organism spread because most patients with invasive disease have not had contact with another patient with invasive disease.
- The prevalence of asymptomatic carriage varies among populations; the average rate is 5% to 15% colonized in nonendemic areas.
- The incubation period is from 2 to 10 days; patients are infectious up to 24 hours after treatment.
- The risk of household transmission is greatest in the first week after contact; 70% of secondary household cases occur in this time frame.
- The annual incidence of all meningococcal disease in the United States is 1.1 per 100,000, with the peak incidence in late winter and early spring.
- It occurs in a worldwide distribution as endemic disease in certain countries or in epidemics; *meningitis belt* is a term used for increased prevalence and outbreaks in sub-Saharan Africa.
- Worldwide, group A strains are responsible for the largest epidemics, but in the United States, recent outbreaks have been increasingly related to serotype C disease.
- Serotype C represents 45% of isolates in the United States; serotype B accounts for another 45%.
- Attack rates are highest in children, with 46% of cases occurring in children 2 years of age or younger.
- Other patients at high risk include splenectomized patients or those with congenital asplenia, terminal complement (C6, C7, C8), or properdin deficiency.
- Immunoglobulin and early complement deficiencies may also be associated with risk.

■ HISTORY

- A prodrome of upper respiratory infection is common.
- Headache, fever, and nausea are reported.
- A rash is noticed by the patient or caregiver.
  1. Rash may at first be faint maculopapular, with rapid change to petechiae with or without larger purpura.
- Rarely, a history of exposure to a known case in a cluster or outbreak setting is reported.
- Obtain history of family members by the following criteria:
  1. Age
  2. Occupations
  3. Day care attendance
  4. School attendance and other extracurricular activities, especially sports teams
     a. Important regarding contacts who may need postexposure prophylaxis (see following section)
- Obtain a history of medication use and prior antibiotic therapy, which may influence the outcome of culture results.

■ PHYSICAL EXAMINATION

- Vital signs usually include a highly febrile patient; blood pressure may be normal, then rapidly drop, or frank hypotension may be seen on presentation.
- Mental status may be normal with rapid obtundation caused by shock with or without meningitis.
- Purpura and petechiae may be minimal or profound with massive skin necrosis and mucosal hemorrhage.
- Petechiae may appear first in areas of pressure.
  1. Blood pressure monitoring
  2. Tourniquets
- Patient may not have a stiff neck; meningococcemia is often seen with early subclinical meningitis, or no meningitis.

🔬 DIAGNOSIS

■ DIFFERENTIAL DIAGNOSIS

- Clinical presentation as described previously, with the presence of purpura and hypotension, is highly suggestive of meningococcemia.
- Many mild viral illnesses may present with fever and petechial exanthems—commonly include enteroviruses and parvovirus B19.
- Other bacterial causes of sepsis and meningitis may present similarly, including the following:
  1. Pneumococci
  2. *Haemophilus influenzae* type b
  3. *Neisseria gonorrhoeae*
- Hemorrhagic fever viruses may be seen.
  1. May present with a similar fulminant shock syndrome, including the following:
     a. Dengue
     b. Hantavirus

- Rickettsial: Rocky Mountain spotted fever and others in the spotted fever group may occur.
- Henoch-Schönlein purpura or anaphylactoid purpura are often preceded by an upper respiratory prodrome.
  1. Palpable purpura
  2. Abdominal pain (does not present with shock unless acute bowel process is involved)
  3. Arthritis
- Drug reaction/rashes can result from the following:
  1. Sulfa drugs
  2. Dilantin
  3. Heparin
  4. Thiazide diuretics
  5. Rifampin
- Thrombocytopenias may be caused by blood disorders.
  1. Immune thrombocytopenia
  2. Aplastic anemia
  3. Leukemias
  4. Wiskott-Aldrich syndrome
- Other vasculitic diseases, such as polyarteritis and Kawasaki disease, may present with fever and petechiae.

■ DIAGNOSTIC WORKUP

- Confirmation of a case is by isolation of *N. meningitidis* from blood, cerebrospinal fluid (CSF), or another normally sterile site.
- All patients with suspected meningococcemia who can tolerate the procedure should have a lumbar puncture (LP) to assess for the presence of meningitis.
- Latex agglutination of CSF may be done if a patient received antibiotics before sampling.
- Petechial skin lesions can be scraped, then Gram stained and cultured.
- Other laboratory workup should include the following tests:
  1. Blood cultures
  2. Complete blood profile with differential and platelet count
  3. Parameters to assess for disseminated intravascular coagulation (DIC)
  4. Clotting studies, such as D-dimer, fibrinogen, prothrombin time, and partial thromboplastin time

■ THERAPY

■ MEDICAL

- Rapid administration of antibiotics is important; obtaining blood cultures and performing an LP should not delay treatment.
  1. Often, antibiotics can be given immediately after obtaining blood.
- The ability to give antibiotics in an outpatient office setting has been documented to decrease adverse outcomes.

- Appropriate antibiotics may be given by the intramuscular or intraosseous route if no intravenous access is available.
  1. Penicillin G: 250,000 to 300,000 U/kg/day divided every 4 to 6 hours (maximum, 24 million U/day)
  2. Cefotaxime: 300 mg/kg/day divided every 6 to 8 hours (maximum, 12 g/day)
  3. Ceftriaxone: 100 mg/kg/day divided every 12 to 24 hours (maximum, 4 g/day)
- Patients should be isolated in the hospital for 24 hours after the first dose of appropriate antibiotic therapy.
- The length of therapy is 7 days.
- Release of endotoxin after administering antibiotics may cause further symptoms of shock, so intensive care support is required for all cases, initially, for fluid resuscitation and often respiratory support, management of blood products, and inotropic support.
- Central venous access is usually necessary.

■ ADJUNCTIVE THERAPY

- Cortisol may be considered if profound shock is present, given in replacement doses with hydrocortisone sodium phosphate or succinate.
- Pharmacologic doses of steroids have not been proven to be beneficial.
- Sympathetic blockade and topical nitroglycerin may be tried to improve perfusion locally.
- A hypercoagulable state may be treated with a heparin infusion.
- Experimental therapies, such as recombinant tissue plasminogen activator and concentrated antithrombin III, have also been tried in DIC.
- Access to wound care units and hyperbaric oxygen therapy is beneficial for patients with extensive tissue necrosis.

■ PROGNOSTIC FACTORS

Poor prognosis is associated with the following conditions:
- Petechiae present for less than 12 hours
- Hypotension (systolic blood pressure lower than 70 mm Hg)
- Absence of meningitis (less than 20 white blood cells [WBCs] in CSF)
- Low peripheral WBCs (less than 10,000) or erythrocyte sedimentation rate (less than 10)
- Thrombocytopenia, coma, seizures, and extremes of age

■ PREVENTIVE TREATMENT

- Chemoprophylaxis for all family members of the index case is warranted.

- Close contacts of the index patient who sleep or eat together should be given prophylaxis.
  1. Close contact with oral secretions
- All day-care contacts in the same care room with close contact should receive prophylaxis.
- The drug of choice for prophylaxis is rifampin.
  1. Penetrates secretions well
  2. Eliminates carriage of the organism if it is not resistant
- Rifampin dosing is 10 mg/kg/dose (up to 600 mg/dose) every 12 hours for four doses.
- Sulfonamides should be used only if resistance testing of the organism is done.
- Ceftriaxone and ciprofloxacin are effective in eradicating carriage and may be used.
- Ceftriaxone dosing is 250 mg intramuscularly as a single dose for adults, 125 mg intramuscularly as a single dose for children younger than 12 years of age.
- Ciprofloxacin dosing is 500 to 750 mg as a single dose for adults.
- The index patient who has received at least one dose of ceftriaxone does not need to receive other prophylaxis.
- Ceftriaxone is the drug of choice for prophylaxis of a pregnant contact.

■ VACCINATION

- Tetravalent vaccine containing capsular polysaccharides of serogroups A, C, Y, and W135 meningococci is licensed in the United States and approved for use in children older than 2 years of age.
- Serotype B capsule is poorly immunogenic, and no vaccine is currently available.
- Meningococcal conjugate vaccines are currently being tested for constructs that contain serotypes C and A, with promising reduction in serotype C disease recently reported from the United Kingdom with a serotype C conjugate vaccine.
- Tetravalent vaccine is indicated for patients in high-risk categories for acquiring disease, which include splenectomized or functionally asplenic patients and patients with terminal complement component or properdin deficiency.
- Immunization of college students living in dormitories has been recommended by the American College Health Association.
- Discussion with students and their families should be provided regarding the moderately increased risk of meningococcal illness of first-year students living in dormitories and the potential benefit of the vaccine, as recommended by the American Academy of Pediatrics and the Advisory Committee on Immuni-

zation Practices (ACIP) of the U.S Department of Health and Human Services.

- Students should be immunized at the request of the student or if required by their institution.
- Travelers to areas with current outbreaks or high background rate of disease should receive vaccine.
- Vaccine may be considered for widespread administration in the setting of an outbreak.
  1. Should always be done in conjunction with local and state public health recommendations
- Meningococcemia is a reportable disease to public health authorities, who will assist in tracking cases and contacts and aid in making postexposure prophylaxis recommendations.
- Revaccination of high-risk patients may be considered.
  1. If the patient was younger than 4 years of age at first vaccination
  2. If exposure occurs 2 to 3 years after the first dose
  3. If patient remains in a high-risk category, in which case a subsequent dose may be given 3 to 5 years after the first dose
  4. Need for revaccination in older children and adults: not established

☼ PEARLS & CONSIDERATIONS

■ CLINICAL PEARLS

- Although patients with fever, hypotension, and shock with petechiae and purpura should be treated emergently, most children with fever and petechiae do not have meningococcemia; the diagnosis must *always* be considered, however, because of the rapidity of deterioration that can occur.
- Most children with meningitis without fulminant meningococcemia fare well; younger infants without shock may present as occult bacteremia (5% to 8% of cases of occult bacteremias).
- Very high WBCs on presentation is usually a good prognostic factor but may be associated with development of postinfectious (immune-mediated) arthritis.
- Pediatric offices should have the ability to rapidly administer antibiotics.

■ WEBSITES

- American College Health Association: www.acha.org/special-prj/men.htm
- Centers for Disease Control and Prevention: www.cdc.gov/travel/vaccinat.html; travel recommendations
- Centers for Disease Control and Prevention: www.cdc.gov/epo/mmwr; recommendations of the ACIP
- Meningitis Foundation of America: www.musa.org

REFERENCES

1. Advisory Committee on Immunization Practices, U.S. Public Health Service: Prevention and control of meningococcal disease and meningococcal disease and college students, *MMWR Morb Mortal Wkly Rep* 49:1, 2000.
2. American Academy of Pediatrics, Committee on Infectious Diseases: *2000 Red Book: report of the Committee on Infectious Diseases,* Elk Grove, Ill, 2000, American Academy of Pediatrics.
3. Harrison LH et al: Risk of meningococcal infection in college students, *JAMA* 281:1906, 1999.
4. Kirsch EA et al: Pathophysiology, treatment and outcome of meningococcemia: a review and recent experience, *Pediatr Infect Dis J* 15:967, 1996.
5. MacLennan JM et al: Safety, immunogenicity, and induction of immunologic memory with a serogroup C meningococcal conjugate vaccine in infants: a randomized controlled trial, *JAMA* 283:2795, 2000.
6. Pollard AJ, Levin M: Vaccines for prevention of meningococcal disease, *Pediatr Infect Dis J* 19:333, 2000.
7. Rosenstein NE et al: The changing epidemiology of meningococcal disease in the United States, 1992-1996, *J Infect Dis* 180:1894, 1999.
8. Salzman MR, Rubin LG: Meningococcemia, *Infect Dis Clin North Am* 10:709, 1996.

Author: **Donna Fisher, M.D.**

II

BASIC INFORMATION

■ **DEFINITION**
- Meningomyelocele is the most complex malformation of the spinal cord and involves all layers. Nerve roots protrude through abnormal vertebral arches and soft tissue.
  1. Lipomas or dermoid cysts may accompany the meningomyelocele.
  2. In encephalocele, the brain and meninges protrude through a midline defect of the skull.
- Syrinx is an accumulation of cerebrospinal fluid within the central spinal canal.
  1. *Syringobulbia* refers to accumulation of fluid in the central canal of the brainstem.
  2. *Syringomyelia* is the accumulation of fluid in the spinal cord.
- A tethered spinal cord is abnormally attached in a more caudal (lower) position than normal.
  1. In children without meningomyelocele, tethering may be caused by a thickened filum terminale or a mass, such as a lipoma.
- See also the section "Occult Spinal Dysraphism."

■ **SYNONYMS**
- Meningomyelocele
  1. Myelomeningocele
  2. Spina bifida aperta
- Syrinx
  1. Syringomyelia, hydromyelia, hydrosyringomyelia
  2. Syringobulbia, hydrosyringobulbia

ICD-9CM CODES
741.0   Meningomyelocele— with hydrocephalus
741.9   Meningomyelocele without hydrocephalus
741.0   Use fifth digit classification with category, unspecified region; 1, cervical; 2, thoracic; 3, lumbar
742.0   Encephalocele
336.0 or   Syrinx
742.51
742.59   Tethered spinal cord

■ **ETIOLOGY**
- Failure of the neural tube to close 23 to 28 days after fertilization of the egg is believed to be caused by an interaction between multiple genes and the environment.
- Maternal exposure to any of the following may play a role: valproic acid, malnutrition (especially folate deficiency), hyperthermia, alcohol, or maternal diabetes and maternal obesity.
- Abnormalities in the gene that regulates methylenetetrahydrofolate reductase, an enzyme associated with folate metabolism, have been associated with neural tube defects.

- Chromosome anomalies, such as trisomy 18 or 13, have been implicated.

■ **EPIDEMIOLOGY & DEMOGRAPHICS**
- The incidence is approximately 1 in 1000 live births in the United States.
- The birth prevalence has been decreasing because of improved maternal nutrition and greater prenatal detection, with elective termination of the pregnancy.
- The risk for a second affected child from the same parents is 2 or 3 per 100; for a third, it is 10 per 100.
- Neural tube defects are more common in females and in persons of British ancestry.

■ **HISTORY**
- Family history of neural tube defects or spontaneous abortions
- Maternal nutrition during gestation and prenatal exposures
- Family functioning (including social support and stress) and parental expectations and understanding of the problem
- Assessment of child's growth, development, mobility, and activities of daily living (personal hygiene, ability to feed self, self-help skills)
- Onset of new neurologic symptoms (e.g., weakness, changes in bowel and bladder function, tripping, clumsiness), which usually indicates treatable conditions such as tethered spinal cord, diastematomyelia, syrinx, or ventricular shunt malfunction
- History of reactions to products made of latex
  1. Up to 50% of children who have meningomyelocele have allergies to latex.

■ **PHYSICAL EXAMINATION**
- The backs of *all* children should be examined for pigmented spots, hairy patches, and sinuses that extend into the spine.
  1. These findings may be signs of occult spinal dysraphism (OSD).
     a. OSD predisposes to meningitis.
     b. Neurologic deterioration may occur as a result of diastematomyelia, lipoma, or tethering of the spinal cord (see the section "Occult Spinal Dysraphism").
  2. Scoliosis is common in patients with myelomeningocele.
- Perform a neurologic examination.
  1. Motor function, sensory level, and anal wink
  2. Upper extremity strength, including grip
     a. Deterioration may indicate syrinx or malfunction of the ventricular shunt

- Evaluate for shunt function.
  1. Head circumference and palpation of the anterior fontanelle
  2. Visualization of the eye grounds
  3. Assessment of the cranial nerves (especially of extraocular movements)
  4. Palpation of the shunt valve and tubing
- Perform an orthopedic examination.
  1. Assessment of posture (scoliosis, lordosis, kyphosis)
  2. Joint mobility and stability
- Perform a dermatologic examination.
  1. Evidence of lesions (e.g., decubitus ulcers) in insensate areas
- Developmental assessments are especially important before school entry to optimize learning.
  1. Visual-spatial functioning
  2. Verbal, performance, and educational measures
  3. Fine motor, gross motor, language, and social-adaptive skills

🔬 **DIAGNOSIS**

■ **DIFFERENTIAL DIAGNOSIS**
Diagnosis is made on physical examination, with little else in the differential diagnosis.

■ **DIAGNOSTIC WORKUP**
- Ultrasound or computed tomography (CT) scan of the head—75% to 85% have hydrocephalus
- Magnetic resonance imaging (MRI) scan of head if stridor and hoarseness, vocal cord paralysis, dysphagia, aspiration, apnea, central hypoventilation, breath-holding spells, opisthotonos, weakness of the upper extremities develop—suggests Chiari II malformation, downward displacement of hindbrain and cerebellum
- MRI of spine if weakness in lower extremities, deterioration of gait, atrophy of muscles in lower extremities, sensory loss or change in lower extremities, change in deep tendon reflexes, change in bladder or bowel function, leg or back pain, new orthopedic contracture, foot or leg length discrepancy, progressive scoliosis in absence of vertebral anomalies, trophic ulceration—tethered spinal cord
- Radiograms of the spine and hips
  1. Abnormal vertebrae such as hemivertebrae, butterfly vertebrae
  2. Scoliosis and kyphosis, especially in those with high spinal lesions
- Renal structure and function
  1. Urine culture
  2. Renal ultrasound
     a. Hydronephrosis
     b. Structural anomalies like duplex collecting system
  3. Serum blood urea nitrogen and creatinine

4. Voiding cystourethrogram if vesicoureteral reflux suspected
5. Urodynamics
   a. Bladder capacity
   b. Outlet pressure
   c. Synergy between detrusor and sphincter

℞ THERAPY

■ NONPHARMACOLOGIC
- Access to interdisciplinary care—pediatrician, nurse, social worker, neurosurgeon, orthopedist, physical therapist, urologist, nutritionist, orthotist
- Referral to early intervention program—physical therapy, occupational therapy, special education services
- Clean intermittent catheterization to manage urinary tract
  1. Contact to latex-containing products should be restricted from the first day of life.
- Braces (like ankle-foot-orthosis) and mobility devices (like the parapodium or wheelchair)
- Casting of the feet for deformities like equinovalgus or calcaneus
- High-fiber diet, regular toileting, and biofeedback to manage bowels

■ MEDICAL
- Antibiotic prophylaxis for recurrent symptomatic urinary tract infection or ureteral reflux
  1. Cephalexin or amoxicillin in infants
  2. Trimethoprim-sulfamethoxazole or nitrofurantoin in older children
- Medications to relax the detrusor muscle or increase sphincter tone to enhance continence
  1. Imipramine
  2. Oxybutynin
  3. Pseudoephedrine
- Laxatives and/or enemas for constipation

■ SURGICAL
- Operative
  1. All operative procedures should be performed in a latex-free environment.
- Neurosurgical
  1. Closure of the lesion on the back within 72 hours after birth
  2. Insertion of ventriculoperitoneal shunt for progressive hydrocephalus
  3. Revision of failed ventricular shunt
  4. Untethering of tethered spinal cord
  5. Posterior fossa decompression for symptomatic Chiari malformation
- Orthopedic
  1. Surgery of fixed joint contractures or deformities

2. Surgery for progressive kyphosis and/or scoliosis
- Urologic
  1. Bladder augmentation with catheterizable stoma if conservative treatment fails
- General
  1. Antegrade colonic enema procedure to enhance bowel management

■ FOLLOW-UP & DISPOSITION
- Regular evaluation by specialty team
- Routine renal ultrasounds
- Routine head CT scans to evaluate ventricular size
- Routine radiograms if kyphosis or scoliosis progress
- Routine urine cultures for children who have ureteral reflux
- Close communication with the school or early intervention program
- Avoidance of all latex

■ PATIENT/FAMILY EDUCATION
- Prescribe folic acid (4.0 mg/day periconceptionally) for mothers and affected females to prevent recurrences.
- Help families and educators with their reactions to the child's condition and with developing realistic expectations for the child.
- Help patients understand their condition and develop increasing independence.
- Offer financial counseling.
- Avoid latex, including in the hospital and operating suite.
- Discuss sexuality issues: Males have difficulty with erection and have retrograde ejaculation.
  1. Consider genetic counseling because affected individuals have a 3% chance of having an affected child.

■ PREVENTIVE TREATMENT
- *All women of childbearing age should receive 0.4 mg of folic acid daily periconceptionally to decrease the occurrence of neural tube defects.*
- Women who have a first-degree relative who has a neural tube defect should receive 4.0 mg folic acid daily.
- Prenatal diagnosis can be made using maternal serum α-fetoprotein at 14 to 16 weeks gestation, combined with high-resolution ultrasonography with or without amniocentesis.
- Prenatal endoscopic surgery to cover the open lesion on the back during the second trimester decreases neurologic involvement and diminishes the severity of the Chiari malformation.

■ REFERRAL INFORMATION
- All children 0 to 3 years of age who have neural tube defects should be

referred to an early intervention program.
- All children older than 3 years of age who have neural tube defects should be referred to their school district's Committee on Special Education or Committee on Preschool Special Education.
- All children who have neural tube defects should be referred to an interdisciplinary specialty program for ongoing care.
- All adolescents who have neural tube defects should be referred to a transition program.

☼ PEARLS & CONSIDERATIONS

■ CLINICAL PEARLS
- Ventricular shunt failure in a child who has hydrocephalus may present with subtle or confusing signs and symptoms that can be mistaken for those of Chiari II malformation, syringomyelia, or tethered cord.
- Neural tube defects are static conditions. Any clinical deterioration should be evaluated for a treatable cause, such as ventricular shunt failure, tethered spinal cord, syrinx, or Chiari II malformation.
- Erythema and swelling of a joint or bone in an area that lacks sensation represent a fracture until proved otherwise.

■ WEBSITES
- Children with Spina Bifida: A Resource Page for Parents: www.waisman.wisc.edu/~rowley/sb-kids/index.html
- Spina Bifida Association of America: www.sbaa.org
- Spina Bifida and Hydrocephalus Association of Canada: www.sbhac.ca

■ SUPPORT GROUPS
- A general spina bifida discussion list: listserv@mercury.dsu.edu
- The SB-Parents list, a forum for parents: listserv@waisman.wisc.edu

REFERENCES
1. Albright AL, Gartner JC, Wiener ES: Lumbar cutaneous hemangiomas as indicators of tethered spinal cords, *Pediatrics* 83:977, 1989.
2. American Academy of Pediatrics, Committee on Genetics: Folic acid for the prevention of neural tube defects, *Pediatrics* 92:493, 1993.
3. Liptak G: Neural tube defects. In Batshaw ML, Perret YM (eds): *Children with disabilities*, ed 4, Baltimore, 1997, Paul H Brookes.

Author: **Gregory S. Liptak, M.D., M.P.H.**

BASIC INFORMATION

■ DEFINITION
Mental retardation is cognitive limitation as characterized by scores greater than 2 standard deviations below the mean on a valid intelligence quotient (IQ) measure, with limitation of adaptive function in communication, self-care, daily living skills at home or in the community, or social skills.

■ SYNONYMS
- Developmental delay
- Slow learner
- Learning disability (in Europe, not in United States)

ICD-9CM CODES
317   Mild mental retardation
318.0 Moderate mental retardation
318.1 Severe mental retardation
318.2 Profound mental retardation
319   Unspecified
783.4 Global delays

■ ETIOLOGY
- Prenatal infections
- Genetic disorders
- Teratogens (e.g., alcohol)
- Embryologic errors
- Post natal injuries
- Birth injuries and prematurity
- Multifactorial

■ EPIDEMIOLOGY & DEMOGRAPHICS
- The incidence is 1% of the population, with a male preponderance.
- Most affected individuals have mild mental retardation (IQ 50/55 to 70).
  1. Moderate mental retardation is defined by a tested IQ of 35/40 to 50/55.
  2. Severe mental retardation is defined by a tested IQ of 20/25 to 35/40.
  3. Profound mental retardation is defined by a tested IQ of less than 20 to 25.
- Approximately 70% of cases with severe to profound mental retardation have a known cause.
- About 24% of cases with IQ in the 50 to 70 range have a specific medical cause identified.

■ HISTORY
- Delays may be global.
- Relative preservation of motor skills may also be noted.
- Initial presentation in early childhood may be language delay if not identified through motor or dysmorphic features.
- Medical and family history help guide the workup for a cause.
- Family history of mental retardation or "slow learners," especially if it follows inheritance of fragile X, suggests that genetic evaluation is needed.
  1. A sibling, parent, grandparent, or aunt/uncle is affected.
  2. Mental retardation predominantly in males on the mother's side of the family would support evaluation for the fragile X syndrome.
- Plateau or loss of skills, behavioral variability (related to dietary intake), refusal of protein foods (as might occur in urea cycle disorders), or specific findings such as smells consistent with organic acidurias (e.g., sweet smell of the urine in maple syrup urine disease) suggests need for a metabolic workup.
- Pica and exposures may suggest the need to evaluate for lead and other toxins.

■ PHYSICAL EXAMINATION
- Syndrome stigmata: look for dysmorphic features
  1. Trisomy 21
  2. Fragile X syndrome
- Careful skin examination to rule out neurocutaneous syndromes
- Hearing and vision assessment
- Motor examination
  1. Up to 60% of children with cerebral palsy also have mental retardation.
- Head circumference: evaluation of both large and small heads necessary
  1. Microcephaly may be caused by early decreased cell proliferation (genetic, embryologic origin), prenatal events with disruption of architecture (viral infections, vascular insults, migrational errors), or early perinatal events (hypoxic encephalopathy, intracranial bleeding).
  2. Macrocephaly may be caused by hydrocephalous, Sotos' syndrome, fragile X syndrome, autism, or chronic subdural bleeding.

DIAGNOSIS

■ DIFFERENTIAL DIAGNOSIS
- Autism
- Language disorders
- Learning disabilities
- Sensory impairment
- Epileptic aphasia
- Mental illness
- Profound environmental deprivation

■ DIAGNOSTIC WORKUP
- The workup is guided by the history and physical examination.
- A hearing test should be performed.
- Karyotype and DNA for fragile X syndrome should be obtained.
- If anomalies of the head (e.g., increased or decreased head circumference) or abnormal neurologic examination are found, consider neuroimaging.
- If history is compatible with seizures or if loss of speech or extreme behavioral variability are present, obtain an electroencephalogram (EEG).
- If loss of milestones, hypotonia, dietary avoidance of protein, suggestive examination, or family history consistent with metabolic or neurodegenerative disease, consider metabolic or neurodegenerative work.
  1. It may be prudent to refer patients to a tertiary care center at this point.
     a. A preliminary workup could include, but not necessarily be limited to, fasting plasma amino acids and urine organic acids.
     b. If hypotonic, lactate, pyruvate, and carnitine levels may be indicated.
  2. Magnetic resonance imaging (MRI) of the head may be indicated with loss of milestones, a distinct change in behavior, cutaneous markings consistent with a neurocutaneous syndrome (e.g., tuberous sclerosis), craniofacial abnormality, or a focal neurologic examination.
- Formal psychologic testing using an appropriate instrument is critical for diagnosis.

THERAPY

■ NONPHARMACOLOGIC
- The primary therapies are educational and behavioral.
- It may be necessary to actively teach social and functional life skills.

■ MEDICAL
- Psychiatric disorders can and do occur in people with mental retardation. Disorder-specific treatments depend on the proper diagnosis.
- Medication is often used for amelioration of specific symptoms such as hyperactivity. Stimulants may be useful in individual cases.
- Medication to treat aggression, self-injury, and stereotyped behaviors, among others, should be coordinated with a structured behavioral plan to teach appropriate behaviors.

■ COMPLEMENTARY & ALTERNATIVE THERAPIES
- Complementary treatments are disorder specific (e.g., megavitamin mixtures for trisomy 21).
  - None are proven efficacious.
  - Some are harmful.

■ FOLLOW-UP & DISPOSITION (IN THE UNITED STATES)

- Children from 0 to 3 years of age receive educational services through the early intervention programs.
- An appropriate public education is provided to students ages 3 to 21 years by home school district.
- School provides triennial formal testing and/or review and at least yearly program review.
- Families need to arrange legal guardianship (if appropriate) at 18 and plan for adulthood.

■ PATIENT/FAMILY EDUCATION

- The risk of recurrence depends on the underlying cause.
- Sexuality issues need to be addressed with education at the appropriate time.
- Families need to work with the agencies that coordinate young adult services well in advance of the anticipated need for them.

■ PREVENTIVE TREATMENT

- Prenatal vitamins (e.g., folic acid) prevent spina bifida.
- Prenatal screening, such as α-fetoprotein and amniocentesis for chromosomal testing, is appropriate for older or high-risk mothers.
- Neonatal metabolic screening, such as phenylketonuria, leads to instituting a preventive diet.
- Education, such as prenatal avoidance of alcohol, should be provided.
- Potential amelioration of some symptoms may occur with early intervention.

■ REFERRAL INFORMATION

- Early intervention is needed for children 0 to 3 years of age.
- School districts provide testing and services for children 3 to 21 years of age.
- Psychologists, developmental/behavioral pediatricians, child neurologists, child psychiatrists, and geneticists may all be consulted for aspects of care.

☼ PEARLS & CONSIDERATIONS

■ CLINICAL PEARLS

- It is difficult to predict the ultimate cognitive outcome from testing in toddlers unless there is a known cause with an established course, such as trisomy 21.
- Children with mental retardation may be well served in inclusive classrooms with appropriate supports.

- Many adults with mental retardation work in competitive or supported employment in the community.
- Institutional care should be considered a thing of the past. Children with mental retardation should anticipate living and working in their communities.

■ WEBSITES

- American Association for Mental Retardation: www.aamr.org
- Association for Retarded Citizens: www.theArc.org/welcome.html

■ SUPPORT GROUPS

- The Association for Retarded Citizens has national and regional chapters.
- Families may prefer disorder-specific support groups.

REFERENCES

1. Accardo PJ, Capute AJ: Mental retardation. In Capute AJ, Accardo PJ (eds): *Developmental disorders in infancy and childhood,* Baltimore, 1996, Paul H Brooks.
2. American Psychiatric Association: *Diagnostic and statistical manual of mental disorders,* ed 4, Washington, DC, 1994, American Psychiatric Association.

Author: **Susan Hyman, M.D.**

BASIC INFORMATION

■ DEFINITION
Both milia and miliaria are common neonatal dermatoses that result from the incomplete differentiation of the epidermis and its appendages at birth. (Nota bene [NB] miliaria can also occur in older children.)
- Milia are tiny 1- to 2-mm pearly white or yellow papules that result from retention of keratin and sebaceous material within the pilosebaceous apparatus of neonatal skin.
- Miliaria results from keratinous plugging of eccrine ducts, with subsequent escape of sweat into the skin below the level of obstruction.
  1. Miliaria crystallina (sudamina) are clear, pinpoint, superficial, thin-walled, noninflammatory vesicles created from sweat retention in the epidermis just below the stratum corneum.
  2. Miliaria rubra (prickly heat) are erythematous, grouped papules or vesicles that result from rupture of the intraepidermal portion of the sweat duct. The vesicle is at the level of the basal layer of the epidermis and may be surrounded by inflammatory cells.
  3. Miliaria pustulosa is rare and involves leukocytic infiltration of the vesicles. Miliaria profunda and miliaria pustulosa are rarely seen in temperate climates.

■ SYNONYMS
- Milia
  1. Single lesions termed *milium*
  2. Epidermal inclusion cyst
- Miliaria
  1. Miliaria crystallina (sudamina)
  2. Miliaria rubra (prickly heat)

ICD-9CM CODE
705.1 Miliaria

■ ETIOLOGY
Incomplete differentiation of the epidermis and its appendages at birth (milia and miliaria) in combination with hot, humid conditions (miliaria)

■ EPIDEMIOLOGY & DEMOGRAPHICS
- Milia
  1. Present in 40% of all races of term infants
  2. Less common in preterm infants
  3. Predilection for the cheeks, nasolabial folds, forehead, nose, ears, chin, and periorbital areas
  4. Rarely found on the arms and legs or penis
- Miliaria
  1. More common before the advent of humidity and temperature control in nurseries
  2. May affect febrile older children or occur with exercise in hot, humid climates
  3. May occur in a neonate exposed to external sources of heat, such as that generated by phototherapy lights or radiant warmers

■ HISTORY
- Milia
  1. Well infant present at birth
  2. Full-term normal pregnancy
  3. Lack of risk factors for bacterial or yeast infection (e.g., prolonged rupture of membranes, maternal fever, chorioamnionitis)
- Miliaria
  1. Sometimes associated with maternal fever during labor
  2. Exposure to hot, humid conditions
  3. Fever, overdressing, ointment use, external sources of heat like phototherapy or infant warmer, exercise in the older child
  4. In older child, may report an itching or a pins-and-needles sensation

■ PHYSICAL EXAMINATION
- Milia
  1. Generally, on face, cheeks, nasolabial folds, forehead, nose, ears, chin, and periorbital areas
  2. Cystic white lesions 1 to 2 mm in size
  3. Expressed contents of lesion resemble tiny white pearls
- Miliaria
  1. Miliaria crystallina (sudamina) are clear, pinpoint, superficial, thin-walled, noninflammatory vesicles in the epidermis.
  2. Miliaria rubra (prickly heat) are erythematous, grouped papules or vesicles. The vesicle is at the level of the basal layer of the epidermis and may be surrounded by inflammatory cells. If inflammation is prominent, the lesion may appear pustular.

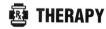

DIAGNOSIS

■ DIFFERENTIAL DIAGNOSIS
- Milia
  1. Large milia (more than 2 mm) are found in the orofacial-digital syndrome (OFD).
  2. Sebaceous gland hyperplasia as a result of exposure to maternal androgens. Lesions are smaller pinpoint lesions, more yellow, and express sebaceous material.
  3. Epstein's pearls are an oral mucosal variant of cutaneous milia.
- Miliaria
  1. Erythema toxicum
  2. Candidal infection
  3. Early pyoderma
  4. Herpes simplex

■ DIAGNOSTIC WORKUP
- Milia: none needed
- Miliaria
  1. Culture, Gram stain, and KOH preparation are done.
  2. Expect no bacteria or yeast.
  3. Erythema toxicum vesicles have eosinophils but no bacteria.

THERAPY

■ NONPHARMACOLOGIC
- Milia
  1. Conservative treatment is indicated because lesions are self-limited. Will exfoliate within a few weeks without scarring. Even the large milia of the OFD syndrome exfoliate in 3 to 4 months, but they do leave pitted scars.
- Miliaria
  1. Conservative treatment is indicated. The infant should be cared for in a cooler, less humid environment.
  2. Give cool-water baths and avoid soap.
  3. Application of calamine lotion to body folds should result in resolution in several days.
  4. Apply 1% hydrocortisone cream to itchy spots three times per day

■ PATIENT/FAMILY EDUCATION
- Miliaria
  1. Avoid hot, humid conditions.
  2. Avoid the use of ointments on neonates.

REFERENCES
1. Behrman RE, Kliegman RM, Arvin AM: *Nelson textbook of pediatrics,* ed 15, Philadelphia, 1996, WB Saunders.
2. Habif TP: *Clinical dermatology: a color guide to diagnosis and therapy,* ed 3, St Louis, 1996, Mosby.
3. Hurwitz S: *Clinical pediatric dermatology: a textbook of skin disorders of childhood and adolescence,* Philadelphia, 1993, WB Saunders.
4. Hurwitz S: Skin lesions in the first year of life, *Contemp Pediatr* 15:110, 1998.
5. Vasiloudes P, Morelli JG, Weston WL: A guide to rashes in newborns, *Contemp Pediatr* 14:156, 1997.
Author: **Cynthia Howard, M.D., M.P.H.**

BASIC INFORMATION

■ DEFINITION
Mitral valve prolapse (MVP) results from focal or diffuse redundancy of mitral valve leaflets with (or without) lengthening of subvalvar chordal structures, leading to abnormal coaptation (closure) of mitral leaflets in systole.

■ SYNONYMS
- Barlow syndrome
- Floppy valve syndrome
- Click-murmur syndrome

ICD-9CM CODE
424 Mitral valve prolapse

■ ETIOLOGY
- "Silent form of congenital heart disease"
- Abnormality of myxomatous matrix of valve leaflets and/or collagenous structure of supportive chordae tendineae
- Redundancy of leaflet tissue similar to Ebstein's anomaly of tricuspid valve

■ EPIDEMIOLOGY & DEMOGRAPHICS
- MVP was first described in 1966 by Barlow and Bosman in the *American Heart Journal*.
- The prevalence in children may be equal to that in adults: 6% to 11%.
  1. Mean age of presentation is 9.9 years.
  2. Female:male ratio is 2:1.
- An increased incidence is seen in patients with atrial septal defects (15% to 41%).
- Also associated with Ebstein's anomaly, L-transposition of great arteries, connective tissue disorders (Marfan's syndrome, Ehlers-Danlos syndrome), Turner syndrome, rheumatic fever, and Kawasaki disease.
- There may be a familial predisposition (developmental malformation).

■ HISTORY
- Atypical auscultatory findings, first noted after febrile illness (34% of patients)
- Abnormality on routine physical examination in asymptomatic child (33% of patients)
- Nonexertional chest pain (18% of patients)
- Arrhythmia, fatigue (each 3%); more common symptoms in adolescents and adults

■ PHYSICAL EXAMINATION
- Examination is best completed with the diaphragm of the stethoscope.
- Abnormalities of other systems (e.g., high-arched palate, increased joint laxity, pectus excavatum, straight back syndrome) may be found.
- Auscultatory findings may vary from examination to examination in the individual patient.
- Midsystolic, "nonejection" click is heard at the left sternal border.
  1. Can vary throughout systole
  2. May have single or multiple clicks
- Second heart sound may be widely split.
- A variable late-systolic crescendo-decrescendo apical murmur that is responsive to postural maneuvers may be found (see "Clinical Pearls"). Murmur may have a "honking" or "whooping" quality.
- There may be an early diastolic sound, which resembles a fixed second heart sound or the opening snap of a second heart sound.

DIAGNOSIS

■ DIFFERENTIAL DIAGNOSIS
- Rheumatic mitral insufficiency (can differentiate by responses to postural maneuvers and lack of click)
- Apical muscular ventricular septal defect (usually lack clicks)

■ DIAGNOSTIC WORKUP
- Diagnosis is based mainly on clinical examination rather than laboratory testing.
- Electrocardiogram (ECG)
  1. Repolarization abnormalities (prolonged QT interval, T-wave inversion in leads II, III, aVF) at rest or during exercise (49% to 63% of patients)
  2. Uniform premature contractions and conduction disturbances (15% to 38% of patients)
  3. Exercise or ambulatory ECG of limited use because neither clinical features nor symptoms correlate with high-grade arrhythmias
  4. Worsening arrhythmias may correlate with increasing mitral regurgitation
- Chest radiograph
  1. Generally normal unless the patient has other associated thoracoskeletal abnormalities
- Echocardiogram
  1. "Prolapsing" systolic movement of mitral valve leaflets (by definition, more than 2 mm superior to annular ring); high rate of false-positive results
  2. Identifies associated anomalies

THERAPY

■ NONPHARMACOLOGIC
Family counseling is crucial to prevent cardiac "neurosis" caused by possible morbidity (see following discussion).

■ MEDICAL
- Antiarrhythmics (e.g., β-blockers) should be administered in the face of ventricular arrhythmias.
- β-Blockers may also improve atypical chest pain associated with this condition.
- Oral antacids may be helpful because of the possible association between MVP and esophageal dysmotility.

■ SURGICAL
- Indicated based on the severity of mitral regurgitation or in the face of severe connective tissue disorders
- Similar to congenital mitral regurgitation (MR): resection of redundant leaflet tissue, annuloplasty ring, repair of chordal attachments

■ FOLLOW-UP & DISPOSITION
- If the patient is asymptomatic, cardiac evaluation should be performed every 1 to 2 years to ascertain changes in examination or appearance of symptoms.
- MVP and MR: Yearly evaluation is needed.

■ PATIENT/FAMILY EDUCATION
- In childhood, MVP is a relatively benign condition. Malignant arrhythmias and near sudden death episodes are anecdotal.
- Uncommon but major complications (i.e., endocarditis, chordal rupture with progressive MR, transient ischemic attacks, ventricular arrhythmias, sudden death) can occur in adulthood.
- Approximately 10% to 15% of patients with MVP undergo significant degenerative changes to their valve over time.
- Morbidity of MVP may increase if the condition is associated with a connective tissue disorder.

■ PREVENTIVE TREATMENT
- Subacute bacterial endocarditis (SBE) prophylaxis is indicated in the face of MR.
- For patients with isolated clicks, MVP, and no valvar regurgitation, the need for SBE prophylaxis is still controversial.

■ REFERRAL INFORMATION
Refer the patient to a cardiologist when concerned about new-onset murmur or click on physical examination, atypical chest pain, or arrhythmias.

⚙ PEARLS & CONSIDERATIONS

■ CLINICAL PEARLS

- The timing of clicks varies with postural maneuvers.
  1. Earlier in systole: Valsalva, squatting to standing position
  2. Later in systole: standing to squatting, sitting to supine positions
- The murmur of MR will also vary with position.
  1. Louder, longer: supine to sitting, squatting to standing positions
  2. Softer, shorter: sitting to supine, standing to squatting positions

■ WEBSITES

- American Heart Association National Center: www.americanheart.org
- The Society for Mitral Valve Prolapse Syndrome: www.mitralvalveprolapse.com

REFERENCES

1. Alpert JS, Sabik J, Cosgrove DM: Mitral valve disease. In Topol EJ (ed): *Textbook of cardiovascular medicine,* Philadelphia, 1998, Lippincott-Raven.
2. Baylen BG, Waldhausen JA: Diseases of the mitral valve. In Adams FH, Emmanouilides GC, Riemenschneider TA (eds): *Moss' heart disease in infants, children and adolescents,* Baltimore, 1989, Williams & Wilkins.
3. Bisset GS III et al: Clinical spectrum and long-term follow-up of isolated mitral valve prolapse in 119 children, *Circulation* 62:423, 1980.
4. Shappell SD et al: Sudden death and the familial occurrence of mid-systolic click, late systolic murmur syndrome, *Circulation* 48:1128, 1973.

Author: **Alan M. Mendelsohn, M.D.**

BASIC INFORMATION

■ DEFINITION
Mitral regurgitation (MR) results from incompetence of the mitral valve and backward ejection of flow into the left atrium during left ventricular systole as a result of a lack of coaptation/closure of anterior and posterior mitral leaflets.

■ SYNONYM
Mitral insufficiency

ICD-9CM CODE
746.6 Mitral regurgitation

■ ETIOLOGY
• Usually associated with other forms of left ventricular outflow tract disease (i.e., atrioventricular canal, ventricular septal defect, coarctation of the aorta, patent ductus arteriosus, anomalous left coronary artery from pulmonary artery, isolated cardiac tumors).
• Acquired: secondary effects of dilated cardiomyopathy, Kawasaki disease, rheumatic or viral myocarditis
• Congenital abnormality of leaflets (e.g., leaflet cleft) or support structures (anomalies of papillary muscles or chordae tendineae)

■ EPIDEMIOLOGY & DEMOGRAPHICS
• MR is a rare event in isolation (less than 1% of children with congenital heart defects).
• MR is the most common manifestation of rheumatic heart disease.
• Mitral valve disease is a common cardiac connective tissue disorder.
  1. Hurler's syndrome
  2. Pseudoxanthoma elasticum
  3. Marfan's syndrome
  4. Ehlers-Danlos syndrome
  5. Homocystinuria
• MR can be associated with rheumatoid diseases:
  1. Systemic lupus erythematosus (SLE)
  2. Ankylosing spondylitis
  3. Systemic sclerosis
• MR may be associated with sickle cell disease.

■ HISTORY
• In most cases, detected because of a murmur in an otherwise asymptomatic patient.
• In the absence of other etiologies, the murmur may represent a remnant of subclinical rheumatic carditis.
• Symptoms include dyspnea on exertion, orthopnea, and paroxysmal nocturnal dyspnea.
  1. These symptoms are more common in patients with chronic, severe disease.

■ PHYSICAL EXAMINATION
• Increased precordial activity, diffuse apical impulse
• Diminished first heart sound, increased pulmonary component of second heart sound
• Second heart sound; may be narrowly split in the face of pulmonary hypertension
• High-frequency, mid to late blowing or harsh holosystolic murmur at apex, with radiation to axilla and back
• With moderate or severe MR, third heart sound, low-frequency apical diastolic murmur, hepatosplenomegaly, peripheral edema

DIAGNOSIS

■ DIFFERENTIAL DIAGNOSIS
• Ventricular septal defect
• Tricuspid insufficiency
• Aortic stenosis, hypertrophic obstructive cardiomyopathy
  1. These murmurs may tend to radiate more to the upper sternal border.
  2. They are more ejection in quality.

■ DIAGNOSTIC WORKUP
• Electrocardiogram
  1. Left atrial and ventricular enlargement is seen with severe insufficiency, otherwise normal voltages.
  2. Changes may be secondary to associated lesions (see previous discussion).
• Chest radiograph
  1. Left atrial and ventricular enlargement
  2. Increased pulmonary vascular markings
• Echocardiogram
  1. Definitive test; confirms diagnosis
  2. Yields information on possible causes (i.e., abnormal mitral anatomy, leaflet clefts, cardiomyopathic changes, coronary abnormalities)
  3. Increased left atrial and ventricular dimensions
• Cardiac catheterization
  1. Primarily indicated for preoperative testing.
  2. Determines angiographic degree of regurgitation
  3. Defines pulmonary artery hemodynamics, left ventricular systolic and diastolic function

THERAPY

■ NONPHARMACOLOGIC
Conservative follow-up (every 1 to 2 years) is indicated in cases of trivial or mild MR, with no electrocardio-graphic, chest radiographic, or echocardiographic evidence of atrial or ventricular dilation.

■ MEDICAL
• Moderate to severe MR
  1. Afterload-reducing agents: angiotensin-converting enzyme inhibitors (i.e., captopril, enalapril, or Monopril)
  2. Positive inotropic agents (i.e., digoxin) and/or diuretic therapy for clinical congestive heart failure

■ SURGICAL
• Only recommended in cases that are unresponsive to medical therapy
• Type of surgery influenced by the anatomic abnormality:
  1. Suture closure of mitral leaflet clef
  2. Resection of redundant leaflet tissue
  3. Annuloplasty ring to improve annular competence
  4. Valve replacement usually with mechanical valve because of short (5- to 7-year) life span of bioprosthetic valve in mitral position

■ FOLLOW-UP & DISPOSITION
• Patients with an annuloplasty ring or a mechanical mitral valve usually require anticoagulation therapy with warfarin.
  1. Ring: 3 to 6 months' anticoagulation
  2. Valve: lifelong anticoagulation
• Valve replacement before adolescence usually requires reoperation in adolescence or adulthood to implant a more appropriately sized valve.

■ PATIENT/FAMILY EDUCATION
• See "Follow-up and Disposition."
• Patients receiving chronic anticoagulation therapy should avoid contact sports and trauma.
• Appropriate group A, β-hemolytic streptococcus prophylaxis (see the section "Rheumatic Fever" and the American Heart Association guidelines) should be administered if the cause of MR was rheumatic fever.
• Subacute bacterial endocarditis (SBE) prophylaxis is always indicated (see "Endocarditis Prophylaxis" in Part III).
• The natural history varies according to the cause.
  1. Rheumatic MR: progressive fibrosis and calcification, worsening MR and/or mitral stenosis
  2. Myxomatous MR (as with connective tissue disorders): higher incidence of spontaneous rupture of subvalvar structures, acute cardiac failure
• Patients with mechanical valves have a higher incidence of hemolysis and vegetations.

II

■ **PREVENTIVE TREATMENT**
• SBE prophylaxis is necessary to prevent worsening of condition.
• Treatment of culture-proven group A, β-hemolytic streptococcal pharyngitis is needed to prevent (worsening) rheumatic carditis.

■ **REFERRAL INFORMATION**
Refer the patient to a pediatric cardiologist for confirmation of diagnosis and grading of MR.

☼ **PEARLS & CONSIDERATIONS**

■ **CLINICAL PEARLS**
• Tricuspid insufficiency murmur: early systolic, ends before second heart sound

• Positional changes: see the section "Mitral Valve Prolapse."

■ **WEBSITES**
• American Heart Association National Center: www.americanheart.org
• drkoop.com: www.drkoop.com
• Oregon Health Sciences University: www.ohsu.edu/bicc-informatics/

REFERENCES
1. Alpert JS, Sabik J, Cosgrove DM: Mitral valve disease. In Topol EJ (ed): *Textbook of cardiovascular medicine,* Philadelphia, 1998, Lippincott-Raven.
2. Baylen BG, Waldhausen JA: Diseases of the mitral valve. In Adams FH, Emmanouilides GC, Riemenschneider TA (eds): *Moss' heart disease in infants, children and adolescents,* Baltimore, 1989, Williams & Wilkins.
3. Davachi R, Moller JH, Edwards JE: Diseases of the mitral valve in infancy: anatomic analysis of 55 cases, *Circulation* 43:565, 1971.

Author: **Alan M. Mendelsohn, M.D.**

BASIC INFORMATION

■ **DEFINITION**

Mitral stenosis is an obstruction to left ventricular inflow (at valvar, subvalvar, or supravalvar levels) secondary to single or multiple etiologies (see "Etiology")

■ **SYNONYMS**

• Mitral valve obstruction
• Mitral stenosis

ICD-9CM CODE

746.5 Mitral stenosis

■ **ETIOLOGY**

• Acquired: rheumatic fever (most patients)
• Associated with other forms of left ventricular disease: hypoplastic left heart syndrome, aortic coarctation, aortic stenosis (valvar, subvalvar), double-outlet right ventricle, atrial septal defect (primum, secundum)
• Congenital
  1. Abnormal deposition of fibrous and myxomatous material in valvar and/or subvalvar components
  2. Commissural fusion
  3. Excessive supravalvar connective tissue ("ring")
  4. Abnormal insertion or fusion or quantity of chordae tendineae
• Inborn errors of metabolism (e.g., Fabry's, Hurler-Scheie)
• Rheumatoid disease (e.g., systemic lupus erythematosus, rheumatoid arthritis)

■ **EPIDEMIOLOGY & DEMOGRAPHICS**

• Rarely, there may be a lesion in isolation (0.4% to 0.5% of congenital cardiac anomalies).
• Median survival (untreated) is $2^{11}/_{12}$ years, mainly related to complicating associated lesions.
• Progression of stenosis is generally slow; the mean time period between acute rheumatic fever episode and symptomatic mitral stenosis is 20 years.
• Poor outcome is associated with presentation in early infancy and signs of low cardiac output and/or heart failure.

■ **HISTORY**

• Mild disease: asymptomatic; approximately 50% of patients
• Moderate disease
  1. Present beyond neonatal period (47%)
  2. Multiple recurrent pulmonary infections
  3. Failure to thrive
  4. Irritability, dyspnea on exertion, diaphoresis with feeds

• Severe disease
  1. Symptoms may begin in early postnatal period (86% within 13 days of life).
  2. Vascular collapse with dyspnea, tachypnea, hypotension, grunting, and ashen color may occur after ductus arteriosus closure.

■ **PHYSICAL EXAMINATION**

• Cardiac examination influenced by the degree of decrease in cardiac output
• Soft first heart sound, absent mitral valve opening sound (findings usually reversed in patients with rheumatic mitral stenosis)
• Second heart sound
  1. Variable splitting
     a. Widely split in mild disease
     b. Narrow split with accentuated pulmonary component secondary to pulmonary hypertension with more severe disease
• Usually low-frequency, low-intensity middiastolic apical murmur; sometimes loud, high-frequency diastolic murmur
• In cases of severe mitral stenosis
  1. Diminished peripheral perfusion, pulses
  2. Jugular venous distention
  3. Hyperdynamic right ventricular impulse
  4. Third, fourth heart sounds: secondary to right ventricular diastolic dysfunction
  5. Variable systolic ejection click, diastolic pulmonary insufficiency murmur (Graham-Steel murmur) in face of severe pulmonary hypertension

🔬 **DIAGNOSIS**

■ **DIFFERENTIAL DIAGNOSIS**

• Primary pulmonary artery hypertension; usually lacks apical diastolic murmur
• Pulmonary venous obstruction/pulmonary vasoocclusive disease
• Cor triatriatum: obstructive membrane within left atrium limiting pulmonary venous drainage
• Atrial myxoma
• Large atrial or ventricular septal defects

■ **DIAGNOSTIC WORKUP**

• Electrocardiogram
  1. Left atrial enlargement
  2. With severe mitral stenosis, findings of right heart disease
     a. Right ventricular enlargement
     b. Right atrial enlargement
     c. Right QRS axis deviation (+90° to 150°)

  3. In adolescents and/or adults, paroxysmal (or chronic) atrial fibrillation
• Chest radiograph
  1. Left atrial enlargement
  2. Increased pulmonary vascular markings
  3. Increased right heart silhouette
• Echocardiogram
  1. Definitive test; confirms diagnosis
  2. Elucidates abnormal Doppler inflow patterns consistent with diagnosis
  3. Demonstrates chamber sizes
  4. Defines all levels of mitral valve apparatus
• Cardiac catheterization
  1. Valuable both as a diagnostic and therapeutic test (see "Therapy")
  2. Defines the degree of mitral valve stenosis, pulmonary hemodynamics, and cardiac index
  3. Helps rule out other pulmonary venous abnormalities
  4. Defines associated left ventricular outflow tract obstruction

💊 **THERAPY**

■ **MEDICAL**

• Standard anticongestive therapy (e.g., diuretics, nitrates) is provided for mild to moderately symptomatic mitral stenosis, although surgical/transcatheter therapy is the treatment of choice.
• Digoxin may be useful in the face of right ventricular failure.
• Antiarrhythmics (e.g., digoxin, β-blockers, calcium channel blockers) should be administered as necessary.
• Chronic anticoagulation should be provided with warfarin.
• Aggressive treatment of pulmonary infections is necessary.

■ **SURGICAL/TRANSCATHETER THERAPY**

• Surgical therapy is indicated for symptomatic relief in the face of inadequate medical relief.
• Optimal age for repair is 3 years.
• Intervention depends on the cause.
  1. Simple commissurotomy (separation of leaflets)
  2. Resection of excessive subvalvar/supravalvar tissue
  3. Mitral valve replacement with mechanical prosthesis for multiple levels of mitral stenosis
• Transcatheter balloon valvuloplasty for congenital mitral stenosis was first proposed by Lock in 1985.
  1. Procedure is of limited utility in very small children or patients with calcified valves.
  2. Approximately 40% to 50% long-term success has been achieved in patients with normal subvalvar

anatomy and adequate annulus size.
3. Complications include mitral regurgitation (rare), transient ischemic attacks, ventricular perforations (anecdotal), and second- or third-degree atrioventricular block (in up to 22% of patients).

■ FOLLOW-UP & DISPOSITION
- Chronic anticoagulation (if necessary) requires close monitoring.
- Chronic pulmonary vascular disease and concomitant pulmonary illnesses also require follow-up every 6 to 12 months.

■ PATIENT/FAMILY EDUCATION
- If mitral stenosis is left untreated (even at mild degree), the patient is at increased risk for cerebral embolic phenomena unrelated to the degree of stenosis.
- Chronic atrial fibrillation occurs in 40% of patients, even with effective gradient relief.
- Pulmonary vascular changes and/or pulmonary hypertension may be slow to resolve even after gradient resolution.

■ PREVENTIVE TREATMENT
- Aggressive antibiotic therapy is indicated for rheumatic fever prophylaxis.
- Subacute bacterial endocarditis prophylaxis should be administered at times of appropriate risk.

■ REFERRAL INFORMATION
Refer the patient to a pediatric cardiologist for full evaluation if the diagnosis is suspected by clinical history or physical examination.

☼ PEARLS & CONSIDERATIONS

■ CLINICAL PEARLS
Short periods of exercise or deep expiration may accentuate the murmur in larger patients.

■ WEBSITES
- Adam.com: www.adam.com/encv/article/00175.htm
- Cardiac Surgery Information Page: www.heart-surgeon.com/mitral-surgery.html
- Emedicine: www.emedicine.com/EMERG/topic.315.htm

REFERENCES

1. Alpert JS, Sabik J, Cosgrove DM: Mitral valve disease. In Topol EJ (ed): *Textbook of cardiovascular medicine*, Philadelphia, 1998, Lippincott-Raven.
2. Baylen BG, Waldhausen JA: Diseases of the mitral valve. In Adams FH, Emmanouilides GC, Riemenschneider TA (eds): *Moss' heart disease in infants, children and adolescents*, Baltimore, 1989, Williams & Wilkins.
3. Mendelsohn AM, Beekman RH: Interventions in congenital heart disease. In Topol EJ (ed): *Comprehensive cardiovascular medicine*, Philadelphia, 1998, Lippincott-Raven.
4. Moore P et al: Severe congenital mitral stenosis in infants, *Circulation* 89:2099, 1994.

Author: **Alan M. Mendelsohn, M.D.**

BASIC INFORMATION

■ DEFINITION
Mixed connective tissue disease (MCTD) is an autoimmune, rheumatic disease with clinical features overlapping systemic lupus erythematosus (SLE), polymyositis, and systemic sclerosis, and associated with anti-UI RNP (ribonucleoprotein) antibodies. Four classification criteria are published, but these are not validated for children.

■ SYNONYMS
- Overlap syndrome
- Undifferentiated connective tissue disease (not all patients qualify by diagnostic serologies)
- MCTD

ICD-9CM CODE
710.9 Connective tissue disease, diffuse (not specifically listed as MCTD)

■ ETIOLOGY
Unknown, as are all autoimmune rheumatic diseases

■ EPIDEMIOLOGY & DEMOGRAPHICS
- No epidemiologic studies have been conducted in the United States.
- The incidence is 0.10 per 100,000 children 0 to 15 years old in Finland, 0.05 per 100,000 in Japan, compared with 0.37 per 100,000 SLE in Finland and 0.47 per 100,000 SLE in Japan.
- The female:male ratio is approximately 4.5:1.
- The youngest reported patient was 5 years old.
- Increased association is observed with HLA DR2/DR4 and anti-UI-70-kd RNP antibodies.

■ HISTORY
- Fever (occasional)
- Fatigue (ubiquitous symptom in connective tissue diseases)
- Arthralgia (arthritis, SLE-like or juvenile rheumatoid arthritis [JRA]-like 97% to 100%)
- Raynaud's phenomenon (approximately 80%)
- Swollen hands (approximately 80%)
- Sclerodactyly (approximately 80%)
- Malar erythema, photosensitivity
- Esophageal dysmotility (dysphagia and reflux symptoms)
- Myositis with proximal muscle weakness
- Abnormal diffusion capacity for carbon monoxide (DL_{co})—may be asymptomatic
- Signs of Sjögren's syndrome: xerostomia, xerophthalmia, swollen parotid glands
- Pericarditis, myocarditis
- Glomerulonephritis, proliferative or membranous (0% to 21%)

- Rare central nervous system (CNS) complications, cerebrovascular accident
- Thrombocytopenia, leukopenia, direct Coombs' positive hemolytic anemia (uncommon)
- Thyroiditis

■ PHYSICAL EXAMINATION
- Malar erythema
- Hand swelling, diffuse induration
- "Sausage digits"
- Sclerodactyly, usually no digital ulcers or pits
- Joint swelling, large and small joints, symmetric distribution
- Proximal muscle weakness
- Rheumatoid nodules (uncommon)
- Swollen parotid glands

🔬 DIAGNOSIS

■ DIFFERENTIAL DIAGNOSIS
- Classification criteria provide systemic signs and symptoms and serologies to establish a provisional diagnosis.
- Any autoimmune disease needs to be considered; however, MCTD manifests overlap components of SLE, scleroderma, polymyositis (dermatomyositis), plus components of JRA and Sjögren's syndrome.
- Anecdotal reports of viral myocarditis and one case of malignancy confused with MCTD.

■ DIAGNOSTIC WORKUP
- Antinuclear antibody test: expect high titer, speckled pattern
- Complete blood count with differential, platelet count
- Positive RNP antibodies (UI-70 kd RNP)
- Much less commonly, also positive ds-DNA, Sm antibodies (Sharp criteria would exclude these patients); these antibodies strongly suggest lupus
- Urine analysis, blood urea nitrogen, creatinine
- Muscle enzymes: creatine kinase, aldolase, aspartate aminotransferase (AST), alanine aminotransferase (ALT), lactate dehydrogenase
- Esophageal studies, barium cine-esophagram
- Pulmonary function tests with routine flow loops and DL_{co}; chest radiograph
- Quantitative immunoglobulins (likely elevated): hypergammaglobulinemia
- C3, C4: occasionally low
- DAT/direct Coombs' test
- Joint radiographs: cumulative may show erosive bone changes over time
- Electrocardiogram, echocardiogram

💊 THERAPY

■ NONPHARMACOLOGIC
- Raynaud's prophylaxis: mittens/gloves, avoidance of cold, no tobacco!
- Physical therapy: range-of-motion exercises, joint/hand protection
- Biofeedback; may be helpful for Raynaud's phenomenon
- Gastroesophageal reflux precautions

■ MEDICAL
- Nonsteroidal antiinflammatory drugs (e.g., naproxen, tolmetin sodium) for arthritis and mild serositis
- Corticosteroids, usually oral administration for myositis, serositis, thrombocytopenia (clinically relevant), pulmonary manifestations
- Raynaud's phenomenon: calcium channel blockers, local nitroglycerine products
- More intense immunosuppression may be needed for serious renal, CNS, cardiac, or pulmonary involvement
- Esophageal protection: H_2 blockers, proton pump inhibitors

■ SURGICAL
Usually none is necessary; however, system-specific intervention may be necessary.

■ FOLLOW-UP & DISPOSITION
- Perform serial evaluation for evolution of disease (i.e., progressive arthropathy, sclerodactyly).
- Surveillance for hematologic, muscular, CNS, renal, and/or pulmonary involvement is necessary.
- Beware of possible development of pulmonary hypertension.
- Watch for growth and nutritional issues, especially in patients with esophageal, intestinal involvement, insidious thyroiditis with hypothyroidism, or corticosteroid treatment.

■ PATIENT/FAMILY EDUCATION & PREVENTIVE TREATMENT
- Protect hands (Raynaud's phenomenon).
- Use sun protection (photosensitive rash).
- Use esophageal reflux precautions.
- Watch for new symptoms.
- Need serial evaluations by physician.
- Maintain all immunizations if not immunosuppressed.

■ REFERRAL INFORMATION
Because MCTD is a complex overlap syndrome, all patients should be evaluated and followed longitudinally by a rheumatologist if possible.

II

☼ PEARLS & CONSIDERATIONS

■ CLINICAL PEARLS
- Anything can happen to MCTD patients; keep your eyes, ears, and fingers tuned-in.
- MCTD patients evolve over time, usually into predominantly lupus or scleroderma characteristics.

■ WEBSITE
Nationwide Internet: www.nationwide.net/~vance/mctd.htm

■ SUPPORT GROUPS
- Arthritis Foundation supported
- Usually lupus group or possible scleroderma or JRA support group
- American Juvenile Arthritis Organization

REFERENCES
1. Michels H: Course of mixed connective tissue disease in children, *Ann Med* 29:359, 1997.
2. Mier R et al: Long-term follow-up of children with mixed connective tissue disease, *Lupus* 5:221, 1996.
3. Singsen BH et al: Mixed connective tissue disease in childhood: a clinical and serologic survey, *J Pediatr* 90:893, 1977.
4. Tiddens HA et al: Juvenile-onset mixed connective tissue disease: longitudinal follow-up, *J Pediatr* 122:191, 1993.

Author: **Murray Passo, M.D.**

BASIC INFORMATION

DEFINITION
Molluscum contagiosum is a benign, asymptomatic, self-limited, cutaneous viral infection caused by poxvirus. It affects children, sexually active adults, and immunocompromised individuals.

ICD-9CM CODE
078.0 Molluscum contagiosum

ETIOLOGY
- The molluscum contagiosum virus is a member of the poxvirus (Poxviridae) family and the sole member of the *Molluscipoxvirus* genus.
- The virus is a large, complex, double-stranded DNA virus that replicates in the cytoplasm of cells.
- The virus is especially adapted to the epidermis and infects only human beings.
- Three types of molluscum contagiosum viruses have been identified (i.e., MCV-I, MCV-II, and MCV-III), with no differences with respect to clinical presentation.

EPIDEMIOLOGY & DEMOGRAPHICS
- Occurs worldwide
- Spread through direct contact with infected individuals and through autoinoculation
- Also spread through contact with contaminated objects (fomites)
- Most commonly affects preschool and school-aged children
- Higher incidence in warm/tropical countries and more commonly seen with poor hygiene
- Higher association with contact sports, such as wrestling, and use of swimming pools
- Commonly involves the genital area in children and may occasionally be spread by sexual abuse
- Also occurs in young adults in the genital area and thighs as a result of sexual transmission
- Commonly seen in immunosuppressed individuals, occurring in 5% to 18% of patients with human immunodeficiency virus (HIV)
- Incubation period 2 weeks to 6 months
  1. Individual lesions last 2 months.
  2. Entire episode lasts 9 months to 2 or more years.

PHYSICAL EXAMINATION
- Individual lesions are flesh-colored or pearly pink dome-shaped papules.
  1. Umbilicated center
  2. Sizes ranging from 1 to 5 mm
- May express cheesy, curdlike material from the center
- May occur anywhere on the body
  1. Tends to cluster in one or two areas, especially skin folds (axillae, neck, inguinal creases)
- Usually fewer than 20 lesions
  1. May see hundreds, especially in immunocompromised individuals
- Usually asymptomatic
  1. Pruritus or surrounding dermatitis may develop.
  2. Occasionally, lesions become inflamed and bleed.
- May be cosmetically disfiguring, especially in advanced acquired immunodeficiency syndrome, when they are numerous on the face and scalp
- May develop conjunctivitis if lesions are present around the eyelids

DIAGNOSIS

DIFFERENTIAL DIAGNOSIS
- Flat warts
- Condyloma acuminata
- Syringoma
- Sebaceous hyperplasia
- Basal and squamous cell carcinoma
- Epidermal inclusion cyst
- Invasive fungal infection (e.g., cryptococcosis) in HIV patients
- Pyogenic granuloma

DIAGNOSTIC WORKUP
- The diagnosis is usually clinically obvious when multiple lesions are present.
- The diagnosis is aided by freezing with liquid nitrogen, which accentuates umbilication.
- Lesions can be removed by curettage or tangential excision.
  1. Crushed onto a microscope slide
  2. Diagnostic intracytoplasmic inclusion bodies (Henderson-Patterson bodies)

THERAPY

NONPHARMACOLOGIC
- May be observed
  1. Disease is usually self-limited, but may continue to spread.
- Best to avoid overly aggressive or traumatic therapy

MEDICAL
- Trichloroacetic acid may be caustic to the skin.
- Cantharidin may cause severe blisters.
- Tretinoin may be applied by the patient daily to individual lesions.
- Topical cidofovir reportedly caused clearing of molluscum in HIV patients in a few studies.
- Podophyllin is minimally effective.

SYSTEMIC
Attempts have been reported to treat with griseofulvin, interferon, and cimetidine but have not been shown to be consistently or universally effective.

SURGICAL
- Cryosurgery with liquid nitrogen is effective but limited by pain and blister formation.
- Cryotherapy followed by curettage with a sharp curette is standard and effective treatment.
- Complications of surgical therapy include the following:
  1. Erythema
  2. Altered pigment (usually hyperpigmentation)
  3. Minor surface depression (usually resolves completely within 3 to 6 months)

FOLLOW-UP & DISPOSITION
- Patients may be treated every 2 to 4 weeks with topical chemical therapy until resolution.
- Following curettage of all lesions, patients should be observed for local recurrence, which usually occurs within 3 to 4 months; any new lesions can be treated similarly.

PATIENT/FAMILY EDUCATION
- Need to be aware of the infectious nature and avoid methods of transmission: contact sports, swimming pools, shared towels.
- Need to be aware of usual spontaneous resolution.
- Patients and parents need to be aware of frequent recurrences, even after successful treatment.

PREVENTIVE TREATMENT
- Avoid known methods of transmission (i.e., contact sports, swimming pools, shared towels).
- Avoid scratching or traumatizing lesions, which can promote spread.

REFERRAL INFORMATION
Referral to a dermatologist is appropriate if lesions are numerous, spreading, or cosmetically disfiguring (on face) and if the primary physician is not trained in curettage of molluscum.

☼ PEARLS & CONSIDERATIONS

■ CLINICAL PEARLS

- It is important to not make the treatment worse than the disease; avoid overly aggressive treatment, especially if painful and/or traumatic to the patient.

- It can be helpful to pretreat the skin with topical anesthetic (EMLA cream) 1 to 2 hours before curettage or cryotherapy.

REFERENCES

1. Lewis E, Lam M, Crutchfield C: An update on molluscum contagiosum cutis, *Cutis* 60:29, 1997.
2. Ordoukhanian E, Lane A: Warts and molluscum contagiosum, *Postgrad Med* 101:223, 1997.
3. Severson J, Tyring S: Viral disease update, *Curr Prob Dermatol* 11:37, 1999.
4. Waugh M: Molluscum contagiosum, *Dermatol Clin* 16:839, 1998.

Author: **Allison L. Holm, M.D.**

BASIC INFORMATION

DEFINITION
Motion sickness refers to nausea and malaise resulting from motion, typically while traveling by boat, airplane, train, or automobile.

SYNONYMS
- Seasickness
- Carsickness
- Airsickness

ICD-9CM CODE
994.6 Motion sickness

ETIOLOGY
- The exact physiologic mechanism is unknown.
- It likely involves overload of peripheral receptors (in semicircular canals) as well as vestibular stimulation.
- An abnormality of neurotransmitter metabolism has been suggested.
- Mechanism results in distended gastric motility, which produces symptoms of nausea and vomiting.

EPIDEMIOLOGY & DEMOGRAPHICS
- The incidence and severity of symptoms vary with the intensity of the stimulus and the susceptibility of the individual.
- The incidence is 100% in rough seas, 25% during moderate turbulence at sea, 3% to 4% in the car, less than 1% in air travelers, and less than 0.2% on trains.
- Motion sickness is most common in children 3 to 12 years old.
- It is more prevalent in females than in males.
- A 55% incidence of motion sickness has been reported in adults with migraines, and 50% of children with childhood migraines experience motion sickness.

HISTORY
- Characteristic symptoms
  1. Nausea, occasionally with vomiting
  2. Malaise
  3. Pallor or flushing
  4. Sweating
  5. Symptoms resolve when stimulus is removed.

PHYSICAL EXAMINATION
Normal

DIAGNOSIS

Typical symptoms in response to motion

DIFFERENTIAL DIAGNOSIS
- Gastroenteritis
- Vasovagal response
- Presyncope
- Ménière's syndrome, other causes of vestibular dysfunction

DIAGNOSTIC WORKUP
- History and physical examination should be performed.
- Symptoms can be recreated using a stimulus such as a rotating optokinetic drum.

THERAPY

NONPHARMACOLOGIC
- Keep children in a central location when traveling on a boat or airplane to reduce head and body movement.
- Focus on a stable horizon or other external object.
- Some studies with adults have suggested that eating less before travel or skipping a meal reduces the incidence of motion sickness.
- Avoid visual stimuli such as reading.

MEDICAL
- Dimenhydrinate (Dramamine, Marmine) has a sedating effect and is generally ineffective if administered after the onset of symptoms.
- Meclizine (Antivert) is also sedating.
- Promethazine (Phenergan) has a sedating effect; can be administered orally, as a suppository, or intramuscularly; and is effective even if symptoms have already begun.
- Scopolamine is effective, but side effects include tinnitus, dizziness, dry mouth, drowsiness, skin rash, and nightmares.

COMPLEMENTARY & ALTERNATIVE THERAPIES
- Ginger root and green tea are reportedly useful, but their efficacy is unproven.
- Biofeedback and acupressure are generally *ineffective*.

FOLLOW-UP & DISPOSITION
Consider the possibility of childhood migraine, particularly in patients with severe motion sickness.

PATIENT/FAMILY EDUCATION
- Most patients adapt to continued motion stimulus over a few days.
- Susceptibility generally diminishes with age, although symptoms may persist into adulthood in some patients.

PREVENTIVE TREATMENT
- See discussion of nonpharmacologic treatment.
- Administer medication before beginning travel.

REFERENCES
1. Barabas G, Matthews WS, Ferrari M: Childhood migraine and motion sickness, *Pediatrics* 72:188, 1983.
2. Kozarsky PE: Prevention of common travel ailments, *Infect Dis Clin North Am* 12:305, 1998.
3. Weinstein SE, Stern RM: Comparison of Marezine and dramamine in preventing symptoms of motion sickness, *Aviat Space Environ Med* 68:890, 1997.

Author: **Michael Visick, M.D.**

II

BASIC INFORMATION

■ DEFINITION
Mumps is a systemic acute viral illness characterized by swelling of one or both parotid glands.

ICD-9CM CODES
072.9 Mumps
072.8 Mumps with complication
072.0 Mumps orchitis

■ ETIOLOGY
Mumps is an RNA virus of the genus *Paramyxovirus* in the *Paramyxovirus* family.

■ EPIDEMIOLOGY & DEMOGRAPHICS
- Humans are the only host.
- The virus is spread by contact with respiratory secretions.
- The disease is generally benign in childhood.
- Severe complications, such as orchitis, may occur in adults.
- The disease should be reported to national regulatory health agencies.
- Death is rare.
- In the prevaccine era, mumps more common
  1. In winter and spring, epidemics every 4 years
- In the postvaccine era, little seasonal variation and a 99% decrease in incidence has been noted since the availability of the vaccine

■ HISTORY
- One third of patients with mumps have subclinical or a mild respiratory illness.
- Parotid swelling is the most common clinical manifestation: It starts on one side and later becomes bilateral in 70% of cases.
- A prodrome lasts 1 to 2 days.
  1. Fever (38.9° to 39.4° C maximum)
  2. Anorexia
  3. Headache
  4. Vomiting
  5. Generalized achiness, vague abdominal pain
- Parotid swelling
  1. Approximately 2 weeks after exposure
  2. In 30% to 40% of cases

■ PHYSICAL EXAMINATION
- Prodrome
  1. Fever
  2. Erythema of parotid ducts (Stensen's duct), which open onto the buccal mucosa near the upper second molar, or Wharton's ducts, the ducts of the submaxillary gland, which open at the base of the tongue

3. Parotid swelling: swelling over lower jaw and cheek, anterior to auricle, extending behind and under the angle of jaw
4. Bilateral in 70% of cases
5. Brawny edema with indiscreet borders
6. May be tender to palpation
7. Maximum swelling at 3 days
8. Resolves slowly after 2 days
9. Possible involvement of submaxillary and subungual glands
10. May have limited jaw opening
- Complications of mumps
  1. Mortality rare
  2. Meningitis
  3. Meningoencephalitis
  4. Epididymitis
  5. Orchitis (14% to 35% of postpubertal males develop this complication)
  6. Pancreatitis
  7. Associated with diabetes mellitus
  8. Nephritis
  9. Hearing loss
  10. Congenital infection
      a. Increased fetal loss in the first trimester
      b. No known congenital syndrome

DIAGNOSIS

■ DIFFERENTIAL DIAGNOSIS
- Bacterial parotitis
- Parotid duct stone
- Drug reaction
- Parotid tumor, Sjögren's syndrome
- Other viral causes of parotitis
  1. Coxsackie A virus
  2. Echoviral
  3. Parainfluenza viruses 1, 2, 3
  4. Human immunodeficiency virus (HIV)
- Lymphadenopathy
  1. Anterior cervical and submandibular lymphadenopathy often confused with parotitis
- Mandibular disease
  1. Tumor of jaw (i.e., neuroblastoma)
  2. Osteomyelitis
- Consider mumps in all cases of the following:
  1. Meningitis
  2. Meningoencephalitis
  3. Encephalitis

■ DIAGNOSTIC WORKUP
- Viral isolation from one of the following:
  1. Saliva
  2. Oropharyngeal swabs
  3. Urine
  4. Cerebrospinal fluid of those with meningitis or meningoencephalitis
- Serum antibody elevation: complement fixation, hemagglutination inhibition, or enzyme-linked

immunosorbent assay to confirm infection or vaccination

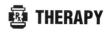

THERAPY

- Supportive and comfort measures are sufficient in uncomplicated cases of mumps.
- No current antiviral agent is available.

■ PRIMARY PREVENTION
- Give mumps virus vaccine (see Table 2-18).
  1. It is a live, attenuated virus.
- Can give monovalent or in combination (measles-mumps-rubella).
- The vaccine produces a subclinical, noncommunicable infection.
- Antibodies develop in 97% of susceptible children.
- Durable protection is afforded.
- The first dose should be administered by 15 months of age, on or after the first birthday.
- By 12 years, a second dose should be received (in accordance with measles vaccine recommendations), preferably between 4 and 6 years.
- Vaccination is important in adolescence if not previously done to prevent increased morbidity associated with disease in this population.
- Consider the patient susceptible if without documentation of vaccination, physician-diagnosed illness, or titers confirming infection.
- Adverse events:
  1. Most often associated with the measles component of the combination vaccine
  2. Fever in 5% to 15%, 7 to 12 days after receiving the vaccine
  3. Rashes in 5% of vaccine recipients
  4. Transient thrombocytopenia
  5. Rare hypersensitivity reactions
  6. Aseptic meningitis associated with the Urabe strain but not with the current U.S. strain (Jeryl-Lynn strain)

■ PRECAUTIONS
- Minor illnesses with fever are not a contraindication.
- Anaphylactic reactions to eggs or neomycin or reactions to gelatin should be evaluated by an allergist before the patient receives the measles vaccine.
- History of receiving immunoglobulin (see the section "Measles") requires special considerations.

■ IMMUNODEFICIENT HOSTS
- Live virus should not be given to severely immunodeficient children.
- An interval of at least 3 months should be observed after cessation of any immunosuppressive therapy.

TABLE 2-18 Mumps Vaccine Recommendations

CATEGORY	RECOMMENDATIONS
Unvaccinated, no history of measles (12-15 mo)	A two-dose schedule (with MMR) is recommended if born after 1956. The first dose is recommended at 12-15 mo; the second is recommended at 4-6 yr.
Children 12 mo in area of recurrent measles transmission	Vaccinate; a second dose is indicated at 4-6 yr (at school entry).
Children 6-11 mo in epidemic situations	Vaccinate (with monovalent measles vaccine or, if not available, MMR); revaccination (with MMR) at 12-15 mo is necessary, and a third dose is indicated at 4-6 yr.
Children 11-12 yr who have received one dose of measles vaccine at 12 mo	Revaccinate (one dose).
Students in college and other post–high school institutions who have received one dose of measles vaccine at 12 mo	Revaccinate (one dose).
History of vaccination before the first birthday	Consider susceptible and vaccinate (two doses).

MMR, Measles-mumps-rubella.

- High-dose corticosteroids necessitate waiting for an interval of 1 month.
- HIV infection is not a contraindication unless the child is severely immunocompromised (low CD4 T-lymphocyte counts).
- Pregnant women should not receive the vaccine.
  1. Counsel to avoid conception for 3 months after mumps vaccination.

■ SECONDARY PREVENTION
- Exclude known infected children from schools and day care.
- Exclude known susceptible children until vaccination occurs.
- Exclude unvaccinated children (for religious, medical, or other reasons) at least 26 days from onset of last case.

■ REFERRAL INFORMATION
Consultation with a pediatric infectious disease specialist may be warranted in complicated cases.

☼ PEARLS & CONSIDERATIONS

■ CLINICAL PEARLS
- Only 30% to 40% of mumps infections produce classic mumps with parotitis.
- Inapparent infection is more common in adults.
- Classic parotitis is most common in children age 2 to 9 years.

■ WEBSITES
- Centers for Disease Control and Prevention: www.cdc.gov/
- *Morbidity and Mortality Weekly Report:* www2.cdc.gov/mmwr

REFERENCES
1. Centers for Disease Control and Prevention (CDC): *MMWR Morb Mortal Wkly Rep* 47:1, 1998.
2. Peter G (ed): *1997 Red Book: report of the Committee on Infectious Diseases,* ed 24, Elk Grove Village, Ill, 1997, American Academy of Pediatrics.
Author: **Maureen Kays, M.D.**

BASIC INFORMATION

DEFINITION
Munchausen syndrome by proxy (MSBP) is a form of child maltreatment in which caretakers exaggerate, feign, or induce symptoms and/or illness in children in search of attention and personal gratification for themselves.

SYNONYMS
- Factitious disorder by proxy
- Meadow's syndrome
- Polle's syndrome

ICD-9CM CODE
301.51 Munchausen syndrome by proxy

ETIOLOGY
- Many practitioners believe that MSBP is symptomatic of a psychiatric disturbance in the perpetrator, who acts in a premeditated way, rather than out of acute frustration or rage.
- Some argue that MSBP is a product of many factors.
  1. A parent who has the capacity for abuse and the potential to be gratified by the medical system
  2. A medical system that is specialized, investigation oriented, fascinated by rare conditions, often ignorant of abusive behaviors, and accepting of reported histories
- Caregivers may do any combination of the following:
  1. Give a false story of illness.
  2. Fabricate a sign of illness.
  3. Interfere with test results.

EPIDEMIOLOGY & DEMOGRAPHICS
- Children are affected equally with respect to gender and birth order.
- No seasonal variation has been noted.
- Perpetrator characteristics are as follows:
  1. Most commonly the patient's mother
  2. Often has had training in a medical field
  3. May have an affective or personality disorder
  4. May have experienced physical or sexual abuse as a child
- Duration from onset of symptoms to diagnosis is months to years.
- Mean age at diagnosis is 20 months.
- Children older than 5 years of age with MSBP are likely to have developmental delay.
- One incidence study from Great Britain found the following:
  1. 2.8 per 100,000 children younger than 1 year of age
  2. 0.5 per 100,000 children younger than 16
- The mortality rate is 9% to 33%.

HISTORY
- Gathering a meticulous history is crucial; poor history taking has been implicated in contributing to the misdiagnosis of MSBP.
- There is no typical history; the most common presentations include the following:
  1. Seizures
  2. Bleeding
  3. Central nervous system depression
  4. Apnea
  5. Vomiting and/or diarrhea
  6. Fever
  7. Rash
- A few generalizations can be made:
  1. The child's medical problems may not have responded as expected to therapy.
  2. The child's medical course may have been unusual in some way.
  3. Family history may elicit numerous medical problems that seem implausible.
  4. Others may have had unexplained illness while under the supervision of the caregiver.

PHYSICAL EXAMINATION
- There may be signs of physical abuse, neglect, or failure to thrive.
- Signs and symptoms of a child's illness may fail to occur in the caregiver's absence.

DIAGNOSIS

The major obstruction in making the diagnosis is failure to consider MSBP.

DIFFERENTIAL DIAGNOSIS
Many medical possibilities may need to be entertained as a cause for the symptoms.

DIAGNOSTIC WORKUP
- Hospitalization is required in most cases to protect the child.
- The workup should be individualized to each patient, remembering that a thorough history, physical examination, and observation alone may exclude many medical diagnoses.
- Videotaping in the hospital has been helpful; however, legal involvement is suggested if covert taping is planned.
- An empiric trial of foster care may be necessary for diagnosis.

THERAPY

NONPHARMACOLOGIC
- Counseling is important for both the patient and the family.
- In most cases of MSBP, removal of

the child from the home is recommended.
- Foster care with an unrelated caregiver is preferred to kinship care, where the perpetrator may still have access to the child after removal.

MEDICAL
Medical therapy is supportive and related to any harm inflicted on the child.

SURGICAL
Indicated only if necessitated because of inflicted harm

FOLLOW-UP & DISPOSITION
- Both the medical stability and the safety of the child must be considered when discussing disposition.
- Mortality and morbidity rates are higher with MSBP than with other forms of child abuse.

PATIENT/FAMILY EDUCATION
- Eight percent of surviving victims of MSBP suffer some kind of long-term morbidity as a result of complications of the induced illness or complications from medical procedures.
- Many more go on to develop psychologic difficulties.

REFERRAL INFORMATION
- Medical consultation with or between specialists is more helpful than referral to specialists.
- Child psychiatry referral may be helpful.
- If MSBP is suspected, a hospital-based child maltreatment team should be involved to ensure the safety of the child and to assist in reporting to state officials.

PEARLS & CONSIDERATIONS

CLINICAL PEARLS
- MSBP often occurs in isolation, unlike other forms of child maltreatment.
- Anticonvulsants and opiates are the most common nonaccidental poisons.

CONSIDERATIONS
- Multidisciplinary team involvement is crucial in MSBP. The team should involve a physician, nurses, and social work members, as well as legal counsel, law enforcement, and a psychologist and/or psychiatrist. A clinical epidemiologist may also be helpful. In the absence of data of commission, relative risk data may be the most compelling evidence available for court proceedings.

- Even with compelling evidence, MSBP is a difficult diagnosis to accept.
- Although diagnosis and intervention is painful for the family, health care providers also find the process extremely stressful and may benefit from counseling.

■ WEBSITES
- Child Abuse Prevention Network: www.child.cornell.edu
- National Clearinghouse on Child Abuse and Neglect: www.calib.com/nccanch
- National Committee to Prevent Child Abuse: www.childabuse.org

REFERENCES
1. Donald L: Munchausen syndrome by proxy, *Arch Pediatr Adolesc Med* 150: 753, 1996.
2. Meadow R: Munchausen syndrome by proxy, *Arch Dis Child* 57:92, 1982.
3. McClure RJ et al: Epidemiology of Munchausen syndrome by proxy, non-accidental poisoning, and non-accidental suffocation, *Arch Dis Child* 75:57, 1996.
4. Rosenberg DA: Web of deceit: a literature review of Munchausen syndrome by proxy, *Child Abuse Negl* 11: 547, 1987.

Author: **Joeli Hettler, M.D.**

II

BASIC INFORMATION

■ **DEFINITION**
Muscular dystrophy (MD) is one of several progressive, degenerative muscle disorders that result in weakness. It is inherited as X-linked recessive or results from de novo, gene mutation. The most common MDs are Duchenne and Becker. Other MDs are Emery-Dreyfuss, congenital muscular dystrophy, facioscapulohumeral, limb girdle, and myotonic dystrophy.

■ **SYNONYMS**
• Dystrophinopathy
• Duchenne MD
• Becker MD

ICD-9CM CODE
359.1 Muscular dystrophy

■ **ETIOLOGY**
• The mutation is a deletion or duplication of the dystrophin gene, which leads to a decrease of dystrophin.
• Dystrophin is a subsarcolemmal cytoskeletal protein that plays a key role in the muscle membrane function and its histologic integrity.
• Decrease or lack of dystrophin can result in various degrees of muscle weakness.
• The dystrophin gene is located in the Xp21 band.
  1. One third of the Duchenne muscular dystrophy (DMD) cases result from de novo gene mutation.

■ **EPIDEMIOLOGY & DEMOGRAPHICS**
• DMD is the most common of all MDs in childhood.
  1. Worldwide incidence is 1 in 4000 newborn boys.
  2. DMD is a lethal disorder that is usually associated with marked deficiency or absence of dystrophin.
• Becker's muscular dystrophy (BMD) occurs in 1 in 30,000 boys.
  1. In some countries, this entity is more common.
  2. BMD is a milder myopathy caused by partial deficiency of dystrophin.

■ **HISTORY**
• A wide variation exists in the age of onset of symptoms, progression of weakness, loss of ambulation, mobility, rate of decline in respiratory status, and age at death.
  1. This heterogeneity is more marked between than within kindreds.
• DMD symptoms usually start before age 3 years.
  1. Delayed onset of walking is caused by symmetric weakness of the hip muscles and calf muscle hypertrophy.
  2. Children never develop the ability to run, hop on one foot, or climb stairs without support.
  3. Most are wheelchair dependent before the age of 13 years.
  4. Approximately one third have an intelligence quotient below 75.
  5. Cardiac symptoms may occur, but progressive heart failure is uncommon.
• BMD has a more variable phenotypic spectrum than DMD.
  1. Symptoms range from slightly less severe than DMD to very mild, with some patients remaining ambulatory until adulthood.
• Other dystrophinopathy phenotypes may present with the following:
  1. Exercise intolerance
  2. Myalgias
  3. Cramps
  4. Minimal limb-girdle weakness
  5. Quadriceps myopathy
  6. Symptoms of congestive heart failure (caused by dilated cardiomyopathy) without muscle weakness
• Incidental creatine kinase elevation may be the presenting feature in some forms.

■ **PHYSICAL EXAMINATION**
• Findings in DMD vary according to the stage of the disease and age of the child.
• A 16-month-old boy may not be walking independently.
  1. He pulls to stand slowly and with assistance.
  2. The neck flexors are weak.
  3. There is hypertrophy of the calf muscles.
• At 5 years of age, the boy has a waddling gait, slow toe-walking, and increased lumbar lordosis.
  1. He cannot run, stand, or hop on one foot.
  2. He has a Gower's sign when rising from supine or sitting.
  3. The heel cords may be tight, and the calf muscles are large.
  4. The proximal muscles in the upper limbs are mildly weak.
  5. The reflexes are depressed in the knees and normal elsewhere.
  6. Mental function may be delayed.
  7. The respiratory muscles have normal strength.
• The sensory examination is normal.
• Symptoms gradually worsen, and progression increases after 8 to 10 years.
  1. Scoliosis increases as the patient becomes wheelchair bound.
  2. The upper limbs and respiratory muscles get weaker.
  3. Deep tendon reflexes are lost.
• Most boys are confined to a wheelchair by 13 years of age.

• Respiratory failure is the most common cause of death.
• The mean age of death in DMD is 20 (± 3.9) years.
• BMD symptoms are milder and often are not noticeable until 8 to 9 years of age.
  1. The mean age of onset is about 12 years.
  2. If symptoms present before 8 years, the disease may be indistinguishable from DMD.
  3. The mean age at loss of ability to walk is in the fourth decade.
  4. Myocardium is often involved.

DIAGNOSIS

■ **DIFFERENTIAL DIAGNOSIS**
• Made on clinical grounds: a male with proximal muscle weakness and enlarged calves in the first 5 years of life
• Inflammatory myopathy (polymyositis)
• Congenital myopathy
• Other MDs: congenital muscular dystrophy, limb-girdle MD, and Emery-Dreyfuss
• Other etiologies of dilated cardiomyopathy

■ **DIAGNOSTIC WORKUP**
• Serum creatine kinase is elevated to more than 10 times the upper-normal levels.
• DNA analysis is done to search for deletions and duplications in the dystrophin gene.
  1. Very sensitive
  2. Identifies 65% of cases
  3. Done on white blood cells
• Muscle biopsy is done for immunoblotting assay of the dystrophin gene in the muscle.
  1. Will show abnormalities in more than 95% of patients with DMD.
  2. Immunostain of the muscle is done to look for absence of or decrease in dystrophin.
• Electromyogram is not necessary.
• Conductive cardiac abnormalities can be present.
  1. Electrocardiogram may show evidence of conduction abnormalities.
• Echocardiogram may show muscle dysfunction or dilation of the heart.

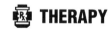 **THERAPY**

Should be provided by a multidisciplinary team with experience in treating children with neuromuscular disorders.

■ NONPHARMACOLOGIC

- Physical and occupational therapy to maintain mobility and independence as long as possible
  1. Provide adaptive equipment at home and school as needed to prolong ambulation.
- Orthopedic therapy
  1. Braces to assist with ambulation
  2. Body jacket to delay development of scoliosis contractures
  3. Prevention of joint contractures
- Respiratory therapy, especially in children who are wheelchair bound
- Special education with adaptive tools as needed
- Psychosocial therapy to provide emotional support and assistance to patients and families

■ MEDICAL

- Prednisone 0.75 mg/kg/day slows progression of weakness and increases the muscle mass.
  1. May begin as early as 5 years or when child is having noticeable difficulty with steps
  2. May stay on medication for years
  3. Side effects generally well tolerated
- Prompt antibiotic coverage for pulmonary infections is needed.
- Gene therapy may be available in the future.

■ SURGICAL

- Spinal fusion decreases progression of restrictive pulmonary disease and prolongs survival.
- Lengthening heel cords improves and maintains standing and walking.
- Be aware that some anesthetics may cause malignant hyperthermia.

■ FOLLOW-UP & DISPOSITION

- Periodic visits to the health care team are important: orthopedic surgeon, physical and occupational therapist, pulmonologist and respiratory therapist, cardiologist, and neurologist.
  1. The need for and timing of procedures, as well as the provision of devices, including a motorized wheelchair, is case based.
  2. Assess the need for adjustments in the orthotic devices, wheelchair, jacket, and so forth, to avoid pressure injuries in the skin.
- Ventilatory support either at night or continuously prolongs life.

■ PATIENT/FAMILY EDUCATION

- Emphasis should be placed on education and group support to the child and family.
- Participation in educational and recreational activities can be sought through nonprofit organizations, such as The Muscular Dystrophy Association.
- Carrier risk may be estimated by the following:
  1. Definite carrier: a female with an affected son and with either an affected brother or maternal uncle
  2. Probable carrier: a female with two or more affected sons without other known affected male relatives
  3. Possible carrier: a female with only one affected son or a female without an affected son but with an affected maternal male relative
- The same DNA, immunoblot, and immunostain tests used to diagnose affected children can be used for carrier detection.

- Prenatal diagnosis can be accomplished.
  1. Prenatal diagnosis can be done with affected sons in subsequent pregnancies of mothers with affected sons.
  2. DNA studies on chorionic villus sample can be done as early as 6 to 8 weeks postconception.

■ REFERRAL INFORMATION

All patients should be referred to a neuromuscular center with experience in treating children with muscular dystrophy.

○ PEARLS & CONSIDERATIONS

■ WEBSITE

Muscular Dystrophy Association: www.mdausa.org

REFERENCES

1. Bakker E, Van Ommen GJ: Duchenne and Becker muscular dystrophy. In Emery AH (ed): *Neuromuscular disorders: clinical and molecular genetics,* Chichester, England, 1998, John Wiley & Sons.
2. Griggs RC, Moxley RT, Mendell JR: Prednisone in DMD: a randomized controlled trial defining the time course and dose response, *Arch Neurol* 48:383, 1992.
3. Sansome A, Royston P, Dubowitz V: Steroids in Duchenne muscular dystrophy: pilot study of low-dosage schedule, *Neuromusc Disord* 3:567, 1993.

Author: **Carlos Torres, M.D.**

BASIC INFORMATION

■ **DEFINITION**
- Acquired myasthenia gravis (MG) is a disorder associated with acetylcholine receptor deficiency at the neuromuscular junction. The main symptoms of weakness and abnormal fatigue on exertion reflect functional failure of the neuromuscular transmission system. These symptoms improve by rest and anticholinesterase drugs.
- Transient neonatal myasthenia occurs in infants of mothers with MG. Symptoms appear within the first few hours after birth and include generalized weakness, poor suck, weak cry, and ptosis.

■ **SYNONYMS**
- Myasthenia
- MG

ICD-9CM CODE
358.0 Myasthenia gravis

■ **ETIOLOGY**
- MG is an autoimmune disorder, with antibodies against the acetylcholine receptors in the muscle that block the neuromuscular transmission. These antibodies are found in the serum in 80% to 90% of patients.
- MG is associated with autoimmune disorders (e.g., systemic lupus erythematosus, rheumatoid arthritis, polymyositis, thyrotoxicosis).
- Thymic hyperplasia is found in most patients; HLA-B8 and DR3 are present in most young females with MG.
  1. Thymoma is commonly seen in older patients with MG.
- Transient neonatal MG is caused by transplacental transfer of acetylcholine receptor antibodies from the mother to the fetus.

■ **EPIDEMIOLOGY & DEMOGRAPHICS**
- MG is the most common disorder of the neuromuscular junction.
- Although sporadic, 2% to 3% have a positive family history.
- Incidence is 1 in 20,000.
  1. In puberty, girls are more often affected than boys.
  2. Approximately 10% to 15% of neonates born to mothers with myasthenia develop symptoms.

■ **HISTORY**
- Insidious onset, chronic muscle weakness, and fatigability of some or all voluntary muscles may be present.
  1. Diplopia; usually the initial symptom and eventually seen in 90% of cases

2. Fatigue with routine physical activities
3. Shortness of breath
4. Difficulty swallowing
5. Slurred speech
- Symptoms may vary from day to day.
  1. Symptoms are usually worse with repeated or sustained exertion; at the end of the day; and with elevation of temperature, illness, emotional upset, and menses.
  2. Symptoms improve after rest.
- Symptoms can be transient, and spontaneous remissions can occur.

■ **PHYSICAL EXAMINATION**
- Unilateral or bilateral weakness of the external ocular muscles is present.
- Ptosis can be provoked by sustained upward gaze.
- Weakness of other voluntary muscles innervated by cranial nerves occurs.
  1. Droopy face
  2. Drooling
  3. Difficulty with chewing and swallowing
  4. Nasal voice, poor elevation of the soft palate
- Respiratory muscle weakness, shortness of breath, and weak cough are seen.
  1. Ask the patient to assume a sitting position and to take a deep breath and start counting as fast as possible without taking another breath.
  2. Normal children older than 10 years of age can count to more than 30.
- Proximal muscle weakness develops.
  1. Difficulty walking upstairs
  2. Difficulty standing from squatting, sitting, or supine position
  3. Note the Gower's sign
- No objective sensory deficits are noted.
- Deep tendon reflexes are normal.

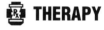 **DIAGNOSIS**

■ **DIFFERENTIAL DIAGNOSIS**
- Myasthenic syndromes
- Infantile botulism
- Oculopharyngeal dystrophy and mitochondrial myopathies
- Hypothyroidism
- Drug induced
  1. Aminoglycoside antibiotics: gentamicin, kanamycin, neomycin, streptomycin
  2. Cardiovascular drugs: quinidine, propanolol, procainamide, lidocaine, calcium channel blockers
  3. Hormonal agents: adrenocorticotropic hormone, thyroxine
  4. Penicillamine

- Hyperkalemic or hypokalemic periodic paralysis
- Guillain-Barré syndrome
- Tick paralysis
- Conversion reaction

■ **DIAGNOSTIC WORKUP**
- Diagnosis is made on clinical grounds and based on confirmatory tests.
- Confirmatory tests include the following:
  1. Elevated plasma acetylcholine receptor antibodies
  2. More than 10% decrement of the compound motor action potential amplitude in the 3 cps repetitive electrical stimulation test
  3. Intravenous edrophonium chloride (Tensilon) test
     a. Watch for immediate improvement of extraocular muscle strength.
     b. Use normal saline as a placebo control and at least two observers.
- Magnetic resonance imaging of the chest and neck is done to look for enlarged thymus and for ectopic locations of the thymus gland.
- Obtain pulmonology and respiratory therapy consultations.
  1. Measure the forced vital capacity.

℞ THERAPY

■ **NONPHARMACOLOGIC**
- Avoid hot environments and showers because heat slows neuromuscular transmission.
- Treat respiratory illness vigorously with physiotherapy.

■ **MEDICAL & SURGICAL**
- Oral pyridostigmine (anticholinesterase agent) may be used.
  1. Effects last for a few hours.
  2. Start with a small dose and gradually increase based on clinical response.
  3. Dose varies with the age.
- Prednisone and other immunosuppressant drugs may be given.
- Intravenous immunoglobulin therapy has replaced the use of plasmapheresis.
  1. Treats acute worsening of symptoms—myasthenic crisis
  2. Stabilizes respiratory function before or after surgery
- Thymectomy may be performed early in treatment.
- Search for ectopic glands and aim for complete resection.
- Treat vigorously, especially during crisis. Therapy may include temporary respiratory assistance, tracheostomy, or even gastrostomy.

1. Avoid drugs that may dampen the neuromuscular transmission (e.g., aminoglycosides, penicillamine, phenytoin, and psychotropic and cardiovascular drugs)
2. Check with a physician or pharmacist before administering drugs.

■ FOLLOW-UP & DISPOSITION
- Periodic visits should be made to monitor respiratory and swallowing functions.
  1. Frequent visits are needed during periods of illness or stress.
- If symptoms become less responsive to medications, check for the presence of residual thymus. A second surgical intervention may be necessary.

■ PATIENT/FAMILY EDUCATION
- Become familiar with the names of drugs that can worsen the symptoms.
- Avoid hot weather and showers.
- Be aware of symptoms associated with overdose of anticholinesterase medications.
  1. Increased weakness
  2. Salivation
  3. Bronchial secretions
- Notify physician of any rapid worsening of weakness or fatigue.

- Be aware of limitations in chewing and swallowing. Do not attempt to swallow solids, which may be difficult.
- Foster a normal life.
  1. Inform the school nurse, teachers, and close friends of the child's condition and possible limitations.
  2. Modify and adapt physical education to the child's needs.
  3. Wear an alert bracelet and have easy access to medical services.
- Enroll the child in recreational activities provided by organizations such as the Muscular Dystrophy Association.

■ REFERRAL INFORMATION
A patient with MG should be referred to a medical center with experience in the management of neuromuscular disorders.

☼ PEARLS & CONSIDERATIONS

■ CLINICAL PEARLS
- Check for the potential effect on the neuromuscular transmission before prescribing a new drug.

- MG should be strongly considered in a child with recent onset of diplopia, ptosis, bulbar muscle weakness, and fatigue.
- MG is a treatable and curable disorder that can be fatal if left untreated.

■ WEBSITE
Muscular Dystrophy Association: www.mdausa.org

■ SUPPORT GROUPS
Myasthenia Gravis Foundation chapters and local groups exist in many major cities.

REFERENCES
1. Drachman DB: Myasthenia gravis, review, *N Engl J Med* 330:1797, 1994.
2. Leshner RG: Myasthenia in infancy and childhood, Course 323, *Am Acad Neurol,* 21:33, 1993.
3. Misulis KE, Fenichel GM: Genetic forms of myasthenia gravis review, *Pediatr Neurol* 5:205, 1989.
4. Papazian O: Transient neonatal myasthenia gravis, *J Child Neurol* 7:135, 1992.

Author: **Carlos Torres, M.D.**

II

BASIC INFORMATION

■ DEFINITIONS
- *Drowning:* death from suffocation in water
- *Near-drowning:* survival, at least temporarily, after suffocation in water
- *Secondary drowning:* death occurring longer than 24 hours after submersion secondary to severe respiratory decompensation (adult respiratory distress syndrome [ARDS], pulmonary edema)
- *Immersion syndrome:* death following submersion in extremely cold water

■ SYNONYM
Submersion injury: injuries resulting from submersion in water

ICD-9CM CODES
994.1 Drowning and nonfatal submersion
518.5 Pulmonary insufficiency after trauma and surgery

■ ETIOLOGY
- Approximately 90% involve aspiration of fluid into lungs—usually less than 20 ml/kg.
- About 10% involve "dry drowning"—laryngospasm occurs, preventing aspiration of fluid.
- Fresh water inactivates surfactant, leading to alveolar collapse and pulmonary dysfunction.
- Salt water dilutes surfactant, leading to alveolar collapse and pulmonary dysfunction.
- Both salt and fresh water damage the basement membrane, leading to fluid shifts, ARDS, and pulmonary edema.
- The steps to death progress from aspiration of fluid to pulmonary dysfunction to hypoxemia to anoxic brain injury and cardiac decompensation to death.

■ EPIDEMIOLOGY & DEMOGRAPHICS
- Near-drowning accounts for 8000 deaths per year in the United States.
- It is the second most common cause of accidental death in children.
- Bimodal distribution is noted, most often affecting toddlers and adolescents.
- Toddlers most commonly drown in pools and bathtubs, occasionally toilets or buckets of water.
- Adolescents most commonly drown in larger bodies of water (e.g., lakes, rivers, ocean).
- Approximately 90% of drownings occur in fresh water.
- About 50% occur in swimming pools.
- Prognosis is poor for patients presenting to the emergency department comatose or with cardiopulmonary resuscitation (CPR) in progress.

■ HISTORY
- The following key historical data need to be obtained:
  1. Last time seen
  2. Estimated length of submersion
  3. Any possibility of diving-related injury (e.g., cervical spine injury)
  4. Any possibility of other associated trauma
  5. Ambient temperatures of water and air
  6. Appearance when pulled from water (e.g., limp, blue, apneic, pulseless)
  7. Resuscitation efforts at the scene and en route to hospital (mouth-to-mouth resuscitation, compressions, medications)
  8. Estimated length of time until CPR begun, length of CPR
  9. Any significant past medical history (e.g., seizures, asthma) or allergies
- Consider abuse or neglect (toddlers)—mechanism proposed in history should match actual physical findings.
- Consider associated drug or alcohol intoxication (adolescents).

■ PHYSICAL EXAMINATION
- Begin with ABCs (airway, breathing, circulation).
- Careful attention should be given to breath sounds, pulse oximetry, respiratory effort, and mental status.
- Serial examination of respiratory status is most important because patients can rapidly decompensate.

DIAGNOSIS

■ DIFFERENTIAL DIAGNOSIS
- Anoxic encephalopathy
- Cerebral edema
- Spinal cord injury
- Suspected child abuse and neglect
- Alcohol or drug intoxication
- Hypothermia
- Pneumonia, bacterial or viral
- Aspiration pneumonia

■ DIAGNOSTIC WORKUP
- Blood should be obtained for a complete blood count, chemistry panel (electrolytes, blood urea nitrogen, creatinine, glucose), and coagulation studies (prothrombin time, partial thromboplastin time, platelets, fibrinogen, and fibrin split products).
- Urine should be obtained for routine urinalysis and, if indicated, a toxicology screen.
- Follow serial chest radiographs.
- Monitor continuous pulse oximetry and, if indicated, obtain serial arterial blood gas analysis.
- If indicated, obtain cervical spine or other skeletal films.
- Computed tomography scan of the brain may be indicated for persistent altered mental status.

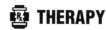

THERAPY

■ NONPHARMACOLOGIC
- Keep the patient warm and dry.
- Intubation and artificial ventilation may be necessary.
- Positive end-expiratory pressure or continuous positive airway pressure is indicated for refractory hypoxemia.

■ MEDICAL
- Give oxygen if warranted.
- Nebulized albuterol is indicated for bronchospasm.
- Furosemide (Lasix) may be indicated in the intensive care unit to maintain urine output and decrease fluid overload (cerebral edema).
- Muscle relaxation and sedation may be beneficial during the early phases of artificial ventilation.
- Advance life support drugs as per standard ACLS/PALS/APLS (Advance Cardiac Life Support/Pediatric Life Support/Advanced Pediatric Life Support) protocols.
- Steroids, prophylactic antibiotics, dexamethasone, and barbiturates *are no longer routinely recommended.*

■ SURGICAL
Extracorporeal membrane oxygenation has occasionally been used as a temporizing measure in extreme cases of refractory hypoxemia.

■ FOLLOW-UP & DISPOSITION
- Symptomatic patients should be admitted for observation.
- Completely asymptomatic patients may be safely discharged after observation for 4 to 6 hours.
- Patients with altered mental status, unstable vital signs, or significant hypoxemia should be admitted to a pediatric intensive care unit (PICU).

■ PATIENT/FAMILY EDUCATION
- Patients and families should be strictly warned against the following activities:
  1. Swimming unsupervised
  2. Using drugs or alcohol
  3. Diving into shallow or unknown waters
- Patients of suitable age should be instructed in swimming and water safety.

■ PREVENTIVE TREATMENT
- *Most drownings are preventable—PREVENTION IS KEY!*
- Toddlers should never be left alone near a body of water. This includes not only the swimming pool, but also the bathtub, toilet, or cleaning bucket of water.
- Residential pools should be surrounded on all four sides by a security fence and have an automatic closing security gate with locking latch.
- Parents and families should be taught CPR, particularly if they own a pool.

■ REFERRAL INFORMATION
PICU referrals described previously

☼ PEARLS & CONSIDERATIONS

■ CLINICAL PEARLS
- Asymptomatic patients should be observed for a minimum of 4 to 6 hours.
- Symptomatic patients should be admitted to the hospital.
- Serial examinations are most helpful.
- In toddlers, consider child abuse and neglect.
- In adolescents, consider cervical spine injury and intoxications.
- Deterioration in respiratory function may be sudden and dramatic.

■ WEBSITES
- Aloha.com: www.aloha.com/~lifeguards/kipc.html; drowning facts and prevention checklist
- City of Pasadena: www.ci.pasadena.ca.us/fire/poolsafety.ASP.html; swimming pool safety
- Department of Boating and Waterways: www.dbw.ca.gov/drown.htm; drowning prevention checklist
- WHHS, Haverford High School: www.whhs.org/NewWJHS/healthathome/drowning.asp; drowning prevention and first aid

■ SUPPORT GROUP
Drowning Prevention Project (Children's Medical Center of Seattle, WA in conjunction with the Head Injury Hotline): www.headinjury.com/linkdrown.htm

REFERENCES
1. American Academy of Pediatrics, Committee on Injury and Poison Prevention: Drowning in infants, children and adolescents, *Pediatrics* 92: 292, 1993.
2. Lavelle JM et al: Ten-year review of pediatric bathtub near drownings: evaluation for child abuse and neglect, *Ann Emerg Med* 25:344, 1995.
3. Modell JH: Treatment of near drowning: is there a role for HYPER therapy? *Crit Care Med* 14:593, 1986.
4. Modell JH: Drowning, *N Engl J Med* 328:253, 1993.
5. Orlowski JP: Drowning, near-drowning and ice water submersion, *Pediatr Clin North Am* 34:75, 1987.
6. Wintemute GJ: Childhood drowning and near-drowning in the United States, *Am J Dis Child* 144:663, 1990.
Author: **Mark A. Hostetler, M.D.**

BASIC INFORMATION

■ **DEFINITION**
Neonatal necrotizing enterocolitis (NEC) is acute inflammation and necrosis involving localized and multifocal areas of the small and large bowel mucosa in the newborn, more commonly preterm, infant.

ICD-9CM CODE
777.5 Necrotizing enterocolitis

■ **ETIOLOGY**
• Unknown, possibly related to one or more of the following factors:
  1. Bacterial invasion or overgrowth
  2. Impaired intestinal perfusion
  3. Rapid advancement of enteral feedings

■ **EPIDEMIOLOGY & DEMOGRAPHICS**
• NEC is primarily a disease of premature infants housed in modern neonatal intensive care units, but it occurs occasionally in term infants.
• NEC is reported in 6% of infants born at 1500 g or less.
• Age of onset is inversely proportional to gestational age at birth.
  1. Occurs in first few days in term infants
  2. Occurs at several weeks of age in premature infants
• Peak incidence is at 32 to 33 weeks' gestational age.
• NEC often occurs sporadically in mini-epidemics during times of high nursery census and acuity.
• Additional risk factors include the following:
  1. History of maternal cocaine use
  2. Hemodynamically significant patent ductus arteriosus
  3. Following double-volume exchange transfusions
  4. Perinatal asphyxia

■ **HISTORY**
• Decreased activity, lethargy
• Apnea, bradycardia, tachypnea, temperature instability, hypotension
• Hypoxemia
• Feeding intolerance, residuals, vomiting
• Occult and gross blood in stools
• Increasing abdominal girth

■ **PHYSICAL EXAMINATION**
• Vital sign instability, hypotension
• Decreased activity and tone
• Abdominal wall redness and discoloration
• Abdominal distention, decreased bowel sounds, and tenderness to palpation
• Decreased peripheral perfusion

■ **DIAGNOSIS**

■ **DIFFERENTIAL DIAGNOSIS**
• Bacterial and viral sepsis
• Midgut malrotation with volvulus
• Isolated ileal perforation

■ **DIAGNOSTIC WORKUP**
• Complete blood count
  1. Low absolute neutrophil count
  2. Increased band count
  3. Low hematocrit secondary to blood loss
  4. Thrombocytopenia
• Blood gas
• Metabolic acidosis
• Elevated C-reactive protein
• Blood culture often positive
• May develop disseminated intravascular coagulation with fibrin-split products and abnormally prolonged coagulation (elevated prothrombin time and partial thromboplastin time)
• Definite radiographic diagnosis: Bell stages II and III
• One or more of the following:
  1. Pneumatosis intestinalis
  2. Portal venous gas
  3. Intestinal perforation: free air in the peritoneum

■ **THERAPY**

■ **NONPHARMACOLOGIC**
• Place patient on "nothing-by-mouth" (NPO) orders with low intermittent suction of stomach.
  1. Use a double-lumen nasogastric tube (Replogle tube).
  2. Maintain NPO orders until at least 7 to 10 days after resumption of normal radiograph.

■ **MEDICAL**
• Pay careful attention to blood pressure, perfusion, and urine output.
• Administer volume expanders (normal saline, fresh frozen plasma, and blood) to maintain hemodynamic stability.
• Administer packed red cells to maintain hematocrit at 40% to 45%.
• Administer platelet transfusions to maintain platelet count greater than 50,000/mm³.
• After blood culture is drawn, initiate antibiotic coverage for gram-positive, gram-negative, and anaerobic organisms.
  1. Combination of ampicillin, aminoglycoside (gentamicin), or cefotaxime, and clindamycin or Flagyl
• Provide parenteral nutrition.
  1. Prolonged period of enteral feeding cessation necessitates parenteral nutrition.

■ **SURGICAL**
• Intestinal perforation requires immediate surgical intervention.
• Failure of medical management with persistent metabolic acidosis, hypotension, and thrombocytopenia may require surgical intervention to remove necrotic gut tissue.
• Surgical interventions depend on distribution, extent, and severity of bowel necrosis.
  1. Intestinal resection followed by primary intestinal anastomosis
  2. Enterostomy with or without intestinal resection

■ **FOLLOW-UP & DISPOSITION**
• Have the patient complete a 10-day course of antibiotic therapy.
• Maintain NPO status for at least 7 to 10 days after documentation of a normal abdominal radiograph.
• Cholestatic jaundice may result from the prolonged use of total parenteral nutrition.
• Intestinal strictures, usually colonic, may develop in patients with or without surgery during the acute phase.
  1. Feeding intolerance develops with reinstitution of feeds.
  2. The diagnosis is made with lower or upper intestinal radiograph contrast studies.
  3. Surgical resection is required.
• Short bowel syndrome may develop after the resection of extensive areas of bowel.

■ **PREVENTIVE TREATMENT**
Breastmilk feedings, when compared with milk formulas, are partially protective for the prevention of NEC.

✪ **PEARLS & CONSIDERATIONS**

■ **CLINICAL PEARLS**
"NEC is a riddle wrapped in a mystery inside an enigma."

REFERENCES
1. Kliegman RM: Pathophysiology and epidemiology of NEC. In Polin RA, Fox WW (eds): *Fetal and neonatal physiology,* Philadelphia, 1999, WB Saunders.
2. Kliegman RM (ed): Issue on NEC, *Clin Perinatol* 2:21, 1994.
3. Neu J, Weiss MD: NEC: pathophysiology and prevention, *J Parent Ent Nutr* 23:S13, 1999.
Author: **James W. Kendig, M.D.**

BASIC INFORMATION

■ **DEFINITION**

Nephrotic syndrome (NS) is characterized by proteinuria (more than 40 mg/m^2/hr), hypoalbuminemia (less than 2.5 g/dl), edema, and hypercholesterolemia. Primary NS is a disease involving only the kidney and is not associated with extrarenal manifestations. Secondary NS occurs as a manifestation of systemic disease, which involves the kidney (e.g., systemic lupus erythematosus [SLE], Henoch-Schönlein purpura [HSP], sickle cell anemia, acute poststreptococcal glomerulonephritis [GN]). This section deals with primary NS.

■ **SYNONYMS**
- Minimal-change nephrotic syndrome
- Minimal-change disease
- Lipoid nephrosis
- Idiopathic nephrotic syndrome
- Nil disease

ICD-9CM CODES
581.9 Nephrotic syndrome, not otherwise specified
581.3 Minimal-change nephrotic syndrome (MCNS)
581.1 Focal segmental glomerulosclerosis (FSGS)
581.2 Membranoproliferative glomerulonephritis (MPGN)
581.1 Membranous nephropathy

■ **ETIOLOGY**
- The cause is unknown in primary NS.
- Evidence suggests abnormal T-cell function in MCNS.
  1. Responds to immunomodulatory medications, such as prednisone
  2. Relapses often associated with upper respiratory and other minor illness
  3. Improves after measles
  4. Increased frequency of atopy and allergies in children with MCNS
  5. Associated with Hodgkin's lymphoma
- Secondary NS
  1. SLE
  2. HSP
  3. Sickle cell anemia
  4. Acute poststreptococcal GN

■ **EPIDEMIOLOGY & DEMOGRAPHICS**
- Incidence is estimated at approximately 5 per 100,000.
- In young children, the male:female ratio is 2:1.
- In adolescents, the male:female ratio is 1:1.
- Eighty percent of nephrotic children are younger than 6 years of age.

- NS is rare in the first year of life.
  1. NS in first year of life: congenital or infantile type
     a. Congenital typically presents in first 3 months of life.
     b. Most are inherited in autosomal recessive fashion.
- MCNS
  1. MCNS accounts for 60% to 90% of NS cases in children.
     a. MCNS accounts for approximately 90% of cases in children younger than 7 years of age.
     b. MCNS accounts for 50% of cases of NS in older children, when other diagnoses become more prevalent.
  2. Gross hematuria is rare with MCNS.
  3. Microscopic hematuria is present in 30%.
  4. Hypertension is present in 30%.
  5. Only 10% have both hematuria and hypertension.
  6. Renal function is usually normal at onset.
  7. Generally, MCNS is steroid responsive.
- FSGS
  1. FSGS is not a single disease but rather represents a reaction of the glomerulus to various insults.
  2. It accounts for approximately 10% of children with NS.
  3. Incidence increases with increasing age.
  4. Thirty percent of patients respond to steroids.
  5. FSGS accounts for approximately 40% of children whose proteinuria persists after 8 weeks of therapy.
- MPGN
  1. Patients often have a low C3.
  2. Likelihood of gross hematuria, azotemia, and hypertension at onset is higher than with MCNS.
  3. A small chance of spontaneous remission exists.
  4. Treatment with steroids is controversial.
  5. Fifty percent of patients progress to renal failure in 10 years.
- Membranous nephropathy
  1. Membranous nephropathy is the most common cause of NS in adults.
  2. It is rare in childhood, accounting for 2% to 5% of children with NS.
  3. Prognosis in children is better than adults; 50% have spontaneous remission.

■ **PATHOPHYSIOLOGY**
- Proteinuria
  1. Alterations in glomerular capillary wall permeability result in increased protein filtration.

  2. The cause of altered permeability varies with disease process.
     a. In MCNS, the negative charge that is normally present on the glomerular capillary wall is lost or neutralized.
     b. The negative charge repels albumin/protein, thereby limiting albumin/protein loss into the urine.
     c. Albumin is the major protein lost in MCNS.
     d. Other proteins that are lost include immunoglobulin G (IgG), thyroxin-binding globulin, transferrin, alternative complement factor B, and antithrombin III.
- Hypoalbuminemia
  1. Results from increased urinary loss of protein
- Edema
  1. Caused by transudation of fluid from the intravascular space to the interstitium
  2. Results from salt and water retention and occurs in combination with hypoalbuminemia (decreased oncotic pressure)
- Hypercholesterolemia
  1. This condition results from increased synthesis as the liver tries to increase albumin production.
  2. Decreased clearance of cholesterol also occurs because of decreased activity of the lipoprotein lipase.

■ **HISTORY**
- Recent history of upper respiratory infection or other viral illness
- History of allergies
- Edema
  1. Insidious onset; often first noted in periorbital region in the morning
  2. May be present for weeks
  3. Often thought to be related to allergies
  4. Progresses to lower extremities, abdomen, and can become generalized
- Respiratory difficulty
  1. Suggests pulmonary edema or pleural effusions
- Decreased urine output
- Gross hematuria: unusual with MCNS
- Weight gain
- Anorexia
- Diarrhea (can result from edema of the intestinal wall)
- Vomiting
  1. May occur and lead to a sudden decrease in intravascular volume, or
  2. May be caused by peritonitis
- Abdominal pain seen with peritonitis
- Headaches
  1. Headaches may suggest associated hypertension.

■ PHYSICAL EXAMINATION
- Signs of intravascular volume depletion
  1. Tachycardia
  2. Hypotension
  3. Poor perfusion
  4. Dry mucous membranes
  5. Orthostatic changes
- Signs of volume overload
  1. Periorbital edema
  2. Decreased breath sounds, which suggest pleural effusions
  3. Rales, which suggest pulmonary edema
  4. Ascites
  5. Presacral edema, scrotal/labial edema
  6. Peripheral edema
  7. Facial edema difficult to assess if you have never seen the child before
     a. Often helpful to compare current appearance with a preillness photograph
- Signs of peritonitis
  1. Abdominal pain
  2. Distention
  3. Rebound
  4. Guarding
  5. Tenderness
  6. Absence of bowel sounds
- Signs of skin breakdown
  1. Infection can spread quickly in nephrotic children.
- Presence of rash or joint swelling
  1. May suggest that the disease is a secondary form of NS

▲ DIAGNOSIS

■ DIFFERENTIAL DIAGNOSIS
- Differential of the various forms of NS is discussed within this section.
- Other renal diseases with edema include acute and chronic renal failure and nephrotic-nephritic syndromes.
- Other causes of edema include the following:
  1. Protein loss states (e.g., protein-losing enteropathy)
  2. Decreased protein production (e.g., liver disease, liver failure)
  3. Congestive heart failure

■ DIAGNOSTIC WORKUP
- Proteinuria
  1. Urinalysis with 3 to 4+ on dipstick
  2. Spot urine protein:creatinine ratio higher than 1.0 suspicious
  3. Protein excretion on timed urine collection of more than 40 mg/m^2/hr
- Hypoalbuminemia less than 2.5 g/dl
- Hyperlipidemia
- Other laboratory markers
  1. Low-normal serum creatinine suggests hyperfiltration secondary to proteinuria.

2. Elevated serum creatinine may be caused by decreased renal perfusion.
3. Hypocalcemia:
   a. Low because of hypoalbuminemia
   b. Ionized calcium normal
4. Hemoglobin may be elevated secondary to hemoconcentration in intravascular volume depletion.
5. C3 is normal.
   a. If low, suggests MPGN
6. Antinuclear antibodies and streptozyme are negative in idiopathic NS.

■ COMPLICATIONS
- Infection
  1. Before 1950, infection accounted for 50% of deaths from NS.
  2. Risk factors include hypogammaglobulinemia and a defect in the alternative complement pathway. Treatment with steroids or other cytotoxic agents is indicated.
  3. Spontaneous bacterial peritonitis:
     a. Most common organism is *Streptococcus pneumoniae,* but gram-negative rods such as *Escherichia coli* are also causative.
     b. If patients have one episode, the risk of recurrence increases.
     c. Antibiotic prophylaxis is not proven effective for prevention.
     d. Patients should receive Pneumovax when they are able to mount an immunologic response.
  4. Cellulitis can spread quickly because edema separates fascial planes.
- Thrombosis: hypercoagulable state results from the following:
  1. Loss of antithrombin III in urine
  2. Increased platelet aggregation
  3. Intravascular volume depletion
  4. Acute renal failure: consequence of acute tubular necrosis secondary to severe hypovolemia

℞ THERAPY

■ NONPHARMACOLOGIC
- Low-salt diet
- Recommended daily allowance (RDA) for protein intake
- Generally not fluid restricted unless severe edema, congestive heart failure, severe hyponatremia
- Relatively low-fat diet for prophylaxis for patients at risk for atherosclerosis

■ MEDICAL
- Corticosteroids may be given.
  1. Initial episode
     a. Dosage is 2 mg/kg/day or 60 mg/m^2/day (maximum,

80 mg) divided two to three times per day for 4 to 6 weeks.
     b. If the patient responded and is in remission and the urine is negative for protein for 3 consecutive days, change regimen to alternate-day steroids: 2 mg/kg every other day or 40 mg/m^2 every other day for 4 to 6 weeks.
     c. Then taper off if the patient continues in remission.
  2. Side effects
     a. Increased appetite, weight gain, change in appearance, moodiness/behavior changes, hypertension, infection, acne, cataracts, poor growth, osteopenia, ulcers, glucose intolerance, avascular necrosis
     b. Rare but serious side effects: pseudotumor cerebri, steroid psychosis, and steroid-related diabetes
  3. Relapses: urine protein excretion 2+ or higher on dipstick for 3 consecutive days
     a. This often occurs with illness and may spontaneously remit within a few days.
     b. Conservatively manage for a few days with close observation without steroids if child is otherwise doing well and has no edema.
     c. If no spontaneous remission, restart prednisone at 60 mg/m^2/day (maximum, 80 mg) divided two to three times per day until urine is protein free for 3 consecutive days. Then change to alternate-day prednisone and begin to taper.
- Other immunosuppressants to consider after consultation with or referral to a pediatric nephrologist include the following:
  1. If frequent relapser: two or more relapses within 6 months of initial response or four or more relapses in a 12-month period
  2. If steroid dependent: two consecutive relapses occurring while on steroids or within 14 days of completion of course
  3. If steroid resistant: no response after 4 weeks of prednisone at dose of 60 mg/m^2/day (maximum, 80 mg/day)
- Alkylating agents may also be considered.
  1. Cytoxan for steroid-dependent NS patients or frequent relapsers with goal of inducing remission and decreasing steroid toxicity
     a. Dosage is 2 mg/kg/day for 8 to 12 weeks
     b. Adverse effects include bone marrow suppression, infection, alopecia, infertility (dose related), risk for neoplasm, hemorrhagic cystitis

c. Instruct patients to drink lots of fluid and void frequently.

d. Check complete blood count with differential each week.

e. Remission may range from days to years.

2. Chlorambucil

a. Dosage is 0.1 to 0.2 mg/kg/day for 8 weeks.

b. Side effects are similar to those of Cytoxan but may have a higher incidence of malignancy.

3. Pulse Solu-Medrol with or without a cytotoxic agent

a. Dosage is 30 mg/kg intravenously Solu-Medrol (maximum, 1 g given three times per week for first 2 weeks and then tapered over 18 months).

b. Side effects are the same as those for prednisone. In addition, a risk of hypertension and arrhythmia during intravenous infusion exists.

- Cyclosporine may be needed.

1. Refer to a nephrologist for consideration of use in patients with steroid toxicity, steroid dependence, or steroid resistance.

2. Results are generally better if given with alternate-day prednisone used initially.

3. Adverse effects include immunosuppression, nephrotoxicity, and hypertension.

4. Perform a renal biopsy before initiation of therapy.

5. Monitor serum creatinine, cyclosporine level, and blood pressure very closely. In addition, potassium may rise and magnesium may fall.

6. May achieve partial or complete remission, but remission tends to be short lived after discontinuation of cyclosporine.

- Edema management is as follows:

1. Diuretics

a. Either furosemide (1 to 2 mg/kg/day) or chlorothiazide (10 mg/kg twice a day) can be used.

b. Furosemide is not as effective if severe hypoalbuminemia is present.

c. Monitor electrolytes for hyponatremia and hypokalemia.

d. A risk of severe intravascular volume depletion exists with aggressive diuresis.

2. Twenty-five percent albumin used for severe edema, hypovolemia, poor renal perfusion

a. The dosage is 0.5 to 1 g/kg intravenously once or twice per day.

b. Give slowly over several hours and monitor patients closely because albumin may precipitate congestive heart failure and pulmonary edema.

c. Albumin often is given in conjunction with 1 to 2 mg/kg furosemide.

- Hypertension management is indicated if blood pressure is persistently greater than 95% for age and height.

1. Consider use of angiotensin-converting enzyme (ACE) inhibitor in a patient with a chronic course.

a. ACE inhibitors can decrease proteinuria in addition to controlling blood pressure.

b. Monitor creatinine and potassium,

c. Be cautious with use in patients with poor renal perfusion.

- Management of hyperlipidemia is as follows:

1. Ideal treatment is to induce remission, which leads to resolution of hyperlipidemia.

2. Provide dietary advice.

3. In patients in whom remission is not achieved, consider use of lipid-lowering agents.

- Infection prophylaxis is as follows:

1. Pneumovax is recommended and should ideally be given once in remission.

a. Revaccination after 3 to 5 years is recommended.

b. Antibody levels may fall during relapse, and patient may be susceptible to pneumococcal infection.

2. Prevnar may also be given.

3. For varicella-zoster exposure:

a. If antibody status is negative, administer varicella-zoster immune globulin (VZIG) within 96 hours of exposure.

b. Decrease prednisone to <1 mg/kg/day during incubation period.

c. If patient develops chickenpox, start acyclovir.

4. Varicella-zoster vaccine (VZV) should be considered in seronegative children.

a. Immunization may occur once the prednisone dose is less than 2 mg/kg/day or 20 mg/day (if patient weighs more than 10 kg).

b. Some experts recommend waiting until the patient is off prednisone for 2 weeks, if possible.

c. The Pediatric Nephrology Panel of the National Kidney Foundation Conference on Proteinuria, Albuminuria, Risk, Assessment, Detection, and Elimination (PARADE) has made no recommendations regarding VZV vaccine.

5. Live vaccines should not be given to patients taking high-dose prednisone or other immunosuppressive medications.

- Consider hospital admission for the following conditions:

1. Hypertension

2. Cardiopulmonary compromise such as congestive heart failure or pleural effusions

3. Oliguria

4. Severe edema or anasarca

5. Skin breakdown

6. Fever because of concern for peritonitis, cellulitis, pneumonia, or other generalized infection

7. Significant intravascular volume depletion

- Consider biopsy for the following situations:

1. Pretreatment

a. Children younger than 1 year of age

b. Children older than 10 years before initiating steroids

c. Presence of low C3

d. Presence of gross hematuria

e. Associated renal failure

2. Posttreatment

a. Steroid resistant

b. Frequent relapser

■ FOLLOW-UP & PATIENT/FAMILY EDUCATION

- Monitor urine for remission and relapses.

1. Check urine at home with dipsticks or sulfosalicylic acid (SSA) daily.

2. Remission occurs when urine is negative to trace for protein for 3 consecutive days.

3. Relapse occurs when urine has 2+ or higher protein by dipstick after a period of remission.

a. Relapses tend to occur with illnesses; therefore it is recommended to check urine daily during illness.

b. Daily testing of urine can allow detection of relapse before patient becomes symptomatic.

- Symptoms and signs requiring medical attention are as follows:

1. Abdominal pain

2. Fever

3. Respiratory distress

4. Poor urine output

5. Increasing edema

- Review the potential medical complications of NS as outlined previously.

- Review the side effects of medications.

- Discuss chickenpox exposure and how to handle this situation.

- Discuss vaccination schedule.

- Provide low-salt dietary counseling.

- Discuss the natural history and course of disease.

1. NS is a chronic illness with remissions and relapses.

2. In MCNS, it may take 1 to 2 weeks to see a response to prednisone therapy.

a. Approximtely 93% respond to

steroids during the initial 8-week course.
 (1) Response by 2 weeks: 70%
 (2) Response by 4 weeks: 90%
 (3) Nonrelapsers: 36%
 (4) Infrequent relapsers: 18%
 (5) Frequent relapsers: 39%
 (6) Become subsequent nonre-sponders and are at risk for having FSGS: 5%
 b. Approximately 7% are initial nonresponders.
 (1) Proteinuria eventually dis-appears, often spontane-ously or with use of medications, in 5%.
 (2) Two percent are nonre-sponders; at risk for FSGS.
 c. Long-term prognosis is gener-ally excellent if patients respond to initial prednisone therapy.
 (1) Approximately 20% of steroid-responsive patients relapse for more than 15 years.
 (2) Patients relapsing into adulthood often had onset before age 6 years.

■ REFERRAL INFORMATION

All children with NS should be referred to a pediatric nephrologist for consul-tation and management in conjunc-tion with the primary care physician.

☼ PEARLS & CONSIDERATIONS

■ CLINICAL PEARLS

Remember that the patient may be total body fluid overloaded and yet be intravascularly hypovolemic.

■ WEBSITE

National Kidney Foundation: www.kidney.org/general/news/nephrotic.cfm

■ SUPPORT GROUPS

• NephKids is an email discussion group for parents of children with kidney disease. To subscribe, email the message "subscribe nephkids" to majordomo@ualberta.ca.
• KidTalk is an email list for children with renal disease: http://home.nycap.rr.com/jazzer/kidtalk.html.

• Local chapters of the National Kidney Foundation can also be found in many areas.

REFERENCES

1. Barratt TM, Clark G: Minimal change nephrotic syndrome and focal seg-mental glomerulosclerosis. In Holliday MA, Barratt TM, Avner ED (eds): *Pedi-atric nephrology*, ed 3, Baltimore, 1994, Williams & Wilkins.
2. Falk RJ, Jennette JC, Nachman PH: Primary glomerular diseases. In Brenner BM, Rector FC (eds): *Brenner and Rector's the kidney*, ed 6, Philadel-phia, 2000, WB Saunders.
3. Hogg RJ et al: Evaluation and manage-ment of proteinuria and nephrotic syndrome in children: recommenda-tions from a pediatric nephrology panel established at the National Kidney Foundation Conference on Proteinuria, Albuminuria, Risk, Assess-ment, Detection, and Elimination (PARADE), *Pediatrics* 105:1242, 2000.
4. Kelsch RC, Sedman AB: Nephrotic syn-drome, *Pediatr Rev* 14:30, 1993.

Author: **Ayesa Mian, M.D.**

BASIC INFORMATION

■ DEFINITION
Neuroblastoma is a highly variable and complex malignancy that arises from primitive neural crest cells populating the adrenal medulla and paravertebral sympathetic ganglion chain. The tumor is highly capricious in its behavior, ranging from spontaneous involution to rapid growth, widespread metastases, and death. Ganglioneuroblastoma and ganglioneuroma are less common, but more benign, differentiated variants of neuroblastoma.

ICD-9CM CODES
M9500/3 Neuroblastoma
194.0   Unspecified site

■ ETIOLOGY
- Embryonal tumor arising from primitive neural crest cells in the distribution of the adrenal medulla and paravertebral sympathetic chain
- Associated with chromosomal changes, including *N-MYC* oncogene amplification, chromosome 1p deletion, and gain of chromosome 16 segment
- No known environmental cause
- Familial variants occur but are rare

■ EPIDEMIOLOGY & DEMOGRAPHICS
- Neuroblastomas account for approximately 8% to 10% of childhood cancers.
- Incidence is 8 per 1 million per year (500 new cases in the United States annually).
- The median age at diagnosis is 22 months.
  1. Younger than 1 year of age: 36%
  2. Younger than 4 years of age: 79%
  3. Younger than 10 years of age: 97%
- Approximately 65% have a primary tumor in the abdomen or pelvis, 15% in the thorax, and 5% in the neck.
- Approximately 35% of patients have localized disease at presentation; 65% have metastases.

■ HISTORY
- Infants: bluish, bruiselike nodules on the skin, rapid breathing, poor oral intake, distended abdomen
- Older children: abdominal pain and distention but otherwise healthy; cough, shortness of breath with thoracic tumor; leg weakness with paravertebral extension of tumor into spinal canal
  1. Occasionally, an asymptomatic child is diagnosed by an incidental finding on chest radiograph.

- Metastatic disease: firm, nontender lumps on the neck, bone pain, proptosis, "raccoon eyes," fever, weight loss, malaise
- Paraneoplastic syndromes: jerking of arms and legs (myoclonus), irregular movements of eyes (opsoclonus), diarrhea

■ PHYSICAL EXAMINATION
- Infants
  1. Respiratory distress
  2. Bluish, palpable subcutaneous nodules
  3. Massive hepatomegaly
  4. Occasionally swollen lower extremities, swollen feet
- Older children
  1. Large, firm, nontender or mildly tender abdominal mass
  2. Decreased lower extremity strength (with spinal cord compression)
- Metastatic disease
  1. Pallor
  2. Cachexia
  3. Petechiae with bone marrow involvement
  4. Horner syndrome with cervical involvement
  5. Firm, nonmobile supraclavicular/cervical adenopathy
  6. Proptosis/periorbital ecchymoses with orbital involvement
- Paraneoplastic syndromes
  1. Myoclonus
  2. Opsoclonus

⚲ DIAGNOSIS

Based on histopathologic diagnosis of neuroblastoma in tumor tissue or presence of tumor cells in bone marrow plus elevated urinary catecholamines

■ DIFFERENTIAL DIAGNOSIS
- Abdominal mass: Wilms' tumor, lymphoma, rhabdomyosarcoma, germ cell tumor
- Lymphadenopathy and bone disease: leukemia, lymphoma, bone metastases
- Diarrhea: infectious causes
- Opsoclonus/myoclonus: primary neurologic disorder

■ DIAGNOSTIC WORKUP
- Radiograph of the chest and abdomen to assess for calcified mass
- Computed tomography scan of the neck/chest/abdomen/pelvis: calcified mass replacing adrenal gland or a long paravertebral sympathetic ganglion chain; extrinsic to kidney; often infiltrative and crossing the midline
- Bone scan/skeletal survey: may reveal lytic lesions caused by bone metastases

- Bone marrow aspirate/biopsy: may reveal bone marrow disease
- Spine magnetic resonance imaging to assess for spinal cord compression resulting from extension of paravertebral tumor through the neural foramina
- MIBG scan: nuclear study that detects primary tumor and metastases
- Laboratory studies: complete blood count, differential, platelet count, chemistries, lactate dehydrogenase, ferritin
- Urine catecholamines: urine homovanillic acid and vanillylmandelic acid elevated in 85% to 90% of children with neuroblastoma

■ STAGING
- The most widely used staging system is the International Neuroblastoma Staging System (INSS), based on surgical staging and examination of lymph nodes:
  1. Stage 1: completely resected, localized disease
  2. Stage 2A: incompletely removed localized tumor
  3. Stage 2B: completely or incompletely removed tumor with positive ipsilateral lymph nodes
  4. Stage 3: tumor crossing the midline
  5. Stage 4: any primary with distant metastases
  6. Stage 4S: localized primary tumor plus metastases to the liver, skin, or bone marrow in a child younger than 1 year of age

■ PROGNOSTIC FACTORS
- Predictors of poor outcome: age older than 1 year, stage 4 disease, and a variety of tumor-specific markers (DNA index 1, amplification of *N-MYC* oncogene, poor risk by Shimada pathology classification)
- Predictors of good outcome: age younger than 1 year; stage 1, 2, or 4S disease; tumor-specific markers (DNA index greater than 1, nonamplification of *N-MYC* oncogene)

▣ THERAPY

- Therapy consists of varying combinations of surgery, radiation, and chemotherapy.
- In addition, newer approaches include high-dose chemotherapy with autologous stem cell rescue, differentiating agents, radiolabeled antitumor monoclonal antibodies, and tumor vaccines.
- Patients are stratified into low-risk, intermediate-risk, and high-risk groups according to age, stage, and *N-MYC* status; treatment is based on the risk group.

II

■ LOW RISK

- Treatment in this group is generally surgery only.
    1. Children of any age with stage 1 or 2A disease
    2. Children younger than 1 year of age with stage 2B or nonamplified N-MYC 4S disease
    3. Children older than 1 year of age with nonamplified N-MYC, favorable histology stage 2B disease
- Chemotherapy and/or radiotherapy in children with stage 4S disease is controversial.

■ INTERMEDIATE RISK

- Treatment is moderately aggressive chemotherapy (cyclophosphamide, doxorubicin, carboplatin [or cisplatin], etoposide).
    1. Children younger than 1 year of age with stage 3, 4, or 4S disease and nonamplified N-MYC
    2. Children older than 1 year of age with stage 3, nonamplified N-MYC
- Radiation is reserved for patients with incomplete response to chemotherapy.
- Treatment of infants with stage 4S disease is controversial, consisting of short-course chemotherapy or low-dose radiation for symptomatic children (e.g., respiratory distress caused by massive hepatomegaly).

■ HIGH RISK

- Treatment is aggressive, consisting of intensive chemotherapy followed by high-dose chemotherapy with autologous stem cell rescue, radiation to sites of residual disease, and cis-retinoic acid.
    1. Children older than 1 year of age with stage 4 disease
    2. Children older than 1 year of age with stage 3 disease and amplified N-MYC
    3. Children younger than 1 year of age with stage 3, 4, or 4S disease with amplified N-MYC

■ FOLLOW-UP & DISPOSITION

- Cure rates are as follows:
    1. Low-risk group: greater than 90% 5-year survival
    2. Intermediate-risk group: 55% to 90% 4-year survival
    3. High-risk group: 40% 4-year survival
- The risk of recurrence is highest in the first 3 years after diagnosis.
- Treatment and follow-up should be a careful, coordinated effort of a tertiary care team consisting of a pediatric surgeon, pediatric oncologist, and pediatric radiation oncologist.
- Imaging studies of sites of disease should be done every 3 to 6 months during the first several years after completion of therapy.

■ PATIENT/FAMILY EDUCATION

- Neuroblastoma is a highly variable and complex disease.
- The treatment plan should be formulated and implemented by a team of pediatric surgeons, pediatric oncologists, and pediatric radiation oncologists.
- Opinions among physicians regarding management may differ because many cases are complex and unique.
- Most children with stage 1 to 3 disease are cured; most older children with stage 4 disease are not.

■ PREVENTIVE TREATMENT

- Screening for neuroblastoma is conducted in several countries, but not routinely in the United States.
- Screening consists of analysis of urine for catecholamines and is typically done in infants at ages 3 weeks, 6 months, and 12 months.
- Screening has been shown to result in increased detection of low-risk disease, but it does not increase detection or improve outcome of children with high-risk disease.

■ REFERRAL INFORMATION

Children suspected of this diagnosis should be referred promptly to a pediatric oncology team (pediatric surgeon, pediatric oncologist, and radiation oncologist).

⚙ PEARLS & CONSIDERATIONS

■ CLINICAL PEARLS

- Neuroblastoma in infants (even with stage 4S disease) can spontaneously regress.
- Heterochromia iridis or Horner's syndrome can be a presentation for neuroblastoma.
- Neuroblastoma can present as hydrops fetalis.

■ WEBSITES

- Association of Cancer Online Resources: www.acor.org
- Children's Cancer Web: www.cancerindex.org/ccw
- The Neuroblastoma Children's Cancer Foundation: www.cncf-childcancer.org

REFERENCES

1. Brodeur GM, Castleberry RP: Neuroblastoma. In Pizzo PA, Poplack DG (eds): *Principles and practice of pediatric oncology*, Philadelphia, 1997, Lippincott-Raven.
2. Constine LS, Schwartz CL, Korones DN: Neuroblastoma. In Williams J, Rubin P (eds): *Pediatric solid tumors in clinical oncology*, ed 8, Philadelphia, 2001, WB Saunders.

Author: **David N. Korones, M.D.**

BASIC INFORMATION

■ DEFINITION
Neurofibromatosis is a neurocutaneous syndrome in which tumors of the central or peripheral nervous system, called *neurofibromas,* are accompanied by a variable degree of pigmentary changes and systemic problems. There are two major types of neurofibromatosis, type I (NF1) and type II (NF2), both of which follow the autosomal dominant mode of inheritance. NF2 is most commonly seen in adults and rarely encountered in the pediatric population and is not included here.

■ SYNONYMS
- von Recklinghausen's disease
- Peripheral neurofibromatosis

ICD-9CM CODE
237.71 Neurofibromatosis

■ ETIOLOGY
- NF1 is caused by mutation in a gene on chromosome 17q11.2 that codes for the protein neurofibromin.
- The NF1 gene is a tumor-suppressor gene, mutation of which results in uncontrolled or poorly controlled cell growth.

■ EPIDEMIOLOGY & DEMOGRAPHICS
- NF1 is the most common neurocutaneous syndrome.
- The incidence is 1 in 4000.
- About 30% of cases are new mutations and therefore have no previous family history.

■ HISTORY
- The most common presentation is the appearance of multiple café-au-lait spots in infancy or early childhood.
  1. Café-au-lait spots may increase in number and intensity with age.
- Cutaneous neurofibromas tend to start during puberty or pregnancy.
- Plexiform neurofibroma, which involves the nerve plexus, often presents early in life.
  1. Symptoms depend on the location.
  2. A large mass on the thigh or a deformation of the face is common.
- Congenital bowing of long bones occurs.
  1. Usually the tibia
  2. May be accompanied by pseudoarthrosis
- There is often a positive family history.
- Peripheral neurofibromas appear.
- Axillary freckling is present.
- Learning disability is possible.

- Ptosis may be seen.
- Visual disturbance may occur.

■ PHYSICAL EXAMINATION
- Diagnosis requires meeting two or more of the following criteria:
  1. Six or more café-au-lait macules over 5 mm in greatest diameter in children, and over 15 mm in adults
  2. Two or more neurofibromas of any type or one plexiform neurofibroma (imaging study may confirm examination finding)
  3. Axillary or inguinal freckling
  4. Optic glioma
  5. Two or more Lisch nodules (iris hamartomas)
  6. Osseous lesion such as sphenoid dysplasia, thinning of the cortex in the long bones, with or without pseudoarthrosis (imaging study confirms suspicious physical examination finding)
  7. A first-degree relative (parent, sibling or offspring) with NF1 by the previously listed criteria
- Other findings may include the following:
  1. Plexiform neurofibroma
     a. Ptosis
     b. Facial asymmetry
     c. Clitoromegaly
  2. Macrocephaly with or without intracranial mass
  3. Areolar neurofibroma
  4. Hypopigmentation
  5. Nevi

🔬 DIAGNOSIS

■ DIFFERENTIAL DIAGNOSIS
Other conditions with café-au-lait (or café-au-lait–like) spots
- NF2 (acoustic neuroma)
- McCune Albright syndrome (polyostotic fibrous dysplasia, precocious puberty)
- Russell-Silver syndrome (short stature, craniofacial disproportion, asymmetry)
- Bloom syndrome (photosensitivity, short stature)
- Ataxia-telangiectasia
- Other neurocutaneous syndromes
- In rare families, café-au-lait spots without any other manifestation of NF1 are inherited in an autosomal dominant fashion

■ DIAGNOSTIC WORKUP
The most common presentation in children is the presence of multiple café-au-lait spots.
- Further workup should include an ophthalmologic examination and imaging when indicated by history and physical examination.

- Head magnetic resonance imaging (MRI) scan often reveals hyperintense signals indicative of intracranial hamartoma, although this finding has not been incorporated as a formal diagnostic criteria.
- A protein truncation assay is available commercially, but its utility is limited because of low sensitivity (60% to 70%).
- To explore if other family members are affected, physical and ophthalmologic evaluation of the parents are always indicated.
- Adults with NF1 have a more than 95% chance of having Lisch nodules on their irides.

💊 THERAPY

- There is no primary treatment for the disease.
- Management is directed toward minimizing the complications, including ophthalmologic, orthopedic, plastic surgery, neurosurgical, dental, educational, developmental, and pharmacologic interventions.

■ SURGICAL
Ophthalmologic, orthopedic, plastic surgery, neurosurgical, and dental management should be provided as needed.

■ FOLLOW-UP & DISPOSITION
- The main focus is surveillance for complications.
  1. A complete physical and ophthalmologic examination should be performed at least once a year.
  2. Particular attention should be directed toward any change in neurofibroma, neurologic status, scoliosis, and/or blood pressure.
- The lifetime risk for malignancy attributable to NF1 is about 5%.
- Routine MRI imaging beyond a baseline study in an otherwise asymptomatic patient is not recommended.

■ PATIENT/FAMILY EDUCATION
- Individuals with NF1 have a 50% chance of having a child with NF1 with each pregnancy.
- Unaffected parents of NF1 patients do not have an increased risk for having additional children with NF1 relative to the general population.
- The severity of NF1 can vary widely even within a family, and there is no available method to predict it.

■ PREVENTIVE TREATMENT
- None is available for prevention of complications.
- A prenatal diagnosis is possible for families with a known mutation in the NF1 gene.

II

■ REFERRAL INFORMATION

The National Neurofibromatosis Foundation has a listing of NF1 clinics around the United States.

☼ PEARLS & CONSIDERATIONS

■ CLINICAL PEARLS

- The most significant burden for NF1 families is psychologic, being always uncertain of what may lie ahead for the affected individual.
  1. This uncertainly is particularly true for families with young children in whom the only manifestation is multiple café-au-lait spots and in whom full diagnostic criteria have not been met.
  2. In these situations, it is often more productive to assume the diagnosis (and to let the family know that this is an assumption, although a highly likely one) and begin the surveillance process.
- The 5% lifetime cancer risk attributable to NF1 is best explained within the context of the lifetime cancer risk for the general population, which is about 25%.
  1. NF1 individuals have a modest increase in cancer risk over the general population.
  2. The kind of malignancy and age of onset for NF1-related malignancy are different.

■ WEBSITE

The National Neurofibromatosis Foundation: www.nf.org

REFERENCE

1. Rubenstein AE, Korf BR: *Neurofibromatosis: a handbook for patients, families and health-care professionals,* New York, 1990, Thieme.

Author: **Chin-To Fong, M.D.**

BASIC INFORMATION

■ DEFINITION
Neuroleptic malignant syndrome (NMS) is a drug-induced disorder, most commonly associated with antipsychotic medications, that results in acute changes in mental status, elevated temperature (38.5° to 42° C), and autonomic and extrapyramidal dysfunction (extreme muscle rigidity).

■ ICD-9CM CODE
333.92 Neuroleptic malignant syndrome

■ ETIOLOGY
- The mechanism of action is unclear.
- Current hypothesis is that there is a decrease in dopamine activity centrally, which leads to multiple dysfunctions based on the anatomic site affected.
  1. Hypothalamus: fever and autonomic instability
  2. Nigrostriatal system: rigidity
  3. Corticolimbal: altered mental status
- Other hypotheses implicate serotonin, catecholamines, and γ-amino butyric acid.
- NMS is a side effect of taking neuroleptic or antipsychotic medications.

■ EPIDEMIOLOGY & DEMOGRAPHICS
- NMS was first described in France.
- No specific genetic or familial component has been identified.
- Incidence rate is 0.2% to 1.9% of patients taking neuroleptic drugs.
- NMS is suspected to be more common in men than in women.
- It is more common with high-potency neuroleptics or dopamine-blocking agents (haloperidol); however, it can occur with lower-potency drugs as well (thioridazine or chlorpromazine).
- The incidence is higher in individuals with human immunodeficiency virus psychosis.
- Mortality rate varies from 4% to 25%, with more recent data showing the lower mortality rates.
- There does not appear to be a direct relationship to malignant hyperthermia (MH).
  1. Key differentiating factors
     a. No genetic or familial link with NMS; however, a genetic component is linked to MH.
     b. Patients with NMS have been given succinylcholine and general inhaled anesthesia without developing MH.
     c. Patients with a history of MH have been given antipsychotic medication without development of NMS.
     d. Neuromuscular blockade with pancuronium and curare causes flaccidity in NMS; however, it does not in MH.

■ HISTORY
- Has there been a recent administration of a neuroleptic, dopamine antagonist, or sedative?
- Time course to onset of symptoms can be dramatic (over hours) or more slowly (presenting over several days).
- NMS can lead to the following complications:
  1. Seizures
  2. Rhabdomyolysis: muscle pain and tenderness
  3. Disseminated intravascular coagulation: easy bleeding, bruising
  4. Aspiration pneumonia: shortness of breath, fever
  5. Pulmonary emboli: chest pain, difficulty breathing
  6. Peripheral nerve and muscle damage
  7. Cardiac, respiratory, and renal failure (anuria)

■ PHYSICAL EXAMINATION
- Altered mental status
  1. Agitation
  2. Irritability
  3. Restlessness
  4. Delirium
  5. Obtundation
  6. Catatonia
  7. Coma
- Muscle rigidity: extreme and progressive-generalized lead pipe rigidity
  1. Cogwheeling
  2. Oculogyric crisis
  3. Retrocollis
  4. Opisthotonos
  5. Trismus
  6. Dysphagia
  7. Choreiform movement
  8. Dyskinesis
  9. Flexor/extensor posturing
- Autonomic instability
  1. Tachycardia (greater than 100 bpm)
  2. Elevated temperature (up to 108° F)
  3. Sweating
  4. Drooling
  5. Hypertension
  6. Urinary incontinence
- Extrapyramidal dysfunction
  1. Dysarthria
  2. Dysphagia
  3. Tremors

DIAGNOSIS

■ DIFFERENTIAL DIAGNOSIS
- Catatonic reaction: lethal catatonia
- Acute encephalitis
- Systemic sepsis
- Thyrotoxicosis
- Pheochromocytoma
- Acute heat stroke
- MH
- Chemical withdrawal (narcotics and cocaine)
- Atropinic drug use
- Stimulants: overdose or high-level ingestion
- Salicylate overdose
- Serotonergic drug use

■ DIAGNOSTIC WORKUP
- Complete blood count; demonstrates a leukocytosis
- Increased creatine phosphokinase
- Metabolic acidosis
- Myoglobinuria

THERAPY

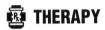

■ NONPHARMACOLOGIC
- Early recognition
- Discontinue provoking medication
- Cooling blankets and ice packs

■ MEDICAL
- Antipyretics such as acetaminophen and ibuprofen can be used.
- Bromocriptine mimics dopaminergic effects and may completely reverse effects of NMS.
  1. 5 to 10 mg doses orally three times per day
- Dantrolene sodium is a muscle relaxant.
  1. Dosage is 100 to 300 mg orally every day.
  2. From 2.5 to 10 mg/kg intravenous is given as a loading dose; then 2.5 mg/kg intravenously every 6 hours is given for maintenance.
  3. Continue for 12 to 48 hours after symptoms resolve.
  4. Use caution with calcium channel blockers because adverse reactions have been noted with co-administration of verapamil.
- Lorazepam, a benzodiazepine, acts as both a sedative and an antianxiolytic agent.
  1. Dosage is 1 mg/kg/dose intravenously every 1 to 2 hours as needed.
  2. Monitor airway and sedation.
- Amantadine use is controversial, with unclear mechanism of action (probable central dopaminergic action).
  1. Dosage is 100 to 200 mg orally two times per day.
- Levodopa is experimental; used to increase dopaminergic activity.
  1. Dosage is 10 to 100 mg orally three times per day.
- Neuromuscular blockade decreases muscle rigidity and temperature.
  1. Titrate dosage for desired effect.

2. Provide airway management: intensive care unit admission and intubation with mechanical ventilation
- Electroconvulsive therapy may reset or help reset dopamine activity.

■ FOLLOW-UP & DISPOSITION
- Thirty percent to fifty percent of patients develop NMS on subsequent administration of medication.
- If neuroleptic medications are required in the future, care must be taken to closely follow clinical course, especially pulse, temperature, and blood pressure.

■ PATIENT/FAMILY EDUCATION & PREVENTIVE TREATMENT
- Avoid neuroleptic medications.
- Be aware of early symptoms.
- Search for family history.

☼ PEARLS & CONSIDERATIONS

■ WEBSITES
- Neuroleptic Malignant Syndrome Information Service: www.nmsis.org
- University of Kansas Medical Center: www.kumc.edu/instruction/sah/nurseanesthesia/nura

■ SUPPORT GROUP
Neuroleptic Malignant Syndrome Information Service, P.O. Box 1069, 32 South Main St., Sherburne, NY 13460-1069; 607-674-7920, 888-776-6747; email: info@nmsis.org

REFERENCES
1. Bone RC: *Pulmonary and critical care medicine,* St Louis, 1998, Mosby.
2. Caroff SN, Mann SC: Neuroleptic malignant syndrome, *Med Clin North Am* 77:185, 1993.
3. Chan TC, Evans SD, Clark RF: *Crit Care Clin* 13:785, 1997.
4. Ellenshorns MJ: *Medical toxicology,* ed 2, Baltimore, 1997, Williams & Wilkins.
5. Keck PE et al: Risk factors for neuroleptic malignant syndrome, *Arch Gen Psych* 46:914, 1989.
6. Tasman A: *Psychiatry,* Philadelphia, 1997, WB Saunders.
Authors: **Stanley Johnsen, M.D., and Reed Shimamoto, M.D.**

BASIC INFORMATION

■ DEFINITION
Neutropenia is not a diagnosis; it is a laboratory finding that signifies that a child may be at increased risk of infection. Neutropenia is an absolute neutrophil count (ANC) of less than 1500/mm^3. The ANC is calculated by multiplying the total white blood cell (WBC) count times the proportion of segmented neutrophils plus band forms. Neutropenia is classified as mild (ANC 1000 to 1500/mm^3), moderate (500 to 1000/mm^3), or severe (0 to 500/mm^3).

■ SYNONYM
Granulocytopenia

ICD-9CM CODE
288.0 Neutropenia

■ ETIOLOGY
- *Acquired:* viral associated, chronic benign neutropenia of childhood, autoimmune disease, autoimmune neutropenia, medications, sepsis
- *Congenital:* Kostmann's syndrome, cyclic neutropenia, Schwachman-Diamond syndrome, metabolic disorders, familial benign neutropenia, immune disorders such as reticular dysgenesis
- *Global bone marrow disorder:* leukemias, aplastic anemia, cancer metastatic to bone marrow, chemotherapy-induced neutropenia
- *Neonatal:* hypoxia, sepsis, pregnancy-induced hypertension, alloimmune neutropenia

■ EPIDEMIOLOGY & DEMOGRAPHICS
- The most common forms are acquired neutropenia caused by viruses, medications, or autoimmune disease.
- Neonatal neutropenias in the setting of hypoxia, sepsis, and pregnancy-induced hypertension are common.
- Congenital neutropenias and neutropenia associated with bone marrow disorders are rare.
- Familial benign neutropenia is identified in African Americans and Yemenite Jews; it is not associated with increased risk of infection.

■ HISTORY
- Frequent infections of mucosal surfaces and skin are common.
  1. Cellulitis
  2. Skin abscesses
  3. Lymphadenitis
  4. Sinusitis
  5. Otitis
  6. Pneumonia

- The patient has frequent mouth sores.
- A previous ANC may help determine whether neutropenia is chronic or new onset.
- Often, it is an incidental finding in asymptomatic children who have a complete blood count (CBC) obtained for unrelated reasons.
- Neonates may have a recent history of sepsis or hypoxia or the mother may have pregnancy-induced hypertension.
- It is more common while taking certain medications (e.g., trimethoprim-sulfamethoxazole, valproate).
- History of bleeding, bruising, fatigue, and pallor suggests a global bone marrow disorder, such as leukemia or aplastic anemia.

■ PHYSICAL EXAMINATION
- Mucosal surfaces are affected.
  1. Skin: cellulitis, abscess
  2. Head/eyes/ears/nose/throat (HEENT): aphthous ulcers, thrush, otitis media, sinus tenderness
  3. Lungs: pneumonia
- Lymph nodes are red, tender, and enlarged.
- Hepatosplenomegaly and disseminated lymphadenopathy suggest systemic disease such as leukemia, autoimmune disease, or infection such as Epstein-Barr virus (EBV) or human immunodeficiency virus (HIV).

DIAGNOSIS

■ DIFFERENTIAL DIAGNOSIS
See "Etiology."

■ DIAGNOSTIC WORKUP
- CBC, differential, platelet count (distinguishes isolated neutropenia from global bone marrow disorder)
- Immunoglobulins (low in some immune disorders associated with neutropenia)
- Antineutrophil antibody (positive in autoimmune and alloimmune neutropenias)
- Serologic studies for viral infection (EBV, cytomegalovirus, HIV)
- Bone marrow aspiration and biopsy
  1. Should be considered for children with associated anemia and/or thrombocytopenia or for children with isolated neutropenia of unknown cause
- Prednisone stimulation test
  1. Children with autoimmune neutropenia or chronic benign neutropenia of childhood respond to prednisone with an acute rise in ANC (this test is rarely used now).

THERAPY

- Treatment depends on the following factors:
  1. How low the ANC is
  2. The cause of the neutropenia
  3. Whether the child is febrile or otherwise ill
- For a previously healthy child with fever who is found to be neutropenic:
  1. *Mild neutropenia* (ANC 1000 to 1500/mm^3):
     a. No further evaluation or special treatment is needed.
     b. Treat focus of infection.
  2. *Moderate neutropenia* (ANC 500 to 1000/mm^3):
     a. Obtain blood, urine cultures, and other cultures as indicated.
     b. Treat focus of infection; empiric antibiotics are not indicated in well children.
     c. Manage as an outpatient if well; consider hospitalization and intravenous antibiotics for the following children:
        (1) Those younger than 2 years old
        (2) Those who are ill appearing
        (3) Those who have high fevers
  3. *Severe neutropenia* (ANC 0 to 500/mm^3):
     a. Obtain blood, urine cultures, and other cultures as indicated.
     b. Hospitalize and treat with broad-spectrum intravenous antibiotics.
     c. Evaluate for cause of neutropenia.
     d. Consider intravenous immune globulin (IVIG), granulocyte colony-stimulating factor (G-CSF) depending on cause of neutropenia and status of child.
- For a child with neutropenia for whom the diagnosis is established:
  1. *Acquired mild to moderate neutropenia*
     a. Specific therapy to increase ANC is not necessary.
     b. Prophylactic antibiotics are not necessary.
     c. If febrile, treat focus of infection.
     d. Empiric antibiotic therapy is not necessary in well-appearing children.
     e. Well-appearing children can be treated as outpatients.
  2. *Acquired severe neutropenia*
     a. Specific therapy to raise ANC is not necessary in well, afebrile children.
     b. Prophylactic antibiotics are reserved for children with frequent pyogenic infections.

c. If febrile:
   (1) Well-appearing children can be managed as outpatients.
   (2) Hospitalization and intravenous antibiotics are reserved for ill-appearing or young children.
   (3) Consider G-CSF for ill-appearing children (IVIG, prednisone, G-CSF effective for autoimmune neutropenia).
3. Congenital neutropenia (e.g., Kostmann's syndrome, cyclic neutropenia, Schwachman-Diamond syndrome)
   a. Chronic G-CSF should be given for Kostmann's syndrome and cyclic neutropenia.
   b. Antibiotic prophylaxis should be considered for children with ANC lower than 500/mm^3.
   c. Febrile children should be hospitalized and treated with intravenous antibiotics.
   d. Use of WBC transfusions is controversial but should be considered for ill, febrile children.
4. Neonatal neutropenia
   a. Treatment to increase ANC is not necessary in the well infant.
   b. Ill infants may benefit from G-CSF or WBC transfusion.

■ FOLLOW-UP & DISPOSITION
• Children with acquired neutropenia should have a CBC checked every few months until the neutropenia resolves, and they should be evaluated for fevers.
• Children with congenital neutropenias should have a CBC checked every few months, should be evaluated for fevers, and need to be monitored for risk of developing leukemia.

■ PATIENT/FAMILY EDUCATION
• Most acquired neutropenias are mild, transient, and not life-threatening.
• Congenital neutropenias are potentially serious chronic illnesses that require close surveillance to prevent or treat infection, poor dentition, poor growth, and risk of leukemia.

■ PREVENTIVE TREATMENT
• G-CSF for children with congenital, profound neutropenia
• Antibiotic prophylaxis for congenital neutropenia, children with frequent pyogenic infections

■ REFERRAL INFORMATION
A child with moderate to severe neutropenia should be referred to a pediatric hematologist/oncologist for further evaluation and treatment.

☼ PEARLS & CONSIDERATIONS

■ CLINICAL PEARLS
• The classic signs of inflammation (i.e., rubor, calor, dolor, turgor) may be subtle or absent in neutropenic children.

• A girl with labial cellulitis should have a CBC checked because this site of infection is unique to neutropenic children.
• Delayed separation of the umbilical cord in a neonate may be associated with neutropenia.

■ WEBSITES
• Neutropenia OnLine Forum: www.delphi.com/Neutropenia
• The Severe Chronic Neutropenia International Registry: http://depts.washington.edu/registry

■ SUPPORT GROUPS
• National Neutropenia Network, Inc.: http://neutropenia.thedomaingame.org/main.html
• Neutropenia Support Association, Inc.: www.neutropenia.ca

REFERENCES
1. Dinauer MC: The phagocyte system and disorders of granulopoiesis and granulocyte function. In Nathan DG, Orkin SH (eds): *Nathan and Oski's hematology of infancy and childhood,* ed 5, Philadelphia, 1998, WB Saunders.
2. Korones DN: Neutropenia and lymphopenia. In Burg FD et al (eds): *Gellis and Kagan's current pediatric therapy,* ed 16, Philadelphia, 1999, WB Saunders.
Author: **David N. Korones, M.D.**

BASIC INFORMATION

DEFINITION

Obesity is having excess body fat or body weight. There is no one accepted standard definition, and because of the difficulty of measuring body fat and the ranges of heights across age, various criteria have been used.

- The most common definition uses body mass index (BMI), which equals weight in kilograms (kg) divided by height in square meters (m^2), a weight-based measure that correlates well with amount of body fat.
  1. Obese/overweight is more than the 95th percentile BMI (generally over 30).
  2. "At risk for becoming overweight" is the 85th to 95th percentile BMI.
  3. Morbid obesity is a BMI more than 100% above the 85th percentile BMI (BMI over 40).

SYNONYMS

- Overweight
- Overfat

ICD-9CM CODES
278.00 Exogenous obesity
259.9 Endogenous obesity
278.01 Morbid obesity

ETIOLOGY

- The etiology is multifactorial, representing an interaction between genetic and environmental influences; relative contributions vary among individuals.
- Only about 5% of patients have underlying specific causes, such as an endocrine problems (3%) or a syndrome (2%).
- Familiar factors are documented by epidemiologic studies; both genetic and environmental factors are involved.
  1. Children and adolescents with one or both obese parents are at significantly higher risk of obesity as adults than those without an obese parent.
- The fat cell theory suggests that fat cells gained early in life, during puberty, or with massive weight gain during adulthood cannot be lost.
  1. Therefore avoid overfeeding during infancy, early childhood, and during puberty to prevent obesity
- Behavioral and lifestyle factors are believed to be key.
  1. Caloric intake is significantly higher in many obese individuals compared with that of nonobese persons.
  2. Sedentary lifestyle, physical inactivity, and large amounts of watching TV and/or playing video games are all implicated.

3. Obese patients often engage in patterns of eating that adversely influence weight.
   a. Eating fast
   b. Skipping meals early in the day and eating large quantities late in the day
   c. Eating in response to anxiety or depression
   d. Eating in front of the TV
   e. Eating when not hungry
4. Eating patterns in the United States have shifted dramatically: 30% of food expenditures are for "take-out" meals, which typically are high in fat and high in calories and are large in quantity.
- Psychologic factors such as early traumatic experiences (i.e., sexual abuse) may be involved.

EPIDEMIOLOGY & DEMOGRAPHICS

- Data from sequential cohorts of national datasets have demonstrated recent and significant increases in the prevalence of obesity in children and adolescents.
- Cycle III of the National Health and Nutrition Examination Survey (NHANES) (1988 to 1994) found 11% overall prevalence of overweight (6- to 18-years-old) and 14% prevalence of those "at risk" for overweight.
- Non-Hispanic African Americans and Mexican Americans have higher rates (14% to 17% range) across all age groups and genders compared with whites (10% to 11%).
- No consistent associations with socioeconomic status or family education are seen.
- Trends in obesity demonstrate that the greatest increases have occurred since the mid-1970s.
  1. Rates are two to three times greater than those seen in surveys done in 1965.
  2. The heaviest cohort of children demonstrate the greatest increase in weight.

INFLUENCES ON HEALTH

- Obesity can cause complications in many organ systems, some of which occur more immediately during childhood and adolescence, whereas others manifest later in adulthood.
- Short-term effects include the following:
  1. Orthopedic complications
     a. Blount's disease (tibia vara)
     b. Slipped femoral capital epiphyses (30% to 50% of cases are obese)
  2. Pseudotumor cerebri
     a. Up to 50% of childhood cases are obese.
  3. Sleep apnea/obesity hypoventilation syndrome
     a. Both obstructive and central

hypoventilation types are seen when patients are morbidly obese.
4. Gallbladder disease and elevated liver enzymes related to steatosis
5. Endocrinologic diseases
   a. Polycystic ovary disease (see the section on this topic)
   b. Glucose intolerance and type 2 diabetes mellitus; associated with acanthosis nigricans and hyperinsulinemia (see the section "Diabetes Mellitus Type 2")
   c. Abnormal lipid profiles: elevated low-density lipoprotein (LDL) cholesterol and triglycerides and decreased high-density lipoprotein (HDL) cholesterol
6. Elevated blood pressure
7. Early physical maturation
   a. Greater height often leads to unrealistic expectations of maturity by adults and peers.
8. Psychosocial consequences most prevalent
   a. Isolation and stigma, poor self-image and self-esteem, depression, and discrimination based on societal norms for thinness
   b. Binge eating disorders in up to 30% of obese female adolescents
- Long-term effects include the following:
  1. Obesity, especially when it occurs or persists until adolescence, will track into adulthood.
     a. Significant increase in adult morbidity and mortality, from all causes and from cardiovascular disease, even after controlling for adult weight status and smoking history
  2. Approximately 80% to 85% of obese adolescents will be obese adults; persistence is greater for females than for males.
  3. Strong associations are found between adolescent obesity and adult chronic diseases, such as cerebrovascular disease, cardiovascular disease, various types of cancers, arthritis, gout, and diabetes mellitus.

HISTORY

Determines potential causes, contributing factors, duration of obesity, and complications

- Abnormal growth or development in early childhood
- Oligomenorrhea or amenorrhea
- Knee pain
- Headaches, blurred vision, vomiting (suggests pseudotumor cerebri)
- Daytime somnolence, breathing difficulty during sleep
- Abdominal pain
- Abnormal eating patterns, binge

eating, purging (may be signs of eating disorder)
- Depressive symptoms (contributing factors or side effects of obesity)
  1. Functioning at school, with family, and with peers to assess degree of social isolation
- History of weight gain from early childhood to present
  1. Point when child began to cross percentiles
  2. Early intervention
  3. Early events that may have coincided with weight change
  4. Periods of extremely rapid weight gain
  5. As a guideline, crossing more than 1 to 2 BMI units per year worrisome
- Family history of obesity, diabetes, cardiovascular disease
- Eating behaviors and diet history
  1. Foods eaten daily
  2. Patterns of eating
  3. Typical meals and snacks
  4. Weekly consumption of high-calorie, high-fat foods, including take-out or convenience meals, fast foods, and caloric beverages (e.g., juices, regular sodas, and sweetened teas)
  5. Eating when not hungry
  6. Eating in front of the TV
  7. Unsupervised eating
  8. Meal skipping
- How foods are prepared and by whom can affect an individual's risk of obesity.
  1. Types of snacks available
  2. Parental behaviors regarding skipping meals
  3. Eating to relieve stress
- Physical activity and exercise habits also play a role.
  1. Organized sports
  2. School-based physical education
  3. Activities done at home and unorganized outdoor play
- Time spent in sedentary activities, such as watching TV, working or playing on a computer, and playing video games increases the risk of obesity.
- Parental involvement and modeling for both active and sedentary patterns affect the child's risk.
- Whether child and parents see obesity as a problem and their readiness to change will affect the ability to overcome obesity.

■ PHYSICAL EXAMINATION
- Plotting of height, weight, and calculated BMI percentile (plot according to current BMI graphs for age available from the Centers for Disease Control and Prevention; see "Growth" in Part III)
- Poor linear growth (seen in endocrine causes such as Cushing's disease or hypothyroidism)

- Triceps skin fold thickness (may be helpful if there is an adequate way to measure it)
- Body fat distribution, concentrating on central versus peripheral
  1. Central obesity correlates with higher visceral adiposity, as seen in adults.
  2. Central obesity predisposes individuals to a higher risk of cardiovascular disease.
- Blood pressure, ensuring that an appropriate-size cuff is used
- Dysmorphic features seen in rare genetic causes, such as Bardet-Biedl and Cohen, and Prader-Willi syndromes
- Acanthosis nigricans (often most apparent at the back of neck, axillae, and intertriginous areas); raises suspicion of insulin resistance
- Violaceous striae, truncal obesity (Cushing's disease), hirsutism (hyperandrogenemic anovulatory states)
- Blurred optic discs and loss of visual acuity (pseudotumor cerebri)
- Abdominal tenderness (especially right upper quadrant, which suggests liver or gallbladder disease)
- Undescended testicle (Prader-Willi syndrome)
- Limited hip range of motion (slipped femoral capital epiphysis)
- Lower leg bowing (Blount's disease)
- Sexual maturity rating (may be accelerated in obese children)

DIAGNOSIS

■ DIFFERENTIAL DIAGNOSIS
Includes rare causes of exogenous obesity versus endogenous obesity, with or without medical complications (outlined previously)
- Exogenous causes
  1. Bardet Biedl and Cohen syndrome
  2. Prader-Willi syndrome
  3. Hypothyroidism
  4. Cushing's disease
  5. Psychologic/eating disorder (i.e., bulimia, depression)
- Endogenous obesity

■ DIAGNOSTIC WORKUP
- Determination of BMI and percentile to identify those who are overweight (more than 95th percentile) and in need of comprehensive medical assessment and intervention versus those at risk for overweight (85th to 95th percentile) who need further assessment and management if there are signs and symptoms of complications from obesity, large recent changes in BMI, or concern about weight (Fig. 2-3)
- Laboratory studies
  1. These are of limited value, except for identifying those rare children

and adolescents with an underlying medical cause and for determining the presence of medical complications of obesity, as outlined previously.
- Thyroid studies, AM cortisol if clinically indicated
- Chromosome studies
- Fasting blood glucose, insulin levels
- Fasting lipid profile: total, LDL, and HDL cholesterol and triglyceride levels
- Electrocardiogram, echocardiogram, chest radiograph, sleep studies
- Follicle-stimulating hormone (FSH), luteinizing hormone (LH), testosterone (free and total)
- Liver function tests, ultrasound of gallbladder

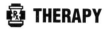 **THERAPY**

■ GOALS OF THERAPY
- The primary goal should be the regulation of body weight and fat through healthy eating and activity levels to provide adequate nutrition for growth and development.
  1. Weight goal may be either maintenance of baseline weight that allows a gradual decline in BMI with linear height growth or weight loss (approximately 1 pound per month) (see Fig. 2-3).
- Secondary goals are to improve any secondary complications and to prevent the development of negative effects of treatment.

■ NONPHARMACOLOGIC
- Principles
  1. Numerous studies have documented positive results in treating children and adolescents, using individualized programs that integrate several components: dietary modification, exercise, behavior change, and family involvement.
  2. Intervention should begin in early childhood when obesity is identified.
  3. Families and children must be ready to make changes; if not, options are to defer treatment or to refer children for counseling using motivational techniques for behavioral change.
  4. Education about the medical consequences of obesity, both short- and long-term, should be included.
  5. All family members and caregivers, as well as the child, need to be involved in any treatment program to create new family behaviors that support the child's goals for eating and activity.
     a. The need for more independent behaviors among adoles-

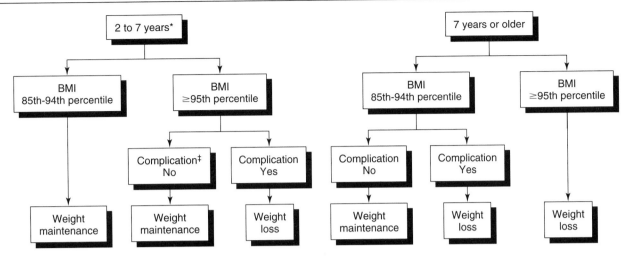

Fig. 2-3 Recommendations for weight goals. *Indicates that children younger than 2 years should be referred to a pediatric obesity center for treatment. ‡Indicates complications such as mild hypertension, dyslipidemias, and insulin resistance. Patients with acute complications, such as pseudo-tumor cerebri, sleep apnea, obesity hypoventilation syndrome, or orthopedic problems, should be referred to a pediatric obesity center. (From Barlow SE, Dietz WH: *Pediatrics* 102, 1998.)

cents needs to be recognized by families.
6. Emphasis is on long-term changes in eating and activity levels rather than a focus on diets or rapid weight loss.
7. Small, gradual changes in behaviors are preferable.
8. Use of a team of professionals, or referral to professionals such as a nutritionist/dietitian or counselor, may enhance the success of the treatment.
- Exercise and physical activity
  1. Efforts to increase physical activity levels are more successful when families incorporate greater activity into daily routines, such as walking to school or doing active chores, rather than starting formal exercise programs.
  2. Making specific efforts to reduce the amount of sedentary activities, such as limiting TV hours, often has the benefit of increasing the child's active time.
- Behavior change methods essential to influencing changes in eating or activity
  1. Most methods involve close input by parents in managing the eating behaviors of their children.
  2. Behavioral choice therapy, such as reducing reinforcements for the child to continue sedentary activities; providing some choice and control over activity and food choices; minimizing a sense of deprivation; and teaching the child how to attend to internal cues of hunger, emotions, and satiety are essential components.

3. Additional techniques, such as goal setting and contracting with both the child/teen and the parents, self-monitoring of caloric intake and weight, and praise, are all beneficial.
- Family involvement
  1. Includes promoting positive parenting skills
     a. Modeling healthy eating behaviors: using praise directed at improved behaviors, not weight loss
     b. Being consistent in messages
     c. Establishing daily meal times: offering only healthy options for snacks and meals
     d. Being observant of the child's behavior
     e. Setting limits when necessary
- Dietary modification
  1. Use the food guide pyramid as a guide to adopting a healthy approach to eating. Separate pyramids are available for 2- to 6-year-olds versus 7-year-olds to adults.
  2. Suggest reducing or eliminating high-calorie, calorie-dense foods or substituting with lower-calorie alternatives to reduce caloric intake.
  3. The "traffic light diet" approach stresses a balance of high-, medium-, and low-calorie foods, rather than counting calories; this is best for children and preadolescents.
- Adjunctive therapies
  1. Support groups or group-oriented programs, especially in the context of school programs or

health education, may be beneficial for some children and teens and provide needed peer support.
2. Groups in which parents are also offered a separate group meeting are more beneficial than those for children and parents together.
3. Commercial programs, such as Jenny Craig and Weight Watchers, are not specifically designed for children and adolescents and have not been evaluated for these ages.

■ **MEDICAL**
- At present, there are no medical therapies that promise long-term significant weight reduction in children and adolescents.
  1. A variety of anorectic drugs are marketed as weight-loss drugs and are available through prescription: schedule II drugs such as methamphetamine HCl (Desoxyn), schedule III drugs such as phendimetrazine tartrate (Bontril, Prelu-2), and the newer schedule IV drugs such as phentermine (Fastin and Ionamin).
  2. Very few studies have been done assessing these drugs' effectiveness in children and adolescents; those that have been done show few differences among those subjects treated with diet control and placebo.
  3. Sibutramine (Meridia, a serotonin, norepinephrine, and dopamine reuptake inhibitor) and orlistat (Xenical, a lipase inhibitor that prevents the absorption of dietary fat) are not currently recom-

mended for use in individuals younger than 16 years of age, although clinical trials are under way.

4. Over-the-counter anorectic agents (e.g., Dexatrim) are not effective and are likely to pose risks from side effects and abuse potential.

- Liquid protein-sparing modified fasts (liquid diets containing 400 to 900 kcal/day) provide enough protein and carbohydrates to keep ketosis and protein loss to a minimum.
  1. These are prescribed through physician-directed programs that typically combine fasting with nutrition education and behavior modification.
  2. Weight loss can be substantial on these programs, but high recidivism rates are typical.
  3. These programs are contraindicated in adolescents who are still actively growing, but they may be recommended in specific cases of extreme obesity and in the presence of secondary complications

■ SURGICAL

- Several surgical gastrointestinal procedures are available, such as gastric balloon placement and gastric-reduction procedures; however, they are used only rarely in cases of extreme obesity in adolescents.
- Generally, surgery is done only when an adolescent is morbidly obese and has tried and failed to lose weight on standard medical/behavioral treatment.
- The few studies that have been done document significant weight loss that is generally overshadowed by the serious side effects of the procedures.
- These procedures are *not* generally recommended for children and adolescents.

■ PREVENTIVE TREATMENT

- Preventive treatment is ideally provided in the course of routine preventive care when monitoring growth and providing information about the avoidance of excessive intake and promotion of physical activity.
- For early prevention or intervention, focus on obese parents of young chil-

dren, even if the children are currently normal weight.

- For older children and adolescents, focus on those who show early signs of increasing weight.

■ FOLLOW-UP & DISPOSITION

- Obesity should be viewed as a chronic disease that requires ongoing and close follow-up to ensure success in treatment.
- Relapse is common, and close follow-up can assist patients in managing relapses.

■ REFERRAL INFORMATION

- For acute medical complications, refer to a specific subspecialist or pediatric obesity center as needed.
- If in the course of treatment, significant conflict between parents and child ensues around eating issues or if signs of an eating disorder or depression emerge, referral to a family therapist or individual counselor may be indicated.
- A nutritionist or registered dietitian may be best able to assess and make recommendations about caloric intake and requirements, especially in cases in which the provider does not have the time or expertise to do this.

☼ PEARLS & CONSIDERATIONS

■ CLINICAL PEARLS

- Because of aromatization of androgens to estrogen that occurs in adipose tissue, obese females have significant amounts of extragonadal estrogen, which may be associated with disruption of normal FSH and LH levels and anovulatory menstrual cycles.
- Many adolescents may use tobacco as a form of weight control, so it is important to ask about this behavior and to counsel the patient regarding the added risk of tobacco use on risks associated with obesity.

■ WEBSITES

- American Dietetic Association: www.eatright.org; provides nutritional information for both parents and children

- Food and Nutrition Information Center, U.S. Department of Agriculture: www.nal.usda.gov/fnic
- Weight Control Information Network: www.niddk.nih.gov//nutritiondocs.html; provides general information on weight control, obesity, and nutritional disorders

REFERENCES

1. Barlow SE, Dietz WH: Obesity evaluation and treatment: expert committee recommendations, *Pediatrics* 102:3, 1998.
2. Dietz WH: Health consequences of obesity in youth: childhood predictors of adult disease, *Pediatrics* 101:518, 1998.
3. Epstein LH et al: A comparison of lifestyle change and programmed aerobic exercise on weight and fitness changes in obese children, *Behav Ther* 13:651, 1982.
4. Epstein LH et al: Treatment of pediatric obesity, *Pediatrics* 101:554, 1998.
5. Long BJ et al. A multi-site field test of the acceptability of physical activity counseling in primary care: project PACE, *Am J Prev Med* 12:73, 1996.
6. Miller WR, Rollnick S: *Motivational interviewing: preparing people to change addictive behavior,* New York, 1991, Guilford Press.
7. Rollnick S, Healther N, Bell A: Negotiating behavior change in medical settings: the development of brief motivational interviewing, *J Mental Health* 1:25, 1992.
8. Troiano RP, Flegal KM: Overweight children and adolescents: description, epidemiology, and demographics, *Pediatrics* 101:497, 1998.
9. US Department of Agriculture: *Childhood obesity: causes & prevention,* Symposium proceeding, October 27, 1998.
10. US Department of Health & Human Services: Obesity in childhood and adolescence: assessment, prevention and treatment, *Int J Obesity* 23:2, 1999.
11. Whitaker RC et al: Predicting obesity in young adulthood from childhood and parental obesity, *N Engl J Med* 337:869, 1997.

Author: **Sheryl Ryan, M.D.**

BASIC INFORMATION

DEFINITION

Obsessive-compulsive disorder (OCD) is recurrent, intrusive, unpleasant thoughts (obsessions) that are not responsive to voluntary suppression, are unrealistic, and are not imposed from without; repetitive behaviors or mental acts (compulsions) occur in response to these thoughts. In OCD, the thoughts or actions are disabling.

SYNONYM

OCD

ICD-9CM CODE

300.3 Obsessive-compulsive disorder

ETIOLOGY

- Involves neurotransmitters (especially serotonin and dopamine) and pathways in the basal ganglia
- Also occurs as an uncommon sequel to streptococcal infection: pediatric autoimmune neuropsychiatric disorders and associated disorders (PANDAs)

EPIDEMIOLOGY & DEMOGRAPHICS

- OCD runs in families and is associated with Tourette's disorder and depression.
- Reported prevalence rates are unreliable, but they range from 0.2% to 1% in children and to 3.6% in adolescents.
- No reliable gender, ethnic, or racial variations have been established.

HISTORY

- Developmental rituals are common but usually disappear by 8 to 10 years of age.
- Onset after a streptococcal infection is reported (PANDAs).

PHYSICAL EXAMINATION

- Chapped, red hands (from excessive washing)
- Patchy hair loss (trichotillomania)

DIAGNOSIS

DIFFERENTIAL DIAGNOSIS

- Tics occur without triggering thoughts.
- Pervasive developmental disorder

and developmental delays may have repetitive behaviors, but these are unaccompanied by ritualized justification.
- Depressed patients' thoughts may be "obsessive," are dysphoric, and do not cause compulsions.
- Psychotic obsessions are "ego syntonic" (make sense to patient), but "ego alien" (perceived as inappropriate by the patient) in OCD.
- Anorexia and bulimia nervosa obsessions and compulsions are limited to weight-losing behaviors.

DIAGNOSTIC WORKUP

- Patients may acknowledge ritualized behavior only reluctantly.
- Parents may observe washing (in 85%), repeating (51%), and checking (46%) rituals.
- Interviewer-administered Yale-Brown Obsessive-Compulsive Scale (YBOCS) may be used in the evaluation of OCD.
- Self-administered Leyton Obsessional Inventory (child version) may also be used.
- Antistreptococcal antibody titers may be elevated in PANDAs.

THERAPY

NONPHARMACOLOGIC

- Cognitive-behavioral therapy works well in older children and adolescents.
  1. Use in combination with medication is even more effective.

MEDICAL

- Several of the selective serotonin reuptake inhibitors are the first choice, with the fewest side effects.
  1. Fluoxetine and fluvoxamine are often effective and are well tolerated.
     a. Start with a low dosage and increase slowly.
     b. Higher dosages than used for depression may be required (80 mg fluoxetine, 200 mg fluvoxamine).
  2. Improvement is cumulative over several months.
- Clomipramine is also effective (up to 3 mg/kg).
  1. Less well tolerated
  2. Anticholinergic
  3. Requires electrocardiographic monitoring for conduction delay

FOLLOW-UP & DISPOSITION

Because recurrence is likely if medication is stopped too soon, continue for at least 1 year and taper very slowly (decrease by 25%, wait 60 days to decrease more).

PATIENT/FAMILY EDUCATION

Reapplication of cognitive-behavioral techniques may forestall recurrence.

PREVENTIVE TREATMENT

Evidence of streptococcal-associated OCD warrants ongoing watch for recurrent streptococcal infection.

REFERRAL INFORMATION

Psychopharmacologic consultations may be appropriate because of the extended treatment needed.

PEARLS & CONSIDERATIONS

CLINICAL PEARLS

- OCD treatment (in adults) changes the basal ganglia blood flow. This occurs with cognitive-behavioral therapy even without medication.
- At least 50% of Tourette's patients develop OCD, with overlapping family histories.

WEBSITES

- American Academy of Child & Adolescent Psychiatry: www.aacap.org/factsfam/index.htm
- Obsessive-Compulsive Foundation, Inc.: www.ocfoundation.org/oofl040.htm

REFERENCES

1. American Psychiatric Association: *Diagnostic and statistical manual*, ed 4, Washington, DC, 1994, American Psychiatric Association.
2. Goodman WK et al: Yale-Brown Obsessive-Compulsive Scale (YBOCS), *Arch Gen Psychiatry* 46:1006, 1989.
3. March J: OCD in children and adolescents. *J Am Acad Child Adolesc Psych* 35:1265, 1996.
4. March J: Treatment of OCD, *J Clin Psych* 58:1, 1997.
5. Leyton Obsessional Inventory: Child version published in *J Am Acad Child Adolesc Psych* 25:84, 1986.
6. Practice Parameters: *J Am Acad Child Adolesc Psych* 37:27S, 1110, 1998.
7. Swedo SE: PANDAs, *Am J Psych* 155: 264, 1998.

Author: **Christopher Hodgman, M.D.**

BASIC INFORMATION

■ DEFINITION

Occult spinal dysraphism (OSD) is a set of malformations that involve defects of neurulation of the spinal cord or a defect in the skeletal investment of neural tube, including malformations of all the tissue layers in the midline of the back. OSD involves incomplete vertebral arch formation, usually in the lumbosacral region, with associated neurologic involvement and an unexposed spinal cord. (For exposed spinal cord, see the section "Meningomyelocele, Syrinx, Tethered Cord.") OSD lesions may include the following:

- Lipomeningomyelocele: spinal lipoma, subcutaneous lipoma
- Spinal cord tethered by a thickened filum terminale
- Dermal sinus tracts with or without dermoid tumors
- Diastematomyelia: split cord malformations, often associated with a hairy patch
- Meningocele manqué: dorsal spinal cord fixation associated with diastematomyelia
- Neurenteric cysts: persistence of the neurenteric canal; occur predominantly anteriorly in the spinal canal and are more common in the cervical region
- Terminal syringomyelia: cerebrospinal fluid–filled cyst involving the lumbar spinal cord, often associated with tethered cord

ICD-9CM CODE
756.17 Occult spinal dysraphism

■ ETIOLOGY
- Open and closed neural tube defects may be genetically related.
- Some lesions cause caudal traction on the conus medullaris, whereas others cause ventral or dorsal traction.
  1. Experimental evidence has shown that traction causes ischemic changes to the spinal cord, which cause neurologic signs and symptoms.
- Spinal cord traction is thought to worsen with growth of the spinal column.
  1. This may explain the progression of neurologic deficits.

■ EPIDEMIOLOGY & DEMOGRAPHICS
- The incidence in the general U.S. population is unknown.
- Female:male predominance is 2:1.

■ HISTORY
- Infectious
  1. Meningitis caused by multiple organisms or that which recurs after appropriate treatment should raise the suspicion of a dermal sinus.
- Urologic/gastroenterologic
  1. Enuresis, frequency, urgency
  2. Urinary tract infections
  3. Bladder and/or bowel incontinence
  4. Constipation
- Orthopedic
  1. Abnormal gait
  2. Back and leg pain (older children and adolescents)
- Neurologic
  1. Lower extremity weakness
  2. Decreased spontaneous leg movement (infants)
  3. Painless foot burns, ulcers

■ PHYSICAL EXAMINATION
- Cutaneous anomalies may occur anywhere along the midline but are seen most often in the lumbar region. Combinations of lesions are common.
  1. Hair tufts (hypertrichosis); strong association with diastematomyelia
  2. Foot ulcers
  3. Capillary hemangioma (pale, flat lesions often pathologic as well)
  4. Lumbosacral dermal sinus; should be distinguished from the common sacrococcygeal pit (see "Pearls and Considerations")
     a. A dermal sinus is an opening in the skin that may connect to a subcutaneous tract lined by epithelium, which can be traced to the dura or spinal cord.
     b. Significant in addition to its role as a sign of intradural pathology, it may become infected and cause meningitis or an intramedullary abscess.
  5. Midline or paraspinal masses, such as a lipoma
  6. Atretic meningocele or "cigarette burn" sign
     a. Thinning of the skin and color changes beneath the skin
     b. Resembles a cigarette burn
- Orthopedic
  1. Foot asymmetry: exaggerated arch, hammer toe
  2. Contracted heel cord
  3. Leg length discrepancy or asymmetry
  4. Progressive scoliosis or kyphosis
- Neurologic
  1. Absent reflexes (infants), especially Achilles tendon
  2. Decreased rectal sphincter tone
  3. Hyperreflexia (older children and adolescents)
  4. Asymmetric motor and sensory dysfunction

DIAGNOSIS

■ DIFFERENTIAL DIAGNOSIS
- Suspicion of diagnosis is based on clinical findings.
- Other neurologic abnormalities may be in the differential for gait disturbances, bowel or bladder dysfunction, and sensory losses or pain.
  1. Spinal injury or tumor, spinal cord abscess
  2. Discitis, epidural or subdural spinal bleeding
  3. Central nervous system injury—bleeding, stroke, tumor
  4. Peripheral neuropathies, heavy metal poisoning
- Bone anomalies or injury may be in the differential of leg length discrepancy, leg pain, and gait disturbances.

■ DIAGNOSTIC WORKUP
- Diagnosis is made with radiographic studies.
- Anteroposterior and lateral plain films
  1. Appropriate initial studies
  2. Useful for identifying vertebral abnormalities
- Spinal magnetic resonance imaging (MRI) scans
  1. Imaging procedure of choice
  2. Most likely to detect subtle anatomic abnormalities
- Ultrasound
  1. Less sensitive in infants older than 2 months of age
  2. Reader dependent

■ THERAPY
- Surgery is indicated in symptomatic patients.
- Observation in these cases usually results in neurologic deterioration.

■ FOLLOW-UP & DISPOSITION
- Patients are followed closely for the first 3 to 4 months after surgery and then with annual visits to the pediatric neurosurgeon.
- Repeat MRI scans in asymptomatic patients are of little value.

■ PREVENTIVE TREATMENT
- It is recommended that women of childbearing age use periconceptional folate (0.4 mg/day) to help reduce the incidence of neural tube defects.
- If the woman has a previous child or a first-degree relative with any neural tube defects (open or closed), 4 mg folate daily is suggested.

☼ PEARLS & CONSIDERATIONS

■ CLINICAL PEARLS

- Coccygeal or sacrococcygeal pits are located in the intergluteal fold over the coccyx; they are of no clinical significance and, if seen in isolation, require no further evaluation.
- Younger children are more likely to present with cutaneous abnormalities, whereas older children are more likely to present with neurologic dysfunction and/or pain.

■ WEBSITES

- Association for Awareness of Occult Spinal Dysraphism (AAOSD): www.novagate.net~imx/assosd/
- Lipomyelomeningocele Family Support Network (LFSN): http://laran.waisman.wisc.edu/fv/www/lib_lipo.html

REFERENCES

1. Gibson PJ et al: Lumbosacral skin markers and identification of occult spinal dysraphism in neonates, *Acta Paediatr* 84:208, 1995.
2. Iskandar B, Oakes WJ: Occult spinal dysraphism. In Albright L, Pollack I, Adelson D (eds): *Principles and practice of pediatric neurosurgery*, New York, 1999, Thieme.
3. Oakes WJ: Lumps, bumps, and holes: a primer on occult spinal dysraphism, http://pedsurg.surgery.uab.edu/cme/lbh/lbh.htm.

Author: **Stephanie Sansoni, M.D.**

BASIC INFORMATION

■ **DEFINITION**
- *Superficial ocular foreign body:* a foreign body on the cornea, conjunctiva, or lid
- *Intraocular foreign body:* a foreign body that penetrates the eye
- *Intraorbital foreign body:* a foreign body that penetrates the orbit

ICD-9CM CODES
930.0   Foreign body, corneal
930.1   Foreign body, conjunctival
374.86 Foreign body, lid retained

■ **HISTORY**
- Usually, there is a history of trauma, but in younger children, there may only be a history of a red eye, tearing, light sensitivity, and irritability.
- Common circumstances are playing in sand, working around cars, and playing with pellet guns.

■ **PHYSICAL EXAMINATION**
- Inspect for the presence of a life-threatening injury.
- Assess the patient's visual acuity.
- Perform a slit-lamp examination and ophthalmoscopy to differentiate a superficial from an intraocular foreign body.

DIAGNOSIS

■ **DIFFERENTIAL DIAGNOSIS**
- Superficial corneal foreign body
  1. Corneal abrasion
  2. Acute conjunctivitis
  3. Uveitis
  4. Congenital glaucoma
- Intraocular foreign body
  1. Uveitis
  2. Intraocular foreign body
  3. Retinal detachment
  4. Vitreous hemorrhage
- Intraorbital foreign body
  1. Orbital cellulitis

■ **DIAGNOSTIC WORKUP**
- Physical examination is key.
- Must rule out an intraocular foreign body.
- If there is a suspicion of an intraocular or intraorbital foreign body, a computed tomography (CT) scan should be ordered. A CT scan is often better for evaluation of trauma and will identify metallic and organic foreign bodies.

THERAPY

■ **NONPHARMACOLOGIC**
- Some superficial foreign bodies may be rinsed out with water or normal saline or tearing.
- A foreign body in or around the eye must be removed.
- If the foreign body is superficial, it may be removed with a cotton-tipped applicator under topical anesthesia.
  1. Use of a forceps or other ophthalmic instruments, particularly with metallic foreign bodies, may be needed.
  2. Remove the entire foreign body.
  3. Use of a slit lamp is often required.
- In a young child, even a superficial foreign body may need to be removed in the operating room with sedation or general anesthesia.
- Organic foreign bodies should be evaluated by an ophthalmologist because there is a greater likelihood of infection from bacterial or fungal organisms.

■ **FOLLOW-UP & DISPOSITION**
Until injury has healed

■ **PATIENT/FAMILY EDUCATION**
- Discuss the dangers of pressurized toys and sports equipment (i.e., "BB" guns, paint ball, bungee cords) at well-child checkup as part of anticipatory guidance.
- Wearing safety glasses for sports and hobbies is encouraged.

■ **REFERRAL INFORMATION**
- Ophthalmologic evaluation is needed for any suspected foreign body not easily removed in the office or to rule out other damage to the eye.
- For intraocular or intraorbital foreign bodies, consult an ophthalmologist.

REFERENCE
1. Hamill MB: Corneal injury. In Krachmer JH, Mannis MJ, Holland JH (eds): *Cornea*, St Louis, 1997, Mosby.
Author: **Anna F. Fakadej, M.D., F.A.A.O.**

BASIC INFORMATION

■ **DEFINITION**
Osgood-Schlatter disease is a condition of adolescence marked by pain, swelling, and tenderness involving the growing tibial tuberosity. It is more specifically characterized by inflammation of the patellar tendon at its insertion site (apophysitis) on the proximal tibial tuberosity.

■ **SYNONYM**
Traction apophysitis of the patellar tendon

ICD-9CM CODE
732.4 Osgood-Schlatter disease

■ **ETIOLOGY**
- Traumatic stress is placed on the proximal tibial tuberosity from repetitive contraction of the patellar tendon by the quadriceps mechanism.
- Repetitive stress causes apophyseal inflammation and heterotopic bone formation at the tibial tuberosity.
- This condition occurs during the developmental period of rapid skeletal growth.

■ **EPIDEMIOLOGY & DEMOGRAPHICS**
- Predominantly a disorder of early adolescent boys (ages 11 to 15) and girls (ages 8 to 13)
- Currently seen in a male:female ratio of 3:1
- More common in adolescents engaging in athletics requiring repetitive quadriceps contraction

■ **HISTORY**
- Anterior knee pain is aggravated by quadriceps stress (ascending and descending stairs, jumping, running) or by direct pressure on the tibial tuberosity.
- Pain improves with rest.
- Bilateral symptoms are present in 30% of patients.

■ **PHYSICAL EXAMINATION**
- Enlargement of tibial tuberosity
- Thickening of patellar tendon
- Absence of synovial inflammation or joint effusion
- Pain increased with quadriceps flexion
- Taut quadriceps mechanism and hamstrings

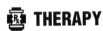 **DIAGNOSIS**

■ **DIFFERENTIAL DIAGNOSIS**
- Proximal tibial stress fracture
- Quadriceps tendon avulsion
- Patellofemoral stress syndrome
- Pes anserinus bursitis
- Proximal tibial neoplasm
- Infection

■ **DIAGNOSTIC WORKUP**
- The diagnosis is made on clinical grounds, often with anteroposterior and lateral radiographs to exclude a neoplastic or infectious process.
- Radiographic findings of soft tissue swelling and irregularity of the tibial tubercle are not specific for Osgood-Schlatter disease.
- Other associated radiographic findings can include calcification or superficial ossicle formation in the patellar tendon.

THERAPY

■ **NONPHARMACOLOGIC**
- Usually responds to limitation of activities that stress the patellar tendon.
- Regular stretching of the quadriceps mechanism and hamstrings
- Knee pads to minimize direct trauma

■ **MEDICAL**
- Nonsteroidal antiinflammatory drugs (NSAIDs) can be prescribed for pain.
- Infrapatellar straps or knee braces may partially alleviate symptoms.
- For severe cases not responding to conservative management, more prolonged tendon rest can be achieved with above-the-knee casting for 3 to 6 weeks.

■ **SURGICAL**
Surgical excision of the tibial tuberosity or the ossicle in tendon is rarely required.

■ **FOLLOW-UP & DISPOSITION**
- The disease is generally self-limited.
- Follow-up is dictated by the degree and persistence of symptoms.
- Complications are rare but can include the following:
  1. Cosmetic deformity of enlarged tibial tuberosity
  2. Genu recurvatum resulting from premature fusion of the anterior tibial tubercle and proximal tibia
  3. Patellofemoral degenerative arthritis
  4. Chondromalacia
  5. Uprising of patella
  6. Patellar tendon avulsion

■ **REFERRAL INFORMATION**
Patients with symptoms not responsive to conservative measures of activity limitation and NSAIDs can be referred to an orthopedic surgeon for bracing or casting.

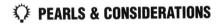 **PEARLS & CONSIDERATIONS**

■ **CLINICAL PEARLS**
Corticosteroid injections into the patellar tendon are rarely indicated and may predispose the patient to tendon avulsion.

■ **WEBSITE**
The Physician and Sports Medicine Online: www.physsportsmed.com; provides strengthening exercises

REFERENCES
1. Dunn J: Osgood-Schlatter disease, *Am Fam Physician* 41:173, 1990.
2. Krause BL et al: Natural history of Osgood-Schlatter disease, *J Pediatr Orthoped* 10:65, 1990.
3. Kujala U et al: Osgood-Schlatter's disease in adolescent athletes, *Am J Sports Med* 13:236, 1985.
4. Tachdjian MO (ed): *Pediatric orthopedics*, ed 2, Philadelphia, 1990, WB Saunders.
Author: **Joseph Nicholas, M.D.**

II

BASIC INFORMATION

■ DEFINITION

Osteogenesis imperfecta (OI) is a generalized disorder of connective tissue manifested by bone fragility, blue sclerae, and other variable soft tissue manifestations. There are at least four clinical subtypes, most of which are autosomal dominantly inherited, but new mutations occur, especially in the lethal forms.

- *OI type I* is the mildest and most common type. Manifestations are bone fragility, with most fractures caused by mild trauma occurring before puberty. The sclera are blue or have a purple or grayish tint.
- *OI type II* is the most severe form and is often lethal in the perinatal period because of respiratory problems. Numerous fractures sustained prenatally, resulting in significant skeletal deformity, contribute to this high mortality. Fractures are also sustained during birth. The sclera are blue or have a purple or grayish tint.
- *OI type III* is manifested by bone fragility and severe deformity. Fractures are present at birth. Short limbs and short stature are common. The sclera are normal but sometimes blue in infancy. Respiratory problems caused by rib deformity can be significant. Inheritance appears to be autosomal recessive in most cases.
- *OI type IV* is intermediate between type I and type III in severity. There is bone fragility, mostly before puberty. Short stature can be present, but sclera are white or near-white. There is mild to moderate bone deformity.
- *Dentinogenesis imperfecta* (brittle teeth) is variable and present in approximately 30% of all types of OI.

ICD-9CM CODE
756.51 Osteogenesis imperfecta

■ ETIOLOGY
- Reduction or abnormality of procollagen I, resulting in abnormal type 1 collagen, is found in patients with OI type I.
- Mutation in the COL1A1 or the COL1A2 gene loci causes different forms of OI.

■ EPIDEMIOLOGY & DEMOGRAPHICS
- OI type I has an incidence of approximately 4 per 100,000 births.
- OI type II has an incidence of approximately 2.5 per 100,000 births.
- OI type III has an incidence of 1.45 per 100,000 births.

■ HISTORY
- Fracture with minimal trauma
- Familial short stature
- Perinatal death (OI type II)
- Presenile hearing loss
- Dentinogenesis imperfecta

■ PHYSICAL EXAMINATION
- Blue sclera in types I, II, and early in III
- Short stature
- Hyperextensible joints
- Hypotonia
- Presenile hearing loss, begins in 20-to 30-year-olds
- Scoliosis
- Deformity
- Brittle teeth
- Barrel chest
- Short limbs

DIAGNOSIS

■ DIFFERENTIAL DIAGNOSIS
- Secondary osteoporosis
- Child abuse
- Hyper-IgE syndrome

■ DIAGNOSTIC WORKUP
- Radiographic
  1. In types I and IV, radiographs usually show osteoporosis.
     a. Fractures can be multiple.
     b. Large calvarium, wormian bones, and hypoplastic dentine are seen.
     c. Kyphoscoliosis is common.
  2. In type II, almost no ossification of the skull or wormian bones is found.
     a. Long bones are short, angulated, and crumpled with thin cortices.
     b. Ribs show a beaded appearance.
     c. Multiple fractures are usually seen.
  3. In type III, severe generalized osteoporosis is seen.
     a. Wormian bones and severe deossification of membranous skull bones are present.
     b. Long bones show mild shortening and marked angulation, with metaphyseal and diaphyseal widening.
- Skin biopsy
  1. Collagen structure is usually normal, but the amount is reduced.
  2. Protein and DNA-based studies are done on skin fibroblast culture derived from a skin biopsy sample and can help confirm the diagnosis in most, but not all, cases.
- Prenatal diagnosis
  1. High-resolution ultrasound in the second trimester can usually identify fetuses with OI type II and type III. The other forms can sometimes be detected late in the pregnancy.
  2. DNA-based prenatal diagnosis using chorionic villus or amniocentesis may be useful in some families.

THERAPY

■ NONPHARMACOLOGIC
- Prevention (see following discussion)
- Dental management in patients with dentinogenesis imperfecta
- Physical therapy to maximize mobility in the more severe types of OI

■ MEDICAL
Experimental therapy with bone marrow transplantation is being conducted.

■ SURGICAL
Orthopedic care relating to fracture and scoliosis management

■ FOLLOW-UP & DISPOSITION
Surveillance for hearing impairment and scoliosis

■ PATIENT/FAMILY EDUCATION
- Types I, II, and IV are autosomal dominantly inherited. Affected individuals have a 50% chance of having a child with the condition with each pregnancy.
- Affected children from families with no previous history of OI usually have new mutations.
  1. Future siblings of the affected child would theoretically not be at an increased risk.
  2. However, gonadal mosaicism in normal parents results in an empirical 6% recurrence risk in offspring of such parents.
- OI type III is autosomal recessively inherited, and parents of affected children have a 25% recurrence risk for each future pregnancy.

■ PREVENTIVE TREATMENT
- Prevent fracture by avoiding high-impact activities.
- Exercise to promote muscle and bone strength.
- Maintain a healthy diet: appropriate vitamin D, calcium, and phosphate intake.
- Avoid steroid use.

■ REFERRAL INFORMATION
- Genetics
- Orthopedics
- Physical therapy
- Dental (as necessary)
- Audiology

☼ PEARLS & CONSIDERATIONS

■ CLINICAL PEARLS
- Families with severe postmenopausal osteoporosis should be considered for OI.

- In suspected child abuse cases because of the presence of recurrent fractures, OI should be considered as part of the diagnostic workup.

■ WEBSITE
The OI Foundation: www.oif.org

REFERENCE
1. Tsipouras P: Osteogenesis imperfecta. In Beighton P (ed): *McKusick's heritable disorders of connective tissue,* ed 5, St Louis, 1993, Mosby.
Author: **Chin-To Fong, M.D.**

II

BASIC INFORMATION

■ DEFINITION
Osteomyelitis is an infection of bone; it is most commonly caused by pyogenic organisms and rarely by fungi and viruses.

ICD-9CM CODES
730.0 Acute osteomyelitis
730.1 Chronic osteomyelitis

■ ETIOLOGY
- Microorganisms are introduced into bone by one of the following three mechanisms:
  1. Hematogenous seeding (most common)
  2. Local invasion from contiguous infection
  3. Direct inoculation from surgery or trauma
- Bacteria localize in the metaphysis of the bone secondary to sluggish blood flow in the area where nutrient arteries send small terminal branches that end at the growth plate.
  1. Secondary thrombosis occurs.
  2. This becomes a nidus for infection.
- Collection of inflammatory cells and exudate causes the following:
  1. Elevation of periosteum and/or rupture into soft tissue
  2. Necrotic bone: sequestrum
  3. Reparative bone laid down over area: involucrum
- Joints with intraarticular metaphysis are predisposed to concomitant septic arthritis as infection ruptures into joint.
  1. Hip
  2. Shoulder
  3. Ankle
  4. Elbow
- A bacterial cause may be responsible.
  1. *Staphylococcus aureus* (70% to 89%), followed by streptococcus (group A β-hemolytic streptococcus, viridans streptococcus, *Streptococcus pneumoniae*)
  2. *Haemophilus influenzae* type b once common, but now greatly decreased in prevalence because of immunization
  3. Other causes: Enterobacteriaceae, *Salmonella, Kingella kingae,* rarely viruses, fungi, mycobacteria
- Special circumstances are as follows:
  1. In patients with sickle cell disease
     a. *Salmonella:* 70%
     b. *S. aureus:* 10%
     c. Gram-negative enterobacteria
  2. Neonates
     a. *S. aureus*
     b. Gram-negative bacteria
     c. Group B streptococcus
     d. Coagulase-negative *S. aureus* (CONS)
     e. *Candida albicans*

  3. Intravenous drug abusers
     a. *Pseudomonas aeruginosa,* especially vertebrae and pelvis
     b. *Serratia marcescens*
  4. Facial and cervical osteomyelitis: actinomyces common
  5. Superinfection of *S. aureus* osteomyelitis: anaerobes
  6. Postvaricella: group A β-hemolytic streptococcus
  7. Puncture wound of foot (especially through sneaker): *Pseudomonas aeruginosa*
- The following locations may be affected:
  1. Femur and tibia most common
     a. Predilection for the most rapidly growing bones, especially the long bones of a lower extremity
     b. Occasionally, nontubular bones involved, such as calcaneus

■ EPIDEMIOLOGY & DEMOGRAPHICS
- The incidence is 1 per 5000 in children younger than 13 years of age.
  1. One third are younger than 2 years.
  2. One half are younger than 5 years.
- It is most common in infants and young children.
- The male:female ratio is 2.5:1.

■ HISTORY
- Bone pain (50%) and fever are common, but presentation varies with age.
- In some cases, systemic signs may be minimal with or without fever.
- Neonate: irritability, poor feeding, pseudoparalysis, red and/or swollen limb, fever, and/or malaise may be present.

■ PHYSICAL EXAMINATION
- Infants and children
  1. Limp or refusal to walk
  2. Tenderness
  3. Limited joint motion
- With extension of infection
  1. Local erythema
  2. Warmth
  3. Swelling more diffuse
- Adolescents
  1. Localized point tenderness and limp

DIAGNOSIS

■ DIFFERENTIAL DIAGNOSIS
- Septic arthritis
- Juvenile arthritis
- Acute rheumatic fever
- Malignancy (leukemia, Ewing's sarcoma, neuroblastoma)
- Bone infarction (sickle cell)
- Toxic synovitis

■ DIAGNOSTIC WORKUP
- Diagnosis requires two of the following conditions:
  1. Purulence of bone
  2. Positive blood or bone culture
  3. Localized erythema, edema, or both
  4. Positive imaging study: radiograph, bone scan, or magnetic resonance imaging (MRI) scan
- Cultures of bone (either surgically or needle aspiration) and blood
  1. Bone culture: positive in 80%
  2. Blood culture: positive in 36% to 67%
- Other blood work
  1. Complete blood count (CBC) is obtained.
     a. Leukocytosis with left shift, but may be normal with normal or only slightly shifted differential
     b. Occasionally thrombocytosis
  2. Erythrocyte sedimentation rate (ESR), a nonspecific sign of inflammation, is usually elevated.
     a. Declines 1 to 2 weeks after therapy started
     b. Normalizes in 3 to 4 weeks
  3. C-reactive protein (CRP), another marker of inflammation, is usually elevated at presentation.
     a. Declines within 6 hours of appropriate therapy
- Imaging studies
  1. Radiograph: may take 10 to 14 days to see changes on radiograph, but useful to exclude fracture or malignancy
     a. Soft tissue swelling: 3 days
     b. Obliteration of fat planes: 3 to 7 days
     c. Metaphyseal irregularities
     d. Periosteal elevation
  2. Bone scan: detects osteomyelitis in the first 24 to 48 hours; three-phase bone scan with technetium MDP (T^{c}MDP) may be used
     a. A *hot spot* is an area of increased uptake in all three phases.
     b. A *cold spot* may occur early in course and is an area of decreased uptake, secondary to bone infarction.
     c. Bone scan sensitivity is 90%; specificity is low; 50% sensitivity in neonates.
  3. Gallium-67 citrate and indium-111 oxide (may be useful if clinical signs are poorly localized)
     a. White cell scan
     b. Limitations of these studies include time, high radiation dose, and low yield
  4. Computed tomography: excellent bony detail
     a. Reserved for select cases
     b. Helpful in spine and pelvis osteomyelitis

5. MRI: detailed anatomic picture
   a. Prospective sensitivity 98%, specificity 75%
   b. Limited usefulness because of low specificity and sedation requirement

℞ THERAPY

■ NONPHARMACOLOGIC
Immobilization or splinting of the extremity may help with pain relief and prevention of a pathologic fracture.

■ MEDICAL
- Initial management is with parenteral antibiotics after bone aspirate and blood culture are completed.
- Antimicrobials should cover *S. aureus*.
  1. β-Lactamase–resistant penicillin, such as oxacillin or nafcillin, or ampicillin-sulbactam, or a first-generation cephalosporin are drugs of choice.
  2. If methicillin-resistant *S. aureus* (MRSA) is suspected and/or if the patient is penicillin or cephalosporin allergic, use vancomycin.
  3. Cefuroxime is empirically used by some with good results.
- *H. influenzae* type b coverage in a very young child includes one of the following:
  1. Cefuroxime
  2. Ampicillin-sulbactam
  3. Third-generation cephalosporin
- The duration of therapy is controversial in hematogenous osteomyelitis.
  1. Treatment is usually for at least 5 to 7 days intravenously, plus
  2. Oral antibiotics for 3 to 4 more weeks at two to three times the usual daily recommended dose.
- Home IV therapy is an alternative to ensure compliance.

- Tailor antimicrobials once the organism and sensitivities have been identified.
- Consider switching to oral antibiotics once the patient is afebrile, local signs/symptoms are reduced, and the patient is maintaining adequate oral intake.
- Check the level of oral antibiotic to ensure absorption and level eightfold to tenfold over mean inhibitory concentration of organism.

■ SURGICAL
- Surgical debridement may be indicated in the following situations:
  1. If purulent drainage is found on aspiration of joint or bone
  2. If signs and/or symptoms fail to improve within 48 hours
  3. If progressive destruction is visible on radiograph

■ FOLLOW-UP & DISPOSITION
- Weekly measurements of CBC, ESR, or CRP should be taken.
- The recommendation to follow peak serial bactericidal titers for desired titer of 1:8 has recently been questioned.
- Repeat films may be indicated in complicated cases or if there is a question of adequate healing.

■ COMPLICATIONS
- Recurrence
- Chronic osteomyelitis
- Leg length discrepancy with lower extremity osteomyopathy
- Risk of complications increases with the following factors:
  1. Polymicrobial infection
  2. Delay in diagnosis and treatment
  3. Short duration of treatment
  4. Neonatal age group

■ PATIENT/FAMILY EDUCATION
Stress the need for compliance and follow-up.

■ REFERRAL INFORMATION
- Orthopedic surgeons for management:
  1. Bone aspiration
  2. Potential need for debridement
- Consult with a pediatric infectious diseases specialist.

☼ PEARLS & CONSIDERATIONS

■ CLINICAL PEARLS
- In the neonate, nutrient vessels transverse the growth plate, ending in the epiphysis. These vessels atrophy by 15 to 18 months; thus more extensive growth plate involvement occurs in this age group.
- Joint aspiration does not significantly alter bone scan.
- Higher yield when suspect *Kingella kingae* with culture aspirate directly into BACTEC bottle.

REFERENCES
1. Karwowska A et al: Epidemiology and outcome of osteomyelitis in the era of sequential intravenous-oral therapy, *Pediatr Infect Dis J* 17:1021, 1998.
2. Krogstad P, Smith AL: Osteomyelitis and septic arthritis. In Feigin R, Cherry J (eds): *Pediatric infectious diseases*, Philadelphia, 1998, WB Saunders.
3. Peltola H et al: Simplified treatment of acute staphylococcal osteomyelitis of childhood, *Pediatrics* 99:846, 1997.
4. Roy DR: Osteomyelitis, *Pediatr Rev* 16: 380, 1995.
5. Sonnen GM, Henry NK: Pediatric bone and joint infections: diagnosis and antimicrobial management, *Pediatr Clin North Am* 43:933, 1996.
Author: **Emma Hughes, M.D.**

II

BASIC INFORMATION

■ DEFINITION
Osteosarcoma is a neoplasm derived from primitive bone-forming mesenchyme. The pathologic appearance is characterized by the production of osteoid and new bone by spindle-shaped tumor cells. Osteogenic sarcoma is a family of tumors that includes osteosarcoma, chondrosarcoma, and fibrosarcoma.

■ SYNONYM
Osteogenic sarcoma

ICD-9CM CODE
170.9 Osteosarcoma

■ ETIOLOGY
- Most cases are sporadic, without an identified cause.
- The only established environmental cause is ionizing radiation, which is implicated in 3% of cases.
- An association exists with Paget's disease, certain benign bone lesions, hereditary retinoblastoma, and Li-Fraumeni syndrome.
- A relationship exists between rapid growth and development of osteosarcoma.
- Trauma often brings patients to medical attention, but evidence of a causal relationship is lacking.

■ EPIDEMIOLOGY & DEMOGRAPHICS
- Osteosarcomas account for 60% of malignant bone tumors.
- The incidence is approximately 5 cases per 1 million children younger than 15 years of age per year in the United States, but the peak incidence is in late adolescence.
- Males are affected more than females.
- Approximately 90% of tumors occur in the extremities.
  1. The most common site of involvement is around the knee.
  2. Metaphyseal sites of the most rapidly growing bones are more commonly involved.

■ HISTORY
- Pain with or without mass or swelling is reported.
- Systemic symptoms such as fatigue and fever are uncommon.
- Pathologic fractures are rare.

■ PHYSICAL EXAMINATION
- Tenderness over the involved bone is elicited.
- A firm mass at the site of involvement is often palpable.

🔬 DIAGNOSIS

■ DIFFERENTIAL DIAGNOSIS
- Other malignancies that occur in the extremities, most commonly the Ewing's family of tumors or rhabdomyosarcoma or other soft tissue sarcomas
  1. Lymphomas may also rarely occur in bone.
- Benign bone tumors
- Traumatic lesions

■ DIAGNOSTIC WORKUP
- Plain films of the involved bone
- Magnetic resonance imaging (MRI) scan of the involved bone
- Bone scan to document the site of disease and assess for bony metastases or synchronous tumors
- Chest roentgenogram
- Computed tomography (CT) scan of the chest to evaluate pulmonary metastases
- Biopsy

■ PATHOLOGY
- Approximately 95% of cases in children are conventional osteosarcomas of high-grade pathology. Other variants, including telangiectatic and small cell osteosarcomas, are also considered high grade.
- Parosteal and periosteal osteosarcomas are rare variants of low-grade and intermediate-grade, respectively.

■ STAGING
- Staging is usually confined to localized or metastatic disease.
- The most common site for metastases is the lungs (85% of patients with metastases).
- Approximately 80% of patients have at least micrometastatic disease.

💊 THERAPY

■ SURGICAL
Local control requires limb salvage or amputation.

■ MEDICAL
- Chemotherapy
  1. Active agents include doxorubicin, cisplatin, methotrexate, ifosfamide, and VP-16.
  2. Patients are usually treated with neoadjuvant chemotherapy before a definitive surgical procedure is performed.
     a. Postoperative adjuvant chemotherapy is administered after recovery from surgery.
     b. Chemotherapy may be adjusted based on the tumor response.
- Radiation therapy (not indicated for front-line therapy of resectable tumors)
  1. Potential role in unresectable tumors
  2. Palliative role in cases of progressive disease

■ PROGNOSIS
- Patients with localized disease have approximately a 70% to 75% 5-year survival rate.
- The overall prognosis for patients with metastatic disease is 20% to 30%.
- Patients with metastatic disease have a better prognosis if metastases can be removed surgically.
- Response to chemotherapy has prognostic significance.
  1. Patients with more than 90% tumor necrosis have a better prognosis.

■ FOLLOW-UP & DISPOSITION
- Plain films and MRI/CT scans of primary tumor are generally obtained every 3 months for a year, then every 4 to 6 months for 2 years, then yearly for 10 years.
  1. Limb salvage hardware may cause an artifact on scans.
- Chest radiograph, CT scan of the chest, and bone scan are performed on the same schedule.
- Potential late effects of chemotherapy may include renal glomerular and tubular dysfunction, hearing loss, and cardiomyopathy.

■ PATIENT/FAMILY EDUCATION
Even bone tumors with a benign radiologic appearance should be evaluated by an experienced orthopedic surgeon.

■ REFERRAL INFORMATION
Patients should be cared for by pediatric oncologists and orthopedic surgeons with experience in bone tumors.

⚙ PEARLS & CONSIDERATIONS

■ CLINICAL PEARLS
- Patients often present with symptoms after minor trauma. Persistent pain should be further evaluated.
- Although trauma is not associated with the development of osteosarcoma, patients often present with symptoms after minor injury. Persistent pain should be further evaluated.

■ **WEBSITES**
- American Cancer Society: www.cancer.org
- National Cancer Institute: www.nci.nih.gov
- OncoLink: www.oncolink.com

■ **SUPPORT GROUPS**
- Pediatric oncologists can refer patients and parents to local or national support organizations for children with cancer and their families.

- National organizations include the American Cancer Society and Candlelighters.

REFERENCES

1. Buckley JD et al: Epidemiology of osteosarcoma and Ewing's sarcoma in childhood, *Cancer* 83:1440, 1998.
2. Crist WM, Kun LE: Common solid tumors of childhood, *N Engl J Med* 324:461, 1991.
3. Halperin EC et al: Osteosarcoma. In Halperin EC et al (eds): *Pediatric radiation oncology*, ed 3, Philadelphia, 1999, Lippincott Williams & Wilkins.
4. Harris MB et al: Treatment of metastatic osteosarcoma at diagnosis: a Pediatric Oncology Group study, *J Clin Oncol* 16:3641, 1998.
5. Link MP, Eilber F: Osteosarcoma. In Pizzo PA, Poplack DG (eds): *Principles and practice of pediatric oncology*, ed 3, Philadelphia, 1997, JB Lippincott.

Author: **Andrea S. Hinkle, M.D.**

II

BASIC INFORMATION

DEFINITION

Otitis externa is inflammation or infection of the external auditory canal and auricle. *Malignant otitis externa* refers to temporal bone osteomyelitis.

SYNONYM

Swimmer's ear

ICD-9CM CODES

380.10 Acute, diffuse, hemorrhagica
380.16 Chronic
380.14 Malignant
380.15 Mycotic

ETIOLOGY

- Disruption of the normal protective barriers (hair in the outer part of the canal, cerumen)
- Mechanisms that disrupt the barriers: high temperature and humidity, allergies, stress, trauma, alkaline pH, cerumen removal, bacterial contamination, swimming
- Factors that may predispose to these mechanisms: impacted cerumen, seborrheic or contact dermatitis, perforated otitis media, congenital or acquired narrowing of the canal, small external canal caused by chromosomal defects (i.e., trisomy 21), infections transmitted from the hands, immersion baths or swimming
- Bacteriologic invasion: *Pseudomonas aeruginosa, Staphylococcus aureus,* other gram-negative bacteria (i.e., *Proteus, Escherichia coli*), pathogenic streptococcus, rarely fungal

EPIDEMIOLOGY & DEMOGRAPHICS

- Uncommon in infants and toddlers
- Accounts for 5% to 20% of pediatric office visits in summer in tropical and subtropical areas

HISTORY

- Ear pain, fullness, possibly itching and conductive hearing loss
- History of swimming
- For malignant otitis externa: chronically ill or immunosuppressed

PHYSICAL EXAMINATION

- Erythema and edema of the canal with clear to seropurulent discharge
- Pain on movement of the tragus of the ear
- In severe cases, periauricular swelling

🔬 DIAGNOSIS

DIFFERENTIAL DIAGNOSIS

- Furunculosis
- Foreign body
- Serous otitis media
- Acute otitis media
- Bullous myringitis
- Mastoiditis
- Malignancies
- Chronic otorrhea secondary to chronic otitis media
- Herpes zoster oticus

DIAGNOSTIC WORKUP

- Imaging is necessary only for complicated cases in which other diagnoses are being ruled out (i.e., mastoiditis).
- Erythrocyte sedimentation rate is necessary if ruling out malignant otitis externa.

℞ THERAPY

NONPHARMACOLOGIC

- Avoid showers, swimming, and excessive exercise until ear edema and pain resolve.
- Lavage and then suction ears with hypertonic saline or 2.5% acetic acid if needed to clear debris.
- Place acetic acid solution 2.5% (white vinegar, 5% acetic acid mixed with 1:1 with water or rubbing alcohol) in the ear (4 to 6 drops in ear every 2 hours while awake) in the inflammatory, preinfected stage. Domeboro otic solution (2% acetic acid) can also be used.
- Ear wick can be used to keep the canal patent and to distribute the medicine (needed only in severe cases).

MEDICAL

- Antibiotic ear drops with or without hydrocortisone may be given.
  1. Polymyxin/neomycin solution or suspension 3 to 4 drops in the affected ear three to four times per day
  2. Ciprofloxacin or ofloxacin solution 3 drops twice daily
  3. Ophthalmic drops such as tobramycin (0.3%) 1 to 2 drops four to six times per day
- Treat 5 to 7 days or until 3 days beyond symptom resolution.
- Including hydrocortisone in the drops speeds symptom resolution.
- Analgesics may be given for pain.
- Systemic antibiotics can be used if secondary complications such as cellulitis develop.
  1. Cover for staphylococcal organisms with oxacillin or nafcillin.
  2. Cover for *Pseudomonas aeruginosa* if malignant otitis suspected.

SURGICAL

Rarely necessary except for severe cases to drain abscesses or chronic cases that are not responding to medical treatment

FOLLOW-UP & DISPOSITION

Reexamination is needed for severe cases, for lack of resolution, or if the diagnosis is uncertain.

PATIENT/FAMILY EDUCATION & PREVENTIVE TREATMENT

- Silicon earplugs, bathing caps, or oil drops should be worn or used before swimming to keep the ears dry.
- Dry ears after swimming with a hair dryer (on low setting), and then apply 70% ethyl alcohol drops.
- Use dilute (2% to 2.5%) acetic acid drops in ear after swimming.
- Avoid manipulation of the ear canal (do not put anything smaller than your elbow inside your ear).

REFERRAL INFORMATION

For treatment failures or severe cases, refer the patient to an otolaryngologist.

💡 PEARLS & CONSIDERATIONS

CLINICAL PEARLS

- Antibiotic ears drops are acceptable even with a perforated eardrum, although there is a small risk of ototoxicity with certain medications (i.e., neomycin).
- Malignant otitis externa (or necrotizing otitis externa) is an osteomyelitis of the temporal bone and is classically caused by *P. aeruginosa.*
- Neomycin drops may cause severe contact dermatitis, which may confuse the diagnosis.
- Ophthalmic drops are less acidic than otic drops and may be tolerated better.
- Unless caused by a perforated otitis media, rarely need to treat for an otitis media even if the tympanic membrane is erythematous.
- In clinical treatment failures, consider Langerhans cell histiocytosis.

REFERENCES

1. Bojrab DI, Bruderly T, Abdulrazzak Y: Otitis externa, *Otolaryngol Clin North Am* 29:760, 1996.
2. Feigin RD, Alexander JJ: Otitis externa. In Feigin RD, Alexander JJ (eds): *Textbook of pediatric infectious diseases,* ed 4, Philadelphia, 1998, WB Saunders.
3. Guthrie RM: Diagnosis and treatment of acute otitis externa, *Ann Otol Rhinol Laryngol* 108:1, 1999.
Author: **Carolyn Cleary, M.D.**

BASIC INFORMATION

■ DEFINITION
Otitis media (OM) is inflammation of the mucoperiosteal lining of the middle ear cavity. OM may be described as suppurative or serous, and acute or chronic. Complications include extension into the adjacent mastoid air cells resulting in mastoiditis or perforation of the tympanic membrane (TM) with otitis externa.

■ SYNONYMS
- Acute otitis media
- Serous otitis media
- Otitis media with effusion
- Suppurative otitis media

ICD-9CM CODES
382.9 Acute otitis media
381.00 Acute otitis media with effusion
382.01 Acute otitis media with spontaneous rupture of tympanic membrane
382.9 Chronic otitis media
381.3 Chronic otitis with effusion

■ ETIOLOGY
- Poor drainage or obstruction of the eustachian tube leads to accumulation of fluid in the middle ear cavity. This fluid can then become infected, resulting in OM.
- Upper respiratory infections lead to edema and hyperemia of the eustachian tubes, obstructing the drainage of fluid.
- The younger child is also anatomically predisposed to ear infections because the eustachian tube is more horizontal than as an adult.
- Causative agents include the following:
  1. *Streptococcus pneumoniae:* 30% to 50% of infections
  2. *Haemophilus influenzae:* 20% to 27%
  3. *Moraxella catarrhalis:* 7% to 23%
  4. Group A β-hemolytic streptococcus, *Staphylococcus aureus,* α-hemolytic streptococcus
  5. Viruses, including respiratory syncytial virus (RSV), influenza A, human rhinovirus, adenovirus, and parainfluenza

■ EPIDEMIOLOGY & DEMOGRAPHICS
- Approximately 62% of children have had one episode of acute otitis media (AOM) by 1 year of age.
- Seventeen percent of children have had more than three episodes by 1 year of age.
- About 42% of antibiotics prescribed for children are written to treat OM.
- Approximately 2 million surgical procedures are performed each year to place tympanostomy tubes.

- Peak incidence coincides with a peak in the upper respiratory infection rate in the winter months. This may be caused by associated edema and hyperemia of the eustachian tube.
- An increased incidence in the disease is associated with the following factors:
  1. Native Americans, North American Eskimos
  2. Cleft palate, cleft uvula
  3. Craniofacial anomalies
  4. Eustachian tube dysfunction
  5. Immune deficiencies, such as chronic granulomatous disease, immunoglobulin deficiencies, malignancies, acquired immunodeficiency syndrome, or immune suppression
  6. Nasopharyngeal tumors
  7. Down syndrome
  8. Connective tissue disorders
  9. Passive smoke exposure
- Breastfeeding longer than 3 months is associated with a decrease in the risk of AOM in the first year of life.

■ HISTORY
- In the older child, ear pain is the hallmark.
- Fever may be present.
- Hearing difficulty occurs.
- In infants and small children, typical symptoms include the following:
  1. Irritability
  2. Decreased feeding
  3. Fever
  4. Difficulty sleeping with frequent arousals

■ PHYSICAL EXAMINATION
- Immobility of TM
- Bulging TM
- Loss of TM landmarks
- Hyperemia of the TM
- Cloudy, clear, or purulent fluid in the middle ear space
- Fever, other signs of systemic illness
- Unsteady gait suggesting vestibular disturbance
- Hearing loss
- Tympanosclerosis, or scarring of the TM
  1. May be visible from previous infections

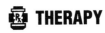 **DIAGNOSIS**

■ DIFFERENTIAL DIAGNOSIS
- Myringitis
- Otitis externa
- Mastoiditis
- Cholesteatoma
- Otorrhea caused by a foreign body in the canal

■ DIAGNOSTIC WORKUP
- Pneumatic otoscopy
  1. An insufflator attached to the otoscope head is used to move the TM.
  2. Fluid in the middle ear space inhibits this movement.
- Tympanometry
  1. Tympanometry incorporates sound energy to determine movement of the TM.
  2. Abnormal movements indicate abnormal pressures in the middle ear.
  3. Tympanometry is used to both evaluate and monitor middle ear effusions.
- Spectral gradient acoustic reflectometry
  1. Reflected sound waves indicate movement of the TM.
  2. This method is helpful when a seal of the canal cannot be achieved.
- Tympanocentesis
  1. Diagnostic culture
  2. Pain relief
  3. Should be considered for the following conditions:
     a. In the seriously ill patient with AOM
     b. Inadequate response to second-line antibiotic
     c. AOM develops while taking prophylactic antibiotics
     d. Neonate with AOM
     e. Immunosuppressed patient
     f. Chronic effusion
- In infants younger than 2 months of age with or without fever
  1. Consider further evaluation for extension of the infection and possible sepsis or meningitis.

THERAPY

■ NONPHARMACOLOGIC
Some experts advocate careful waiting and not treating with antibiotics because many cases are viral and resolve on their own.

■ MEDICAL
- Amoxicillin is given at 40 mg/kg/day divided two to three times (regular dose) or 80 to 90 mg/kg/day divided two to three times per day (high dose) if suspect resistant *Streptococcus pneumoniae* (age younger than 2 years, recent antibiotic therapy, recurrent otitis, day-care attendance).
- Pain relief is achieved with oral analgesics (e.g., acetaminophen, ibuprofen).
- Topical otic analgesics may be used to temporarily ease pain.
  1. Care should be taken not to mask the symptoms and allow extension of the infection.

- Antihistamines and decongestants have not been useful in the treatment or prevention of OM.
- If no improvement is seen after 3 days, change to a second-line antibiotic:
  1. Augmentin 45 mg/kg/day divided two times per day
  2. Cefuroxime axetil 30 mg/kg/day divided two times per day
  3. Cefprozil or cefpodoxime
  4. Azithromycin or clarithromycin
  5. Ceftriaxone 50 mg/kg intramuscularly as a single dose or three daily doses for more recalcitrant cases
  6. Clindamycin (30 mg/kg/day divided every 6 hours); may also be used in culture-confirmed pneumococcal disease
  7. Trimethoprim-sulfamethoxazole
  8. Fluoroquinolones—not be used in the routine treatment of OM

■ SURGICAL
Tympanocentesis as indicated previously for diagnostic culture and pain relief

■ FOLLOW-UP & DISPOSITION
- Persistence of initial symptoms on the third day of appropriate treatment implies resistance, and a second-line antibiotic should be instituted. After the acute infection has been successfully treated, an effusion may persist for the following periods:
  1. One month in 30% to 50%
  2. Two months in 15% to 25%
  3. Three months in 8% to 15%
- Tympanocentesis or a second course of antibiotics may be tried if an effusion persists for more than 3 months. Adding a short course of corticosteroids results in a temporary and limited benefit. The effectiveness of intranasal steroids has not been studied.

■ PATIENT/FAMILY EDUCATION
- Parents should be counseled on the adverse effects of bottle propping and passive cigarette smoke exposure in the development of OM.

- Breastfeeding should be recommended to families whose children have recurrent OM.
- Day-care attendance is also associated with an increased risk.

■ PREVENTIVE TREATMENT
- Recurrent AOM is defined as three or more episodes in 6 months *or* four episodes in 1 year. The following prophylactic antibiotics may be considered:
  1. Sulfisoxazole: 75 mg/kg/day divided two times per day
- Pneumococcal vaccine: The new conjugated polysaccharide-protein vaccine may be a preventive measure.

■ REFERRAL INFORMATION
- Indications for referral to an otolaryngologist are as follows:
  1. Development of AOM despite prophylactic antibiotics
  2. Presence of an effusion for 4 to 6 months
  3. Persistent effusion with documented hearing loss
  4. Tympanocentesis
- Tympanostomy tubes are indicated if the effusion persists longer than 4 to 6 months and is associated with a documented hearing loss.

⚙ PEARLS & CONSIDERATIONS

■ CLINICAL PEARLS
- A red TM is not an indication of OM without concurrent fluid in the middle ear space. Comparison between ears is useful. The tympanic membrane will become injected with crying and fever.
- Children have shorter, more horizontal eustachian tubes with less cartilaginous support that results in

poor ventilatory function. Nearly all children younger than 2 years of age who spend time in a day-care setting have some middle ear fluid collection with each upper respiratory infection.
- AOM with purulent conjunctivitis is associated with nontypeable *H. influenzae* infection.
- AOM with hemorrhagic conjunctivitis and pharyngitis may indicate an adenovirus infection.

■ WEBSITES
- Multiple websites are available with parental information, visual examples, and recent practice guidelines.
- American Academy of Pediatrics (AAP): www.aap.org/policy/otitis.htm; AAP practice parameters
- Kids-ENT.com: www.Kids-ENT.com; parent information, including frequently asked questions

REFERENCES
1. Dowell SF et al: Acute otitis media: management and surveillance in an era of pneumococcal resistance—a report from the Drug-resistant *Streptococcus pneumoniae* Therapeutic Working Group, *Pediatr Infect Dis J* 18:1, 1999.
2. Feigin RD et al: Otitis media. In Klein JO, Bluestone CD (eds): *Textbook of pediatric infectious diseases*, ed 4, Philadelphia, 1992, WB Saunders.
3. Maxson S, Yamauchi T: Acute otitis media, *Pediatr Rev* 17:191, 1996.
4. Scott F et al: Acute otitis media: management and surveillance in an era of pneumococcal resistance, *Pediatr Infect Dis J* 18:1, 1999.
Author: **Lora L. Pak, M.D.**

BASIC INFORMATION

■ DEFINITION
An ovarian mass is an abnormal growth on one or both ovaries.

■ SYNONYMS
- Adnexal mass
- Ovarian tumor
- Adnexal tumor
- Ovarian cyst

ICD-9CM CODES
654.4 Ovary tumor
620.0 Ovary cyst

■ ETIOLOGY
- The cause depends on the ultimate tissue diagnosis of the mass.
- Ovarian masses can be neoplastic or nonneoplastic, cystic or solid, or benign or malignant, and they can arise from ovarian tissue or from other tissues that implant on the ovary.
- Those arising from the ovary differentiate from the oocyte, the follicular cells, or the stroma.
- They are classified into functional, epithelial, germ cell, and sex cord stromal.

■ EPIDEMIOLOGY & DEMOGRAPHICS
- The incidence of all childhood/adolescent ovarian lesions is 2.6 per 100,000 girls per year.
- Sixty-five percent of ovarian masses in this age group are benign.
- From 58% to 67% of ovarian tumors in patients younger than 20 years are germ cell in origin.
- From 20% to 35% of ovarian masses or tumors are epithelial.
  1. Benign follicular cysts make up approximately one third of these cysts.
- Approximately 2% to 18% of ovarian masses are sex cord stromal.
- There does not appear to be a racial or geographic predisposition.
- Masses can arise at any age, including before birth.

■ HISTORY
- The most common presenting symptom is abdominal or pelvic pain; this may be acute or chronic.
- If prepubescent, the pain is midabdominal because the ovaries have not descended deep into the pelvis.
- Ovarian or ovarian mass torsion may be associated with nausea and vomiting.
- Rupture or torsion can mimic an acute abdomen.
- An abdominal mass may also be found incidentally.
- Uncommonly, precocious puberty or virilization may be the presenting sign.

- Important information to obtain includes family or personal history of ovarian masses, pubertal stage, sexual activity, menstrual history (if appropriate), vaginal discharge, fevers, or bowel changes.

■ PHYSICAL EXAMINATION
- Vital signs
- Abdominal examination for the following:
  1. Palpation of mass
  2. Localization of tenderness
  3. Presence or absence of rebound tenderness
  4. Referred rebound pain
  5. Guarding
  6. Rigidity
  7. Psoas and obturator signs
  8. Bowel sounds
- Pelvic and/or rectal examination for the following:
  1. Cultures
  2. Size of uterus
  3. Location of mass
  4. Tenderness
  5. Studding or induration of the pouch of Douglas
- If the patient is not sexually active or is prepubescent: rectal examination may be sufficient to palpate a mass

DIAGNOSIS

■ DIFFERENTIAL DIAGNOSIS
- Benign functional cysts are the most common in any ovulating female.
  1. Follicular, theca-lutein, and corpus luteal
  2. Ultrasound characteristics: a thin-walled, uniocular cyst less than 6 cm in diameter
- Other tumors are classified by cell derivation; these are solid, any size, and persistent.
  1. Germ cell
     a. Mature teratoma
     b. Immature teratoma
     c. Endodermal sinus tumor
     d. Dysgerminoma
     e. Choriocarcinoma
     f. Mixed germ cell tumor
  2. Epithelial
     a. Cystadenoma (mucinous or serous)
     b. Borderline epithelial tumors
     c. Cystadenocarcinoma
  3. Sex cord stromal
     a. Fibrothecoma
     b. Androblastoma
     c. Granulosa cell tumor
- Differential also includes other causes of abdominal and pelvic masses:
  1. Pregnancy
  2. Ectopic pregnancy
  3. Endometrioma
  4. Tubo-ovarian abscess
  5. Pelvic kidney
  6. Bowel, renal, and adrenal masses

■ DIAGNOSTIC WORKUP
- The diagnostic test of choice is ultrasound. Ultrasound will determine the following:
  1. Location of mass: ovarian, other
  2. Size of mass
  3. Consistency of mass: thin-walled cyst, multiloculated cyst, solid
- Doppler ultrasound of the ovarian vasculature should be done if torsion is suspected.
- Computed tomography and magnetic resonance imaging rarely add information to the ultrasound unless a malignancy is highly suspected.
- Other laboratory data include the following:
  1. Complete blood count
  2. Urine pregnancy test if appropriate
  3. Tumor markers including the following:
     a. β-Human chorionic gonadotropin (β-hCG)
     b. α-Fetoprotein (AFP)
     c. Carcinoembryonic antigen
     d. Cancer antigen 125
- There is no need for extensive metabolic laboratory workup unless a malignancy is suspected.

THERAPY

- The following are treatments for functional cysts:
  1. Simple cysts are most likely follicular (in adolescents) and resolve over time.
     a. If less than 6 cm, they can be observed over a few months for resolution.
        (1) If no resolution, operative intervention (removal) is indicated.
     b. If greater than 6 cm, surgery is indicated.
     c. If simple cysts rupture, transient peritonitis can occur but usually resolves within several hours without surgical intervention.
        (1) Other causes of peritonitis must be ruled out before conservative management.
  2. Corpus luteal cysts may rupture and cause hemoperitoneum.
     a. These can be managed conservatively.
     b. Operative management is indicated if the patient is hemodynamically unstable.
  3. Theca-lutein cysts are rare.
     a. They are associated with pregnancy, choriocarcinoma, or molar pregnancy.
     b. They can be quite large and resolve spontaneously.
     c. Operative removal is not indicated.

II

4. Mature cystic teratomas are the most common germ cell tumor.
   a. They can be discerned by ultrasound.
   b. Surgical removal is indicated; the ovary is left in situ, when possible.
- Malignant masses are managed surgically.
   1. Every attempt is made to perform conservative surgery.
   2. Provided the disease is not on the contralateral ovary or uterus, unilateral salpingo-oophorectomy and surgical staging are performed.
   3. Chemotherapeutic agents are adjunctive.
- Other cysts not mentioned here generally require surgical intervention at some point for appropriate diagnosis and treatment.
   1. Rarely is surgery emergent.
- Ovary or ovarian mass torsion is a surgical emergency.

■ FOLLOW-UP & DISPOSITION
- For simple cysts, observation with or without oral contraceptive pills can be done on an outpatient basis for a few months.
- Patients with ruptured simple cysts can be watched in an outpatient (emergency department) setting or in the hospital until symptom resolution while the workup is being completed.

- Hemorrhagic cysts can sometimes be watched conservatively in the hospital with serial abdominal examinations.
- Operative management for benign disease is usually via laparoscopy but may require laparotomy.
- Masses suspected of being malignant should be referred to a gynecologic oncologist.

■ PATIENT/FAMILY EDUCATION
- Patients with simple cysts who are being observed should understand the following:
   1. The benign nature of these cysts
   2. The potential for rupture
   3. The risk of torsion
   4. The likelihood of spontaneous resolution

✷ PEARLS & CONSIDERATIONS

■ CLINICAL PEARLS
- The vast majority of ovarian masses in patients younger than 20 years old are benign.
- Ultrasound is the diagnostic test of choice.
- Cystic teratomas (dermoids) have a high risk of torsion, and 15% are bilateral.

- The tumor markers noted previously can help differentiate between the following germ cell tumors:
   1. Dysgerminoma (−) AFP (−) β-hCG
   2. Choriocarcinoma (−) AFP (++) β-hCG
   3. Endodermal sinus tumor (+) AFP (−) β-hCG
   4. Immature teratoma (−) AFP (−) β-hCG

REFERENCES
1. Berek JS, Hacker NF (eds): *Practical gynecologic oncology*, ed 3, Philadelphia, 2000, Lippincott Williams & Wilkins.
2. Droegemueller W: Benign gynecologic lesions. In Droegemueller W et al (eds): *Comprehensive gynecology*, St Louis, 1987, Mosby.
3. Freud E et al: Ovarian masses in children, *Clin Pediatr* 38:573, 1999.
4. Lavvorn HN, Tucci LA, Stafford PW: Ovarian masses in the pediatric patient, *AORN* 67:3, 1998.
5. Skinner MA et al: Ovarian neoplasm's in children, *Arch Surg* 128:849, 1993.
6. Templeman C et al: Non-inflammatory ovarian masses in girls and young women, *Obstet Gynecol* 96:229, 2000.
Authors: **Elizabeth K. Cherot, M.D., and Fletcher R. Wilson, M.D.**

BASIC INFORMATION

DEFINITION
Pancreatitis is inflammation in the pancreas, which can be acute or chronic. *Acute pancreatitis* usually resolves without functional sequelae. *Chronic pancreatitis* involves ongoing structural and functional changes, which may be manifest clinically with chronic persistent symptoms or recurrent exacerbations. *Chronic obstructive pancreatitis* can be considered a subset of chronic pancreatitis and either improves with relief of the obstruction or progresses to chronic pancreatitis if untreated. Acute pancreatitis is not common in children, and progression to chronic pancreatitis is rare.

ICD-9CM CODES
577.0 Acute pancreatitis
577.1 Chronic pancreatitis

ETIOLOGY
- Acute pancreatitis
  1. The most common cause of acute pancreatitis in adults is gallstones.
  2. Alcohol can cause acute episodes of pancreatitis, but there is usually already underlying chronic damage.
  3. As many as 50% of cases of acute pancreatitis in children are considered idiopathic.
  4. Other causes include the following:
     a. Drugs and toxins
     b. Infections
        (1) Viral
        (2) Bacterial
        (3) Parasites
     c. Mechanical/structural
        (1) Trauma
        (2) Pancreatic outflow obstruction (pancreas divisum, strictures, cholelithiasis)
        (3) Bile reflux (choledochal cyst, strictures, choledocholithiasis)
        (4) Duodenopancreatic reflux (duodenal obstruction)
     d. Systemic disease
        (1) Vasculitis and inflammatory disorders
        (2) Sepsis
        (3) Shock
        (4) Reye's syndrome
     e. Metabolic/inherited abnormalities
        (1) Hypercalcemia
        (2) Hyperlipidemia
        (3) Hypothermia
        (4) Uremia
        (5) Malnutrition with refeeding
        (6) Cystic fibrosis
        (7) Hereditary pancreatitis
        (8) Diabetes mellitus
- Chronic pancreatitis
  1. The most common cause of chronic pancreatitis in adults is alcohol.
  2. In children, chronic pancreatitis is rare and usually results from hereditary pancreatitis, cystic fibrosis, or a structural abnormality such as pancreas divisum. Clinically, these conditions cause recurrent bouts of acute pancreatitis, which result in chronic inflammation and damage.
- Pathophysiology of the inflammation
  1. The exact mechanism is still unclear, but the general process is one of autodigestion resulting from premature activation of proenzymes to active digestive enzymes within the pancreas, beginning with activation of trypsin.

EPIDEMIOLOGY & DEMOGRAPHICS
- Specific diseases
- Hereditary (familial) pancreatitis
  1. Hereditary pancreatitis is characterized by recurrent bouts of acute pancreatitis, which can eventually result in pancreatic insufficiency.
  2. This disease is suggested by a family history and radiographic evidence of pancreatic calcifications.
  3. Inheritance is autosomal dominant.
  4. A genetic defect has been identified—mutation(s) in the trypsinogen gene render trypsin resistant to hydrolysis by pancreatic enzymes designed to protect the pancreas from autodigestion initiated by excess trypsin.
  5. Screening tests for the mutation are available.
  6. This condition is associated with pancreatic insufficiency and pancreatic cancer later in life.
- Cystic fibrosis
  1. Chronic pancreatitis has recently been associated with a specific genotype of cystic fibrosis.
  2. Each allele may have a different mutation.
  3. Sweat tests are often normal.
  4. Diagnosis is made by identifying abnormalities in the genotype and measuring nasal potential difference (PD), which is abnormally high.
- Pancreas divisum
  1. The dorsal and ventral pancreatic ducts do not fuse during development, resulting in drainage of the pancreas through the dorsal duct alone.
  2. This is considered a normal variant but may cause pancreatitis by obstruction.

  3. Management is controversial but may involve surgery or interventional endoscopy.

HISTORY
- Presenting symptoms include the following:
  1. Abdominal pain (may be mild or severe), often worse with meals
  2. Vomiting (common)
  3. Nausea
  4. Anorexia
- Identify predisposing factors:
  1. Drugs or toxins
  2. Trauma
  3. Infections
- Ask about a family history of cystic fibrosis or pancreatitis.

PHYSICAL EXAMINATION
Physical signs vary with the degree of pancreatic inflammation and systemic involvement.
- Abdominal tenderness (epigastric)
- Peritoneal signs (rebound, guarding)
- Abdominal distention
- Decreased or absent bowel sounds
- Fever (low grade)
- Hypotension, shock
- Ascites
- Respiratory distress
- Cullen's sign: ecchymoses around the umbilicus (hemorrhagic pancreatitis)
- Turner's sign: ecchymoses along the flank (hemorrhagic pancreatitis)

DIAGNOSIS

DIFFERENTIAL DIAGNOSIS
- Hepatobiliary disease
  1. Hepatitis
  2. Hepatic abscess
  3. Cholecystitis
  4. Cholangitis
  5. Biliary colic (choledocholithiasis)
- Peptic acid disease
  1. Gastritis
  2. Duodenitis
  3. Ulcers
- Intestinal disease
  1. Appendicitis
  2. Perforation/peritonitis
  3. Obstruction
  4. Acute gastroenteritis
- Renal disease
  1. Nephrolithiasis
  2. Pyelonephritis

DIAGNOSTIC WORKUP
- *Step 1:* Establish the presence of pancreatitis.
- Laboratory: The most commonly used tests to establish the diagnosis of pancreatitis are amylase and lipase.
  1. Amylase
     a. Increases within hours of onset of pancreatitis and remains elevated for 4 to 5 days.

b. Other causes for increased amylase include the following:
  (1) Biliary obstruction
  (2) Perforation
  (3) Intestinal obstruction
  (4) Trauma
  (5) Appendicitis
  (6) Mesenteric ischemia
  (7) Parotitis
  (8) Salivary duct obstruction
  (9) Tuboovarian disease
2. Lipase
  a. More specific for pancreatitis than amylase
  b. Increases within hours of onset of pancreatitis and remains elevated for 8 to 14 days and is therefore better for verifying the presence of pancreatitis later in the course of illness
  c. Nonpancreatic sources of lipase: salivary glands, stomach, breastmilk
3. Results
  a. Either the amylase or the lipase may be falsely normal or falsely elevated in the presence of pancreatitis.
  b. An increase of at least threefold in both of these tests is highly suggestive of pancreatitis.
  c. They are rarely *both* falsely normal or elevated.
- Radiographic studies: A kidney, ureter, and bladder (KUB) examination can suggest the presence of pancreatic inflammation, whereas ultrasound and computed tomography (CT) can confirm the presence of pancreatic inflammation and identify potential causes and complications.
  1. KUB
    a. Nonspecific findings that suggest the presence of pancreatitis include the following:
      (1) Sentinel loop (distended loop of small bowel near the pancreas)
      (2) Colon cutoff sign (dilated transverse colon with termination of the gas pattern at the level of the splenic flexure)
  2. Ultrasound
    a. Usually the initial study performed
    b. Will show changes consistent with pancreatitis in 70% to 80% of patients
      (1) Diffuse or focal enlargement
      (2) Decreased echogenicity
    c. Identifies potential causes, including stones and biliary tract disease
    d. Identifies complications of pancreatitis, specifically phlegmonous and pseudocysts

3. CT
  a. CT is useful if ultrasound is nondiagnostic or does not adequately visualize the pancreas.
  b. As many as 20% of adults with pancreatitis may have a normal CT.
  c. CT with intravenous contrast is particularly useful for identifying necrotizing pancreatitis, which has a higher association with infection and poor outcome.
- *Step 2:* Assess the severity of pancreatic inflammation.
- Determining the severity of the pancreatitis is important to anticipate complications and predict course. This determination is based on several clinical and laboratory parameters:
  1. Ranson's criteria (see references)
  2. APACHE II score (see references)
  3. Interstitial versus necrotizing pancreatitis
    a. This is determined by CT with intravenous contrast.
    b. If the pancreas is perfused, the process is interstitial, usually mild and sterile.
    c. Areas that are not perfused represent necrotizing pancreatitis, a more severe process that may be sterile or infected.
- *Step 3:* Determine the cause of pancreatitis.
- Initial episode of pancreatitis: If the cause is not apparent by history and presentation, the evaluation should include laboratory tests for metabolic causes and imaging studies.
  1. Laboratory
    a. Calcium
    b. Lipid profile (triglycerides)
    c. Genetic screening for hereditary pancreatitis and cystic fibrosis under the following conditions:
      (1) If supported by family history
      (2) If pancreatic calcifications are identified on imaging studies (hereditary pancreatitis)
- Recurrent pancreatitis: With the second episode of pancreatitis, if the cause has not been established, the evaluation should include the following:
  1. Laboratory
    a. Perform genetic screening for hereditary pancreatitis and cystic fibrosis, regardless of family history.
  2. Radiographic studies
    a. Repeat ultrasound and/or CT scan.
    b. Perform endoscopic retrograde cholangiopancreatography (ERCP).

💊 THERAPY

Therapy is directed toward the following:
- Decreasing inflammation
  1. Eliminate any cause or potential contribution to inflammation (e.g., drugs or impacted gallstones).
- Providing supportive care
  1. Close clinical monitoring (in the intensive care unit if pancreatitis is severe) is necessary.
  2. Laboratory tests include a complete blood count, blood urea nitrogen, creatinine, glucose, electrolytes, calcium, magnesium, and liver function tests.
  3. Eliminate oral intake (minimize pancreatic exocrine function).
  4. Place a nasogastric tube (in the presence of protracted vomiting or ileus).
  5. Provide intravenous fluid hydration and correction of electrolyte imbalances.
  6. Administer nutritional support (parenteral nutrition or nasojejunal feedings) if oral feedings cannot be initiated within a few days.
  7. Provide pain management.
- Assessing for and treating complications
  1. Metabolic complications include hypocalcemia and hyperglycemia.
  2. Infections: Phlegmon, fluid collections, and areas of pancreatic necrosis may become infected.
    a. Incidence of infection in necrotizing pancreatitis is 30% to 50% compared with 1% in interstitial (mild) pancreatitis.
    b. Infection significantly increases morbidity and mortality.
    c. In the presence of necrotizing pancreatitis and signs and symptoms of infection, antibiotic therapy with imipenem is recommended.
    d. If there is deterioration or no improvement, CT-guided aspiration can verify the presence of infection, which then requires surgical debridement and antibiotics.
  3. Pseudocysts are collections of fluid and debris that are encapsulated but do not contain an epithelial lining.
    a. Identified by ultrasound or CT
    b. Found in 10% to 20% of patients with pancreatitis
    c. Common in traumatic pancreatitis
    d. Require surgical or percutaneous drainage if they exhibit the following conditions:
      (1) Cause severe pain

(2) Cause obstruction (common bile duct, duodenum)

(3) Bleed

(4) Leak or rupture

(5) Become infected

(6) Persist longer than 16 weeks, expand rapidly

■ PATIENT/FAMILY EDUCATION

- This condition is not common in children, and specific causes of pancreatic inflammation should be identified and addressed if possible.
- Therapy is supportive and usually includes having nothing to eat or drink by mouth for a period to rest the pancreas. A nasogastric tube may also be necessary in the presence of protracted vomiting or an ileus.
- Assessing the severity of the inflammation with clinical observation, laboratory tests, and radiographic studies guides subsequent therapy and predictions of outcome.

■ REFERRAL INFORMATION

Patients should be referred to a gastroenterologist if they have the following conditions:

- Mild pancreatitis without a clear cause

- Pancreatitis severe enough to require hospitalization
- Recurrent pancreatitis

⚙ PEARLS & CONSIDERATIONS

■ CLINICAL PEARLS

- Clinical signs and symptoms may be nonspecific, and a high index of suspicion is necessary to make the diagnosis.
- The diagnosis can be established in most cases with an amylase, lipase, and an ultrasound.
- A family history of recurrent pancreatitis or cystic fibrosis should raise the possibility of pancreatitis in a child with abdominal pain.

■ WEBSITES

There are several websites with general information about pancreatitis. Search for "pancreatitis" on an Internet browser.

REFERENCES

1. Baron TH, Morgan DE: Acute necrotizing pancreatitis, *N Engl J Med* 340:1412, 1999.

2. Gorry MC et al: Mutations in the cationic trypsinogen gene are associated with recurrent acute and chronic pancreatitis, *Gastroenterology* 113:1063, 1997.

3. Moyer MS, Jenson HB: Acute pancreatitis. In Jenson HB, Baltimore RS (eds): *Pediatric infectious diseases: principles and practice,* New York, 1995, Appleton & Lange.

4. Ranson JHC et al: Prognostic signs and the role of operative management in acute pancreatitis, *Surg Gynecol Obstet* 139:69, 1974.

5. Sharer N et al: Mutations of the cystic fibrosis gene in patients with chronic pancreatitis, *N Engl J Med* 339:645, 1998.

6. Werlin SL: Pancreatitis. In Wyllie R, Hyams JS (eds): *Pediatric gastrointestinal disease: pathophysiology, diagnosis and management,* Philadelphia, 1999, WB Saunders.

7. Wilson C, Heath DI, Imrie CW: Prediction of outcome in acute pancreatitis: a comparative study of APACHE II, clinical assessment and multiple factor scoring systems, *Br J Surg* 77:1260, 1990.

Author: **M. Susan Moyer, M.D.**

II

BASIC INFORMATION

DEFINITION

Patent ductus arteriosus (PDA) is the abnormal persistence of an open lumen in the ductus arteriosus after birth.

SYNONYMS

- Persistent ductus arteriosus
- Patency or persistence of the arterial duct

ICD-9CM CODE

747.0 Patent ductus arteriosus

ETIOLOGY

- The exact mechanisms for normal postnatal closure are not fully understood.
- With advancing gestation, the constrictive response to rising Po_2 increases, hence the high incidence in preterm infants.
- Failure of constriction in the term infant is probably secondary to a structural abnormality, with underdevelopment of smooth muscle.
- Increased incidence exists with maternal rubella.
- PDA is more common in individuals born at a high altitude.

EPIDEMIOLOGY & DEMOGRAPHICS

- Incidence in the preterm infant is strongly influenced by birth weight and gestational age.
- Approximately 45% of infants less than 1700 g and approximately 80% less than 1000 g birth weight have clinical signs of PDA.
- Surfactant therapy, resulting in improved lung function and more rapid decrease in pulmonary vascular resistance, has led to earlier and more frequent clinical emergence of PDA.
- In the term infant, the incidence is approximately 1 per 2500 live births.
- A female : male predominance of approximately 2.5-3:1 exists in term infants.

HISTORY

- Preterm: surfactant therapy, labile blood pressure, worsening pulmonary status
- Term infant and older child: highly variable, dependent on the size of the shunt
  1. Large shunt: failure to thrive, poor feeding associated with tachypnea and diaphoresis
  2. Small shunt: asymptomatic

PHYSICAL EXAMINATION

- Large shunt (term infant and older child)
  1. Bounding, poorly sustained pulses, reflecting a wide pulse pressure
  2. Hyperdynamic apical impulse with inferolateral displacement
  3. Decreased splitting of S2 (paradoxical splitting has been documented with a very large shunt)
  4. Increased intensity of S2p
  5. Harsh, rough continuous murmur, loudest at left infraclavicular area, with decrescendo during systole
  6. May have multiple systolic clicks
- Small shunt (term infant and older child)
  1. Normal pulses
  2. Normal precordium
  3. Normal to slightly decreased splitting of S2, with normal S2p
  4. Grade 2/6 murmur, which is typically still continuous, although the diastolic portion may be difficult to auscultate
- Large shunt (preterm infant)
  1. Bounding, poorly sustained pulses ("Ninja" pulses) strike fast and fade away
  2. Hyperdynamic apical impulse with inferior displacement (often visible and palpable in the left paraxiphoid area)
  3. Narrowly split S2 with prominent S2p
  4. Murmur often nonspecific (or even absent), with the diastolic portion rarely audible
  5. Note: The physical findings are much less reliable in the small (less than 1200 g) infant, particularly if there is hemodynamic compromise. In this group of patients, the activity and displacement of the left ventricular impulse is the most reliable physical finding in terms of assessing the magnitude of the shunt.

DIAGNOSIS

DIFFERENTIAL DIAGNOSIS

- Based on physical findings alone, the differential diagnosis could include the following:
  1. Tetralogy of Fallot with pulmonary atresia and large aortic-pulmonary collaterals
  2. Coronary cameral fistula
  3. Large arteriovenous fistula
- In the older child, the continuous murmur of a venous hum has less variability in intensity during the phases of the cardiac cycle, tends to disappear in the supine position, and can be extinguished by changes in neck position or compression of the jugular vein.

DIAGNOSTIC WORKUP

- Electrocardiogram (ECG): depends on patient age and the size of the shunt
  1. Criteria for left atrial enlargement and left ventricular hypertrophy may be present.
  2. In the preterm infant with hemodynamic compromise, repolarization changes consistent with ischemia may be present.
- Chest radiograph
  1. Cardiomegaly may be noted.
  2. Increased pulmonary vascular markings are seen.
  3. Signs of pulmonary edema may be present in the preterm infant.
  4. Differentiation between worsening lung disease is difficult in the preterm infant.
- Echocardiography: uniformly diagnostic and obviates the need for ECG and/or chest radiograph
  1. The actual structure can typically be imaged and measured two-dimensionally.
  2. Color-flow mapping demonstrates the direction of shunting.
  3. Pulsed or continuous-wave Doppler is helpful in identifying the exact timing of bidirectional shunting.
  4. Color-flow mapping can detect trivial left-to-right shunts that are not detectable by two-dimensional imaging or by physical examination.

THERAPY

MEDICAL

- Indomethacin has been available since 1976.
- This drug is an effective alternative to surgery and has greatly decreased the need for surgical ligation in preterm infants.
- An initial clinical response may not be permanent, and a second course may be required.
- It is most effective in children younger than 10 days of age and in less mature infants.
- Indiscriminate and prophylactic use are not advisable.
- Early detection and treatment reduce morbidity.
- Renal side effects are usually transient.
- Prolonged treatment, especially in very-low-birth-weight infants, has been associated with an increased risk of necrotizing enterocolitis.

■ SURGICAL

- Ligation is extremely safe and essentially 100% effective.
- It is the preferred therapy in most institutions for the older infant and child.
- In some institutions, catheter closure with detachable coils is becoming an effective alternative.
  1. Proper selection of patient and coil is critical.
  2. Less effective for PDA larger than 3.5 mm in diameter.

☼ PEARLS & CONSIDERATIONS

■ CLINICAL PEARLS

- The magnitude of the left-to-right shunt depends on the following:
  1. Physical size of the PDA
  2. Relationship of pulmonary and systemic vascular resistance
  3. Left ventricular ejection performance
- Each of these factors is highly variable in the extremely preterm infant in the first few days of life.
- After successful treatment with indomethacin, smooth muscle constriction at the origin of the left pulmonary artery may result in a short, high-pitched systolic ejection murmur at the upper left sternal border radiating to the left axilla.
- The older infant with a hemodynamically important PDA is more predisposed to congestive heart failure than with a comparable shunt at the ventricular level because of the potential for compromise of coronary perfusion secondary to decreased diastolic aortic perfusion pressure.

■ WEBSITE

Congenital Heart Diseases: www. bharatonline.com/heart/htcod8.html

REFERENCES

1. Moss AJ, Adams FH: *Heart disease in infants, children, and adolescents*, ed 5, Baltimore, 1995, Williams & Wilkins.
2. Ramsay JM et al: Response of the patent ductus arteriosus to indomethacin treatment, *Am J Dis Child* 141: 294, 1987.
3. Tammela O et al: Short versus prolonged indomethacin therapy for patent ductus arteriosus in preterm infants, *J Pediatr* 134:552, 1999.
Author: **Dennis Steed, M.D.**

II

BASIC INFORMATION

DEFINITION
- Pelvic inflammatory disease (PID) is an acute clinical syndrome caused by the spread of microorganisms from the lower genital tract (vagina/endocervix) to the upper genital tract (endometrium, fallopian tubes, and/or adjacent structures).
- Any combination of endometritis or salpingitis is included.
- Clinical pictures varying from milder forms, such as salpingitis, to more severe pictures, such as tuboovarian abscess (TOA) and pelvic peritonitis.

SYNONYMS
- Salpingitis
- Endometritis

ICD-9CM CODES
614.9 Pelvic inflammatory disease
381.51 Acute salpingitis
615.9 Endometritis
614.2 Tuboovarian abscess

ETIOLOGY
- PID is a polymicrobial infection, although sexually transmitted organisms, particularly *Chlamydia trachomatis* (25% to 50% of cases) and *Neisseria gonorrhoeae* (33% to 50% of cases), are often implicated.
- Any of the microorganisms that are part of the vaginal flora, as well as those typically causing sexually transmitted diseases (STDs), can be involved:
  1. Facultative anaerobes (*Escherichia coli, Gardnerella vaginalis, Streptococcus* species including enterococci and *Haemophilus influenzae*) and anaerobes (anaerobic streptococci and staphylococci, *Bacteroides* species, *Actinomyces*) are both implicated, especially with TOA.
  2. Genital mycoplasmas responsible for bacterial vaginosis, such as *Ureaplasma urealyticum* and *Mycoplasma hominis,* are implicated as a contributing factor in "non-STD" cases of PID.

EPIDEMIOLOGY & DEMOGRAPHICS
- Adolescent age is a strong risk factor for the development of PID; females aged 15 to 19 years are 10 times more likely to develop PID than those aged 25 to 29 years.
- Increased risk in adolescents is related to numerous factors:
  1. Higher numbers of multiple partners
  2. Cervical ectopy (presence of columnar epithelium on exocervix); *C. trachomatis* and *N. gonorrhoeae* infect columnar epithelial cells
  3. Lower use of barrier methods of contraception

- PID is a serious consequence of STDs and an important cause of infertility, ectopic pregnancy, and chronic pelvic pain.

HISTORY
- PID is difficult to diagnose and manage because of the wide variations in clinical signs and symptoms and the lack of precise criteria for diagnosis and treatment.
- Diagnosis is generally made on the basis of history and clinical findings.
- Specific genitourinary symptoms may include the following:
  1. Lower abdominal pain or cramping, generally bilateral, worse with movement and sexual intercourse; peritoneal signs in severe cases
  2. Vaginal discharge
  3. Abnormal vaginal bleeding
  4. Any change in previous menses, such as being heavier, of longer duration, or accompanied by worse cramping
  5. Dysuria
- PID involving gonococcus is more likely to develop within 1 week of menses and to have rapid onset of symptoms.
- Chlamydial or anaerobic PID is more likely to be insidious in onset.
- Although uncommon, systemic signs include the following:
  1. Anorexia
  2. Nausea
  3. Vomiting
  4. Fever
  5. Generalized malaise
- To generate differential diagnoses, it is essential to obtain information about sexual activity, including the following:
  1. The number of current and most recent sexual partners
  2. Any STD symptoms in partners
  3. Use of barrier methods of contraception
  4. History of STDs or PID

PHYSICAL EXAMINATION
- Abdominal examination findings:
  1. Lower abdominal tenderness
  2. Peritoneal signs, such as rebound, guarding (in severe cases)
  3. Right upper quadrant pain; may be present with associated perihepatitis (Fitz-Hugh-Curtis syndrome)
- Pelvic examination findings key for diagnosis:
  1. Uterine tenderness
  2. Adnexal tenderness
  3. Cervical motion tenderness
- Additional physical examination findings that support the diagnosis:
  1. Fever of greater than 38.3° C
  2. Abnormal cervical or vaginal discharge

🔬 DIAGNOSIS

DIAGNOSTIC CRITERIA
- Minimal requirements:
  1. Lower abdominal tenderness
  2. Adnexal tenderness (unilateral or bilateral)
  3. Cervical motion tenderness
- Additional criteria to increase specificity:
  1. Oral temperature greater than 38.3° C (101° F)
  2. Leukocytosis (white blood cell [WBC] count greater than 10,000/mm³) or elevated erythrocyte sedimentation rate (ESR) greater than 15 mm/hr
  3. Gram-negative intracellular diplococci evident in Gram stain of endocervix
  4. Laboratory evidence of *N. gonorrhoeae* or *C. trachomatis* at cervix
- Specificity enhanced but sensitivity reduced by requiring more of these additional criteria.

DIFFERENTIAL DIAGNOSIS
- Ectopic pregnancy
- Ovarian cyst (with or without torsion)
- Acute appendicitis
- Endometriosis
- Pyelonephritis
- Septic abortion
- Pelvic thrombophlebitis
- Functional pain

DIAGNOSTIC WORKUP
- Laboratory tests (assist in ruling out differential diagnoses)
  1. Pregnancy test (to rule out ectopic pregnancy)
  2. Tests for elevated acute phase reactants, such as WBC, ESR, or C-reactive protein
  3. Tests for gonorrhea and chlamydial cervical infection
- Ultrasound
  1. May be helpful if diagnosis is in question, ectopic pregnancy is a strong consideration, or TOA is being considered as part of the clinical picture
  2. Increased adnexal volume the most discriminating finding
- Laparoscopy
  1. Not recommended on a routine basis, although it provides a definitive diagnosis with findings of hyperemia, edema, or purulent exudate of tubal surfaces
  2. May be required for evaluation of treatment failures, to exclude surgical emergencies, or if TOA ruptures or does not respond to medical management within 48 to 72 hours

THERAPY

■ TREATMENT PRINCIPLES

- Treatment is generally empiric and must be broad spectrum.
- All regimens should be effective against *N. gonorrhoeae* and *C. trachomatis,* even when endocervical cultures are negative.
- Evidence also suggests that providing coverage against anaerobes and other gram-negative organisms is important.
- Treatment should be initiated as soon as the presumptive diagnosis is made.
  1. Prevention of long-term sequelae is linked directly to prompt administration of appropriate antibiotics.
  2. Delays in initiating antibiotic treatment until culture results are available should be avoided.
- Indications for hospitalization are as follows:
  1. Strong consideration of surgical emergencies as possible diagnoses
  2. Severely ill or immunocompromised patient
  3. Pregnancy
  4. TOA
  5. Failure to respond to outpatient therapy
  6. Adherence to therapy or close follow-up within 72 hours cannot be reasonably ensured (often the case with adolescents).

■ THE CENTERS FOR DISEASE CONTROL AND PREVENTION RECOMMENDED REGIMENS

- Parenteral regimens in inpatient setting (one of the following):
  1. Cefotetan 2 g intravenously every 12 hours *or* cefoxitin 2 g intravenously every 6 hours *plus* doxycycline 100 mg intravenously or orally every 12 hours. (Because intravenous doxycycline is extremely painful, it should be given orally when possible. Administer for 24 to 48 hours after clinical improvement.)
  2. Clindamycin 900 mg intravenously every 8 hours *plus* gentamicin loading dose intravenously or intramuscularly (2 mg/kg body weight), followed by a maintenance dose (1.5 mg/kg) every 8 hours. Single daily dosing of gentamicin may be substituted. (Administer for 24 to 48 hours after clinical improvement.)
  3. Following parenteral therapy,

doxycycline 100 mg orally twice a day for 14 days. Clindamycin 450 mg orally four times per day should be instituted to complete a total of 14 days of therapy. When TOA is present, clindamycin is preferred to doxycycline because of its better anaerobes coverage.
- Alternative parenteral regimens (one of the following):
  1. Ofloxacin 400 mg intravenously every 12 hours *plus* metronidazole 500 mg intravenously every 8 hours *or* ampicillin/sulbactam 3 g intravenously every 6 hours *plus* doxycycline 100 mg intravenously or orally every 12 hours *or* ciprofloxacin 200 mg intravenously every 12 hours *plus* doxycycline 100 mg orally every 12 hours *plus* metronidazole 500 mg intravenously every 8 hours
- Oral regimens in outpatient setting (one of the following):
  1. Ofloxacin 400 mg orally twice per day for 14 days *plus* metronidazole 500 mg orally twice per day for 14 days
  2. Ceftriaxone 250 mg intravenously single dose *or* cefoxitin 2g intramuscularly, *plus* probenecid 1 g orally in a single dose once, *plus* doxycycline 100 mg orally twice per day for 14 days
  3. Other parenteral third-generation cephalosporin (ceftizoxime or cefotaxime) *plus* doxycycline 100 mg orally twice per day for 14 days
- Follow-up
  1. Close follow-up of adolescents is essential when treated as outpatients.
  2. A repeat visit within 48 to 72 hours is necessary to ascertain adequate clinical improvement versus the need for hospitalization.
- Sex partners
  1. Sex partners of patients with PID should be examined and treated to reduce the risk of reinfection.

■ PATIENT/FAMILY EDUCATION

- The risks of unprotected sexual intercourse should be explained.
- Infertility rates increase with number of PID episodes:
  1. 13% to 20% with one episode
  2. 35% with two episodes
  3. 55% to 75% with three or more episodes
- The risk of ectopic pregnancy is increased 6 to 10 times after one episode of PID.

- Because of the role of *Chlamydia* and the high frequency of asymptomatic infections, all sexually active adolescents need routine screening for STDs every 6 to 12 months.

☼ PEARLS & CONSIDERATIONS

■ CLINICAL PEARLS

- Reported changes in menstrual pattern (e.g., heavier periods, more painful cramps, menses occurring earlier or later than expected) should raise suspicion of early endometrial infection, even in the absence of other symptoms.
- Unilateral adnexal tenderness or swelling is suggestive of TOA, as well as other differential diagnoses. Ultrasound should be done to rule out TOA.
- Much information is available demonstrating the efficacy of each of the treatment regimens listed in this section, although no specific data are available directly comparing parenteral with oral regimens.
- Cervical specimen tests for gonorrhea and *Chlamydia* are often negative because active infection occurs in the upper genital tract.
- A positive gonorrhea or *Chlamydia* test at follow-up is more likely a result of reinfection by an untreated sex partner than treatment failure.

■ WEBSITE

Centers for Disease Control and Prevention: www.cdc.gov/epo/mmwr/preview/mmwrhtml/00050909.htm

REFERENCES

1. Centers for Disease Control and Prevention: 1998 guidelines for treatment of sexually transmitted diseases, *MMWR Morb Mortal Wkly Rep* 47:RR-14, 1998.
2. Lawson MA, Blythe MJ: Pelvic inflammatory disease in adolescents, *Pediatr Clin North Am* 46:767, 1999.
3. Wald ER: Pelvic inflammatory disease in adolescents, *Curr Prob Pediatr* 26:86, 1996.
4. Walker CK et al: Anaerobes in pelvic inflammatory disease: implications for the Centers for Disease Control and Prevention's guidelines for treatment of sexually transmitted diseases, *Clin Infect Dis* 28:29, 1999.
Authors: **Sheryl Ryan, M.D., and Gale R. Burstein, M.D., M.P.H.**

BASIC INFORMATION

■ DEFINITION

Pericarditis is a syndrome caused by inflammation (either acute or chronic) of the pericardium, resulting in an increase in the normal volume of pericardial fluid surrounding the heart.

ICD-9CM CODES

420.99 Pericardial effusion, bacteriologic
420.90 Acute pericarditis, infective, hemorrhagic (acute nonrheumatic)
423.8   Chronic pericarditis
423.2   Constrictive pericarditis
423.9   Cardiac tamponade

■ ETIOLOGY

- Idiopathic: no cause identified, uncommon
- Viral infections: Coxsackie A and B virus, echovirus, adenovirus, Epstein-Barr virus, cytomegalovirus, varicella-zoster virus, mumps, hepatitis B, human immunodeficiency virus (HIV)
- Acute bacterial infections: *Streptococcus pneumoniae, Staphylococcus aureus, Streptococcus* species, gram-negative septicemia
- Tuberculous, fungal: toxoplasmosis, echinococcus, Lyme disease
- Autoimmune and other inflammatory disorders: juvenile rheumatoid arthritis, systemic lupus erythematosus, acute rheumatic fever, inflammatory bowel disease
- Chest trauma
- Postoperative: postpericardiotomy syndrome, Fontan procedure
- Neoplastic disease: leukemia, Hodgkin's disease, lymphoma
- Drugs and toxins: radiation and chemotherapy, hydralazine, procainamide, penicillin
- Uremia
- Hypothyroidism (especially in trisomy 21)

■ EPIDEMIOLOGY & DEMOGRAPHICS

Primary pericardial disease is rare in infants and children.

■ HISTORY

- If acute onset, sudden onset of malaise, anorexia, dyspnea, orthopnea, chest or shoulder pain
- If chronic onset, discovered incidentally on physical examination
- May have a history of recent infectious disease, autoimmune disease, neoplastic disease, and/or treatment of such, chest trauma or surgery, renal disease

■ PHYSICAL EXAMINATION

- Vital signs should be obtained.
  1. Pulsus paradoxus: a greater than 10-mm inspiratory decline in aortic systolic and pulse pressures
  2. Tachycardia
- Patient is ill appearing, pale, dyspneic, tachypneic, and tachycardic; prefers to sit up and lean forward, will not lie supine.
- Patient is usually febrile.
- Pericardial friction rub over precordium or distant heart sounds may be heard.
- Occasionally, jugular venous distention and hepatomegaly are present.
- Diminished perfusion and pulses coupled with pulsus paradoxus is a sign of extension of effusion with progression to tamponade.
- Chronic pericarditis may present with no symptoms (incidental chest radiograph finding) but may have a rub or distant heart sounds.

 DIAGNOSIS

■ DIFFERENTIAL DIAGNOSIS

- Dilated cardiomyopathy
- Restrictive cardiomyopathy
- Respiratory illnesses
- Aortic dissection

■ DIAGNOSTIC WORKUP

- Chest radiograph: enlarged cardiac silhouette, loss of landmarks, "water bottle" appearance, may show pulmonary venous congestion
- Electrocardiogram: variable ST-T wave changes, depends on the evolution of the effusion; voltages may be diminished
- Echocardiogram: the most accurate, rapid, and widely used technique for initial evaluation and monitoring of the effusion over time
- Blood tests:
  1. Inflammation: there may be nonspecific indicators of inflammation such as leukocytosis and elevation of the sedimentation rate
  2. Cardiac isoenzymes: may be mildly elevated
  3. Bacterial, viral, and fungal cultures: should be obtained
  4. Electrolytes, blood urea nitrogen, and creatinine
  5. HIV antibody
  6. Thyroid studies
  7. ASO
  8. Antinuclear antibody and other markers for lupus and juvenile arthritis
- Pericardial fluid: chemical composition, cell counts, Gram stains, cell block if malignancy suspected, and bacterial, viral, and fungal cultures

 THERAPY

The first step involves establishing the relationship of pericarditis to an underlying problem that requires specific therapy.

■ NONPHARMACOLOGIC

- Prescribe bed rest until the pain and fever disappear.
- Even if the patient is not in significant pain, limit activity until the effusion resolves.
- Monitor vital signs closely.
  1. Hospitalization is advocated with the first episode of acute pericarditis.
- Allow the patient to sit upright.

■ MEDICAL

- Not all pericardial effusions require intervention—monitor for signs of tamponade.
  1. Fifteen percent develop tamponade.
- Supplemental oxygen is required for dyspnea.
- Avoid diuretics.
- Give volume at early signs of tamponade.
- Pain may respond to nonsteroidal antiinflammatory drugs (NSAIDs) such as aspirin, indomethacin, and ibuprofen.
  1. NSAIDs are most efficacious for postpericardiotomy syndrome.
- If the patient does not respond to NSAIDs, glucocorticosteroids may be initiated for 5 to 7 days.
- If purulent pericarditis is present, antibiotics should be administered and surgical drainage is required.
- Avoid anticoagulation therapy.

■ SURGICAL

The clinical significance of any pericardial effusion depends on hemodynamic compromise and the nature and progression of the underlying disease.

- Pericardiocentesis is recommended for the following conditions:
  1. Evidence of cardiac compression (tamponade)
  2. Analysis of pericardial fluid if necessary for establishing diagnosis
- Hemodynamic support for pericardial effusion with or without drainage should include administration of fluid in the form of blood, plasma, or saline.
- Volume expansion delays the right ventricular diastolic collapse and improves hemodynamic function.
- Avoid positive-pressure ventilation.
- Pericardiocentesis or surgical drainage may be necessary with recalcitrant pericardial effusions or purulent or sanguineous effusions that may progress to restrictive peri-

carditis (e.g., staphylococcal pericarditis).

■ FOLLOW-UP & DISPOSITION
Patients with underlying diseases such as autoimmune disease, which predispose them to pericarditis, should have long-term supervision by a cardiologist.

■ PATIENT/FAMILY EDUCATION
- Pericarditis can recur depending on the cause.
- Treat the cause of pericarditis.
- Vigilance for signs and symptoms of pericardial effusion should be maintained.

■ PREVENTIVE TREATMENT
Treatment of underlying condition

■ REFERRAL INFORMATION
Regular follow-up with a cardiologist

☼ PEARLS & CONSIDERATIONS

■ CLINICAL PEARLS
Patients are characteristically uncomfortable, are dyspneic, may complain of pain on swallowing, and prefer to sit forward.

■ WEBSITE
Congenital Heart Diseases: www. bharatonline.com/heart/htcod8.html

REFERENCES
1. Fyler DC: Pericardial disease. In Fyler DC (ed): *Nadas' pediatric cardiology,* St Louis, 1992, Mosby.
2. Lorell BH: Pericardial disease. In Braunwald E (ed): *Heart disease,* Philadelphia, 1997, WB Saunders.
3. Rheuban KS: Diseases of the pericardium. In Emmanouilides GC et al (eds): *Heart disease in infants, children, and adolescents: including the fetus and young adult,* Baltimore, 1995, Williams & Wilkins.

Author: **Michelle A. Grenier, M.D.**

II

BASIC INFORMATION

DEFINITION
Peritonitis is inflammation of the peritoneal lining of the abdominal cavity.

SYNONYM
Primary peritonitis
• Spontaneous bacterial peritonitis (SBP)

ICD-9CM CODES
567.9 Acute peritonitis
567.2 Bacterial peritonitis, general, generalized acute
540.0 With appendicitis

ETIOLOGY
• Primary peritonitis is infection in the peritoneal cavity without an intraabdominal source.
  1. The most common organisms include the following:
     a. Pneumococci
     b. Group A streptococci
     c. Gram-negative enteric organisms
     d. Staphylococci
     e. Enterococci
• Secondary bacterial peritonitis is caused by abdominal viscous rupture or extension of an intraperitoneal organ infection or abscess.
  1. Etiologies include the following:
     a. Ruptured appendix
     b. Incarcerated hernia
     c. Midgut volvulus
     d. Meckel's diverticulum
     e. Intussusception
     f. Necrotizing enterocolitis
     g. Hemolytic uremic syndrome
     h. Peptic ulcer disease
     i. Traumatic perforation
     j. Other (e.g., meconium in preterm infant)
  2. Peritonitis may be seen with genital tract infection from fallopian tube extension of pelvic inflammatory disease (PID).
     a. *Neisseria* gonococci
     b. Chlamydia
• Foreign body (e.g., ventriculoperitoneal shunt, peritoneal dialysis catheter) may contribute to peritonitis.
• Autoimmune or chemical process may lead to noninfectious peritonitis.
  1. Systemic lupus erythematosus
  2. Mediterranean fever

EPIDEMIOLOGY & DEMOGRAPHICS
• Most cases are primary and occur in children with nephrotic syndrome or, much less often, cirrhosis.
• An uncommon cause of acute abdomen, SBP without underlying renal disease, occurs in children younger than 7 years of age.
• A complication of appendicitis is the most common cause of peritonitis in older children.

HISTORY
• Renal (or liver) disease in most children
• Insidious or rapid onset
• Fever
• Abdominal pain
• Anorexia, vomiting, diarrhea

PHYSICAL EXAMINATION
• "Toxic" appearance (common)
• Hypotension, tachycardia
• Shallow, rapid respirations
• Absent or decreased bowel sounds
• Rebound tenderness
• Rigid abdomen
• Indwelling catheter

DIAGNOSIS

DIFFERENTIAL DIAGNOSIS
• Appendicitis with or without perforation, peritonitis, or localized abscess
• PID, Fitz-Hugh-Curtis syndrome
• Tuboovarian abscess
• Liver, splenic, or renal abscess
• Psoas abscess
• Bowel perforation
• Pneumonia

DIAGNOSTIC WORKUP
• Complete blood count shows increased white blood cell (WBC) count with polymorphonuclear predominance.
• Proteinuria is noted in patients with nephrotic syndrome.
• If known renal or liver disease or ascites, a paracentesis should be done. Findings include the following:
  1. Increased WBC count (greater than 250 cells/mm^3)
  2. Increased lactate
  3. Decreased pH (less than 7.35)
  4. Positive Gram stain for organisms

THERAPY

MEDICAL
• Fluid resuscitation should be provided if the patient is unstable.
• Ampicillin or ceftriaxone and an aminoglycoside should be administered while awaiting definitive culture results and sensitivities.
• Include anaerobic coverage (metronidazole or clindamycin) if secondary peritonitis is suspected (e.g., appendicitis with rupture).
• Treatment is generally for 10 to 14 days.

SURGICAL
• Drainage if abscess
• Repair of perforated viscous
• Excision of gangrenous bowel
• Removal of foreign body

FOLLOW-UP & DISPOSITION
Depends on primary cause

REFERRAL INFORMATION
• A nephrologist or gastroenterologist may be involved for underlying disease consultation.
• A pediatric surgeon will be involved for most forms of secondary peritonitis, catheter-related peritonitis, and if an acute abdomen is suspected.

PEARLS & CONSIDERATIONS

CLINICAL PEARLS
• If no underlying renal or liver disease is present, think bowl perforation.
• Treat peritonitis emergently.

REFERENCES
1. Hyans JS: Peritonitis. In Behrman RE, Kliegman RM, Arvin AM (eds): *Nelson textbook of pediatrics*, Philadelphia, 1998, WB Saunders.
2. Shandling B: Peritonitis. In Walker WA et al (eds): *Pediatric gastrointestinal disease: pathophysiology, diagnosis, management*, ed 3, Philadelphia, 2000, BC Decker.
Author: **Lynn C. Garfunkel, M.D.**

BASIC INFORMATION

■ DEFINITION
Peritonsillar abscess is a fascial space abscess complicating tonsillitis.

■ SYNONYM
Quinsy

ICD-9CM CODE
475 For both peritonsillar abscess and peritonsillar cellulitis

■ ETIOLOGY
- A complication of acute tonsillar pharyngeal infection
- Cultures often polymicrobial with aerobes (e.g., *Streptococcus pyogenes*, α-hemolytic streptococci) and anaerobes (e.g., *Bacteroides* species, *Fusobacterium*)

■ EPIDEMIOLOGY & DEMOGRAPHICS
- Peritonsillar abscess is the most common cervical fascial space abscess in pediatric patients.
- The incidence is 30 per 100,000 in the United States among patients 5 to 59 years of age.
- The percentage of patients who are 20 years of age or younger ranges from 33% to 39%.
  1. Rare in children younger than age 5

■ HISTORY
- From 2 to 4 days of the following:
  1. Sore throat
  2. Dysphagia
  3. Fever
  4. Muffled "hot potato" voice

■ PHYSICAL EXAMINATION
- Fever, unilateral tonsillar erythema (often without an exudate)
- Bulging of the superior aspect of the tonsil, often with palpable fluctuance
- Uvular deviation
- Trismus
- Fetid breath
- Ipsilateral cervical adenopathy

DIAGNOSIS

■ DIFFERENTIAL DIAGNOSIS
- Peritonsillar cellulitis
- Parapharyngeal space abscess

■ DIAGNOSTIC WORKUP
- Clinical differentiation of peritonsillar cellulitis from peritonsillar abscess can be difficult.
- Traditionally, the diagnosis is confirmed by needle aspiration.
- Noninvasive imaging techniques of intraoral ultrasound or computed tomography with contrast are reliable in differentiating peritonsillar cellulitis from abscess.
- Culture does not seem to be necessary, except possibly for immunocompromised patients.
  1. Culture results do not affect the management.
  2. Culture results do not change the outcome.

THERAPY

■ NONPHARMACOLOGIC
- Most patients (more than 80%) can be managed as outpatients.
- Hydration (oral or parenteral) should be maintained.

■ MEDICAL
- Pain relief
- Antibiotics
  1. No clear consensus has been reached regarding penicillin (oral or intravenous) versus broad-spectrum antibiotics, such as clindamycin, penicillin plus metronidazole, or amoxicillin/clavulanate.
  2. Penicillin alone is as effective as broad-spectrum antibiotics.

■ SURGICAL
- Drainage of the abscess can be accomplished either by needle aspiration, incision and drainage, or abscess tonsillectomy.
- Studies (see Herzon references) suggest that initial surgical management should be needle aspiration because the success rate is 94%.
- For the 6% who fail needle aspiration, incision and drainage is recommended.
- For the 20% to 30% of children with a history of prior recurrent tonsillitis (two to three episodes of tonsillitis in the past year), the recommended surgical management is either abscess tonsillectomy or needle aspiration, followed by delayed tonsillectomy because these patients are at greater risk for recurrence.

■ FOLLOW-UP & DISPOSITION
- Approximately 4% of patients who are initially managed with needle aspiration require a second aspiration.
- Most recurrences of peritonsillar abscess occur in patients younger than 30 years of age and within 2 months of the initial peritonsillar abscess.

■ PATIENT/FAMILY EDUCATION
Approximately 10% of patients have a recurrence after needle aspiration.

■ PREVENTIVE TREATMENT
Early antimicrobial treatment of streptococcal pharyngitis may decrease the likelihood of developing a peritonsillar abscess.

■ REFERRAL INFORMATION
Otolaryngologist for surgical management

PEARLS & CONSIDERATIONS

■ CLINICAL PEARLS
- Response to parenteral antibiotics in patients who will not tolerate needle aspiration (5% or less) can help differentiate peritonsillar abscess from peritonsillar cellulitis.
  1. Patients with cellulitis had improvement of at least one clinical factor (sore throat, fever, trismus, or tonsillar bulge) within 24 to 48 hours of parenteral antibiotics.
  2. Children with peritonsillar abscess had no symptomatic change.
- The incidence of abscess within the contralateral tonsil ranges from 2% to 24%.

■ WEBSITES
For patients
- HealthAnswers: www.healthanswers.com/centers/body/overview.asp?id=throat&filename=000986.htm
For physicians
- Pediatric Infectious Diseases: www.pedid.uthscsa.edu/057.htm
- University of California, San Diego Medical Center, Department of Surgery: www–surgery.ucsd.edu/ent/davidson/Pathway/Tonsil.htm

REFERENCES
1. Herzon FS: Peritonsillar abscess: incidence, current management practices, and a proposal for treatment guidelines, *Laryngoscope* 105:1, 1995.
2. Herzon FS, Nicklaus P: Pediatric peritonsillar abscess: management guidelines, *Curr Prob Pediatr* 26:270, 1996.
3. Kieff DA et al: Selection of antibiotics after incision and drainage of peritonsillar abscesses, *Otolaryngol Head Neck Surg* 120:57, 1999.
4. Scott PM et al: Diagnosis of peritonsillar infections: a prospective study of ultrasound, computed tomography and clinical diagnosis, *J Laryngol Otol* 113:229, 1999.
Author: **Robert R. Wittler, M.D.**

BASIC INFORMATION

■ **DEFINITION**
Pertussis is an acute bacterial respiratory illness usually associated with significant paroxysmal cough, with associated "whoop," caused by *Bordetella pertussis* and less commonly by *Bordetella parapertussis*.

■ **SYNONYM**
Whooping cough

ICD-9CM CODE
033.9 Pertussis

■ **ETIOLOGY**
B. pertussis is a fastidious gram-negative aerobic pleomorphic bacillus.

■ **EPIDEMIOLOGY & DEMOGRAPHICS**
• Humans are the only known host.
• Transmission is via respiratory secretions.
• Cases are endemic with periodic outbreaks.
• Adolescents and adults are currently major reservoirs.
• A 90% transmission rate exists among nonimmune household contacts.
• The highest risk of disease is in young infants and children.
• In the prevaccine era:
   1. An attack rate of 157 per 100,000 population existed.
   2. Epidemics occurred in 2- to 5-year intervals; these cycles continue today, although immunization has controlled disease.
   3. Approximately 85% of all cases occurred in children between ages 1 and 9 years, and pertussis was a major cause of mortality in infants.
• In the postvaccine era:
   1. The attack rate has decreased significantly to 2 to 3 per 100,000, from 1982 to 1993.
   2. Epidemic cycles continue in unvaccinated populations, with adolescents and adults remaining a reservoir of infection.
   3. Mortality has significantly decreased.
      a. Most deaths occur in unimmunized infants younger than 6 months old.
      b. In the United States, approximately 10 deaths per year are caused by pertussis.

■ **HISTORY**
• Catarrhal stage (lasts 1 to 2 weeks)
   1. Classically seen in children 1 to 10 years of age
   2. Rhinorrhea
   3. Lacrimation
   4. Mild cough
   5. Afebrile
   6. Cough severity gradually increases
• Paroxysmal stage (lasts about 4 weeks)
   1. Repetitive cough
      a. Five to ten coughs occur per expiration, followed by a large inspiration. Whoop occurs as inhaled air is forced through the narrowed glottis.
      b. Paroxysms occur throughout the day and night. Between episodes, patients may appear normal.
   2. Associated symptoms with cough
      a. Cyanosis
      b. Eye bulging
      c. Tongue protrusion
      d. Salivation
      e. Lacrimation
      f. Posttussive emesis
• Convalescent stage (lasts 1 to 2 weeks)
   1. Improvement of coughing spasms
   2. Decreased frequency and forcefulness

■ **PHYSICAL EXAMINATION**
• Afebrile
• Observation of paroxysms
• Otherwise usually unremarkable: normal respiratory rate, normal lung examination

■ **COMPLICATIONS**
• Pneumonia
   1. Caused by pertussis
   2. Secondary bacterial infection
• Otitis media
   1. Caused by *Streptococcus pneumoniae*
• Apnea
   1. Can occur at any time, usually within the paroxysmal phase
• Seizures
   1. Believed to be caused by hypoxia
• Encephalopathy
   1. May be caused by *B. pertussis*
   2. May be secondary to hypoxia associated with cough
• Rare complications
   1. Subconjunctival hemorrhage
   2. Epistaxis
   3. Alveolar hemorrhage and /or rupture
   4. Dehydration
   5. Cerebral asphyxia
      a. Seizures
      b. Coma

🔬 **DIAGNOSIS**

■ **DIFFERENTIAL DIAGNOSIS**
• Respiratory syncytial virus bronchiolitis
• Common upper respiratory infection
• *Chlamydia*
• Allergy
• Cough equivalent asthma
• ALTE: an episode that is frightening to the observer and is characterized by some combination of apnea (central or obstructive), change in color (pallor, cyanosis, or suffusion), change in muscle tone (usually diminished), choking, or gagging; in some cases, the observer fears that the infant has died
• Classic disease
   1. Clinical picture is diagnostic.
   2. Epidemiology is important.
      a. History of ill contact is reported.

■ **DIAGNOSTIC WORKUP**
• Leukocytosis with lymphocytosis
   1. High white blood cell count (greater than 15,000/mm^3 with 80% lymphocytes)
   2. Nonspecific and not sensitive
• Culture
   1. Nasopharyngeal mucus from aspiration or on a Dacron swab should be inoculated onto Bordet-Gengou media.
   2. Incubation lasts for 10 to 14 days.
   3. Recovery is best in the early stages of illness, with recovery after the fourth week rare.
   4. A positive culture is diagnostic.
   5. Negative cultures are common in the following scenarios:
      a. In vaccinated patients
      b. In patients on antibiotics
      c. Late in the illness
• Nonculture methods
   1. Poorly standardized
   2. Direct fluorescent antibody
      a. Low sensitivity
      b. Variable specificity
      c. Culture confirmation
   3. Polymerase chain reaction
      a. Still investigational, but promising
• Serologic methods
   1. Heterogeneous antibody response makes use of this test problematic and not diagnostic.
   2. Research laboratories include the following:
      a. IgG to *B. pertussis* toxin
      b. IgA to *B. pertussis* filamentous hemagglutinin

℞ **THERAPY**

• Primary prevention
   1. Whole cell vaccination
      a. Suspension of inactivated *B. pertussis* cells with multiple antigens
      b. Efficacy: 50% to 90%
      c. Immunity: persists 3 years and diminishes with time
      d. Combined with diphtheria and tetanus toxoids as intramuscular injection

2. Acellular vaccine
   a. Preferred vaccine because of decreased vaccine-associated reactions
   b. One or more immunogens, but minimal to no endotoxin
   c. Combined with diphtheria and tetanus toxoids as intramuscular injection
   d. Less local and systemic reactions than whole cell vaccine
   e. Use same DTaP vaccine product for first three doses
   f. Total of five doses recommended by school entry: first dose at 2 months of age, next two doses at 2-month intervals, fourth dose at 12 to 18 months, and fifth dose at 4 to 6 years of age (If fourth dose is delayed until after fourth birthday, no fifth dose is necessary. Pertussis immunization is not currently recommended for children older than 7 years of age.)
3. Precautions
   a. Children who have had well-documented pertussis should still complete the immunization schedule with at least DT; some experts recommend including the pertussis component as well.
   b. In outbreaks, immunization of adult contacts is not recommended.
   c. Adverse immunization reactions: Fever, erythema, induration, and pain at injection site are much less common with acellular pertussis than with the whole cell vaccine.

- Contraindications to vaccination
  1. Anaphylaxis
  2. Encephalopathy within a week of immunization
- Deferral of vaccination
  1. In children with a progressive neurologic disorder characterized by developmental delay or neurologic findings
  2. History of recent seizure until the cause is known or seizures are well controlled

■ **TREATMENT**
- Supportive care
  1. Hydration, oxygenation, nutrition
  2. Antibiotics to decrease further spread
     a. Not efficacious in changing course of illness once established
     b. Erythromycin (40 to 50 mg/kg/day divided four times a day for 14 days), or
     c. Clarithromycin (15 mg/kg/day orally in two divided doses for 10 days), or
     d. Trimethoprim-sulfamethoxazole (10 mg/kg/day of trimethoprim in two divided doses for 14 days); efficacy is unproven
  3. Might consider corticosteroids to decrease coughing
  4. Albuterol
  5. Pertussis-specific immunoglobulin (investigational)
- Exposed contact treatment
  1. Immunize contacts younger than 7 years who are unimmunized.
  2. Chemoprophylaxis should be instituted as follows:
     a. Erythromycin for all household contacts regardless of age or

immunization status (40 to 50 mg/kg/day divided in four doses; maximum, 2 g/day for 14 days, see alternatives listed previously)

■ **REFERRAL INFORMATION**
Pediatric infectious disease consultation may be warranted in complicated cases.

☼ **PEARLS & CONSIDERATIONS**

■ **WEBSITES**
- Centers for Disease Control and Prevention: www.cdc.gov
- *Morbidity and Mortality Weekly Report:* www2.cdc.gov/mmwr

REFERENCES
1. American Academy of Pediatrics: *1997 Red Book: report of the Committee on Infectious Diseases,* ed 24, Elk Grove Village, Ill, 1997, American Academy of Pediatrics.
2. Centers for Disease Control and Prevention (CDC): Notice to readers: FDA approval of a fourth acellular pertussis vaccine for use among infants and young children, *MMWR Morbid Mortal Wkly Rep* 47:934, 1998.
3. Cherry J, Heininger U: Pertussis and other *Bordetella* infections. In Feigin RD, Cherry JD (eds): *Textbook of pediatric infectious diseases,* ed 4, Philadelphia, 1998, WB Saunders.
Author: **Maureen Kays, M.D.**

II

BASIC INFORMATION

DEFINITIONS

- Streptococcal pharyngitis is the inflammation of the tonsils/pharynx caused by infection with group A streptococcus (GAS).
- Scarlet fever is a systemic illness characterized by a typical "sandpaper" rash that results from erythrogenic toxins produced by GAS.
- Acute rheumatic fever (ARF) is a late, autoimmune complication of GAS infection and is characterized by carditis, arthritis, chorea, erythema marginatum rash, and subcutaneous nodules. (See the section "Rheumatic Fever.")
- Acute poststreptococcal glomerulonephritis (APSGN) is an immune complex–mediated complication of GAS infection and is characterized by hematuria, proteinuria, edema, and acute renal failure. (See the section "Glomerulonephritis, Acute.")

SYNONYMS

- Streptococcal pharyngitis
  1. Infective sore throat
  2. Strep throat
- Scarlet fever
  1. Streptococcal fever
  2. Strep rash
  3. Scarlatina (rash)
  4. Scarlatiniform eruption

ICD-9CM CODES
463 Tonsillitis
462.9 Pharyngitis
465.8 Tonsillopharyngitis
034.0 Streptococcal tonsillitis or pharyngitis
034.1 Scarlet fever

ETIOLOGY

- Multiple serotypes of GAS (*Streptococcus pyogenes*) are distinguished by distinctive surface proteins called *M-proteins*.
- GAS associated with tonsillopharyngitis and scarlet fever differs from that causing skin infection.
- Certain serotypes are associated with ARF: The specific rheumatogenic factor has not been identified.
- Other serotypes are associated with APSGN: nephritogenic strains.

EPIDEMIOLOGY & DEMOGRAPHICS

- Acute GAS infection
  1. Tonsillopharyngitis and scarlet fever result from direct contact with respiratory tract secretions from a GAS-infected person.
  2. Neither fomites nor household pets are vectors.
  3. Epidemic outbreaks occur in crowded conditions (e.g., schools, day-care facilities, and military installations).
  4. Foodborne outbreaks have also occurred.
  5. Incidence is most common among school-age children, but can occur at any age.
  6. Occurs more frequently in late autumn, winter, and spring in temperate climates.
  7. Communicability is highest during the acute infection, then diminishes over several weeks even without treatment, but abruptly declines within 24 to 48 hours after antibiotic therapy.
  8. Asymptomatic prevalence rates of 15% to 50% during outbreaks include both children who are infectious but not ill and those with pharyngeal carriage who are not infectious.
  9. Local complications (e.g., otitis media, sinusitis, peritonsillar, retropharyngeal abscesses, cervical adenitis) are more likely to occur in untreated patients.
  10. Scarlet fever usually occurs with GAS pharyngitis but may be seen with skin or wound infections ("surgical scarlet fever").
  11. Scarlet fever is rare in infancy.
     a. Possibly because of placental transfer of maternal antibody to the erythrogenic toxins
     b. More likely rare because of the need for the development of hypersensitivity to these exotoxins through prior exposure
  12. Streptococcal toxic shock syndrome is a rare and severe form of scarlet fever with shock and systemic toxicity that has a high mortality rate despite timely and high doses of antibiotics.
  13. The incidence of severe, invasive GAS infections (including bacteremia, toxic shock, necrotizing fasciitis, and pneumonia) has increased, although such infections rarely follow GAS pharyngitis.
- Late sequelae of GAS infection: ARF and APSGN
  1. The incidence of ARF has declined sharply from 3% in the 1950s to the current attack rate presumed to be as low as 0.3%.
     a. Outbreaks of ARF have continued.
     b. Emphasize both the importance of accurate diagnosis and of compliance with the recommended duration of therapy.
  2. APSGN may follow either GAS throat or skin infection.
     a. The latent period for nephritis is longer after skin infection (3 weeks) than after throat infection (10 days).

HISTORY

- This is a brief, acute illness occurring after a short incubation period (1 to 4 days).
- There is wide variation in morbidity: subclinical form (30%) to a very toxic form (less than 10%).
- Extreme toxicity is most common in epidemic foodborne outbreaks.
- Acute and sudden onset of fever, sore throat, headache (usually nonspecific and frontal), and abdominal pain (especially in children) that is not associated with diarrhea are present.
  1. Absence of other respiratory symptoms (e.g., sneezing, cough, coryza, rhinorrhea, conjunctivitis) and diarrhea in the typical case
- History of exposure to an infected classmate or other close contact is reported.
- Subsequent symptoms may include halitosis and neck pain and stiffness.
- Clinical manifestations subside spontaneously in 3 to 5 days unless complications occur.
- Scarlet fever usually presents as a more severe illness with the following symptoms:
  1. High fever and mild toxicity
  2. Abdominal pain with nausea and vomiting 12 to 24 hours before the onset of rash
  3. Appearance of the typical rash on day 2 of the illness
- Young children (1 to 3 years of age) with GAS rarely develop the classic acute pharyngitis or scarlet fever.
  1. Present with moderate fever and serous, serosanguinous, or mucopurulent rhinitis
  2. Illness is more protracted, with persistent low-grade fever, irritability, and anorexia
  3. Referred to as *streptococcal fever* or *streptococcosis*

PHYSICAL EXAMINATION

- Variable toxicity and fever
- Erythema and inflammation of the posterior pharynx
  1. Pharyngeal exudate in 50% to 80% by day 2, whitish to yellowish in color, may become confluent
  2. Absence of oral ulcers and vesicles, nasal discharge, conjunctivitis, or other respiratory signs
- Swollen and tender anterior cervical lymphadenopathy in 30% to 60%
- Palatal petechiae possible
- Pathognomonic rash of scarlet fever
  1. Fine, erythematous, confluent punctate rash that begins on trunk and spreads peripherally
  2. Sandpaper texture, often described as "goose pimples on sunburn"
  3. Facial flushing with circumoral pallor

4. Rash fades with pressure
5. Deep red lines, with petechiae in folds of the joints (Pastia lines)
6. Rash; ultimately desquamates after 7 to 21 days; commonly on palms, soles but may be diffuse
7. Strawberry tongue (white coated or red in color) with enlarged papillae
- Young children (1 to 3 years of age) with GAS infection
  1. Generally have low-grade fever, generalized lymphadenopathy, persistent nasal discharge, and appear ill but not toxic

DIAGNOSIS

DIFFERENTIAL DIAGNOSIS
- Viral throat infections are more common than GAS and are clinically indistinguishable.
  1. Adenovirus
  2. Epstein-Barr virus
  3. Cytomegalovirus
  4. Herpes simplex virus
  5. Influenza
  6. Parainfluenza
  7. Coxsackie and possibly other enteroviruses
- Other streptococcal groups (C and G) have been associated with pharyngitis and nephritis but not with acute rheumatic fever.
- Other bacterial infections of the pharynx are uncommon in children, although bacterial cultures can reveal other streptococci (nonβ-hemolytic) and *Haemophilus influenzae,* which are generally thought to be normal inhabitants of the upper respiratory tract and need not be treated.

DIAGNOSTIC WORKUP
- In the nontoxic child, diagnostic testing should be limited to differentiating GAS infection from viral causes because of the need to treat GAS to prevent complications and sequelae.
  1. Laboratory confirmation of GAS in the form of a throat culture is recommended.
     a. A specimen should be obtained by vigorous swabbing of the tonsils and posterior pharynx.
     b. Cultures on sheep blood agar with appropriate use of a bacitracin disk allows a presumptive identification of GAS.
     c. A false-negative rate of less than 10% is achieved if the swab is obtained and processed properly.
  2. Several rapid diagnostic tests are available.
     a. Most of these tests have high specificity but lower sensitivity.
     b. A throat culture should be sent

in any patient suspected of having GAS who has a negative rapid diagnostic test.
- Factors to be considered in the decision to obtain a throat swab for testing in children with pharyngitis are the patient's age, clinical signs and symptoms, the season, and the family and community epidemiology, including contact with a known case, potential exposure to a family member with a history of ARF or PSGN.
- In the rare, toxic child, the extent of the workup depends on the clinical presentation and may include a white cell count and differential, blood and throat cultures, and radiographic studies (e.g., computed tomography scan of soft tissues of the neck, chest radiographs, and a sinus series).
- In a nontoxic child with tonsillitis/pharyngitis and classic scarlet fever, diagnostic evaluation is not thought to be required because the rash is pathognomonic of GAS infection.
- GAS is unlikely in patients younger than 3 years of age and in those with signs of viral infection (e.g., coryza, conjunctivitis, hoarseness, cough, anterior stomatitis, diarrhea, discrete oral ulcers).
  1. GAS testing is not recommended in these patients.
- All symptomatic contacts should be tested for GAS, although symptomatic household contacts are often treated presumptively.
  1. Asymptomatic contacts should be tested only if the contact or a family member of the contact has a history of ARF or PSGN.
  2. Individuals testing positive under these circumstances should be treated.
- Patients in whom repeated episodes of pharyngitis occurring at short intervals and associated with positive cultures or tests for GAS pose a special problem.
  1. These individuals are often GAS carriers who are experiencing frequent viral illnesses.
  2. Noncompliance or treatment failure should be considered.

THERAPY

MEDICAL
- Although GAS infection is a self-limited disease, treatment prevents spread, complications, and latent sequelae and shortens the clinical course.
- A brief delay in initiating antibiotic therapy to process a throat culture does not increase the risk of latent sequelae.

- Penicillin V is the drug of choice for GAS tonsillopharyngitis and scarlet fever. Amoxicillin is often used instead but offers no microbiologic advantage.
  1. The dosage of penicillin is 250 mg (400,000 U) two to three times per day for children and 500 mg two to three times per day for adolescents and adults.
  2. Medication should be continued for 10 days to prevent ARF, regardless of the promptness of clinical recovery.
- Intramuscular benzathine penicillin G is also appropriate therapy.
  1. It ensures adequate blood concentrations and avoids the problem of compliance, but administration is painful.
  2. A single dose of 600,000 U is appropriate for children weighing less than 60 pounds, and 1.2 million U is recommended for larger children, adolescents, and adults.
  3. Mixtures with shorter-acting penicillins (e.g., procaine penicillin) are less painful, as is warming benzathine penicillin G to room temperature before administration.
- Orally administered erythromycin is indicated for patients who are allergic to penicillin.
  1. Treatment can be given as either the estolate (20 to 40 mg/kg per day in two to four divided doses), or
  2. Erythromycin ethylsuccinate (40 mg/kg per day in two to four divided doses)
  3. Continued for 10 days
- Other macrolides (clarithromycin and azithromycin) are also effective.
- Penicillin-allergic individuals can also be treated with a cephalosporin or clindamycin.
- Penicillin- and erythromycin-resistant strains of GAS are uncommon in the United States.
- Tetracycline and sulfonamides should not be used to treat GAS pharyngitis.
- Infected individuals remain infectious until they have had 24 hours of appropriate therapy; thus they should stay home for that period.

SURGICAL
- Surgical management in the child with acute GAS tonsillopharyngitis is reserved for the acute complication of associated peritonsillar abscess, which may require surgical drainage.
- Tonsillectomy for recurrent GAS infection is not done as commonly as it was in the past.
  1. Experts remain conflicted about whether tonsillectomy alters the course of recurrent disease or

lessens the possibility of latent sequelae.

2. Only children with more than seven documented episodes of streptococcus tonsillitis in a year or five episodes each in 2 consecutive years should be referred for evaluation for possible tonsillectomy.

■ **FOLLOW-UP & DISPOSITION**

- A follow-up visit and repeat culture or rapid test to document resolution of disease is not indicated for most children with GAS infection, with or without scarlet fever.
- The clinical response to antimicrobial treatment is usually prompt, so failure to respond within 48 hours would suggest a viral cause or may indicate a need for reevaluation to search for suppurative complications.
- Therapy should be continued for a total of 10 days to prevent latent sequelae.
- In patients who develop sequelae, there is a latent period of several days to weeks in which the child or adult seems completely well.
- The development of new symptoms after the usual latency periods (average of 10 days for ARF and 3 weeks for PSGN) necessitates an immediate and appropriate investigation.
- The management and follow-up of patients with recurrent symptomatic episodes of pharyngitis and repetitively positive tests for GAS are problematic and controversial.
  1. Most experts recommend trying to document the clearance of the strep by culture when the child is asymptomatic between episodes.
  2. Failure to obtain a negative test for strep suggests that the patient is a streptococcal carrier. Treatment of such patients is usually not necessary.

■ **PATIENT/FAMILY EDUCATION**

- Parents should be informed about the following:
  1. Natural history, communicability, and usual clinical course of the disease
  2. The importance of prompt follow-up if symptoms have not resolved in 3 days

3. The importance of finishing all of the treatment to prevent latent sequelae
4. The importance of recognizing symptoms of the late sequelae of GAS (ARF and PSGN) and seeking immediate treatment

- Patients with a history of ARF and their family members must be vigilant and prompt in seeking diagnosis and treatment of possible GAS infection because they are at risk for recurrence.

■ **PREVENTIVE TREATMENT**

- Preventive, prophylactic antibiotics are not indicated for patients at low risk for rheumatic fever.
- Patients with a well-documented history of ARF and those with rheumatic heart disease should be given continuous antibiotic prophylaxis to prevent recurrent attacks.
- Some experts recommend oral penicillin prophylaxis during the period of the year of greatest risk for children with repeated episodes of GAS pharyngitis. The effectiveness of such an approach is unsubstantiated and should be limited because of concerns of antimicrobial resistance.

■ **REFERRAL INFORMATION**

- Most cases of GAS tonsillopharyngitis and scarlet fever can be easily recognized and treated on an outpatient basis by primary care physicians.
- Inpatient treatment may be initially required for toxic-appearing patients suspected of having associated invasive disease.
- Certain complications (e.g., peritonsillar abscess) may necessitate referral for surgical comanagement.
- Referral of patients for tonsillectomy should be infrequent.
- Patients who develop latent sequelae of GAS infections, including ARF and PSGN, generally require referral to a pediatric subspecialist for diagnosis, initial management, and subsequent comanagement.

■⃰ **PEARLS & CONSIDERATIONS**

■ **CLINICAL PEARLS**

- Most cases of tonsillopharyngitis in childhood are caused by viruses. Clinicians need to detect those cases

caused by GAS in order to provide therapy that will lessen both transmission and the possibility of acute and latent complications. Diagnostic testing is readily available but should be used with discretion to detect only those patients with disease who need treatment and not those with GAS carriage.

- Patients with classic scarlet fever can be diagnosed purely on clinical grounds and do not require diagnostic studies.

■ **WEBSITES**

All sites listed here are sponsored by the Centers for Disease Control and Prevention.

- General and technical information: www.cdc.gov/ncidod/dbmc/diseaseinfo/groupastreptococcal_g.htm
- "The ABCs of Safe and Healthy Child Care," information on strep throat and scarlet fever: www.cdc.gov/ncidod/hip/abc/facts39.htm
- "Trends in Bacteremic Infection Due to *Streptococcus pyogenes*, 1986-1995": www.cdc.gov/ncidod/EID/vol2no1/strepyro.htm

REFERENCES

1. American Academy of Pediatrics: Group A streptococcal infections. In Peter G (ed): *2000 Red Book: report on the Committee of Infectious Diseases,* ed 25, Elk Grove Village, Ill, 2000, American Academy of Pediatrics.
2. Darmstadt GL: Scarlet fever and its relatives, *Contemp Pediatr* 15:44, 1998.
3. Gerber MA: Streptococcal pharyngitis: update on management, *Contemp Pediatr* 14:156, 1997.
4. Group A streptococcal infections: proceedings of a conference held January 20-22, 1995, in Tampa, Florida, *Pediatrics* 97:S945, 1996.
5. Kaplan EL: Group A streptococcal infections. In Feigin RD, Cherry JD (eds): *Textbook of pediatric infectious diseases,* ed 3, Philadelphia, 1992, WB Saunders.

Author: **Lynn R. Campbell, M.D.**

BASIC INFORMATION

DEFINITION
Pityriasis rosea (PR) is an acute, benign skin disorder affecting mostly adolescents and young adults. It is most common in the cooler months and is self-limited.

ICD-9CM CODE
696.3 Pityriasis rosea

ETIOLOGY
- The cause is unknown, but a viral etiology is suspected based on the self-limiting course, epidemics with seasonal clustering, and tendency for lifelong immunity.
- Human herpesvirus (HHV) types 6 and 7 (HHV-6 and HHV-7, respectively) and parvovirus B19 are among the specific viruses being investigated as possible causative agents.

EPIDEMIOLOGY & DEMOGRAPHICS
- Slight female predominance, with a female:male ratio of 1.2:1
- More common in fall, winter, and spring
- Usually occurs in adolescents and young adults (uncommon in children younger than 5 years of age)

HISTORY
- There is occasionally a nonspecific prodrome (headache, pharyngitis, lymphadenitis, malaise).
- Approximately 70% to 80% retrospectively recall a *herald patch.*
  1. Isolated lesion
  2. Usually on trunk, upper arms, neck, or thigh, in order of decreasing frequency
- Generalized eruption begins 5 to 10 days after development of the herald patch.
  1. Spares face (85%), scalp, and distal extremities
- Peaks 2 to 7 days after onset of generalized eruption.
- In 25% of cases, lesions are moderately pruritic.
- Resolution of lesions begins after 2 to 4 weeks.
- Lesions fade over 4 to 6 weeks.
- Patients may have postinflammatory hypopigmentation or hyperpigmentation (especially in dark-skinned individuals) for weeks to months after healing is complete.

PHYSICAL EXAMINATION
- A *herald patch* is a sharply defined round or oval area (2 to 5 cm) with a flat, pink or brown center and a red, finely scaled, slightly elevated border.
- Secondary generalized eruption occurs in crops.
  1. Lesions may resemble the herald patch but are smaller and more ovoid.
  2. Lesions on the trunk have a characteristic Christmas tree pattern—the long axis of individual lesions is parallel to lines of skin, with the trunk of the tree along the spine.
  3. Secondary lesions typically have a fine, scaly edge with a cigarette paper–like collarette of scale.
- Young children may have lesions that are papular, vesicular, pustular, urticarial, or purpuric in the early stages.
  1. Atypical lesions are more common in very young children, dark-skinned individuals, and pregnant women.
  2. Children may also have lesions on the face and neck.
  3. Uncommonly, the lesions may be found on oral mucosal surfaces.
- Atypical presentations may show an inverse distribution of lesions affecting the face, wrists, and extremities and sparing the trunk.

DIAGNOSIS

DIFFERENTIAL DIAGNOSIS
- The differential diagnosis of the herald patch includes tinea corporis.
- The differential of the secondary eruption includes the following:
  1. Drug eruption
  2. Seborrheic dermatitis
  3. Nummular eczema
  4. Guttate psoriasis
  5. Secondary syphilis
  6. Acute form of pityriasis lichenoides (Mucha-Habermann disease)

DIAGNOSTIC WORKUP
- The diagnosis is based on clinical recognition of lesions and distribution pattern.
- The fine, peripheral collarette of scale is characteristic of pityriasis rosea.

THERAPY

NONPHARMACOLOGIC
There is no specific therapy for PR, which is a self-limited disease.

MEDICAL
- Pruritus, if present, may be treated with mild, topical corticosteroids and/or oral antihistamines.
- Exposure to sunshine or ultraviolet light tends to hasten resolution of lesions but may accentuate postinflammatory hypopigmentation.

FOLLOW-UP & DISPOSITION
See "Therapy."

PATIENT/FAMILY EDUCATION
- The disease is self-limited, including the postinflammatory changes.
- Resolution will not occur for many weeks.
- Patient may need physician note to return to work or school.
- Contagion pattern is not known.
- No short- or long-term untoward effect has been identified.

PEARLS & CONSIDERATIONS

CLINICAL PEARLS
- Herald patch is followed by similar (and usually smaller) lesions in the typical Christmas tree distribution.
- Individual lesions have a *collarette* of fine scale.

REFERENCES
1. Darmstadt GL, Lane A: Diseases of the epidermis. In Behrman RE, Kliegman RM, Arvin AM (eds): *Nelson textbook of pediatrics,* ed 15, Philadelphia, 1996, WB Saunders.
2. Drago F et al: Human herpesvirus 7 in patients with pityriasis rosea: electron microscopy investigations and polymerase chain reaction in mononuclear cells, plasma and skin, *Dermatology* 195:374, 1997.
3. Hurwitz S: *Clinical pediatric dermatology,* ed 2, Philadelphia, 1993, WB Saunders.
4. Marcus-Farber BS et al: Serum antibodies to parvovirus B19 in patients with pityriasis rosea, *Dermatology* 194:371, 1997.
5. Zitelli BJ, Davis HW: *Atlas of pediatric physical diagnosis,* ed 3, St Louis, 1997, Mosby.
Author: **Lisa Loeb Colton, M.D.**

II

BASIC INFORMATION

■ DEFINITION
Pleural effusion is a pathologic collection of fluid or pus between the parietal and visceral pleura.

ICD-9CM CODES
511.9 Unspecified
511.1 Bacterial
012.0 Tuberculous, fifth digit dependent on laboratory diagnosis
862.29 Traumatic
For others, primary disease code.

■ ETIOLOGY
- Pleural effusions can be categorized as transudates or exudates based on their cellular and chemical composition (see "Diagnostic Workup").
- Transudates are caused by decreased oncotic or increased hydrostatic pressure in capillaries.
- Exudates are caused by increased permeability (inflammation) of pleura or impaired lymphatic drainage.
  1. Parapneumonic effusion is associated with underlying pneumonia; this is the most common pleural effusion in childhood.
  2. Empyema is pus in the pleural space.

■ HISTORY
- Recent respiratory symptoms: cough, shortness of breath, difficulty breathing, chest pain
- Symptoms of systemic illness: fever, fatigue, loss of appetite, decreased activity
- Tuberculosis exposure

■ PHYSICAL EXAMINATION
- Increased respiratory rate
- "Splinting" of chest
- Dullness to percussion on affected side(s)
- Egophony
- Decreased breath sounds on affected side(s)

DIAGNOSIS

Examination should prompt chest x-ray evaluation and then, unless the effusion is small and the cause known, thoracentesis.

■ DIFFERENTIAL DIAGNOSIS
- Pneumonia
- Chest mass

■ DIAGNOSTIC WORKUP
Imaging
- Chest radiograph, posteroanterior and lateral views, may be diagnostic.
  1. Small effusions may be visible

only as blunting of costophrenic angles.
  a. Easily missed on supine film
  2. With increasing effusion size, the radiograph demonstrates the following:
    a. Obscuration of hemidiaphragm
    b. Mass effect with shift of mediastinum away from affected side
    c. "White out" of affected side
  3. Decubitus film with affected side down may help demonstrate mobility of small or moderate-sized effusion; not helpful for very large effusion.
- Ultrasound
  1. Useful for determining if fluid is free flowing or loculated
  2. May help distinguish a solid mass from a large effusion
  3. May provide guidance for thoracentesis
- Computed tomography (CT) scan: most helpful in the following situations:
  1. In complicated effusion
  2. If question of chest mass and effusion exists

Thoracentesis
- Therapeutic
  1. For relief of respiratory distress
- Diagnostic
  1. To assist in diagnosing the type of pleural effusion at time of recognition
  2. To facilitate radiographic examination of underlying lung and thorax
- Studies to obtain at the time of thoracentesis (those in bold distinguish exudate and transudate or assist in determining whether a chest tube will be required for drainage of an exudate):

Pleural Fluid	Blood	Other
pH	Electrolytes	Purified protein derivative
Protein	**Protein**	
Lactate dehydrogenase (LDH)	**LDH**	
Glucose	**Glucose**	
Cell counts, cytology	Complete blood count, erythrocyte sedimentation rate	
Cultures, antigen detection	Cultures	
Lipids	Serologies	

- An **exudate** has 1 or more of the following characteristics:
  1. Protein: pleural/serum more than 0.5
  2. LDH: pleural/serum more than 0.6
  3. LDH: pleural more than two-thirds upper limit of serum normal

■ DIFFERENTIAL DIAGNOSIS—EXUDATE
- Infection (generally pneumonia with parapneumonic effusion or empyema): *Streptococcus pneumoniae* (including penicillin-resistant strains), group A streptococcus, *Mycoplasma, Staphylococcus, Haemophilus influenzae* (rare since immunization in North America); consider anaerobes
- Pancreatitis (left-sided)
- Collagen vascular diseases
- Chylothorax (lipid 1 to 4 g/dl but may be low before feeding in newborn)
- Malignancy: most commonly lymphoma (cytology may be diagnostic *if* positive)
- Trauma
- A transudate has none of the chemical characteristics of an exudate.

■ DIFFERENTIAL DIAGNOSIS—TRANSUDATE
- Congestive heart failure
- Hypoalbuminemia
- Nephrosis
- Hepatic cirrhosis
- Iatrogenic: central line, ventriculopleural shunt complication

THERAPY

- Therapy is directed toward the underlying disease process.
- Chest tube placement is controversial because of the following:
  1. Pediatric recommendations have been drawn from data obtained in adults.
  2. Recent follow-up series of children suggest good long-term results even in empyema without chest tube placement.
- The most common practice is to insert a chest tube in parapneumonic effusion under the following conditions:
  1. For relief of respiratory distress
  2. If there is pus at thoracentesis or organisms on Gram stain
  3. More controversial is chest tube placement in parapneumonic effusions meeting "Light" criteria (pH less than 7.0, LDH more than 1000 IU/dl, or glucose less than 40 mg/dl)
- Fibrinolysis with urokinase via the chest tube appears safe for loculated effusions.
- Video-assisted thoracoscopic surgery may be considered when the effusion is loculated at presentation.
- Surgical decortication practice varies: Some centers prefer early operative management, whereas others reserve the procedure for unremitting fevers despite antibiotics and chest tube drainage.

■ FOLLOW-UP & DISPOSITION

- Complicated pleural effusion and empyema may resolve slowly.
  1. Staff, patient, and family should be prepared for prolonged therapy.
  2. Intravenous access and nutritional issues should be addressed early.
- A chest radiograph showing resolution is desirable.
  1. If patient is improving clinically, wait 4 to 6 months.
- Follow-up studies in children are encouraging.
  1. Recent studies have not demonstrated the restrictive defects reported earlier.

■ PREVENTIVE TREATMENT

- None is available for most causes.
- Influenza vaccine and vaccination against *S. pneumoniae* may decrease those infections underlying some parapneumonic effusions.

☼ PEARLS & CONSIDERATIONS

■ WEBSITE

Virtual Hospital: www.vh.org/ Providers/TeachingFiles/TAP/ Thoracopedia.html; brief case descriptions with chest radiographs and CT scans.

REFERENCES

1. Givan DC, Eigen H: Common pleural effusions in children, *Clin Chest Med* 19:63, 1998.
2. Kkrishnan S et al: Urokinase in the management of complicated parapneumonic effusions in children, *Chest* 112:1579, 1997.

Author: **Debbie Toder, M.D.**

II

BASIC INFORMATION

■ DEFINITION
Pneumonia is inflammation of the lung caused by a variety of pathogens.

ICD-9CM CODE
486.00 Pneumonia

■ ETIOLOGY
- Determination of the precise cause for pneumonia in children is often difficult.
- The more common pathogens include the following:
  1. Virus: respiratory syncytial virus (RSV), parainfluenza, influenza, adenovirus
  2. Bacteria: *Streptococcus pneumoniae, Streptococcus pyogenes, Staphylococcus aureus, Streptococcus agalactiae, Haemophilus influenzae* type B
  3. *Mycoplasma pneumoniae*
  4. *Chlamydia trachomatis, Chlamydia pneumoniae*
  5. *Mycobacteria tuberculosis*
- In the immunocompromised patient, also consider organisms such as *Pneumocystis carinii*, fungi (*Candida*, aspergillus), *Legionella pneumophilia*, and cytomegalovirus

■ EPIDEMIOLOGY & DEMOGRAPHICS
- Pneumonia is more prevalent in the winter months.
- It is more common in younger children.
- Viruses are the most common cause of pneumonia.
- Viral pneumonias are often observed in epidemics.
- Children who are immunocompromised or who have underlying lung disease are at greater risk for significant pneumonia.

■ HISTORY
- Pneumonia is often preceded by symptoms of an upper respiratory tract infection.
- Symptoms include fever, malaise, anorexia, and chest pain.
- Cough may be associated with vomiting.
- Some infants may have associated apnea.

■ PHYSICAL EXAMINATION
- Child may only have nonspecific signs, such as fever and general ill appearance.
- Signs suggestive of pneumonia include tachypnea, nasal flaring, retractions, grunting, dullness to percussion of chest, decreased breath sounds, rales, and egophony.
- Infants may have episodes of cyanosis.

■ DIAGNOSIS

■ DIFFERENTIAL DIAGNOSIS
- Sepsis
- Asthma
- Atelectasis
- Lung sequestration
- Hypersensitivity reaction
- Pulmonary hemorrhage
- Sarcoidosis
- Wegener's granulomatosis
- Foreign body aspiration
- Congestive heart failure
- Malignancy

■ DIAGNOSTIC WORKUP
- A complete blood count and differential and chest roentgenograph are initial tests.
- Blood cultures are recommended in young, febrile children and children who are seriously ill.
- Computed tomography may better delineate chest pathology and may be useful in the severely ill or immunocompromised host.
- Sputum for Gram stain and culture in children who can produce an adequate specimen. Most young children, however, cannot provide such a specimen.
- Thoracentesis should be considered if a pleural effusion is present. The specimen is sent for Gram stain and culture, pH, cell count, protein, and cytology to differentiate transudate from exudate and to provide drainage.
- Bronchoscopy or open lung biopsy (for culture and histology) may be necessary in the evaluation of pneumonia in the seriously ill and immunocompromised patient.

■ SPECIFIC TESTING
- Virus
  1. Rapid testing is generally available for RSV and influenza.
  2. Shell viral cultures may be read within a few days (used for influenza A and B, RSV, parainfluenza, and adenovirus).
  3. Traditional viral cultures are kept longer.
- Bacteria
  1. Gram stain and culture
  2. Antigen testing in urine samples may be helpful for *S. pneumonia, H. influenzae*, and group B streptococci.
- *M. pneumoniae*
  1. Elevated serum cold agglutinins may be present, but this test has low specificity.
  2. Organism may be cultured in some laboratories.
  3. Mycoplasma-specific antibody titers may be tested.
- *Chlamydia*
  1. Fluorescent antibody staining is available for *C. trachomatis*.
- *M. tuberculosis*
  1. Mantoux skin test (5 TU of PPD) is done for determination of infection.
  2. In young children, an early morning gastric aspirate is the preferred specimen for acid-fast stain and culture.
  3. Sputum or bronchoscopy specimens may also identify the organism.
- *P. carinii*
  1. Sputum samples and specimens obtained by bronchoscopy or lung biopsy are examined for organisms with a silver stain.
  2. Fluorescent antibody staining may also be performed.
- Fungi
  1. Organism may be cultured from lung biopsy or observed on histology.
  2. Sputum cultures alone may be difficult to interpret.
- *Legionella pneumophilia*
  1. Organism may be cultured using special media.
  2. Urine antigen detection and serology are also available.

■ THERAPY

- Supportive care should be initiated, with maintenance of adequate oxygenation, hydration, nutrition, and fever control.
- Pulse oximetry is helpful to access level of oxygenation.
- Mechanical ventilation may be necessary in severely ill children.

■ ANTIMICROBIAL THERAPY
- Virus: Most viral pneumonias are treated symptomatically, but specific antiviral therapy may be beneficial in certain situations.
  1. RSV: Ribavirin given by aerosol should be considered in children at high risk for serious RSV disease (i.e., children with congenital heart disease, chronic lung disease, or immunocompromised state; some infants born prematurely or with chronic medical conditions; infants hospitalized with severe illness).
  2. Influenza: Amantadine has activity against influenza A. It should be considered for children with severe illness or children at risk for developing severe disease (i.e., children with chronic lung disease, immunocompromised children, and children with certain chronic medical condi-

tions). It is also used in some healthy children for those desiring specific therapy. It should be started early in the illness. Amantadine may have central nervous system side effects. The antiviral zanamivir has been approved for treatment of uncomplicated influenza (A and B) in children 12 and older.
3. Cytomegalovirus: Ganciclovir and cytomegalovirus (CMV) intravenous immune globulin (IVIG) have been used in CMV pneumonia in bone marrow transplant patients.
• Bacteria
1. Numerous antibiotics have activity against the usual bacterial pathogens. Commonly used oral antibiotics include amoxicillin (with or without clavulanate acid), the second- and third-generation cephalosporins, and the macrolides. Intravenous antibiotics are indicated for children who are seriously ill or vomiting. For the common bacterial pathogens, the duration of antibiotic therapy is usually 10 to 14 days. Longer courses of therapy are often required for children with pneumonia complicated by empyema or abscess, and in the immunocompromised patient.
2. Macrolides and trimethoprim/sulfamethoxazole (TMP/SMX) should not be used for treatment of penicillin-resistant *S. pneumoniae*.
• *M. pneumoniae*
1. Macrolides (erythromycin, clarithromycin, and azithromycin)
2. Tetracycline; may be used in children 8 years and older
• *C. trachomatis, C. pneumoniae*
1. Macrolides
2. Tetracycline; may be used in children 8 years and older
• *M. tuberculosis:* Multidrug therapy is given for at least 6 months. Therapy depends on organism sensitivity. Unless drug resistance is suspected, usual therapy consists of isoniazid, rifampin, and pyrazinamide for the first 2 months, followed by isoniazid and rifampin for an additional 4 months. Therapy is extended to a minimum of 1 year in children infected with human immunodeficiency virus (HIV).
• *P. carinii:* TMP/SMX; pentamidine is

an alternative drug. Corticosteroids should be considered in children with moderate to severe illness. The duration of therapy is at least 2 to 3 weeks.
• Fungal (*Candida,* aspergillus): Amphotericin B is the drug of choice. Higher dosages are used for aspergillosis. Liposomal amphotericin preparations should be considered if renal insufficiency, intolerance to amphotericin B, or need for very high dosing is present. An extended course of therapy is usually required.
• *Legionella pneumophilia:* Macrolides are given. The addition of rifampin is recommended in cases of severe illness, immunocompromised patients, or poor response to macrolide. Treatment is for 3 weeks.

■ **SURGICAL**
Empyemas require drainage. Thoracoscopy or thoracotomy with decortication may be necessary.

■ **FOLLOW-UP & DISPOSITION**
Close follow-up is essential. A repeat chest roentgenograph several weeks after completion of antibiotics helps verify the absence of an underlying abnormality.

■ **PATIENT/FAMILY EDUCATION**
• Parents of neonates should be counseled about the spread of respiratory viruses and the importance of good handwashing and decreased exposures to ill individuals.
• Preventive therapy against RSV may be recommended.
• Children who are immunocompromised or who have certain chronic illnesses should also be appropriately educated about exposures and recommended preventive therapies.

■ **PREVENTIVE TREATMENT**
• Children should receive the usual recommended vaccines unless they have a specific contraindication.
• Other available immunizations for selected high-risk children include vaccines against influenza, pneumococcus, and meningococcus.
• Penicillin prophylaxis against pneumococcal disease is recommended in many asplenic children.
• Young children who are at high risk for RSV may receive monthly prophylaxis during RSV season with palivizumab or RSV immune globulin.

• Children who have infection with mycobacterial tuberculosis, but without disease, should receive prophylactic isoniazid for 6 to 9 months.
• Prophylaxis against *P. carinii* with TMP/SMX is indicated for children who are significantly immunocompromised, including some HIV-infected children, some children with primary immunodeficiencies, and some children receiving immunosuppressive therapy. HIV-infected children who have had prior *P. carinii* pneumonia usually receive lifelong prophylaxis.

■ **REFERRAL INFORMATION**
Referral to a pediatric infectious disease specialist is suggested for children with unusual or complicated pneumonias.

☼ PEARLS & CONSIDERATIONS

■ **CLINICAL PEARLS**
• Respiratory viruses are the most common cause of pneumonia.
• The etiologic diagnosis is difficult. Bacterial cultures of upper respiratory tract secretions are usually not helpful. Blood cultures are often not positive.
• Think of pneumonia in febrile children younger than 5 years old with significant leukocytosis (white blood cell count 20,000/mm^3 or higher).

REFERENCES
1. American Academy of Pediatrics: Pneumonia. In Pickering LK (ed): *2000 Red Book: report of the Committee on Infectious Diseases,* ed 25, Elk Grove Village, Ill, 2000, American Academy of Pediatrics.
2. Bachur R, Perry H, Harper MB: Occult pneumonias: empiric chest radiographs in febrile children with leukocytosis, *Ann Emerg Med* 33:166, 1999.
3. Boyer KM: Nonbacterial pneumonia. In Feigin RD, Cherry JD (eds): *Textbook of pediatric infectious diseases,* ed 4, Philadelphia, 1998, WB Saunders.
4. Klein JD: Bacterial pneumonias. In Feigin RD, Cherry JD (eds): *Textbook of pediatric infectious diseases,* ed 4, Philadelphia, 1998, WB Saunders.
Author: **Carol McCarthy, M.D.**

BASIC INFORMATION

■ DEFINITION

A spontaneous pneumothorax is an accumulation of air in the pleural space.

■ SYNONYM

Collapsed lung

ICD-9CM CODES

512.8 Acute, spontaneous
512.1 Iatrogenic/postoperative/
  procedural complication
770.2 Newborn
860.0 Traumatic
512.0 Tension

■ ETIOLOGY

- Primary pneumothorax (PTX)
  1. PTX is most often secondary to rupture of subpleural blebs or bullae on apical portion of upper lobes.
  2. Blebs may be secondary to abnormalities of connective tissue, inflammation of bronchioles, or overdistention of alveoli.
  3. PTX leads to a decrease in vital capacity and an increase in the alveolar-arterial oxygen gradient (with consequent hypoxemia).
- Secondary PTX; occurs in patients with preexisting lung disease
  1. Airway disease (asthma, cystic fibrosis [CF])
  2. Infectious disease (*Pneumocystis carinii* pneumonia; anaerobic, gram-negative, or staphylococcal pneumonia)
  3. Interstitial lung disease
  4. Connective tissue disease (Marfan's disease, Ehlers-Danlos syndrome)
- Traumatic
  1. Most commonly these are complications (which develop within 24 hours) of a procedure
     a. Transthoracic needle aspiration
     b. Subclavian catheterization
     c. Thoracentesis
     d. Transbronchial biopsy
     e. Tracheostomy
  2. Mechanical ventilation
  3. Penetrating or nonpenetrating chest injury
  4. Blunt trauma to chest
- Catamenial
  1. Rare form of recurrent pneumothorax within 48 to 72 hours of onset of menses
  2. Most occur in the right hemithorax
  3. Associated with pelvic endometriosis

■ EPIDEMIOLOGY & DEMOGRAPHICS

- Age-adjusted incidence: 7 to 18 per 100,000 in males; 1 to 6 per 100,000 in females
- Male:female ratio of 3:1 to 6:1
- Familial tendency
- Risk factors
  1. Tobacco smoking: quantity of cigarettes per day and length of time exposed
  2. Tall and thin body habitus
  3. Males aged 10 to 30 years
- Recurrence rate
  1. Approximately 20% to 30% after first pneumothorax; usually occurs within 2 years and on the same side
  2. From 50% to 60% following the second pneumothorax
  3. More than 80% after the third
  4. Risk of subsequent contralateral pneumothorax 5% to 10%

■ HISTORY

- Approximately 95% of patients complain of acute, localized and pleuritic chest pain associated with dyspnea and tachycardia.
- Cough, hemoptysis, and orthopnea are uncommon manifestations.
- Less than 10% occur during strenuous exercise.
- Ipsilateral shoulder pain is common.

■ PHYSICAL EXAMINATION

- Small pneumothoraces (less than 20%) usually not detectable on physical examination
- Vital signs usually normal except for moderate tachycardia
- Lung examination
  1. Hyperresonant to percussion
  2. Decreased or absent breath sounds on affected side
  3. Enlargement or depressed respiratory movement on affected side
- Hypoxemia usually mild when pneumothorax is less than 25%
  1. Hypoxemia, when present, is caused by shunting
- Hypercapnia rare because underlying lung function is normal

DIAGNOSIS

■ DIFFERENTIAL DIAGNOSIS

- Based on history
  1. Pleuritis
  2. Asthma
  3. Cardiac or psychogenic pain
- Based on examination
  1. Empyema
  2. Pleural effusion
  3. Bullae or lung cyst
- In neonates
  1. Congenital lobar emphysema

  2. Congenital adenomatoid malformation
  3. Diaphragmatic hernia

■ DIAGNOSTIC WORKUP

- Chest radiograph
  1. Outer margin of visceral pleura is separated from the parietal pleura by lucent gas space devoid of pulmonary vessels or lung markings.
  2. In upright position, air collects at the apex.
  3. In supine position, air collects juxtacardiac, at the lateral chest wall, or in the subpulmonic region.
  4. Lateral decubitus or end-expiratory film can highlight air collection.
  5. Signs of tension pneumothorax include the following:
     a. Mediastinal shift
     b. Diaphragmatic depression
     c. Rib cage expansion
- Quantification of pneumothorax by two different techniques
  1. $100 - [(\text{Diameter of collapsed lung})^3/(\text{Diameter of affected hemithorax})^3]$
  2. Nomogram
     a. Interpleural distance at the apex and at midpoints of both upper and lower lung fields
     b. Average three values and apply to nomogram
- Computed tomography scan
  1. Identifies presence of bullae
  2. Controversial whether this is predictive of recurrence

THERAPY

- Management centers on evacuating air from the pleural space and preventing recurrence.
- Choice of therapy depends on the clinical status of the patient, the cause of pneumothorax, evidence for concomitant lung disease, prior history, risk of recurrence, and technology available to the physician.

■ NONPHARMACOLOGIC

- Observation
  1. Requires evidence that air leak is sealed
  2. Generally reserved for asymptomatic patients with less than 20% primary, unilateral pneumothorax
  3. Serial chest radiographs over 24 hours to ensure no progression
  4. Can be outpatient with close observation, limited physical activity, and ability to obtain emergency services quickly
  5. Five percent mortality reported as

a result of the development of tension pneumothorax from unrecognized pleural leak
6. Gas reabsorbed spontaneously
   a. In closed pleural space, gas is at atmospheric pressure (760 mm Hg).
   b. Systemic venous blood has total pressure of 720 mm Hg.
   c. Positive-pressure gradient drives gas reabsorption.

■ MEDICAL
- Supplemental oxygen
  1. Partial pressure of nitrogen is greater in pneumothorax than in venous blood.
  2. Supplementation of oxygen increases this gradient as nitrogen is "washed out" of venous blood.
  3. As nitrogen diffuses out of pneumothorax across this gradient, the total volume of gas in pleural space decreases.
- Oxygen will accelerate reabsorption by a factor of 4 above room air.

■ SURGICAL
- Thoracentesis or chest tube drainage should be considered for all pneumothoraces 25% or greater, in patients with continued air leak, and in incomplete reexpansion or respiratory distress.
- Simple aspiration is successful in 70% of patients with moderate-sized PTX.
  1. Tube or needle is placed in the second anterior intercostal space in midclavicular line.
  2. Recurrence rate is 25% to 40%.
- Chest tube has a success rate of 90% for treatment of first PTX; success rates decrease with recurrences.
  1. Insertion is done through the fifth intercostal space in midaxillary line.
- All secondary PTX should be managed with chest tubes because of the risk of respiratory compromise.
- If the duration of pneumothorax is unknown, initial management is through a water-seal rather than negative pressure to minimize risk of reexpansion pulmonary edema;

negative pressure is used if lungs fail to reexpand after 12 to 24 hours.
- Complications include pain, pleural infection, incorrect placement of tube, hemorrhage, and reexpansion pulmonary edema.
- Continued air leak after 72 hours should prompt consideration of more invasive intervention.
  1. Pleurodesis
  2. Mechanical or chemical pleural abrasion leading to inflammatory response and subsequent adhesion formation
  3. Low success rate in patients with persistent air leak
  4. Goal to achieve adhesion of visceral and parietal pleura in order to obliterate pleural space
  5. Generally performed after second recurrence or after first pneumothorax in patients who plan to continue high risk activities (i.e., flying or diving)
  6. Future surgical procedures, such as pulmonary resection, open lung biopsy, and lung transplantation, may be hampered by process
- Thoracoscopy is indicated for patients who fail noninvasive intervention, have persistent or recurrent pneumothorax, or have a risk of significant morbidity should recurrence occur.
  1. Most often, it is performed via video-assisted thoracoscopic surgery under general anesthesia; it may also be an open procedure.
  2. Recurrence rate is 0.6% to 2%.
- Other surgical interventions include the following:
  1. Bullectomy: stapling or oversewing of bullae
  2. Pleurectomy
  3. Removal of fibrotic "peel"

■ COMPLICATIONS
- Tension pneumothorax
  1. This is defined as the point when intrapleural pressure is greater than atmospheric throughout expiration and often during inspiration.
  2. It is more common after traumatic or mechanical ventilation–induced pneumothorax.

3. Clinical picture includes labored breathing, tachypnea, marked tachycardia, profuse diaphoresis, and cyanosis.
4. Distended neck veins, tracheal deviation to side opposite the pneumothorax, subcutaneous emphysema, and hypotension are noted on physical examination.
- Bronchopleural fistula
  1. Approximately 3% to 5% of patients with pneumothorax will have persisting air leak.
  2. Patients with CF are at increased risk.
  3. Generally, surgical intervention is required.
- Reexpansion pulmonary edema
  1. Unilateral pulmonary edema following rapid reexpansion of lung
  2. Appears to be caused by increased permeability of pulmonary capillaries damaged by mechanical stress during reexpansion
  3. Based on animal models, occurs when PTX is present for more than 3 days and lung is expanded with greater than -20 cm H_2O pleural pressure
  4. Symptoms usually progress over 24 to 48 hours

☼ PEARLS & CONSIDERATIONS

■ CLINICAL PEARLS
- Pleural effusions occur coincident in 20% to 25% of cases.
- In room air, a pneumothorax is absorbed by 1% to 6% per 24 hours.
- Pneumothorax is associated with cocaine inhalation and marijuana smoking.

REFERENCES
1. Mahfood S et al: Re-expansion pulmonary edema, *Ann Thorac Surg* 45:340, 1988 (review).
2. Sahn SA, Heffner JE: Spontaneous pneumothorax, *N Engl J Med* 342:868, 2000.

Author: **Ann Marie Brooks, M.D.**

BASIC INFORMATION

■ DEFINITION
Polio is an acute viral infection of the brainstem and spinal cord. It is caused by an enterovirus and leads to irreversible motor neuron damage and paralysis. Endemic wild-type viral illness has been eradicated in North America as a result of the high rates of vaccination.

■ SYNONYMS
- Paralytic polio
- Infantile paralysis
- Poliomyelitis

ICD-9CM CODES
045.9 Polio
V04.0 Polio immunization

■ ETIOLOGY
- Poliovirus serotypes 1, 2, and 3 are in the group Enterovirus.
- Polio is transmitted by the fecal-oral route.
- Patients are contagious as long as fecal shedding persists, which can be weeks to months.
- Incubation is as follows:
  1. Three to six days for mild, nonspecific illness (abortive polio)
  2. Seven to 21 days for paralytic polio
- Postpolio syndrome may develop 30 to 40 years after initial childhood infection.

■ EPIDEMIOLOGY & DEMOGRAPHICS
- Before widespread immunization, outbreaks of polio occurred in the late summer and fall, with the largest epidemic (more than 57,000 cases) occurring in the United States in 1952.
- 1955: Inactivated (Salk) vaccine (IPV) was introduced.
- 1964: Trivalent oral (Sabin) vaccine (OPV) was introduced.
- 1978: Enhanced-potency inactivated vaccine (E-IPV) was developed.
- 1979: Last case of wild-type poliomyelitis was reported in the United States.
- Fewer than 10 cases per year of vaccine-associated paralytic poliomyelitis (VAPP) cases continue to occur in the United States, about 1 case for every 2.4 million doses.
- 1997: Advisory Committee on Immunization Practices (ACIP) changed the recommendation for the schedule of polio immunization to a sequential dosing of two inactivated doses followed by two oral vaccine doses.
- 1999: ACIP voted to change the recommendation for childhood polio vaccination beginning in 2000 to a schedule using only the E-IPV to eliminate the occurrence of VAPP.
- IPV should be administered at 2, 4, and 6 to 18 months of age, and a booster dose should be given at 4 to 6 years of age.

■ HISTORY
- VAPP: antecedent administration of OPV from 1 week to 1 month before symptoms; recent administration of DTP may enhance paralysis in active poliovirus infection
- Immunocompromise and/or exposure to a person recently vaccinated with OPV
- Abortive or aseptic meningitis: nonspecific signs and symptoms of a febrile illness, diarrhea, headache, meningismus, vomiting, and photophobia
- Paralytic poliomyelitis (spinal type): ascending paralysis, may occur without antecedent prodrome, especially in young infants; weakness and paralysis progress through the febrile period of the illness
- Respiratory difficulties occurring with paralysis of the intercostal muscles or with bulbar polioencephalitis affecting the brainstem medullary respiratory center
  1. Symptoms include shallow or spasmodic breathing, other cranial nerve involvement, and paralysis of pharyngeal or laryngeal muscles.
- Constipation and voiding abnormalities (urinary retention and overflow incontinence caused by bladder paresis)

■ PHYSICAL EXAMINATION
- Tremor upon sustained effort may present before weakness.
- Paralysis: Muscle tightness and intense muscle pain without true paralysis may be noted early in the presentation.
- Superficial and deep muscle reflexes are absent on the affected side.
- Cranial nerve paralysis presents in the bulbar form.

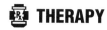 **DIAGNOSIS**

■ DIFFERENTIAL DIAGNOSIS
- Guillain-Barré syndrome
- Peripheral neuritis (herpes zoster, Bell's palsy of other etiologies)
- Rabies
- Botulism
- Tetanus
- Transverse myelitis
- Tick paralysis
- Various viral encephalitis/arbovirus infections

■ DIAGNOSTIC WORKUP
- Lumbar puncture: cerebrospinal fluid (CSF) may be normal in 10% to 15% of patients, pleocytosis as in viral meningitis
- Viral culture: stool and throat specimens for enterovirus culture, rarely grown from CSF
- Seroconversion of antibody titer to specific serotype
- Nerve conduction studies: asymmetric loss of stretch reflex is the hallmark of poliomyelitis

THERAPY

No medical or surgical therapies are available for polio, although patients with paralytic polio may need ventilatory support (e.g., intubation, tracheostomy) and appropriate antibiotics for potential associated pneumonias.

■ NONPHARMACOLOGIC
- Supportive care for respiratory support, including mechanical ventilation if required
- Nutritional support
- Physical therapy

■ PREVENTIVE TREATMENT
- Polio vaccine has been highly effective in eradicating wild-type polio circulation in the Western hemisphere and dramatically reducing its circulation in other areas of the world.
- OPV contains live, attenuated poliovirus types 1, 2, and 3 in monkey kidney cell lines and generates intestinal immunity.
- OPV viruses are excreted in the stool for several weeks after vaccination.
- IPV contains the same three virus types grown in human diploid cells or monkey kidney cells and inactivated with formaldehyde.
- IPV generates high rates of seroconversion but a lesser degree of mucosal immunity than OPV.
- Trace amounts of streptomycin, neomycin, and polymixin B may be in IPV preparations and may cause rare allergic reactions.
- Both vaccine types are highly immunogenic and effective in preventing polio.
- The only significant adverse reaction to OPV is VAPP, with risk being highest after the first dose of vaccine (1 case per 760,000 doses) and lower risk with each subsequent dose.
  1. For immunocompromised persons, the risk is 3200- to 6800-fold greater.
     a. Patients with antibody deficiency syndromes are at highest risk for acquiring VAPP from contact with a vaccinee or from primary vaccination.
- Immunodeficient persons should receive only IPV; household contacts

of such persons should also receive only IPV.

- Recent recommendations for the United States were to switch to a schedule of IPV only for all doses beginning January 2000.
- Routine immunization should occur at 2, 4, and 6 to 18 months of age, with a booster dose at 4 to 6 years of age.
- OPV would be acceptable in the following circumstances:
  1. Mass vaccination campaigns to control outbreaks
  2. Unvaccinated children who will be traveling in less than 4 weeks to areas where polio is endemic
  3. Children of parents who do not accept the multiple vaccine injections to complete the recommended vaccine schedule
  4. A recommendation is that OPV be administered as the third or fourth doses or both after discussion with the family of the risk of VAPP
  5. OPV still the recommended vaccine to eradicate polio in other countries where polio is still endemic
- Combination vaccines are in development to help reduce the number of injections in the first year of life
- Any suspected case of poliomyelitis should be reported to state health departments so that proper investigation can be initiated.
  1. If wild-type virus is isolated, OPV may need to be administered in a possible epidemic area.
  2. If OPV virus is implicated, no vaccination campaign is necessary because outbreaks with vaccine strains have not been seen.

☼ PEARLS & CONSIDERATIONS

Immunization with IPV should eliminate the occurrence of VAPP.

■ WEBSITES
- American Academy of Pediatrics: www.aap.org
- Centers for Disease Control and Prevention: www.cdc.gov/nip
- Food and Drug Administration: www.fda.gov/cber/vaers
- *Morbidity and Mortality Weekly Report:* www2.cdc.gov/mmwr

REFERENCES

1. American Academy of Pediatrics: Poliovirus infections. In Peter G (ed): *1997 Red Book: report of the Committee on Infectious Diseases,* Elk Grove Village, Ill, 1997, American Academy of Pediatrics.
2. American Academy of Pediatrics, Committee on Infectious Diseases: Poliomyelitis prevention: revised recommendations for use of inactivated and live oral poliovirus vaccines, *Pediatrics* 103:171, 1999.
3. Impact of the sequential IPV/OPV schedule on vaccination coverage levels, *MMWR Morb Mortal Wkly Rep* 47:1017, 1998.
4. Plotkin SA, Mortimer EA (eds): *Vaccines,* ed 2, Philadelphia, 1994, WB Saunders.
5. Recommendations of the Advisory Committee on Immunization Practices: Revised recommendations for routine poliomyelitis vaccination, *MMWR Morb Mortal Wkly Rep* 48:590, 1999.
Author: **Donna Fisher, M.D.**

BASIC INFORMATION

■ **DEFINITION**

Polycystic kidney diseases are hereditary disorders involving the development of innumerable fluid-filled cysts throughout the cortex and medulla of the kidneys. The following two main types are seen:
- Autosomal dominant polycystic kidney disease (ADPKD)
- Autosomal recessive polycystic kidney disease (ARPKD)

■ **SYNONYMS**
- Adult polycystic kidney disease (ADPKD)
- Infantile polycystic kidney disease (ARPKD)

ICD-9CM CODES
753.13 ADPKD
753.14 ARPKD

■ **ETIOLOGY**
- Cysts increase in number and size throughout life and compress normal kidney tissue, causing inflammation leading to destruction of renal parenchyma.
- ADPKD: Approximately 85% of cases are linked to chromosome 16p and an inherited mutation of one *PKD-1* gene allele.
  1. The *PKD-1* gene product, polycystin, is a large membrane-associated protein.
  2. A cyst appears to develop from a renal epithelial cell carrying this inherited abnormal *PKD-1* gene when a spontaneous mutation occurs in the other normal, but highly mutagenic, *PKD-1* allele.
  3. This leads to two abnormal *PKD-1* genes in the same cell and apparently to cyst formation.
- Most of the remaining cases are linked to the *PKD-2* gene on chromosome 4q, but a few families appear to have a third form.
- ARPKD: Linked to a locus on chromosome 6p. Dilated collecting ducts form small fusiform cysts that can enlarge with age.

■ **EPIDEMIOLOGY & DEMOGRAPHICS**
- ADPKD
  1. ADPKD affects approximately 1 in 1000 individuals.
  2. Onset usually occurs in adulthood.
  3. Fifty percent develop end-stage renal failure by age 60 to 70.
  4. All racial groups are affected.
  5. Clinical symptoms appear usually in the third to fifth decades of life, although PKD1 may present in childhood. PKD2 tends to have a milder course.

- ARPKD
  1. ARPKD affects between 1 in 10,000 and 1 in 55,000 children.
  2. Onset usually occurs in infancy and younger childhood.
  3. It is invariably associated with congenital hepatic fibrosis.
  4. Fifty percent of patients live beyond 10 years of age.

■ **HISTORY**
- ADPKD
  1. Positive family history
  2. Abdominal and flank pain
  3. Gross or microscopic hematuria
  4. Urinary tract infections
  5. Kidney stones
  6. Hypertension
  7. Renal cysts may be discovered, even on prenatal ultrasound
- ARPKD
  1. Parents unaffected
  2. Respiratory distress
  3. Oligohydramnios
  4. Spontaneous pneumothoraces
  5. Severe hypertension
  6. Portal hypertension with age
  7. Urinary tract infections are common.

■ **PHYSICAL EXAMINATION**
- ADPKD
  1. Hypertension
  2. Abdominal or flank masses
  3. Hepatomegaly (rare)
- ARPKD
  1. Flank masses (common)
  2. Potter syndrome (oligohydramnios sequence: flattened nose, micrognathia, low-set ears, pulmonary hypoplasia, limb deformities)
  3. Respiratory distress (in the neonatal period)
  4. Hypertension (common)
  5. Hepatosplenomegaly (usually presents in toddlers to school-aged children)
  6. Signs of portal hypertension
  7. Growth retardation

🔬 **DIAGNOSIS**

- ADPKD
  1. Diagnosis is made by finding large bilateral renal cysts (may be unilateral early on) in the presence of a family history of ADPKD.
  2. In affected families, prenatal and presymptomatic diagnosis can be made by DNA linkage analysis.
- ARPKD
  1. Massively enlarged kidneys are detected at birth or in an older child with congenital hepatic fibrosis.
  2. Congenital hepatic fibrosis is invariably found.
  3. Renal cysts are absent in parents.

  4. In affected families, prenatal diagnosis can be made by DNA linkage analysis.

■ **DIFFERENTIAL DIAGNOSIS**
- ADPKD
  1. Multiple simple renal cysts
  2. von Hippel-Lindau disease
  3. Tuberous sclerosis
  4. Bardet-Biedl syndrome
- ARPKD
  1. Bilateral Wilms' tumor
  2. Meckel syndrome
  3. Jeune syndrome
  4. Ivemark syndrome

■ **DIAGNOSTIC WORKUP**
- ADPKD
  1. Renal ultrasonography detects macroscopic cysts of various sizes.
  2. Because the course of ADPKD may be mild and 30% of adults may be unaware that they have the disease, renal ultrasonography should be performed on the parents of a child with bilateral renal cysts and a negative family history of ADPKD.
     a. Of patients, 83% have renal cysts by 30 years of age.
  3. Urinalysis reveals overt proteinuria in 23% of children.
     a. This may portend a worse prognosis.
  4. Magnetic resonance angiography is used to detect intracerebral aneurysms that may be associated with ADPKD in high-risk older children (those with a family history of ruptured cerebral aneurysm, symptoms suggestive of cerebral aneurysm).
  5. Hepatic ultrasound may show hepatic cysts are rare in children, but increase with age.
  6. Mitral valve prolapse occurs in 12% of children and may be seen on echocardiogram.
- ARPKD
  1. Renal ultrasonography: massive enlargement of the kidneys with loss of corticomedullary differentiation and diffuse marked increased echogenicity of the renal parenchyma from microcysts; cysts may enlarge as the child grows older
  2. Liver ultrasound
  3. Liver biopsy to document congenital hepatic fibrosis

💊 **THERAPY**

- No specific treatments are available for either of these disorders.
- Treat symptoms as they arise.

■ NONPHARMACOLOGIC
- ADPKD
  1. Bed rest, hydration, and analgesics for gross hematuria and cyst hemorrhage
  2. Segmental renal arterial embolization for massive bleeding
  3. Dialysis for patients reaching end-stage renal failure
- ARPKD
  1. Dialysis for patients reaching end-stage renal failure

■ MEDICAL
- ADPKD
  1. Antihypertensive agents are used for hypertension.
  2. Nonsteroidal antiinflammatory drugs are given for pain control (carefully monitoring renal function).
  3. Antibiotics are given for urinary tract infection.
     a. Many antibiotics penetrate into cysts poorly, and infections may prove refractory even in the face of sensitive organisms.
     b. Trimethoprim/sulfamethoxazole, ciprofloxacin, and tetracyclines tend to gain better entry into cysts than other agents, although the use of the latter agents may be problematic in young children.
     c. Prolonged treatment may be required.
- ARPKD
  1. Antihypertensive agents are given for blood pressure control. Several agents may be necessary.
  2. Antibiotics are given for urinary tract infections.

■ SURGICAL
- ADPKD
  1. Cyst reduction for chronic pain
  2. Cyst drainage for refractory cyst infection
  3. Kidney transplantation for patients reaching end-stage renal failure
  4. Nephrectomy; may be indicated before transplantation in the face of recurrent urinary tract infections, recurrent severe hematuria, or massively enlarged kidneys interfering with allograft placement
- ARPKD
  1. Kidney transplantation for end-stage renal failure
  2. Unilateral nephrectomy; suggested for severe respiratory compromise related to compression of the lungs by massively enlarged kidneys
  3. Portocaval anastomosis for severe portal hypertension
  4. Liver transplantation for severe congenital hepatic fibrosis

■ FOLLOW-UP & DISPOSITION
- ADPKD
  1. Monitor urinalysis and blood pressure closely in at-risk children.
  2. A high index of suspicion is required for urinary tract infections and kidney stones.
  3. Monitor renal function in patients with known ADPKD.
- ARPKD
  1. Monitor renal function.
  2. Monitor blood pressure.
  3. A high index of suspicion is required for urinary tract infections.
  4. Monitor for evidence of hypersplenism (e.g., splenomegaly, anemia, thrombocytopenia) secondary to hepatic disease.

■ PATIENT/FAMILY EDUCATION
- ADPKD: Presymptomatic evaluation and diagnosis may label an at-risk child early on in a disorder that may remain asymptomatic well into adulthood.
- ARPKD: It was initially thought that all patients died in infancy; however, more recent studies have shown that children who survive the neonatal period have a relatively good prognosis (67% are alive without end-stage renal disease at 15 years).

■ REFERRAL INFORMATION
- Involvement by a pediatric nephrologist should be obtained in the care of children with these disorders.
- Pediatric gastroenterology involvement is needed for children with ARPKD.

☼ PEARLS & CONSIDERATIONS

■ CLINICAL PEARLS
- ADPKD
  1. Onset of clinical symptoms, extrarenal manifestations, and progression of renal disease can vary significantly, even within families.
- ARPKD
  1. Children presenting early tend to have more severe renal involvement and less severe hepatic involvement at presentation than children presenting at an older age.
  2. Approximately 30% to 50% die from pulmonary hypoplasia in the newborn period.
  3. Twenty-three percent develop bleeding esophageal varices.
  4. Approximately 50% of children require antihypertensive treatment by age 5 years.
  5. For those surviving the neonatal period, 25% reach end-stage renal failure by age 5 years.

■ WEBSITES
- GeneTests Laboratory Directory: www.genetests.org; lists laboratories performing genetic testing; search the laboratory directory for ADPKD or ARPKD
- Online Mendelian Inheritance in Man (OMIN): www.ncbi.nlm.nih.gov/Omim/; contains summaries and links related to inherited disorders; search for ADPKD or ARPKD

■ SUPPORT GROUPS
- The Polycystic Kidney Research Foundation: www.pkdcure.org
- NEPHKIDS is an email discussion group for parents of children with kidney disease. To subscribe, email the message "subscribe nephkids" to majordomo@ualberta.ca
- KidTalk is an email list for children with renal disease: http://home.nycap.rr.com/jazzer/kidtalk.html
- Local chapters of the National Kidney Foundation

REFERENCES
1. Bennett WM, Elzinga LW: Clinical management of autosomal dominant polycystic kidney disease, *Kidney Int* 44:S74, 1993.
2. Perrone RD: Extrarenal manifestations of ADPKD, *Kidney Int* 51:2022, 1997.
3. Sushmita R et al: Autosomal recessive polycystic kidney disease: long-term outcome of neonatal survivors, *Pediatr Nephrol* 11:302, 1997.
4. Zeres K, Rudnik-Schönenborn S, Mücher G: Autosomal recessive polycystic kidney disease: clinical features and genetics, *Adv Nephrol* 25:147, 1996.

Author: **William S. Varade, M.D.**

BASIC INFORMATION

■ DEFINITION
Polycystic ovary syndrome (PCOS) is a disorder of the hypothalamic-pituitary-ovarian axis that leads to temporary or persistent anovulation and hyperandrogenism, which encompasses a spectrum of clinical variability. Polycystic ovaries are a sign, not a diagnosis, and are associated with several endocrinopathies.

■ SYNONYMS
- PCOS
- Polycystic ovary syndrome
- Stein-Leventhal syndrome
- Sclerocystic ovarian disease
- Polycystic ovarian disease (PCOD)

ICD-9CM CODE
256.4 Polycystic ovaries

■ ETIOLOGY
- The exact cause is unknown.
- Possible causes include the following:
  1. Abnormal hypothalamic-pituitary function
     a. Increased frequency or amplitude of secretory pulse of luteinizing hormone (LH)
     b. Increased inhibition of follicle-stimulating hormone (FSH) secretion by estrogens
     c. Insensitivity of FSH to gonadotropin-releasing hormone (GnRH) stimulation
  2. Abnormal ovarian function
     a. Suboptimal androgen aromatization by aromatase enzyme, which is influenced by FSH
     b. Subsequent androgen excess, which leads to self-enhancement
     c. More theca cells, more androgen production
     d. Reduced number of granulosa cells secondary to androgen-induced follicular atresia
  3. Abnormal adrenal androgen metabolism
     a. Adrenarche important to premenarchal onset of PCOS
     b. Elevation of androgen-forming enzyme at level of the adrenals and ovary
     c. Adrenal androgen gets peripherally converted into estrogen
     d. Peripheral estrogen induces inappropriate gonadotropin secretion
  4. Insulin resistance
     a. Increase in insulin and insulin resistance at puberty
     b. Insulin may affect glycosylation of LH and alter bioactivity
     c. Subsequent stimulatory effect of LH on ovarian secretion of androstenedione

■ EPIDEMIOLOGY & DEMOGRAPHICS
- PCOS affects 5% to 10% of reproductive women.
- Approximately 50% of women who have PCOS are obese.
- Signs of PCOS begin in adolescence.
  1. Maturing pattern of LH secretion
  2. Increased adrenal androgen production
  3. Increase in body mass
  4. Onset of adult pattern of insulin resistance

■ HISTORY
- Ask about the following:
  1. Amenorrhea or oligomenorrhea 2 years or more postmenarche
  2. Signs of virilization
     a. Acne
     b. Hirsutism
     c. Male-pattern baldness
     d. Deepening voice
     e. Clitoromegaly
     f. Increased muscle mass
     g. Darkening of the skin
- Obtain family history:
  1. Menstrual abnormalities
  2. Infertility
  3. Hirsutism
  4. Diabetes mellitus

■ PHYSICAL EXAMINATION
- General appearance: obesity
- Skin
  1. Acne
  2. Alopecia
  3. Evidence of hirsutism: standardized Ferriman and Gallwey scoring system (i.e., upper lip, chin, chest, upper back, lower back, upper abdomen, lower abdomen, arm, forearm, thigh, and leg)
     a. Each body area is graded 0 to 4.
     b. Score of 8 or higher indicates hirsutism.
  4. Acanthosis nigricans of neck, groin, or axilla
  5. Abdominal striae
- Deepening of voice
- Thyromegaly
- Chest
  1. Upper body muscle mass
  2. Galactorrhea
- Abdominal or pelvic masses
- Clitoromegaly
- Pelvic examination: cystic ovaries

DIAGNOSIS

- Criteria for PCOS diagnosis:
  1. Chronic anovulation with early onset of menstrual irregularities
  2. Evidence of androgen excess
- Supportive but not necessary criteria:
  1. Obesity
  2. Inappropriate gonadotropin secretion
  3. Cystic ovaries
  4. Normal level of prolactin

■ DIFFERENTIAL DIAGNOSIS
- Cushing's syndrome
- Hypothyroidism
- Androgen-producing ovarian and adrenal tumors: characteristic rapid-onset virilization
- Congenital adrenal hyperplasia (CAH): late-onset 21-hydroxylase deficiency
- Stromal hyperthecosis: similar to PCOS but high testosterone levels
- Hyperprolactinemia
- Familial hirsutism

■ DIAGNOSTIC WORKUP
- At initial screening:
  1. LH, FSH
  2. Thyroid-stimulating hormone (TSH), T_3, T_4
  3. Total and free testosterone
  4. DHEAS
  5. Prolactin
  6. Fasting total cholesterol and high-density lipoprotein (HDL) cholesterol
- If patient is obese and/or has acanthosis nigricans:
  1. Fasting glucose and insulin level
- Pelvic ultrasound

Expected results are as follows:
- LH:FSH ratio is greater than 3.
  1. LH higher than 21 mIU/ml
  2. FSH low to normal
- DHEAS is elevated.
- Insulin levels may be elevated.
- HDL cholesterol may be low.
- Pelvic ultrasound may show enlarged ovary with multiple small cysts and a thickened capsule.

Interpretation of abnormal results is as follows:
- Very elevated free testosterone and DHEAS: Suspect ovarian or adrenal tumor.
  1. Pelvic ultrasonography
  2. Abdominal computed tomography or magnetic resonance imaging
- Elevated TSH: Suspect hypothyroidism.
- Elevated prolactin: Suspect prolactinoma.

Further workup includes the following:
- Suspect Cushing's syndrome.
  1. Fasting cortisol
  2. 24-hour urinary cortisol levels
- Suspect late-onset CAH.
  1. Obtain morning sample of DHEAS and 17-OHP.
  2. If 17-OHP is 200 to 1000 ng/dl, perform adrenocorticotropic hormone stimulation test.

⟨Rx⟩ THERAPY

■ NONPHARMACOLOGIC
- Weight loss
- Smoking cessation
- Cosmetic enhancement of hirsute features
  1. Waxing
  2. Shaving
  3. Electrolysis
  4. Bleaching

■ MEDICAL
- Hormonal therapy should be considered.
  1. Combination oral contraceptive pills (OCPs) containing progestins like norethindrone, norgestimate, or desogestrel
     a. Demulen 1/35
     b. Ortho-Cyclen
     c. Ortho Tri-Cyclen
  2. Provera 10 mg daily for 10 to 12 days every 1 to 2 months to promote withdrawal bleeding
  3. Depomedroxyprogesterone acetate (Depo-Provera) 150 mg intramuscularly
- Antiandrogen agents include the following:
  1. OCPs are given for pregnancy prevention; avoid feminization of male fetus.
  2. Spironolactone dosing is 100 to 200 mg orally every day.
  3. Finasteride dose is 5 mg orally every day.
- Dermatologic agents for acne include the following:
  1. Benzoyl peroxide (topical gel or cream)
  2. Topical or oral antibiotics, depending on severity of acne
     a. Erythromycin 500 mg orally two times per day
     b. Tetracycline 500 mg orally two times per day
  3. Retin-A 0.025% apply to affected areas at bedtime
  4. Accutane 0.5 mg/kg orally two times per day

- Controversial medical therapies used in PCOS include the following:
  1. GnRH agonists: may decrease bone density
  2. Insulin-resistant adolescents
     a. Metformin 500 mg orally two times per day
     b. Roglitazone 200 mg orally two times per day
  3. Antihyperlipidemic medication for adolescents with high lipid profiles
  4. More research needed

■ FOLLOW-UP & DISPOSITION
- No specific follow-up guidelines are available for PCOS.
- For adolescents who require OCPs, see the adolescent in 1 month, again at 3 months, and then every 6 months.
- Provide particular attention and follow-up to cosmetic implications because they affect self-esteem.
- Provide supportive counseling.

■ PATIENT/FAMILY EDUCATION
- Explain the diagnosis and cause.
- Explain the risk for pregnancy despite the chronic anovulation.

■ PREVENTIVE TREATMENT
- Smoking cessation
  1. Decreased risk of thromboembolic disease, which is increased for women taking OCPs who smoke
  2. Decrease hirsutism secondary to androgens (smoking elevates androstenedione levels)
  3. Decreased risk of cardiovascular disease, which may be independently increased by obesity, hyperinsulinism, hyperandrogenism, and of course, tobacco
- Provera for prevention of endometrial hyperplasia

■ REFERRAL INFORMATION
- Endocrine consultation for associated endocrinopathies
- Dermatology consultation for more severe acne
- Psychological consultation, if indicated

- Reproductive gynecology consultation for infertility issues

✷ PEARLS & CONSIDERATIONS

■ CLINICAL PEARLS
- Although ovulation is uncommon, these patients can still become pregnant.
- Unopposed estrogen of PCOS increases the risk for the following:
  1. Endometrial cancer
  2. Breast cancer
- Elevated lipoprotein profile may lead to future risk of cardiovascular disease.
- Obesity and insulin resistance may result in development of type 2 diabetes.

■ WEBSITES
- InteliHealth: www.intelihealth.com/IH/
- National Women's Health Resource Center: www.healthywomen.org/
- Support-Group.com: www.support-group.com; several chat rooms for PCOS

REFERENCES
1. Gordon CM: Menstrual disorders in adolescents, *Pediatr Clin North Am* 46: 519, 1999.
2. Neinstein L: Menstrual problems in adolescents, *Med Clin North Am* 74: 1181, 1990.
3. Neinstein L: Polycystic ovary syndrome and ovarian cysts and tumors. In Neinstein LS (ed): *Adolescent health care: a practical guide,* Baltimore, 1996, Williams & Wilkins.
4. O'Connell B: The pediatrician and the sexually active adolescent, *Pediatr Clin North Am* 44:1391, 1997.
5. Wild RA: Hyperandrogenism in the adolescent, *Obstet Gynecol Clin North Am* 19:71, 1992.

Author: **Cheryl M. Kodjo, M.D.**

BASIC INFORMATION

■ DEFINITION
Posterior urethral valves (PUV) are congenital membranes or tissue folds within the posterior urethra that obstruct urine outflow.

■ SYNONYM
Congenital obstructing posterior urethral membrane (COPUM)

ICD-9CM CODE
753.6 Posterior urethral valves

■ ETIOLOGY
- Persistent remnants of the cloacal membrane that normally regress upon interaction with the mesonephric duct
- The classic description of PUV
  1. Type I, 95%, fibroepithelial leaflets that extend distally from the verumontanum toward the external urinary sphincter
  2. Type II, 5%, musculoepithelial folds commonly seen in prunebelly syndrome (PBS) (The obstructing nature of this lesion is a point of some controversy.)
  3. Type III, rare, diaphragm with pinpoint lumen anatomically not in relation to verumontanum
- Current concern about the accuracy of these descriptive categories
  1. A higher incidence of type III valves is noted if endoscopy is performed before catheter passage.
  2. There is the implication that type III valves are converted to type I iatrogenically.
     a. Likely, catheter passage causes some alterations in valve appearance.
     b. The original description, however, specifies that type III valves lack continuity with the verumontanum.

■ EPIDEMIOLOGY & DEMOGRAPHICS
- Incidence is 1 in 8000 to 1 in 25,000 males.
- Up to one third of children with PUV have renal insufficiency or failure.

■ HISTORY
- Prenatal
  1. Ultrasound showing hydronephrosis
  2. Oligohydramnios
  3. Ascites (urine)
- Newborn
  1. Urine leakage
  2. Delayed voiding
- Any age
  1. Straining to void
  2. Weak or intermittent urinary stream

  3. History of urinary tract infections (UTIs)
  4. History of gross or microscopic hematuria
- Older child
  1. Dysuria
  2. Incontinence
  3. Enuresis
  4. Failure to thrive
- Renal failure

■ PHYSICAL EXAMINATION
- Hypertension
- Bladder distention, suprapubic mass
- Leakage of urine with increased abdominal pressure
- Abdominal fluid wave or dullness
- Palpably enlarged kidneys
- Undescended testes
- Patent urachus

🔬 **DIAGNOSIS**

■ DIFFERENTIAL DIAGNOSIS
- Prenatal
  1. PBS
  2. Ectopic ureterocele
  3. Neurogenic bladder
  4. Nonneurogenic neurogenic bladder
  5. Megaureter (reflux, obstruction)
- Postnatal based on specific signs or symptoms
  1. Dysuria, enuresis, incontinence: UTIs, neurogenic bladder, reflex, dysfunctional voiding, constipation
  2. Hematuria: glomerular diseases, trauma, cystitis
  3. Abdominal mass: Wilms' tumor, duplication, hydronephrosis of other causes, lymphoma, neuroblastoma, congenital mesoblastic nephroma

■ DIAGNOSTIC WORKUP
- Ultrasound of kidneys and bladder
  1. Hydronephrosis is often the first sign of abnormality.
     a. Seventy percent of infants with PUV have hydronephrosis.
  2. Approximately 50% of patients also have other findings, including the following:
     a. Megacystis (huge bladder)
     b. Oligohydramnios
     c. Dilated posterior urethra ("keyhole" sign)
  3. Renal dysplasia may be suggested by increased renal parenchymal echogenicity, loss of corticomedullary distinction, and the presence of renal cortical cysts and calcifications.
- Voiding cystourethrogram (VCUG)
  1. A fluoroscopic VCUG is done for definitive diagnosis of PUV.
  2. In PUV, type I, the posterior

urethra is elongated, dilated, and "sausage" shaped.
  3. In contrast, PBS shows a triangular defect.
  4. A persistent indentation at the bladder neck (internal sphincter) may be present in either condition.
  5. Concurrent vesicoureteral reflux occurs in at least 50% of patients.

💊 **THERAPY**

■ NONPHARMACOLOGIC
- Acute management: prenatal
  1. In utero treatment of valves with either ablation or vesicoamniotic shunting may be considered in the face of oligohydramnios to aid in pulmonary development.
  2. Despite anecdotal successes, universal application of these measures to maximize ultimate renal function awaits a reliable measure of fetal renal potential.
- Acute management: postnatal
  1. Many newborns with PUV present with a prenatal diagnosis, pulmonary immaturity, renal insufficiency, or urinary ascites.
  2. The initial management depends on bladder drainage via a urethral catheter.
     a. Placement in the bladder must be verified.
     b. Positioning of the catheter within the urethra, a common occurrence, will not provide adequate decompression of the urinary tract.
  3. Creatinine measurement, after the first few days of life, reflects the baby's renal status.
     a. A rising value necessitates reassessment of catheter position and degree of hydronephrosis.
     b. Surgical drainage may be warranted.

■ MEDICAL
- Antibiotics
  1. Initially sterile catheters are unlikely to remain sterile after 48 hours.
  2. Prophylactic antibiotics (amoxicillin, penicillin, Keflex) may not maintain sterility of the urine but may limit colony count and prevent early symptomatic UTI.
  3. Periodic instillation of intravesical gentamicin (every other day to achieve minimum inhibitory concentration for *Escherichia coli*) may prevent pyelonephritis when continuous catheterization is prolonged.
  4. Antibiotics are not routinely used in children with vesicostomies or

in those who are receiving intermittent catheterization.

- Anticholinergics/antimuscarinics
  1. Some bladders maintain such high pressures that they adversely affect either renal function or continence.
  2. Anticholinergic medications such as oxybutynin, tolterodine, and imipramine may be useful adjuncts in overall care.

■ SURGICAL

- Valve ablation
  1. Once the patient is stable medically, valve ablation (incision, resection, vaporization, disruption) is the primary treatment choice.
  2. Endoscopic techniques allow treatment to be performed safely in the 8- to 9.5-Fr urethra (approximately 3 mm in diameter).
  3. Smaller urethrae can be manipulated with excellent success in trained hands.
- Vesicostomy
  1. This procedure is a safe approach to the infant with a small urethra, prior vesicoamniotic shunt, urinary ascites, or need for other neonatal surgery.
  2. Neonates, with increasing creatinine levels, progressive hydronephrosis, and poor voiding dynamics, may benefit from vesicostomy even after successful primary valve ablation.
     a. There is a potential benefit of bladder cycling (i.e., repeated filling and emptying) to maximize bladder function in PUV.
     b. These pathophysiologic benefits are still anecdotal.
     c. Bladders after vesicostomy still cycle to some degree.

■ FOLLOW-UP & DISPOSITION

- Renal function
  1. Children with creatinine levels of greater than 1.0 mg/dl at 12 months of age are likely to develop renal failure.
  2. One in ten children demonstrate VURD (valves, unilateral ureteral reflux, renal dysplasia), in which one kidney appears to be sacrificed for the preservation of the contralateral renal unit. The sanctity of the opposite kidney, in cases of PUV, is unfortunately not absolute. Therefore all children require monitoring of their renal status well into adulthood.
- Bladder function
  1. Normal bladder function in PUV is rare.
  2. Overall, 50% to 80% of boys have their continence delayed significantly.
  3. Almost all achieve continence by their teenage years.
  4. Detrusor hyperreflexia, poor bladder compliance with small capacity, and myogenic failure all occur with PUV.
     a. These conditions may represent sequential stages in the development of bladder dysfunction.
     b. Although manageable, bladder dysfunction is a source of considerable long-term disability in PUV.

■ PATIENT/FAMILY EDUCATION

- The primary goals are to preserve and maximize renal function.
- PUV is treated with valve ablation, but long-term effects from this congenital lesion, particularly on renal and bladder function, are likely. Follow-up is essential.

■ REFERRAL INFORMATION

The pediatric urologist and nephrologist are critical members of the team in caring for children with PUVs.

☼ PEARLS & CONSIDERATIONS

■ CLINICAL PEARLS

- Urinary diversion above the bladder is rarely indicated but may be lifesaving or kidney saving in select cases.
- Transplantation in children with PUV has equal patient and graft survival rates (100%, 81%) when compared to transplant survival rates for other causes of end-stage renal disease in children.
- Increasing hydronephrosis may be seen despite good surgical results in cases of nephrogenic diabetes insipidus.

■ WEBSITES

- Society for Fetal Urology: www.fetalurology.org
- Society of Pediatric Urology: www.spu.org

REFERENCES

1. Chevalier RL, Klahr S: Therapeutic approaches in obstructive uropathy, *Semin Nephrol* 18:652, 1998.
2. Close CE et al: Lower urinary tract changes after early valve ablation in neonates and infants: is early diversion warranted? *J Urol* 157:984, 1997.
3. Holmdahl G et al: Four-hour voiding observation in young boys with posterior urethral valves, *J Urol* 160:1477, 1998.
4. Indudhara R et al: Renal transplantation in children with posterior urethral valves revisited: a 10-year follow-up, *J Urol* 160:1201, 1998.
5. Nguyen HT, Peters CA: The long-term complications of posterior urethral valves, *Br J Urol Int* 83:23, 1999.

Authors: **R.A. Mevorach, M.D., William C. Hulbert, M.D., and Ronald Rabinowitz, M.D.**

BASIC INFORMATION

DEFINITION

Posttraumatic stress disorder (PTSD) is a specific psychiatric diagnosis based on abnormal or unusual feelings or behaviors that occur subsequent to a traumatic stressor and that interfere with daily functioning.

ICD-9CM CODE

309.81 Posttraumatic stress disorder

ETIOLOGY

- The main risk factor for the development of PTSD is the severity and length of exposure to the stressor. Typical stressors include the following:
  1. Sexual and/or physical abuse
  2. Natural disasters
  3. Violence in school and/or community
  4. Witnessing domestic violence
  5. Chronic life-threatening diseases, especially those with painful treatment procedures
- The recovery environment, especially the level at which the parents are able to function emotionally and in day-to-day living in order to provide for their child's needs, is especially important to the following:
  1. Child's response to the stressor, and
  2. Potential development of PTSD
- The presence of preexisting psychiatric conditions increases the risk of developing PTSD.
  1. The onset of PTSD often precedes or coincides with development of other disorders (e.g., depression, substance abuse).
  2. According to one study, 80% of adolescents with PTSD met the criteria for at least one other psychiatric disorder, and 40% had two or more other disorders, especially depression.
- Presentation of symptoms may be triggered by a medical examination (e.g., gynecologic visit for an adolescent who was or is being sexually abused).

EPIDEMIOLOGY & DEMOGRAPHICS

- In the United States, more than 3 million children and adolescents experience some form of trauma annually (e.g., sexual abuse, physical abuse, exposure to domestic and/or community violence).
- Depending on the severity and number of traumatic events, 27% to 100% of children and adolescents develop PTSD with exposure.
- Children exposed to sudden, unexpected, manmade violence are at greatest risk.
  1. As many as 45% to 60% develop PTSD according to some reports.

- Girls are at higher risk than boys. Reportedly, girls are six times more likely to develop PTSD.
  1. Boys tend to report fewer symptoms than needed to meet the criteria for PTSD.

HISTORY

- Infants and toddlers may show the following:
  1. Regressive symptoms
     a. Thumb-sucking
     b. Enuresis
     c. Loss of newly acquired developmental skills
  2. Irritability
  3. Sleeping and/or eating disturbances
- Preschool children reenact the traumatic event through play.
  1. New fears may develop:
     a. Fear of the dark
     b. Separation anxiety
- Elementary school children typically experience the following:
  1. Nightmares
  2. Preoccupation with the traumatic event
  3. Hyperarousal symptoms
     a. Difficulty concentrating
     b. Irritability
     c. Angry outbursts
  4. Somatic complaints
     a. Headaches
     b. Stomachaches
  5. Restriction in range of expressed emotions
  6. Avoidance of situations, places, or people that remind the child of the traumatic event
- Adolescents may present as compliant and withdrawn or, conversely, act out aggressively.
  1. They may seek premature independence.
     a. Move out from home
     b. Act out sexually
  2. They may become more dependent.
  3. They are at risk for delinquency, substance abuse, and self-endangering reenactment behavior.
- Chronic PTSD may present with several symptoms that mask PTSD:
  1. Dissociation
  2. Self-injurious behaviors
  3. Substance abuse
  4. Conduct problems

DIAGNOSIS

DIFFERENTIAL DIAGNOSIS & COMORBID CONDITIONS

- Adjustment disorder: Stressor is not extreme in nature.
- Acute stress disorder: Posttrauma symptoms appear and resolve within 4 weeks.

- Simple phobia: Avoidance behavior is not limited to trauma-related stimuli.
- Obsessive-compulsive disorder: Intrusive thoughts are unrelated to a traumatic event.
- Mood disorder: Symptoms present before exposure to the extreme stressor.
- Psychotic disorders: Flashbacks associated with PTSD should be distinguished from illusions, hallucinations, and other perceptual disturbances unrelated to the trauma.
- Attention deficit/hyperactivity disorder (AD/HD): Hypervigilance, which may appear as distractibility, and hyperarousal present before exposure to trauma.
- Other anxiety disorders: Symptoms present before exposure to an extreme stressor.
- Many of these conditions can develop in addition to PTSD, necessitating dual or multiple diagnoses and comprehensive treatment plans.

DIAGNOSTIC WORKUP

- At least one of the following reexperiencing symptoms:
  1. Recurrent and intrusive distressing memories of the event, including images, thoughts, perceptions, or repetitive play in which traumatic theme(s) occur(s)
  2. Recurrent distressing dreams about the trauma or frightening dreams without recognizable content (for younger children)
  3. Acting or feeling as if the trauma were recurring, including flashbacks (more common for adolescents), illusions, hallucinations, or trauma-specific reenactment
  4. Intense distress at exposure to cues that symbolize or resemble an aspect of the trauma
  5. Physiologic reactivity at exposure to internal or external cues that symbolize or resemble an aspect of the traumatic event
- At least three of the following avoidance/numbing symptoms, which are the most common symptoms for children (not present before the trauma):
  1. Efforts to avoid thoughts, feelings, or conversations associated with the trauma
  2. Efforts to avoid reminders of the trauma
  3. Amnesia for an important aspect of the trauma
  4. Diminished interest or participation in normal activities
  5. Feelings of detachment or estrangement from others
  6. Restricted range of affect (blunted emotions)
  7. A foreshortened sense of future (e.g., life will be too short to live to adulthood)

- At least two of the following indications of increased arousal (new since the trauma):
  1. Sleep difficulties
  2. Irritability or angry outbursts
  3. Difficulty concentrating
  4. Hypervigilance
  5. Exaggerated startle response
- The symptoms from these three categories must be present for at least 1 month and cause clinically significant distress or impairment in functioning.
- Specification of onset and duration of the symptoms of PTSD include the following:
  1. Acute: duration of symptoms is less than 3 months
  2. Chronic: duration of symptoms is 3 months or longer
  3. Delayed onset: at least 6 months have passed between the traumatic event and the onset of symptoms

TREATMENT

■ NONPHARMACOLOGIC
- Outpatient cognitive-behavioral psychotherapy is generally considered the preferred initial treatment.
- Essential components to treatment include the following:
  1. Use of specific stress management techniques
     a. Deep breathing
     b. Thought-stopping and positive imagery
  2. Direct exploration of the trauma after mastering stress management techniques
  3. Exploration and correction of inaccurate attributions regarding the trauma (e.g., inappropriate guilt)
  4. Inclusion of nonabusing parent(s) or appropriate caretakers in treatment

  5. Addressing grief when loss was experienced

■ MEDICAL
- There is a lack of empirical data supporting pharmacologic intervention.
- Psychoactive medications should be considered as adjunctive treatment for children and adolescents with symptoms of the following:
  1. Depression
  2. AD/HD
  3. Panic disorder
  4. Unsuccessful outpatient psychotherapy: may also be an indication for medication

■ FOLLOW-UP & DISPOSITION
Close collaboration with mental health professionals and follow-up visits to monitor symptom severity and treatment progress should be maintained.

■ PREVENTIVE TREATMENT
Children's Safety Network, National Injury and Violence Prevention Resource Center: www.edc.org/HHD/csn/

☼ PEARLS & CONSIDERATIONS

■ CLINICAL PEARLS
- The interviewer should follow these guidelines:
  1. Be direct while providing a supportive environment.
  2. Use developmentally appropriate language with the child.
  3. Ask specific questions about PTSD symptoms.
- Although some children and adolescents may not meet the full criteria for PTSD, cognitive-behavorial therapy should be provided.

- Address the family's need for intervention when indicated.

■ WEBSITES
- American Academy of Child and Adolescent Psychiatry: www.aacap.org
- Traumatic Incident Reduction: www.healing-arts.org/tir/links.htm
- Trauma information site with hundreds of links: www.trauma-pages.com

■ SUPPORT GROUP
National Council on Anxiety Disorders, Rte. 1, Box 1364, Clarkesville, GA 30523; 706-947-3854

REFERENCES
1. American Psychiatric Association: *Diagnostic and statistical manual of mental disorders,* ed 4, Washington, DC, 1994, American Psychiatric Association.
2. Cohen JA: AACAP official action: summary of the practice parameters for the assessment and treatment of children and adolescents with posttraumatic stress disorder, *J Am Acad Child Adolesc Psychiatry* 37:997, 1998.
3. Cooley-Quille MR, Turner SM, Beidel DC: Emotional impact of children's exposure to community violence: a preliminary study, *J Am Acad Child Adolesc Psychiatry* 34:1362, 1995.
4. Pfefferbaum B: Postraumatic stress disorder in children: a review of the past 10 years, *J Am Acad Child Adolesc Psychiatry* 36:1503, 1997.
5. Schwartz E, Perry BD: The posttraumatic response in children and adolescents, *Psych Clin North Am* 17:311, 1994.
6. Wintgens A, Boileau B, Robaey P: PTSD and medical procedures in children, *Can J Psychiatry* 42:611, 1997.
Author: **Tina McCann, Ph.D.**

BASIC INFORMATION

■ DEFINITIONS
- Lower age limits for onset of normal pubertal development have traditionally been defined as follows:
  1. Girls: 7.5 to 8.5 years of age for breast development and 9.5 years for menarche
  2. Boys: 9.0 years of age
- These ages were based on small, nonrepresentative samples. Age of onset of girls has recently been reexplored in a large-scale office based study (Pediatric Research in the Office Setting [PROS]–American Academy of Pediatrics). Evaluation for precocious puberty (as advised by statement from Lawson Wilkins Pediatric Endocrine Society) based on the review of the PROS data is now recommended for the following:
  1. White girls with breast or pubic hair before age 7 years, *or*
  2. African-American girls with breasts or pubic hair before age 6 years, *or*
  3. Girls with early puberty and rapid pubertal progression (including rapidly advancing bone age), central nervous system (CNS) abnormalities, or behavioral issues associated with the early puberty

Puberty is the period during and process by which sexual maturation occurs, leading to reproductive capacity. Gonadarche and adrenarche (see following discussion) lead to the acquisition of commonly noted secondary sexual characteristics (e.g., thelarche and pubarche). *Thelarche* is the beginning of breast development, associated with estrogen effects. *Adrenarche* is the beginning of the maturational increase in adrenal androgen secretion that accompanies (and slightly precedes) puberty. *Pubarche* is the beginning of pubic hair growth, indicating androgen effects. *Gonadarche* is the beginning of gonadal hormonal activity, associated with marked increases in androgens in boys and estrogens in girls.

ICD-9CM CODE
259.1 Precocious puberty/adrenarche/thelarche

■ ETIOLOGY
Varies as function of age and gender
- True precocious puberty of central (hypothalamic/pituitary) origin
  1. Girls
     a. About 95% idiopathic, presumably premature activation of the usual mechanism
     b. Other causes: central nervous system damage from trauma, irradiation, or infection; hypothalamic hamartoma; rarely pineal tumor; hypothalamic mass; optic glioma (often associated with neurofibromatosis [NF]-1)
  2. Boys
     a. Less likely than girls to be idiopathic
     b. Hypothalamic hamartoma most common abnormal finding
     c. Other CNS causes: germinomas, astrocytomas, optic nerve gliomas, septo-optic dysplasia, NF-1
- Precocious puberty associated with independent (autonomous) gonadal function
  1. Girls
     a. Simple ovarian cyst: transient estrogen secretion
     b. McCune-Albright syndrome (multiple ovarian cysts) caused by G-protein mutation, which results in café-au-lait spots, polyostotic fibrous dysplasia, and autonomous ovarian estrogen secretion
  2. Boys
     a. Familial male precocious puberty: G-protein mutation causes luteinizing hormone (LH) receptor abnormality resulting in increased testosterone but only minimal testicular enlargement
- Premature pubarche: androgen effects only (pubic and axillary hair, adult body odor, acne, skin oiliness) without estrogen effects or other signs of true puberty
  1. Girls
     a. Premature adrenarche
        (1) Mechanism controlling adrenarche is still not clear.
        (2) It is more common in overweight, African-American, and Latino girls.
        (3) Girls who are more severely affected (e.g., have higher androgen levels) often have hyperinsulinism as a result of insulin resistance, which is believed to stimulate adrenal androgen production.
     b. Nonclassic congenital adrenal hyperplasia (CAH) mild enough not to have congenital genital abnormalities
     c. Masculinizing tumors
  2. Boys: androgen effects without testicular enlargement (as found in true puberty)
     a. CAH results in adrenal production of androgens with subsequent signs of virilization, including growth acceleration, bone age advancement, and pubic hair growth
- Premature thelarche
  1. Appears to be caused by subtle overfunctioning of the pituitary-ovarian axis, with mild increases in follicle-stimulating hormone (FSH)

■ EPIDEMIOLOGY & DEMOGRAPHICS
- Premature puberty is found in approximately 3% of girls (by definition) using the recommendations from the PROS study.
- Premature pubarche is more common in girls with increased insulin resistance, including those who are obese, have a family history of type II diabetes, and are minorities.
- Premature thelarche occurs in 21 per 100,000 patient years.
  1. Sixty percent occur between 6 and 18 months.

■ HISTORY
- True central precocious puberty in girls and boys—history compatible with normal, albeit early, puberty
  1. Estrogen effects (girls): unilateral or bilateral breast development, vaginal leukorrhea, growth acceleration, and ultimately menstruation
  2. Low-level androgen effects (girls and early puberty in boys): increased body odor, axillary hair, pubic hair, skin oiliness, and mild acne
  3. Higher-level androgen effects (boys with mid or late puberty): change in voice, growth acceleration, and facial hair
- Careful review of systems for complaints referable to CNS masses
- Premature pubarche from premature adrenarche
  1. Increased body odor, pubic hair, and axillary hair
  2. No report of estrogen effects such as breast development, vaginal secretions, or menarche
- Premature thelarche
  1. Unilateral or bilateral breast development without evidence of other signs of puberty
     a. Usually regresses over time
  2. Typical in first 2 years of life

■ PHYSICAL EXAMINATION
- True puberty—girls
  1. Increased growth velocity is seen early in puberty.
  2. Other changes include pubic hair growth, axillary hair, change in color of vaginal mucosa from red to pink, vaginal leukorrhea, and menarche.
  3. Café-au-lait spots are seen in McCune-Albright syndrome (autonomous ovarian function).
- True puberty—boys
  1. Early changes include testicular enlargement (greater than 2.2 cm

in length), pubic hair, axillary hair, and skin oiliness.
2. Midpubertal and later changes include maximum growth acceleration, voice change, penile growth, increase in muscle bulk, and facial hair growth.

DIAGNOSIS

■ DIFFERENTIAL DIAGNOSIS
It is important to distinguish thelarche, pubarche, autonomous gonadal function, and true (central) puberty because causes, evaluation, and therapies differ.

■ DIAGNOSTIC WORKUP
- Bone age: appropriate to obtain in all disorders of early puberty and variations
  1. True puberty: advanced significantly beyond chronologic age
  2. Premature adrenarche and premature thelarche: not abnormally advanced, although girls with premature adrenarche associated with obesity often have moderately accelerated bone age
- Gonadotropins (LH and FSH)
  1. Random daytime levels are often within normal prepubertal range in early puberty.
  2. Levels are low in cases of autonomous gonadal function.
- Estrogen and testosterone
  1. These levels are measurably elevated in true puberty.
  2. Early-morning levels are typically higher than late-afternoon determinations and are thus a more sensitive indicator.
- 17-Hydroxyprogesterone (OHP) and androstenedione: often elevated in nonclassic CAH and should be measured in boys with isolated pubarche and in girls and boys with pubarche and advanced bone ages
- DHEA-s: often mildly elevated in typical premature pubarche because of premature adrenarche
- Gonadotropin-releasing hormone (GnRH) stimulation test: helpful in distinguishing central precocious puberty from autonomous gonadal function
  1. Rise in LH over FSH after GnRH administration indicates central (hypothalamic/pituitary) activation.
- Magnetic resonance imaging of head with hypothalamic/pituitary protocol: normal in most pubertal disorders, except those associated with structural abnormalities, such as hamartomas, germinomas, astrocytomas, optic nerve gliomas, or septo-optic dysplasia
  1. This test is not necessary in simple premature adrenarche or in most cases of mildly advanced pubertal development in girls.
- Ultrasound of ovaries and uterus: can be helpful in determining whether pubertal process is currently active, as indicated by enlarged uterus and endometrial stripe
  1. Useful in visualizing solitary ovarian cysts or multiple cysts (as in McCune-Albright syndrome)

THERAPY

■ NONPHARMACOLOGIC
Psychologic counseling should be considered for select children.

■ MEDICAL
- True central precocious puberty
  1. Administration of long-acting GnRH agonists (e.g., Lupron-Depo) results in suppression of pituitary gonadotropin secretion.
- Autonomous ovarian function
  1. Aromatase inhibitors such as ketoconazole and testolactone have been used but are not uniformly totally effective.
- CAH is treated with hydrocortisone replacement (see the section "Congenital Adrenal Hyperplasia").

■ SURGICAL
- Surgery is useful when a discrete tumor results in precocity, such as a gonadal tumor or some intracranial tumors.
  1. Hypothalamic hamartomas are generally not removed.

■ FOLLOW-UP & DISPOSITION
- The frequency of follow-up depends on the condition and specific circumstances, but in general, careful monitoring of pubertal status every 3 to 6 months is appropriate.
- Reevaluation of bone age is typically done once yearly unless rapid progression is noted.

■ PATIENT/FAMILY EDUCATION
- Many cases of premature development wax and wane over time; thus clinical status could unexpectedly change between routine visits.
- Parents should be instructed to notify physician whenever they note any significant change in pubertal development in child who is being monitored.

■ REFERRAL INFORMATION
- The decision to consult a pediatric endocrinologist is based on many considerations, including the experience of primary care physician, the age of the child, and the presence of other medical conditions.
- In general, very young children with evidence of true puberty, boys with precocious puberty, children with known or suspected CNS abnormalities, and children with significantly advanced bone ages should be referred.

PEARLS & CONSIDERATIONS

■ CLINICAL PEARLS
- A bone age is good to obtain in any situation in which there is doubt about whether significant premature development has occurred.
- Obese girls with a small amount of pubic hair, adult body odor, and borderline advanced bone ages rarely have significant treatable pathology. These girls are often initially thought to have true precocious puberty because, in addition to the aforementioned findings, increased subcutaneous adiposity is often confused with true breast tissue.
- Boys presenting with pubic hair at ages 3 to 8 years may have non–salt-losing CAH and should be evaluated with a bone age, serum 17-OHP, and androstenedione.

■ WEBSITES
- Craniofacial & Skeletal Disease Branch, Division of Intramural Research, NIDCR: http://csdb.nidcr.nih.gov/csdb/info_mas.htm; good link for information regarding McCune-Albright syndrome
- KeepKidsHealthy.com: www.keepkidshealthy.com/welcome/conditions/precocious_puberty.html
- TooSoon.com: www.toosoon.com; good information for parents, children, and physicians, although run by pharmaceutical company

REFERENCES
1. Herman-Giddens ME et al: Secondary sexual characteristics and menses in young girls seen in office practice: a study from the pediatric research in office setting network, *Pediatrics* 99: 505, 1997.
2. Ibanez L, De Zegher F, Potau N: Anovulation after precocious pubarche: early markers and time course in adolescence, *J Clin Endocrinol Metab* 84: 2691, 1999.
3. Kaplowitz PB, Oberfield SE, the Drug and Therapeutics and Executive Committees of the Lawson Wilkins Pediatric Endocrine Society: Reexamination of the age limit for defining when puberty is precocious in girls in the United States: implications for evaluation and treatment, *Pediatrics* 104:936, 1999.

4. Lee PA: Central precocious puberty: an overview of diagnosis, treatment, and outcome, *Endocrinol Metab Clin North Am* 28:901, 1999.

5. Miller WL: Pathophysiology, genetics, and treatments on hyperandrogenism, *Pediatr Clin North Am* 44:375, 1997.

6. Root AW: Precocious puberty, *Pediatr Rev* 21:10, 2000.

7. Rosenfield RL: The ovary and sexual maturation. In Sperling MA (ed): *Pediatric endocrinology*, Philadelphia, 1996, WB Saunders.

8. Styne DM: New aspects in the diagnosis and treatment of pubertal disorders, *Pediatr Clin North Am* 44:505, 1997.

Author: **Craig Orlowski, M.D.**

BASIC INFORMATION

■ DEFINITION
Premenstrual syndrome (PMS) is a constellation of physical and psychologic symptoms that start during the luteal phase of the menstrual cycle or 1 to 2 weeks before the onset of menses. The symptoms usually abate at the onset of menses.

■ SYNONYMS
- PMS
- Premenstrual tension
- Premenstrual dysphoria

ICD-9CM CODE
625.4 Premenstrual tension syndromes

■ ETIOLOGY
- The cause is unknown.
- There are several theories:
  1. Change in endocrine homeostasis: progesterone deficiency, hyperprolactinemia, estrogen excess, imbalance of estrogen:progesterone ratio
  2. Vitamin B_{12} deficiency
  3. Change in glucose metabolism: hypoglycemia
  4. Change in neurotransmitters: endorphins, serotonin

■ EPIDEMIOLOGY & DEMOGRAPHICS
- The prevalence of PMS in adult women ranges from 20% to 40%, with 5% to 10% of women demonstrating severe symptoms.
- The prevalence among adolescents is unknown.
  1. A longitudinal study conducted by Raja (1992) documents a prevalence of 14%.
  2. A study by Fisher (1989) found that 89% of their subjects reported at least one symptom of moderate severity, 59% reported symptoms of severe degree, and 43% reported symptoms of extreme degree.

■ HISTORY
- Adolescents experience the same symptoms as adult women.
- More than 150 symptoms are described in the literature.
- When obtaining a patient's history, one should include questions about the following physical and psychologic symptoms:

Physical	Psychologic
Headaches	Irritability
Edema: breasts, abdomen, legs	Depression
	Anxiety
Increased appetite	Mood swings
Food cravings	Anger
Increased acne	
Constipation	
Dizziness	
Fatigue	
Muscle aches and pains	
Palpitations	

■ PHYSICAL EXAMINATION
No specific physical findings

🔬 DIAGNOSIS

■ DIFFERENTIAL DIAGNOSIS
- Diagnosis of exclusion: No other physical or psychologic factors are involved.
- This is purely a clinical diagnosis remarkable for history of cyclical onset.
- Symptoms occur over several menstrual cycles.
- Assessment tools include the following:
  1. PMS symptom calendar
  2. Self-Assessment Disk
  3. Premenstrual Assessment Form (PAF)
  4. Prospective Record of the Impact and Severity of Menstrual Symptoms (PRISM)

■ DIAGNOSTIC WORKUP
No specific laboratory findings

💊 THERAPY

■ NONPHARMACOLOGIC
- Most adolescents do not have symptoms severe enough to warrant medication.
- Dietary changes: Avoid salty foods, alcohol, caffeine, chocolate, and concentrated sweets.
  1. Increase calcium intake.
- Exercise regularly.
- Maintain a routine sleep schedule.
- Stress management techniques include the following:
  1. Biofeedback
  2. Self-hypnosis
  3. Relaxation

■ MEDICAL
- Consider the severity of symptoms.
- No consistent benefits with any of the pharmacologic therapies have been proven (anecdotal).
  1. Hormonal therapy to inhibit ovulation
     a. Combination oral contraceptives
     b. Depomedroxyprogesterone acetate (Depo-Provera) 150 mg intramuscularly
  2. Nonsteroidal antiinflammatory drugs, especially if the patient also has dysmenorrhea
     a. Naproxen 500 mg orally twice per day on days 17 to 28 of menstrual cycle
     b. Naproxen sodium 550 mg orally twice per day on days 17 to 28 of menstrual cycle
     c. Mefenamic acid 250 mg orally three times per day on days 24 to 28 for bloating, 500 mg orally three times per day on days 19 to 28 for pain
  3. Vitamin B_6 50 to 100 mg orally every day throughout cycle
     a. Rare side effect: sensory neuropathy in doses as low as 50 to 200 mg every day over several months
  4. Consider: benzodiazepine, serotonin reuptake inhibitor, β-blocker, or calcium channel blocker if the adolescent continues with psychologic symptoms not relieved by other modalities
     a. Alprazolam 0.25 mg orally two to three times per day for approximately 1 week before menses
     b. Prozac 20 to 60 mg orally every day

■ COMPLEMENTARY & ALTERNATIVE THERAPIES
Evening primrose oil (gamma-linolenic acid) 1.5 g orally two times per day on day 15 to onset of menses

■ CONTROVERSIAL MEDICAL THERAPIES
- No clinical trials have been done in adolescents.
- Drugs that have been used in adults are as follows:
  1. Diuretics (i.e., hydrochlorothiazide and spironolactone) have been used for management of bloating or weight gain; they may cause dizziness and nausea.
  2. Gonadotropin-releasing hormone agonists (i.e., bromocriptine) have been used for management of breast symptoms and may decrease bone density.

II

3. Tamoxifen, used for breast pain, may cause hot flashes, nausea and/or vomiting, and liver function abnormalities.
4. Danazol decreases cyclic hormonal responses; it may cause liver dysfunction, weight gain, acne, and menstrual disturbances.
- Side effects may outweigh the benefits.

■ FOLLOW-UP & DISPOSITION
- No specific follow-up guidelines are available for PMS.
- For adolescents who require oral contraceptives, see the adolescent at 1 month, again at 3 months, and every 6 months.
- The adolescent should maintain a premenstrual changes calendar.
- Significant mood changes warrant psychologic or psychiatric consultation.

■ PATIENT/FAMILY EDUCATION
- Explain the menstrual cycle, possible causes of PMS, and the cyclic nature of PMS.
- Give reassurance.

⚙ PEARLS & CONSIDERATIONS

■ CLINICAL PEARLS
- Older adolescents tend to have more intense symptoms than younger adolescents.
- Dysmenorrhea and PMS symptoms are strongly correlated in adolescents.

■ WEBSITES
- Excite: excite.netscape.com/health
- InteliHealth: www.intelihealth.com/IH

REFERENCES

1. Coupey SM, Ahlstrom P: Common menstrual disorders, *Pediatr Clin North Am* 36:551, 1989.
2. Fisher M, Trieller K, Napolitano B: Premenstrual symptoms in adolescents, *J Adolesc Health Care* 10:369, 1989.
3. Freeman EW, Rickels K, Sondheimer SJ: Premenstrual symptoms and dysmenorrhea in relation to emotional distress factors in adolescents, *J Psychosomatic Obstet Gynecol* 14:41, 1993.
4. Kaplan DW, Mammel KA: Adolescence. In Hay W et al (eds): *Current pediatric diagnosis and treatment*, New York, 2001, Appleton & Lange.
5. Neinstein L: Menstrual problems in adolescents, *Med Clin North Am* 74: 1181, 1990.
6. Neinstein L: Dysmenorrhea and premenstrual syndrome. In Neinstein LS (ed): *Adolescent health care: a practical guide*, ed 6, Philadelphia, 1996, Lippincott Williams & Wilkins.
7. O'Connell B: The pediatrician and the sexually active adolescent, *Pediatr Clin North Am* 44:1391, 1997.
8. Raja SN et al: Prevalence and correlates of the premenstrual syndrome in adolescence, *J Am Acad Child Adolesc Psychiatry* 31:783, 1992.

Author: **Cheryl M. Kodjo, M.D.**

BASIC INFORMATION

■ DEFINITION

Prolonged QT syndrome (LQTS) is a familial but clinically and genetically heterogeneous ion channel cardiac disorder leading to syncope, "seizures," and sudden death as a consequence of ventricular tachyarrhythmias.

■ SYNONYMS

- Romano-Ward (R-W) syndrome (heterozygotic mutations)
- Jervell-Lange-Nielsen (J-L-N) syndrome (homozygotic mutations)
- Long QT syndrome

ICD-9CM CODE

794.31 Abnormal electrocardiogram

■ ETIOLOGY

- LQT_1: gene mutation on chromosome 11 ($KvLQT_1$)
- LQT_2: gene mutation on chromosome 7 (HERG)
  1. Gene mutations in LQT_1 and LQT_2 reduce the outward, repolarizing potassium channel function, causing prolongation of the action potential and, consequently, the QT interval.
- LQT_3: gene mutation on chromosome 3 (SCNSA)
  1. LQT_3 is caused by persistent or repetitive patency of the inward sodium channel during the plateau phase of the action potential, thereby prolonging the QT interval.

■ EPIDEMIOLOGY

- Incidence is 1 in 10,000 individuals.
- No gender preference exists.
- Inheritance pattern is familial in 80%: autosomal dominant in R-W syndrome and autosomal recessive in J-L-N syndrome.
- New mutations occur in 20% of cases.
- Mortality is 5% to 20% per year after onset of symptoms in untreated patients.
- A nearly 10% risk of sudden death as the initial symptom has been reported.

■ HISTORY

- Syncope, commonly during physical or emotional stress
- "Seizures" with abrupt onset and paucity of postevent confusion
- Cardiac arrest also related to exercise or emotion
- Sudden death in the same circumstances
- Congenital deafness in most but not all J-L-N patients
- Family history

■ PHYSICAL EXAMINATION

- Often normal
- Bradycardia
- Deafness in J-L-N patients

DIAGNOSIS

■ DIAGNOSTIC WORKUP

- QTc: QT corrected for heart rate
  1. Bazett's formula:

$$QTc = \frac{QT \ (sec)}{\sqrt{Preceding \ R\text{-}R \ interval \ (sec)}}$$

  a. A corrected QT interval more than 460 msec is abnormal.
  b. Borderline QTc is 440 to 460 msec.
- Family history
  1. Variable penetrance; QTc may be normal
  2. Electrocardiogram (ECG) on first-degree relatives; consider other family members as well
- Genetic screening for gene mutations
- Appearance of T waves may identify type: LQT_1, LQT_2, or LQT_3
- T-wave alternans: appearance of T-wave alternates in a bigeminal pattern
- Polymorphic ventricular tachycardia (PVT): torsades de pointes
- In general, the longer the QTc, the greater the risk of PVT

■ DIFFERENTIAL DIAGNOSIS

- Drug-induced QT prolongation (intravenous erythromycin, cisapride, imipramine, pentamidine)
- Mild QTc prolongation related to myocardial ischemia or injury
- Acute central nervous system events
- Cardiomyopathies
- Hypokalemia
- Hypocalcemia
- Hypomagnesemia

THERAPY

■ NONPHARMACOLOGIC

Avoidance of competitive sports

■ MEDICAL

- β-Blockers (propranolol, nadolol, atenolol)
- Future use of mexiletine for LQT_3
  1. Antiarrhythmic agent
  2. Class IB: sodium channel blocker
- Avoidance of drugs capable of prolonging the QTc and sympathomimetics
- Avoidance of, and rapid correction of, electrolyte abnormalities

■ SURGICAL

- Pacing for native or β-blocker–induced bradycardia
- Left stellate ganglionectomy if medications or pacing insufficient
- Implantable cardioverter-defibrillator if previous therapies insufficient
- Cardiac transplantation (rarely done)

■ FOLLOW-UP & DISPOSITION

All LQTS patients require lifelong cardiac follow-up and therapy.

■ PATIENT/FAMILY EDUCATION

- Compliance with therapeutic regimens is essential.
- With appropriate therapy, mortality should be 3% or less *per year.*
- Advancements in gene-directed therapy (e.g., potassium channel openers in LQT_1 or LQT_2) should further reduce the risk of symptoms including sudden death.
- Obtain a list of contraindicated medications from the cardiologist.

■ REFERRAL INFORMATION

All patients with documented or suspected LQTS should be referred to a pediatric cardiologist with expertise in arrhythmias.

PEARLS & CONSIDERATIONS

■ CLINICAL PEARLS

- All patients with syncope, atypical "seizures," unexplained life-threatening events, or a family history of premature sudden death should have screening ECGs.
- At present, sufficient evidence to incriminate QTc prolongation as an etiology of the sudden infant death syndrome is not available.

■ WEBSITE & SUPPORT GROUP

Sudden Arrhythmia Death Syndromes Foundation (SADS): www.sads.org

REFERENCES

1. Ackerman MJ: The long QT syndrome, *Pediatr Rev* 79:232, 1998.
2. Moss AJ et al: ECG T-wave patterns in genetically distinct forms of the hereditary long QT syndrome, *Circulation* 95:2929, 1995.
3. Schwartz PJ: The long QT syndrome. In Camm A (ed): *Clinical approach to tachyarrhythmia series,* Armonk, NY, 1997, Futura.
4. Zareba W et al: Influence of the genotype on the clinical course of the long-QT syndrome, *N Engl J Med* 339: 960, 1998.

Author: **J. Peter Harris, M.D.**

II

BASIC INFORMATION

■ DEFINITION

Pseudotumor cerebri is a diagnosis of exclusion characterized by increased intracranial pressure in the absence of other intracranial pathology, such as infection, mass lesions, hydrocephalus, or hypertensive crisis.

■ SYNONYMS

- Idiopathic intracranial hypertension
- Serous meningitis
- Otic hydrocephalus
- Benign intracranial hypertension

ICD-9CM CODE
348.2 Pseudotumor cerebri

■ ETIOLOGY

The cause is unclear; however, several mechanisms have been proposed:
- Decreased cerebrospinal fluid (CSF) absorption into the sagittal sinus
  1. Blockage at the arachnoid villi
  2. Increased venous pressure
- Decreased absorption leading to increased pressure
  1. Increased intraparenchymal volume
- Decreased CSF production, a less likely mechanism

■ EPIDEMIOLOGY & DEMOGRAPHICS

- More common in females (female:male ratio of 2:1 to 4:1)
- Obesity the most common overall factor
- Vitamins A and D overuse
- Anemia
- Cardiac disease with increased venous pressure
- Chronic pulmonary disease with increased venous pressure

■ HISTORY

- Headache that is aggravated by cough, strain, or Valsalva and worse in morning
- Blurred vision
- Unilateral or bilateral visual loss, which may be transient or fixed
  1. Blindness
  2. Enlargement of blind spot
- Diplopia
- None

■ PHYSICAL EXAMINATION

- Papilledema
- Retinal hemorrhages
- Normal neurologic examination
- Well-appearing individual

DIAGNOSIS

■ DIFFERENTIAL DIAGNOSIS

- Must rule out other causes of increased intracranial pressure
- Infection
  1. Meningitis (bacterial, viral, or fungal)
  2. Encephalitis
- Intracranial tumor, especially frontal or temporal lobes
- Obstructive hydrocephalus
- Pickwickian syndrome (obesity-induced obstructive pulmonary disease)
- High-altitude cerebral edema
- Hypertensive encephalopathy
- Chronic subdural hematomas

■ DIAGNOSTIC WORKUP

- Computed tomography (CT) or magnetic resonance imaging (MRI) of the head
- Magnetic resonance venography to rule out venous occlusion
- Lumbar puncture
  1. Perform after the ventricular system is evaluated by CT or MRI.
  2. Opening pressure in pseudotumor cerebri ranges from 250 to 600 mm Hg.
  3. Protein is in the low-normal range 10 to 20 mg/dl.
  4. Glucose is normal.
  5. Cell count and cytology are normal.

THERAPY

■ NONPHARMACOLOGIC

- Treatment of obesity: weight loss, decreased caloric intake, increased exercise
- Frequent ophthalmologic evaluations

■ MEDICAL

- Treatment is continued until physical signs and symptoms are resolved.
  1. As patients improve, trials off medication may be attempted.
- Many of the following medications are long term:
  1. Carbonic anhydrase inhibitor
     a. Acetazolamide, decreases CSF production
        (1) 5 mg/kg dose one to four times per day either orally or intravenously
  2. Loop diuretics
     a. Furosemide, decreases CSF production in animal models
        (1) 0.5 to 2 mg/kg/dose intravenously, intramuscularly, or orally one to four times per day

3. Hypertonic solutions
   a. Mannitol 25% intravenously, acutely decreases intracranial parenchymal volume
      (1) 0.25 g/kg/dose intravenously over 20 to 30 minutes
      (2) Maximum total, 1 g/kg/day
   b. Glycerol orally, decreases intracranial parenchymal volume
      (1) High caloric load
4. Systemic steroids
   a. Dexamethasone, reduces intracranial edema and thereby reduces volume
      (1) Last-resort treatment because it causes adrenal suppression
      (2) 1 to 2 mg/kg/dose orally, intravenously, or intramuscularly every day to every 6 hours in intensive care unit setting

■ SURGICAL

- Lumbar puncture (LP)
  1. Removal of 15 to 30 ml of fluid to normalize pressure
     a. Effects may last for several days to weeks to months.
     b. Repeat LP may need to be done.
- Lumbar peritoneal shunt
  1. May prove helpful in cases of intractable headache and visual loss
- Optic nerve decompression/optic nerve sheath fenestration
  1. Creation of a window in the optic nerve sheath to allow an outlet for CSF and to protect the optic nerve from compression

■ FOLLOW-UP & DISPOSITION

- Vision needs to be monitored carefully, including visual fields examination.
- This condition is often self-limited and may undergo spontaneous remission in weeks or months.
- Recurrent episodes are noted in 5% to 10% of patients.

■ PATIENT/FAMILY EDUCATION

- Patients should have frequent examinations by an ophthalmologist to evaluate the optic nerves.
- Patients should have follow-up with a neurologist to evaluate symptoms and/or changes in neurologic examination.

PEARLS & CONSIDERATIONS

■ WEBSITES

- National Institute of Neurological Disorders and Stroke: www.ninds.nih.gov/patients/disorder/pseudo/pseudo.htm

- National Organization of Rare Diseases (NORD), Pseudotumor Cerebri: www.rarediseases.org
- Pseudotumor Cerebri Support Network: www.pseudotumorcerebri.com

■ SUPPORT GROUPS

- Pseudotumor Cerebri Support Network, 6632 Kennington Square South, Pickerington, OH 43147; 614-759-7760.
- Pseudotumor Cerebri Society, 1319 Butternut Street #3, Syracuse, NY 13208; 315-464-3937.

- National Organization for Rare Disorders (NORD), P.O. Box 8923, New Fairfield, CT 06812-1783; 203-746-6518, 800-999-6673.

REFERENCES

1. Baker R et al: Idiopathic intracranial hypertension (pseudotumor cerebri) in pediatric patients, *Pediatr Neurol* 5:5, 1989.
2. Duncan FJ, Corbett JJ, Wall M: The incidence of pseudotumor cerebri, *Arch Neurol* 45:875, 1988.
3. Eggenberger ER: Lumboperitoneal shunt for the treatment of pseudotumor cerebri, *Neurology* 46:1524, 1996.
4. Fishman RA: Pseudotumor cerebri. In Fishman RA (ed): *Cerebrospinal fluid in diseases of the nervous system*, ed 2, Philadelphia, 1992, WB Saunders.
5. Fishman RA: *Merritt's textbook of neurology*, ed 9, Baltimore, 1995, Williams & Wilkins.
6. Wall M: Idiopathic intracranial hypertension, *Neurol Clin* 9:73, 1991.

Authors: **Stanley Johnsen, M.D., and Reed Shimamoto, M.D.**

II

BASIC INFORMATION

■ DEFINITION
Psittacosis is a systemic infection with *Chlamydia psittaci,* named for the organism's earliest identified natural hosts—psittacine birds (parrots, parakeets).

■ SYNONYMS
- Ornithosis
- Parrot fever
- Pneumotyphus
- Chlamydiosis
- Bird breeder's disease
- Bird fancier's lung

ICD-9CM CODE
073.9 Psittacosis

■ ETIOLOGY
Systemic infection caused by *C. psittaci*

■ EPIDEMIOLOGY & DEMOGRAPHICS
- Transmission occurs from infected birds to humans via the respiratory route by direct contact or inhalation of infectious organisms in aerosolized dust or secretions.
- Most commonly infected birds include parrots, parakeets, finches, turkeys, gulls, pigeons, ducks, and chickens.
- Most infected birds display minimal symptoms, but some may be more severely affected, displaying ruffled feathers, closed eyes, shivering, anorexia, emaciation, dyspnea, serous or mucopurulent ocular or nasal discharge, and diarrhea.

■ HISTORY
- Greatest at-risk individuals include pet bird owners, pigeon handlers, pet shop employees, poultry farmers, veterinarians, and poultry abattoir (slaughterhouse) workers.
- There are several manifestations of infection:
  1. Subclinical infection or mild, nonspecific symptoms resembling a viral illness
  2. Mononucleosis-like syndrome of fever, chills, malaise, pharyngitis, photophobia, and myalgia
  3. Typhoidal form, including fever and malaise
  4. Atypical pneumonia may present with nonproductive cough, dyspnea, fever, and headache
  5. Seizure, headache, lower extremity weakness

■ PHYSICAL EXAMINATION
- Fever, pharyngeal erythema, adenopathy, rales/crackles on chest auscultation, and hepatomegaly in more than 50% of patients

- Splenomegaly and bradycardia with typhoidal form
- Less commonly:
  1. Tachycardia (pericarditis, myocarditis, culture-negative endocarditis) or new murmur
  2. Right upper quadrant tenderness and jaundice (hepatitis)
  3. Cranial nerve palsy, ataxia, neck stiffness (meningitis)
  4. Diminished or absent reflexes, decreased strength, and sensory level (transverse myelitis)
  5. Joint pain and swelling (reactive arthritis)
  6. Horder's spots (pink, maculopapular rash resembling rose spots of typhoid fever)

🔬 DIAGNOSIS

■ DIFFERENTIAL DIAGNOSIS
- Viral lower respiratory tract infection
- Atypical pneumonia with *Mycoplasma pneumoniae, Chlamydia pneumoniae,* or *Legionella pneumophila*
- Infectious mononucleosis
- Typhoid fever
- Q fever
- Brucellosis
- Tularemia
- Mycobacterial or fungal pneumonia

■ DIAGNOSTIC WORKUP
- Chest radiograph is abnormal in 75% of patients, with findings striking in comparison to degree of illness; consolidation is seen in single lower lobe in 90% of abnormal chest radiographs. However, diffuse miliary or ground-glass appearance and hilar adenopathy are also reported.
- Isolation of organism can be done only in a research laboratory setting and is not indicated because of the danger to laboratory personnel; therefore diagnosis is usually confirmed by demonstration of antibodies in patient serum by complement fixation (CF) or by microimmunofluorescence (MIF).
- Chlamydial CF antibody is not species–specific; therefore high CF titers also may result from infection with *C. pneumoniae* and *Chlamydia trachomatis;* polymerase chain reaction assay may distinguish between species but is not commercially available.
- Confirmed case:
  1. Clinical illness compatible with psittacosis, plus
  2. Laboratory confirmed by one of the following methods:
     a. *C. psittaci* is cultured from respiratory secretions.
     b. Antibody against *C. psittaci* is increased fourfold or greater to a reciprocal titer of 32 be-

tween paired (i.e., acute- and convalescent-phase) serum samples obtained at least 2 weeks apart, as demonstrated by CF or MIF.
     c. Immunoglobulin M antibody against *C. psittaci* is detected by MIF to a reciprocal titer of 16.
- Probable case:
  1. Clinical illness compatible with psittacosis, or
  2. Clinical illness epidemiologically linked to a confirmed case of psittacosis, or
  3. Single antibody titer of 1:32 (demonstrated by CF or MIF) found in at least one serum sample obtained after onset of symptoms

💊 THERAPY

■ MEDICAL
- Drug of choice is tetracycline hydrochloride 500 mg orally four times per day
- Alternative therapeutic agents (particularly for children younger than 8 years of age) include the following:
  1. Erythromycin 2 g/day; azithromycin and clarithromycin also are effective
- Because of the high probability of relapse after shorter courses of therapy, the usual recommended duration of therapy is 10 to 21 days, or until the patient is afebrile for 10 to 14 days.

■ FOLLOW-UP & DISPOSITION
- Symptoms should begin to abate within 48 to 72 hours of initiation of appropriate therapy.
- Infection does not confer long-term immunity, so reinfection is a possibility.

■ PATIENT/FAMILY EDUCATION
Pet birds should be purchased only from a reputable dealer complying with U.S. Department of Agriculture 30-day quarantine and chlortetracycline treatment regulations.

■ PREVENTIVE TREATMENT
Treatment of infected and sick birds with tetracycline, chlortetracycline, or doxycycline for at least 45 consecutive days

■ REFERRAL INFORMATION
- Patients suspected of having psittacosis should be referred to an infectious disease specialist to consider other possible similar illnesses included in the differential diagnosis of psittacosis.
- Consultation with a veterinarian or the state health department may also be helpful.

☼ PEARLS & CONSIDERATIONS

■ CLINICAL PEARLS
- Splenomegaly in a patient with acute pneumonitis should raise the diagnostic consideration of psittacosis.
- Person-to-person transmission of psittacosis is uncommon, but secondary cases can be severe.

■ WEBSITES
- American Veterinary Medicine Association Compendium of Psittacosis (Chlamydiosis) Control, 1999: www.avma.org/pubhlth/psittacosis.htm
- Centers for Disease Control and Prevention updated case definition: www.cdc.gov/epo/mmwr/other/case_def/psitta97.html

REFERENCES

1. US Department of Agriculture, Animal and Plant Health Inspection Service: Importation of certain animals, birds, and poultry, and certain animal, bird, and poultry products; requirements for means of conveyance and shipping containers. In *Code of federal regulations,* Washington, DC, 1997, USDA Animal and Plant Health Inspection Service.
2. US Department of Health and Human Services, Centers for Disease Control and Prevention: Case definitions for infectious conditions under public health surveillance, *MMWR CDC Surveill Summ* 46:27, 1997.
3. US Department of Health and Human Services, Centers for Disease Control and Prevention: Summary of notifiable diseases, United States, 1997, *MMWR CDC Surveill Summ* 46:3, 1998.

Author: **Chris Nelson, M.D.**

II

BASIC INFORMATION

■ DEFINITION
Psoriasis vulgaris is a chronic skin disorder with a waxing and waning course. Abnormally rapid turnover of the epidermis results in the accumulation of thick scale over sites of frequent trauma and irritation.

ICD-9CM CODE
696.1 Psoriasis vulgaris

■ ETIOLOGY
- The exact pathogenesis and relative importance of genetic and environmental factors are still unknown.
- Family studies, epidemiologic studies, and human leukocyte antigen (HLA) studies suggest that psoriasis is genetically determined.
  1. The prevalence of psoriasis is higher among first- and second-degree relatives of patients with psoriasis than in the general population.
  2. There is an increased frequency of some HLA haplotypes (HLACw6, B13, B17) in patients with psoriasis.
  3. Twin studies show higher concordance rates among monozygotic than dizygotic twin pairs.
     a. Concordance rates amongst monozygotic twins is at most 70%, suggesting a role for environmental factors.
- A variety of local and systemic stimuli have been reported to trigger the onset of psoriasis.
  1. Medications such as nonsteroidal antiinflammatory drugs, antimalarials, and systemic corticosteroids
  2. Pregnancy and use of progesterone-containing oral contraceptive pills
  3. Streptococcal infections (especially with guttate psoriasis)

■ EPIDEMIOLOGY & DEMOGRAPHICS
- Approximately 0.5% to 1.5% of the U.S. population is affected.
- The female:male ratio in children is 2:1; in adults, the ratio is 1:1.
- Psoriasis vulgaris is more common in Caucasians, and less common in African Americans, Japanese, and North/South American Indians.
- Most cases occur during the fall and winter months.

■ HISTORY
- Guttate psoriasis occurs most often in children and young adults.
  1. The term is derived from the Latin for *gutta* (a drop), which describes the type of lesions seen.
- Guttate psoriasis appears abruptly, often 1 to 2 weeks after a streptococcal infection.
- Plaques of psoriasis may be pruritic or painful.
- Both streptococcal pharyngitis and perianal infections have been described.
- Guttate psoriasis usually persists for 3 to 4 months and then resolves spontaneously.

■ PHYSICAL EXAMINATION
- Guttate psoriasis
  1. Guttate lesions are round and oval erythematous plaques with silvery scale, measuring from 2 to 10 mm in diameter.
  2. Guttate lesions are symmetrically distributed over the trunk and proximal extremities.
- Plaque psoriasis
  1. Plaque psoriasis in children is similar to that seen in adults.
  2. Lesions are sharply demarcated, round, erythematous plaques with silvery scale.
  3. Plaque size is highly variable, but individual lesions are bigger than those seen in guttate psoriasis.
  4. Lesions are often symmetrically distributed.
  5. Common sites of involvement include the scalp, eyebrows, elbows, knees, umbilicus, genitalia, and gluteal cleft.
  6. May be induced in areas of local injury, such as scratches or insect bites (Koebner phenomenon).
  7. Nail findings include pitting, oil spots (yellowish brown discolorations), onycholysis (separation of nail-plate from nailbed), subungual distal hyperkeratosis (debris), and nail dystrophy (crumbling).

DIAGNOSIS

■ DIFFERENTIAL DIAGNOSIS
- Plaque psoriasis
  1. Seborrheic dermatitis
  2. Atopic dermatitis
  3. Lichen planus
  4. Pityriasis rubra pilaris
- Guttate psoriasis
  1. Pityriasis rosea
  2. Secondary syphilis

■ DIAGNOSTIC WORKUP
- The diagnosis is usually made on the basis of the characteristic clinical picture.
- Biopsy is rarely needed and avoided in children.
- Specific histologic findings can be used if the diagnosis is in question.

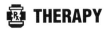

THERAPY

■ NONPHARMACOLOGIC
- Mild soap one to two times per day (e.g., Dove, Purpose, Neutrogena, Basis)
- Thick emollients two to three times per day (e.g., petroleum jelly, Aquaphor ointment, Theraplex emollient, Eucerin cream)

■ MEDICAL
- Topical corticosteroids should be applied twice a day to individual plaques for several weeks.
- Oral corticosteroids are contraindicated.
- Patients with severe or extensive disease should be referred to a dermatologist.
- Acute guttate forms, associated with streptococcal infection, should be treated with appropriate antibiotics, which sometimes resolves the lesions.

PEARLS & CONSIDERATIONS

■ CLINICAL PEARLS
- Most patients with guttate psoriasis experience a recurrence of some type of psoriasis within the next 3 to 5 years.
- More than one third of patients with psoriasis experience their first episode by age 20.
- Psoriatic arthritis is rare in children.

■ WEBSITES
- American Academy of Dermatology: www.aad.org
- National Psoriasis Foundation: www.psoriasis.org (Patient oriented)
- Society for Pediatric Dermatology: www.spdnet.org

REFERENCES
1. Chapel KL, Rasmussen JE: Pediatric dermatology: advances in therapy, *J Am Acad Dermatol* 36:513, 1997.
2. Farber EM: Juvenile psoriasis: early interventions can reduce risks for problems later, *Postgrad Med* 103:89, 1998.
3. Howard R, Tsuchiya A: Adult skin disease in the pediatric patient, *Dermatol Clin* 16:593, 1998.
Author: **Susan Haller Psaila, M.D.**

BASIC INFORMATION

■ DEFINITION

Pulmonary embolism (PE) is the result of acute blockage of a pulmonary artery by a thrombus formed at another anatomical site, usually a deep vein of the leg.

■ SYNONYMS

• PE
• Pulmonary thromboembolism

■ ICD-9CM CODE

415.11 Pulmonary embolism

■ ETIOLOGY

• A thrombus is formed at a distant site (see the section "Deep Venous Thrombosis").
• Pieces of the thrombus detach and travel through the right heart to the pulmonary vasculature.
• The resulting pulmonary arterial obstruction and the release of vasoactive agents by platelets elevates pulmonary vascular resistance.

■ EPIDEMIOLOGY & DEMOGRAPHICS

• The incidence is 1 per 1000 per year, more common in men.
• More than 250,000 patients are hospitalized annually in the United States with venous thromboembolism.
• The 3-month mortality rate ranges from 10% to 15%.
• As many as 40% of patients who have deep venous thrombosis (DVT) but no symptoms of PE have small PEs on lung scanning.

■ HISTORY

• Typical symptoms include the acute onset of pleuritic chest pain, shortness of breath, cough, and hemoptysis.
• Other symptoms include fever, diaphoresis, wheezing, and syncope.
• Ask about the following risk factors:
  1. Surgery within the past 12 weeks
  2. Recent immobilization for 3 or more days
  3. Previous DVT or PE
  4. Fracture and immobilization within the past 12 weeks
  5. Strong family history of DVT or PE
  6. Cancer, postpartum, and lower extremity paralysis

■ PHYSICAL EXAMINATION

• Classically tachycardia, tachypnea, and hypoxia
• Other signs may be loud pulmonary component of S_2, murmur of tricuspid insufficiency, right ventricular heave, or evidence of DVT (see the section "Deep Venous Thrombosis")

DIAGNOSIS

■ DIFFERENTIAL DIAGNOSIS

• Musculoskeletal chest pain (costochondritis)
• Pleurisy
• Cardiac chest pain
• Esophageal spasm
• Pneumothorax

■ DIAGNOSTIC WORKUP

• Available tests include chest computed tomography (CT), ventilation/perfusion lung scanning, Doppler ultrasonography or venography of the legs, and the gold standard of pulmonary angiography.
• Decide whether the patient has a low, moderate, or high pretest probability of PE based on history, physical examination, and results of arterial blood gas (ABG) and electrocardiogram (ECG) as well as more likely alternative diagnoses.
• If the patient has a low pretest probability of PE, a normal chest CT scan or D-dimer blood assay effectively rules out PE.
• If the patient has a high pretest probability of PE, a high-probability lung scan confirms PE.
• If the patient has a moderate pretest probability or the results of your initial test are equivocal or not confirmatory, a series of tests, including compression ultrasonography and venography of the leg, lung scanning, and chest CT, are indicated, reserving invasive pulmonary angiography for the most difficult cases.
• Chest radiograph is usually normal or shows a small pleural effusion on the affected side. Classically, it has a wedge-shaped infiltrate consistent with pulmonary infarction.
• ABG reveals respiratory alkalosis with hypoxia.
• ECG most commonly reveals sinus tachycardia, right ventricular strain, right bundle branch block, or the "$S_IQ_{III}T_{III}$" pattern of large S wave in lead I, and large Q and T waves in lead III.

THERAPY

■ MEDICAL

• First, provide supportive measures, including oxygen, pain control, and hemodynamic stabilization.
• The mainstay of therapy is anticoagulation with heparin. Low-molecular-weight heparin (LMWH) can be given subcutaneously (1 mg/kg twice a day) and does not need activated partial thromboplastin time monitoring. Outcomes with LMWH are equivalent to those with

intravenous unfractionated heparin in PE.
• Oral anticoagulation with warfarin is begun the first day to prevent delays in hospitalization. A target International Normalized Ratio (INR) of 2 to 3 is desired.
• Thrombolytic therapy should be reserved for patients with acute, massive PE because bleeding risk is estimated at close to 50%, intracranial hemorrhage is estimated at 1%, and mortality rates are equal to placebo in randomized controlled trials.

■ SURGICAL

• Inferior vena caval (Greenfield) filters should be reserved for patients with contraindications to anticoagulation or for patients with recurrent PE on anticoagulation.
  1. They do prevent PE in patients with DVT.
  2. They carry an increased risk for recurrent DVT after placement.

■ FOLLOW-UP & DISPOSITION

• Anticoagulation should be continued for 3 to 12 months.
• Lifelong anticoagulation is recommended for patients with recurrent PE or for those at high risk of recurrence (i.e., patients with active cancer).

■ PATIENT/FAMILY EDUCATION

• Patients should understand that PE is a potentially fatal disease.
• Treatment with anticoagulants reduces the fatality rate to minimal levels.
• Treatment with oral warfarin necessitates intense education about the risks of bleeding (5% per year) and dietary restrictions.

■ PREVENTIVE TREATMENT

Early ambulation after surgical procedures, subcutaneous heparin (both LMWH and unfractionated), and pneumatic compression stockings are the mainstays of DVT and PE prophylaxis in high-risk patients.

■ REFERRAL INFORMATION

If a hypercoagulable state is found, referral to a hematologist is indicated to map out initial management and follow-up.

PEARLS & CONSIDERATIONS

■ CLINICAL PEARLS

In the presence of a patent foramen ovale or atrial septal defect, paradoxic embolism may occur with signs of systemic arterial embolization, including stroke and threatened limb.

II

REFERENCES

1. Dalen J et al: Thrombolytic therapy for pulmonary embolism, *Arch Intern Med* 157:2550, 1997.
2. Decousus H et al: A clinical trial of vena caval filters in the prevention of pulmonary embolism in patients with proximal deep-vein thrombosis, *N Engl J Med* 12:409, 1998.
3. Ginsberg J et al: Sensitivity and specificity of a rapid whole-blood assay for d-dimer in the diagnosis of pulmonary embolism, *Ann Intern Med* 129:1006, 1998.
4. Goldhaber S: Pulmonary embolism, *N Engl J Med* 8:93, 1998.
5. Hyers T et al: Antithrombotic therapy for venous thromboembolic disease, *Chest* 114:561S, 1998.
6. Moser KM et al: Frequent asymptomatic pulmonary embolism in patients with deep venous thrombosis, *JAMA* 271:223, 1994.
7. Remi-Jardin M et al: Diagnosis of pulmonary embolism with spinal CT: comparison with pulmonary angiography and scintigraphy, *Radiology* 200:699, 1996.
8. Shulman S et al: A comparison of six weeks with six months of oral anticoagulant therapy after a first episode of venous thromboembolism, *N Engl J Med* 22:1661, 1995.
9. Simonneau G et al: A comparison of low-molecular-weight heparin with unfractionated heparin for acute pulmonary embolism, *N Engl J Med* 4:663, 1997.
10. Teigen CL et al: Pulmonary embolism: diagnosis with contrast-enhanced electron-beam CT and comparison with pulmonary angiography, *Radiology* 194:313, 1995.
11. Wells P et al: Use of a clinical model for safe management of patients with suspected pulmonary embolism, *Ann Intern Med* 129:997, 1998.

Author: **Brett Robbins, M.D.**

BASIC INFORMATION

■ **DEFINITION**

Pulmonary hypertension is the abnormal elevation of pulmonary arterial pressure or pulmonary vascular resistance. Some authors specify a mean pulmonary arterial pressure greater than 25 mm Hg to define abnormal. Both primary and secondary pulmonary hypertension occur in children and adolescents.

ICD-9CM CODES

416.0 Primary forms
416.8 Secondary forms

■ **ETIOLOGY**

- Primary forms include the following:
  1. Primary or idiopathic pulmonary hypertension
  2. Familial pulmonary hypertension
- Secondary forms include the following:
  1. Increased pulmonary blood flow from congenital heart lesions
     a. Ventricular septal defect
     b. Atrioventricular septal defect
     c. Patent ductus arteriosus
     d. Isolated atrial septal defect; can result in pulmonary hypertension, but usually only after many decades
  2. Irreversible pulmonary hypertension (with cyanosis); occurs after years of increased pulmonary blood flow; also called *Eisenmenger syndrome*
  3. Pulmonary venous obstruction
     a. Obstructed anomalous pulmonary venous return
     b. Pulmonary venoocclusive disease
     c. Cor triatriatum (obstructive left atrial membrane)
  4. Left-sided heart failure
     a. Dilated cardiomyopathy
     b. Mitral valve stenosis or severe incompetence
  5. Chronic pulmonary emboli
     a. Collagen vascular diseases, including scleroderma, systemic lupus erythematosus, and systemic juvenile rheumatoid arthritis
     b. Protein S deficiency and other thrombophilias
     c. Ventriculoatrial shunts for hydrocephalus
  6. Other conditions
     a. Human immunodeficiency virus infection
     b. Anorexic drug use
     c. Cocaine abuse
     d. High-altitude exposure
  7. Chronic parenchymal lung disease
  8. Chronic airway obstruction
  9. Musculoskeletal disorders with hypoventilation
  10. Pulmonary hypertension resulting from lung disease, airway obstruction, or hypoventilation often termed *cor pulmonale*
      a. This indicates right ventricular hypertrophy or signs of right-sided heart failure secondary to lung or airway disease.
      b. Etiologies of cor pulmonale are discussed in the section "Cor Pulmonale."

■ **EPIDEMIOLOGY & DEMOGRAPHICS**

- Primary (idiopathic) pulmonary hypertension, isolated or familial, is rare in children.
- Incidence in all ages is 2 per 1,000,000 in Western countries.
  1. A female preponderance exists.
  2. Approximately 5% to 6% are familial with dominant incomplete penetrance pattern.
     a. One gene for familial primary pulmonary hypertension has been found on chromosome 2q 31-32.
- Reversible pulmonary hypertension secondary to a large left-to-right shunt is not uncommon in patients with congenital heart disease, but Eisenmenger syndrome has become rare since early surgical repair is standard practice.

■ **HISTORY**

- Fatigue and effort intolerance
- Dyspnea and shortness of breath
- Syncope and near sudden death episodes
- Look for family history of the following:
  1. Pulmonary hypertension
  2. Sickle cell disease
  3. Thrombotic disorders

■ **PHYSICAL EXAMINATION**

- Pulmonic component of second heart sound is loud (loud P_2 or loud S_2).
- Cyanosis is usually found only in secondary forms with intracardiac shunting (Eisenmenger syndrome) or severe pulmonary disease (e.g., cystic fibrosis).
- Lung examination is abnormal only in cases secondary to pulmonary parenchymal disease.

DIAGNOSIS

■ **DIFFERENTIAL DIAGNOSIS**

See "Etiology."

■ **DIAGNOSTIC WORKUP**

- Right ventricular hypertrophy on electrocardiogram may suggest pulmonary hypertension.
- Echocardiography may be diagnostic if significant pulmonary hypertension can be demonstrated and cardiac causes of pulmonary hypertension (e.g., left-to-right shunts, pulmonary venous obstruction, left ventricular failure) ruled out.
- Cardiac catheterization documents elevated pulmonary arterial pressure and excludes the secondary causes noted previously.
- If family history suggests inherited disorders causing pulmonary emboli or infarction, the following tests should be considered:
  1. Hemoglobin electrophoresis is done to look for sickle cell disease (SS).
  2. Obtain protein S, protein C, and antithrombin levels. The role of other thrombophilic disorders may be considered, including abnormal factor V (factor V Leiden, factor V Arg506->Gln mutation), and the G20210A mutation in the prothrombin gene.
  3. In some cases, radionuclide perfusion studies may be needed to diagnose or exclude multiple pulmonary emboli.
- Chest radiography and pulmonary function testing may exclude serious lung disease causing secondary pulmonary hypertension.
- Laboratory testing may confirm systemic disorders (e.g., collagen vascular disease) that history or clinical features suggest in cases of secondary pulmonary hypertension.

THERAPY

■ **MEDICAL**

- Pulmonary vasodilator therapy
  1. Home oxygen treatment
  2. Oral calcium channel blocker treatment (e.g., nifedipine)
  3. Continuous intravenous prostacyclin (PGI_2) infusion
  4. Inhaled nitric oxide
  5. Prostacyclin and nitric oxide used as "bridges" to lung transplantation
- Anticoagulation/chronic warfarin treatment if possible thrombotic or embolic component

■ **SURGICAL**

- Lung transplantation may be an option for patients with primary lung disease.
- Palliative atrial septostomy may alleviate symptoms of syncope or resuscitated sudden death and serve as a bridge to transplantation.
- Secondary forms of pulmonary hypertension may respond well to therapeutic interventions (e.g., surgical closure of cardiac shunts) before irreversible vascular changes occur.

■ **PROGNOSIS**
- For primary pulmonary hypertension, the prognosis is much worse than for secondary forms; 2- to 3-year survival with current treatment is approximately 50%.
- For some secondary forms, the prognosis may be as poor as with primary pulmonary hypertension (e.g., progressive pulmonary vein stenosis not amenable to surgical repair). Other secondary forms may have significantly better long-term prognosis (e.g., Eisenmenger syndrome in which survival into the fourth and fifth decades is possible).

■ **FOLLOW-UP & DISPOSITION**
- Specialized, usually intensive, follow-up of children with severe pulmonary hypertension is indicated, especially those with primary pulmonary hypertension.
- Referral to a lung transplantation center may be warranted.

☼ **PEARLS & CONSIDERATIONS**

■ **CLINICAL PEARLS**
- Patients with Eisenmenger physiology and unrepaired congenital heart disease have a longer survival than those with no heart disease and severe primary pulmonary hypertension.
- Right-to-left shunting across intracardiac defects causes cyanosis but may prevent or delay sudden death caused by a sudden lack of systemic cardiac output during periods of increased pulmonary hypertension.
- Syncope is an ominous sign and may predict sudden death.

■ **WEBSITES**
- American College of Chest Physicians Consensus Statement on Primary Pulmonary Hypertension: www.chestnet.org/health.science. policy/chest.104.236.html
- Executive summary from the World Symposium on Primary Pulmonary Hypertension 1998: www.who.int/ncd/cvd/pph.html
- PHCentral Website: www.phcentral. org/med/links.html

■ **REFERENCES**
1. Barst RJ: Recent advances in the treatment of pediatric pulmonary artery hypertension, *Pediatr Clin North Am* 46:331, 1999.
2. Haworth SG: Primary pulmonary hypertension in childhood, *Arch Dis Child* 79:452, 1998.

Author: **David Hannon, M.D.**

BASIC INFORMATION

■ DEFINITION
Hypertrophic pyloric stenosis (HPS) is an acquired condition in which the circumferential muscle of the pyloric sphincter becomes thickened, resulting in elongation and obliteration of the pyloric channel.

■ SYNONYMS
- Hypertrophic pyloric stenosis
- Congenital hypertrophic pyloric stenosis
- Pyloric stenosis (PS)
- HPS

ICD-9CM CODE
750.5 Pyloric stenosis, hypertrophic

■ ETIOLOGY
- Many theories exist regarding the cause of HPS:
  1. Gastric hyperacidity
  2. Abnormal innervation with decreased ganglion cell density
  3. Decreased nitric oxide production
- No direct cause has ever been confirmed.

■ EPIDEMIOLOGY & DEMOGRAPHICS
- The incidence of HPS is up to 3 of every 1000 live births.
- HPS is five times more common in males than in females.
- It is most common in Caucasian children and rare in Asian infants.
- Firstborn males are not necessarily more frequently afflicted than other siblings.
- Children of women who had HPS in childhood more commonly develop HPS than children from fathers who were affected.
  1. HPS develops in 19% of male offspring and 7% of female offspring born to mothers who had HPS.
  2. Approximately 5% and 2.5% of boys and girls, respectively, were born to a father who had pyloric stenosis have HPS.

■ HISTORY
- HPS presents between 2 weeks and 2 months of age.
  1. Case reports of both younger and older children
- Several days to weeks of projectile, nonbilious emesis is reported.
- Vomitus can be coffee ground or blood streaked as a result of gastritis or esophagitis.
- Patients have often been followed with a diagnosis of feeding intolerance.
- Patients may have had several changes in formula.
- Parents report child hunger.
- Weight loss or no weight gain may be reported.

- Urine output decreases.
  1. These children can present with profound dehydration, lethargy/apathy, or irritability.

■ PHYSICAL EXAMINATION
- The examination may be unremarkable or the patient may be severely malnourished and dehydrated.
- Palpable "olive" is felt just under the epigastrium.
  1. If palpated, there is no need for further diagnostic tests.
  2. Palpation of this pyloric "tumor" is extremely difficult in an agitated, crying infant with a full stomach.
- Diagnostic aids to physical examination include the following:
  1. Pass a nasogastric tube and empty the stomach.
  2. Quiet the child by allowing him or her to suck on a "sweet" pacifier.
     a. Made by taking a bottle nipple, enlarging the hole and passing a 4×4 gauze through it.
     b. Gauze is then soaked in Pedialyte, which has been sweetened with table sugar.
  3. Have mother hold infant.
  4. Examination may take 15 to 30 minutes; be patient.
  5. Apply firm, gentle, steady pressure with the flat part of the first three to four digits.
  6. Hold the baby's legs up in a bent position.
     a. For right-handed examiners, the legs are held up at the ankles with the left hand.
     b. The right hand is placed between the legs with the fingertips in the epigastrium.
  7. Apply pressure posteriorly toward the vertebral bodies until the child strains and flexes the abdominal muscles.
     a. Pressure should be kept steady until the child relaxes.
     b. The common mistake is to relax pressure when the child strains.
  8. Gentle palpation under the epigastrium will reveal an acornlike mass that rolls under the fingers with respirations and palpation.
     a. Be careful not to mistake the liver edge or rectus muscle for the olive.

DIAGNOSIS

■ DIFFERENTIAL DIAGNOSIS
The differential diagnosis of nonbilious emesis in nonfebrile infants includes the following:
- Pylorospasm
- Feeding/milk intolerance

- Gastroesophageal reflux disease
- Salt-wasting adrenogenital syndrome
- Central nervous system conditions resulting in elevated cerebrospinal fluid pressures (e.g., hydrocephalus, subdural hemorrhage)
- Less common diagnoses:
  1. Duodenal or antral webs
  2. Gastric tumors

■ DIAGNOSTIC WORKUP
- If an olive is palpated, there is no need for further diagnostic tests.
- In an infant with suspected HPS who does not have a palpable olive, further radiographic testing is essential.
- Historically, the diagnostic test of choice is an upper gastrointestinal series.
  1. HPS is confirmed by finding a narrowed pyloric channel, known as the *string sign*.
  2. Shouldering of the pyloric muscle with bulging into the proximal duodenum is also common.
- Currently, the gold standard for diagnosing HPS is an ultrasound.
  1. Pyloric muscular wall thickness is greater than 4 mm.
  2. Channel length is greater than 17 mm.
  3. Together, these have greater than 90% positive predictive value.
- Laboratory values that are highly suggestive of a gastric outlet obstruction include the following:
  1. Hypochloremic, hypokalemic metabolic alkalosis
  2. Paradoxic aciduria; may occur with significant dehydration
- Unconjugated hyperbilirubinemia is common.
  1. Believed to be secondary to a decrease in hepatic glucuronosyltransferase activity

THERAPY

■ MEDICAL
- Medical therapy of HPS is solely for stabilization for operation.
- The most important component of preoperative preparation is to correct hypovolemia.
- Correction of electrolyte abnormalities is also critical.
- Because the primary electrolyte abnormality in the child with HPS is a chloride deficiency, these patients should initially be bolused with normal saline.
  1. A bolus of 20 ml/kg normal saline is given.
  2. $D_5\frac{1}{2}NS$ or D_5NS follows at 1 to 1.5 times the maintenance rate.
  3. Potassium should not be added to the maintenance intravenous fluid until the child has voided.

II

- Serum electrolytes should be repeated and repeat boluses of normal saline given if needed.
  1. The serum bicarbonate should be less than 30 mmol/L
  2. The serum chloride should be greater than 95 mmol/L
- Surgery for HPS is not an emergency; correcting the metabolic abnormalities associated with this condition is imperative.

■ SURGICAL

- Surgical correction consists of pyloromyotomy.
- This may be performed through several types of incisions, including umbilical, right upper quadrant, and supraumbilical.
- Laparoscopic approach is also in practice in many institutions.
- Laparoscopic and umbilical approaches may offer a cosmetic advantage.
- Regardless of the operative approach chosen, successful treatment of HPS ensures that the hypertrophied muscle is split the entire length of the pylorus.
- Incomplete myotomy can result in failure to relieve symptoms and may require reoperation.

■ COMPLICATIONS

- Wound infection
- Hemorrhage
- Incomplete myotomy
- Incisional hernia
- Accidental mucosal injury—potentially the most serious complication
  1. Of the few reported cases of operation related deaths after pyloromyotomy, almost all are secondary to an unrecognized mucosal injury.
  2. If recognized at the time of operation, mucosal injury is treated by primary repair and remyotomy at another site on the pylorus with minimal, if any, morbidity.

■ FOLLOW-UP & DISPOSITION

- Postoperatively, patients are kept NPO (nothing by mouth) for 4 to 6 hours.
- They are begun on small volumes of Pedialyte or breastmilk after 4 to 12 hours.
- Gradually, volume is increased over 12 to 16 hours until the baby is taking full, maintenance feeds.
- It is not uncommon for children to vomit once or twice postoperatively.

- Emesis is often projectile in nature.
- Parents are encouraged to continue with feeding regimen.

◯ PEARLS & CONSIDERATIONS

■ CLINICAL PEARLS

- Children with presumed formula intolerance who have had their formulas changed several times may have HPS.
- Careful examination by an experienced surgeon or evaluation by ultrasound may prove helpful in deciding further treatment plans in these patients.

REFERENCES

1. Ascraft KW et al (eds): *Pediatric surgery,* ed 3, Philadelphia, 2000, WB Saunders.
2. Odham KT, Colombani PM, Foglia RP: *Surgery of infants and children,* Philadelphia, 1997, Lippincott-Raven.
3. Rowe MI et al: *Essentials of pediatric surgery,* St Louis, 1994, Mosby.
Authors: **Mark Arkovitz, M.D., and Frederick Ryckman, M.D.**

BASIC INFORMATION

■ DEFINITION
Rabies is a viral infection of the central and peripheral nervous systems, causing encephalitis with or without paralysis that is uniformly fatal.

■ SYNONYMS
- Hydrophobia
- Mad dog disease

ICD-9CM CODES
071 Rabies
V04.5 Rabies immune globulin
V04.5 Rabies vaccinations
V01.5 Rabies exposure

■ ETIOLOGY
- Rabies is caused by the rabies virus—genus *Lyssavirus,* family Rhabdoviridae.
- It is a bullet-shaped RNA virus with three major components:
  1. Surface glycoprotein (G protein)
  2. Outer envelope protein (M or matrix protein)
  3. Nucleocapsid
- It is transmitted by bite or saliva of an infected mammal or by contamination of mucosa or skin lesions by infectious material.
- Any mammal can carry and potentially transmit rabies, but it is usually transmitted by carnivorous species and bats.

■ EPIDEMIOLOGY & TRANSMISSION
- Terrestrial rabies:
  1. In the United States, terrestrial rabies is most common in raccoons on the eastern coast, skunks, foxes and coyotes, and dogs on the Texas-Mexican border.
- Bat (avian) rabies:
  1. Widespread in the 49 continental states
- Five antigenic variants of rabies strains exist in the United States.
  1. The single raccoon strain is predominant.
- No cases of human rabies have resulted from the raccoon rabies strain to date in the United States.
- Domestic animals usually succumb to the virus strain predominant in their geographic region.
- The only rodent in the United States that can carry rabies long enough to transmit to humans is the groundhog.
- Other small rodents and lagomorphs (e.g., rabbits, hares) usually die before transmitting the virus to humans.
- Human-to-human transmission has occurred only with corneal transplants.

- Cases of rabies have been reported in humans exposed to aerosols of bat guano in caves or aerosolized laboratory strain virus.
- Transmission of virus in saliva through mucous membranes, open wounds, or scratches is possible but rarely documented.
- Cats are the most common domestic animals reported by health departments as being rabid.
  1. High number of unvaccinated strays, with possible contacts to bats and other mammals
- Human cases: Since 1980, most endemic rabies cases in humans have been associated with bat strains.
- From 1990 to 1998, bats caused 20 of 22 cases of human rabies in the United States.
- Other cases have been associated with dog or animal bites in travelers returning from abroad, especially in countries where wild canine rabies is endemic.
- When rabies virus enters muscles, it replicates locally; then it is transported through peripheral sensory nerves to the spinal ganglia, replicates, and travels up the spinal cord to the brain. The virus migrates to the gray matter of the brain, predominantly in the neurons of the limbic system, midbrain, and hypothalamus. Efferent nerves transport the virus to the acinar glands of the submaxillary salivary glands, where it achieves high concentrations.
- This transit time is presumably shorter if the initial wound is severe with a high load of virus and is close to the head.
- The incubation period in human beings is as short as 5 days to many years; the average is 1 to 3 months before onset of symptoms.

■ HISTORY
- Determine the nature of the interaction with the animal (i.e., provoked attack or unexpected?).
- Was there any strange animal behavior? Was the animal typically nocturnal but out during the daytime?
- Determine the vaccination status of the animal for rabies (see following section).
- Document the nature of the presentation of illness in the animal and possible human case:
  1. Most common in humans is the "furious" form.
     a. Classic symptoms of paresthesias at site of bite, hypersalivation, and hydrophobia—spasms and contractions of the neck muscles. This form is also common in cats.
- Many other animals, including bats, exhibit "dumb" rabies—paralytic form.

- Both forms progress to paralysis of pharyngeal and respiratory muscles, seizures, and coma, with death in 1 to 3 weeks.
- Age of the injury: Rabies postexposure prophylaxis should be given in a true exposure instance no matter how old the injury.

■ PHYSICAL EXAMINATION
Examination of a patient who has been bitten by an animal should include the following:
- Localization and documentation of the extent of the wound
- Neurologic examination looking for signs of altered mental status, anxiety, hyperactivity, or bizarre behaviors with interspersed calm periods
- Autonomic instability: hypertension, hypersalivation, hyperthermia, hyperventilation
- Muscle fasciculations, priapism, focal or generalized convulsions
- Paralysis
  1. May be present only in the bitten limb at first; usually becomes diffuse
  2. May ascend (similar to Guillain-Barré syndrome)

■ COMPLICATIONS
- Secondary complications such as bacterial superinfection and tissue destruction may occur.
- Coma may last for hours to months with active intensive care support.
- Cardiac arrhythmias, myocarditis, and further autonomic dysfunction lead to cardiopulmonary arrest.

DIAGNOSIS

■ DIFFERENTIAL DIAGNOSIS
- Other encephalitides should be ruled out, especially herpes simplex encephalitis because it is treatable.
- Guillain-Barré syndrome, transverse myelitis, and poliomyelitis may present with similar paralytic features.
- Tetanus: The rigidity of tetanus contractions are more prolonged, and mental status is usually normal.
- Other forms of epilepsy and poisoning with atropine-like compounds should be ruled out.

■ DIAGNOSTIC STUDIES
- Brain biopsy with immunohistochemical or fluorescent antibody staining is definitive; wild animals that have been captured after biting should be euthanized and have testing of the unfixed brain tissue done by state health departments.
- Skin or corneal biopsy should be done for similar specific stains.

- Serologic diagnosis: A rise in specific neutralizing antibodies by rapid fluorescent focus inhibition test (RFFIT) is often not documented in true rabies cases because the victims succumb before mounting a response. This test is more useful to ascertain serostatus in immunized animals and humans.
- Viral culture of saliva, cerebrospinal fluid, and brain can also be done in specialized laboratories.

THERAPY

■ MEDICAL
Postexposure prophylaxis
- Major components of bite wound management include the following:
  1. Cleansing of the wound with soap and water or preferably povidone-iodine solution for at least 10 minutes, with debridement of devitalized tissue as necessary–
     a. Failure of adequate cleansing has caused failure of passive and active immunoprophylaxis in human rabies cases.
  2. Tetanus status and updating of immunization and antibiotics as necessary
  3. Determination of rabies immune status of biting animal
     a. In many instances, determination of the nature of the interaction may be critical. Was the attack provoked?
  4. Prophylaxis
     a. If the domestic animal (e.g., cat, dog, ferret) is known and can be observed for 10 days, prophylaxis can be postponed.
     b. Similarly, prophylaxis can be postponed if a wild animal is caught and will be tested for rabies in a timely fashion. If the animal was not captured, prophylactic immunization should proceed.
  5. Postexposure prophylaxis
     a. Recommendations for postexposure prophylaxis have changed regarding bat exposure: Any person who had direct contact with a bat should be considered for prophylaxis, and any person who was sleeping or who may be unaware of contact with a bat who awakes to find a bat nearby, and the bat cannot be tested for rabies, should be considered for prophylaxis.
- Human rabies immune globulin (HRIG) should be administered to any person not previously vaccinated against rabies in a dose of 20 IU/kg (for adults and children). Half the dose or more should be given at the injury site. The other half of the dose

should be given as a deep intramuscular (IM) injection in the gluteal area. HRIG may be given up to the seventh day after the first dose of vaccine if it is not immediately available when the patient presents for evaluation.
- Equine rabies immune globulin may be available in other countries; it has minimal side effects if it is in the purified form, but if unpurified, it may cause serum sickness and anaphylaxis.
- Three different inactivated rabies vaccines are licensed in the United States:
  1. Human diploid cell vaccine (HDCV) comes as an intradermal (ID) preparation for use only as preexposure prophylaxis, and as regular dosing to be given as an IM injection.
  2. Rabies vaccine adsorbed (RVA) is made and distributed in Michigan for IM use only.
  3. Purified chick embryo cell vaccine (PCEC) was licensed in the United States in 1997 for IM use only.
  4. Doses of all the vaccines for postexposure prophylaxis are 1.0 ml intramuscularly in the deltoid or upper outer thigh in infants.
  5. The five-dose schedule is the same for all three vaccine products: day 0, day 3, day 7, day 14, and day 28 after exposure.
  6. Postexposure antibody testing is not necessary in normal individuals.
  7. Mild local and systemic adverse reactions to these vaccines and immune globulin may occur; reactions are usually treatable with supportive care, antihistamines, and antiinflammatory medications. Local pain, erythema, headache, nausea, and abdominal pain may occur. Treatment should not be postponed or discontinued because of mild side effects if prophylaxis is warranted.
  8. Pregnancy and immunosuppression are not contraindications to vaccination; immunosuppressed individuals, including those taking corticosteroids, should have antibody testing after vaccination to determine their immune response.
  9. In previously vaccinated individuals who have a subsequent rabid exposure injury, rabies immune globulin does not need to be administered; vaccine should be given on days 0 and 3 only.
  10. Immune complex–like reactions have occurred in 6% of persons receiving booster doses of

vaccine after having completed the primary vaccine series; none have been life-threatening.
Preexposure prophylaxis
- Certain occupations or travel destinations pose a risk for possible rabies exposure (e.g., rabies laboratory workers, animal control officers, veterinarians, spelunkers, travelers to areas where rabies is enzootic and where immediate access to medical care may not be available), and these people should all receive preexposure rabies vaccine.
- The preexposure immunization schedule consists of three shots.
- The IM preparation is given as a 1.0-ml dose in the deltoid on days 0, 7, and 21 or 28.
- The ID preparation of HDCV is given as a 0.1-ml dose intradermally over the lateral deltoid on days 0, 7, and 21 or 28.
- If a person is to receive malarial prophylaxis during the period of immunization, the ID route should not be chosen because chloroquine interferes with the immune response to the ID preparation; IM dosing should be given.
- Postvaccination antibody titers are recommended for rabies laboratory workers and animal care workers every 6 months or every 2 years, depending on the level of exposure during their occupations, with readministration of booster doses when titers are less than 1:5 by RFFIT antibody testing.

■ PREVENTIVE TREATMENT & PATIENT/FAMILY EDUCATION
- Domestic animal vaccination programs have effectively limited canine rabies in the United States; families should be encouraged to keep their pet vaccinations up to date and to limit the reproduction of domestic animals to prevent stray populations.
- Education efforts at home and at schools should be supported that teach children to observe pet animal and wild animal safety procedures—not to handle strays or wildlife.
- Report animals that are sick or acting strangely to local authorities.
- Keep pets indoors at night, pet dishes indoors, and pets fenced or leashed when possible.
- Remove bat colonies from homes and barns.
- Sick or dead animals should be handled with heavy gloves and shovels.
- Trash container lids should be tight, and compost piles should be kept away from dwellings.
- Veterinarians and public health officials are excellent resources for concerns regarding animal rabies prevention.

- Massachusetts and Texas have active oral recombinant rabies vaccine drop programs to immunize wildlife to limit the geographic spread of terrestrial rabies.

☼ PEARLS & CONSIDERATIONS

■ CLINICAL PEARLS
New recommendations concerning bat exposure: Any person with direct contact with a bat or any person who was sleeping and finds a bat nearby should be considered for rabies prophylaxis.

■ WEBSITES
- Centers for Disease Control and Prevention: Human rabies prevention guidelines, 1999: www.cdc.gov/epo/mmwr
- Centers for Disease Control and Prevention: Travel vaccination recommendations: www.cdc.gov/travel/vaccinat.html
- New York State Laboratory site: www.wadsworth.org/rabies; many state health departments have websites with local rabies data and educational materials
- World Health Organization data on worldwide surveillance of human and animal rabies: www.who.int/m/topics/rabies/en/index.html

REFERENCES

1. Advisory Committee on Immunization Practices, US Public Health Service: Human rabies prevention— United States, 1999, *MMWR Morb Mortal Wkly Rep* 48(RR-1):1, 1999.
2. American Academy of Pediatrics: *2000 Red Book: report of the Committee on Infectious Diseases,* ed 25, Elk Grove Village, Ill, 2000, American Academy of Pediatrics.
3. Centers for Disease Control and Prevention: Compendium of animal rabies control, 2000: National Association of State Public Health Veterinarians, Inc., *MMWR Morb Mortal Wkly Rep* 49(RR-8):19, 2000.
4. Fishbein DB, Robinson LE: Rabies, *N Engl J Med* 329:1632, 1993.
5. Fisher DJ: New developments: epidemiology and prevention of rabies, *Curr Probl Pediatr* 25:304, 1995.
6. Fisher DJ: Resurgence of rabies, *Arch Pediatr Adolesc Med* 149:306, 1995.
7. Krebs JW et al: Rabies surveillance in the United States during 1998, *J Am Vet Med Assoc* 215:1786, 1999.

Author: **Donna Fisher, M.D.**

BASIC INFORMATION

■ DEFINITION

Raynaud's disease is an idiopathic vascular disorder characterized by episodic attacks of a triphasic color reaction of the digits and sometimes of the ears or nose.
- Initial pallor followed by cyanosis and hyperemia
- Induced by cold or emotional distress
- Not associated with identifiable underlying disease or anatomic abnormality

■ SYNONYMS
- Primary Raynaud's disease
- Idiopathic Raynaud's disease
- Paroxysmal digital cyanosis

ICD-9CM CODE
443.0 Raynaud's disease

■ ETIOLOGY
- The cause is unknown.
- Pathophysiology is presumably similar to that of Raynaud's phenomenon.
- Significant familial aggregation exists, suggesting a genetic or constitutional basis.

■ EPIDEMIOLOGY & DEMOGRAPHICS
- In proband studies, no significant differences in age or sex were observed between proband and control families.

- Raynaud's disease can occur at any age, but it most often appears in the second through fourth decades of life.

■ HISTORY
Negative for predisposing associated diseases (see the section "Raynaud's Phenomenon")

■ PHYSICAL EXAMINATION
- Initial pallor is followed by cyanosis and reactive hyperemia in a well-demarcated distribution.
  1. Most commonly distal digits, usually bilaterally
  2. May involve feet, ears, and nose
- Color changes and pain/paresthesias are relieved by warming.
  1. Immerse hands in warm water.

THERAPY

■ NONPHARMACOLOGIC
- Protection from and avoidance of cold exposure
- Prompt attention to warming
- Avoidance of trauma to affected areas
- Avoidance of vasoconstricting medications and smoking

PEARLS & CONSIDERATIONS

■ CLINICAL PEARLS
Raynaud's disease is a benign disorder.

■ RESOURCES
- National Organization for Rare Disorders, Inc. (NORD), P.O. Box 8923, New Fairfield, CT 06812-8923; 203-746-6518, fax: 203-746-6481, toll-free: 800-999-6673, TDD: 203-746-6927; email: orphan@ nord-rdb.com; www.rarediseases.org
- American Heart Association, 7272 Greenville Avenue, Dallas, TX 75231-4596; 214-373-6300; email: inquire@heart.org; www. americanheart.org
- NIH/National Heart, Lung and Blood Institute Information Center, P.O. Box 30105, Bethesda, MD 20824-0105; 301-251-1222; email: nhlbiic@dgsys.com
- Scleroderma Info Exchange, Inc., 150 Hines Farm Road, Cranston, RI 02921; 401-943-3909; email: hshinc@yahoo.com

REFERENCES
1. Blacklow RS: *MacBryde's signs and symptoms: applied pathologic physiology and clinical interpretation,* ed 6, Philadelphia, 1983, JB Lippincott.
2. Callen JP: Office dermatology, part II collagen vascular diseases, *Med Clin North Am* 82:1217, 1998.
3. *French's index of differential diagnosis,* ed 13, London, 1996, Butterworth-Heinemann.

Author: **Carmelita Britton, M.D.**

BASIC INFORMATION

■ DEFINITION

Raynaud's phenomenon is a vascular disorder characterized by episodic attacks of a triphasic color reaction of the digits, and sometimes of the ears or nose. It presents initially with pallor, followed by cyanosis and hyperemia. It is induced by cold or emotional distress and is associated with an underlying disease or anatomic abnormality. In the absence of identifiable underlying disease or anatomic abnormality, this condition is termed *Raynaud's disease*.

■ SYNONYMS

- Secondary Raynaud's phenomenon
- Raynaud's syndrome
- Paroxysmal digital cyanosis

ICD-9CM CODE
443.0 Raynaud's phenomenon

■ ETIOLOGY

In the presence of underlying disease, Raynaud's phenomenon is likely caused by one or more local defects in a complex interactive system involving:
- Neural signals
- Circulating hormones (e.g., epinephrine, vasopressin)
- Mediators released from circulating cells and the blood vessel itself (e.g., bradykinin, histamine, leukotrienes)

■ EPIDEMIOLOGY & DEMOGRAPHICS

Depends on the underlying disease/condition
- Most commonly associated with a form of rheumatologic or connective tissue disease
- In general, less common in children with these diseases than in adults
- May be the presenting symptom of systemic lupus erythematosus (SLE)
- May antedate onset of cutaneous manifestations of systemic scleroderma by several years

■ HISTORY

- Triphasic color changes of skin when exposed to cold
- Sometimes pain and/or paresthesias
- Episodic, inconsistent; may be stress related
- Difficult to reproduce with deliberate exposure (e.g., ice water immersion)
- May be associated with ergots, β-blockers, or chemotherapeutic agents.

■ PHYSICAL EXAMINATION

- Classic manifestation of Raynaud's phenomenon as described is initial pallor followed by cyanosis and reactive hyperemia.
- Well-demarcated distribution, most commonly in the distal digits, is usually seen bilaterally.
- The feet, ears, and nose may be involved.
- Color changes and pain and paresthesias are relieved by warming, such as immersing hands in warm water.
- Distal fingertip pitting is observed.
- Other physical findings depend on the underlying disease process:
  1. Fever
  2. General pallor
  3. Lymphadenopathy
  4. Lung disease
  5. Hepatosplenomegaly
  6. Polyarthritis
  7. Rash suggestive of SLE or dermatomyositis
  8. Scleroderma-like skin changes

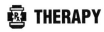 **DIAGNOSIS**

■ DIFFERENTIAL DIAGNOSIS

- The differential diagnosis of possible underlying diseases or disorders is less extensive in children than in adults:
  1. Systemic scleroderma
  2. SLE
  3. Dermatomyositis
  4. Fibromyalgia syndrome (Raynaud's phenomenon in 13% of patients)
  5. Drug associated (ergots, β-blockers, or chemotherapy agents)
  6. Hepatitis B
- All of these conditions are uncommon in children.

■ DIAGNOSTIC WORKUP

- No one laboratory test exists to prove the diagnosis of Raynaud's phenomenon.
- Laboratory assessment is aimed at determining the underlying disease.
- General screening tests may include the following:
  1. Complete blood count: anemia, leukopenia
  2. Platelet count: thrombocytopenia

  3. Erythrocyte sedimentation rate
  4. Urine analysis: red cells, white cells, casts suggestive of nephritis
  5. Antinuclear antibody, anti-dsDNA
  6. Rheumatoid factor
  7. Coombs' test
  8. Hepatitis panel

■ THERAPY

■ NONPHARMACOLOGIC

- Protection from and avoidance of cold exposure and prompt attention to warming
- Avoidance of trauma to affected areas
- Avoidance of vasoconstricting medications and smoking

■ MEDICAL

- Role of sympatholytic drugs and vasodilators has not been well studied. Enthusiasm for a given agent is generally determined by an individual's experience.
  1. Response depends on the underlying cause.
  2. Severe cases may benefit from the following:
     a. A calcium channel blocker such as nifedipine or amlodipine (Norvasc) (scleroderma, fibromyalgia syndrome)
     b. Topical nitroglycerin paste (scleroderma)

■ SURGICAL

The role of digital sympathectomy or other invasive interventions in pediatric patients has not been studied.

■ FOLLOW-UP & DISPOSITION

Depends on known or suspected underlying disease

■ PATIENT/FAMILY EDUCATION

Aside from managing underlying disease, treatment of Raynaud's phenomenon consists of anticipatory guidance.

TABLE 2-19 Occurrence of Raynaud's Phenomenon with Other Rheumatologic Diseases

DISEASE	INCIDENCE IN OUTPATIENT RHEUMATOLOGY CLINICS (%)	OCCURRENCE OF RAYNAUD'S PHENOMENON (%)
Dermatomyositis	5	15
Systemic lupus erythematosus	10	25
Systemic scleroderma	2	70-75

II

■ REFERRAL INFORMATION
Consultation with rheumatology and other specialists is indicated for underlying disease.

☼ PEARLS & CONSIDERATIONS

■ CLINICAL PEARLS
When Raynaud's phenomenon is diagnosed, search for the associated disease.

■ RESOURCES
• National Organization for Rare Disorders, Inc. (NORD), P.O. Box 8923, New Fairfield, CT 06812-8923; 203-746-6518, fax: 203-746-6481, toll-free: 800-999-6673, TDD: 203-746-6927; email: orphan@nord-rdb.com; www.rarediseases.org

• American Heart Association, 7272 Greenville Avenue, Dallas, TX 75231-4596; 214-373-6300; email: inquire@heart.org; www.americanheart.org
• NIH/National Heart, Lung and Blood Institute Information Center, P.O. Box 30105, Bethesda, MD 20824-0105; 301-251-1222; email: nhlbiic@dgsys.com
• Scleroderma Info Exchange, Inc., 150 Hines Farm Road, Cranston, RI 02921; 401-943-3909; email: hshinc.@yahoo.com

REFERENCES

1. Callen JP: Office dermatology, part II collagen vascular diseases, *Med Clin North Am* 82:1217, 1998.
2. DeSilva TN, Kress DW: Pediatric dermatology management of collagen vascular diseases in childhood, *Dermatol Clin* 16:579, 1998.
3. Maricq HR et al: Geographic variation in the prevalence of Raynaud's phenomenon: Charleston, SC, USA, versus Tarentaise, Savoie, France, *J Rheumatol* 20:70, 1993.
4. Siegel DM, Janeway D, Baum J: Fibromyalgia syndrome in children and adolescents: clinical features at presentation and status at follow-up, *Pediatrics* 101:377, 1998.
5. Wigley FM, Flavahan NA: Scleroderma Raynaud's phenomenon, *Rheum Dis Clin North Am* 22:765, 1996.

Author: **Carmelita Britton, M.D.**

BASIC INFORMATION

■ **DEFINITION**

Rectal prolapse is a protrusion of the rectal wall through the anal opening. It can be partial, involving only a portion of the circumference of the rectum (uncommon), or complete, involving the entire circumference of the rectum. This is distinguished from prolapse of mucosal abnormalities within the rectum, such as polyps or hemorrhoids, in which the rectal wall remains in its normal position.

ICD-9CM CODE

569.1 Rectal prolapse

■ **ETIOLOGY**

- Weakening of the rectal-supporting muscular elements occurs.
- Pressure at defecation is increased.
- As prolapse occurs, further stretching of the supporting ligaments and mesentery of the rectum makes subsequent prolapse more likely to occur.
- Factors that predispose to weakness of the pelvic floor muscles include the following:
  1. Myelomeningocele
  2. Debilitation
  3. Malnutrition
  4. Exstrophy of the bladder
- Factors that cause excess force in defecation include the following:
  1. Chronic constipation
  2. Cystic fibrosis
  3. Acute or chronic diarrhea

■ **EPIDEMIOLOGY & DEMOGRAPHICS**

- Boys are affected slightly more often than girls.
- Most patients present before 4 years of age.

■ **HISTORY**

- Parent observes bloody mucus in the diaper and may see prolapsed mucosa/bowel wall.
- There is often one or several of predisposing factors.

■ **PHYSICAL EXAMINATION**

- Complete prolapse presents with an intussuscepted segment of rectum outside of the anal verge.
- Pattern is similar to concentric rings formed by the mucosal folds of the rectum.
- Prolapsed segment can become quite congested when chronic; it appears as a blue or red mass at or near the anal opening.
- Irritation of the mucosa leads to local bleeding and mucus formation.
- Rectal examination to exclude a polyp, rectal mass, or constipation is necessary.

🔬 **DIAGNOSIS**

■ **DIFFERENTIAL DIAGNOSIS**

- Hemorrhoidal tissue
- Anal tag
- Prolapsed rectal polyp

■ **DIAGNOSTIC WORKUP**

- Sweat chloride or genetic screen to exclude cystic fibrosis
- Contrast enema to exclude a rectal polyp in recurrent cases

℞ **THERAPY**

■ **NONPHARMACOLOGIC**

- Reduction of the prolapsed segment is possible with simple sustained pressure on the prolapsed segment.
- The prolapse is often uncomfortable, but it is rarely painful; thus sedation is not usually necessary.

■ **MEDICAL**

- Long-term prevention requires attention to correction of constipation or diarrhea, both of which enhance recurrence risk.

- Most cases are successfully resolved with these medical measures.

■ **SURGICAL**

- Operative therapy for rectal prolapse is used only in refractory cases.
- Many procedures described lack of consensus on which is most successful.
  1. Retrorectal packing, injection of sclerosing substances, or electro-fulguration may be tried.
  2. Most surgeons now use a form of posterior suspension of redundant rectum to the sacrum.
     a. Resection of redundant bowel
     b. Posterior reconstruction of normal rectal musculature

■ **PATIENT/FAMILY EDUCATION**

- Most patients with single episode of prolapse do not need surgical treatment.
- Control of abnormal bowel habits is the best cure.

■ **REFERRAL INFORMATION**

Refer to a general pediatric surgeon if recurrent prolapse or concern regarding rectal mass or polyp.

🔆 **PEARLS & CONSIDERATIONS**

■ **CLINICAL PEARLS**

Careful examination, including a digital examination of the rectum

REFERENCES

1. Ashcraft KW: Acquired anorectal disorders. In Holder TM, Ashcraft KW (eds): *Pediatric surgery*, ed 3, Philadelphia, 2000, WB Sanders.
2. Keighley MRB, Williams NS: *Surgery of the anus, rectum and colon*, ed 2, Philadelphia, 1997, WB Sanders.

Author: **Frederick Ryckman, M.D.**

II

BASIC INFORMATION

■ DEFINITION
Acute renal failure (ARF) is sudden decline in renal function with increasing blood urea nitrogen (BUN) and creatinine, with or without changes in urine output. *Oliguria* in infants and younger children is a urine output of less than 1 ml/kg/hr. In older children, *oliguria* is a urine output of less than 200 ml/m²/24 hr. *Anuria* is a complete absence of urine output. *Polyuria* is urine output of more than 2000/ml/ 1.73 m²/day.

■ SYNONYMS
- Azotemia
- Uremia
- Renal insufficiency

■ ICD-9CM CODES
584.5 Acute renal failure with acute tubular necrosis
584.6 Acute renal failure with cortical necrosis
584.8 Acute renal failure with other associated disease
788.9 Extrarenal uremia

■ ETIOLOGY
- Prerenal
  1. Dehydration
  2. Congestive heart failure
  3. Shock
- Renal
  1. Hemolytic uremic syndrome (HUS)
  2. Acute tubular necrosis (ATN)
  3. Glomerulonephritis (GN)
  4. Pyelonephritis
  5. Nephrotoxin exposure (e.g., drugs, hemolysis, rhabdomyolysis)
  6. Malignant hypertension
- Postrenal
  1. Obstruction
  2. Bilateral ureteral atresia
  3. Posterior ureteral valves
  4. Nephrocalcinosis

■ EPIDEMIOLOGY & DEMOGRAPHICS
- Prerenal azotemia is probably the most common overall cause of acute renal failure in children.
- ATN is the most common cause of ARF in hospitalized patients.
- HUS is the most common intrinsic cause of ARF.

■ HISTORY
- Varies depending on the cause of ARF
- Prerenal ARF
  1. Diarrhea and vomiting
  2. Poor oral intake
  3. Severe burns because of excessive fluid losses
  4. Orthopnea and dyspnea caused by congestive heart failure
  5. Recent surgery leads to third-spacing and loss of effective circulating volume
- Intrinsic ARF
  1. ATN: hypotension, previous use of nephrotoxic drugs, ischemia
  2. HUS: bloody diarrhea, pallor, bruising, irritability, abdominal pain
  3. GN: gross hematuria, swelling, headache, recent streptococcal infection
  4. Pyelonephritis: fever, dysuria, urgency, frequency, foul-smelling urine
- Postrenal (obstructive) ARF
  1. Decreased urine output
  2. Suprapubic pain if obstruction is distal to bladder
  3. History of stones

■ PHYSICAL EXAMINATION
- Prerenal ARF
  1. Tachycardia
  2. Hypotension
  3. Decreased skin turgor
  4. Poor perfusion
  5. Sunken eyes and dry mucosa
- Intrinsic ARF
  1. HUS: pallor, petechiae, flow murmur, hypertension
  2. GN: periorbital edema, hypertension
  3. Pyelonephritis: fever, costovertebral tenderness, suprapubic tenderness
- Postrenal ARF
  1. Distended bladder
  2. Abdominal mass

🔬 DIAGNOSIS

■ DIFFERENTIAL DIAGNOSIS
- Dehydration with appropriately decreased urine output
- Ketoacidosis: acetoacetate can cause false increase in creatinine
- Increased protein catabolism: causes increased BUN, not creatinine
  1. Gastrointestinal (GI) bleeding
  2. Excessive protein feeding (incorrectly diluted infant formulas)
- GI hemorrhage: causes increased BUN without change in creatinine
- Syndrome of inappropriate antidiuretic hormone secretion with decreased urine output, edema, and increased vascular volume

■ DIAGNOSTIC WORKUP
- Urinalysis
  1. Specific gravity higher than 1.020 suggests prerenal ARF.
  2. Gross hematuria with or without proteinuria suggests GN.
  3. Gross hematuria without red cells is concerning for HUS because of hemolysis.
  4. Pyuria with or without bacteriuria suggests pyelonephritis.
- Serum electrolytes
  1. Hyperkalemia and acidosis common in all forms of ARF
  2. Hypernatremia more common in prerenal ARF
- Serum BUN and creatinine
  1. BUN:creatinine ratio higher than 20 suggests prerenal ARF.
     a. Interpretation may be complicated with associated GI bleeding
  2. Creatinine clearance can be estimated using plasma creatinine.
     a. kL/P_{Cr} = estimated glomerular filtration, where k is constant, L is height (cm), and P_{Cr} is serum creatinine
        (1) $k = 0.33$ for low-birth-weight infants during first year of life
        (2) $k = 0.45$ for term infant during first year of life
        (3) $k = 0.55$ for children and adolescent girls
        (4) $k = 0.7$ for adolescent boys
- Normal creatinine clearance: depends on age and renal maturity
  1. Neonates younger than 1 month old: average creatinine clearance = 40 ml/min/1.73 m²
  2. Infants 1 to 6 months old: average creatinine clearance = 70 ml/min/1.73 m²
  3. Infants 6 to 12 months old: average creatinine clearance = 100 ml/min/1.73 m²
  4. Children older than 1 year: average clearance = 120 ml/min/1.73 m²
- A child should be considered to have ARF if there is a doubling of the serum creatinine or a halving of the creatinine clearance
- Urinary sodium and creatinine
  1. Allows calculation of fractional excretion of sodium
     a. $FE_{Na} = U_{Na}/P_{Na} \times U_{Cr}/P_{Cr} \times 100$.
     b. FE_{Na} less than 1.0% suggests prerenal ARF.
     c. FE_{Na} greater than 1.0% suggests intrinsic ARF.
  2. FE_{Na} in neonates higher because of tubular immaturity
     a. FE_{Na} less than 2.0% suggests prerenal ARF.
     b. FE_{Na} greater than 2.0% suggests intrinsic ARF.
- Complete blood count and platelets
  1. Anemia can be seen in HUS and GN.
  2. HUS also has schistocytes on blood smear and thrombocytopenia.
  3. Prerenal ARF may be associated with polycythemia.
- Serum calcium and phosphorus
  1. Hyperphosphatemia can be seen in severe ARF.
  2. Profound calcium and phosphorus abnormalities are concerning for a chronic component to renal failure.

- Renal ultrasound: can demonstrate obstruction

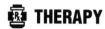 THERAPY

- Prevention of ARF is the best therapy.
- ARF with urine output is much easier to treat than oliguria or anuria.
- Unless evidence of volume overload is present (i.e., gallop, hepatomegaly, signs of congestive heart failure), all patients can be given a 10 ml/kg normal saline bolus.
- Once volume status is restored, if urine output has not normalized, furosemide, 3 to 5 mg/kg/dose, with or without a thiazide diuretic, can be given to try to restore urine output.
- Therapy is directed toward maintaining volume status and correcting electrolyte abnormalities.
- Intravenous fluid should be calculated based on insensible water loss (10 to 15 ml/kg/day for children and adolescents; 15 to 20 mg/kg/day for infants) plus urine output.

- Hyperkalemia can be treated with sodium polystyrene sulfonate (Kayexalate), correction of acidosis, insulin/glucose drips, or the use of β-agonists (see the section "Hyperkalemia").
- Hypocalcemia should be corrected before correcting acidosis to prevent tetany.
- Hyperphosphatemia can be treated using nonaluminum phosphate binders such as calcium carbonate.
- Dialysis may be needed in patients with volume overload, severe electrolyte abnormalities, or prolonged oliguria to allow nutrition.

■ PREVENTIVE TREATMENT
- Patients with multiple risk factors for ARF (e.g., sepsis, hypotension, use of nephrotoxins) should have close monitoring of urine output, fluid balance, and weight.
- Patients with impaired renal function who require exposure to nephrotoxic drugs should be well hydrated before drug administration.
- Nonsteroidal antiinflammatory drugs should be avoided in volume-depleted patients because prostaglandin inhibition can lead to ARF.

■ REFERRAL INFORMATION
All patients with persistent abnormality in renal function should be referred to a pediatric nephrologist.

☿ PEARLS & CONSIDERATIONS

■ CLINICAL PEARLS
- Serum creatinine is based on muscle mass. The smaller the child, the lower the normal serum creatinine.
- A doubling of the serum creatinine roughly corresponds to a halving of renal function.

REFERENCES
1. Sehic A, Chesney RW: Acute renal failure: diagnosis, *Pediatr Rev* 16:101, 1995.
2. Sehic A, Chesney RW: Acute renal failure: therapy, *Pediatr Rev* 16:137, 1995.

Author: **Melissa J. Gregory, M.D.**

II

BASIC INFORMATION

■ DEFINITION
Chronic renal failure (CRF) is a stage of renal dysfunction in which the glomerular filtration rate (GFR) has been reduced to below 25% of normal for at least 3 months (see the section "Renal Failure, Acute"). *Chronic renal insufficiency* (CRI) is a reduction in GFR of between 25% and 50%. CRF almost invariably progresses to end-stage renal disease (ESRD), despite correction or arrest of the primary cause. *ESRD* is a GFR of less than 10%.

■ ICD-9CM CODE
585 Chronic renal failure

■ ETIOLOGY
Diseases leading to CRF in combined series of 4136 children are as follows:
- Glomerulopathy: 33%
  1. Henoch-Schönlein purpura nephritis
  2. Lupus nephritis
  3. Membranoproliferative glomerulonephritis
  4. Focal segmental glomerulonephritis
- Reflux or obstruction: 25%
  1. Obstructive nephropathy
     a. Ureteropelvic junction obstruction
     b. Hydroureter
     c. Posterior urethral valves
     d. Meatal stenosis
     e. Urethral strictures
     f. Vesicoureteral reflux
     g. Urinary tract malformations
        (1) Ectopic kidneys
- Hereditary nephropathies: 16%
  1. Polycystic kidney disease
  2. Alport's syndrome
  3. Congenital nephrotic syndrome
  4. Cystinosis
- Hypoplasia/dysplasia: 11%
- Vascular disorders: 5%
  1. Renal vein thrombosis
  2. Hemolytic uremic syndrome
  3. Arteritis
  4. Diabetes
- Other: 10%
  1. Renal tumors
  2. Drash syndrome

■ EPIDEMIOLOGY & DEMOGRAPHICS
- In the United States, 10 to 12 per million children have CRF.
- Asians and Native Americans have lower rates than African-American and Caucasian children.
- Rates are highest in African-American children.

■ HISTORY
In contrast to acute renal failure, the signs and symptoms of CRF are more subtle. As GFR decreases, symptoms of CRF increase.
- Failure to thrive (occurs in more than 50% of children with CRF)
  1. Anorexia, nausea, and gastroesophageal reflux are common.
  2. Morning nausea and vomiting are particularly common.
  3. Prolonged unexplained vomiting may occur.
- Fatigue, malaise
- Salt craving
- Enuresis, nocturia, polyuria
- Bone diseases as a sign of renal osteodystrophy include the following:
  1. Rickets
  2. Valgus deformity of legs
  3. Fractures after minimal trauma
- Poor school performance, fatigue, inattention
- Family history of renal disease

■ PHYSICAL EXAMINATION
- Physical examination may be surprisingly unrewarding:
  1. Growth parameters to identify growth failure
  2. Blood pressure to identify hypertension
  3. Edema
  4. Signs of volume status, including weight, skin turgor, and perfusion

DIAGNOSIS

■ DIFFERENTIAL DIAGNOSIS
See "Etiology"

■ DIAGNOSTIC WORKUP
- Laboratory evaluation includes the following:
  1. Electrolytes, blood urea nitrogen (BUN), creatinine, calcium, magnesium, phosphorus, urate, albumin, and total protein
  2. Urinalysis to identify proteinuria, hematuria, casts, crystals, and cell morphology
  3. Timed urine collection to measure creatinine and total protein levels
  4. Urinary sodium, creatinine, osmolality, urea, and urinary indices, including the fractional excretion of sodium
  5. Complete blood count, differential, blood smear
     a. Normochromic normocytic anemia
        (1) Caused by a deficiency of erythropoietin, a hormone manufactured in the kidney
- Additional laboratory evaluation may include the following:
  1. Complement levels (C3, C4, CH50): these are low in some forms of glomerulonephritis and rheumatologic diseases.
  2. Antinuclear antibodies and antineutrophil cytoplasmic antibodies are seen in vasculitis.
- Imaging studies may include the following:
  1. Hand and wrist roentgenograms to determine bone age and evidence of renal osteodystrophy
  2. Chest roentgenograms for evidence of cardiomegaly and the severity of CRF
  3. Renal ultrasonography with Doppler flow
     a. Should be routine in all patients who have renal failure
     b. Assists in assessing kidney size, shape, and number
     c. Determines the adequacy of renal blood flow and obstruction
- Additional imaging studies may include the following:
  1. Computed tomography, voiding cystourethrogram, magnetic resonance imaging, and echocardiogram
- A renal biopsy may be valuable for making the diagnosis, assessing prognosis, and/or providing basis for treatment.

THERAPY

■ NONDIALYTIC THERAPY
- Close monitoring of the patient's clinical and laboratory status
  1. Blood pressures
  2. Routine blood studies, including the following:
     a. Hemoglobin to identify anemia
     b. Electrolytes for evidence of hyponatremia, hyperkalemia, and acidosis
     c. BUN and creatinine to determine nitrogen accumulation and level of renal function
     d. Calcium, phosphorus, and alkaline phosphatase for evidence of hypocalcemia, hyperphosphatemia, and osteodystrophy
- Diet
  1. Provide at least 100% recommended daily allowance (RDA) caloric intake with unrestricted carbohydrates.
  2. Provide 1.5 g/kg/day of high-quality protein (i.e., all amino acids provided), such as eggs, meat, and fish.
  3. Provide water-soluble vitamins, which may be lost because of inadequate intake and/or dialysis.
- Renal osteodystrophy
  1. Hyperphosphatemia may be controlled with low-phosphate formula.
  2. Oral calcium carbonate will bind phosphate and enhance excretion and increase serum calcium.

3. Vitamin D supplements are indicated for persistent hypocalcemia despite aforementioned therapy.
4. Recombinant human growth hormone may accelerate growth in children with persistent growth failure despite adequate calories.
- Anemia
  1. Recombinant human erythropoietin can be administered subcutaneously.
  2. Iron may be needed because of poor dietary intake of iron.
- Hypertension
  1. Control sodium intake.
  2. Antihypertensives, including diuretics and/or angiotensin-converting-enzyme inhibitors, are often necessary.
- Acidosis
  1. May improve with reduced protein intake
  2. Usually treat with Bicitra or sodium bicarbonate tablets if serum bicarbonate falls below 20 mEq/L
- Water and electrolyte management
  1. Water restriction is usually not necessary until the development of ESRD.
  2. Hyperkalemia may be controlled by reducing dietary potassium.
- Drug dosage
  1. Because many drugs are excreted in the kidneys, the dose and frequency may need to be changed in patients with CRF.

■ **DIALYSIS**
- ESRD necessitates renal replacement therapy, whether it be dialysis or transplantation.
- Continuous ambulatory peritoneal dialysis:
  1. This uses gravity to instill individual prefilled bags of dialysate into the peritoneal cavity four or five times a day, allowing for mobility and excellent extracellular fluid control.
  2. Disadvantages include the need for repeated connections and disconnections.
     a. Time-consuming
     b. Increased risk of infection
- Continuous cycler-assisted peritoneal dialysis
  1. This uses an automated cycler to instill and drain dialysate fluid via repeated exchanges overnight.
  2. The connection and disconnection are needed only once a day, reducing the risk of infection.
- Hemodialysis
  1. Typical hemodialysis prescriptions call for dialysis three times per week.
  2. Treatment sessions last 3 to 4 hours.
  3. Hypotension and muscle cramping are the most common complications.

■ **TRANSPLANTATION**
- Chronic dialysis therapy is often associated with failure to thrive, social maladaptation, and lack of sexual maturation
- Optimal treatment for children with ESRD is early renal transplantation from a living-related donor or cadaveric donor. A well-functioning graft may fully rehabilitate the patient.
- Renal transplantation is rarely a permanent cure for ESRD.

☼ **PEARLS & CONSIDERATIONS**

■ **CLINICAL PEARLS**
- Measure blood pressure and interpret readings carefully.
- Carefully interpret the results of urinalysis.

- Given the relative infrequency of CRF, there is no need to search for renal disease in every child with vomiting, fatigue, or enuresis because these are common pediatric problems. It is important to keep renal disease in the differential, especially if several symptoms are present.

■ **WEBSITES**
- National Kidney Foundation: www.kidney.org
- Kidney Dialysis Foundation: www.kdf.org.sg
- Kidney Transplant/Dialysis Association, Inc.: www.ultranet.com/~ktda
- American Association of Kidney Patients: www.aakp.org

REFERENCES
1. Bergstein J: Chronic renal failure. In Behrman RE, Kliegman RM, Arvin AM (eds): *Nelson's textbook of pediatrics,* ed 15, Philadelphia, 1996, WB Saunders.
2. Evans E, Greenbaum L, Ettenger R: Principles of renal replacement therapy in children, *Pediatr Clin North Am* 42:1579, 1995.
3. Harmon WE: Chronic renal failure. In Barratt TM, Avner ED, Harmon WE (eds): *Pediatric nephrology,* ed 4, Baltimore, 1999, Lippincott Williams & Wilkins.
4. Vogt B: Identifying kidney disease: simple steps can make a difference, *Contemp Pediatr* 14:115, 1997.
5. Warady B: New hormones in the therapeutic arsenal of chronic renal failure, *Pediatr Clin North Am* 42:1551, 1995.

Author: **Stephanie Sansoni, M.D.**

II

BASIC INFORMATION

■ DEFINITION

Renal tubular acidosis (RTA) is a defect in the renal tubular handling of bicarbonate and/or protons, which results in a persistent nonanion gap metabolic acidosis in an otherwise normal child (serum anion gap = [Na] − ([Cl] + [HCO₃]), normally less than 12 mEq/L).

■ SYNONYMS

- Type 1 or classic RTA = distal renal tubular acidosis (DRTA)
- Type 2 RTA = proximal renal tubular acidosis (PRTA)
- Type 3 RTA = infantile DRTA with bicarbonate wasting ("hybrid" RTA, classification no longer used)
- Type 4 RTA = aldosterone-dependent RTA

ICD-9CM CODES

588.8 Other specified disorders resulting from impaired renal function
276.2 Acidosis

■ ETIOLOGY

- PRTA is caused by a defect in proximal tubular bicarbonate reabsorption.
  1. PRTA may be isolated or associated with multiple tubular defects (Fanconi syndrome).
- DRTA is caused by a defect in distal renal acidification (proton and ammonium excretion).
  1. May be primary (autosomal recessive or dominant)
  2. May be secondary (associated with systemic or renal conditions, drugs, and toxins)
- Aldosterone-dependent RTA is caused by aldosterone deficiency or renal tubular unresponsiveness to aldosterone effect.

■ EPIDEMIOLOGY & DEMOGRAPHICS

- PRTA and aldosterone-dependent RTA may be transient in infancy.
  1. Transient PRTA is more likely in male than in female infants.
- DRTA is almost always permanent.
  1. Sporadic forms are more common than familial forms.
- There is no sex predominance in DRTA or in aldosterone-dependent RTA.

■ HISTORY

- Failure to thrive, particularly beyond early infancy
  1. Length is the first criteria to fall below the 5th percentile.
- Recurrent and excessive vomiting
- In DRTA, the following symptoms may be found:
  1. Polyuria, polydipsia
  2. Poor feeding

3. Weakness
4. Recurrent dehydration
5. Constipation
6. Myalgias and arthralgias

■ PHYSICAL EXAMINATION

- Length is below the 5th percentile.
- Weight may also be below the 5th percentile.
- Signs of dehydration are often seen with DRTA (i.e., sunken eyes, fontanelle, dry mucous membranes, tachycardia, skin tenting).
- Signs of volume depletion and circulatory collapse are also seen in some forms of aldosterone-dependent RTA.
- Kussmaul respiration with severe acidosis is observed.
- Central nervous system (CNS) depression, ranging from fatigue, weakness, and lethargy to stupor and coma is present.
- Rickets may be seen with PRTA in association with Fanconi syndrome.
- Sensorineural deafness is often associated with DRTA.

⚗ DIAGNOSIS

■ DIFFERENTIAL DIAGNOSIS

For hyperchloremic metabolic acidosis (normal anion gap)
- Renal loss of bicarbonate (proximal tubule)
  1. PRTA
  2. Administration of carbonic anhydrase inhibitors
  3. Posthypocapnia
- Gastrointestinal loss of bicarbonate
  1. Diarrhea
  2. Ileostomy drainage, digestive fistulas
  3. Ureterosigmoidostomy, ileal bladder, or conduits
  4. Cholestyramine resin
- Renal acid secretion defects (distal nephron)
  1. Chronic renal insufficiency (early phase)
  2. DRTA
  3. Aldosterone-dependent RTA
- Acid load
  1. Ammonium chloride, calcium chloride, or arginine chloride
  2. Hyperalimentation fluids (excessive cationic amino acids)
  3. Diabetic ketoacidosis (recovery phase)
- Miscellaneous
  1. Dilutional
  2. Laboratory artifact

■ DIAGNOSTIC WORKUP

- Salt wasting may be seen with aldosterone-dependent RTA.
- Venous, or preferably arterial, blood gas should be done to confirm the presence of acidosis, and simultaneous urinalysis should be done to check pH (by electrode, not dipstick)

and anion gap ([Na] + [K] − [Cl]) so that the urine ammonium concentration can be estimated.
1. If urine anion gap is negative {[Cl] > ([Na] + [K])} and urine pH is less than 5.5, there is appropriate ammonium excretion, so consider the following:
   a. Gastrointestinal bicarbonate wasting
   b. Acid (hydrogen chloride) ingestion
   c. Type 2 RTA (PRTA) with serum bicarbonate below threshold
2. If urine anion gap is positive {([Cl] < ([Na] + [K])}, there is inadequate ammonium excretion, so consider a defect in distal tubular acidification.
3. If urine pH is more than 5.5 during acidosis, DRTA is most likely.
- Serum electrolytes should be done to determine anion gap {[Na] − ([Cl] + HCO₃])}, calcium, phosphorus, magnesium, and creatinine.
  1. To estimate glomerular filtration rate (GFR) in children by Schwartz formula: GFR (ml/min/1.73m²) = 0.55 × Height (cm)/Creatinine
     a. Normal in children is greater than 100 ml/min per 1.73m².
  2. In infants, estimation of GFR = 0.45 × Length (cm)/Creatinine
     a. Normal in infants is greater than 60 ml/min per 1.73 m².
  3. When serum potassium is elevated and urine pH is more than 5.5, consider aldosterone-dependent RTA: Measure plasma renin and aldosterone excretion and renal sodium handling.
- Do a urinalysis to look for proximal tubule dysfunction (e.g., proteinuria, glycosuria, low-molecular-weight proteinuria).
  1. Confirm other proximal tubular transport defects by measuring serum glucose, phosphate, and urate and by performing urine screen for amino acids.
- Obtain a renal ultrasound to determine the presence of nephrocalcinosis/nephrolithiasis.
  1. Hypercalciuria, nephrocalcinosis, and nephrolithiasis are seen primarily with DRTA.

Interpretation of abnormal results
- In PRTA, there is a depression in the renal bicarbonate threshold with urinary bicarbonate wasting at lower than normal age-related plasma bicarbonate levels.
  1. Urine pH is less than 5.5 and urine anion gap is negative when below the renal bicarbonate threshold.
  2. In the absence of hypophosphatemia, rickets, osteomalacia, nephrocalcinosis, and urolithiasis are not observed in PRTA.

- In DRTA, urinary pH is more than 5.5 and urine anion gap is positive during systemic acidosis.
  1. This indicates a defect in distal renal acidification, resulting in continued bone buffering of acid.
  2. Osteomalacia, hypercalciuria, nephrocalcinosis, and/or urolithiasis occur.
- In "hybrid" RTA, infants cannot acidify the urine (DRTA) and waste bicarbonate in the urine (PRTA).
  1. The bicarbonate wasting usually disappears after infancy.
- In aldosterone-dependent RTA, urine is acidic during systemic acidosis, but rates of ammonium and potassium excretion are decreased out of proportion to any decrease in GFR.
  1. There may be problems with sodium retention.

THERAPY

MEDICAL
- Acute
  1. Children with plasma pH below 7.25 should be given intravenous sodium bicarbonate.
     a. Correct serum bicarbonate to 15 mEq/L over 1 to 4 hours.
     b. Calculate dose of bicarbonate needed [(0.5 × weight) × (15 − patient's serum bicarbonate)]
  2. Hypokalemia and hypocalcemia (seen with most forms of DRTA) should be corrected before correction of acidosis to prevent severe muscle weakness, respiratory muscle paralysis, arrhythmia, or painful tetany during bicarbonate infusion.
- Chronic
  1. Sodium bicarbonate is effective therapy and corrects acidosis caused by any form of RTA.
  2. A preferred alternative is citrate of sodium or potassium, which is converted by the liver to bicarbonate.
     a. Citrate is more palatable than bicarbonate.
     b. It is not associated with bloating and belching.
     c. Potassium citrate does not result in the volume expansion as do sodium salts.
     d. Citrate can be given as a liquid (e.g., Polycitra or Polycitra-K, ALZA) or as a tablet (e.g., Urocit-K, Mission Pharmacal).
  3. Initial therapeutic dosages of alkali are as follows:
     a. DRTA: 1 to 3 mEq/kg/day
     b. PRTA: 5 to 20 mEq/kg/day
     c. Hybrid RTA of infancy: 5 to 15 mEq/kg/day
     d. Aldosterone-dependent RTA: 1 to 4 mEq/kg/day

4. Infants and children may need higher dosages to start to neutralize acid that is released from bone and other buffers.
   a. Once the buffers are neutralized and catch-up growth ceases, the dosage can be decreased.
5. The hyperkalemia of aldosterone-dependent RTA caused by chronic renal disease with hyporeninemic-hypoaldosteronism usually responds to periodic furosemide plus fludrocortisone.
6. Infants with aldosterone-dependent RTA caused by primary pseudohypoaldosteronism (aldosterone resistance) are treated with salt supplements, low-potassium diets, and sodium bicarbonate.

FOLLOW-UP & DISPOSITION
- Some cases, particularly of infantile proximal and aldosterone-dependent RTAs, may remit spontaneously.
- DRTA with hypokalemia responds well to potassium citrate.
- PRTA responds well to a mixture of sodium and potassium citrate.
  1. This reduces the volume expansion caused by sodium salts.
  2. Treatment with sodium salts alone results in hypokalemia.
- Successful treatment results in catch-up skeletal growth and subsequent maintenance of normal growth, prevention of bone disease, and arresting of nephrocalcinosis.
- Dosage needs to be adjusted during rapid growth spurts.
- Some cases of PRTA are refractory to alkali therapy alone because of rapid urinary losses.
  1. Such cases may require concomitant thiazide diuretic treatment to reduce volume expansion.

PATIENT/FAMILY EDUCATION
- Acute treatment of the acidosis and concomitant electrolyte disorders rapidly reverses weakness, Kussmaul breathing, and CNS abnormalities.
- Chronic treatment is almost always successful in restoring and maintaining skeletal growth.
- Treatment may be needed for life.
- Failure to continue treatment of DRTA is likely to result in renal damage caused by nephrolithiasis.
- In PRTA associated with Fanconi syndrome, additional treatment and management of phosphate, sugar, and amino acid wasting may be required.

REFERRAL INFORMATION
- Formal diagnosis of any form of RTA should be referred to a pediatric nephrologist.

- Subsequent management of alkali therapy can be shared with a pediatric nephrologist, provided that growth is maintained and there is no risk of nephrolithiasis/nephrocalcinosis.

PEARLS & CONSIDERATIONS

CLINICAL PEARLS
- The astute clinician will take advantage of spontaneous acidosis to examine renal acidification ability (urine pH and anion gap).
  1. It is important for volume depletion and electrolyte disorders to be corrected before formal testing of renal acid and bicarbonate handling.
- Low serum bicarbonate can be an artifact when a small amount of blood (1 ml) is obtained with difficulty and stored in a large-capacity (10-ml) tube before measurement.
- Serum bicarbonate should agree within 10% of bicarbonate concentration calculated from simultaneous venous blood gas.
  1. A larger disagreement may be the result of a laboratory artifact, which requires repeating electrolytes and blood gas determinations.
- Urine pH measurement is not useful in the absence of a near-simultaneously obtained serum bicarbonate or blood pH.
- DRTA should be considered, in addition to an inborn error of metabolism, when a patient presents with hyperammonemia and severe acidosis (acidosis leads to increased ammonia synthesis, but there is inadequate renal excretion with the high urine pH of DRTA).
- Gastroesophageal reflux has been observed with severe DRTA; electrolytes should be checked when such reflux is refractory to therapy.
- Urine anion gap is inaccurate when there is a large concentration of non-chloride anions (e.g., ketoacids, penicillin, salicylate).
- Urinary citrate excretion is decreased in DRTA (leading to stone formation and nephrocalcinosis), and successful treatment of the acidosis increases urinary citrate excretion.

WEBSITES
Description and distinctions of the different forms of RTAs:
- eMedicine: www.emedicine.com/EMERG/topic312.htm
- National Institute of Diabetes & Digestive & Kidney Diseases: www.niddk.nih.gov/health/kidney/pubs/rta/rta.htm

II

- The WorldWide Anaesthetist: Proximal RTA: www.anaesthetist.com/icu/elec/nagacid.htm#prox Description of Fanconi syndrome, which includes PRTA:
- Icon Data Systems: Fanconi Syndrome—Renal: www.icondata.com/health/pedbase/files/Fanconis.htm

REFERENCES

1. Gregory MJ, Schwartz GJ: Diagnosis and treatment of renal tubular disorders, *Semin Nephrol* 18:317, 1998.
2. Herrin JT: Renal tubular acidosis. In Barratt TM et al (eds): *Pediatric nephrology,* ed 4, Philadelphia, 1999, Lippincott Williams & Wilkins.
3. Karet F et al: Mutations in the gene encoding B1 subunit of H^+-ATPase cause renal tubular acidosis with sensorineural deafness, *Nat Genet* 21:84, 1999.
4. Miller S, Schwartz GJ: Hyperammonemia with distal renal tubular acidosis, *Arch Dis Child* 77:441, 1997.
5. Rodriguez-Soriano J: Renal tubular acidosis. In Edelmann CM (ed): *Pediatric kidney disease,* ed 2, Boston, 1992, Little Brown.
6. Rodriguez-Soriano J: Renal tubular acidosis, *Pediatr Nephrol* 4:268, 1990.
7. Schwartz GJ: Potassium and acid-base. In Barratt TM et al (eds): *Pediatric nephrology,* ed 4, Philadelphia, 1999, Lippincott Williams & Wilkins.

Author: **George J. Schwartz, M.D.**

BASIC INFORMATION

DEFINITION
Respiratory syncytial virus (RSV)/bronchiolitis is an acute wheezing-associated illness in early life preceded by an upper respiratory infection, resulting in obstruction of small airways.

SYNONYM
RSV bronchiolitis

ICD-9CM CODE
466.1 Acute bronchiolitis

ETIOLOGY
- RSV in 45% to 75% of cases
- Parainfluenza viruses the second most common cause (type 3 > 1 > 2)
- Other: influenza virus, rhinovirus, adenovirus, and mycoplasma pneumoniae

EPIDEMIOLOGY & DEMOGRAPHICS
- RSV occurs in yearly epidemics in winter to spring.
- Parainfluenza type 3 occurs primarily spring to fall, type 1 occurs in epidemics in the fall every other year, and type 2 occurs in the fall.
- It is most common in infants younger than 1 year of age.
- The male:female ratio is 1.5:1.
- The incidence in the United States is 11.4 cases per 100 children in first year of life.
- Fifty percent of all infants will be infected with RSV by the end of the first year of life; nearly all infants will be infected by the end of the second year.
- Transmission occurs predominantly from direct contact rather than aerosol.
- Viral shedding occurs from 1 to 2 days before symptoms and continues for 1 to 2 weeks after symptoms abate.

HISTORY
- Upper respiratory infection with rhinorrhea and cough for several days
  1. Low-grade fever common
  2. Increasingly productive cough and increasing respiratory distress
- Decreased feeding
- Otitis media common (RSV and/or bacteria)
- Hypoxemia in severe cases; cyanosis often not evident
- Contact with older siblings or children at day care who have viral respiratory symptoms
- Apnea: may occur in former premature infants and infants younger than 4 months old

PHYSICAL EXAMINATION
- Tachypnea and tachycardia are noted.
- Hyperinflated chest with increased anteroposterior diameter, hyperresonance on percussion, or intercostal retractions may be seen.
- Wheezing is often detectable without a stethoscope.
- On auscultation, wheezing occurs frequently, with inspiratory crackles and prolonged expiration.
- The liver and spleen may be palpable secondary to a hyperinflated chest.
- Signs of dehydration (e.g., dry mucous membranes, sunken eyes, sunken fontanelle, fatigue) occur secondary to posttussive emesis and poor oral intake.

DIAGNOSIS

DIFFERENTIAL DIAGNOSIS
- Broadly, the differential diagnosis includes all causes of wheezing.
- Often, it may not be differentiated from asthma, especially if this is the first episode of wheezing.
- Other possibilities include the following:
  1. Gastroesophageal reflux with aspiration
  2. Foreign body aspiration
  3. Vascular rings
  4. Congestive heart failure
  5. Cystic fibrosis
- Cough must also be differentiated from pertussis syndromes.

DIAGNOSTIC WORKUP
- Diagnosis is made on the combination of clinical and epidemiologic findings.
- Chest roentgenograms typically show hyperinflation with flattened diaphragms and hyperlucency of the parenchyma, prominent bronchovascular markings, and multiple areas of atelectasis (right upper and middle lobes), which are difficult to differentiate from infiltrates.
- Rapid antigen tests detecting RSV are available.
  1. Sensitivities of 78% to 91%
  2. Specificities varying from 94% to 98%
  3. Negative predictive values of 75% to 98%
- Nasopharyngeal washings or a nasal and pharyngeal swab combined in one transport media vial are the most effective means of collecting a sample.
- Although viral isolation is the standard in reference laboratories, the technical difficulty, cost, and in-

creased time to detection are disadvantages compared with the rapid antigen tests.
1. Sensitivity of viral isolation (60% to 97%) varies according to the laboratory's experience and methods.
2. Specificity is nearly 100%.

THERAPY

NONPHARMACOLOGIC
- Considerations for hospitalization include the following:
  1. Premature infants
  2. Those with underlying heart or lung abnormalities, age younger than 3 months
  3. Poor feeding
- Infants who need to be hospitalized include those with the following conditions:
  1. Low initial oxygen saturation
  2. Dehydration
  3. Concern regarding parental observational skills or inability to return to the hospital in a timely fashion
- Oxygen and supportive care with fluid replacement are the mainstays of treatment.

MEDICAL
- Bronchodilator use is controversial.
  1. Nebulized albuterol demonstrates short-term improvement in clinical scores but not in reduction of admissions or length of hospital stay.
  2. Nebulized epinephrine improves clinical scores, improves oxygenation in the emergency department, decreases time spent in the emergency department, and reduces admission rates.
  3. Current practice is to try a bronchodilator and continuation of bronchodilators for those patients who respond favorably.
     a. Remember that epinephrine may be more effective.
- In multiple controlled studies, corticosteroids have not been beneficial.
- Treatment with ribavirin is controversial because of its high cost and inconsistent findings in some outcome measures, such as duration of hospitalization. Consider in patients with the following criteria:
  1. Premature
  2. Chronic pulmonary or cardiac disease
  3. Compromised immunity
  4. Younger than 6 weeks old
  5. Pao_2 less than 65 mm Hg or increasing $Paco_2$

■ FOLLOW-UP & DISPOSITION
- Up to 75% of hospitalized patients have recurrent bronchospasm and wheezing, especially in the first 2 years after discharge. Episodes decrease in number and severity over time.
- Subsequent wheezing and/or long-term pulmonary function abnormalities occur in some patients.
  1. This depends on multiple factors, including the following:
     a. Genetic or atopic predisposition
     b. Environmental exposures (e.g., cigarette smoke)
     c. Direct viral effects on lung tissue

■ PATIENT/FAMILY EDUCATION
- Avoid exposing infants to cigarette smoke.
- Provide parents with instruction on the use of bronchodilators if indicated.
- Refer to "Follow-Up & Disposition."

■ PREVENTIVE TREATMENT
- Vaccines are being investigated; none is currently available.
- Monoclonal antibody (Palvizumab) and polyclonal antibody (RSV-IVIG)

to RSV have been given once per month as prophylaxis to high-risk, premature infants and have resulted in a significant decrease in the rate of hospitalization. These products have not been effective as therapy.

■ REFERRAL INFORMATION
Severe cases may necessitate referral to a pulmonologist.

☼ PEARLS & CONSIDERATIONS

■ CLINICAL PEARLS
- Auscultatory examination changes often.
- Apnea occurs early or at onset of disease process.
- Secondary bacterial infections rarely occur (1.2%).

REFERENCES
1. Hall CB: Respiratory syncytial virus. In Feigin RD, Cherry JD (eds): *Textbook of pediatric infectious diseases,* ed 4, Philadelphia, 1997, WB Saunders.
2. Hall CB et al: Risk of secondary bacterial infection infants hospitalized with respiratory syncytial viral infection, *J Pediatr* 113:266, 1988.
3. The Impact-RSV Study Group: Palivizumab, a humanized respiratory syncytial virus monoclonal antibody, reduces hospitalization from respiratory syncytial virus infection in high-risk infants, *Pediatrics* 102:531, 1998.
4. Klassen TP: Recent advances in the treatment of bronchiolitis and laryngitis, *Pediatr Clin North Am* 44:249, 1997.
5. Michaels MG et al: Respiratory syncytial virus: a comparison of diagnostic modalities, *Pediatr Infect Dis J* 11:613, 1992.
6. PREVENT Study Group: Reduction of respiratory syncytial virus hospitalization among premature infants and infants with bronchopulmonary dysplasia using respiratory syncytial virus immune globulin prophylaxis, *Pediatrics* 99:93, 1997.
7. Rodriquez WJ et al: Respiratory syncytial virus (RSV) immune globulin intravenous therapy for RSV lower respiratory tract infection in infants and young children at high risk for severe RSV infections, *Pediatrics* 99:454, 1997.
8. Welliver JR, Welliver RC: Bronchiolitis, *Pediatr Rev* 14:134, 1993.
Author: **Sharon Chen, M.D.**

BASIC INFORMATION

DEFINITION
Retinoblastoma is a malignant tumor of neuroepithelial origin that arises from embryonic neural retina. It is the most common ocular tumor of childhood.

ICD-9CM CODE
190.5 Retinoblastoma

ETIOLOGY
- All tumors are associated with mutation in the retinoblastoma (Rb) gene (located at chromosome 13q14). The Rb gene is a tumor-suppressor gene (i.e., a gene whose function is to stop cell division).
- Patients with familial (inherited) retinoblastoma have an inherited mutation in one Rb gene and develop retinoblastoma when there is a spontaneous mutation in the second gene of the Rb gene pair.
- Patients with nonfamilial retinoblastoma develop spontaneous mutation in both Rb genes.

EPIDEMIOLOGY & DEMOGRAPHICS
- Retinoblastoma occurs in 1 per 14,000 to 1 per 34,000 live births (200 to 350 per year in the United States).
- Approximately 65% to 80% are unilateral (in one eye); 20% to 35% are bilateral (in both eyes).
- The median age of detection for bilateral disease is 4.5 months; for unilateral disease, the median age is 22 months.
- Most cases are detected by age 3 years.
- Although only 10% of patients have a family history, 25% to 40% of cases are familial (inherited): Parent has retinoblastoma, parent has Rb gene but asymptomatic, or parent has new germline mutation of Rb gene.

HISTORY
- Most commonly, parents notice something in the eye (leukocoria) or notice "white reflex" in a flash picture.
- Less commonly, "lazy eye" (esotropia or exotropia) is noted.
- Approximately 10% of patients have a family history of retinoblastoma.

PHYSICAL EXAMINATION
- Leukocoria
- Less often esotropia, orbital inflammation, hyphema, fixed pupil, or heterochromia iridis
- Ophthalmologic examination:
  1. White-yellow-pink mass with associated tortuous vessels
  2. Sometimes associated with retinal detachment and/or vitreous hemorrhage
  3. Vitreous seeding of tumor
  4. Multifocal, bilateral masses

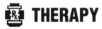

DIAGNOSIS

The diagnosis is usually straightforward and can be made based on the ophthalmologic examination without a biopsy.

DIFFERENTIAL DIAGNOSIS
- For a mass
  1. Hamartoma
  2. Granuloma
  3. Uveitis
  4. Emboli caused by subacute bacterial endocarditis
- For associated retinal detachment
  1. Coats' disease
  2. Retinopathy of prematurity
  3. Persistent hyperplastic vitreous

DIAGNOSTIC WORKUP
- Ophthalmologic examination under anesthesia to assess for vitreous seeding, multifocal disease, bilateral disease
- Head computed tomography or magnetic resonance imaging scan to assess for extension of disease through optic nerve and the presence of a pineal region tumor (trilateral retinoblastoma)
- Lumbar puncture (indicated for patients with locally advanced or metastatic disease)
- Bone marrow aspirate and biopsy (indicated for patients with locally advanced or metastatic disease)

STAGING
- Because retinoblastoma is usually confined to the orbits and is such a curable disease, the most commonly used staging system is based on the likelihood of saving vision in the affected eye or eyes.
  1. Group I (very favorable): single or multiple tumors less than 4 disc diameters (1 disc diameter = 1.5 mm)
  2. Group II (favorable): single or multiple tumors 4 to 10 disc diameters
  3. Group III (doubtful): any tumor anterior to the equator or single lesion more than 10 disc diameters
  4. Group IV (unfavorable): multiple tumors, some more than 10 disc diameters, any tumor extending anterior to ora serrata
  5. Group V (very unfavorable): large tumors involving more than half the retina; vitreous seeds

- There is no universally agreed-upon system for disease beyond orbit. One proposed system is the St. Jude Children's Research Hospital Staging System:
  1. Stage 1: tumor confined to the retina
  2. Stage 2: tumor confined to globe, involving up to or beyond cut end of optic nerve
  3. Stage 3: extraocular extension into the central nervous system, including tumor cells in cerebrospinal fluid
  4. Stage 4: distant metastases

PROGNOSTIC FACTORS
Adverse factors include the following:
- Tumor involvement in optic nerve beyond lamina cribrosa or beyond cut end of optic nerve
- Tumor involvement in scleral emissaria veins and episcleral tissues
- Trilateral retinoblastoma (retinoblastoma plus ectopic retinoblastoma in pineal region)
- Distant metastases

THERAPY

- The goal of therapy is cure.
- Because disease is so often localized and so often curable, a second goal is preservation of vision.

SURGICAL
- Enucleation is reserved for the following cases:
  1. Unilateral retinoblastoma when eye is blind
  2. Bilateral retinoblastoma when one eye is blind
  3. Glaucoma with visual loss
  4. Local recurrence uncontrolled by less aggressive measures
- Local therapy includes the following:
  1. Photocoagulation: "Burn" vessels around small tumors. This is effective for tumors less than 4.5 mm in diameter. It is not effective when the tumor is near the optic disc, near the macula, or in vitreous because of the risk of vision loss.
  2. Cryotherapy: This treatment is indicated for small tumors anterior to equator or for recurrences after radiotherapy; sometimes given with chemotherapy.
  3. Radioactive plaque application: Radiation implant is done for larger tumors 2 to 16 mm.

MEDICAL
- External beam radiation
  1. Indicated for multifocal tumors, tumors too close to the optic nerve or macula, larger tumors, vitreous seeding

II

- Chemotherapy
  1. May be effective adjunct in infants with multifocal disease, allowing for delay in external beam radiotherapy
  2. Indicated for children with metastatic disease
  3. Effective agents: carboplatin, VP-16, cyclophosphamide, vincristine

■ **FOLLOW-UP & DISPOSITION**
- The 5-year overall survival is approximately 90%, higher for children with local disease and much lower for children with advanced local disease or metastatic disease.
- Recommended follow-up includes examination under anesthesia periodically over the first 5 years, with decreasing frequency over time.
- Late effects include the following:
  1. The risk of a second malignancy in children with retinoblastoma is high.
  2. Risk is greatest in children with familial retinoblastoma who received external beam radiotherapy.
  3. Risk is increased with increasing dose of radiation, with younger age at radiation, and with treatment with cyclophosphamide.
  4. Most second malignancies are in the radiation field and include osteosarcoma, fibrosarcoma, and other spindle cell neoplasms.
  5. Overall risk of second malignancy with 50 years' follow-up is as high as 50% in familial retinoblastoma; it is only 5% in children with sporadic retinoblastoma.
  6. With 40 years' follow-up, there is 30% mortality from second malignancy in patients with familial retinoblastoma who received radiation (versus 6% in those who did not receive radiation).
  7. Ocular complications include increased risk of cataracts, decreased tearing, and orbital bone hypoplasia with external beam radiation.

■ **PATIENT/FAMILY EDUCATION**
- Retinoblastoma is a very curable disease; thus treatment goals are aimed at preservation of vision as well as cure.
- A child can have familial (inherited) retinoblastoma even without a family history of the disease.
- Children with familial retinoblastoma are at increased risk of second malignancies.

■ **PREVENTIVE TREATMENT**
- An infant with a family history of retinoblastoma should undergo periodic screening ophthalmologic examinations under anesthesia to look for retinoblastoma.
- Infants and children with retinoblastoma should continue to undergo screening examinations under anesthesia to look for recurrent or new lesions.
- Genetic counseling should be a part of the evaluation of the families of children with retinoblastoma, and siblings should be examined for the disease.

■ **REFERRAL INFORMATION**
Children with retinoblastoma should be evaluated and treated by an ophthalmologist with experience in treating this disease, and it should be done in conjunction with a pediatric oncologist and pediatric radiation oncologist.

✵ PEARLS & CONSIDERATIONS

■ **CLINICAL PEARLS**
- Familial (inherited) retinoblastoma usually occurs in infants and is usually multifocal and bilateral.
- Although only 10% of children with retinoblastoma have a family history of the disease, another 15% to 30% have inherited disease.
- Children with familial retinoblastoma have an increased risk of ectopic pineal region retinoblastoma (trilateral retinoblastoma).

■ **WEBSITES**
- Retinoblastoma.com: A Parent's Guide to Understanding Retinoblastoma: www.retinoblastoma.com/guide/guide.htm
- CancerNet: Retinoblastoma (PDQ) Treatment—Health Professionals: www.cancernet.nci.nih.gov

REFERENCES
1. Halperin EC et al: Retinoblastoma. In Halperin EC et al (eds): *Pediatric radiation oncology*, ed 3, Philadelphia, 1999, Lippincott Williams & Wilkins.
2. Donaldson SS et al: Retinoblastoma. In Pizzo PA (ed): *Principles and practice of pediatric oncology*, Philadelphia, 2001, Lippincott Williams & Wilkins.
Author: **David N. Korones, M.D.**

BASIC INFORMATION

■ **DEFINITION**

Retropharyngeal abscesses are deep neck infections involving either the retropharyngeal space or the parapharyngeal (lateral pharyngeal) region.

■ **SYNONYMS**

- Deep neck infections
- For retropharyngeal abscess:
  1. Retrovisceral space abscess
  2. Posterior visceral space abscess
  3. Retroesophageal space abscess
- For lateral pharyngeal abscess:
  1. Pterygomaxillary abscess
  2. Parapharyngeal abscess
  3. Pharyngomaxillary abscess

■ **ICD-9CM CODES**

478.29 Abscess, lateral pharyngeal
478.24 Abscess, retropharyngeal

■ **ETIOLOGY**

- Retropharyngeal abscesses in children usually result from suppurative adenitis of retropharyngeal lymph nodes.
  1. Often, the patient has had a recent episode of nasopharyngitis, adenoiditis, or otitis media.
- In both children and adults, infection may also reach the retropharyngeal space from contiguous or distant sites.
- Sources include the following:
  1. Traumatic perforation from a foreign body, endotracheal intubation, or endoscopy
  2. Dental abscess
  3. Peritonsillar abscess
  4. Extension from the lateral pharyngeal space
- Infections of the lateral pharyngeal space may arise from several sources:
  1. Dental infections are most common.
  2. Occasionally, lateral pharyngeal space infections complicate other processes:
     a. Peritonsillar abscess
     b. Retropharyngeal abscess
     c. Infection in the submandibular or parotid glands
     d. Infection in the tongue
     e. Mastoiditis
     f. Otitis media
     g. Following penetrating trauma
- Deep infections are often caused by a variety of aerobic and anaerobic bacteria:
  1. Aerobes are only rarely found without anaerobes.
  2. Occasional infections are caused only by anaerobes.
  3. The most common aerobic isolates from these infections include the following:
     a. α- and γ-hemolytic streptococci

  b. Group A β-hemolytic streptococcus
  c. *Staphylococcus aureus*
  4. Less common isolates include the following:
     a. *Neisseria* species
     b. *Moraxella catarrhalis*
     c. *Haemophilus* species
     d. Members of the Enterobacteriaceae family
  5. The predominant anaerobes are as follows:
     a. *Bacteroides* species
     b. *Fusobacterium* species
     c. *Peptostreptococcus* species
  6. Rarely, *Mycobacterium tuberculosis,* the atypical mycobacteria, or fungi have been linked to these infections.

■ **EPIDEMIOLOGY & DEMOGRAPHICS**

- Retropharyngeal infections are at least tenfold more common in children than lateral pharyngeal infections.
- Because the retropharyngeal nodes tend to atrophy with age, retropharyngeal abscesses primarily occur in young children (younger than age 5 years).
  1. Approximately 55% occur in children younger than age 2 years.
  2. About 35% occur in those younger than age 1 year.
- However, retropharyngeal abscesses may occur in older children and adults.
- Lateral pharyngeal abscesses are most likely to occur in older children and adults rather than young children.

■ **HISTORY**

- With both infections, there is often a history of a preceding upper respiratory infection.
- Children with an infection in the retropharyngeal space may present with the following:
  1. Fever
  2. Restlessness
  3. Limited motion of the neck
  4. Sore throat
  5. Poor oral intake
  6. Dysphagia
  7. Drooling
  8. Dyspnea
  9. Muffled speech and cry
  10. Stridor
- In contrast to the child with a peritonsillar abscess or cellulitis, trismus is usually not present.
- Children with lateral pharyngeal space infections often have many of the same symptoms as those with retropharyngeal space infections.
  1. Trismus is more common, particularly if the anterior (muscular) compartment is involved.

■ **PHYSICAL EXAMINATION**

- The child with a retropharyngeal abscess may demonstrate variable symptoms, such as the following:
  1. Toxicity
  2. Fever
  3. Stridor
  4. Tachypnea
  5. Dyspnea
  6. Evidence of pharyngitis
  7. Pain or stiffness with active or passive movement of the neck
  8. Torticollis
  9. Midline or unilateral swelling of the posterior pharynx
  10. Ipsilateral, mildly tender cervical lymphadenopathy
- The patient with a lateral pharyngeal abscess may demonstrate variable symptoms, such as the following:
  1. Toxicity
  2. Fever
  3. Stridor
  4. Tachypnea
  5. Trismus
  6. Perimandibular induration and erythema
  7. Tender, high cervical mass
  8. Other
     a. Intraoral examination may reveal unilateral swelling and medial displacement of the lateral pharyngeal wall, with displacement of the tonsil medially and anteriorly.
     b. When there is involvement of the posterior compartment, there may be evidence of involvement of one of the cranial nerves (IX, X, XII) or the cervical sympathetic trunk. The latter may produce Horner's syndrome:
        (1) Meiosis
        (2) Ptosis
        (3) Enophthalmos
        (4) Ipsilateral anhidrosis of the face

■ **DIAGNOSIS**

■ **DIFFERENTIAL DIAGNOSIS**

Both of these infections must be distinguished from the following:
- Each other
- Cervical lymphadenitis
- Peritonsillar abscess
- Viral laryngotracheobronchitis (croup)
- Bacterial tracheitis
- Epiglottitis
- Prevertebral abscess

■ **DIAGNOSTIC WORKUP**

- Laboratory studies
  1. The white blood cell count is usually elevated, with a predominance of polymorphonuclear leukocytes.

2. Gram stain, aerobic, and anaerobic cultures should be done on any material obtained at the time of needle aspiration or incision and drainage.
- Radiographic studies
  1. Computed tomography (CT) scan of the neck, with and without administration of a contrast agent, has evolved as the imaging study of choice for patients suspected of having a deep neck infection.
     a. Advantages over conventional radiography include the following:
        (1) Ease of interpretation in the presence of normal variation in the appearance of the soft tissues of the neck with phases of respiration and neck position
        (2) Ability to determine the extent of the infection, including involvement of adjacent spaces
        (3) Ability to visualize vascular structures and potential complications (like venous thrombosis)
        (4) Potential to help distinguish cellulitis of deep structures from abscess formation
     b. The sensitivity of CT scanning in detecting abscess formation is 88% to 91%, with a specificity of approximately 87%.
  2. Conventional anteroposterior and lateral radiographs of the neck may be done.
     a. If done, these should be taken with the neck in the neutral or fully extended position.
     b. In retropharyngeal space infections, the lateral neck radiograph may demonstrate the following:
        (1) Increased thickness of the prevertebral soft tissues (anteroposterior diameter of the soft tissue exceeds that of the contiguous vertebral bodies, a retropharyngeal space more than 7 mm, or a retrotracheal space more than 14 mm)
        (2) Air or an air-fluid level in the soft tissues
        (3) Loss or reversal of the normal cervical lordotic curvature
        (4) Presence of a foreign body
     c. In lateral pharyngeal space infections, the anteroposterior neck radiograph may reveal the following:
        (1) Ipsilateral pharyngeal fullness
        (2) Obliteration of the pyriform sinus

d. Use of conventional radiography has largely been supplanted by CT scanning.

💊 THERAPY

■ NONPHARMACOLOGIC
- Patients with deep neck infections should be monitored carefully for the development of significant respiratory distress secondary to upper airway obstruction.
- If significant respiratory distress develops, the patient should be transferred to a pediatric intensive care unit.
- Endotracheal intubation to secure the airway may be necessary pending incision and drainage of an abscess in the operating room.

■ MEDICAL
- Empiric antimicrobial therapy of deep neck infections is directed at the usual offending pathogens.
- If aspiration or incision and drainage become necessary, antimicrobial therapy may be altered on the basis of results of the Gram stain as well as aerobic and anaerobic bacterial cultures.
- Infections are often caused by β-lactamase–producing organisms.
  1. If the patient is not allergic to penicillin, the combination of ampicillin and the β-lactamase inhibitor sulbactam (Unasyn) is considered a regimen of choice.
     a. Good clinical efficacy is achieved in mixed aerobic-anaerobic infections.
  2. Clindamycin would be an acceptable alternative in the penicillin-allergic patient if gram-negative aerobes are not likely pathogens.
     a. However, it is usually only bacteriostatic against *S. aureus*.
  3. Cefuroxime with an agent active against more anaerobes, such as clindamycin or metronidazole, is another alternative.
- Therapy is given intravenously initially, although once the patient has improved sufficiently, a change to a suitable oral agent is reasonable.
  1. For patients who were treated with ampicillin/sulbactam (Unasyn), amoxicillin/clavulanic acid (Augmentin) is usually used.
- Therapy is usually continued for 10 to 14 days, with hospitalization usually recommended until the patient is ready to be switched to oral antibiotic therapy.

■ SURGICAL
- It was previously believed that only a minority (10% to 25%) of patients could be cured with medical therapy alone.

- Now it is increasingly recognized that most patients with deep neck infections, including many of those with small abscesses by CT scan, will respond to antibiotic therapy and not require surgical drainage.
- Patients with a CT scan consistent with cellulitis, without abscess formation, will almost always respond to empiric antibiotic therapy directed against the usual pathogens.
  1. Needle aspiration of the affected area could be performed in an effort to identify the etiologic agent, but it is not essential.
- Patients who appear to have an abscess by CT scan and have significant airway compromise, hemorrhage, subcutaneous emphysema, or cranial nerve involvement should be taken to the operating room to secure the airway, followed by incision and drainage.
- Patients who appear to have an abscess by CT scan but who do not have significant airway compromise, hemorrhage, subcutaneous emphysema, or cranial nerve involvement can be managed in two ways:
  1. Needle aspiration can be attempted in an effort to recover the etiologic agent and drain purulent material.
     a. Parenteral antibiotic therapy should be administered, and the patient's response to therapy can be assessed clinically and with follow-up CT scans.
     b. If an unsatisfactory response occurs, repeat needle aspiration or incision and drainage can be performed.
        (1) Needle aspiration is safer and more feasible in patients with lateral pharyngeal abscess than in those with retropharyngeal abscess.
        (2) Patients with retropharyngeal abscesses are more likely to be treated with incision and drainage.
  2. Empiric antibiotic therapy can be begun and the patient can be closely observed clinically and radiographically with follow-up CT scans.
     a. If there is no improvement with 48 hours or if there is apparent progression of infection, a drainage procedure is mandatory.
- Patients with retropharyngeal abscesses who require incision and drainage can usually have the procedure done via a transoral approach, particularly if the mass is relatively small. Some patients, however, will need drainage via an external approach.

• Patients with lateral pharyngeal abscess who require incision and drainage will have the procedure done via an external approach.

■ FOLLOW-UP & DISPOSITION

• Patients require close follow-up after therapy is instituted to assess whether they are responding adequately to therapy. This is particularly true for patients who are initially managed medically; if improvement is seen within 48 hours or if infection progresses, a drainage procedure is indicated.

• The patient should be monitored closely for the development of one or more of the potentially serious complications of deep neck infections, including the following:
  1. Severe upper airway obstruction
  2. Rupture of the abscess into the pharynx or trachea, resulting in asphyxiation, pneumonia, empyema, or lung abscess
  3. Suppurative descending mediastinitis
  4. Thrombophlebitis with thrombosis of the internal jugular vein
  5. Erosion of the carotid or vertebral arteries resulting in hemorrhage
  6. Cranial nerve palsies (VI, IX, X, XI, XII)
  7. Horner's syndrome
  8. Septic pulmonary emboli

■ PATIENT/FAMILY EDUCATION

Patients and their families should be informed about the seriousness of these infections, the potential for complications, the need for close monitoring once antibiotic therapy is initiated, and the potential need for surgical drainage.

■ PREVENTIVE TREATMENT

Because deep neck infections may follow selected upper respiratory tract infections, appropriate management of these infections may help prevent the development of a deep neck infection.

■ REFERRAL INFORMATION

• In view of the potential for airway compromise and other serious complications of deep neck infections, patients with these infections should be admitted to hospitals where they can be monitored closely and where complications can be dealt with.

• Ready access to a pediatric intensive care unit is essential, as is access to an infectious disease specialist and an otolaryngologist experienced in the medical and surgical management of these infections.

☼ PEARLS & CONSIDERATIONS

■ CLINICAL PEARLS

• A deep neck infection should be considered in a child with a preceding upper respiratory tract infection or oral or neck trauma who develops fever, irritability, limited motion of the neck, torticollis, dysphagia, drooling, dyspnea, muffled speech or cry, stridor, neck swelling, or displacement of the posterior or lateral pharyngeal wall.

• CT scanning of the neck has evolved as the imaging modality of choice in assessing these infections.

• Patients should be hospitalized and treated with parenteral antimicrobials initially; some patients require surgical drainage, but most respond to medical therapy alone.

■ WEBSITES

• The Bobby R. Alford Department of Otorhinolaryngology and Communicative Sciences: www.bcm.tmc.edu/oto/grand/10694.html; includes information about deep neck space infections and changing trends

• Pediatric Infectious Disease: www.pedid.uthscsa.edu/057.htm; includes information about infections of the deep fascial spaces of the neck

REFERENCES

1. Bluestone CD: Retropharyngeal and lateral pharyngeal space infections. In Kaplan SL (ed): *Current therapy in pediatric infectious diseases,* ed 3, St Louis, 1993, Mosby.
2. Broughton RA: Nonsurgical management of deep neck infections in children, *Pediatr Infect Dis J* 11:14, 1992.
3. Chow AW: Life threatening infections of the head and neck, *Clin Infect Dis* 14:991, 1992.
4. Hammerschlag PE, Hammerschlag MR: Peritonsillar, retropharyngeal, and parapharyngeal abscesses. In Feigin RD, Cherry JD (eds): *Textbook of pediatric infectious diseases,* ed 4, Philadelphia, 1998, WB Saunders.

Author: **Robert A. Broughton, M.D.**

BASIC INFORMATION

DEFINITION
Rhabdomyolysis is injury to the skeletal muscle with release of cellular contents into the circulation. The classic triad of muscle weakness, myalgias, and darkened urine may be present. Increased serum intracellular contents such as myoglobin, creatinine phosphokinase (CPK), potassium, phosphorus, glutamic oxaloacetic transaminase, and lactate dehydrogenase serve as clinical markers to the syndrome.

SYNONYMS
- Myoglobinuria (much less descriptive for the clinical syndrome)
- Meyer-Betz disease

ICD-9CM CODE
728.89 Rhabdomyolysis

ETIOLOGY
- Damage to the muscle cell membrane (sarcolemma) results in liberation of intracellular contents. Etiologic agents cause damage to the sarcolemma secondary to sodium pump dysfunction, energy demand/supply mismatch, defective energy utilization, or direct injury to the muscle cell and its membrane.
- Many causes exist, including the following:
  1. Toxins, drugs, venoms
  2. Intrinsic muscle dysfunction: trauma, genetic disorders affecting carbohydrate or lipid metabolism, immunologic disorders, or excessive muscle activity
  3. Endocrine and metabolic disorders: thyroid dysfunction, diabetic ketoacidosis, electrolyte abnormalities
  4. Infections
  5. Tissue hypoxia: vascular obstruction, external compression, vasculitis, sickle cell disease
  6. Temperature-related injury
  7. Idiopathic

EPIDEMIOLOGY & DEMOGRAPHICS
- The exact incidence in children is unknown.
- Of all cases of renal failure, 9% are caused by rhabdomyolysis.

HISTORY
- Clinical suspicion is the key to diagnosis.
- History taking should be directed at identifying a causative agent.
- Clinical presentation often reflects an underlying disease.
- Patients will complain of pain if a compartment syndrome is present.

PHYSICAL EXAMINATION
- Localized or diffuse muscle tenderness
- Focal muscle weakness
- Edema
- Skin changes secondary to pressure necrosis
- Findings suggestive of a compartment syndrome
  1. Pain
  2. Pulselessness
  3. Paresthesias
  4. Pallor
  5. Pain on passive range of motion
- Other
  1. Sources suggest that tenderness and weakness are present in 50% of cases, with the addition of edema in 4% to 15% of cases.

DIAGNOSIS

DIFFERENTIAL DIAGNOSIS
A significant overlap exists between etiology and differential diagnoses.
- Autoimmune
  1. Polymyositis
  2. Dermatomyositis
- Genetic disorders
  1. Muscular dystrophies
  2. Abnormal carbohydrate/lipid metabolism
- Infection
  1. Pyomyositis
  2. Abscess

DIAGNOSTIC WORKUP
- An abnormal serum CPK level is considered the gold standard for the diagnosis of rhabdomyolysis.
  1. This test is the most sensitive marker of myocyte injury.
  2. MM fraction accounts for at least 95% of elevated CPK, MB fraction as the remainder.
  3. Some sources suggest that five times the normal level of CPK is required for diagnosis.
  4. Conflicting data exist as to whether CPK levels correlate with the severity of disease.
- Urinalysis with microscopy reveals tea-colored urine.
  1. Dipstick is positive for blood.
  2. No (or few) red blood cells (RBCs) are seen on microscopic evaluation.
  3. Muddy casts are also seen.
- Serum electrolytes may reveal an anion-gap metabolic acidosis, increased potassium, increased PO_4, increased blood urea nitrogen (BUN), and increased creatinine.
- Serum and urine myoglobin are not reliable markers for diagnosis because of the rapid clearance of myoglobin from plasma and the poor correlation of myoglobinuria with myoglobinemia.
  1. Fifty percent of patients with rhabdomyolysis have myoglobinuria.
- Magnetic resonance imaging may be useful in diagnosis with 90% to 95% sensitivity.
- Further studies are guided by suspicions for etiology.

COMPLICATIONS
- Renal failure secondary to acute tubular necrosis and obstruction from pigment casts
  1. Myoglobin is not directly toxic to renal parenchyma.
  2. Its breakdown product, ferriheme, has direct nephrotoxic effects.
  3. Injury is accentuated by acidic urine.
- Metabolic abnormalities: hyperkalemia, hyperphosphatemia, hypocalcemia, hypercalcemia, hyperuricemia, metabolic acidosis
- Compartment syndrome: damage to a compartment with subsequent leakage of cellular contents result in increased pressure
- Disseminated intravascular coagulation: secondary to release of thromboplastin from myocytes
- Respiratory insufficiency: from damage to respiratory muscles
- Hepatic insufficiency
- Peripheral neuropathy

THERAPY

NONPHARMACOLOGIC
Search for any reversible cause.

MEDICAL
- Early aggressive therapy appears to lower the risk of complications.
- Administer intravenous (IV) fluids (saline) at a rate to maintain high urine output.
  1. Suggested IV rates of 100 to 300 ml/hr in adults
- Administer sodium bicarbonate to maintain a urine pH higher than 6.5.
- Treat electrolyte abnormalities.
- Consider dialysis for patients who do not respond to fluid therapy.
- Most patients can be managed in an outpatient setting and respond to aggressive fluid therapy.
- Consider hospital admission for very high levels of CPK, any evidence of renal failure, and significant electrolyte abnormalities.

REFERRAL INFORMATION
Nephrology referral is indicated with any evidence of renal failure.

☼ PEARLS & CONSIDERATIONS

■ CLINICAL PEARLS
- The classic triad of muscle weakness, myalgias, and darkened urine is *not* present in most patients, especially early in the disease course.
- Myoglobinuria occurs only in the presence of rhabdomyolysis, but rhabdomyolysis may occur without detectable myoglobin in the urine.
- CPK is present in the serum immediately after muscle injury and peaks within 36 hours.
- The urine will be tea-colored with a positive dipstick for blood, although few RBCs are seen on microscopic analysis.
- Acute renal failure is the primary determinant of morbidity and mortality.
- Serum creatinine is elevated to a greater extent than BUN because of creatinine release from injured muscle.
- Levels of CPK, phosphate, albumin, and potassium or the presence of sepsis or hypotension may have some value as a predictive tool for renal failure.
- Suspect rhabdomyolysis in any patient with a history of prolonged immobilization or unconsciousness.

■ WEBSITE
Open Directory Project: www.dmoz.org/Health/Conditions_and_Diseases; search under "rhabdomyolysis"

REFERENCES
1. Moghtader J, Brady WJ, Bonadio W: Exertional rhabdomyolysis in an adolescent athlete, *Pediatr Emerg Care* 13: 382, 1997.
2. Rosen P, Barkin R: *Emergency medicine,* ed 4, St Louis, 1998, Mosby.

Author: **Heather Chapman, M.D.**

II

BASIC INFORMATION

■ **DEFINITION**
Rhabdomyosarcoma (RMS) is a neoplasm derived from primitive mesenchymal cells of striated muscle lineage. It may occur anywhere in the body, including sites that do not normally contain striated muscle.

ICD-9CM CODE
171.9 Rhabdomyosarcoma

■ **ETIOLOGY**
• Most cases are sporadic.
• No environmental risk factors have been identified.
• RMS is associated with neurofibromatosis and Li-Fraumeni syndrome.
• Insulin-like growth factor II may play a role in pathogenesis.
• Molecular lesion may involve lack of activity of MyoD family of proteins, which function to commit mesenchymal cells to a skeletal muscle lineage.

■ **EPIDEMIOLOGY & DEMOGRAPHICS**
• RMS is the most common soft tissue sarcoma.
• It accounts for 2% to 4% of pediatric cancers.
• Incidence is 4 to 7 cases per year per 1 million children younger than 15 years of age.
• Approximately 250 new cases are diagnosed per year in the United States.
• Incidence in males is greater than in females.
• Incidence in African Americans and Asians is less than Caucasians.
• Approximately 60% to 70% of patients are younger than 10 years of age; second smaller incidence peaks in early to midadolescence.
• Approximately 35% to 40% of rhabdomyosarcomas arise in the head and neck region, 25% in the genitourinary (GU) tract, 20% in extremities, and the remainder from truncal and other sites.

■ **HISTORY**
• A mass or swelling develops, with or without pain, or a disturbance of normal body function occurs because of the presence of a mass (e.g., bowel or bladder dysfunction).
• Orbital masses usually present with proptosis, limited eye movement, or diplopia.
• Nasopharyngeal tumors often present with nasal discharge, which may be bloody.
• Bladder tumors may present with hematuria.
• Tumors of the female genital tract may present with vaginal discharge or extrusion of tumor.

• Parameningeal sites with central nervous system extension may present with cranial nerve palsies or headache and vomiting.
• Systemic complaints such as fatigue or weight loss may occur.

■ **PHYSICAL EXAMINATION**
• The mass may be palpable, usually firm with indistinct margins.
• The mass may be tender or nontender.
• No mass may be apparent on examination.
• Examination may reveal only signs as described in history (e.g., proptosis, limited extraocular movements, cranial nerve palsies).
• Lymphadenopathy may be palpable if rhabdomyosarcoma has metastasized to lymph nodes.
• Tenderness may be elicited in sites of bony metastases, if present.

🔬 **DIAGNOSIS**

■ **DIFFERENTIAL DIAGNOSIS**
• Other malignancies
  1. Other sarcomas
  2. Neuroblastoma
  3. Wilms' tumor
  4. Germ cell tumors
  5. Lymphoma
• Trauma
• Benign tumors
• Infection (may present with mass lesions similar to rhabdomyosarcoma)

■ **DIAGNOSTIC EVALUATION**
• Computed tomogram (CT) and/or magnetic resonance imaging (MRI) scan of primary is generally done.
• Metastatic evaluation includes the following:
  1. Chest CT
  2. Skeletal survey
  3. Bone scan
  4. Bilateral bone marrow aspirates and biopsies
  5. Cerebrospinal fluid cytology for parameningeal tumors
• No diagnostic laboratory test is available.
• Baseline complete blood count and chemistries, including renal and liver function tests, should be obtained.
• Pathology is as follows:
  1. Embryonal: more likely in GU sites and orbital sites, more common in younger children. Botryoid tumors are polypoid variants. A characteristic loss of heterozygosity is seen at 11p15.
  2. Alveolar masses are seen more often in extremity and trunk primaries and older patients. Characteristic chromosomal translocation occurs at t(2;13).

  3. Undifferentiated sarcomas express no lineage markers and are traditionally treated with rhabdomyosarcoma regimens.
• Staging is as follows:
  1. Stage 1 to 4 is determined by clinical and radiologic evaluation, based on location and size of primary, evidence of lymph node involvement, and presence or absence of metastases.
• Grouping for surgical assignment, based on extent of resection, is as follows:
  1. Group I: completely resected tumor
  2. Group II: microscopic residual, either at margins of tumor or in regional lymph nodes
  3. Group III: unresectable or incompletely resected tumor with gross residual
  4. Group IV: metastatic disease

💊 **THERAPY**

■ **MEDICAL**
• Chemotherapy includes the following:
  1. Vincristine and actinomycin D, with cyclophosphamide, administered for higher-risk disease.
  2. Other active agents include ifosfamide, VP-16, doxorubicin, and topotecan.
• Radiation therapy can be instituted for high-risk disease, including groups II, III, and IV and stages 2, 3, and 4.
• There may be a role for high-dose therapy with autologous peripheral blood stem cell rescue in metastatic or recurrent disease.

■ **SURGICAL**
Surgical resection should be performed if possible, but cosmetic result and function need to be considered in assessing resectability.

■ **PROGNOSIS**
• With current therapy, histology does not affect survival.
• Current studies demonstrate 65% survival at 5 years.
  1. Relapses after 5 years are rare.
• Patients with orbital or nonbladder, nonprostate GU tract tumors have the best outcome, with 80% to 84% survival at 5 years.
• Patients with metastatic disease continue to fare poorly, with 25% to 30% 5-year survival.

■ **FOLLOW-UP & DISPOSITION**
• CT or MRI of primary tumor site is generally performed every 3 months the first year off therapy, then repeated at increasing intervals. Also, surveillance chest CT scans and bone scans are performed.

- Late effects of radiation depend on radiation field but may include the following:
  1. Hypoplasia
  2. Linear growth impairment
  3. Bowel or bladder dysfunction
  4. Gonadal failure
  5. Second malignancies including skin, thyroid, brain, bone, and breast
- Late effects of chemotherapy are usually secondary to alkylating agents (cyclophosphamide or ifosfamide) and may include the following:
  1. Infertility
  2. Renal tubular dysfunction
  3. Secondary malignancies including leukemia and bladder cancer

■ PATIENT/FAMILY EDUCATION

In the case of advanced-stage disease, earlier detection would not necessarily have correlated with lower-stage disease.

■ REFERRAL INFORMATION

- Patients should be referred to pediatric specialists, including pediatric surgeons, pediatric oncologists, and pediatric radiation therapists.
- Patients should ideally be cared for at institutions that enroll patients in Intergroup Rhabdomyosarcoma Studies.

☼ PEARLS & CONSIDERATIONS

■ CLINICAL PEARLS

- Malignancy should be considered in the differential diagnosis of usually benign conditions such as epistaxis, chronic sinusitis or otitis, and persistent pain.
- Boys should be encouraged from an early age to report any change in testes.
- Patients at the highest risk for developing secondary malignancies are those with neurofibromatosis or a family history of cancer.

■ WEBSITES

- American Cancer Society: www.cancer.org
- National Cancer Institute: nci.nih.gov
- OncoLink: www.oncolink.com

■ SUPPORT GROUPS

- Pediatric oncologists can refer patients and parents to local or national support organizations for children with cancer and their families.
- National organizations include the American Cancer Society and Candlelighters.

REFERENCES

1. Crist WM, Kun LE: Common solid tumors of childhood, *N Engl J Med* 324:461, 1991.
2. Halperin EC et al: Rhabdomyosarcoma. In Halperin EC et al (eds): *Pediatric radiation oncology*, ed 3, Philadelphia, 1999, Lippincott Williams & Wilkins.
3. Wexler LH, Helman LJ: Rhabdomyosarcoma and the undifferentiated sarcomas. In Pizzo PA (eds): *Principles and practice of pediatric oncology*, Philadelphia, 2001, Lippincott Williams & Wilkins.

Author: **Andrea S. Hinkle, M.D.**

II

BASIC INFORMATION

■ **DEFINITION**

Rheumatic fever is an acute, noninfectious, inflammatory sequela to a virulent group A β-hemolytic streptococcal pharyngitis with joint, skin, subcutaneous, and cardiac symptoms appearing 2 to 3 weeks after infection. Neurologic symptoms of choreoathetosis are generally delayed by weeks to months.

ICD-9CM CODES

390 Acute rheumatic fever
391 Acute rheumatic fever with carditis
392 Rheumatic (Sydenham's) chorea

■ **ETIOLOGY**

- Follows group A β-hemolytic streptococcal pharyngitis
- Genetic component present
- Specific pathologic pathway unknown

■ **EPIDEMIOLOGY & DEMOGRAPHICS**

- Formerly epidemic in inner-city, crowded, lower-class neighborhoods
  1. Now sporadic, clinically milder, and more common in middle class, suburban, and rural areas
  2. Reasons for the change not known
- Formerly more severe
  1. Now with fewer joints involved, less severe carditis clinically, but more valve involvement by echocardiography
  2. Difficult to interpret these finding in view of the introduction of the echocardiogram

■ **HISTORY & PHYSICAL EXAMINATION**

Modified Jones criteria are used for the diagnosis.

- Major criteria
  1. Arthritis
     a. Abrupt onset of hot, red, swollen, very tender middle-sized joints
        (1) Elbows, wrists, knees, and ankles are involved.
        (2) Involvement of other joints is less common.
        (3) Typically, the arthritis is multiple and migratory: Individual joints resolve without residual in 24 hours as other joints are affected.
  2. Carditis
     a. Mitral valve involvement is most common.
        (1) Acute annular valvulitis with dilation leading to mitral insufficiency/regurgitation

        (2) Pansystolic, pure-toned, high-pitched murmur at the apex
        (3) Accentuated by maneuvers that increase systemic vascular resistance, such as hand grip, squat
        (4) Important not to confuse with normal vibratory (Still's) murmur (i.e., early and midsystolic; musical and low-pitched with multiple overtones; heard at the lower left sternal border)
     b. Aortic insufficiency is the second most common cardiac abnormality.
        (1) An early diastolic, high-pitched murmur
        (2) Metallic, echoing quality
        (3) Heard over midsternum and toward the apex (over the left ventricular cavity)
        (4) Important not to confuse with the diastolic component of a venous hum (i.e., more hollow; heard below the right clavicle; completely eradicated by maneuvers that affect venous inflow, such as change in head position, lying supine, jugular vein distention)
     c. Severe degrees of mitral and/or aortic regurgitation may lead to left-sided congestive heart failure.
     d. Tricuspid or pulmonic valve involvement is rare.
  3. Chorea
     a. A progressive increase in uncontrolled and uncontrollable writhing, choreiform movements
        (1) "St. Vitus Dance"
        (2) Particularly the extremities
        (3) Facial grimacing or truncal choreiform movements also seen
     b. Progressive clumsiness
     c. Irritability and mood swings
     d. Prolonged course of weeks to months
     e. Eventual resolution without neurologic residual
  4. Erythema marginatum
     a. Evanescent, reasonably symmetric, smoothly irregular rash
     b. Primarily over the trunk and proximal extremities
     c. Pale pink borders and clear centers
     d. Considered diagnostic for acute rheumatic fever
  5. Subcutaneous nodules
     a. Small, lentil-sized, nontender nodules beneath the skin
     b. Found on extensor surfaces of joints and occiput

        c. Considered diagnostic for acute rheumatic fever
- Minor criteria
  1. Arthralgia: similar to arthritis except without objective findings of inflammation
  2. Fever: moderate
  3. Family history: usually positive for another family member with acute rheumatic fever

🔬 **DIAGNOSIS**

- Laboratory data
  1. White blood cell (WBC) count: moderate elevation to 12,000 to 18,000 cells/mm^3, with little if any left shift
  2. Erythrocyte sedimentation rate (Westergren method) elevated
     a. Without carditis, 60 to 80 mm/hr
     b. With carditis, greater than 100 mm/hr
  3. Evidence of a preceding virulent streptococcal pharyngitis—required for diagnosis
     a. Elevated ASO titer and/or elevated streptozyme
     b. Elevated C-reactive protein
     c. Positive throat culture
     d. History, if convincing
     e. Positive culture in a sibling
- Electrocardiogram
  1. Tachycardia
  2. Loss of sinus arrhythmia with carditis
  3. Prolonged PR interval
     a. Indicative of vagus nerve involvement, not carditis
  4. Left atrial and/or left ventricular enlargement may be apparent
- Chest radiograph
  1. Usually normal
  2. If significant carditis, evidence of left atrial and left ventricular dilation
  3. May show pulmonary venous congestion
- Echocardiography
  1. Useful for confirming valve leak and assessing significance
  2. Left ventricular size
  3. Myocardial function
  4. Difficult to assess minimal degrees of valve dysfunction

■ **DIFFERENTIAL DIAGNOSIS**

- Rash
  1. Urticaria
  2. Viral exanthems
  3. Serum sickness
  4. Acute streptococcal infection
  5. Staphylococcal scalded skin syndrome
  6. Toxic shock syndrome
- Arthritis/arthralgias
  1. Septic joint
  2. Juvenile arthritis

3. Serum sickness
4. Any collagen vascular disease
- Cardiac finding
  1. Cardiomyopathy
  2. Myocarditis, endocarditis
  3. Congenital valve abnormalities

THERAPY

■ NONPHARMACOLOGIC

Bed rest, formerly considered essential, should probably be continued during the period of acute inflammation.
- Improves comfort of patients with arthritis
- Decreases cardiac demands in patients with carditis

■ MEDICAL

- A full therapeutic course of an antistreptococcal antibiotic should be administered to eradicate any remaining streptococci.
  1. Oral penicillin V
     a. Children: 250 mg two to three times daily for 10 days
     b. Adolescents and adults: 500 mg two to three times daily for 10 days
  2. Benzathine penicillin, one dose intramuscularly
     a. 600,000 units for children who weigh less than 60 pounds
     b. 1.2 million units for children who weigh more than 60 pounds
- Antiinflammatory therapy with aspirin 100 mg/kg/day, divided in four doses, may be given.
  1. This is adequate therapy for all except severe carditis.
  2. Therapy is continued until signs of active inflammation have disappeared.
  3. Decrease dosage if needed to avoid symptoms of abdominal pain or tinnitus.
- Patients with severe or life-threatening carditis and congestive heart failure should be treated with prednisone (2 mg/kg/day, divided in four doses) and conventional treatment for heart failure.

■ SURGICAL

- Intervention is rarely necessary during acute rheumatic fever.
- Intervention should be considered, however, if valve dysfunction is severe.

■ FOLLOW-UP & DISPOSITION

- All patients who have had acute rheumatic fever should receive antistreptococcal prophylaxis.
  1. No carditis with initial episode: prophylaxis for 5 years or until age 21 years

  2. Carditis with no residual heart disease: prophylaxis into adulthood or at least 10 years
     a. Both groups need careful throat culturing and treatment for any sore throat and fever.
  3. Carditis with residual heart disease: prophylaxis at least until age 40, possibly lifelong
- Choice of antistreptococcal prophylactic regimens:
  1. Intramuscular benzathine penicillin 1.2 million units monthly
     a. Excellent antistreptococcal protection
     b. Therapeutic for acquired infection
     c. Painful
  2. Oral penicillin V 250 mg twice daily
     a. Requires patient cooperation, difficult to enforce
     b. Well tolerated
  3. Penicillin-sensitive patients
     a. Sulfadiazine or sulfisoxazole daily
        (1) Children who weigh less than 60 pounds: 0.5 g
        (2) Children who weigh more than 60 pounds: 1.0 g
  4. Penicillin- and sulfa-sensitive patients
     a. Erythromycin 250 mg twice daily
- Antibacterial prophylaxis at times of possible bacteremia is needed in the presence of rheumatic heart disease.
  1. The drug chosen should be different from the prophylactic antistreptococcal agent.
- Careful attention to protection against infective endocarditis is needed for patients with residual rheumatic heart disease, and particularly for those who have required artificial valve implantation.
  1. Choose an antibiotic in conformity with the American Heart Association recommendations (see Part III).
  2. Drug should be different from that used for antistreptococcal prophylaxis.

■ PATIENT/FAMILY EDUCATION

- Patients with rheumatic arthritis and rheumatic chorea recover without residual.
  1. Patients remain susceptible to recurrences, particularly in first 3 years after initial episode.
  2. Patients should receive antistreptococcal prophylaxis during that time.
  3. Emphasize appropriate throat culturing and therapy for illnesses with fever and sore throat lifelong.

- Patients with rheumatic carditis may recover or have significant cardiac damage.
  1. Mitral valve regurgitation may progress to mitral valve stenosis.
  2. Aortic valve regurgitation may progress, uncommonly accompanied by aortic stenosis.
  3. Surgical repair or valve replacement may be needed.
  4. Cardiac damage is more severe with each recurrent episode.

■ PREVENTIVE TREATMENT

See "Follow-Up & Disposition" and "Patient/Family Education."

■ REFERRAL INFORMATION

Acute and long-term follow-up with a cardiologist is appropriate.

PEARLS & CONSIDERATIONS

■ CLINICAL PEARLS

- Normal sinus arrhythmia is lost during acute rheumatic carditis.
- Mitral regurgitation murmurs increase in intensity with isometric contraction, such as hand grip or squat.
- Aortic valve regurgitation is best heard over the sternum and the left ventricular cavity.
  1. Accentuated by leaning forward, by holding the breath in deep expiration, and by crouching on hands and knees
- A patient with rheumatic chorea has the following conditions:
  1. When told to raise the hands over the head, the patient will have the palms facing out, which is not seen normally.
  2. The patient demonstrates milkmaid's grip, a rhythmic squeezing of the fingers when grasping an object.
  3. Rheumatic chorea may be one-sided, a condition called *hemichorea.*
  4. Handwriting may deteriorate severely in rheumatic chorea.
  5. Choreiform movements may be brought out or intensified by intention, holding the hands with fingers spread and counting backward from 10 to 1.
  6. Chorea rarely occurs with the other manifestations of acute rheumatic fever.
- Acute rheumatic arthritis is extremely painful.
- Recurrent episodes of rheumatic fever are usually similar to the first (i.e., if there is carditis during the first episode, subsequent episodes are likely to have carditis as well).

II

- "Modern" rheumatic fever is significantly different, with less severe arthritis, fewer joints involved, and more common carditis if echocardiography findings are used as diagnostic.

■ **WEBSITE**

American Heart Association National Center: www.americanheart.org; look under Head and Stroke A-Z Guide: Rheumatic Heart Disease/Rheumatic Fever and Scientific Publications: AHA Scientific Statements: Treatment of Acute Streptococcal Pharyngitis and Prevention of Rheumatic Fever

REFERENCE

1. Park M: *Pediatric cardiology for practitioners,* ed 3, St Louis, 1996, Mosby.

Author: **Chloe Alexson, M.D.**

BASIC INFORMATION

■ DEFINITION
Failure in mineralization of growing bone or osteoid tissue with characteristic changes of the growth plate cartilage in children before closure of growth plate is referred to as *rickets*.

ICD-9CM CODE
268.0 Rickets

■ ETIOLOGY
- Abnormalities of vitamin D
  1. Deficiency: sunshine or nutritional deprivation, intestinal malabsorption, anticonvulsant drugs, chronic renal disease
  2. Metabolic defects: absence of renal 25-hydroxyvitamin D-1αhydroxylase, abnormal $1,25(OH)_2D$ receptor
- Deficiency of calcium
  1. Nutritional deprivation (in preterm infants)
  2. Malabsorption
  3. Excessive loss
     a. Hyperphosphaturia: familial hypophosphatemia, renal tubular acidosis, oncogenic
     b. Hypercalciuria
- Hypophosphatasia

■ EPIDEMIOLOGY & DEMOGRAPHICS
- Fortification of infant formulas and/or routine supplementation of infants with vitamin D has significantly decreased the incidence of rickets during the first 2 to 4 years of life.
- "At-risk" populations include the following:
  1. Unsupplemented exclusively breastfed infants for extensive periods
  2. Formula-fed infants in countries where infant milk is not supplemented with vitamin D
  3. Infants fed macrobiotic or strictly vegetarian diets
- Children with a higher risk of rickets include the following:
  1. Recent emigrants to industrial areas
  2. Those who have restricted outdoor activities or clothing that precludes sun exposure
  3. Poorly fed infants and children
  4. Those who escape regular medical surveys
  5. Those born to vitamin D–deficient mothers

■ HISTORY
- Osseous changes of rickets can be recognized after several months of vitamin D deficiency.
  1. Florid rickets can appear toward the end of the first and during the second year of life.

2. Later in childhood, manifest vitamin D deficiency rickets is rare.
- Muscular hypotonia, skeletal changes, and bone pain are the main features of vitamin D deficiency during infancy.

■ PHYSICAL EXAMINATION
- Early skeletal signs of rickets
  1. Rachitic rosary (palpable costochondral beading) and epiphyseal enlargement at the wrists, knees, and ankles—the most reliable signs of rickets
  2. Craniotabes (thinning of the outer table of the skull)
- Other signs (not specific)
  1. Large anterior fontanelle with delayed closure
  2. Delayed tooth eruption
- Signs of advanced rickets
  1. Deformities of the head with frontal bossing and parietal or occipital flattening
  2. Deformities of the chest
     a. Pigeon chest
     b. Harrison's groove
  3. Deformities of the spinal column and pelvis
     a. Scoliosis
     b. Kyphosis
     c. Lordosis
     d. Coxa vara
  4. Bowlegs or knock-knees and overextension of the knee joints (caused by relaxation of ligament)
- Other clinical signs
  1. Failure to thrive
  2. Delay in standing or walking

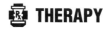

DIAGNOSIS

- Diagnosis based on a history of inadequate sunshine exposure and intake of vitamin D
  1. Often noted in African Americans or immigrant populations who are breastfeeding for prolonged periods
  2. Seen in cultures where extensive clothing cover precludes sun exposure
- Clinical observation
- Confirmed chemically and by roentgenographic examination

■ DIFFERENTIAL DIAGNOSIS
- Nonrachitic craniotabes: physiologic, hydrocephalus, osteogenesis imperfecta
- Enlargement of costochondral junction
  1. Scurvy
  2. Chondrodystrophy
- Epiphyseal lesions: congenital epiphyseal dysplasia, cytomegalic inclusion disease, syphilis, rubella, and copper deficiency

- Other metabolic disturbances with osseous lesions resembling rickets
  1. Hereditary or acquired hyperphosphaturia
  2. Hypophosphatasia
  3. Gastrointestinal malabsorption
  4. Renal diseases (primary renal tubular acidosis, type II proximal)

■ DIAGNOSTIC WORKUP
- Wrist radiograph: the distal ends of long bone
  1. Widened, cupped, and frayed
  2. Decreased shaft density
  3. Increased distance of distal ends to the metacarpal bones
- Serum minerals
  1. Normal or low serum calcium
  2. Low serum phosphorus (less than 4 mg/dl)
  3. Elevated serum alkaline phosphatase
  4. Serum 25-hydroxyvitamin D low in vitamin D deficiency but normal in metabolic disturbances of vitamin D metabolism

THERAPY

■ MEDICAL
- Cure of simple rickets: Daily doses of 400 to 800 IU/day (10 to 20 µg/day) vitamin D for 3 to 6 months result in the following:
  1. An increase of serum $25(OH)_2D$ and correction of calcium and phosphorus within 6 to 10 days
  2. Normalization of parathyroid hormone levels within 1 to 2 months
  3. Normalization of alkaline phosphatase activity
  4. Healing of radiologic signs of rickets within 3 to 6 months depending on the severity of the deficiency
- In countries where follow-up care is difficult, traditional 5 mg vitamin D single-day therapy repeated in 3 months could be given, but care should be taken to observe for hypercalcemia.
- Sufficient calcium for correction of the demineralization defect and to avoid the complication of hypocalcemia
  1. Children should have daily intakes of calcium of at least 1 g/day during the first months of treatment, via either dietary intake or oral calcium supplements.
  2. In children with very low serum calcium (less than 7.0 mg/dl), if large doses of vitamin D are given, calcium infusion may be needed from a few hours before the first administration of vitamin D, not to exceed daily total doses of 50

II

mg/kg/day, up to normalization of serum calcium, to avoid the occurrence of clinical signs of hypocalcemia.

■ FOLLOW-UP & DISPOSITION
- See "Therapy."
- If therapy is appropriate, healing begins within a few days and progresses slowly until normal bone structure is restored.
- Enlargement of the epiphyses of the long bones disappears only after months or years of treatment.
  1. Severe bowing of the legs may disappear within several years without osteotomies.
- In developing countries, intercurrent infections (i.e., pneumonia, tuberculosis, and enteritis) may cause death in rachitic children.

■ PREVENTIVE TREATMENT
- Regular sun exposure is the most physiologic way to prevent vitamin D deficiency.

- Food should be enriched with vitamin D to compensate for the lack of sun exposure during pregnancy and early life.
- "At-risk" infants who are exclusively breastfed or who live in countries where infant milk is not supplemented with vitamin D should be given daily vitamin D supplementation.
  1. Oral doses of vitamin D 400 IU/day, all year up to the age of 2 years
  2. During the winter up to 5 years
- Prevention of maternal vitamin D deficiency: Daily oral doses of vitamin D 400 IU/day during pregnancy is recommended.
- Prevention in preterm infants requires fortification of formula or human milk with calcium and phosphate (commercial mineral fortified formulas or milk fortifiers are available).

⚙ PEARLS & CONSIDERATIONS

■ CLINICAL PEARLS
- Rickets and osteopenia in preterm infants are usually unrelated to vitamin D deficiency.
  1. These conditions are related to calcium and phosphate deficiency.
  2. Phosphate deficiency is of particular concern in preterm infants who are fed human milk.

REFERENCES
1. Garabedian M, Ben-Mekhbi H: Rickets and vitamin D deficiency. In Holick MF (ed): *Vitamin D: physiology, molecular biology, and clinical applications,* Totowa, NJ, 1999, Humana Press.
2. Koo WWK, Tsang RC: Building better bones: calcium, magnesium, phosphorus, and vitamin D. In Tsang RC (ed): *Nutrition during infancy: principles and practice,* ed 2, Cincinnati, 1997, Digital Educational Publishing.
Authors: **Ran Namgung, M.D., Ph.D., and Reginald Tsang, M.B.B.C.**

BASIC INFORMATION

■ **DEFINITION**
Obstruction of outflow of blood from the right ventricle to the pulmonary artery, which occurs at the level of the pulmonary valve, the subpulmonic area (right ventricular outflow tract [RVOT] or infundibulum), or the supravalve or main pulmonary artery area or that which occurs in the branch pulmonary arteries, is referred to as *RVOT obstruction.*

■ **ICD-9CM CODES**
746.02 Pulmonary valve stenosis
746.02 Critical pulmonary valve stenosis/atresia
746.83 Infundibular or subvalve pulmonary stenosis
747.3   Supravalve pulmonary stenosis
747.3   Peripheral pulmonary artery stenosis, peripheral pulmonary stenosis

■ **SYNONYMS**
• Pulmonary artery stenosis
• Infundibular pulmonary stenosis
• Pulmonic (or pulmonary) valve stenosis
• Peripheral pulmonary stenosis (PPS)

■ **ETIOLOGY**
• In some instances, RVOT obstruction may be acquired or may develop in utero secondary to altered patterns of fetal blood flow.
• Subvalve obstruction is either hypertrophied infundibular muscle or isolated intraventricular muscle bands.
• A stenotic pulmonic valve may have a normal annulus diameter with commissural fusion of the leaflets, narrowing the orifice.
• In severe or "critical" neonatal pulmonic valve stenosis, the annulus may be hypoplastic and the valve leaflets thickened, dysplastic, and immobile, or the valve may be atretic with no opening.
• Supravalve pulmonary stenosis may be a localized narrowing of the artery or arteries or may be generalized hypoplasia of the distal pulmonary arterial tree.

■ **EPIDEMIOLOGY & DEMOGRAPHICS**
• RVOT obstruction is not commonly familial.
• PPS is part of Williams syndrome (infantile hypercalcemia syndrome) and is seen in Alagille's syndrome.
• RVOT obstruction may occur after some kinds of cardiac surgery (i.e., Norwood procedure).
• Occasionally, RVOT obstruction exists as an isolated anomaly.

• Infundibular pulmonary stenosis is uncommon as an isolated anomaly.
1. Part of tetralogy of Fallot
2. May be seen in severe pulmonary valve stenosis

■ **HISTORY**
• Neonatal "critical" or severe pulmonary valve stenosis or atresia
1. Presents shortly after birth with cyanosis secondary to right-to-left atrial shunt
2. Right-sided congestive heart failure
• Noncritical pulmonary valve stenosis
1. Murmur usually heard at birth or shortly thereafter
2. Rarely symptomatic
• Subvalve (infundibular) obstruction
1. Rarely occurs as isolated anomaly
• Supravalve pulmonary stenosis (main pulmonary artery stenosis)
1. Usually seen with recognizable syndromes such as Williams syndrome, congenital rubella syndrome
• PPS
1. Normal in newborns through approximately 8 months of age

■ **PHYSICAL EXAMINATION**
• Neonatal "critical" or severe pulmonary valve stenosis or atresia
1. Generalized cyanosis
2. Tachypnea without distress
3. Marked hepatomegaly
4. Peripheral edema: usually seen in periorbital area in infants
5. Peripheral pulses: normal unless cardiac output severely diminished
6. Cardiac examination
   a. May have ejection murmur in the pulmonic area
   b. May have murmur of tricuspid valve regurgitation
   c. May have continuous murmur of patent ductus arteriosus
   d. Ejection click uncommon in neonates
   e. Pulmonic component of second sound at base usually absent
• Noncritical pulmonary valve stenosis
1. Well-developed, well-nourished child
2. Wide atrioventricular oxygen difference: may give appearance of duskiness.
3. Normal peripheral pulses
4. Cardiac examination
   a. Ejection (crescendo-decrescendo) murmur can be heard at the upper left sternal border.
      (1) Murmur tends to increase in intensity and to peak later in systole as the severity of the obstruction increases.

   b. A prominent ejection click is heard unless the valve is significantly dysplastic.
   c. The pulmonic component of second sound at the base is delayed and diminished, sometimes absent.
• Subvalve (infundibular) obstruction
1. A systolic ejection murmur is heard in the mid to upper left sternal border; it peaks in midsystole.
2. No ejection click is audible.
3. The pulmonic component of second sound at base is usually normal.
• Supravalve pulmonary stenosis (main pulmonary artery stenosis)
1. An ejection murmur is heard high along the left sternal border and may be transmitted to lung fields.
2. No ejection click is audible.
3. The pulmonic component of second sound at base may be accentuated.
4. Assess for syndromes (e.g., Williams syndrome, congenital rubella)
• Peripheral pulmonary artery stenosis (branch pulmonary artery stenosis)
1. A physiologic murmur is often heard in infants.
2. Soft ejection murmurs, more prominent over lung fields, are heard.
3. Murmurs disappear by 8 months to 1 year of age.
4. Anatomic PPS has soft ejection murmurs over the lung fields.

🔬 **DIAGNOSIS**

■ **DIFFERENTIAL DIAGNOSIS**
• Careful attention to location and characteristics helps differentiate pulmonary stenosis from other systolic murmurs.
• Aortic stenosis murmur is heard at the mid-left sternal border and aortic area.
• Ventricular septal defect murmur is heard at the lower left sternal border; it is harsh and pansystolic.
• These murmurs are rarely confused with mitral regurgitant or tricuspid regurgitant murmurs because the location is wrong.
• Shunting defects (atrial septal defect) have soft flow murmur rather than true ejection.

■ **DIAGNOSTIC WORKUP**
• Neonatal "critical" or severe pulmonary valve stenosis or atresia
1. Electrocardiogram
   a. Variable findings
   b. May show either right ventric-

ular hypertrophy or less than expected right ventricular forces
  c. May show right atrial hypertrophy P_{II} less than 3 mm
2. Chest radiograph
  a. Marked cardiomegaly
  b. Prominent right atrium
  c. Diminished pulmonary blood flow
3. Echocardiogram
  a. Identifies site of obstruction
  b. Size of pulmonary annulus
  c. Gradient across valve
  d. Right ventricular size
  e. Right and left ventricular function elucidated
  f. Atrial shunt (via foramen ovale or atrial septal defect) and direction of flow across the atrial septum
  g. Identifies abnormal coronary artery communications with right ventricle
4. Cardiac catheterization and angiocardiography
  a. Should be delayed until response to prostaglandin infusion
  b. May not be indicated unless to be combined with balloon valvuloplasty
  c. If done, gives specific anatomic details
- Noncritical pulmonary valve stenosis
1. Electrocardiogram
  a. Right ventricular hypertrophy
    (1) Increases with increasing right ventricular hypertension, increasing degrees of obstruction
2. Chest radiograph
  a. Normal heart size
  b. Prominent pulmonary artery segment reflecting poststenotic dilation
  c. Normal pulmonary blood flow, although the pulmonary artery branches are not prominent
  d. Apex possibly rounded and uptilted off the diaphragm
3. Echocardiogram
  a. Localizes obstruction
  b. Estimation of gradient
  c. Nature of valve leaflets (e.g., thin, mobile, doming)
  d. Size and function of right ventricle
4. Cardiac catheterization and angiocardiography
  a. Not necessary in mild pulmonic stenosis
  b. Noninvasive methods give adequate data
  c. Gives specific anatomic data, gradient, annulus size
  d. May be combined with balloon valvuloplasty

- Subvalve (infundibular) obstruction
1. Electrocardiogram, chest roentgenogram, echocardiogram, catheterization, and angiography per primary diagnosis (e.g., tetralogy of Fallot)
- PPS
1. Electrocardiogram, chest roentgenogram, echocardiogram, cardiac catheterization, and angiography same as pulmonary valve stenosis; localization of obstruction may be difficult

⊞ THERAPY

■ NONPHARMACOLOGIC
- Noncritical PS
1. Routine follow-up with mild degrees of obstruction
  a. No activity restriction needed
  b. No need for antibiotic prophylaxis at times of bacteremia (generally accepted)

■ MEDICAL
- Neonatal "critical" or severe pulmonary valve stenosis or atresia
1. Immediate prostaglandin infusion
  a. Reopens ductus arteriosus
  b. Increases pulmonary blood flow
  c. Continue after surgery
- Supravalve pulmonary stenosis (main pulmonary artery stenosis)
1. Treatment should be as for primary diagnosis.

■ SURGICAL
- Neonatal "critical" or severe pulmonary valve stenosis or atresia
1. Balloon valvuloplasty for some infants—individualized therapy
  a. Tricuspid annulus may be too small.
  b. Pulmonic annulus may be too small.
  c. Pulmonary valve may be too thick and dysplastic to tear.
  d. Right ventricular chamber may be too small for adequate function.
2. Surgical pulmonary valvotomy/valvectomy and/or RVOT reconstruction
3. Systemic-pulmonary anastomosis: may be the most reasonable procedure, followed by direct approach to the RVOT
- Noncritical pulmonary valve stenosis
1. More severe obstruction—definitive therapy with balloon valvuloplasty or surgical valvotomy
2. Repeat balloon dilation occasionally necessary

3. Repeat surgical valvotomy rarely necessary
- Supravalve pulmonary stenosis (main pulmonary artery stenosis)
1. May be amenable to balloon dilation and stenting
2. Surgery delayed until obstruction severe, but some not repairable
- Peripheral pulmonary artery stenosis (branch pulmonary artery stenosis)
1. Difficult; most not amenable to surgical repair
2. Stenting possible in some

■ FOLLOW-UP & DISPOSITION
- Neonatal "critical" or severe pulmonary valve stenosis or atresia
1. Long term may recur
  a. May need further relief of obstruction
  b. May need pulmonary valve insertion
    (1) Less likely with more cosmetic approach to RVOT in neonatal period
- Noncritical pulmonary valve stenosis
1. Follow-up for possible restenosis
2. No need for activity restriction
3. No need for antibiotic prophylaxis at times of bacteremia beginning 6 months after procedure (generally accepted)

■ PATIENT/FAMILY EDUCATION
- The prognosis for valve pulmonic stenosis after balloon valvuloplasty or surgery is excellent.
- The need for repeat repair is not common if the initial repair was done after early infancy.
- The prognosis is less favorable if nonvalve obstruction.
1. Depends on associated defects and anatomy
- Antibiotic prophylaxis at times of possible bacteremia is not usually recommended for valve stenosis; all others require prophylaxis.
- Activity restriction depends on adequacy of relief of RVOT obstruction.

☼ PEARLS & CONSIDERATIONS

■ CLINICAL PEARLS
- The later the peak in the murmur, the more severe the obstruction.
- An ejection click means a thin, mobile valve.
- Physical growth is excellent with pulmonic stenosis.
- A wide atrioventricular oxygen difference may mimic cyanosis.
- Ejection murmurs are crescendo-decrescendo.
- Regurgitant murmurs are pansystolic and constant.

- The location of the murmur is critical for differentiating etiology.
  1. Pulmonic valve upper left sternal border
  2. Infundibular pulmonary stenosis, mid-upper left sternal border
  3. Supravalve pulmonary stenosis

high left sternal border, lung fields

■ WEBSITE

American Heart Association National Center: www.americanheart.org/children

REFERENCE

1. Park M: *Pediatric cardiology for practitioners,* ed 3, St Louis, 1996, Mosby.

Author: **Chloe Alexson, M.D.**

II

BASIC INFORMATION

■ DEFINITION
Rocky Mountain spotted fever (RMSF) is an infection caused by *Rickettsia rickettsii*. RMSF is the most common rickettsial illness in the United States; it is a multisystem disease with significant mortality if untreated.

ICD-9CM CODE
082.0 Rocky Mountain spotted fever

■ ETIOLOGY
R. rickettsii—a small gram-negative obligately intracellular bacterium

■ EPIDEMIOLOGY & DEMOGRAPHICS
- Ticks are both the vector and the reservoir in nature (dog tick, *Dermacentor variabilis,* in eastern two thirds and western coast of United States; wood tick, *D. andersoni,* in Rocky Mountain states; other ticks in Mexico, Central and South America).
- Modes of transmission are as follows:
  1. Tick bites, with transmission from tick salivary glands after at least 6 to 10 hours of attachment
  2. Rare transmission by direct contact with tick fluid during removal
- RMSF is strongly seasonal.
  1. Approximately 90% of cases occur between April and September.
  2. Approximately 10% of cases are sporadic year-round.
  3. About 600 cases per year are reported in the United States (the true number is likely higher).
- RMSF is strongly geographic.
  1. It was once most common in Rocky Mountain states; now, most U.S. cases occur in Oklahoma, North Carolina, Virginia, Missouri, and Arkansas.
  2. Case distribution may be focal—restriction to small "islands" or "hot spots" in some rural counties or even urban neighborhoods is well documented.
- Roughly two thirds of reported cases in the United States are in children younger than 15 years of age.
  1. Peak incidence is between 5 and 9 years of age.
- Risk groups for infection include the following:
  1. Age 5 to 9 years
  2. Exposure to wooded areas with high grass
  3. Exposure to dogs with ticks
  4. Residence in or travel to known endemic areas during April to September
  5. Slight predominance among males, Caucasians

- Risk factors for fatal outcome include the following:
  1. African Americans with glucose-6-phosphate dehydrogenase deficiency
  2. Delay in treatment beyond fifth day of illness
  3. Atypical symptoms
     a. Lack of history of tick bite
     b. Late-appearing or negligible rash (spotless fever)
     c. Prominent gastrointestinal symptoms suggesting alternative diagnosis
  4. Age older than 40 years

■ HISTORY
- There are risk factors for exposure, as discussed previously (residence in or travel to endemic area, dog exposure, tick bite [50% to 60%]).
- Most common initial presentation is as follows:
  1. Fever, commonly higher than 38.9° C (70% to 80%)
  2. Severe headache (80% to 90%)
  3. Myalgia (80%)
  4. Nausea (50%)
  5. Rash (develops after 2 to 3 days)
- "Classic triad" of fever, rash, and history of tick bite eventually evident in 60% to 70% of cases, but only in 3% to 18% of cases at the initial physician visit—history (and physical examination) must be repeated serially.
- Incubation period is 2 to 14 days after tick bite, with a mean of 7 days.

■ PHYSICAL EXAMINATION
- Fever: nearly uniformly present after third day
- Rash
  1. Appears after 2 to 3 days
     a. On day 1: 14% of patients
     b. By day 3: 42% of patients
     c. By day 6: 80% to 95% of patients
  2. Begins as blanching, erythematous, 1- to 4-mm macules on ankles and wrists, moving inward to trunk; palms and soles involved in 50% to 80%; within a few days, macules progress to maculopapules and then nonblanching petechiae
  3. Rash less likely to be recognized or present in African Americans and in older men
- Later complications as disease progresses
  1. Widespread vasculitis, edema; may progress to skin necrosis
  2. Encephalitis (25% to 30%): confusion, lethargy or stupor, delirium, coma, cerebrospinal fluid lymphocytic pleocytosis
  3. Noncardiogenic pulmonary edema, adult respiratory distress syndrome (10% to 20%)

  4. Cardiac arrhythmia
  5. Coagulopathy, gastrointestinal hemorrhage
  6. Anemia
- Death: usually occurs at 8 to 15 days after onset if no treatment is given or if treatment is begun too late

DIAGNOSIS

■ DIFFERENTIAL DIAGNOSIS
- In the early stages of RMSF
  1. Enteroviral infection
  2. Infectious mononucleosis
  3. Scarlet fever
  4. Ehrlichiosis
  5. Gastroenteritis
  6. Acute abdomen
  7. Leptospirosis
  8. If late in the year, influenza a possibility
- After 3 to 5 days
  1. Meningococcemia
  2. Measles
  3. Kawasaki syndrome
  4. Ehrlichiosis
  5. Other rickettsial infection (e.g., murine typhus)
  6. Immune complex vasculitis
  7. Thrombotic thrombocytopenic purpura

■ DIAGNOSTIC WORKUP
- Diagnosis is based on history and physical examination.
  1. Culture is not routinely available.
  2. Serologic tests become positive only after 7 to 10 days of illness, after the time at which treatment should be begun.
- Common nonspecific laboratory abnormalities include the following:
  1. Thrombocytopenia (less than 150,000/µl in 67% of cases)
  2. Normal white blood cell count with left shift
  3. Hyponatremia (less than 134 mEq/L in 50% to 80%)
  4. Elevated transaminases
- Specific diagnostic tests are as follows:
  1. Standard assay is indirect immunofluorescent antibody titer (IFA) in serum, with sensitivity of 94% to 100% and specificity approaching 100%.
  2. Titers of more than 1:64 are usually detectable after 7 to 10 days of illness.
  3. A fourfold rise in IFA antibody titer in paired acute and convalescent samples, or a single titer of more than 1:64 in the presence of a compatible illness is diagnostic.
- Other antibody tests are available but less standardized or perform less well (e.g., latex agglutination, enzyme im-

munoassay, polymerase chain reaction assay).
1. None reveal antibodies earlier than the IFA test.
2. The classic Weil-Felix agglutination titers have poor sensitivity and specificity (less than 70% to 80%) and are no longer suggested for use.
- Direct immunofluorescence staining of vascular endothelium in skin-punch biopsies for detection of *R. rickettsii* is 70% to 90% sensitive and very specific, but it is useful only in patients with rash. In addition, the time spent obtaining a proper specimen and shipping it to one of the few reliable laboratories capable of correctly performing this assay often precludes its theoretical advantage of rapid diagnosis.

THERAPY

■ MEDICAL
- Empiric antimicrobial therapy for RMSF is necessary because delaying treatment until confirmation of the diagnosis can lead to death.
- The only drugs proven to be effective in the treatment of RMSF are tetracyclines (including doxycycline) and chloramphenicol.
  1. Chloramphenicol toxicities include dose-related bone marrow suppression, idiosyncratic aplastic anemia, and the need to monitor drug levels to avoid "gray-baby syndrome" in ill children who may have decreased hepatic function. In addition, oral chloramphenicol is no longer available in the United States.
  2. Doxycycline is associated with much less staining of the teeth of children younger than 8 years of age than are other tetracyclines, and tooth staining is now believed to be a consequence of frequently repeated longer courses of therapy than would be required for RMSF treatment. Doxycycline is also the drug of choice for ehrlichiosis, which may be a diagnostic consideration in patients thought to have RMSF.

3. *Hence, doxycycline is the drug of choice for RMSF even in children younger than 8 years of age.* Parents should be informed of the small, theoretical risk of tooth staining with doxycycline therapy compared with the greater risk of fatal RMSF if therapy is not provided.
- Doxycycline dosage is 4 mg/kg/day in two divided doses, up to a maximum of 100 mg two times per day (may be administered orally or, if seriously ill, intravenously).
- Therapy is recommended for 7 days or until patient is afebrile for more than 2 days (whichever is longer).

■ PREVENTIVE TREATMENT & PATIENT/FAMILY EDUCATION
- Careful checking for ticks and removal of entire tick without crushing may prevent RMSF transmission.
- Wearing long clothing, applying insect repellent when outdoors, and spraying tick repellent on pet dogs are also appropriate preventive measures.
- Even in endemic areas, most ticks are not infected with rickettsia, so prophylactic antibiotics are not indicated for asymptomatic individuals after a bite.
- No vaccine is available.

PEARLS & CONSIDERATIONS

■ CLINICAL PEARLS
- Rocky Mountain "spotless fever" or "near spotless" or "abortive" fever is rarely observed (less than 5% to 10% of cases of RMSF). Some of these cases have been even harder to diagnose because of the prominence of less typical symptoms (e.g., encephalitis, acute abdomen).
- If a child from the southeastern or south-central United States (e.g., Oklahoma, Arkansas, Missouri, North Carolina, South Carolina, Virginia) develops an RMSF-like illness characterized by few or no macular lesions, rare to absent petechiae, and relatively more prominent leukope-

nia, ehrlichiosis may actually be the cause. *Ehrlichia* are rickettsia-like bacteria that are transmitted either by the bite of the Lone Star tick, *Amblyomma americanum,* or the deer tick, *Ixodes scapularis* (the Lyme disease tick), depending on the *Ehrlichia* species and region of the country. Fortunately, doxycycline treats both RMSF and ehrlichiosis.
- *Borrelia burgdorferi* (the Lyme disease spirochete) and *Ehrlichia* can coinfect the same deer tick and thus cause dual human infections. Lyme disease is not transmitted by ticks that carry *R. rickettsi.*
- Long-term sequelae of survivors of severe RMSF are common, including gangrene and loss of limbs; impaired hearing, motor, and intellectual function; and incontinence.

■ WEBSITE
Centers for Disease Control and Prevention: www.cdc.gov/health/diseases.htm

REFERENCES
1. American Academy of Pediatrics: Rocky Mountain spotted fever. In Pickering LK (ed): *2000 Red Book: report of the Committee on Infectious Diseases,* ed 25, Elk Grove Village, Ill, 2000, American Academy of Pediatrics.
2. Lochary ME, Lockhart PB, Williams WT Jr: Doxycycline and staining of permanent teeth, *Pediatr Infect Dis J* 17:429, 1998.
3. Thorner AR, Walker DH, Petri WA Jr: Rocky Mountain spotted fever, *Clin Infect Dis* 27:1353, 1998.
4. Walker DH: Rocky Mountain spotted fever: a seasonal alert, *Clin Infect Dis* 20:1111, 1995.
5. Walker DH, Raoult D: *Rickettsia rickettsi* and other spotted fever group rickettsiae (Rocky Mountain spotted fever and other spotted fevers). In Mandell GL, Bennett JE, Dolin R (eds): *Mandell, Douglas, and Bennett's principles and practice of infectious diseases,* ed 5, Philadelphia, 2000, Churchill Livingstone.

Author: **Geoffrey A. Weinberg, M.D.**

II

BASIC INFORMATION

■ DEFINITION

Impingement of the shoulder is classically defined as an obstruction of the subacromial outlet space, anatomically defined by the coracoacromial arch above and upper humerus below, which results in irritation of the supraspinatus tendon. Current classifications divide impingement syndrome into the following three categories: external (subacromial), primary and secondary, and internal (glenoid).

■ SYNONYM

Shoulder impingement syndrome

ICD-9CM CODE

726.1 Rotator cuff syndrome

■ ETIOLOGY

- Primary external (subacromial) category: This is seen in patients older than 35 years. Pathologic mechanisms secondary to aging compromise the subacromial space.
- Secondary external (subacromial) category: This is impingement secondary to anterior instability (chronic stresses from overhead motions change the static anterior stabilizers of the shoulder and subsequently fatigue the dynamic muscle stabilizers). The progressive forward movement of the humeral head compromises the subacromial space outlet.
- Internal (glenoid) category: This results from repetitive microtrauma to the undersurface of the tendon, impinging on the posterior superior part of the glenoid; it is seen mostly in late cocking stage of throwing. Sometimes it is associated with anterior instability.

■ EPIDEMIOLOGY & DEMOGRAPHICS

- Athletes whose sport involves repetitive overhead motions (e.g., baseball pitch, tennis serve, volleyball serve, swimming strokes) commonly exhibit this condition.
- Adolescent athletes mainly exhibit secondary external impingement problems.

■ HISTORY

- Exacerbation of pain with overhead throwing motions may be associated with weakness, stiffness, or loss of range of motion.
- Pain at night associated with lying on shoulder is *not* commonly reported with secondary impingement.
- "Dead arm" syndrome (arm heaviness without neurologic deficits) is associated with instability and hence possible secondary impingement.

■ PHYSICAL EXAMINATION

- Inspection
  1. Shoulder asymmetry or bony abnormalities from the following:
     a. Acromioclavicular (AC) separations
     b. Shoulder dislocations
     c. Clavicular fractures
- Palpation
  1. AC joint for separation
  2. Biceps tendon and supraspinatus tendon for tendinitis
  3. Clavicle for fractures
  4. Anterior acromial, coracoid, or coracoacromial ligament tenderness: indicates possible impingement problems
- Range of motion, active and passive
  1. Complete forward flexion
  2. External rotation with arm at side and at 90 degrees abduction
  3. Internal rotation
  4. Painful arc between 70 and 120 degrees abduction: indicates some type of impingement
- Provocative testing for impingement
  1. Neer test: Standing behind or beside the patient, the patient's arm is passively elevated (forward flexion) while stabilizing the scapula with downward digital pressure on the coracoacromial arch. A positive test demonstrates pain with increasing arm elevation.
  2. Hawkins/Kennedy test (may be more accurate): Passively elevate (forward flex) the arm to 90 degrees in adduction, then forcibly internally rotate the humerus. A positive test elicits pain.
  3. Impingement is likely if either of these tests is positive.

� DIAGNOSIS

■ DIFFERENTIAL DIAGNOSIS

- Anterior subluxation of the shoulder
- AC joint separation
- Suprascapular nerve injury
- Traumatic tendinitis
- Cervical spine pathology

■ DIAGNOSTIC WORKUP

- The workup is based on clinical grounds with suggestive history and physical examination, as described previously.
- Plain radiographs are not helpful in secondary impingement. If obtained, anteroposterior, outlet Y, and axillary views are recommended and will delineate any anatomic variant or calcific deposits.

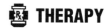 **THERAPY**

■ NONPHARMACOLOGIC

- Relieve inflammation by restricting aggravating activities.
- It is very important to maintain range of motion through passive range-of-motion exercises performed below the shoulder level.
- Once inflammation has subsided, a *supervised* strengthening and stretching program for the rotator cuff and periscapular muscles should be started.
- In the latter stages of rehabilitation, a sport-specific interval return program may be used to gradually transition the athlete to full participation with no restrictions.

■ MEDICAL

- Nonsteroidal antiinflammatory drugs can be used to help alleviate initial pain and inflammation.
- Subacromial steroid injections are controversial and should be used with caution because intratendonous injections and chronic steroid exposure can be deleterious to the tendon.

■ SURGICAL

In general, surgery is not considered until a supervised rehabilitation program has been attempted for 3 to 6 months or increased pain and decreased function occurs after 2 months of rehabilitation.

■ FOLLOW-UP & DISPOSITION

Conservative therapy as outlined earlier in a supervised rehabilitation program should be followed for 6 months before failure can be considered.

■ PATIENT/FAMILY EDUCATION

- Impingement responds to conservative therapy in about 80% of cases.
- Secondary external impingement can be self-limited.

■ PREVENTIVE TREATMENT

- Stretching before activities
- Maintaining strength of rotator cuff and periscapular muscles
- Gradual increase in intensity and frequency of activity to minimize injury or reinjury

■ REFERRAL INFORMATION

Sports medicine specialist, physical therapist, orthopedic surgeon if surgery is indicated

☼ PEARLS & CONSIDERATIONS

■ CLINICAL PEARLS
- Most adolescent athletes whose sport involves an overhead motion exhibit *secondary external* type impingement with rotator cuff syndrome.
  1. Rotator cuff tears are seen in more advanced impingement problems and occur mostly in adults older than 35 years.
- Signs and symptoms of biceps tendinitis are usually secondary to the impingement syndrome and are not a separate diagnosis.
- Cervical spine pathology must be ruled out with chief complaints of shoulder pain.

■ WEBSITE
Sportsrehab.com: www.sportsrehab. com; includes numerous links to sports medicine–related sites

REFERENCES
1. Butters KP, Rockwood CA Jr: Office evaluation and management of the shoulder impingement syndrome, *Orthoped Clin North Am* 19:755, 1998.
2. Cavallo RJ, Speer KP: Shoulder instability and impingement in throwing athletes, *Med Sci Sports Exercise* 30: S18, 1998.
3. Fongemie AE, Buss DD, Rolnick SJ: Management of shoulder impingement syndrome and rotator cuff tears, *Am Fam Physician* 57:667, 1998.
4. Lyons PM, Orwin JF: Rotator cuff tendinopathy and subacromial impingement syndrome, *Med Sci Sports Exercise* 30:S12, 1998.

Author: **Sharon Chen, M.D.**

II

BASIC INFORMATION

■ **DEFINITION**
Rubella is a mild disease characterized by a rash, generalized lymphadenopathy, and fever. Congenital rubella syndrome consists of anomalies of ophthalmologic, cardiac, auditory, and neurologic systems.

■ **SYNONYMS**
• Three-day measles
• German measles

ICD-9CM CODES
056.9 Rubella without mention of complication
771.0 Congenital rubella

■ **ETIOLOGY**
An RNA virus classified as a Rubivirus of the Togaviridae family

■ **EPIDEMIOLOGY & DEMOGRAPHICS**
• In the prevaccine era, rubella circulated in an epidemic pattern of 6- to 9-year cycles.
• The last pandemic period in the United States was in 1964.
• The virus is transmitted by droplet secretions or direct contact with infected human or contaminated fomite.
• The peak incidence is in late winter and early spring.
• Approximately 25% to 50% of infections are asymptomatic.
• Maximum infectivity occurs from 5 days before and continues for 5 to 6 days after rash starts.
• The incidence has decreased by 99% from prevaccine era (vaccination started in 1966-1968).
• The incubation period for postnatal rubella is 14 to 21 days, usually 16 to 18 days.
• The attack rate was highest in 5- to 9-year-olds.
• The incidence is high in preschool children.

■ **HISTORY**
Immunization status

■ **PHYSICAL EXAMINATION**
• Postnatal illness
  1. Prodromal complaints of malaise, fevers (rarely last beyond first day of rash), anorexia for a few days
  2. Rash: erythematous, maculopapular; starts on face with centrifugal spread toward hands and feet
    a. Involves entire body during first day, begins to fade the next day, and lasts 3 to 5 days

3. Lymphadenopathy (suboccipital, postauricular, and cervical): precedes exanthem and may last several weeks
4. Complications may include the following:
  a. Arthritis, arthralgia
  b. Encephalitis
  c. Thrombocytopenia
  d. Rarely myocarditis and pericarditis
• Congenital rubella
  1. This disease occurs as a result of in utero infection during the first trimester of pregnancy.
  2. Fetal infection may be subacute, chronic, or may result in abortion, stillbirth, or malformations.
  3. Congenital anomalies include the following:
    a. Auditory: sensorineural deafness
    b. Cardiac: patent ductus arteriosus, peripheral pulmonary artery stenosis
    c. Neurologic: behavioral problems, meningoencephalitis, mental retardation
    d. Ophthalmologic: cataracts, retinopathy, congenital glaucoma

🔬 **DIAGNOSIS**

■ **DIFFERENTIAL DIAGNOSIS**
• Febrile illness with rash
  1. Measles
  2. Toxoplasmosis
  3. Scarlet fever
  4. Roseola
  5. Parvovirus B19 (fifth disease)
  6. Adenoviruses
  7. Enteroviruses
  8. Other common respiratory viruses

■ **DIAGNOSTIC WORKUP**
• Cell culture: Virus can be isolated from throat, blood, urine, or cerebrospinal fluid
  1. Laboratory technicians need to know to look for rubella virus (not done routinely now).
• Acute and convalescent serology by enzyme immunoassay and latex agglutination assays for group A rubella virus antigen detection
  1. A fourfold or greater rise in titer or seroconversion is diagnostic.
• Rubella-specific immunoglobulin M (IgM) antibody testing is available.
  1. Useful in babies with intrauterine growth retardation and nonimmune mothers

2. Mothers with suspected rubella during pregnancy

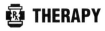 **THERAPY**

• No specific therapy is available.
• Symptomatic therapy is indicated.

■ **PATIENT/FAMILY EDUCATION**
• Immune status should be assessed in early pregnancy.
• Seronegative pregnant women should be immunized in postpartum period.

■ **PREVENTIVE TREATMENT**
• Live-virus rubella immunization (RA 27/3 strain) is usually combined with measles and mumps vaccines (MMR).
• Serum rubella antibody develops in 95% after a first dose at 12 months of age or older.
• Two doses of measles vaccine are now recommended.
  1. Second dose should be given at 4 to 6 years and no later than 11 to 12 years of age.

🔆 **PEARLS & CONSIDERATIONS**

■ **CLINICAL PEARLS**
• Rubella is now rare in immunized children: Think of it in underimmunized and older populations.
• Rubella is the third childhood febrile exanthem. (Measles and scarlet fever are first and second, respectively.)

■ **WEBSITES**
• Centers for Disease Control and Prevention: www.cdc.gov
• Yahoo!: dir.yahoo.com/Health/ Diseases_and_Conditions/Rubella

REFERENCES
1. American Academy of Pediatrics: Rubella. In Pickering LK (ed): *2000 Red Book: report of the Committee on Infectious Diseases,* ed 25, Elk Grove Village, Ill, 2000, American Academy of Pediatrics.
2. Centers for Disease Control and Prevention: Rubella among Hispanic adults—Kansas, 1998 and Nebraska, 1999, *MMWR Morb Mortal Wkly Rep* 49:225, 2000.
3. Cherry JD: Rubella virus. In Feigin RD, Cherry JD (eds): *Textbook of pediatric infectious diseases,* ed 4, Philadelphia, 1998, WB Saunders.
Author: **Cynthia Christy, M.D.**

BASIC INFORMATION

DEFINITION
Typhoid fever is a bacteremic, febrile illness that can result in chronic carriage, self-limited illness, shock, or death. Nontyphoidal *Salmonella* causes gastroenteritis and locally invasive infections.

SYNONYM
Enteric fever

ICD-9CM CODES
003.9 Salmonella
002.0 Typhoid

ETIOLOGY
- Salmonella are non–spore-forming, motile, usually non–lactose-fermenting gram-negative rods.
- Bacteria invade the intestinal wall; fecal leukocytes are present.
- A cholera-like enterotoxin causes secretory diarrhea.
- Bacteremia leads to sepsis, typhoid fever, or focal invasive infections in 10% (e.g., meningitis, osteomyelitis, suppurative arthritis, urinary tract infection, pericarditis, peritonitis, pneumonia, empyema).
- Typhoid fever (usually *Salmonella typhi* and several other *Salmonella* serotypes) presents with gradual-onset fever, constitutional symptoms, abdominal pain, hepatomegaly, splenomegaly, rose spots, altered mental status, shock, and coma.

EPIDEMIOLOGY & DEMOGRAPHICS
- Incidence
  1. Nontyphoidal: 50,000 cases per year in the United States
  2. Typhoid fever: fewer than 500 cases per year in the United States (usually foreign travelers)
- Peak incidence
  1. Infants (younger than 12 months) and children younger than 5 years, adults older than 70 years
  2. Higher incidence in warmer months
- Transmission
  1. Nontyphoidal: contaminated food (especially poultry, red meat, raw eggs, dairy) or contact with infected reptiles, pets, or human carriers; occurs in outbreaks
  2. Typhoid fever: no animal reservoir; transmission by food or water contaminated with human feces
- Carriage
  1. Bacteria is excreted in stool for a mean of 5 weeks, up to 1 year (longer in children younger than 5 years).
  2. Chronic carriers (excretion for more than 1 year) often have gallbladder disease.

- Incubation
  1. Gastroenteritis: 6 to 72 hours (mean 24 hours)
  2. Typhoid fever: 3 to 60 days (usually, 7 to 14 days)

HISTORY
- Ill contacts, geographic location, season, travel, child care, breastfeeding (protective)
- Risk factors
  1. Decreased acid production (neonates and children taking antacids)
  2. Impaired cellular immunity (chronic granulomatous disease, hemoglobinopathy, cancer, immunosuppressive therapy, human immunodeficiency virus [HIV])
  3. Sickle cell disease (osteomyelitis)
  4. Age younger than 12 months
  5. Concurrent infections (malaria, schistosomiasis, bartonellosis)
- Gastroenteritis
  1. Potential contaminated foods or water
  2. Travel
  3. Fever
  4. Nausea, vomiting, and diarrhea (with blood and mucus)
  5. Abdominal pain, cramps, and tenderness
- Typhoid fever
  1. Travel outside the United States or household contact with carrier
  2. Constipation early in the illness; fever, constitutional symptoms, abdominal pain
  3. Altered mental status (can progress to lethargy or nonresponsiveness)
- Focal infection
  1. Previous anatomic abnormalities or in areas of trauma are typical sites.

PHYSICAL EXAMINATION
- Fever, elevated heart rate, assess blood pressure
- Abdominal tenderness without discrete mass
- Hepatosplenomegaly
- Rose spots
- Altered mental status

DIAGNOSIS

DIFFERENTIAL DIAGNOSIS
- Viral: rotavirus, astrovirus, adenovirus, caliciviruses (Norwalk agent), hepatitis A
- Bacterial: *Campylobacter, Shigella, Escherichia coli,* staphylococcal food poisoning, *Vibrio* species, *Yersinia*
- Parasitic: *Giardia, Cryptosporidia,* others
- Other: antibiotic-associated colitis, chemical colitis

DIAGNOSTIC WORKUP
- Culture of *Salmonella* from stool, blood, urine, or foci of infection is diagnostic.
- Serologic tests are not recommended (high false-positive and false-negative rates).
- Fecal leukocytes are usually present (often mononuclear cells with *S. typhi*).
- Serotyping is important in outbreak evaluation: A through E cause human disease; *S. typhi* is group D.
- Blood culture should be obtained for all febrile or toxic-appearing patients.

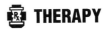 THERAPY

NONPHARMACOLOGIC
- Rehydration and electrolyte management are the mainstays of therapy.
- Lactobacillus preparations may help decrease pH and bacterial growth (evidence-based studies not available).
- Hospitalize patients with "toxic" appearance, severe dehydration, or grossly bloody stools, or if immunocompromised.

MEDICAL
- Noninvasive disease
  1. Antibiotics are *not recommended* for noninvasive gastroenteritis because they may prolong the carrier state.
  2. Antibiotics are recommended for patients younger than 3 months old and those with immunocompromise, chronic gastrointestinal disease, or hemoglobinopathy: amoxicillin or trimethoprim-sulfamethoxazole (TMP-SMX) for 5 to 7 days.
  3. Antimotility agents are *not recommended* because they may worsen disease.
- Typhoid fever and invasive disease
  1. Bacteremia: Treat for 14 days; provide parenteral therapy for severely ill patients.
  2. Bacteremia in patients with HIV: 4 to 6 weeks of therapy may help prevent relapse.
  3. Osteomyelitis or abscess: Treat for 4 to 6 weeks; surgical intervention as indicated.
  4. Meningitis: Treat for at least 4 weeks with third-generation cephalosporin.
  5. Multidrug-resistant *S. typhi* (suspect in travelers to India, Pakistan, and Egypt): Treat 7 to 10 days with third-generation cephalosporin.
  6. Give corticosteroids for typhoid fever with severe mental status changes.

- Selection of antibiotics
  1. Multiple resistance is common.
  2. Treat according to susceptibility results but interpret with caution.
  3. Empiric therapy includes third-generation cephalosporin (fluoroquinolones only if benefits outweigh risks).
- Relapse common and warrants retreatment

■ SURGICAL

Focal purulent collections should be surgically drained.

■ FOLLOW-UP & DISPOSITION

- Follow-up cultures are indicated only for infection control.
- Chronic (1 year or longer) *S. typhi* carriage may be eradicated by high-dose amoxicillin and probenecid.

■ PATIENT/FAMILY EDUCATION

- Use proper handwashing technique, sanitary water supplies, and food preparation techniques.
- Discourage keeping reptiles as pets.
- Do not eat raw eggs or foods containing raw eggs.

■ PREVENTIVE TREATMENT

- Isolation: contact precautions for diapered/incontinent children
  1. *S typhi:* Follow contact precautions and maintain exclusion from child care until three consecutive negative stool cultures (off antibiotics) are obtained.
  2. Stool cultures from asymptomatic *S. typhi* contacts should be obtained.
  3. Other species: Exclude only symptomatic children from child care; asymptomatic contacts do not need to be cultured.

4. Infected persons should be excluded from food handling.
- Vaccines
  1. No vaccine is currently available for nontyphoidal *Salmonella.*
  2. *S. typhi:* Vaccinate only children traveling in endemic areas with prolonged exposure, especially in areas with multidrug-resistant *S. typhi* (India, Pakistan, and Egypt); consider vaccinating household contacts of chronic carriers.
     a. Ty21a live-attenuated vaccine (oral): Children older than 6 years, variable efficacy in younger children; do not administer while patients are taking antibiotics or are immunocompromised. Capsule given every other day for four doses; booster is required every 5 years.
     b. Vi capsular polysaccharide vaccine (intramuscular): Children older than 2 years, single dose, booster is required every 2 years.
     c. Heat-phenol–inactivated vaccine (subcutaneous): Children older than 6 months to 2 years, least preferred because of more frequent side effects (e.g., fever, headache, pain and swelling at site, hypotension, shock); requires two doses at least 4 weeks apart; booster is required every 3 years.

■ REFERRAL INFORMATION

- All documented cases of *Salmonella* should be reported to the local health department.
- Refer complicated or severely ill patients to pediatric infectious

disease or pediatric gastroenterology specialists.

☼ PEARLS & CONSIDERATIONS

■ CLINICAL PEARLS

- Inoculum size determines incubation period, symptoms, and severity.
- Typhoid fever can present with constipation.

■ WEBSITES

- Centers for Disease Control and Prevention: Safe Food and Water: www.cdc.gov/travel/foodwater.htm
- Centers for Disease Control and Prevention: Salmonellosis: www.cdc.gov/ncidod/dbmd/diseaseinfo/salmonellosis_g.htm
- Centers for Disease Control and Prevention: Salmonella Enteritidis: www.cdc.gov/ncidod/dbmd/diseaseinfo/salment_g.htm

REFERENCES

1. American Academy of Pediatrics: Salmonella infections. In Pickering L (ed): *2000 Red Book: report of the Committee on Infectious Diseases,* ed 25, Elk Grove Village, Ill, 2000, American Academy of Pediatrics.
2. Gomez HF, Cleary TG: *Salmonella* species. In Long SS et al (eds): *Principles and practice of pediatric infectious disease,* New York, 1997, Churchill Livingstone.
3. Gomez HF, Cleary TG: *Salmonella.* In Feigin RD, Cherry JD (eds): *Textbook of pediatric infectious diseases,* ed 4, Philadelphia, 1998, WB Saunders.

Author: **Melanie Wellington, M.D.**

BASIC INFORMATION

DEFINITION
Scabies is a skin infestation by small parasites called itch mites *(Sarcoptes scabiei)*, derived from the Latin word *scabere,* meaning "to scratch."

ICD-9CM CODE
133.0 Scabies

ETIOLOGY
- The female mite burrows into stratum corneum, sucking tissue for nutrition.
- It lays approximately 40 to 50 eggs over 4 to 6 weeks.
- Immune-mediated sensitivity to mites, their feces, and eggs causes the intense pruritic reaction.

EPIDEMIOLOGY & DEMOGRAPHICS
- Immune reaction occurs 10 to 30 days after exposure.
  1. Time to develop immune-mediated sensitivity
- Humans are main infection source via close human physical contact.
- Transmission from dogs and other animals is rare.
- Infants and young children have a more varied presentation.
- Approximately 50% to 66% of family members will become clinically infected.
- Mites die within 2 to 3 days without human contact.
- African Americans are less commonly infected.

HISTORY
- Intense pruritic rash appears, which is worse at night.
- Other household members often report similar symptoms.
- Severity varies within a household.

PHYSICAL EXAMINATION
- Classic lesion is a burrow.
  1. Fairly linear, ranging from a few millimeters to a centimeter with a black dot at the leading edge (mite)
  2. Typically in webs of fingers and toes and sides of hands and feet
- Children younger than 5 years are often infected from head to toe, including palms and soles with more variable and eczematous lesions.
- Older children and adults have lesions in webs of fingers, axilla, flexor surfaces of arms, belt line, nipples, buttocks, and genitals. Facial involvement is rare.

- Secondary lesions are common as a result of scratching and possibly secondary infection and include the following:
  1. Crusted papules
  2. Vesicles
  3. Pustules
  4. Excoriations
  5. Eczematous areas

DIAGNOSIS

DIFFERENTIAL DIAGNOSIS
- Atopic dermatitis (commonly misdiagnosed as this in infancy)
- Papular urticaria
- Acropustulosis of infancy
- Dyshidrotic eczema on hands

DIAGNOSTIC WORKUP
- Often based on clinical findings
- Scabies scraping
  1. Locate a burrow.
  2. Put a drop of mineral oil on the lesion.
  3. Scrape with a No. 15 blade to produce a speck of blood.
  4. Scrape several lesions and place them on a slide, with a cover slip, and examine under low power.

THERAPY

MEDICAL
- Permethrin 5%
  1. Apply from head (including scalp) to toe and leave on 8 to 14 hours and then rinse.
  2. This may be used in children older than 2 months of age.
- 1% gamma benzene hexachloride lotion (Lindane or Kwell)
  1. Apply for 8 to 12 hours and then rinse.
  2. This lotion is less preferable because of central nervous system toxicity with prolonged skin contact.
  3. Use is contraindicated in persons with a seizure disorder, infants (younger than 2 years old), and pregnant women.
- Necessary to treat all household contacts
- May need to cover infants' and toddlers' hands and body with clothing to prevent licking of scabicide
- Oral antihistamines for antipruritic effect worth trying to decrease itching, scratches
- Topical corticosteroids worth trying to relieve pruritus, but only after scabicide treatment is complete

FOLLOW-UP & DISPOSITION
In severe cases, a follow-up visit may be warranted in 2 weeks to assess the success of the therapy.

PATIENT/FAMILY EDUCATION
- Instructions on the use of scabicides should be clear.
- Emphasize need to treat all close household contacts.
- Persistence of itching 1 to 2 weeks after successful treatment is normal because of sensitivity to degenerating mites.
- Vacuum furniture and mattresses.
- Wash, in hot water, bed linens, towels, and clothing worn next to skin in the past 4 days, including jackets, sweaters, and hats.
- Children may return to day care or school 24 hours after treatment.

PEARLS & CONSIDERATIONS

CLINICAL PEARLS
- Prior use of topical steroids may produce some improvement and mask clinical findings.
- When it is difficult to identify a burrow for scraping, apply a washable marker over web spaces and rinse with water. Retained ink after rinsing may identify a burrow.
- Norwegian scabies is an intense infestation with widespread crusted hyperkeratotic lesions. It is uncommon and generally occurs in disabled or immunocompromised patients.

WEBSITE
HeadLice.org: www.headlice.org; common questions and answers about scabies and lice

REFERENCES
1. American Academy of Pediatrics: Scabies. In *1997 Red Book: report of the Committee on Infectious Diseases,* ed 24, Elk Grove Village, Ill, 1997, American Academy of Pediatrics.
2. Pomeranz AJ, Fairley JA: The systematic evaluation of the skin in children, *Pediatr Clin North Am* 45:61, 1998.
3. Weston WL, Lane AT, Morelli JG: *Color textbook of pediatric dermatology,* ed 3, St Louis, 1996, Mosby.
4. Zabawski EJ et al: A potpourri of parasitic infestations, *Cutis* 63:81, 1999.
Author: Kristen Smith Danielson, M.D.

BASIC INFORMATION

■ DEFINITION
Idiopathic scoliosis is an abnormal lateral curvature of spine when looking front to back. In fact, it is a three-dimensional abnormality and includes angulation and rotational deformities as well. Scoliosis is a common complication of some neuromuscular and vertebral abnormalities. Other forms of spinal deformity include kyphosis and Scheuermann's kyphosis.

■ SYNONYMS
- Crooked back
- Spinal deformity

ICD-9CM CODE
737.30 Scoliosis

■ ETIOLOGY
- The cause is unknown; hence, the term *idiopathic*. As yet, unsubstantiated hypotheses include the following:
  1. Differential growth rate as a result of growth hormone secretion abnormalities
  2. Central nervous system (CNS) abnormalities of proprioception and vibratory sensation
  3. Insufficiency of costovertebral ligaments and biomechanical abnormalities
  4. Asymmetric weakness of spinal support muscles, possibly caused by calcium transport defect resulting from abnormal calmodulin
  5. Collagen abnormality
- Forms related to underlying neuromuscular abnormalities are caused by the inability to maintain posture because of muscle weakness or laxity.
  1. Osteogenesis imperfecta (OI)
  2. Muscular dystrophy
  3. Cerebral palsy
- Bony anomalies are rarely responsible for scoliosis.
  1. Vertebral collapse (e.g., resulting from leukemia)
  2. Injury of vertebrae
- Progression of idiopathic scoliosis depends on the amount of growth left after diagnosis.
  1. Progression more likely with the following:
     a. Younger age at diagnosis
     b. Lower Risser sign (rating of skeletal maturity) at diagnosis
        (1) Risser 0-1 with spinal curve 20 degrees: 22% progressed
        (2) Risser 4-5 and same curve abnormalities; less than 2% progressed
        (3) Risser 0-1 with curve 20° to 30°: 68% progressed
        (4) Risser 4-5 with this larger curve: 23% progressed
     c. Longer time to onset of menarche from diagnosis
     d. Female gender
- Large curves, greater than 50 degrees, often progress, even in skeletally mature persons.

■ EPIDEMIOLOGY & DEMOGRAPHICS
- Infantile (birth to 3 year), rare
  1. Associated with plagiocephaly, bat ear deformity, congenital muscular torticollis, developmental dysplasia of the hip
  2. Mental retardation also associated
  3. Congenital heart disease in 2.5%
  4. Inguinal hernia in 7.5%
- Juvenile (3 to 10 years)
  1. Equal male:female ratio
  2. Course may be severe, but not uniformly
- Adolescent (older than 10 years), idiopathic, 90% of all scoliosis
  1. Approximately 2% to 3% prevalence of greater than 10-degree curve at 16 years old
  2. Up to 2% prevalence of curves greater than 20 degrees
  3. Approximately 0.2% prevalence of curves greater than 30 degrees
  4. Girl:boy ratio of 5:1 to 8:1
- Female:male ratio of 3:1 to 6:1 for curves less than 10 degrees and 10:1 for curves greater than 30 degrees in adolescent idiopathic scoliosis
- No increased risk of early mortality in mild to moderate adolescent idiopathic scoliosis
- Dominant or multiple gene inheritance pattern likely
  1. Increase risk in offspring of parents with idiopathic scoliosis
  2. High concordance rates in monozygotic twins

■ HISTORY
- Age at onset: typically during puberty in idiopathic scoliosis
- Gradual or sudden
  1. Sudden onset is atypical for idiopathic scoliosis.
  2. Sudden onset may indicate trauma, infection, or tumor of the spine.
- Age of menarche to help predict progression
- Back pain: ominous sign; suggests not idiopathic scoliosis
- Other congenital anomalies
  1. Increased scoliosis with musculoskeletal diseases
  2. Increased association of spine deformities with congenital cardiac and urologic abnormalities
  3. Spinal defects seen after radiation to chest or abdomen
- Family history
  1. Genetic associations
     a. Marfan's syndrome
     b. Osteogenesis imperfecta
     c. Neurofibromatosis
  2. Idiopathic scoliosis in one or both parents

■ PHYSICAL EXAMINATION
- Less than 10-degree curvature is normal.
- Flexibility of spine measured with twisting and rotation: Stiffness indicates irritating lesions (e.g., spondylolysis, spinal cord tumor).
- Posture: Shoulder and pelvic symmetry should be noted.
- Characteristic paravertebral rib hump is seen.
  1. Truncal rotation
  2. Apical rib prominence
- Leg length: Inequality may lead to secondary scoliosis, which will be corrected with shoe lifts.
- Plumbline, dropped from T1 spinal process, should be 2.7 cm or less from gluteal cleft.
- Angle of trunk rotation should be measured with a scoliometer (an inclinometer).
  1. Adam's forward-bending test: Have bend forward with knees extended until the spine is parallel to the floor.
  2. Place the scoliometer over the spine at the apex of the curve.
  3. Scoliometer measurement of more than 7 degrees is abnormal.
- Skin pigmentation, spinal skin dimpling, or nevi over spine may be seen.
  1. Neurofibromatosis
  2. Spinal dysraphism
- Gait should be assessed.
- A neurologic examination should be performed to look for the following:
  1. Ankle clonus, Babinski, abdominal reflexes; asymmetry may indicate intraspinal process:
     a. Intraspinal tumor
     b. Lipoma
     c. Syringomyelia, hydromyelia
     d. Tethered cord
     e. Neurofibromatosis
  2. Muscle weakness
     a. Cavus foot indicates neurologic process.
- Height should be measured over time, obtaining both sitting and standing measurements.
  1. Upper-lower body segment and arm span if considering Marfan's syndrome

■ COMPLICATIONS
- Restrictive lung disease, but only with marked scoliosis of more than 100 degrees in the absence of kyphosis
- Secondary rib and sternum rotational displacement
- Cardiac restriction (very rare except in infantile scoliosis)
- No increased prevalence of back pain compared with that of the general population

- Degenerative joint disease increased only in those whose vertebrae shift translaterally in thoracolumbar and lumbar curves
- Neurologic function interference (rare)

DIAGNOSIS

■ DIFFERENTIAL DIAGNOSIS
- Neuromuscular diseases
  1. Muscular dystrophy
  2. Spinal muscular atrophy
  3. Cerebral palsy
- Neurofibromatosis
- Spinal tumors, lipoma
- Vertebral body bony anomalies or fractures
- Marfan's syndrome
- Syringomyelia

■ DIAGNOSTIC WORKUP
- Radiograph of entire spine—occiput to sacrum
  1. Including pelvis to determine Risser stage (skeletal maturity rating)
  2. Triradiate cartilage
  3. Standing anteroposterior and lateral views
- Seated radiograph if patient not ambulatory
- If leg length discrepancy, blocks used under feet to assess curvature better
- Special views: may be warranted as directed by orthopedic surgeon or neurosurgeon(s)
- Computed tomography, magnetic resonance imaging, or computed tomographic myelography
  1. Performed in all infantile scoliosis because of the significant association with CNS abnormalities
  2. To rule out spinal dysraphism
  3. If new or progressive neurologic abnormalities that require investigation
- Bone scan
  1. May be used in patients with pain if source of symptoms is not obvious
- Congenital deformity
  1. Approximately 25% associated with genitourinary (GU) anomalies, so consider GU visualization
  2. Associated with cardiac disease 10% to 15% of the time

THERAPY

■ NONPHARMACOLOGIC
- Follow-up every 4 to 6 months if greater than 10-degree curve in skeletally immature child or adolescent.
- No specific exercises are proven to be beneficial.
- For kyphosis, reassurance and observation or exercise are generally indicated.

■ MEDICAL
- If 20- to 30-degree curvature or greater and more than 5 degrees of progression, bracing is indicated.
- If initial curve is greater than 25 degrees, even without evidence of progression, some would brace, especially in the skeletally immature patient.
- Bracing does not change torsional deformities such as rib prominence.
- Bracing:
  1. Bracing is 40% effective in adolescents with thoracic curves.
  2. Under-arm brace is worn 23 hours per day.
  3. Girls are weaned from brace gradually when skeletal maturity is reached (Risser score of 4 or higher) and 2 years past menarche.
  4. Boys are treated until achieving a Risser score of 5 as progression continues for longer.
- If scoliosis is associated with other processes, other specific treatments may be needed.

■ SURGICAL
- If greater than 40-degree curvature, surgical correction is recommended.
- If greater than 50-degree curvature, even if skeletally mature, surgery is also recommended.
- Anterior fusion, posterior fusion, or both, may be done depending on degree of curvature and skeletal maturity, may require surgical intervention.
- Instrumentation may also be appropriate, and instrumentation without fusion with progressive rod lengthening may be appropriate for infantile scoliosis.

■ FOLLOW-UP & DISPOSITION
- The patient must be followed by orthopedic surgeon and pediatrician until progression is no longer occurring.
- Back pain is common after fusion.

■ PATIENT/FAMILY EDUCATION
- This is a common abnormality.
- Idiopathic scoliosis is not associated with pain or neurologic abnormalities.
- Activity restriction is not indicated for most patients with idiopathic adolescent scoliosis.

■ PREVENTIVE TREATMENT
Bracing may halt progression, but it does not improve curvature.

■ REFERRAL INFORMATION
- Orthopedic surgeon for large, progressive, or atypical courses
- Orthopedic referral for any cases of preadolescent scoliosis

PEARLS & CONSIDERATIONS

■ CLINICAL PEARLS
- Rapid onset or progression of scoliosis indicates a neurologic or vertebral process.
- Idiopathic adolescent scoliosis should be neither painful nor activity limiting.

■ WEBSITES
General
- Scoliosis Research Society: http://srs.org/
- Virtual Hospital: www.vh.org/Providers/Textbooks/AIS/AIS.html
Patient information
- Familydoctor.org: Familydoctor.org/handouts/107.html
- KidsHealth: www.Kidshealth.org/teen/health_problems/diseases/scoliosis.html
- MIT Artificial Intelligence Laboratory: www.ai.mit.edu/extra/scoliosis//scoliosis.html

■ SUPPORT GROUP
National Scoliosis Foundation, 5 Cabot Place, Stoughton, MA 02072; 800-NSF-myback; 718-341-6333, email: scoliosis@aol.com

REFERENCES
1. Boachie-Adjei O, Lonner B: Spinal deformity, *Pediatr Clin North Am* 43:883, 1996.
2. Miller NH: Cause and natural history of adolescent idiopathic scoliosis, *Orthop Clin North Am* 30:343, 1999.
3. Roach JW: Adolescent idiopathic scoliosis, *Orthop Clin North Am* 30:353, 1999.
Author: **Lynn C. Garfunkel, M.D.**

II

BASIC INFORMATION

■ DEFINITION
Scorpions are arachnids that sting with the tip of their flexible tail. A scorpion sting can be incapacitating.

ICD-9CM CODE
989.5 Toxic effect of venom

■ ETIOLOGY
- The scorpion of medical importance in the United States is *Centruroides exilicauda*.
- Its venom is a neurotoxin that causes severe systemic symptoms.
- Other U.S. species cause only local reactions.

■ EPIDEMIOLOGY & DEMOGRAPHICS
- Scorpions are found mostly outdoors in the southwestern United States.
- Scorpions were responsible for almost 14,000 stings worldwide in 1997.

■ HISTORY
- Very painful sting
- Blurred vision
- Difficulty breathing

■ PHYSICAL EXAMINATION
- Severe local pain and significant tenderness with no redness at site
- No erythema or swelling
- Extremity movements similar to convulsions
- Tongue and muscle fasciculations
- Disconjugate gaze and nystagmus
- Tachycardia
- Respiratory distress from poor respiratory muscle coordination

DIAGNOSIS

- The diagnosis of a scorpion sting is made from history and physical examination.
- It is important to know the offending species because *C. exilicauda* has the only native sting with systemic sequelae.
- The lack of swelling and erythema at the sting site, as well as exaggerated pain to a firm finger tap (tap test), indicate a sting by this species.

THERAPY

Airway management is the cornerstone of therapy for victims of a scorpion sting, especially small children and the elderly, who are more likely to have respiratory difficulty.

■ NONPHARMACOLOGIC
- Ice pack
- Elevation
- Tourniquet use: controversial

■ MEDICAL
- In small children, the risks associated with antivenin therapy are overshadowed by the risks from an untreated scorpion sting.
  1. Prompt antivenin administration may prevent the need for endotracheal intubation in children.
- In adults, the converse is true because symptoms are relatively short lived (12 to 48 hours).
  1. The risk of antivenin administration is too great because serious sting sequelae are rare.

- Benzodiazepines may be used for sedation.
- Barbiturates are helpful to control fasciculations and spasms.
- Symptomatic relief, such as analgesia, corticosteroids, and antihistamine therapy, should be provided as needed.

■ FOLLOW-UP & DISPOSITION
Patients are usually monitored closely until a patent airway is ensured and symptoms are under control.

PEARLS & CONSIDERATIONS

■ CLINICAL PEARLS
- Airway compromise is of greatest concern in children younger than 1 year of age.
- Airway management is the first step in the care of scorpion stings.

■ WEBSITE
Desert USA: www.desertusa.com/oct96/du_scorpion.html

REFERENCES
1. Bond GR: Snake, spider, and scorpion envenomation in North America, *Pediatr Rev* 20:147, 1999.
2. Kemp ED: Bites and stings of the arthropod kind: treating reactions that can range from annoying to menacing, *Postgrad Med* 103:88, 1998.
3. Litovitz TL et al: 1997 Annual Report of the American Association of Poison Control Centers Toxic Exposure Surveillance System, *Am J Emerg Med* 16:443, 1998.

Author: **Robert Freishtat, M.D.**

See also the section "Febrile Seizures."

 BASIC INFORMATION

■ DEFINITIONS
- A *seizure is a* paroxysmal discharge of cortical neurons. Manifestations may include changes in motor function, sensory function, alertness, perception, or autonomic function.
- *Seizure type* is defined by the International Classification of Epileptic Seizures (not including neonatal seizures):

I. **Partial seizures: Clinical and electroencephalogram (EEG) indicate initial activation of neurons related to a specific part of the cerebral cortex. May be simple or complex.**
  A. Simple partial seizure: Consciousness is not impaired. Usually very brief and stereotyped. May include motor, somatosensory, psychic, or autonomic features. Transient motor weakness is common.
  B. Complex partial seizures: Most common seizure type in children and adults. Consciousness is always impaired. May start as simple partial seizure and progress or may begin as complex seizure. Usually lasts 30 seconds to minutes. Often includes automatisms. May have affective, psychic, and somatosensory symptoms.
  C. Complex partial seizures evolving to secondarily generalized seizures.

II. **Generalized seizures: All have abrupt onset and involve alteration of consciousness. Begin with abnormal discharges in both hemispheres simultaneously.**
  A. Absence seizures: Usually brief (less than 10 seconds). Most untreated children have more than 10 seizures a day; some may have hundreds. May have impaired consciousness only or may include tonic, atonic, and clonic components. May also have automatisms.
  B. Tonic-clonic seizures: Most generalized tonic-clonic seizures in children are really secondarily generalized partial seizures. Presence of an aura suggests focal onset.
- *Epilepsy* is a condition of recurrent (two or more), unprovoked seizures in an individual with a predisposition because of underlying brain dysfunction.
- *Epilepsy syndrome* is an episodic disorder characterized by a cluster of clinical characteristics. Within a syndrome, seizures have similar etiology, natural history, genetic predisposition, and prognosis. A few examples include the following:
  1. Benign centrotemporal epilepsy (benign rolandic epilepsy)
  2. West syndrome (infantile spasms)
  3. Lennox-Gastaut syndrome
  4. Landau-Kleffner syndrome
  5. Juvenile myoclonic epilepsy

■ SYNONYMS
- Convulsions
- Epilepsy (see previous definition)

ICD-9CM CODE
345.90 Epilepsy, unspecified

■ ETIOLOGY
- There is a disruption in the normal balance between excitation and inhibition in part or all of the brain.
- Ultimately, there must be hyperexcitability and hypersynchrony of involved neurons. Many different conditions can lead to such a state, including the following:
  1. Central nervous system malformation
  2. Genetic and hereditary factors (e.g., benign rolandic epilepsy, idiopathic generalized tonic-clonic seizures, benign familial neonatal convulsions, juvenile myoclonic epilepsy)
  3. Head trauma
  4. Neoplasm or space-occupying lesion
  5. Cerebrovascular disease
  6. Metabolic disease (e.g., urea cycle defects, disorders of amino acid and organic acid metabolism, B_6 dependency, mitochondrial diseases)
    a. These typically present in the neonatal period.
  7. Toxins, including alcohol and pharmacologic agents
  8. Fever

■ EPIDEMIOLOGY & DEMOGRAPHICS
- Annual incidence from birth to 20 years is 0.56 per 1000.
- Cumulative risk during first 20 years is 1%.
- Prevalence in the pediatric population is 4 to 6 cases per 1000 children.

■ HISTORY
- If possible, obtain history from the patient and someone who witnessed the event.
- Determine the patient's premorbid status.
  1. Any known neurologic disorder, cognitive or developmental delay, other medical conditions with increased incidence of seizure disorders
  2. Developmental and behavioral history of child
  3. Age at onset
  4. Family history
  5. Current medications
  6. History of toxin exposure or drug or alcohol use
  7. History of hypoglycemia, breath-holding, hyperventilation
  8. Where the child was and what he or she was doing just before the event
  9. History of recent head trauma
  10. Health at time of seizure: ill, febrile, sleep deprived
- Determine what occurred during the seizure:
  1. Was there an aura (olfactory, gustatory, sensory, emotional, perceptual)?
  2. Was there mood or behavior change during the seizure?
  3. Were any preictal symptoms reported by the patient?
  4. Was there a cry, gasp, slurring of words, or garbled speech?
  5. Was there motor activity?
    a. Focal or generalized in onset
    b. Spread
    c. Head or eye turning
    d. Eye deviation
    e. Jerking (clonic activity)
    f. Stiffening (tonic activity)
    g. Symmetric movement
    h. Posturing
    i. Automatisms (purposeless repetitive movements such as picking at clothes, lip smacking)
  6. Were there autonomic signs?
    a. Pupillary dilation
    b. Drooling
    c. Change in heart rate or respiratory rate
    d. Pallor
    e. Incontinence
    f. Piloerection
  7. Respiratory: Was there a change in breathing pattern, apnea, or cyanosis?
  8. Did the child lose consciousness or the ability to understand or speak (at onset of seizure or later)?
  9. How long did the event last?
- Was there a postictal state?
  1. Amnesia for events
  2. Confusion
  3. Lethargy
  4. Sleepiness
  5. Headache
  6. Transient focal weakness (Todd's paralysis)

■ PHYSICAL EXAMINATION
- Assess stability of the patient.
  1. If actively seizing, signs suggestive of meningitis, history of recent head trauma, deteriorating mental status, prolonged alteration of

mental status, or new focal neurologic findings, refer immediately to emergency department for assessment and treatment.
- If patient is stable and seizure has stopped:
  1. Look for clues to the cause.
     a. Dysmorphic features
     b. Head circumference, fontanelle
     c. Skin findings
        (1) Pigmentary abnormalities, including café-au-lait spots, hypopigmented macules
        (2) Port-wine stain
        (3) Adenoma sebaceum
        (4) Neurofibromas, periungual fibromas
        (5) Signs of recent trauma
     d. Retina
        (1) Papilledema
        (2) Abnormal pigmentation
        (3) Retinal hemorrhages
     e. Ears
        (1) Hemotympanum
     f. Cardiac
        (1) Rhythm
        (2) Murmurs
  2. Perform a complete neurologic examination, with emphasis on mental status and focal findings.

🔬 DIAGNOSIS

■ DIFFERENTIAL DIAGNOSIS
- Paroxysmal movements
  1. Tics
  2. Benign sleep myoclonus
  3. Startle response
  4. Paroxysmal torticollis
  5. Paroxysmal choreoathetosis
  6. Pseudoseizures
  7. Infantile masturbation
  8. Self-stimulation
- Loss of tone or consciousness
  1. Syncope
  2. Narcolepsy
  3. Attention deficit/hyperactivity disorder or daydreaming
  4. Migraine
- Respiratory disorders
  1. Apnea
  2. Breath-holding spells
  3. Hyperventilation
- Behavior disorders
  1. Head banging
  2. Rage attacks
- Sleep disorders
  1. Sleep terrors
  2. Sleep walking
  3. Nightmares
- Psychiatric disorders
  1. Fugue
  2. Hallucinations
  3. Panic attack
- Perceptual disorders
  1. Vertigo
- Specific disorders with episodic events
  1. Hypoglycemia
  2. Hypocalcemia

3. Periodic paralysis
4. Cardiac arrhythmia
5. Tetralogy spells
6. Hydrocephalic spells
7. Gastroesophageal reflux (including Sandifer syndrome)
8. Acute intoxication
9. Migraine

■ DIAGNOSTIC WORKUP
- Beyond the neonatal period, the workup will depend on the type of seizure, the patient's age, and the patient's history.
- An EEG should be done after the first unprovoked seizure. It should include wake and sleep tracing, hyperventilation, and photic stimulation.
  1. Interictal EEG will show an abnormality in only about 60% of patients with epilepsy.
  2. It is most likely to show abnormalities if obtained within 24 to 48 hours of the seizure, but this may be nonspecific slowing.
  3. It is not diagnostic; however, it is helpful in determining seizure type, epilepsy syndrome, and risk for recurrence.
  4. Absence epilepsy: Interictal EEG should show typical spike-and-wave pattern with sleep, hyperventilation, or photic stimulation.
  5. Prolonged EEG recording and simultaneous video monitoring may help capture ictal EEG and clarify focus.
  6. Surface EEG may not detect seizure activity from deep cortical structures. Invasive monitoring may be required.
- Consider neuroimaging studies.
  1. Neuroimaging is not necessary in benign epilepsy syndromes, including benign partial epilepsy of childhood (benign rolandic epilepsy, primary generalized epilepsy, absence epilepsy).
  2. Magnetic resonance imaging (MRI) is the preferred study.
     a. Significant cognitive or motor impairment of unknown origin, unexplained abnormalities on neurologic examination, seizure with focal onset, children younger than 12 months of age, adolescents
  3. In emergent situations, computed tomography (CT) may be more readily available.
     a. CT may clarify the cause of the seizure.
     b. A negative study does not rule out a seizure disorder.
     c. Emergent neuroimaging should be done for any child with postictal focal deficit or altered sensorium that does not resolve within several hours of seizure, high suspicion of central nervous system

trauma, or increased intracranial pressure.
  4. CT in nonemergent situations may be helpful if MRI is unavailable.
     a. Especially helpful in diagnosing tuberous sclerosis and congenital cytomegalovirus
- Laboratory tests may be helpful.
  1. Based on clinical history, consider glucose, calcium, and phosphorus.
  2. In an infant with seizures, especially infantile spasms, assess for a metabolic disturbance.
     a. Amino acids
     b. Organic acids
     c. Biotinidase
     d. Ammonia
     e. Lactate/pyruvate
  3. Genetic studies are based on the clinical diagnosis.

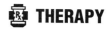 **THERAPY**

■ NONPHARMACOLOGIC
- Avoid specific triggers such as sleep deprivation and fever.
  1. Some seizures may be triggered by light, reading, or minor trauma.
- Ketogenic diet may be helpful in select cases.
  1. This diet is reserved for children who have refractory seizures or intolerable side effects to medication.
  2. If the child responds, it may be possible to significantly decrease use of antiepileptic drugs.
  3. There must be rigorous adherence to this diet, which is very restrictive and is very high in fat content.
  4. Valproate is contraindicated with a ketogenic diet (diet increases risk of valproate-induced hepatotoxicity).

■ MEDICAL
General considerations
- Most recommend no treatment after the first nonfebrile seizure. However, if the first seizure is absence, infantile spasm, or myoclonic, initiate treatment.
- Choice of medication depends on the seizure type, epileptic syndrome, and age of the patient.
- The goal is for seizure control with monotherapy, but this is not always possible.
- Drug half-life is variable, depending on the age of the patient.
- Drug interactions (especially with phenytoin, lamotrigine, valproic acid, and phenobarbital) are common, and it is imperative to be aware of these and monitor carefully. A few examples are as follows:
  1. Carbamazepine, primidone, phenytoin, and phenobarbital induce

enzymes. When used together, they may increase metabolism and lower plasma levels.

2. Erythromycin inhibits the enzyme system that metabolizes carbamazepine, potentially leading to toxic levels.

3. Valproic acid may increase serum levels of phenytoin and phenobarbital.

4. Valproic acid prolongs the clearance of lamotrigine.

- Antiepileptic drugs can have significant behavioral and cognitive side effects. Many are also associated with cosmetic or hormonal disturbances.
- Adverse reactions to anticonvulsant drugs are common and are most likely during the first 3 months of therapy.
- Refer to a pediatric neurologist if seizures persist despite trying two antiepileptic drugs as monotherapy and in cases of malignant epilepsy syndromes (e.g., infantile spasms, Lennox-Gastaut syndrome, early myoclonic encephalopathy, Rasmussen syndrome, continuous spike waves during slow sleep).

Suggested medication by seizure type

- Partial seizures with or without secondary generalization
  1. First line: carbamazepine/oxcarbazepine, phenytoin
  2. Second choice: topiramate, gabapentin, lamotrigine, valproate
- Generalized tonic-clonic (make sure not secondary generalization)
  1. First choice: valproate, carbamazepine, phenytoin
  2. Second choice: topiramate, lamotrigine
- Absence seizures
  1. First choice: valproate (can use ethosuximide if younger than 10 years of age)
  2. Second choice: lamotrigine
- Juvenile myoclonic epilepsy
  1. First choice: valproate
  2. Second choice: lamotrigine
- Benign epilepsy with centrotemporal spikes
  1. First choice: valproate, gabapentin (no treatment may be first choice in some)
  2. Second choice: carbamazepine, phenytoin

Prescribing information on selected antiepileptic drugs

- Carbamazepine
  1. Indications: partial epilepsy, partial seizure with secondary generalization
  2. Dosage: begin 10 mg/kg/24 hr; increase by 5 mg/kg per day each week to total dosage of 20 to 30 mg/kg/day in two or three divided doses
  3. Half-life: 3 to 35 hours; autoinduction of enzyme, meaning over time, metabolism of drug increases

4. Laboratory follow-up: blood level (trough), complete blood count (CBC), liver function tests (LFTs) at 1 month, 2 months, 4 months, and then every 6 months

5. Therapeutic trough range: 4 to 12 µg/ml

6. Contraindications: patients taking monoamine oxidase (MAO) inhibitors, patients with sensitivity to tricyclic antidepressants

7. Interactions
   a. Increases metabolism of other antiepileptic drugs
   b. Erythromycin, verapamil, cimetidine, and isoniazid (INH) may increase serum levels
   c. May decrease activity of doxycycline, theophylline, phenytoin, ethosuximide, and valproic acid

8. Some side effects: transient diplopia, ataxia, nausea, vomiting, rash, anemia, leukopenia

- Valproic acid
  1. Indications: generalized tonic-clonic, absence, myoclonic, partial epilepsy, tonic seizures
  2. Dosage: start with 5 to 10 mg/kg/day divided in one to three doses; gradual increase by 5 to 10 mg/kg per day each week to 20 mg/kg/day in two to three divided doses; average dosage for child: 20 to 60 mg/kg/day
  3. Half-life in children: 4 to 14 hours
  4. Therapeutic range (trough): 50 to 100 µg/ml
  5. Laboratory tests
     a. CBC, aspartate aminotransferase (AST), alanine aminotransferase (ALT) before beginning therapy
     b. Drug levels 5 days after 20 mg/kg/day and 5 days after each subsequent increase
     c. Monitoring of LFTs, CBC at 2 weeks, then monthly for 6 months; subsequently every 3 to 6 months
     d. Amylase, check for polycystic ovaries if abdominal pain
     e. Ammonia if mental status changes
  6. Interactions: increases phenytoin, lamotrigine, phenobarbital, felbamate, ethosuximide; increases levels of carbamazepine epoxide
  7. Cautions
     a. Severe hepatotoxicity is more likely to occur in developmentally delayed or neurologically impaired children younger than 2 years old who are treated with multiple anticonvulsants. Risk is also increased if there is an underlying metabolic disorder. Therefore in children younger than 2 years, assess serum

lactate and pyruvate, carnitine, ammonia, amino acids, and urinary organic acids before using valproic acid.

- Phenytoin
  1. Indications: partial epilepsy, generalized tonic-clonic seizures
  2. Dosage: start with 5 mg/kg/day divided twice daily (this is usual dose); may need increased dosage in children younger than 6 years
  3. Half-life: quite variable and dose dependent, ranging 7 to 42 hours
     a. Nonlinear kinetics imply that once hepatic saturation occurs, very small increments in dosage result in significant elevations of blood level. Therefore, when blood level in low therapeutic range, increase dosage only by very small increments.
  4. Laboratory tests
     a. Monitor trough level after 5 to 10 days of steady administration, then every 6 months or whenever new medication is added.
     b. Therapeutic blood level is 10 to 20 µg/ml.
  5. Interactions
     a. Phenytoin levels may be increased by cimetidine, chloramphenicol, INH, sulfonamides, and trimethoprim.
     b. Phenytoin leads to decreased effectiveness of oral contraceptives, valproic acid, and theophylline.
  6. Common side effects: gingival hyperplasia, hirsutism, coarsening of facial features, ataxia, nystagmus, rash, Stevens-Johnson syndrome
  7. Contraindications: patients with heart block or sinus bradycardia; relatively contraindicated in pregnancy
- Gabapentin
  1. Indications: generally add-on therapy for partial epilepsy, tonic-clonic seizures, benign rolandic epilepsy
  2. Dosage
     a. For children older than 12 years: begin with 300 mg/24 hr; increase by 300 mg/24 hr each day to maximum 900 to 1200 mg (or higher) per 24 hours in three divided doses
     b. For children younger than 12 years: begin with 10 mg/kg/day; increase daily by 5 mg/kg/day to 20 mg/kg/day in three or four daily doses
     c. Dosage adjustment necessary in renal impairment
  3. Half-life: 5 to 8 hours
  4. Laboratory tests: therapeutic level not established

5. Interactions: no serious drug interactions
6. Common side effects: behavior problems (e.g., tantrums, aggression, hyperactivity, defiance), weight gain, somnolence, dizziness, ataxia

■ SURGICAL

- Reserved for children with focal seizures unresponsive to anticonvulsant therapy
- Assessment and treatment in tertiary centers where detailed studies aid in localization
- Types of surgery (depending on indication and seizure type): lobectomy, hemispherectomy, corpus callosotomy, multiple subpial transections
- Vagal nerve stimulation
  1. Indicated as adjunct therapy to reduce frequency of seizures in individuals older than 12 years of age with partial-onset seizures that are refractory to antiepileptic medications
  2. Works by intermittent stimulation of vagal nerve via surgically implanted battery and electrodes

■ FOLLOW-UP & DISPOSITION

- Provide frequent follow-up until symptom free, then every 6 months.
- If seizure free for 2 years, consider weaning from antiepileptic drugs.
  1. If EEG still shows paroxysmal pattern, do not stop medication.
  2. There is an increased risk of recurrence if the patient has a developmental delay or motor handicap, onset of seizures after 12 years of age, history of multiple seizures, or partial complex seizures. Consult a neurologist.
- Careful monitoring of psychosocial adjustment of family and patient

■ PATIENT/FAMILY EDUCATION

- Educate parents and child about causes and treatment for epilepsy.
- Carefully educate concerning medication side effects, interactions, and necessity for compliance.
- Review first aid for seizures: Loosen clothing around neck, remove harmful objects from environment, and maintain an airway.
- Refrain from swimming and bathing alone.
- Patient may participate in all sports, including contact sports, using appropriate protective equipment.
- Check state laws concerning driving and epilepsy.
- Alert teachers and school officials, review first aid, and monitor for learning disorders.
- Provide information about child bearing.

■ PREVENTIVE TREATMENT

- Factors that may exacerbate seizures: fever, undue stress, lack of sleep, video games, menstruation
- Careful consideration of other medications concerning possible lowering of seizure threshold (e.g., bupropion, phenothiazines)

■ REFERRAL INFORMATION

- Referral to a pediatric neurologist is necessary in the following cases:
  1. Patient is a neonate.
  2. Seizures are not responsive to monotherapy treatment after trying two agents.
  3. A malignant epilepsy syndrome (early infantile epileptic encephalopathy, myoclonic epilepsy of infancy, infantile spasms, Lennox-Gastaut syndrome, Doose syndrome, Landau-Kleffner syndrome, epilepsy with electrical status epilepticus of sleep or continuous spike waves of sleep) is suspected.
  4. Medication discontinuation is being considered in a patient at risk for recurrence (see "Follow-Up & Disposition").
- Refer to tertiary epilepsy center if the patient has refractory seizures so that the center can determine the patient's candidacy for surgery, whether to institute a ketogenic diet, and whether to use vagal nerve stimulation.
- Refer for family or individual counseling as necessary.
- Refer to appropriate community education and support groups.

☼ PEARLS & CONSIDERATIONS

■ CLINICAL PEARLS

- Blood levels of carbamazepine, phenobarbital, primidone, ethosuximide, and phenytoin correlate fairly well with seizure control. Blood levels of valproate, lamotrigine, gabapentin, felbamate, and clonazepam are less helpful.
- Blood levels of antiepileptic drugs should be obtained in steady state (i.e., after five half-lives on the current dose)
- EEG correlation with the clinical picture is essential. A patient may have epilepsy with a normal EEG, and an abnormal EEG may occur in a patient without epilepsy.
- With complex partial seizures, the clinical features are usually stereotyped from one seizure to the next, do not typically have directed violence, and have no obvious provocation.
- Rage attacks often have different manifestations from episode to episode, have a component of directed violence, and are usually provoked.
- A child with epileptic staring spells occurring less than once a day is likely to have partial complex seizures and not absence seizures.
- Abdominal epilepsy is rare. When it does occur, it is associated with partial complex seizures and impaired consciousness.
- Staring as a sole manifestation of absence epilepsy is unusual. There are usually associated symptoms such as eye blinking or clonic arm movements.

■ WEBSITES

- Epilepsy Education Association, Inc.: www.iupui.edu/~epilepsy
- Epilepsy Foundation of America: www.epilepsyfoundation.org

■ SUPPORT GROUPS

Local support groups may be found through the aforementioned resources and pediatric neurologists.

REFERENCES

1. Haslam RHA: Non-febrile seizures, *Pediatr Rev* 18:39, 1997.
2. Hirtz D et al: Practice parameter: evaluating a first non-febrile seizure in children, *Neurology* 55:616, 2000.
3. Pellock JM: Treatment of seizures and epilepsy in children and adolescents, *Neurology* 51:S8, 1998.
Author: **Ellen Gellerstedt, M.D.**

BASIS INFORMATION

DEFINITION
Serum sickness is a systemic vasculitis induced by introduction of foreign antigen.

ICD-9CM CODE
999.5 Serum sickness

ETIOLOGY
- Serum sickness is a type III hypersensitivity reaction (immune complex mediated).
- Immune complexes are deposited on endothelial tissue and initiate an inflammatory process.
- Known antigens include equine sera (including *Centruroides* antivenom, which is produced in horses), drugs (typically antibiotics), human gamma globulin, *Hymenoptera* stings, and hepatitis viruses.

EPIDEMIOLOGY & DEMOGRAPHICS
- Incidence varies depending on the specific antigen; for each antigen, the quoted rates vary greatly from source to source.
- Incidence and severity increase with age.
- Antibiotics are the leading cause of serum sickness; cefaclor and penicillin have the highest incidence rates.
- Horse serum produces a very high rate of severe serum sickness.

HISTORY
- Symptoms begin 4 to 21 days after administration of the antigen; if previously sensitized to the antigen, symptoms may begin within 1 to 2 days.
- After an injection, serum sickness typically begins as erythema and pain at the injection site before systemic manifestations.
- Rash is the first systemic sign.
- Common complaints include low-grade fever, malaise, myalgia, arthralgia, arthritis of multiple joints (most often ankles and knees), generalized pruritus, and gastrointestinal distress such as cramping and nausea.

PHYSICAL EXAMINATION
- Physical findings
  1. The incidence of physical findings varies greatly from patient to patient; no standardized criteria exist for diagnosis.
- Skin
  1. Lesions typically begin as erythematous rash with serpiginous border.
  2. Lesions occur along the junction of palmar and plantar surfaces of hands, fingers, feet, and toes.
  3. They may progress into generalized urticaria or morbilliform-like lesions.
- Extremities
  1. Edema and pain involves multiple joints.
  2. Hands and feet swell.
- Lymphadenopathy near injection site
- Facial flushing and edema
- Retinal and palpebral hemorrhages

DIAGNOSIS

DIFFERENTIAL DIAGNOSIS
- Lupus erythematous
- Erythema multiforme
- Urticaria

DIAGNOSTIC WORKUP
- This is a clinical diagnosis; no specific criteria exist.
- Commonly noted laboratory data may include the following:
  1. Hematology: thrombocytopenia, initial leukocytosis followed by leukopenia, eosinophilia (typically late in course)
  2. Nephrology: proteinuria, hemoglobinuria, microscopic hematuria
  3. Immunology: slightly elevated erythrocyte sedimentation rate, low compliment levels C3 and C4 (more notable with disease secondary to horse serum)
  4. Skin biopsy of a lesion: immune deposits of IgM, IgG, IgE, and C3, along with perivascular infiltration of lymphocytes, histiocytes, and rarely neutrophils

THERAPY

MEDICAL
- Discontinue suspect medications.
- Typically, it is a 7- to 10-day self-limited course that requires only symptomatic treatment with antihistamines and nonsteroidal antiinflammatory drugs.
- Severe cases respond well to 1 to 2 mg/kg/day of prednisone for 7 to 14 days.

FOLLOW-UP & DISPOSITION
- For typical self-limited course, no follow-up is needed.
- Rare complications include Guillain-Barré syndrome, permanent neuritis (most commonly involving brachial plexus), myocarditis, arteritis of coronary arteries, laryngeal edema, and pleuritis.

PATIENT/FAMILY EDUCATION
Patients need to be aware that exposure to the same antigen may trigger another episode of serum sickness.

REFERRAL INFORMATION
Most cases can be managed by a primary care physician with appropriate referrals for any significant complications.

PEARLS & CONSIDERATIONS

CLINICAL PEARLS
- Horse serum produces the most significant symptoms.
- Today, most reactions are secondary to drugs and are relatively benign.
- Although skin testing can predict anaphylactic reactions to drugs, there is no way of predicting who will develop serum sickness.
- Some experts believe that administering prophylactic antihistamines may reduce the rate of serum sickness.

REFERENCES
1. Bielory L et al: Human serum sickness: a prospective analysis of 35 patients treated with equine anti-thymocyte globulin of bone marrow failure, *Medicine* 67:40, 1988.
2. Erffmeyer J: Serum sickness, *Ann Allergy* 56:105, 1986.
3. Lawley TJ et al: A prospective clinical and immunologic analysis of patients with serum sickness, *N Engl J Med* 311:1407, 1984.
4. Martin J, Abbott J: Serum sickness like illness and antimicrobials in children, *NZ Med J* 108:123, 1995.
5. Naguwa SM, Nelson BL: Human serum sickness, *Clin Rev Allergy* 3:117, 1985.
6. Roujeau JC, Stern RS: Severe adverse cutaneous reactions to drugs, *N Engl J Med* 331:1272, 1994.

Author: **Christopher Copenhaver, M.D.**

BASIC INFORMATION

DEFINITION
Sexual abuse is the exposure of a child to or engagement in sexual activities that are inappropriate for the child's developmental level or chronologic age by an older or more mature person. These activities may include the following:
- Fondling of genitalia or breasts
- Orogenital contact
- Vaginal or anal penetration
- Exploitation in pornography or prostitution
- Exhibitionism or voyeurism

SYNONYMS
- Molestation
- Sexual assault
- Rape

ICD-9CM CODE
995.53 Sexual abuse

ETIOLOGY
- Why children are sexually abused is unclear. Factors related to the perpetrator, the victim, and the environment set the stage for potential abuse.
- Whether the abuse is intrafamilial or occurs outside the family structure, moral inhibitions must be overcome by the perpetrator in a setting where the child is not adequately protected or supervised.
- Individual factors (e.g., developmental or physical disabilities or risk-taking behaviors) may predispose some children to sexual abuse.

EPIDEMIOLOGY & DEMOGRAPHICS
- Sexual abuse makes up 10% to 15% of all abuse cases.
- Reported cases rose to more than 400,000 nationally in the early 1990s but fell to 200,000 in the mid-1990s.
  1. Approximately 1 in 2 to 1 in 3 reports are substantiated.
- An estimated 12% to 25% of girls and 8% to 10% of boys have been sexually abused.
- Perpetrators have the following characteristics:
  1. More than 90% are males (at least 20% are adolescents).
  2. Up to 90% are known to the victims (approximately one third are relatives).
- Sexual abuse is most common in school-age children but has occurred at all ages.
- Sexual abuse occurs in all socioeconomic groups.

HISTORY
- Sexual abuse classically develops along the following pattern:
  1. The victim is engaged in a relationship with the perpetrator.
  2. Sexual interaction is gradually established.
  3. Secrecy is established through threats or rewards.
  4. Disclosure may occur depending on the receptiveness of the caretakers.
  5. Suppression may occur if abuse is not disclosed or when there is inadequate therapy.
- Focus on the genitourinary system (rectal or genital bleeding or other complaints) as well as behavioral issues (e.g., phobias, sleep disorders).
- Use a nonleading interview style, with attention to the child's spontaneous utterances.
- Anatomically correct dolls or line drawings may be helpful to the experienced interviewer.

PHYSICAL EXAMINATION
- If less than 72 hours since the assault, rape protocol with collection of forensic material is critical (physical findings are more likely to be seen, although not common).
- If more than 72 hours since the abusive episode, the examination should include the following:
  1. A thorough pediatric examination, noting signs of trauma (digital or speculum exams are not necessary in the prepubertal child)
  2. Genital examination using the supine and knee-chest positions in females
  3. Anal evaluation, although abnormalities are uncommon
  4. Visualization of the hymen: child supine, gentle traction on the labia majora with moderate separation, often combined with the prone knee-chest position
     a. Hymenal appearance is annular, crescentic, fimbriated (redundant), septate, and imperforate.
     b. Transverse diameter of the opening varies with position and age of child.
     c. Foley catheter technique may be helpful in adolescents.
     d. Culdoscopy is helpful.
     e. Tears, abrasion, or other trauma is present in only 10% to 20% of cases.
- Interpretation of examination findings is as follows:
  1. Most children proven to be sexually abused have normal examinations or nonspecific findings after normal examinations.
  2. Minor variations of the hymen or anus are often seen in non-abused children.

3. A normal examination should not deter a physician from reporting a history of sexual abuse.

DIAGNOSIS

Based largely on the history that may or may not be supported by physical findings

DIFFERENTIAL DIAGNOSIS
- Genital findings may be caused by the following:
  1. Lichen sclerosis
  2. Prolapsed urethra
  3. Streptococcal rash
  4. Congenital hemangiomas
  5. Straddle injuries
  6. Molluscum contagiosum
- Anal findings, including fissures or dilation, may be caused by the following:
  1. Postmortem dilation
  2. Crohn's disease
  3. Constipation
  4. Neurogenic problems

DIAGNOSTIC WORKUP
- Laboratory evaluation is centered on sexually transmitted diseases (STDs).
  1. Prevalence is 2% to 7%.
- Screening for STDs should be considered in the following situations:
  1. Historical factors: perpetrator with STD, patient with STD or genital discharge, sibling with an STD, other high-risk situations such as prostitution or multiple perpetrators
  2. Examination factors: vaginal discharge, genital injuries, adolescent
- The most common STDs are gonorrhea, *Chlamydia*, and genital warts.
- Interpretation of positive tests for STDs and their relationship to sexual abuse (excluding congenital infections) are as follows:
  1. Gonorrhea, syphilis, human immunodeficiency virus (HIV), *Chlamydia*: almost always
  2. Genital warts, *Trichomonas*, genital herpes: possible
  3. Bacterial vaginosis: unclear
- Forensic analysis involves the following:
  1. Swabs of mouth, rectum, vagina, and any suspicious staining on skin (identified by Wood's lamp) for sperm, semen, acid phosphatase, blood, or other antigens, and screen for STDs
  2. Saliva specimen of victim to determine secretor status
  3. Collection of underwear and any clothing with suspicious staining
  4. Collection of combed pubic hair as well as cut or plucked pubic hair
- Expected results: Forensic evidence is most likely to be recovered when collected close to the time of assault. It

is not useful to attempt collection of forensic evidence after 72 hours.
- Interpretation of abnormal results is as follows:
  1. Definitive evidence of sexual contact: sperm, seminal fluid, or pregnancy
  2. Highly suspect for sexual contact: acute injuries of the genitalia or an STD

THERAPY

■ NONPHARMACOLOGIC
Mental health assessment and therapy

■ MEDICAL
- STDs should be treated with appropriate agents when identified.
- STD prophylaxis is acceptable in sexually active adolescents.
- Antiretroviral therapy should be considered if patient is at high risk to acquire HIV.
- Postcoital contraception should be discussed with adolescent if less than 72 hours since the assault.

■ SURGICAL
Intervention is required only with significant vaginal or rectal injuries requiring repair.

■ FOLLOW-UP & DISPOSITION
- Medical personnel are mandated reporters by law in all states in suspected or known cases of sexual abuse.
  1. Be familiar with your jurisdiction's reporting agencies.
  2. Positive tests may need follow-up for test of cure or repeat testing, as with HIV.

■ PATIENT/FAMILY EDUCATION
- The caretakers should understand that protecting the child from further abuse is paramount.
- Mental health therapy is critical.
- The child should be informed of his or her normal examination or the likelihood that his or her body will heal to a normal state even if injuries are present.

■ REFERRAL INFORMATION
- Acute rape cases should be seen immediately.
- Less acute cases of abuse should be evaluated in a judicious manner.

PEARLS & CONSIDERATIONS

■ CLINICAL PEARLS
It is normal to be normal (i.e., on the physical examination) after sexual abuse.

■ WEBSITES
- American Humane Association: www.amerhumane.org
- National Benevolent Association Colorado Christian Home Tennyson Center for Children & Families: www.childabuse.org

■ SUPPORT GROUPS
- Parents Anonymous Inc.: www.parentsanonymous.org
- Call the local United Way referral line.

REFERENCES
1. American Academy of Pediatrics Committee on Child Abuse and Neglect: Guidelines for the evaluation of sexual abuse of children, *Pediatrics* 103:186, 1999.
2. Atabaki S, Paradise JE: The medical evaluation of the sexually abused child: lessons from a decade of research, *Pediatrics* 104:178, 1999.
3. Reece RM: *Child abuse: medical diagnosis and management,* Baltimore, 1994, Lea & Febiger.
Author: **Charles Schubert, M.D.**

BASIC INFORMATION

■ DEFINITION
Shigellosis is a gram-negative bacillary dysentery caused by members of the genus *Shigella* (family Enterobacteriaceae).

■ SYNONYM
Bacillary dysentery

ICD-9CM CODE
004 Shigellosis

■ ETIOLOGY
- Shigellosis is caused by nonmotile, gram-negative, nonencapsulated rods, usually non–lactose-fermenting and non–gas-producing.
- *Shigella* are serologically grouped (A to D) on the basis of the carbohydrate antigen of their lipopolysaccharide.
  1. Group A: *Shigella dysenteriae:* 10 serotypes (widespread in rural Africa and the Indian subcontinent)
  2. Group B: *Shigella flexneri:* 14 serotypes (most common in tropical countries, second most common in the United States)
  3. Group C: *Shigella boydii:* 18 serotypes (uncommon in the United States)
  4. Group D: *Shigella sonnei:* 1 serotype (causes most shigellosis in the United States; mildest disease)

■ EPIDEMIOLOGY & DEMOGRAPHICS
- Shigellosis is spread from human feces by the fecal-oral route.
  1. No natural animal reservoirs are known.
- This is most commonly a pediatric disease infecting children 6 months to 5 years of age.
  1. Crowded areas with poor hygiene and sanitation are predisposing factors.
- It is most commonly transmitted from person to person.
  1. Ingestion of contaminated food and water and contact with a contaminated object can transmit *Shigella*. Transmission also can occur with anal intercourse.
  2. Houseflies are considered vectors, transporting infected feces.
- Foodborne transmission represents 20% of *Shigella* transmission in the United States.
  1. Shigellosis accounts for 2% of foodborne illness–related hospitalizations and 0.8% of total foodborne illness deaths.
- Transmission in feces ceases when the organism is no longer present in

stool, which usually occurs within 4 weeks of illness.
  1. *Shigella* carriers are rare, but they can have intermittent bouts of the disease and can harbor the organism for more than 1 year.

■ HISTORY
- The incubation period is usually 2 to 4 days.
- Shigellosis classically presents with crampy abdominal pain; rectal burning; and multiple small, bloody, mucoid bowel movements. Severity can vary greatly and may or may not include constitutional symptoms.
- Fever presents in 40% of cases. The classic presentation of blood and mucus in the stool is seen in only 33% of cases.
- Children usually have mild infections lasting 1 to 3 days (as opposed to 7 days in adults).
- It is often biphasic:
  1. Phase one is secondary to enterotoxin.
     a. Symptoms include fever, watery diarrhea, and abdominal pain.
  2. Phase two is secondary to invasion of colonic epithelium, leading to tenesmus and small-volume bloody stools.
- A variety of extraintestinal manifestations may be seen:
  1. Bacteremia
  2. Colonic perforation
  3. Neurologic (not related to direct central nervous system infection) manifestations particularly common in children and include seizures and meningismus
     a. Fulminant toxic encephalopathy (ekiri) is rare.
  4. Hemolytic uremic syndrome (usually from *S. dysenteriae* type 1)
  5. Reiter's syndrome or asymmetric large joint arthritis: may develop 2 to 3 weeks after onset (*S. flexneri*)

■ PHYSICAL EXAMINATION
Guaiac-positive stool is helpful in identifying enteroinvasive diarrheal illnesses.

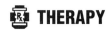

DIAGNOSIS

■ DIFFERENTIAL DIAGNOSIS
- Invasive (bacterial) diarrheal illnesses include the following:
  1. *Salmonella, Campylobacter,* and *Yersinia*
  2. Invasive amoebic illness (*Entamoeba histolytica*)
  3. Colonic mucosal-damaging organisms, including *Escherichia coli* O157:H7
- Subacute illness can be confused with ulcerative colitis.

■ DIAGNOSTIC WORKUP
- Methylene blue wet mount of stool can help identify erythrocytes and sheets of polymorphonuclear cells, but it is not specific.
- Rectal swabs or fecal specimens can be sent for culture. This organism is fastidious, and samples should be placed in fecal transport medium or cultured directly within 2 to 4 hours.
- Blood cultures are rarely helpful because bacteremia is uncommon in immunocompetent hosts.

THERAPY

■ NONPHARMACOLOGIC
Rehydration and electrolyte management

■ MEDICAL
- Medical management is indicated in most cases. With dysentery, antibiotics shorten the duration of diarrhea and eliminate organisms from stool. In mild illness, antibiotics can help limit the spread of the organism.
- Ampicillin *(not amoxicillin because it is less effective)* is the drug of choice for U.S.-acquired *sensitive* strains (12.7% resistance).
- For shigellosis of unknown susceptibility or ampicillin-resistant strains, trimethoprim-sulfamethoxazole (TMP-SMX) is the drug of choice. *Shigella* acquired from developing countries is more likely to have multiple resistances (often plasmid acquired) and may be resistant to both TMP-SMX and ampicillin.
- A 5-day course of antibiotics is usually considered adequate therapy.

■ FOLLOW-UP & DISPOSITION
The disease is usually self-limited. Hydration/electrolyte disturbances may require close monitoring.

■ PATIENT/FAMILY EDUCATION
Handwashing, as well as control measures for sanitary water and food handling, should be emphasized.

■ PREVENTIVE TREATMENT
- Infected individuals should not return to food preparation occupations or child care until treatment has been provided and diarrhea has ceased.
- Symptomatic contacts of infected individuals (whether child care providers or household contacts) should be cultured.

■ REFERRAL INFORMATION
There are few indications for referral.

☼ PEARLS & CONSIDERATIONS

■ CLINICAL PEARLS
- Narcotic-related antimotility agents may prolong excretion and course of symptoms.
- Symptoms of mild diarrhea and cramps may persist after adequate treatment secondary to mucosal injury.

■ WEBSITE
Centers for Disease Control and Prevention: www.cdc.gov/ncidod

REFERENCES
1. American Academy of Pediatrics: *Shigella* infections. In Pickering LK (ed): *2000 Red Book: report of the Committee on Infectious Diseases,* ed 25, Elk Grove Village, Ill, 2000, American Academy of Pediatrics.
2. Edwards B: Salmonella and shigella species, *Clin Lab Med* 19:469, 1999.
3. Feldman M et al: *Sleisenger and Fordtran's gastrointestinal and liver disease: pathophysiology/diagnosis/ management,* ed 6, Philadelphia, 1998, WB Saunders.
4. Green S, Tillotson G: Use of ciprofloxacin in developing countries, *Pediatr Infect Dis J* 16:150, 1997.
5. Mead PS et al: Food-related illness and death in the United States, *Emerg Infect Dis* 5:607, 1999.

Author: **Gus G. Emmick, M.D.**

II

BASIC INFORMATION

■ **DEFINITION**
Short bowel syndrome refers to a foreshortened bowel with subsequent nutrient malabsorption. Neither the absolute length nor the percent of resection or reduction in surface area is part of the definition.

■ **SYNONYM**
Short gut (syndrome)

ICD-9CM CODE
579.2 Blind loop syndrome
579.3 Short bowel syndrome number

■ **ETIOLOGY**
Any disease or abnormality that decreases the absorptive area of the intestines can lead to short bowel syndrome.
• Inflammatory diseases
  1. Crohn's disease
  2. Necrotizing enterocolitis
  3. Radiation enteritis
• Anatomic disorders
  1. Bowel atresia
  2. Volvulus
  3. Gastroschisis
  4. Omphalocele
  5. Hirschsprung's disease
  6. Congenital short bowel
• Vascular insufficiency
  1. Thrombosis
  2. Volvulus
  3. Vascular disease

■ **EPIDEMIOLOGY & DEMOGRAPHICS**
• No known ethnic distribution
• Prematurity (necrotizing enterocolitis)
• True incidence unknown

■ **HISTORY**
• Previous bowel resection
• Poor weight gain
• Diarrhea
• Multiple nutrient deficiency states

■ **PHYSICAL EXAMINATION**
• Muscle wasting
• Abdominal distention
• Succession splash
• Scars from previous surgery

🔬 **DIAGNOSIS**

■ **DIFFERENTIAL DIAGNOSIS**
• Steatorrhea: fecal fat coefficient of absorption less than 90%
  1. Liver disease
  2. Pancreatic insufficiency (cystic fibrosis)
• Impaired xylose absorption

• Malabsorption from disaccharidase deficiency
  1. Low-pH stools with positive reducing substances
• Chronic infections: can present with short gut–like syndrome
  1. Acquired immunodeficiency syndrome
  2. Parasites
• Celiac disease
• Milk-protein intolerance

■ **DIAGNOSTIC WORKUP**
Radiographic demonstration of shortened gut must be abnormal, but extent of resection varies.

💊 **THERAPY**

■ **MEDICAL**
• Parenteral nutrition
  1. Use exclusively only for 1 to 2 weeks.
  2. Institute enteral feedings as early as possible.
  3. Monitor volume and electrolyte losses in diarrheal stool.
    a. Replace milliliter per milliliter with solution containing electrolyte concentrations equal to losses.
• Enteral nutrition
  1. Begin early.
  2. Begin slowly.
  3. Use continuous infusions, not bolus feedings.
  4. Use amino acid or protein hydrolysate formula, preferably with a high percentage of long-chain fat content to stimulate gut adaptation and reduce osmotic fluid losses.
  5. Advance enteral and decrease parenteral nutrition in an isocaloric fashion on a daily basis.
    a. Base transition on tolerance, with periodic adjustments for growth and metabolic needs.
    b. Use weight gain as the primary endpoint, not calculations of needed caloric intake.
• Monitoring
  1. Stool output is primary endpoint for advancing or reducing enteral feedings.
  2. Do not monitor stool fat content.
  3. Do not monitor for occult blood, but observe for gross blood.
  4. Advance enteral feedings as long as stool or ostomy output is reasonable (less than 20 to 40 ml/kg/day).
  5. Monitor electrolytes, minerals, trace minerals, vitamins, and liver enzymes based on institutional total parenteral nutrition (TPN) guidelines.
  6. Monitoring for nutritional deficiencies becomes more crucial once TPN is discontinued.

• Dietary therapy
  1. Use amino acid or hydrolysate formula during the first year to reduce the risk of allergic inflammation in the gut.
  2. Start infant on solids at a normal developmental age, but begin feedings with meat because high fat content will reduce osmotic stool losses and increase the stimulus for adaptation of the bowel.
  3. Avoid hypertonic liquids (e.g., Kool-Aid, juices, soda).
  4. Introduce oral feedings of liquids and solids early (i.e., during the first 2 to 3 weeks) in small quantities to stimulate sucking and swallowing reflexes.
• Once TPN has been weaned
  1. Monitor carefully for deficiencies of minerals and fat-soluble vitamins.
  2. Use continuous enteral infusion during the nighttime and bolus or oral feeding during the daytime as a transition to oral feeding.
  3. Avoid hypertonic beverages and high-carbohydrate diets.
  4. Avoid high oxylate-containing foods, such as chocolate.
  5. Caloric needs may rise during puberty, necessitating transient return to parenteral nutrition.

■ **SURGICAL**
• Consider tapering enteroplasty or intestinal lengthening procedure (Bianchi procedure) in the case of dilated bowel with bacterial overgrowth when otherwise unable to advance feedings or manage condition medically.
• Do not attempt artificial valves, reverse segments, or other means designed to reduce intestinal transit in children because these procedures often induce bacterial overgrowth.
• Consider intestinal transplantation only in the presence of irreversible liver disease or life-threatening recurrent sepsis or loss of central venous access.

■ **COMPLICATIONS**
• TPN liver disease
  1. Prevent with aggressive use of enteral feedings, avoidance of septic episodes, and treatment of small bowel bacterial overgrowth.
  2. Ursodeoxycholic acid has been used but has not been definitively shown to be helpful.
• Nutritional deficiency states
  1. Fat-soluble vitamins (A, D, E, K) and minerals, such as calcium, magnesium, and zinc, are the most common deficiencies.
  2. Usually, deficiencies develop after patient has been weaned from parenteral nutrition.

3. B_{12} deficiency is common with extensive ileal resection and requires parenteral or nasal therapy.
- Biliary tract disease
  1. Gallstones
  2. More common in TPN-dependent patients who are intolerant of enteral feedings
  3. Often requires cholecystectomy if present
- Small bowel bacterial overgrowth
  1. This is common if motility is slow or the bowel is dilated.
  2. Diagnosis based on increased urine indicans, elevated breath hydrogen after glucose administration, increased serum D-lactate level.
  3. Bacterial overgrowth is common but usually only a problem when inflammation exists; therefore culture demonstration of increased bacterial organisms is not generally helpful.
  4. Demonstration of inflammation in the distal small bowel endoscopically is often suggestive of pathologic bacterial overgrowth and may respond to antiinflammatory therapy (i.e., aspirin, glucocorticosteroids)
- Anastomotic ulcerations
  1. May result in severe blood loss and anemia
  2. Requires endoscopic diagnosis
  3. Medical therapy usually not helpful; often requires resection

■ FOLLOW-UP & DISPOSITION
- Patients with less than 40 cm of small bowel at the time of neonatal resection and those who lack an ileocecal valve have a poor prognosis for becoming independent of parenteral nutrition.
  1. Exceptions common
- Patients with less extensive resection may eventually over a period of years no longer need parenteral nutrition.
  1. If patients are not independent of

parenteral nutrition by age 5 years, they will likely need parenteral nutrition lifelong.
- Intestinal transplantation has been advocated for children with irreversible TPN liver disease, loss of central venous access, or severe recurrent sepsis.
  1. The prognosis for long-term survival off TPN is little better than 50% with transplantation.
  2. Long-term parenteral nutrition in the stable patient probably carries a better ultimate prognosis.

☼ PEARLS & CONSIDERATIONS

■ CLINICAL PEARLS
- If a patient is previously doing well and then starts doing poorly with no changes, look for bacterial overgrowth or nutritional deficiency states.
- Avoid antidiarrheal agents such as loperamide in children with stasis and bacterial overgrowth.
- Encourage use of diets high in fat and low in simple carbohydrates.

■ WEBSITES
- Healthtouch Online: www.healthtouch.com
- MCW HealthLink: www.Healthlink.mcw.edu
- National Institute of Diabetes & Digestive & Kidney Diseases: www.niddk.nih.gov/health/digest/summary/shortbo/shortbo.htm

REFERENCES

1. Kaufman SS et al: Magnesium acetate vs. magnesium gluconate supplementation in short bowel syndrome, *J Parenter Gastroenterol Nutr* 16:104, 1993.
2. Kaufman SS et al: Influence of bacterial overgrowth and intestinal inflammation on duration of parenteral nutrition in children with short bowel syndrome, *J Pediatr* 131:356, 1997.
3. Thompson JS, Vanderhoof JA, Antonson DL: Intestinal tapering and lengthening for the short bowel syndrome, *J Parenter Gastroenterol Nutr* 4:495, 1985.
4. Thompson JS et al: Experience with intestinal lengthening for the short bowel syndrome, *J Pediatr Surg* 26:721, 1991.
5. Thompson JS et al: Surgical approach to short bowel syndrome: experience in a population of 160 patients, *Ann Surg* 222:600, 1995.
6. Vanderhoof JA: Short bowel syndrome: smoothing the road to recovery, *Contemp Pediatr* 9:19, 1992.
7. Vanderhoof JA: Short bowel syndrome in children, *Curr Opinion Pediatr* 7:560, 1995.
8. Vanderhoof JA: Short bowel syndrome, *Clin Perinatol* 23:377, 1996.
9. Vanderhoof JA: Short bowel syndrome and intestinal transplantation, *Pediatr Clin North Am* 43:533, 1996.
10. Vanderhoof JA, Langnas AN: Short bowel syndrome in children and adults, *Gastroenterology* 113:1767, 1997.
11. Vanderhoof JA et al: Invited review: short bowel syndrome, *J Parenter Gastroenterol Nutr* 14:359, 1992.
12. Vanderhoof JA et al: Treatment strategies for small bowel bacterial overgrowth in short bowel syndrome, *J Parenter Gastroenterol Nutr* 27:155, 1998.

Authors: **Jon A. Vanderhoof, M.D.,** and **Rosemary J. Young, R.N., M.S.**

II

BASIC INFORMATION

■ DEFINITION
Short stature is height below the 3rd percentile or greater than 2 standard deviations (SD) below the mean height for chronologic age.

■ SYNONYM
Dwarfism (severe form of short stature with height below 3 SD from the mean)

ICD-9CM CODES
783.43 Short stature
783.4   Constitutional delay

■ ETIOLOGY
Normal variant
- Familial or genetic short stature
  1. Child is normal weight and length at birth.
  2. Growth velocity may be decreased in the first 2 to 3 years of life ("catch down") but normal thereafter.
  3. Onset and progression of puberty are normal.
  4. Final adult height is short but appropriate for parental heights.
  5. Bone age is consistent with chronologic age.
- Constitutional delay of growth and adolescence
  1. Normal or near-normal growth velocity
  2. Delayed skeletal growth and maturation and delayed onset of puberty
  3. Final adult height and progression of sexual development normal
  4. Often with family history of delayed growth and onset of sexual development
Pathologic causes of short stature
- Proportionate: normal upper:lower body segment ratio for age
  1. Endocrinopathies: usually associated with an increased weight:height ratio.
     a. Growth hormone (GH) deficiency/insensitivity
     b. Hypothyroidism
     c. Cushing's syndrome
  2. Malnutrition
  3. Gastrointestinal pathology: malabsorption, inflammatory bowel disease, celiac disease
  4. Renal disease: renal tubular acidosis, chronic renal failure, nephrogenic diabetes insipidus
  5. Other chronic diseases: cardiac, pulmonary, liver, chronic infection
  6. Intrauterine growth retardation
     a. Infants with birth weight more than 2 SD below the mean for gestational age, sex, and race
     b. Causes: placental insufficiency, fetal infections, teratogens, chromosomal abnormalities

- Disproportionate: abnormal upper:lower body segment ratio for age
  1. Skeletal dysplasia: achondroplasia, hypochondroplasia
  2. Metabolic bone disease: rickets
  3. Abnormalities of vertebral bodies
- Associated with dysmorphic features
  1. Trisomy 21 (Down syndrome)
  2. Prader-Willi syndrome
  3. Turner syndrome
     a. Short stature is the most consistent and sometimes the only clinical sign of this syndrome.
  4. Russell-Silver syndrome

■ HISTORY
- Prenatal history: maternal infection, consumption of alcohol, use of drugs
- Pattern of growth (height and weight): include birth weight and length in relation to gestational age
- Family history: parental heights, onset of puberty of parents and immediate relatives
- Profile of patient's pubertal development: include onset of breast development, menarche, onset of penile enlargement, pubic hair development
- Nutrition
- Evidence of systemic disease: gastrointestinal, cardiac, pulmonary, renal
- Drug administration: steroids, methylphenidate
- Neurologic symptoms: headache, visual disturbance, recent history of enuresis
- Psychosocial milieu

■ PHYSICAL EXAMINATION
Full physical examination with special emphasis on the following:
- Accurate measurements of height, weight, head circumference, arm span, and upper and lower body segments
- Nutritional state, fat distribution
- Pubertal stage
- Dysmorphic features
- Complete neurologic examination, including funduscopy and visual fields
- Examination of the thyroid gland

DIAGNOSIS

■ DIFFERENTIAL DIAGNOSIS
See "Etiology."

■ DIAGNOSTIC WORKUP
- Growth curve analysis
  1. Reliability of measurements
     a. Inaccurate plotting of measurements on the growth chart and measurement error are common reasons for misdiagnosis of growth disorders and inappropriate referral.

2. Height velocity
   a. This is the most important aspect of growth evaluation.
   b. Accurate determination requires a minimum of 6 months of observation.
   c. Normal height velocity for chronologic age at any absolute height is unlikely to be associated with pathologic causes.
   d. Normal average yearly growth rates are 8 cm at 2 years, 7 cm at 3 years, and 5 to 6 cm from 4 to 9 years.
3. Absolute height
   a. This bears some relationship to the likelihood of a pathologic condition.
   b. Absolute height of 3 SD below the mean is more likely to be pathologic than height of 1 SD below the mean.
4. Weight:height ratio
   a. Endocrine disorders are usually associated with relatively preserved weight gain or frank obesity in a short child.
   b. Systemic disorders (e.g., gastrointestinal, renal, pulmonary, cardiac) are associated with greater impairment of weight gain than linear growth.
- Other helpful parameters
  1. Target height
     a. Males = [father height (cm) + mother height (cm) +13] ÷ 2
     b. Females = [father height (cm) + mother height (cm) – 13] ÷ 2
     c. Child's height is appropriate for the family if the projected adult height is within the target height by 8 cm.
  2. Upper:lower segment body ratio
     a. Lower segment is measured from symphysis pubis to the floor.
     b. Upper segment = height – lower segment
     c. Useful to assess whether the short stature is proportionate or disproportionate.
     d. Mean upper:lower segment ratio is 1.7 at birth, 1.3 at 3 years, 1.0 after 7 years, and 0.9 as an adult.
- Bone age
  1. Skeletal maturity assessment is done by comparing the appearance of epiphyseal centers on radiography with age-appropriate published standards.
  2. This assessment is more prognostic than diagnostic; its main use is in prediction of final height.
  3. Normal or advanced bone age in a child with short stature is of greater concern than delayed bone age. Linear growth will continue until epiphyseal fusion is complete.

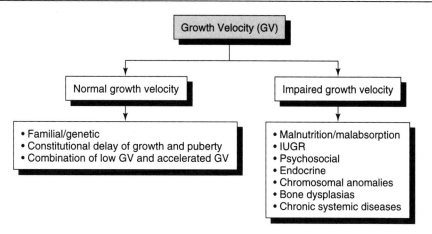

Fig. 2-4   Growth velocity.

- Laboratory screening tests
  1. Well-nourished or obese child with deceleration in linear growth
     a. Thyroid-stimulating hormone (TSH) and free T_4: Elevated TSH and low free T_4 indicate primary hypothyroidism.
     b. Insulin-like growth factor I (IGF-I, somatomedin C) and insulin-like growth factor binding protein-3 (IGF-BP): Low levels are suggestive of GH deficiency.
        (1) Provocative GH stimulation test (arginine insulin tolerance test) is the accepted gold standard method for confirming the diagnosis of GH deficiency.
     c. Urinary free cortisol level: if Cushing's syndrome is suspected.
  2. Thin child with deceleration of linear growth
     a. Complete blood count and sedimentation rate: helpful to identify patients with inflammatory bowel disease or chronic inflammatory process
     b. Urinalysis, serum creatinine, and electrolytes: to exclude renal disorder
     c. Sweat chloride test: indicated if suspect cystic fibrosis
     d. Serum calcium, phosphorus, alkaline phosphatase: to exclude subtle forms of rickets or other disorders of mineral metabolism
  3. Short child with dysmorphic features or disproportionate short stature
     a. Karyotype should be obtained if features suggest chromosomal abnormalities or a syndrome. Also indicated in most female children with short stature to exclude Turner syndrome even in the absence of classical physical stigmata.
     b. Skeletal dysplasia radiologic survey should be done, especially in disproportionate short stature.

■ THERAPY

- If specific cause is identified, treat the underlying disease.
- Specific hormone replacement should be considered for hypothyroidism and GH deficiency.
- In Turner syndrome, consider GH treatment.
- Constitutional delay of growth and adolescence:
  1. Reevaluate every 6 to 12 months.
  2. Treatment with short course of testosterone is an option in some patients.

☼ PEARLS & CONSIDERATIONS

■ CLINICAL PEARLS

- Deceleration of height velocity after 2 to 3 years of life indicates a pathologic condition unless proven otherwise.

- Systemic disorders are usually associated with greater impairment of weight gain than linear growth.
- For a short child with preserved weight gain, think of endocrine disorders.
- Longitudinal determination of height velocity is the most important factor in evaluating short stature.

■ SUPPORT GROUPS

- Little People of America, National Headquarters, P.O. Box 745, Lubbock, TX 79408; 888-572-2001; www.lpaonline.org
- Human Growth Foundation, Inc., 997 Glen Cove Avenue, Glen Head, NY 11545; 800-451-6434; www. hgfound.org
- Turner's Syndrome Society of the U.S., 1313 Southeast 5th Street, Suite 327, Minneapolis, MN 55414;800-365-9944; www. turner-syndrome-us.org

REFERENCES

1. Lifshitz F, Cervantes C: Short stature. In Lifshitz F (ed): *Pediatric endocrinology,* ed 3, Philadelphia, 1995, WB Saunders.
2. Rosenfeld R: Disorders of growth hormone and insulin-like growth factor secretion and action. In Sperling MA (ed): *Pediatric endocrinology,* Philadelphia, 1996, WB Saunders.
3. Vogiatzi M, Copeland K: The short child, *Pediatr Rev* 19:92, 1998.
Authors: **Marlah M. Tomboc, M.D., and Ram K. Menon, M.D.**

BASIC INFORMATION

DEFINITION

The term *sickle cell disease* describes hemoglobin SS (Hb SS), hemoglobins resulting from the production of Hb S in concert with another abnormal hemoglobin (e.g., Hb SC, SD, SO), and the sickle β-thalassemia syndromes in which Hb S is accompanied by either reduced (β^+) or absent (β°) production of normal adult hemoglobin (Hb Sβ thalassemia). Vasoocclusion and chronic hemolytic anemia characterize the disease.

SYNONYM

Sickle cell anemia applies to Hb SS

ICD-9CM CODE

282.60 Sickle cell anemia

ETIOLOGY

- A single nucleotide change (A to T) in the β globin gene results in substitution of valine for glutamic acid in the sixth position of the β globin chain of hemoglobin; this change leads to the synthesis of Hb S.
- When exposed to low oxygen tension, Hb S tends to polymerize within the red cell, resulting in alterations of membrane shape and function, increased cell density, and reduced deformability.
- Distorted "sickled" cells obstruct blood flow in small vessels, leading to tissue ischemia (vasoocclusion).
- Red cell alterations lead to reduced cell life span (hemolytic anemia).
- Young reticulocytes express receptors that make them more adherent to endothelial cells lining blood vessels; increases in cytokines enhance these interactions.
- Abnormalities of clotting are noted and may contribute to stroke, chest crises, and the like.

EPIDEMIOLOGY & DEMOGRAPHICS

- In the United States, African Americans and Hispanics are most commonly affected.
- The disease severity is quite variable.
- The sickle cell trait is identified in 8% of the African-American population.
- If the sickle mutation (S trait) is carried by both parents, there is a 25% chance of an offspring having Hb SS, a 50% chance of the essentially benign condition S trait, and a 25% chance of having normal hemoglobin (Hb AA).
- Many states provide universal hemoglobinopathy screening shortly after birth.

HISTORY

- Anemia and reticulocytosis generally present in Hb SS by 4 months of age and are not detected in newborn; baseline anemia intensified with aplastic crises or splenic sequestration
- Pain crises
  1. These are experienced as deep, throbbing pain, usually without physical findings; children younger than 5 years may experience pain in the form of the "hand-foot syndrome," with swelling and tenderness of hands and/or feet.
- Increased susceptibility to infection with encapsulated organisms
- Acute chest syndrome with pulmonary infiltrate; restrictive lung disease
- Symptoms of stroke; subtle cognitive abnormalities
- Delayed growth and sexual development
- Scleral icterus, cholelithiasis, acute pancreatitis
- Hyposthenuria (usually seen by age 3) with urinary frequency and enuresis. Papillary necrosis, nephrotic syndrome, priapism
- Cortical thinning, bony expansion, aseptic necrosis of femoral/humoral heads, osteomyelitis
- Skin ulcers
- Retinal neovascularization resulting in blindness, vitreous hemorrhage, retinal detachment; hyphema

PHYSICAL EXAMINATION

- Short stature, evidence of delayed sexual maturation
- Bony distortion secondary to bone marrow expansion
- Scleral icterus, funduscopic abnormalities
  1. Nonproliferative retinopathy with adjacent hemorrhage
  2. Proliferative retinopathy stages 1 to 5
- Systolic murmur
- Splenomegaly in infants and children; also seen in adolescents with Hb SC or Sβ⁺
- Pain with weight bearing or with rotation of hip or arm
- Skin ulcers
- Neurologic deficits secondary to stroke

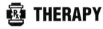

DIAGNOSIS

DIFFERENTIAL DIAGNOSIS

Other causes of anemia, primarily hemolytic

DIAGNOSTIC WORKUP

- Preferably on child and his or her parents; interpret with aid of a hematologist, if possible (following ranges apply to children older than 5 years)
- Complete blood count (CBC): Hb (g/dl) = 6 to 11 (SS), 6 to 10 (Sβ⁰ thalassemia), 9 to 12 (Sβ⁺ thalassemia), 10 to 15 (SC)
- Indices: mean corpuscular volume (fL) = more than 80 (SS), less than 80 (Sβ⁰ thalassemia), less than 75 (Sβ⁺ thalassemia), 75 to 95 (SC)
- Reticulocyte count (%) = 5 to 20 (SS, Sβ⁰ thalassemia), 5 to 10 (Sβ⁺ thalassemia, SC)
- Blood film: sickle cells, targets, Howell-Jolly bodies, nucleated red cells, polychromasia
- Solubility test (e.g., the Sickledex): positive in sickle cell trait, disease; negative in Hb C, D, O, and so forth, β-thalassemia trait
- Hemoglobin electrophoresis, quantitative measurements of Hb A_2 and F

THERAPY

- Anemia
  1. Red cell transfusion may be needed when anemia is exacerbated by aplastic crises or splenic sequestration.
  2. Patient should be transfused preoperatively (consult a hematologist for guidelines) if general anesthesia is to be used.
- Infection
  1. Examine the child and obtain cultures and appropriate laboratory studies.
  2. Emergently treat any febrile or ill-appearing child with antibiotics effective against *Streptococcus pneumoniae* and *Haemophilus influenzae*.
     a. Use additional antibiotic in areas where resistant organisms are identified.
     b. National Institutes of Health (NIH) guidelines for admission are as follows:
        (1) Temperature higher than 40° C
        (2) Seriously ill appearance
        (3) Hypotension
        (4) Poor perfusion and dehydration
        (5) Pulmonary infiltrate
        (6) Corrected white blood cell count of more than 30,000/mm³ or less than 5000/mm³
        (7) Platelet count less than 100,000/mm³
        (8) Hemoglobin less than 5 g/dl
        (9) History of *S. pneumoniae* sepsis
     c. Admit all children whose follow-up cannot be guaranteed.

3. If treated as an outpatient:
   a. Examine the child and obtain cultures and obtain appropriate laboratory studies.
   b. Give ceftriaxone intravenously or intramuscularly.
   c. Have patient return within 24 hours or sooner if ill appearing.
   d. Administer a second dose of ceftriaxone at 24 hours.
   e. If blood cultures are negative at 48 hours, may discontinue antibiotics or treat identifiable source orally.
- Pain
  1. Provide hydration, nonsteroidal antiinflammatory drugs, codeine, and oral morphine.
  2. Administer intravenous hydration and morphine in the emergency department.
  3. Continued therapy as an inpatient may be required.
     a. Anticipate pain with regular, not as-needed, dosing.
     b. Patient-controlled analgesia pump to administer morphine may be useful.
  4. Hydroxyurea, given under the supervision of a hematologist, is useful for selected children with frequent debilitating pain episodes.
  5. Behavioral modification techniques and hypnosis may be helpful.
- Acute chest syndrome: admit to hospital
  1. May need antibiotics
  2. May require transfusion
  3. Bedside spirometer helpful
- Stroke: immediate intervention in an intensive care unit
  1. Administer an exchange transfusion under the supervision of a hematologist.
  2. The goal is to reduce the Hb S level to less than 20%.
  3. Subsequent chronic transfusion therapy will be needed.

■ FOLLOW-UP & DISPOSITION
Regular visits to a comprehensive sickle cell disease center, primary physician, dentist, and ophthalmologist are needed.

■ PATIENT/FAMILY EDUCATION
- Anticipatory guidance should be age and syndrome appropriate.
  1. Topics for discussion and reinforcement include the following:
     a. Need to seek medical attention for fever or ill appearance
     b. Regular penicillin administration
     c. Appropriate hydration
     d. Thermometer use
     e. Spleen palpation
     f. Recognition of signs of sequestration, aplastic crises, stroke, priapism, aseptic necrosis, and chest crises
- Genetic counseling and diagnostic testing should be made available to all families of children with sickle cell disease.
- Emphasis should be on preventing complications.

■ PREVENTIVE TREATMENT
- Immunizations
  1. Standard series, including hepatitis B if not immunized
  2. Pneumococcal vaccine (age 2 years and again at age 4 to 6 years)
  3. Annual influenza vaccine
  4. Meningococcal vaccine (offered by some centers)
- Penicillin prophylaxis: 125 mg orally two times per day until age 3 years, then 250 mg orally two times per day
- Folic acid: optional (recently published data show patients are actually folate replete)
  1. Age 2 to 6 months: 0.1 mg
  2. Age 6 to 12 months: 0.25 mg
  3. Age 1 to 5 years: 0.5 mg
  4. Age 5 years or older: 1 mg orally per day
- Regular laboratory studies, including a full CBC, reticulocyte count, platelet count, urinalysis, tests of liver and kidney function, hepatitis/human immunodeficiency virus antibodies if transfused, and tests to assess pulmonary status
- Regular transcranial Doppler ultrasound screening to assess stroke risk

■ REFERRAL INFORMATION
May require referral to a pediatric nephrologist, cardiologist, pulmonologist, orthopedist, urologist, neurologist, gastroenterologist, and/or surgeon for evaluation and treatment of various complications

☼ PEARLS & CONSIDERATIONS

■ CLINICAL PEARLS
The documented decrease in the mortality rate for children with sickle cell disease is likely related to preventive strategies, including early diagnosis, penicillin prophylaxis, comprehensive care, and the recognition and treatment of life-threatening events.

■ WEBSITE
Emory University: www.emory.edu/PEDS/SICKLE

■ SUPPORT GROUP
Sickle Cell Disease Association of America, Inc.; local chapters in many cities

REFERENCES
1. Lane PA: Sickle cell disease, *Pediatr Clin North Am* 43:639, 1996.
2. Platt OS et al: Mortality in sickle cell disease: life expectancy and risk factors for early death, *N Engl J Med* 330:1639, 1994.
3. Reid CD et al: *Management and therapy of sickle cell disease,* ed 3, NIH Publication No. 95-2117, Bethesda, Md, 1995, National Institutes of Health, National Heart, Lung and Blood Institute.
Author: **Norma B. Lerner, M.D.**

BASIC INFORMATION

DEFINITION
- *Sinusitis* is inflammation of one or more of the paranasal sinuses. The most common cause of sinusitis is infection.
- *Acute sinusitis:* Symptoms for more than 10 days and up to 3 to 4 weeks (some clinicians would suggest to consider up to 8 weeks), consisting of some or all of the following: persistent upper respiratory infection (URI) symptoms, purulent rhinorrhea, postnasal drainage, anosmia, nasal congestion, facial pain, headache, fever, cough, and vomiting.
- *Chronic sinusitis:* Symptoms for more than 3 to 4 (or up to 8) weeks of varying severity, consisting of the same symptoms as seen in acute sinusitis.
- *Recurrent sinusitis:* Three or more episodes of acute sinusitis per year. Patients with recurrent sinusitis may be infected by different organisms at different times.

SYNONYMS
- Rhinosinusitis
- Acute rhinosinusitis
- Acute bacterial sinusitis
- Infectious sinusitis

ICD-9CM CODE
461.9 Acute sinusitis

ETIOLOGY
- Infants have patent maxillary and ethmoid sinuses, which continue to grow until late adolescence. Sphenoid sinuses begin development at 2 years of age. Frontal sinuses begin to form by age 6 and complete development by 12 years.
- During an acute viral respiratory tract infection, the epithelium of the sinus ostia, ostiomeatal complex, and with sinuses undergo inflammatory response.
  1. Altered ciliary function
  2. Increased secretory activity
- Obstruction of an ostium during an acute viral process creates the conditions for a secondary bacterial infectious sinusitis.
- Sinusitis occurring in the first week of a respiratory infection is usually viral in origin.
- In patients with acute sinusitis, about 75% of maxillary sinus aspirates contain bacteria, usually *Streptococcus pneumoniae,* nontypable *Haemophilus influenzae,* or *Moraxella catarrhalis.* Group A streptococcus or *Staphylococcus aureus* may also be present.
- These organisms are also common in patients with chronic sinusitis, al-

though *S. aureus,* coagulase-negative staphylococci, α-hemolytic streptococci, and enteric bacilli are more common in this condition.
- Fungal infections may rarely be observed as a nonfulminant, chronic sinusitis in older children and adolescents.
- Conditions that predispose children to chronic sinusitis include the following:
  1. Allergic and nonallergic rhinitis
  2. Anatomic abnormality of the ostiomeatal complex
  3. Nasal anatomic variations (septal deviation, concha bullosa, abnormality of the middle turbinate)
  4. Cystic fibrosis
  5. Common variable immunoglobulin deficiency
  6. Immunoglobulin A (IgA) deficiency
  7. Ciliary dyskinesia, Kartagener syndrome, Young syndrome
  8. Aspirin sensitivity
  9. Acquired immunodeficiency syndrome
  10. Bronchiectasis
  11. Cocaine abuse
  12. Wegener's granulomatosis
  13. Rhinitis medicamentosa

EPIDEMIOLOGY & DEMOGRAPHICS
- URIs are the most common clinical problems for primary practitioners who care for children.
- Approximately 5% to 10% of URIs in early childhood are complicated by acute sinusitis.

HISTORY
- Bacterial sinusitis causes a spectrum of nonspecific symptoms and is likely underdiagnosed.
- Classic symptoms reported in adults include nasal congestion, purulent rhinorrhea, postnasal drainage, facial or dental pain, headache, hyposmia, and cough.
- Unlike adults, children do not usually report sinus congestion, pain, or headache.
- Some children may not even appear to be ill, and if fever is present, it is low grade.
- Some children may have a cold that seems more severe than usual, with high fever, purulent and copious nasal discharge, periorbital swelling, and facial pain.
- Important symptoms in a child could include daytime and nighttime cough (particularly when first lying down) and nasal discharge. A persistent daytime cough is often the symptom that brings a child to medical attention.

PHYSICAL EXAMINATION
- In general, for children younger than 10 years of age, the physical examination is of little value in making a specific diagnosis of acute sinusitis.
- *Visualization:* nasal mucosa: Characterize nasal secretions, polyps, and the structure of the nasal septum; inspect tympanic membranes because concomitant otitis media is common.
- *Palpation:* Check tenderness over maxillary and frontal sinuses; tap maxillary teeth with tongue blade.
- *Transillumination* is best when determined to be either normal or absent; difficult in children younger than 10 years of age.
- When present, periorbital swelling, facial tenderness, and malodorous breath (in the absence of dental disease) are probably the most specific findings in acute sinusitis.

DIAGNOSIS

DIFFERENTIAL DIAGNOSIS
- *Infectious:* acute viral infection, acute or chronic bacterial sinusitis
- *Allergic:* seasonal allergic rhinitis (pollens), perennial allergic rhinitis (dusts, molds)
- *Vasomotor:* idiopathic (vasomotor rhinitis), abuse of nose drops (rhinitis medicamentosa), drugs (reserpine, guanethidine, prazosin, cocaine), psychologic stimulation (anger, sexual arousal)
- *Mechanical:* foreign body, polyps, tumor, deviated septum, crusting, hypertrophied turbinates, central nervous system leak, enlarged tonsils and adenoids
- *Hormonal:* pregnancy, hypothyroidism, hyperthyroidism

DIAGNOSTIC WORKUP
- Standard radiographic projections include an anteroposterior, a lateral, and for the maxillary sinuses, an occipitomental view.
  1. Remember that in simple URI, sinus radiographs may be abnormal.
- Radiographic findings in patients who have acute sinusitis include diffuse opacification, mucosal thickening of at least 4 mm, or an air-fluid level.
- In a patient with suggestive signs and symptoms, the radiologic evaluation provides supportive information and often is unnecessary.
- In addition to mucosal thickening and complete opacification, radiographic changes seen in chronic sinusitis may include an actual decrease in sinus size caused by increased wall thickness.

- Although computed tomography scans of the sinuses are superior at delineating sinus abnormalities, they are not necessary for management of children with uncomplicated acute sinusitis and should be reserved for the evaluation of complicated or chronic sinusitis.
  1. If available, a limited coronal view reduces radiation exposure and cost.
- Current indications for maxillary sinus aspiration include the following:
  1. Failure to respond to multiple courses of antibiotics
  2. Severe facial pain
  3. Orbital or intracranial complications
  4. Evaluation of an immunocompromised host

THERAPY

■ MEDICAL
- *Antibiotics* are the primary therapy for bacterial sinusitis.
  1. Antibiotics chosen should be based on predicted effectiveness, cost, and side effects.
- In general, treat acute sinusitis for 10 to 14 days and chronic sinusitis for 21 days minimum (at least 7 asymptomatic days on treatment).
  1. Drugs of choice include the following:
     a. Amoxicillin
     b. Amoxicillin/clavulanate
  2. Other antibiotics include the following:
     a. Cephalosporins such as cefuroxime, cefpodoxime, and cefdinir
     b. Macrolide antibiotics such as azithromycin and clarithromycin
     c. Clindamycin
     d. Metronidazole
- *Antihistamines:* No data are presently available to recommend their use in acute sinusitis; they may have a role in chronic sinusitis, particularly in patients with allergic rhinitis.

- *α-Adrenergic decongestants* are commonly used in both acute and chronic sinusitis, but no studies have demonstrated efficacy.
- *Glucocorticoids:* Intranasal steroids may be beneficial as an adjunct to antibiotics, but the use of systemic steroids is not well delineated.
- *Adjunctive therapies:* Saline nose drops or spray appear to be useful for symptomatic treatment, but prophylactic use is empiric and not supported by clinical data.
- *Intravenous immune globulin* is indicated for use in patients with impaired humoral immunity.

■ SURGICAL
- Antral puncture and irrigation may be useful in acute ethmomaxillary sinusitis refractory to medical therapy.
- For immunosuppressed patients, identification of the pathogenic organism may be warranted via antral puncture.

■ REFERRAL INFORMATION
- Referral to an otolaryngologist should be considered when complications such as bronchiectasis, fungal sinusitis, or multiple antibiotic allergies occur, and/or when quality of life is compromised.
- Referral to an allergist should be considered if an underlying allergic or immunologic process is suspected.
- An otolaryngologic surgeon should be consulted when anatomic factors impair optimal medical management, biopsy and/or cultures are required, or severe complications ensue.

PEARLS & CONSIDERATIONS

■ CLINICAL PEARLS
- Sinusitis is insidious in children, and concurrent otitis media is common.
- For children older than 10 years of age, the combination of maxillary toothache, poor response to nasal de-

congestants, abnormal transillumination, and colored nasal discharge by history or examination are the most useful clinical findings in primary care populations.
  1. When all five features are present, the odds of sinusitis rise sharply (positive likelihood ratio of 6.4).
  2. When none are present, sinusitis is virtually ruled out.
- Transillumination of the maxillary sinuses requires a completely darkened room, adequate time for dark adaptation, and practice.
- Quantitative sweat chloride tests for diagnosis of cystic fibrosis should be considered in children with nasal polyps and/or colonization of the nose and sinuses with *Pseudomonas* species.

■ WEBSITES
For health care providers
- Joint Council of Allergy, Asthma, and Immunology; www.jcaai.org/param/sinusitis/complete_text.htm
For patients:
- Western Michigan University: www.wmich.edu/healthquest/patientedu/earnosethroat.htm

REFERENCES
1. Blumer J: Clinical perspectives on sinusitis and otitis media, *Pediatr Infect Dis J* 17:S68, 1998.
2. Hopp R, Cooperstock M: Medical management of sinusitis in pediatric patients, *Curr Probl Pediatr* 27:178, 1997.
3. Spector SL et al: Sinusitis practice parameters, *J Aller Clin Immun* 102:S107, 1998.
4. Wald ER: Sinusitis, *Pediatr Rev* 14:345, 1993.
5. Wald ER: Sinusitis in children, *N Engl J Med* 326:319, 1992.
6. Williams JW, Simel DL: The rational clinical exam: does this patient have sinusitis? Diagnosing acute sinusitis by history and physical exam, *JAMA* 270:1242, 1993.

Author: **Marc A. Raslich, M.D.**

II

BASIC INFORMATION

■ DEFINITION
Obstructive sleep apnea is disordered breathing during sleep characterized by periods of partial and/or complete upper airway obstruction with disruption of normal sleep and ventilatory patterns.

ICD-9CM CODE
780.57 Sleep apnea

■ ETIOLOGY
- Anatomic (structural blockage of nasopharyngeal/laryngeal airway)
  1. Nasal/nasopharyngeal
     a. Adenoid hypertrophy
     b. Septal hematoma/deviation
     c. Choanal atresia/stenosis
     d. Nasal polyps/sinonasal tumors
  2. Oropharyngeal
     a. Tonsillar hypertrophy (pharyngeal/lingual)
     b. Macroglossia
     c. Tumors in floor of mouth/tongue (especially vascular malformations)
  3. Laryngeal
     a. Laryngomalacia
     b. Laryngeal tumors/cysts
  4. Craniofacial (e.g., Down, Crouzon, Apert, and Treacher-Collins syndromes)
     a. Mandibular hypoplasia/retrognathia (e.g., Pierre-Robin sequence)
     b. Midface hypoplasia
- Neuromuscular (poor muscle tone/pharyngeal support)
  1. Cerebral palsy
  2. Myotrophic dystrophy
  3. Arnold-Chiari malformation
- Miscellaneous
  1. Obesity: causes redundant pharyngeal tissue
  2. Mucopolysaccharidoses (Hunter and Hurler's syndrome): nasal congestion, redundant pharyngeal tissue, poor pharyngeal support, fatty soft tissue deposits
  3. Achondroplasia: small pharynx, poor muscle tone, relative macroglossia
  4. Prader-Willi syndrome (mental retardation, obesity, hypogonadism)
  5. Gastroesophageal reflux disease: airway irritation and swelling with associated laryngospasm

■ EPIDEMIOLOGY & DEMOGRAPHICS
- It occurs in 1% to 3% of children.
- Of those affected, 75% to 90% are male.
- Incidence has increased over the last 20 years.

■ HISTORY
- Snoring (continuous or intermittent, changes with position)
- Mouth breathing, retractions, gasping respirations, pauses in breathing
- Behavior disturbances, declining school performance
- Excessive daytime sleepiness
- Morning headaches
- Enuresis
- Failure to thrive (poor weight gain)
- Search for history of cor pulmonale and/or congestive heart failure
  1. Shortness of breath
  2. Dyspnea
  3. Orthopnea
  4. Easy fatigue
  5. Poor exercise tolerance

■ PHYSICAL EXAMINATION
- Tonsillar enlargement
- Mouth breathing
- Craniofacial anomalies: adenoid facies (opened mouth posture, flat midface, dull appearance)
- Body habitus: obesity

DIAGNOSIS

■ DIFFERENTIAL DIAGNOSIS
- Benign snoring must be differentiated from apnea (see definitions under "Diagnostic Workup")
- Apnea may be obstructive (blockage of upper airway) or central (decreased respiratory drive from central neurologic origin)

■ DIAGNOSTIC WORKUP
- Diagnosis is often based on clinical history and examination.
- Flexible nasopharyngoscopy/laryngoscopy will identify anatomic obstruction.
- Lateral airway film can be obtained to identify adenoid hypertrophy.
- Polysomnography monitors oxygen, respirations, air flow, electroencephalogram, sleep stages, and electrocardiogram.
  1. Done if the diagnosis or severity of the problem is unclear, if no obvious anatomic obstruction is present, or if symptoms are not resolved after initial treatment.
  2. Definitions are as follows:
     a. Apnea: cessation of air flow for 10 seconds
     b. Hypopnea: 50% reduction in air flow with decreased oxygen saturation
     c. Respiratory disturbance index: number of apneas (greater than 1 is normal) and hypopneas (apnea hypopnea index greater than 5 is abnormal) per hour

     d. Sleep disturbance index: number of arousals per hour (no normative data, number is nonspecific)
- Home videotapes or cassette recordings may help identify questionable apneic events.
- Chest radiograph or echocardiogram can identify cor pulmonale and congestive heart failure.

THERAPY

■ NONPHARMACOLOGIC
Weight loss

■ MEDICAL
- Continuous positive airway pressure (CPAP) is effective but poorly tolerated by some children.
- Allergy and infection treatment should be considered.

■ SURGICAL
- Adenotonsillectomy is often the only intervention necessary.
- Tracheostomy is the gold standard, bypasses area of obstruction.
- Septoplasty or removal of obstructive nasal tissue can be effective.
- Uvulopalatopharyngoplasty is more common in adults. This process removes excessive uvulae and redundant pharyngeal/soft palatal tissue. Tonsillectomy is often performed as well.
- Tongue reduction and mandibular advancement can be helpful.

■ FOLLOW-UP & DISPOSITION
- Patients often need to be monitored postoperatively.
- Risk is respiratory problems and postobstructive pulmonary edema.

■ PATIENT/FAMILY EDUCATION
- Teach parents about pulmonary and cardiac risks if symptoms are severe.
- Provide weight loss education when appropriate.

■ REFERRAL INFORMATION
- Otolaryngologists assist in the diagnosis of anatomic obstruction and provide surgical therapy if needed.
- Pulmonologists perform sleep studies, help with diagnosis of central sleep apnea, and assist in the use of CPAP.

PEARLS & CONSIDERATIONS

■ CLINICAL PEARLS
- Not all snoring is obstructive sleep apnea. Look for gasping, frequent positional changes, neck extension, or

brief awakenings to help differentiate the two.
- Most obstructive sleep apnea is from adenotonsillar hypertrophy and is easily treated.
- Sleep apnea in children is different from that in adults. Children are less likely to have sustained apneic events but are more susceptible to hypopneas and repeated desaturations.

■ WEBSITE
American Sleep Apnea Association: www.sleepapnea.org

REFERENCES
1. Guilleminault C et al: Recognition of sleep disordered breathing in children, *Pediatrics* 98:871, 1996.
2. Potsic WJ: Obstructive sleep apnea, *Pediatr Clin North Am* 36:1435, 1989.
3. Suen JS et al: Adenotonsillectomy for the treatment of obstructive sleep apnea in children, *Arch Otolaryngol Head Neck Surg* 121:525, 1995.
Authors: **L. Mark Gustafson, M.D., and Charles M. Myer III, M.D.**

II

BASIC INFORMATION

■ DEFINITION
Sleep problems include difficulty sleeping through the night, disturbance in the amount or timing of sleep (including refusal and night wakings), and abnormal behaviors that occur during sleep (night terrors, nightmares, sleep talking and sleepwalking).

■ SYNONYMS
- Sleep disorders
- Sleep disruption

ICD-9CM CODES
307.40 Nonorganic sleep disorder, unspecified
307.41 Transient disorder of initiating or maintaining sleep
307.42 Persistent disorder of initiating or maintaining sleep
307.43 Transient disorder of initiating or maintaining wakefulness
307.44 Persistent disorder of initiating or maintaining wakefulness
307.45 Phase-shift disruption of 24-hour sleep-wake cycle
307.46 Somnambulism or night terrors
307.47 Other dysfunction of sleep stages or arousal from sleep
307.48 Repetitive intrusions of sleep
307.49 Other sleep disorder

■ ETIOLOGY
- Physical factors such as upper respiratory infections or injuries may lead to a temporary sleep problem.
- Developmental factors such as separation anxiety may also be a cause.
- Behavioral factors such as children remaining dependent on parents and parents who continue to be overinvolved may be an issue.
  1. Other possible behavioral aspects include anxiety, depression, and posttraumatic stress.
- Environmental and interactional factors include the following:
  1. Bedtime and nighttime feedings
  2. Use of objects that are associated with falling asleep, including the presence of the parents, that may not be available to the child throughout the night
  3. Overprotective or overinvolved parents
  4. Parents who have difficulty setting limits
  5. Family stresses

■ EPIDEMIOLOGY & DEMOGRAPHICS
- This is one of the most common complaints of parents to pediatricians.
- Frequent night waking occurs in 25% of 6- to 12-month-olds and 20% of 1- to 2-year-olds.
- Difficulty settling occurs in 50% of 4-year-olds.
- Nightmares occur from 5% in 1-year-olds to 39% in 4-year-olds.

■ HISTORY
- Familial causes of nonorganic sleep problems are uncommon.
- Questions to ask include the following
  1. Are there evening activities and a bedtime ritual?
  2. How are difficulties at bedtime handled?
  3. What is the time and length of wakening?
  4. What are the time, ease, and spontaneity of morning waking?
  5. What is the daytime schedule for weekdays and weekends?
  6. What are the timing and length of daytime sleeping?
  7. How do the parents view the problem?
- History of snoring may be suggestive of obstructive sleep apnea
- Determine whether the child experiences sleep terrors.
- Determine whether the child experiences sleepwalking.
- Obtain a description of the sleep environment: noise (TV), lighting, with other people (parents, siblings), pets.
- Ask about medications and other medical conditions.
- Ask about recent illnesses.
- Determine whether there is a history of seizures.

■ PHYSICAL EXAMINATION
- Airway
- Nasal air flow
- Tonsil size
- General physical condition
- Neurologic examination

🔬 DIAGNOSIS

■ DIFFERENTIAL DIAGNOSIS
- Diagnosis is based on the history, with physical examination used to rule out other abnormalities.
- Obstructive sleep apnea is often caused by enlarged tonsils and adenoids in children.
- Seizure disorder, anxiety, and/or depression may be present.

■ DIAGNOSTIC WORKUP
- Have parents keep a sleep log (diary) for at least 1 week to obtain the current pattern of difficulties.
- The use of a polysomnogram and the multiple sleep latency test may be useful if no other explanation is obtained for a child with a significantly shorter nighttime sleep pattern (less than 5 hours) and no additional daytime sleep.

💊 THERAPY

■ NONPHARMACOLOGIC
- Difficulty initiating sleep
  1. Set limits.
  2. This is done by a gradual ignoring procedure.
     a. Increase length of time before each return to child's room.
     b. Spend a brief time in room to reassure the child.
- Difficulty with nighttime waking
  1. Review sleep associations.
  2. Assist the child in self-soothing behaviors.
  3. Good sleep hygiene is essential.
     a. Consistent schedule
     b. Consistent pattern
  4. Wait for progressively longer periods before checking on, or briefly visiting with, the child.
- Night terrors
  1. Explain that they are not harmful.
  2. Night terrors occur in a sleep state that is not a dream state (non–rapid eye movement).
  3. Child has no memory of the event.
  4. Night terrors last minutes to half an hour.
  5. Parents should provide protection if the child is thrashing wildly.
  6. Usually, terrors resolve in days to months.
- Nightmares
  1. These are managed by comforting the child.
  2. Any additional discussion about the nightmare should occur during the day.
  3. Nightmares can be caused by watching scary movies or TV shows or by family stress.
  4. Eliminate or manage stress to help relieve additional nightmares.
- Sleep phase-shift
  1. Managed by an incremental shift back to the normal night shift, then rigidly adhering to the schedule
- Transient sleep problems
  1. Generally no need for specific treatment

■ MEDICAL
- Benadryl use for sleep initiation has been recommended and may result in brief, limited improvement.
- For serious sleep terrors (high frequency or extreme disruption to family), benzodiazepines or tricyclic antidepressants have been recommended for use.

■ FOLLOW-UP & REFERRAL INFORMATION
- Most of the aforementioned sleep problems are well managed behaviorally.
  1. If difficulty persists, a behavioral specialist can be consulted.

2. Organic sleep problems should be treated and referred as medically indicated.

- Concerns of serious emotional disturbance related to sleep problems should be referred for evaluation of the emotional disturbance.

■ PATIENT/FAMILY EDUCATION

- Focus on understanding of the following:
  1. Normal patterns and length of sleep based on age
  2. The stages of sleep
  3. The normal occurrence of nightly partial awakenings
  4. Sleep associations and how to establish bedtime rituals with positive sleep associations
  5. Use of a "transitional object" (e.g., a special toy or favorite blanket) to assist a child in falling asleep.
- Typically, nighttime feedings are not needed after 3 months of age.
- By 6 months, most children are capable of sleeping through the night.

■ PREVENTIVE TREATMENT

Anticipatory guidance about normal sleep patterns, positive sleep associations, good sleep hygiene, and good behavioral limit setting can significantly reduce or prevent sleep problems.

☼ PEARLS & CONSIDERATIONS

■ CLINICAL PEARLS

- Behavioral solutions of sleep problems can lead to other successful behavioral changes.
- Common sleep problems can often be relieved in 2 weeks or less.
- Sleep initiation problems and nighttime waking solutions using a progressive ignoring procedure allow parents to gain control.
- Solving basic sleep problems should be presented to parents as a way of providing the child with appropriate developmental guidance.

■ WEBSITES

- Sleep Medicine Home page: www.users.cloud9.net/~thorpy
- Sleepnet.com: www.sleepnet.com
- Behavioral Sleep Medicine Network list serve, send subscription to majordomo@maillist.urmc.rochester.edu; Command:Subscribe Behavsleepmed; in body of email, type email address

REFERENCES

1. Blum NJ, Carey WB: Sleep problems among infants and young children, *Pediatr Rev* 17:87, 1996.
2. Ferber RA: *Solve your child's sleep problems,* New York, 1985, Simon & Schuster.
3. Ferber RA, Kryger MH (eds): *Principles and practice of sleep medicine in the child,* Philadelphia, 1995, WB Saunders.
Author: **Roger Yeager, Ph.D.**

II

BASIC INFORMATION

■ DEFINITION
Slipped capital femoral epiphysis (SCFE) is the most common adolescent orthopedic hip disorder. The femoral head separates from the femoral neck at the epiphysis.

■ ICD-9CM CODES
820.01 Epiphysis
731.1 Femoral capital epiphysis

■ ETIOLOGY
- The cause has not been completely determined. Current theory involves interaction of both biomechanical forces and biochemical events.
  1. The growth plate is known to be in a weakened state during puberty.
  2. Slipping, even with minor shearing forces, can occur with a combination of the following:
     a. Weakened growth plate
     b. Large body mass
     c. Hormonal changes: thyroid, growth hormone, testosterone, and estrogen
- Endocrine disorders with possible association include hypothyroidism, growth hormone deficiency, and hypogonadism.
  1. Hypothyroidism is the most common endocrine disorder associated with SCFE.
- Obesity is seen in 60% to 70% of patients.
  1. Obese children have decreased femoral anteversion.
  2. Femoral retroversion is found to be associated with SCFE.
- Genetic factors include HLA-B12 in two case reports of identical twins and HLA-DR4 in a separate study of six patients.
- Significant trauma is not common.

■ EPIDEMIOLOGY & DEMOGRAPHICS
- The general incidence is 1 to 3 per 100,000.
- It is more prevalent in boys than girls; ratio reported at 1.43 to 2:1.
- Ages range from 12 to 14 years old for Caucasian boys and 11 to 13 years old for Caucasian girls.
  1. During adolescent growth spurts
     a. Early puberty for girls
     b. Midpuberty for boys
- Most common in Native Australians and Pacific Islanders, then African Americans, then Caucasians (Europeans).
- Left hip is involved more often.
- Bilateral involvement occurs in 18% to 25% for Caucasians and 31% to 51% for African Americans.
  1. Occurs more commonly sequentially (61%) than simultaneously (39%)

2. Average time of 1 year (range, 1 to 4 years) between recognition of first and second hip involvement

■ HISTORY
- Presentation is classified as stable versus unstable.
- Stable: Symptoms may last weeks to months.
  1. Pain or discomfort at hip, groin, or knee (from referred pain)
  2. Complaints of "pulled muscle"
  3. Limping after strenuous exercise
- Unstable: Symptoms are acute.
  1. Patient is not able to bear weight, even with use of crutches.
  2. Pain seems excessive relative to a presumed associated traumatic event (e.g., tripping over curb).

■ PHYSICAL EXAMINATION
- Limited internal rotation and abduction of hip are noted.
- Flexion rotation test is positive: external rotation of the hip upon passive flexion of hip.
- Pain is felt with internal and external rotation.
- If chronic, leg will be externally rotated with associated antalgic limp and abductor lurch.
- Always evaluate the contralateral (normal) hip for comparison.

🔬 DIAGNOSIS

■ DIFFERENTIAL DIAGNOSIS
- Legg-Calvé-Perthes
- Avascular necrosis of femoral head
- Juvenile arthritis
- Toxic synovitis

■ DIAGNOSTIC WORKUP
- Anteroposterior and cross-table lateral hip radiographs: Abnormalities include the following:
  1. Widened irregular epiphyseal plate
  2. Osteopenia of femoral neck and head
  3. Abnormal Klein line (drawn along superior femoral neck) will not transect epiphysis (should transect about 20% of epiphysis)
- Classification of femoral head slippage is as follows:
  1. Minimal: slight to one third epiphyseal diameter (of femoral neck)
  2. Moderate: one third to two thirds epiphyseal diameter
  3. Severe: greater than two thirds epiphyseal diameter

💊 THERAPY

■ NONPHARMACOLOGIC
- No known nonpharmacologic therapy is available.
- Discuss weight loss in all obese children.

■ MEDICAL
Treat underlying endocrinopathies.

■ SURGICAL
- Proper therapy is immediate surgery.
  1. Slipping will continue to progress.
  2. Minor trauma can increase the severity of the displacement and the potential for development of avascular necrosis.
- Surgery consists of pin fixation to stabilize the femoral head onto the femoral neck.

■ FOLLOW-UP & DISPOSITION
- After surgery, weight bearing should be with crutches until pain free, approximately 2 to 6 weeks.
- Patient can resume sports after growth plates fuse, which takes 6 weeks to 6 months.
- Contralateral hip should be followed and pinned early if symptoms occur.

■ PATIENT/FAMILY EDUCATION
- Avascular necrosis (up to 50%) and chondrolysis (up to 40%) are possible complications.
  1. Avascular necrosis is seen secondary to stretching of vessels during slipping of the femoral head.
  2. Chondrolysis is seen mostly with penetration of the femoral head articular cartilage during surgical correction. It can also be seen with severe slips.
- The possibility of contralateral hip involvement should be discussed.

■ PREVENTIVE TREATMENT
- Early diagnosis is important for management.
- Patient must not bear weight on the affected leg once the diagnosis is made.

■ REFERRAL INFORMATION
All patients should be referred to an orthopedic surgeon.

☼ PEARLS & CONSIDERATIONS

■ CLINICAL PEARLS
- If the patient is younger than 9 years or older than 16 years, think of endocrinopathies (e.g., hypothyroidism).
  1. The abnormality seen on plain anteroposterior radiograph in hypothyroidism will be an epiphysis not overlapping the metaphysis, usually present by age 10.

- In girls, SCFE occurs before menarche (growth spurt early in puberty for girls).
- Presentation at a younger age increases the possibility of future contralateral hip involvement (more time involved until epiphyseal closure).

REFERENCES

1. Bielak KM, Henderson JM: Slipped capital femoral epiphysis. In Birrer RB (ed): *Sports medicine for the primary care physician,* ed 2, Boca Raton, Fla, 1994, CRC Press.
2. Gunal I, Ates E: The HLA phenotype in slipped capital femoral epiphysis, *J Pediatr Orthopaed* 17:655, 1997.
3. Loder RT: The demographics of slipped capital femoral epiphysis, *Clin Orthopaed Related Res* 322:8, 1996.
4. Richards BS: Slipped capital femoral epiphysis, *Pediatr Rev* 17:69, 1996.
5. Schwend RM, Geiger J: Outpatient pediatric orthopedics: common and important conditions, *Pediatr Clin North Am* 45:943, 1998.
6. Weiner D: Pathogenesis of slipped capital femoral epiphysis: current concepts, *J Pediatr Orthopaed* 5:67, 1996.
7. Weisman DS: Personal communication, Department of Orthopaedics, University of Rochester School of Medicine and Dentistry, Rochester, New York.

Author: **Sharon Chen, M.D.**

BASIC INFORMATION

■ DEFINITION
Snake bites are of particular medical significance in children. Although fatalities are rare, the clinical condition of a child after a snake bite tends to be worse than that of an adult because of a larger per kilogram dose of venom.

ICD-9CM CODE
989.5 Toxic effect of venom

■ ETIOLOGY
- Most snake bites on this continent are from the *Crotalidae,* which include such species as rattlesnakes, copperheads, and water moccasins.
- Their venom contains a variety of toxins that have a wide array of effects.

■ EPIDEMIOLOGY & DEMOGRAPHICS
- Snake bites can occur in any area of North America, especially because many snakes are kept as pets or for entertainment purposes.
- Adolescents and adults are most commonly bitten.

■ HISTORY
- Usually witnessed bite
- Local pain and inflammation
- Nausea
- Metallic taste
- Fasciculations

■ PHYSICAL EXAMINATION
- Spectrum of possible reactions ranging from very mild local inflammation to death
- Variable local edema
- Fang marks (may or may not be visible)
- Ecchymosis at site
- Bullae (may be hemorrhagic)
- Necrotic areas later
- Possible compartment syndrome
- Regional lymphadenitis
- Generalized bleeding
- Hypovolemic shock from capillary leak syndrome

DIAGNOSIS

■ DIFFERENTIAL DIAGNOSIS
The diagnosis of a snake bite is typically made based on history and physical examination alone.
- Snake bite
- Spider bite
- Anaphylaxis
- Sepsis

■ DIAGNOSTIC WORKUP
- Check for coagulopathy and bleeding.
  1. Complete blood count with platelet count
  2. Prothrombin time
  3. Fibrinogen
- Check for electrolyte abnormalities.

THERAPY

Therapy is aimed at managing local damage, capillary leak syndrome, and possible coagulopathic and neurotoxic effects.

■ NONPHARMACOLOGIC
- Minimize movement.
- Remove clothing, bracelets, and any other restrictive items.
- Apply a circumferential rubber band (not a tourniquet) to occlude venous and lymphatic drainage of venom.
- Elevate the affected area.

■ MEDICAL
- Provide intravenous fluid resuscitation.
- Administer narcotic analgesia.
- Update tetanus status.
- Antivenin administration is indicated for all but mild local reactions and is dosed according to severity. The regional poison control center should be consulted regarding the specifics of administration.
  1. Anaphylaxis can occur.
  2. A delayed serum sickness occurs in almost all patients after antivenin administration.

■ SURGICAL
- Serial extremity circumference measurements should be taken every 20 minutes.
  1. Increasing values of greater than 0.5 cm per hour should warrant concern and frequent assessment of perfusion distal to the bite.
- Although compartment syndrome is relatively rare since the advent of antivenin, any compromise of distal perfusion requires surgical consultation.

■ FOLLOW-UP & DISPOSITION
- Discharge can occur when the patient is managed with oral analgesics and systemic symptoms have ceased. Edema must be stable as well.
- Physical therapy is often indicated during the recovery phase.

■ REFERRAL INFORMATION
The regional poison control center can answer any questions about the treatment of snake bite victims.

PEARLS & CONSIDERATIONS

■ CLINICAL PEARLS
- Maintain vital signs.
- Ensure distal perfusion.
- Consult regional poison control center regarding antivenin administration.

■ WEBSITE
Queensland Ambulance Service: www.ambulance.qld.gov.au/firstaid/hints.asp; select "Bites and Stings"

REFERENCES
1. Bond GR: Reptile envenomation. In Reisdorff EJ, Roberts MR, Wiegenstein JG (eds): *Pediatric emergency medicine,* Philadelphia, 1993, WB Saunders.
2. Bond GR: Snake, spider and scorpion envenomation in North America, *Pediatr Rev* 20:147, 1999.
Author: **Robert Freishtat, M.D.**

BASIC INFORMATION

■ DEFINITION
Hereditary spherocytosis is the most common inherited abnormality of the red cell membrane that can cause hemolytic anemia.

■ ICD-9CM CODE
282.0 Hereditary spherocytosis

■ ETIOLOGY
- Hereditary spherocytosis is transmitted as an autosomal dominant and, much less often, as an autosomal-recessive disorder.
- The spheroid red cells most commonly result from abnormalities of spectrin or ankyrin, which are structural proteins of the red cell membrane.
- The spherocytic red cells are destroyed prematurely in the spleen.

■ EPIDEMIOLOGY & DEMOGRAPHICS
- Hereditary spherocytosis affects approximately 1 in 5000 individuals.
- It is most common in persons of Northern European ancestry.

■ HISTORY
- Affected individuals may have minimal hemolysis and therefore may not be diagnosed as children or may have a severe hemolytic anemia with pallor, jaundice, fatigue, and exercise intolerance.
  1. Because of the shortened red cell life span, patients are susceptible to aplastic crises associated with parvovirus and other infections.
  2. Patients can present in the newborn period with anemia and hyperbilirubinemia.
- Positive family history of jaundice, anemia, or gallbladder stones may be reported.

■ PHYSICAL EXAMINATION
- Tachycardia, pallor
- Icterus
- Right upper quadrant tenderness (bilirubin cholelithiasis)
- After infancy, the spleen usually is enlarged

■ DIAGNOSIS

■ DIFFERENTIAL DIAGNOSIS
- Other inherited disorders of the red cell membrane include hereditary elliptocytosis, hereditary stomatocytosis, and hereditary pyropoikilocytosis. These disorders can be distinguished from each other by evaluating the blood film for their distinctive morphology.
- Immune hemolysis also may cause a large number of spherocytes on the blood film. This may be distinguished from hereditary spherocytosis by a positive direct Coombs' test.

■ DIAGNOSTIC WORKUP
- The diagnosis of hereditary spherocytosis is suggested by the presence of a positive family history, splenomegaly, reticulocytosis, and spherocytosis of red cells.
- The hemoglobin level is usually 6 to 10 g/dl, depending on individual severity.
- The reticulocyte count is increased to 6% to 20%.
- Spherocytes are found on the blood film, usually accounting for 15% to 20% of the cells.
- The presence of spherocytes in the blood can be confirmed by an osmotic fragility test.
- A Coombs' test should be performed to ensure that the clinical findings are not secondary to immune hemolytic anemia.
- Other evidence of hemolysis may include elevated indirect bilirubin and decreased haptoglobin.
- Gallstones can be seen on abdominal ultrasonography.

■ THERAPY

■ NONPHARMACOLOGIC
Hematocrit and reticulocyte percentage should be obtained early during febrile illnesses to detect aplastic crises.

■ MEDICAL
- Patients with hereditary spherocytosis who maintain a hemoglobin greater than 10 g/dl and a reticulocyte percentage less than 10 should be treated expectantly with folic acid 1 mg/day.
- In infants with severe anemia, chronic transfusion therapy may be necessary to delay splenectomy until at least 2 years of age to reduce the highest risk of postsplenectomy sepsis.

■ SURGICAL
- Splenectomy eliminates the hemolysis in hereditary spherocytosis but should be delayed until age 6 years to minimize the risk of postsplenectomy sepsis.
- Splenectomy should be reserved for the following patients:
  1. Patients who cannot sustain a hemoglobin of 10 g/dl
  2. Those who have experienced repeated aplastic crises
  3. Those with markedly enlarged spleens who may be at risk for splenic rupture

■ FOLLOW-UP & DISPOSITION
- Hematocrit and reticulocyte percentages should be monitored every 6 to 12 months.
- Immunizations for encapsulated bacteria before splenectomy and penicillin prophylaxis after splenectomy are recommended.

REFERENCES
1. Hassoun H, Palek J: Hereditary spherocytosis: a review of the clinical and molecular aspects of the disease, *Blood Rev* 10:129, 1996.
2. Nathan DG, Orkin SH (eds): *Nathan and Oski's hematology of infancy and childhood*, ed 5, Philadelphia, 1998, WB Saunders.

Authors: **Jill S. Halterman, M.D., and George B. Segel, M.D.**

II

BASIC INFORMATION

■ DEFINITION
Spiders belong to the class Arachnida, which includes animals with four pairs of legs and no wings or antennae.

ICD-9CM CODE
989.5 Toxic effect of venom

■ ETIOLOGY
- Although most spider bites cause no more than a local reaction, the bites of two species of spiders in the United States can cause severe symptoms.
- The two spiders of medical significance are the brown recluse and the black widow.
- Other spiders are discussed here as well.

■ CLINICAL COURSE
- Brown recluse
  1. Bite is initially usually painless.
  2. One hour later or more, the site becomes erythematous, urticarial, and edematous.
  3. The center of the bite, which begins pale and macular, becomes purpuric and then vesicular.
  4. It may progress to necrosis.
  5. Induration at the site and regional lymphadenopathy may be present.
  6. Young children are at the greatest risk for systemic symptoms (i.e., nausea, vomiting, arthralgias, hemolysis, and thrombocytopenia).
  7. Resolution of the lesion may take months.
- Black widow
  1. Bite begins with a pinprick sensation at the site.
  2. The bite develops into a wheal.
  3. Within an hour, muscle cramping spreads throughout the body.
  4. Abdominal pain can be severe.
  5. Systemic symptoms peak at 3 hours.
  6. Symptoms resolve slowly without antivenom and may take 2 days.
  7. Headaches and other vague symptoms may persist for weeks without antivenom.

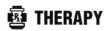

DIAGNOSIS

■ DIFFERENTIAL DIAGNOSIS
- The change in a bite lesion over time helps determine the species responsible.
- Knowing the region of the country that the bite occurred in helps identify the specific spider.
- Differentiate from snake bite.
- Vascular diseases, coagulopathy, and embolic phenomenon are in the differential.

■ DIAGNOSTIC WORKUP
Complete blood counts should be followed frequently for signs of hemolysis in a brown recluse bite.

THERAPY

■ NONPHARMACOLOGIC
- Except as listed here, other spider bites are treated symptomatically.
- Brown recluse therapy is as follows:
  1. Therapy is limited to treating the

TABLE 2-20 Signs and Symptoms of Spider Bites

ETIOLOGY	DEMOGRAPHICS	HISTORY	PHYSICAL EXAMINATION
Brown recluse Disease: loxoscelism Toxin: phospholipase D Size: ~25 mm	Midwest through Texas, southern U.S.	Painless bite, rarely catch spider; thin spider body with "violin" shape on its back	Two fang marks; initial purpuric urticarial macule becomes vesicular; central necrosis late
Black widow Disease: latrodectism Toxin: neurotoxin Size: 12-16 mm	Most common in southern U.S., occasionally in northern climates	Pinprick bite sensation, red hourglass on its back; usually bite after web is disturbed	Two fang marks; target lesion early; sore lymph nodes and severe muscle and abdominal pain
Tarantula Size: 10-50 mm	Southwest U.S.	Large and hairy; bite after provoked; hairs can cause hives themselves	Two fang marks; wheal and flare; local pain; usually short-lived symptoms
Running spider Yellow sac spiders Toxin: necrotic Size: 5-12 mm	Indoors throughout the U.S., especially in northeast U.S.	Yellow sack on back; localized irritation	Two fang marks; wheal and flare; necrotic crust; nausea
Hobo spider Toxin: necrotic Size: ~10-18 mm	Pacific northwest	Found in sheet webs in the home; headaches and nausea	Warm swelling at site turns to blistering and necrosis
Wolf spider Nonvenomous Size: 14-15 mm	Very common in North America; many are nocturnal	Dark in color	Two fang marks; wheal and flare
Black jumping spider Nonvenomous Size: 5-15 mm	Common in North America; diurnal	Bright colors	Two fang marks; wheal and flare; local urticaria

local lesion and hematologic problems.
2. Ice packs can be used.
3. Site should be elevated.
• Black widow therapy is as follows:
1. Antivenom causes a rapid resolution of symptoms.
2. Antivenom use is limited because of the possibility of severe anaphylactic reactions and serum sickness.
3. Hospitalization is the norm for black widow spider bite patients except those adequately managed with oral pain relievers.
4. Ice packs can be used.
5. The site should be elevated.

■ MEDICAL
• Tetanus immunization status should be updated in all spider bite patients.
• Brown recluse treatment is as follows:
1. Oral dapsone can inhibit skin necrosis.
2. Corticosteroids are controversial.
• Black widow treatment is as follows:
1. Antivenom is indicated only for extreme hypertension or uncontrollable pain.
2. Narcotic pain management with morphine or meperidine should be initiated.

3. Intravenous calcium is falling out of favor because of its transient effect.
4. Benzodiazepines or muscle relaxants are useful adjuncts to analgesia.
5. Nitroprusside or antivenom can be provided for persistent hypertension after adequate pain relief.

■ SURGICAL
• Brown recluse
1. Early excision is controversial.
2. Cosmetic issues predominate after the initial period.
3. Skin grafting is common later.

■ FOLLOW-UP & DISPOSITION
All patients should be monitored for signs of anaphylaxis.

■ REFERRAL INFORMATION
Referral of a brown recluse spider bite to a plastic surgeon is prudent.

☼ PEARLS & CONSIDERATIONS

■ CLINICAL PEARLS
• Anaphylaxis, although rare, is a possibility as with any bite or sting.
• Proper identification of the spider is

helpful in predicting systemic symptoms.
• Pain relief with narcotics is the foundation of therapy.
• All victims of a spider bite need to have their tetanus immune status updated.

■ WEBSITE
Sparks Health System: www.sparks.org/pma/bugbite.htm

REFERENCES
1. Anderson PC: Spider bites in the United States, *Dermatol Clin* 15:307, 1997.
2. Bond GR: Snake, spider, and scorpion envenomation in North America, *Pediatr Rev* 20:147, 1999.
3. Kemp ED: Bites and stings of the arthropod kind: treating reactions that can range from annoying to menacing, *Postgrad Med* 103:88, 1998.
4. Koh WL: When to worry about spider bites: inaccurate diagnosis can have serious, even fatal, consequences, *Postgrad Med* 103:235, 1998.
5. Levi H, Levi L: *Spiders and their kin*, New York, 1990, Golden Books.
Author: **Robert Freishtat, M.D.**

II

BASIC INFORMATION

■ **DEFINITION**

Spinal muscular atrophy (SMA) is an inherited neuromuscular disorder resulting in anterior horn cell degeneration with resultant disuse and atrophy of voluntary muscles.

- The classic infantile disease (type I) presents before age 5 months and is generally severe, leading to death before 2 years of age.
- A milder form (type III) may present after age 3 years and progress slowly, with survival into adulthood.
- An intermediate form is also relatively common (type II), typically presents between 3 to 24 months of age, and is associated with a variable prognosis.

■ **SYNONYMS**

- SMA type I—Werdnig-Hoffman disease, acute SMA
- SMA type II—subacute, proximal SMA
- SMA type III—Kugelberg-Welander disease, Wohlfart-Kugelberg-Welander disease, chronic SMA

ICD-9CM CODES

335.0　Werdnig-Hoffman disease
335.1　Spinal muscular atrophy, nonspecified
335.11 Kugelberg-Welander disease
335.19 Other—adult spinal muscular atrophy

■ **ETIOLOGY**

- Homozygous mutations occur in the telomeric survival motor neuron (SMN1) gene on chromosome 5q13.
  1. The most common mutation (90% to 95%) is a homozygous deletion of exon 7.
     a. The abnormal gene product fails to self-oligomerize into nuclear bodies called gems.
     b. These gems appear to be important in mRNA processing.
  2. Early reports suggest a relationship between ability of the SMN1 protein to self-oligomerize and disease severity, but the genotype-phenotype correlations are poorly understood at this time.
     a. Other genetic factors appear to modify the severity of the disease because the phenotype is fairly consistent within a single sibship.
     b. When one child is affected with the type I form, subsequent affected siblings are highly likely to also present with the type I form.

3. A centromeric survival motor neuron (SMN2) pseudogene nearby on the same chromosome complicates genetic analysis, especially heterozygote prediction.
   a. The product of the pseudogene typically skips exon 7.
- Another nearby gene locus, the neuronal apoptosis inhibitory protein (NAIP), appears deleted in about half of severe SMA type 1 cases, and the NAIP and/or SMN2 locus may be involved in the modification of the SMA phenotype.

■ **EPIDEMIOLOGY & DEMOGRAPHICS**

- Disease frequency is approximately 1 in 10,000.
- Carrier frequency is 1 in 50.
- SMA is the most common genetic cause of death in infancy.

■ **HISTORY**

- Progressive weakness
  1. Generalized, including bulbar muscles, in the acute forms
  2. More proximal in the chronic forms
- Delayed or absent motor milestones or loss of motor milestones/skills

■ **PHYSICAL EXAMINATION**

- Weakness
- Hypotonia
- Respiratory and bulbar weakness
- Hyporeflexia
- Fasciculations, especially tongue and/or fingers
- Occasional skeletal deformities
- Scoliosis

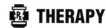 **DIAGNOSIS**

■ **DIFFERENTIAL DIAGNOSIS**

- Congenital myotonic dystrophy
- Maternal myasthenia gravis
- Acquired anterior horn cell disease (e.g., poliomyelitis, which is usually asymmetric)
- Kennedy spinal-bulbar neuronopathy
- Amyotrophic lateral sclerosis
- Muscular dystrophies

■ **DIAGNOSTIC WORKUP**

- Muscle biopsy is usually definitive and shows large, round atrophic fibers and clumps of hypertrophic type Ia fibers.
- Genetic testing (white blood cell DNA) is now available.
- Creatine kinase may be normal to slightly elevated.
- Nerve conduction velocity and cerebrospinal fluid protein are normal.
- Sensory nerves are normal.

THERAPY

■ **NONPHARMACOLOGIC**

Careful attention should be paid to pulmonary toilet and nutritional needs.

■ **MEDICAL**

- Treatment with antibiotics for respiratory illnesses should be initiated.
- Influenza immunization should be provided at 6 months of age or older and then yearly.
- Some families have elected intubation and long-term ventilation for children with type I disease.
  1. The ethics of this choice are highly debated.

■ **FOLLOW-UP & DISPOSITION**

- Follow-up depends on the age of presentation, rate of progression, and severity of symptoms.
- This disease is usually rapidly fatal in infants. Older patients with milder disease may have slow progression with variable, occasionally even relatively normal, survival.

■ **PATIENT/FAMILY EDUCATION**

- Genetic counseling is important for affected individuals and family members.
  1. Inheritance is autosomal recessive in most cases.
  2. As noted, heterozygote detection may be difficult.
  3. Prenatal diagnosis, including pre-implantation diagnosis, has been accomplished in a few cases.
- Phenotype (severity of disease) appears to cluster in families.
- Discussion of nutritional, pulmonary, and habilitative issues should be addressed early.
- Course and progress can be anticipated and reviewed.
  1. Planning for long-term care should begin at diagnosis.

■ **REFERRAL INFORMATION**

- A neurologist will most likely make this diagnosis.
- Patients may require the assistance of a nutritionist, gastroenterologist, pulmonologist, respiratory therapist, and nursing care specialist.
- The local muscular dystrophy association clinic may be of assistance in patient management (see "Support Groups").

PEARLS & CONSIDERATIONS

■ **CLINICAL PEARLS**

- The combination of weakness and areflexia or hyporeflexia should prompt serious concern for SMA.

- Fasciculations, especially tongue fasciculations, are highly suggestive of SMA.
- The understanding of the molecular genetic pathophysiology of SMA is evolving at a rapid rate. The reader is referred to the genetic literature or Online Mendelian Inheritance in Man for periodic updates in this field.

■WEBSITES
- Family Village: Spinal Muscular Atrophy: www.familyvillage.wisc.edu/lib_spma.htm

- Families of Spinal Muscular Atrophy: www.fsma.org/
- Muscular Dystrophy Association: www.mdausa.org/disease/sma1
- Online Mendelian Inheritance in Man: www3.ncbi.nlm.nih.gov

■ SUPPORT GROUPS
- Families of SMA, P.O. Box 196, Libertyville, IL 60048-0196; 800-886-1762; email: sma@interaccess.com
- Muscular Dystrophy Association, 3300 East Sunrise Drive, Tucson, AZ 85718-3208; 800-572-1717; email: mda@mdausa.org

REFERENCES
1. Bundey S: *Genetics and neurology,* Edinburgh, 1992, Churchill Livingstone.
2. Dreesen JC et al: Preimplantation genetic diagnosis of spinal muscular atrophy, *Mol Hum Reprod* 4:881, 1998.
3. Lorson CL et al: A single nucleotide in the SMN gene regulates splicing and is responsible for spinal muscular atrophy, *Proc Natl Acad Sci USA* 96: 6307, 1999.

Author: **Georgianne Arnold, M.D.**

BASIC INFORMATION

■ DEFINITION
Staphylococcal scalded skin syndrome (SSSS) is a blistering skin disease caused by exfoliative (epidermolytic) toxins of some strains of *Staphylococcus aureus*.

■ SYNONYMS
- SSSS
- Scalded skin syndrome
- Ritter's disease (first described by Gottfried Ritter von Rittersheim in the nineteenth century as *dermatitis exfoliativa infantum*)
- Pemphigus neonatorum

ICD-9CM CODES
695.1 Scalded skin syndrome
695.81 Ritter's disease

■ ETIOLOGY
- Responsible *S. aureus* usually belong to phage group II.
- The exfoliative toxin reaches skin via circulation.
- Two known epidermolytic toxins exist: ET-A and ET-B.
- Toxins cause intraepidermal lysis at the granular layer (zona granulosa) of the epidermis.
- No or few inflammatory cells are involved.

■ EPIDEMIOLOGY & DEMOGRAPHICS
- SSSS usually occurs in neonates, infants, and young children.
  1. Perianal and periumbilical lesions are common in neonates.
  2. Children usually have extremity lesions.
  3. Very ill infants and children have diffuse skin involvement.
- Occasionally, SSSS is seen in adults.
- Immature renal function with reduced ability to clear bacterial exotoxin may be the reason why neonates are susceptible.
- Renal and/or immunologic dysfunction may lead to this disease in adults.
- Approximately 5% of *S. aureus* isolates produce exfoliative toxins.
- About 32% of patients with exfoliative toxin-producing strains develop SSSS.
- Caucasian children are more susceptible than African-American children.
- Mortality rate is less than 4% in pediatric cases but greater than 50% in the adult population.
- *Ritter's disease* is the term used to describe generalized SSSS in neonates.
- Pemphigus neonatorum is a milder, self-limited disease of infants and causes few blisters.

■ HISTORY
- Neonatal presentation:
  1. Febrile illness presents at 3 to 16 days of life.
  2. Rapid skin changes with redness, blistering, and peeling are noted.
  3. Skin changes may be diffuse or focal with periumbilical or perianal distribution.
- Older children may have local or diffuse disease.
  1. Early febrile stage followed by generalized erythema
  2. Rapid onset of flaccid blister formation
  3. Peeling of large sheets of skin

■ PHYSICAL EXAMINATION
- Fever
- Generalized erythema for less than 10 to 18 hours
- Skin diffusely tender
- Rapid development of flaccid bullae and vesicles that rupture, leaving painful, denuded red base
  1. Positive Nikolsky's sign
     a. Gentle pressure or force on intact skin leads to blister formation at plane of cleavage within upper epidermis.
  2. Develops over large areas
  3. Common in flexural creases in those with more limited skin involvement
- Perioral erythema and peeling is common with sparing of the mucous membranes
- Conjunctival erythema common
- In neonates with mild or limited disease bullae, more periumbilical and perineal

DIAGNOSIS

■ DIFFERENTIAL DIAGNOSIS
- Toxic epidermal necrolysis (TEN), also known as *Lyell disease:* usually drug induced
- Burns
- Epidermolysis bullosa (congenital bullous disorder)
- Listeriosis
- Stevens-Johnson syndrome, also known as *erythema multiforme major*
- Staphylococcal or streptococcal scarlet fever
- Bullous impetigo (may be a limited form of SSSS)
- Atopic dermatitis
- Staphylococcal toxic shock syndrome (TSS)

■ DIAGNOSTIC WORKUP
- Clinical recognition of blistering exanthem, with sparing of the mucous membranes is necessary.

- Blisters themselves are usually culture negative.
- Other areas may be culture positive.
  1. Umbilicus
  2. Conjunctivae
  3. Breast
  4. Nasopharynx
  5. Blood (rare)

THERAPY

■ NONPHARMACOLOGIC
Keep exposed denuded skin covered and clean.

■ MEDICAL
- Antistaphylococcal antibiotics
  1. β-Lactamase–resistant penicillins, or
  2. First-generation cephalosporins (not in jaundiced newborn, however)
- Isolation, especially in nursery settings
- Fever control
- Fluid support if necessary

■ FOLLOW-UP & DISPOSITION
- Fluid losses through skin can be significant.
- Recovery is generally rapid in the absence of secondary infection.

■ PATIENT/FAMILY EDUCATION
Full reepithelialization without scarring usually takes 1 to 2 weeks.

■ PREVENTIVE TREATMENT
- Surveillance of potential carriers especially in nurseries
- Good handwashing
- Meticulous umbilical cord care

■ REFERRAL INFORMATION
- Rarely indicated
- Dermatology consultation if diagnosis is questionable

PEARLS & CONSIDERATIONS

■ CLINICAL PEARLS
- Differentiating from TEN is critical because SSSS requires antibiotic therapy.
- No mucous membrane involvement is seen in SSSS.

■ WEBSITES
- eMedicine: www.emedicine.com/ EMERG/topic782.htm
- Rutgers: www.eden.rutgers.edu/ ~dessi/SSSS.html
- Virtual Hospital: www.vh.org

REFERENCES

1. Farrell AM: Staphylococcal scalded-skin syndrome, *Lancet* 354:880, 1999.
2. Ladhani S, Evans RW: Staphylococcal scalded skin syndrome, *Arch Dis Child* 78:85, 1998.
3. Ladhani S, Newson T: Familial outbreak of staphylococcal scalded skin syndrome, *Pediatr Infect Dis J* 19:578, 2000.
4. Ladhani S et al: Clinical, microbiological, and biochemical aspects of the exfoliative toxins causing staphylococcal scalded-skin syndrome, *Clin Micro Rev* 12:224, 1999.
5. Pollack S: Staphylococcal scalded skin syndrome, *Pediatr Rev* 17:18, 1996.

Author: **Lynn C. Garfunkel, M.D.**

II

BASIC INFORMATION

■ DEFINITION

Stevens-Johnson syndrome (SJS) involves severe erosions of at least two mucosal surfaces, with extensive necrosis of lips and mouth and a purulent conjunctivitis. It is also known as *erythema multiforme major.*

ICD-9CM CODE

695.1 Stevens-Johnson syndrome

■ ETIOLOGY

- Drugs are a major precipitating factor, although many other factors have been implicated.
- Nonsteroidal antiinflammatory drugs (ibuprofen, naproxen) are the most common offenders, followed by sulfonamides, anticonvulsants (hydantoins and barbiturates), penicillins, tetracycline, and doxycycline.
- It has been postulated that in children with drug-induced SJS, genetic differences in detoxification of drugs may be responsible.

■ EPIDEMIOLOGY & DEMOGRAPHICS

- The exact incidence is unknown.
- Peak incidence is in the second decade of life.
- SJS is more common in the spring and summer.

■ HISTORY

- Most children have a prodrome of upper respiratory infection with fever, cough, rhinitis, sore throat, headache, vomiting, diarrhea, and malaise.
- SJS has a prolonged course of 4 to 6 weeks, with mortality up to 30% and significant morbidity.

■ PHYSICAL EXAMINATION

- One to fourteen days after the prodrome, abrupt-onset symmetric red macules develop, which progress to central blister formation and extensive epidermal necrosis.
- The extent of skin involvement is variable.

- Lips develop hemorrhagic crusts with loss of the mucosa and severe stomatitis.
- Purulent conjunctivitis with photophobia and pseudomembrane formation may develop.
- Anogenital mucosa may be involved as well.
- Esophageal, respiratory, and nasal mucosa are occasionally involved.
- Generalized lymphadenopathy and hepatosplenomegaly are usually present.
- Signs of dehydration (tachycardia, hypotension) may be noted.
- Signs of electrolyte abnormalities (edema, arrhythmias) may be seen.

DIAGNOSIS

■ DIFFERENTIAL DIAGNOSIS

- Kawasaki disease
- Acute graft-versus-host disease
- Staphylococcal scalded skin syndrome
- Paraneoplastic pemphigus

■ DIAGNOSTIC WORKUP

- The diagnosis is usually made by the characteristic prodrome followed by the abrupt onset of extensive areas of mucocutaneous necrosis, with at least two mucosal sites involved.
- Children develop fluid and electrolyte imbalances.
- A complete blood count will demonstrate leukocytosis (65%), eosinophilia (20%), and anemia (15%).
- All children with SJS have an increased erythrocyte sedimentation rate.

THERAPY

■ MEDICAL

- Prolonged hospitalization in a burn or intensive care unit is usually necessary.

- All possible offending agents should be stopped.
- Provide fluid and electrolyte management.
  1. Involves intravenous volume and electrolyte repletion, maintenance, and ongoing loss replacement
- Protection from secondary infection includes wound dressing and burn care.
- Ophthalmologic care is closely monitored by an ophthalmologist.
- Pulmonary toilet must be monitored.
- Nutritional supplementation is critical.
- Pain management should be provided.
- Physical therapy to prevent contractures.
- Use of systemic steroids is controversial.

■ SURGICAL

Possible early skin grafting or use of biologic dressings

PEARLS & CONSIDERATIONS

■ CLINICAL PEARLS

SJS is often complicated by dehydration; electrolyte imbalance; and secondary bacterial infection of skin, mucosa, or lungs, as well as cutaneous scarring and dyspigmentation.

■ WEBSITES

- American Academy of Dermatology: www.aad.org
- Society for Pediatric Dermatology: www.spdnet.org

REFERENCES

1. Brice SL, Huff JC, Weston WL: Erythema multiforme, *Curr Prob Dermatol* 2:3, 1990.
2. Weston WL: What is erythema multiforme? *Pediatr Ann* 252:106, 1996.
Author: **Susan Haller Psaila, M.D.**

BASIC INFORMATION

■ **DEFINITION**
Strabismus is misalignment of the eyes.

■ **TYPES**
• Nonparalytic (most common type in children), including esotropia, exotropia, hypertropia, and hypotropia
• Paralytic, including third, fourth, and sixth nerve palsies
• Strabismic syndromes, including Duane's, Brown, and Möbius syndromes

Esotropia and exotropia are the emphasis of this section because they account for 75% of all cases of strabismus.
• Esotropia: eyes turn inward (medialis)
  1. Congenital (onset younger than 6 months)
  2. Accommodative (onset usually 6 months to 7 years)
• Exotropia: eyes deviate out (temporally)
  1. Congenital (rare, onset younger than 6 months)
  2. Acquired (onset 6 months to 6 years)

■ **SYNONYMS**
• Convergent/divergent strabismus
• Lazy or wandering eye
• "Wall-eyed," "cross-eyed"
• Squint
• Esotropia
• Exotropia

ICD-9CM CODES
378.50 Paralytic strabismus
378.9 Nonparalytic strabismus
378.41 Esotropia
378.42 Exotropia
378.3 Hypertropia

■ **ETIOLOGY**
• Most cases of strabismus have no known cause.
  1. There may be an absence of fusion potential at the cortical level.
• Accommodative esotropia, however, is caused by overconvergence in an attempt to focus on objects.

■ **EPIDEMIOLOGY & DEMOGRAPHICS**
• Strabismus affects approximately 4% of children younger than age 6.
• Esotropia is three times more common than exotropia.
• Esotropia has no gender predilection.
• The incidence of strabismus increases in children born prematurely, those with developmental delay, and those with a first-degree relative with strabismus.

■ **HISTORY**
• Birth and developmental history
• Age of onset of strabismus (younger than 6 months = congenital, older than 6 months = acquired)
• One eye or both
• Associated with fatigue or illness
• Intermittent or constant
• Previous surgery, patching, or glasses

■ **PHYSICAL EXAMINATION**
• Visual acuity of each eye or fixation preference (up to 50% of patients with strabismus have reduced vision)
• Ocular motility (oblique muscle overreaction, A or V pattern strabismus, nystagmus)
• Bruckner test
  1. A deviated eye gives a brighter red reflex.
• Hirschberg test: examines corneal light reflex
  1. If reflex is centered on both pupils, eyes are aligned.
  2. If reflex is displaced temporally, that eye is esotropic.
  3. If reflex is displaced nasally, that eye is exotropic.
• Cover test: examination of the uncovered eye
  1. If no movement, eyes are aligned.
  2. If the eye moves out to take up fixation, that eye was esotropic.
  3. If the eye moves in to take up fixation, that eye was exotropic.
• Full dilated eye examination to rule out significant refractive error or ocular lesion (i.e., retinoblastoma) as the cause of strabismus

DIAGNOSIS

■ **DIFFERENTIAL DIAGNOSIS**
• Pseudostrabismus
  1. Wide nasal bridge gives esotropic appearance (pinch skin over bridge and note symmetric light reflexes and ocular alignment)
  2. Hypertelorism gives exotropic appearance (note symmetric light reflexes and ocular alignment)

THERAPY

• Potential therapies depend on the type of strabismus and include glasses, miotic eyedrops, prisms, eye exercises, and surgery.
  1. Congenital esotropia usually requires surgery (usually after age 6 months).
  2. Accommodative esotropia usually requires glasses and less often surgery.
  3. Exotropia may require surgery, but therapy may also include glasses, prisms, and eye exercises.
  4. Amblyopia is common with strabismus and requires treatment.

■ **FOLLOW-UP & DISPOSITION**
Follow-up is determined by the eye specialist and depends on the type of strabismus, presence of amblyopia, and method of treatment.

■ **PATIENT/FAMILY EDUCATION**
• Children do not outgrow true strabismus.
• Children usually do not complain of diplopia.
• Early detection and treatment yield the best outcome.

■ **PREVENTIVE TREATMENT**
Strabismus usually cannot be prevented. Theoretically, however, it could be if a potential cause of strabismus such as hyperopia is detected and treated.

■ **REFERRAL INFORMATION**
All children with strabismus require referral to an eye care provider.

PEARLS & CONSIDERATIONS

■ **CLINICAL PEARLS**
• Children do not outgrow strabismus.
• Strabismus may indicate a blind eye (i.e., retinoblastoma).
• If pseudostrabismus is suspected, pinch the skin of the nasal bridge to reveal symmetric light reflexes and ocular alignment.

■ **WEBSITE**
• Yahoo! Health: http://health.yahoo.com/health

REFERENCES
1. Diamond GR: Esotropia. In Yanoff M, Duker JS (eds): *Ophthalmology,* London, 1999, Mosby.
2. Lavrich JB, Nelson LB: Diagnosis and treatment of strabismus disorders, *Pediatr Clin North Am* 40:737, 1993.
3. Olitsky SE, Nelson LB: Strabismus disorders. In Nelson LB (ed): *Harley's pediatric ophthalmology,* ed 4, Philadelphia, 1998, WB Saunders.
Author: **Kristina Lynch-Guyette, M.D.**

II

BASIC INFORMATION

■ DEFINITION

- "Disorders in the rhythm of speech, in which the individual knows precisely what he or she wishes to say, but at the same time is unable to say it because of an involuntary, repetitive prolongation or cessation of sound." (*International Classification of Diseases*, The World Health Organization, 1977, p. 202).
- Developmental stuttering is brief periods of stuttering that cease by the time a child enters school. In general, these are repetitions of whole words and phrases; they may include simple comments and changes to previously spoken thoughts. Part-word repetitions and sound prolongations occur much less commonly.

■ SYNONYMS

- Stammering
- Dysfluency
- Developmental stuttering
- Idiopathic or pathologic stuttering
- Acquired stuttering

ICD-9CM CODE
307.0 Stammering and stuttering

■ ETIOLOGY

- The cause remains controversial.
- The current understanding describes subtle neurophysical dysfunctions that disrupt the precise timing required to produce speech.
- Stutterers have difficulty coordinating air flow, articulation, and resonance. Small asynchronies are even found in stutterers' fluent speech.
- There is a genetic role in stuttering. The specific mode or modes of transmission are unknown.
- A higher concordance for stuttering is observed in monozygotic twins (77%) than in dizygotic same-sex twins (32%) or same-sexed siblings (18%).
- First-degree relatives of people who stutter have more than a threefold higher risk of developing stuttering than the general population.
- Male relatives of female stutterers are at the highest risk—greater than a fourfold risk of stuttering.
- The severity of stuttering is not related to the extent of the family history of stuttering.
- For men who ever stuttered, 9% of their daughters and 22% of their sons will stutter.
- For women who ever stuttered, 17% of their daughters and 36% of their sons will be affected.
- Perinatal brain damage is the only environmental factor known to be associated with some cases of idiopathic stuttering.
    1. Perinatal brain damage is also associated with epilepsy, cerebral palsy, and other neurologic syndromes.
    2. All are associated with stuttering at a higher-than-expected prevalence rate.
- Deafness is the only "factor" resulting in a reduced prevalence of stuttering.
- Acquired stuttering may develop in a previously fluent speaker after brain damage, usually vascular or traumatic in origin. The symptoms are clinically identical to idiopathic stuttering.

■ EPIDEMIOLOGY & DEMOGRAPHICS

- The prevalence of stuttering in prepubertal schoolchildren is 1.0% but generally drops in postpubertal school children. The prevalence seems to remain constant from school entry to age 12 and declines slowly thereafter. The prevalence after puberty is 0.8%.
- The prevalence in children is elevated because of the high incidence of developmental dysfluency.
- The male:female ratio is approximately 3:1 overall but increases with age.
- The age of onset of stuttering is the same for both sexes.
- Stuttering is present in all cultures, races, languages, and historical periods.
- The incidence varies among cultures and socioeconomic groups—more common in the upper socioeconomic classes (this may be a function of increased surveillance of this group).
- Famous people who stuttered include Moses, Aristotle, Sir Isaac Newton, Winston Churchill, John Updike, King George VI, James Earl Jones, Marilyn Monroe, and Jimmy Stewart.

■ PROGNOSIS

- Almost 80% of school-aged children who stutter recover fluency spontaneously or with minimal speech therapy by the age of 16 years.
- Even with more severe stuttering, the prognosis is favorable if treatment starts early.
- The outcome is less favorable for those who continue to stutter into adulthood.

■ HISTORY

- Patient has a past medical history of perinatal asphyxia or trauma, associated seizure disorder, cerebral palsy, head trauma, or cerebral vascular injury.

- Stuttering onset is between toddlerhood and puberty.
    1. Highest onset is between 2 to 5 years of age.
    2. Mean age of onset is 5 years, median age is 4 years.
- Stuttering develops gradually.
- A family history of stuttering in a twin or first-degree relative increases the risk.

■ PHYSICAL EXAMINATION

- Evaluation of motor skills, auditory skills, and language level is indicated, in addition to the child's speech performance.
- Assess the type and degree of word dysfluencies.
- More than 90% of stuttering occurs on the initial syllable of the utterance.
- The incidence is greater on words starting with consonants, words located early in a sentence, and longer words.
- In general, there is concern if the child has five or more "breaks" per 100 words spoken.
- "Breaks" may include any of the following:
    1. Whole word, phrase, or syllable repetitions and sound prolongations
    2. Presence of silent pauses before, after, or within a word
    3. Inappropriate articulating postures
- Also make note of the following:
    1. Normal or excessive speaking rate
    2. Tendency toward more dysfluencies in response to stress
- Assess the stutterer's and parents' attitude toward the problem.
- People almost never stutter when singing, whispering, speaking together in a group, or when they cannot hear their own voice.

🔬 DIAGNOSIS

■ DIFFERENTIAL DIAGNOSIS

- Developmental stuttering
- Idiopathic stuttering
- Acquired stuttering

■ DIAGNOSTIC WORKUP

- A certified speech and language pathologist should perform a formal evaluation after the appropriate referral.
- The presence of repetitions, together with prolongations, are both necessary and sufficient for the disorder to be diagnosed.
- Referral to a speech-language pathologist is indicated if a child meets the following criteria:
    1. Is older than 4 years

2. Shows consistent stuttering behaviors
3. Has been stuttering at least 3 months
4. Demonstrates tension or struggle behavior when stuttering
5. Is aware that his or her stuttering is abnormal

- Referral is also necessary if the child's parents show great concern about the problem, regardless of the child's awareness or secondary behaviors.
- Speech and language development is delayed in stutterers by about 6 months.
- Articulation errors are three times more common in children who stutter.
  1. Errors are noted before the child's stuttering behaviors.
  2. Errors are independent of the age of onset of the stuttering.
- Intelligence tests have revealed a significantly lower score for stutterers compared with nonstutterers (half a standard deviation).
  1. Both verbal and nonverbal tests of intelligence have demonstrated the same difference.
- Stutterers have been described as having "difficulty with social adjustment," but this condition is probably a consequence rather than a cause of stuttering.

℞ THERAPY

■ NONPHARMACOLOGIC

- Mild stuttering can be self-limited, but behaviorally oriented therapy is effective in young children.
- Delaying direct stuttering therapy for the "mild" stutterers may actually interfere with their ability to establish fluency.
- Many practitioners believe that speech therapy for stuttering should begin with the onset of stuttering to maximize the efficiency and cost-effectiveness of therapy.
- More severe stuttering requires speech therapy directed at the behavioral, cognitive, and affective aspects of speech, as well as counseling.
- There are seven conditions in which stuttering frequency can be immediately reduced or eliminated: (1) chorus reading, (2) lipped speech,

(3) prolonged speech and delayed auditory feedback, (4) rhythmic speech, (5) shadowing, (6) singing, and (7) slowed speech.
- Several treatment methods increase the fluency of stutterers' speech: (1) prolonged speech, (2) precision fluency-shaping, (3) rhythmic speech, (4) airflow therapy, (5) electromyogram (EMG) biofeedback of the speech musculature, and (6) attitude change. Of these methods, only prolonged speech, precision fluency-shaping strategies, and EMG biofeedback have been shown critically to provide long-lasting fluency.
- In general, the goal of speech therapy is to establish and maintain the feeling of fluency control, rather than to attain an arbitrarily determined level of fluency.
- "Self-acceptance" is the treatment of choice of the National Stuttering Project rather than working to directly change the stutterers' speech behaviors.

■ MEDICAL

- Haloperidol (Haldol) is the only drug that has demonstrated consistent improvement in stuttering.
  1. This drug cannot be used long term, however, because of its unacceptable side effects.

■ PREVENTIVE TREATMENT

- When dysfluencies are first detected in children, parents are commonly advised to speak more slowly to children and avoid interrupting them, in an effort to decrease the dysfluencies. These strategies have not been proven to help, however.
- Stuttering Prevention Programs: 519-675-0449 or 905-682-6388; email: twray@prevent-stuttering.com

☼ PEARLS & CONSIDERATIONS

■ CLINICAL PEARLS
How to Talk to People Who Stutter*
- Try not to finish sentences for people who stutter. This can make them feel more frustrated, and you might not say the same words they were thinking.

---

*Taken from *Current Health* 1:29, 1998.

- Avoid saying things such as, "relax" and "slow down." It doesn't help.
- Be extra patient, especially on the telephone, which can be the hardest place to talk smoothly.
- If you didn't understand what was said, say, "I'm sorry, I didn't get that." This is always better than just pretending to understand or making a wild guess.
- Use a relaxed tone of voice yourself, and don't talk extra slowly. There is nothing wrong with the hearing of people who stutter!
- Keep eye contact with them; don't drop your eyes in discomfort or embarrassment, because this will only make them feel worse.
- Show in every way that you are listening to what they are saying and how they are saying it.

■ WEBSITES
- American Speech-Language-Hearing Society: www.asha.org
- The National Center for Stuttering: www.stuttering.com

■ SUPPORT GROUPS
- Stuttering Foundation of America, P.O. Box 11749, 3100 Walnut Grove Road, Suite 603, Memphis, TN 38111; 800-992-9392
- National Stuttering Project, 5100 E. LaPalma Avenue, #208, Anaheim Hills, CA 92807; 800-364-1677
- The National Center for Stuttering, The National Stutterers' Hotline: 800-221-2483; email: executivedirector@stuttering.com

REFERENCES
1. Andrews G et al: Stuttering: a review of research findings and theories circa 1982, *J Speech Hearing Disord* 48:226, 1983.
2. Hancock K et al: Two- to six-year controlled-trial stuttering outcomes for children and adolescents, *J Speech Lang Hearing Research* 41:1242, 1998.
3. Lawrence M, Barclay DM III: Stuttering: a brief review, *Am Fam Physician* 57:2175, 1998.
4. Nippold MA, Rudzinski M: Parents' speech and children's stuttering: a critique of the literature, *J Speech Lang Hearing Research* 38:978, 1995.
Author: **Dorothy M. Delisle, M.D.**

II

BASIC INFORMATION

DEFINITION
Sudden infant death syndrome (SIDS) is the sudden and unexpected death of an infant younger than 1 year of age, which remains unexplained after a thorough case investigation, including performance of a complete autopsy, examination of the death scene, and review of the clinical history.

SYNONYMS
- SIDS
- Crib death
- Cot death

ICD-9CM CODE
798.0 Sudden infant death syndrome

ETIOLOGY
- The cause or causes of SIDS remain unknown and are likely to be multifactorial.
- SIDS is believed to occur among vulnerable infants during a critical period of development following exogenous (environmental) stressors.
- In some SIDS victims, neuropathologic findings include subtle structural and neurochemical abnormalities within brain regions that are believed to be important to arousal and cardiorespiratory control, located especially within chemosensing and effector regions of the ventrolateral medulla.

EPIDEMIOLOGY & DEMOGRAPHICS
- SIDS is the single most common cause of death for infants 1 month to 1 year of age.
- In 1997, a total of 2991 SIDS deaths were recorded in the United States, corresponding to an incidence of 0.77 deaths per 1000 live births (National Center for Health Statistics).
- The U.S. incidence has fallen 50% since the 1994 "Back to Sleep" campaign.
- Males outnumber females at a ratio of 3:2.
- A higher incidence is seen among African-American and Native American infants; a lower incidence is seen among Hispanic and Asian infants.
- Deaths occur more often during from September through April.

HISTORY
- The infant is typically healthy, feeding well, and growing normally.
- Approximately 12% to 20% of SIDS victims are former preterm or low-birth-weight infants.
- The infant is discovered lifeless associated with a period of sleep.
- The age at death is characteristic: 60% of victims are 2 to 4 months of age, 90% are younger than 6 months, and 95% are younger than 8 months of age.

AUTOPSY FINDINGS
- The infant typically appears well nourished and well cared for.
- Rigor mortis and postmortem lividity are generally present.
- The absence of a lethal lesion is noted.
- The thymus and adrenal glands are typically normal.
- A minor microscopic inflammatory change within the distal airways may be evident.

DIAGNOSIS

- Diagnosis follows analysis of data history, and scene of death.
- Death is attributed to SIDS once known (natural or nonnatural, i.e., accident or homicide) causes of unexpected infant death are ruled out.

PATIENT/FAMILY EDUCATION & FOLLOW-UP
- Contact the family to offer condolence, support, and sympathy.
- Meet with the family to review the autopsy results (if they are ready) and answer questions pertaining to the death.
  1. Families harbor many questions reflecting self-blame and irrational fears that their care of the infant caused the death. These fears or concerns can be addressed in follow-up.
- Counsel the family about subsequent children and the risk for SIDS, if appropriate.
  1. A twofold to fivefold increased risk of SIDS exists in subsequent siblings.
  2. Asymptomatic siblings do not need polysomnography or cardio-respiratory monitoring unless indicated by individualized factors.

PREVENTIVE TREATMENT
- SIDS is unpredictable. At present, no medical tests are predictive of risk.
- The "Back to Sleep" campaign has been successful in reducing the incidence of SIDS.
  1. Measures that may modify an infant's risk for SIDS include the following:
     a. Place the infant on his or her back (supine) for sleep.
     b. Place infant on a firm surface for sleep.
        (1) Avoid placing the infant on soft or padded sleep surfaces (e.g., waterbeds, beanbag cushions, quilts, comforters).
     c. Do not overbundle the infant or dress him or her too warmly.
     d. Avoid cigarette smoke exposure.
     e. Seek early prenatal care and regular well-child care after the birth.

PEARLS & CONSIDERATIONS

CLINICAL PEARLS
The "Back to Sleep" campaign has been successful.

WEBSITES
- Association of SIDS and Infant Mortality Programs (ASIP): www.asip1.org; national association of statewide SIDS information and counseling programs providing direct service to families after SIDS and other infant deaths; ASIP members also participate in SIDS research, education, and training initiatives
- National SIDS Resource Center: www.circsol.com/SIDS; federally funded clearinghouse providing information on all aspects of SIDS
- SIDS Alliance: www.sidsalliance.org, national organization of parent-sponsored chapters

SUPPORT GROUPS
Bereavement support groups exist in most states in the United States and can be located through the ASIP website.

REFERENCES
1. Guidelines for death scene investigation of sudden, unexplained infant deaths: recommendations of the interagency panel on sudden infant death syndrome, *MMWR Morb Mortal Wkly Rep* 45:RR-1, 1996.
2. Krous HF et al: Instruction and reference manual for the international standardized autopsy protocol for sudden unexpected infant death, *J SIDS Inf Mort* 1:203, 1996.
3. Kattwinkel J et al: Positioning and SIDS: an update, *Pediatrics* 98:1216, 1996.
4. Willinger M et al: Defining the sudden infant death syndrome: deliberations of an expert panel convened by the National Institute of Child Health and Human Development, *Pediatr Pathol* 11:677, 1991.
Author: **Patrick L. Carolan, M.D.**

BASIC INFORMATION

■ DEFINITION

Suicidal behavior is intention to end one's own life, most often accompanied by intense feelings of hopelessness, helplessness, and/or self-destructive behaviors and attitudes. Increasing levels of severity include suicide *gesture* (a serious "cry for help or attention"), suicide *attempt* (a more serious event in which the intent is to kill one's self), and *completed* suicide (death occurs).

ICD-9CM CODES
300.9 Risk, tendencies
959.9 Trauma

■ ETIOLOGY

Complex behaviors that generally involve multiple exacerbating risk factors combined with an imbalance of central nervous system neurotransmitters, in a biopsychosocial interaction may lead to suicide or a suicide attempt. Such risk factors include the following:
- Feelings of hopelessness or desperation
- Excessive drug or alcohol use or abuse
- History of emotional illness or disruptive behavior problems
- Extreme anxiety, agitation, or rage
- Feelings of shame or humiliation

■ EPIDEMIOLOGY & DEMOGRAPHICS
- Adolescent females are three times more likely to attempt suicide than males, usually by toxic ingestion.
- Males, however, are five times more likely to complete suicide because they are more likely to use violent means such as firearms, hanging, jumping from heights, or placing themselves in front of moving vehicles.
- Completed suicide occurs in 1.7 per 100,000 10- to 14-year-olds and 11 per 100,000 15- to 19-year-olds.
- Suicide is the third leading cause of death in 15- to 24-year-olds, following accidents and homicide; it is the fourth leading cause of death in 10- to 14-year-olds.
- Although suicide rates are highest for Caucasian males, the suicide rate has increased 105% for 15- to 19-year-old African-American males in the past 15 years, almost entirely attributed to firearms.

■ HISTORY
Factors associated with an increased risk of suicide include the following:
- Family history of emotional disorder, especially with suicide attempt
- Previous personal suicide attempt
- Current talk of suicide or making a plan
- Strong wish to die, preoccupation with death, giving away prized possessions
- Signs of depression, including moodiness, hopelessness, or social withdrawal
- Anxiety, agitation, or rage
- Increased alcohol or drug use
- Recent suicide attempt by friend or family member or media attention to suicide
- Access to firearms
- Impulsiveness with risk taking
- Isolation, including recent losses within social support system
- Suddenly cheerful after a period of depression

■ PHYSICAL EXAMINATION
- Bodily injuries caused by risk taking
- Intentional cutting or scarring, especially of wrists
- Mental status examination revealing dysphoria or depression

DIAGNOSIS

- Suicide risk is best determined by direct inquiry about current and past suicidal ideation, intent, and plans, as well as access to means, such as firearms, knives, or drugs.
- Such questioning should be included in routine comprehensive visits for adolescents, especially if risk factors are present.
- Assessing recent suicide or death of family or friends, recent losses (e.g., social failures, breakup with a girlfriend or boyfriend), and family history of mental health problems can collectively be beneficial in making a determination about disposition.
- Homosexual adolescent males are at increased risk of suicide.
- The combination of clinical interview with self-report measures may provide sufficient information to determine the level of suicidal risk and/or need for a specialty evaluation.
  1. Instruments that may facilitate assessment include the Beck Depression Inventory and Kovacs' Child Depression Inventory; however, no depression measure is highly sensitive or specific.
  2. Some providers prefer a more broad-based assessment across a range of behavioral and emotional functioning, such as in *Bright Futures* or the *Guidelines for Adolescent Preventive Services* (GAPS), to put the individual in context, rather than focusing only on suicidality.

THERAPY

■ NONPHARMACOLOGIC
- Therapeutic alliance with health care providers is a critical task because acute risk of suicide correlates inversely with meaningful personal and therapeutic relationships.
- Some communities have mobile teams that provide excellent urgent care and transport at times of acute crisis.
- For urgent care, planning for immediate transport to a local hospital's emergency department for further evaluation can be lifesaving.
- For youth who have risk factors, but no active suicidal thoughts, referral to a mental health specialist may be helpful.
  1. It is important to emphasize to the child or adolescent that the referral is not because he or she is "crazy," but rather to provide help with feelings of sadness, boredom, isolation, or other emotions that are interfering with their health.
  2. Specific suicide prevention programs have been developed, but targeted programs are less beneficial than those that focus on more global social competencies, communication, coping, and self-esteem.
- Therapy for children can be in group, family, or individual formats, each of which is appropriate for different situations, preferences, and needs. With few exceptions, effective child therapy incorporates some family or parenting component.
  1. Strategies for treating depression vary by provider philosophy, as well as by patient characteristics.
  2. Adolescents are more likely than children to benefit from individual treatment, but family and group therapy may also be helpful.
- Regardless of the patient's age, common elements of therapy include an emphasis on the patient being a proactive participant in therapy. This includes assignments and activities that are completed between sessions to facilitate progress toward one's goals.

II

- Cognitive-behavioral therapy is one of the most effective approaches to treat depression.
  1. This approach focuses on the mutual influence exerted amongst thoughts, behaviors, and emotions.
  2. Therapeutic goals and efforts facilitate changes toward healthier functioning in cognitive and behavioral arenas that are expected to result in more positive emotional outcomes.
  3. Based on the patient's needs, skills training may be included such as with problem-solving, social, or communication skills.
- Effective treatment is associated with symptom reduction, including an absence of suicidal thoughts.
  1. This recovery is often accompanied by an increase in coping skills and an increase in functioning for areas that were disturbed during the course of illness (e.g., school, sleep, appetite, energy, interest in activities and friends), but recovery may be slow and marked by improvements and relapses.
  2. Because of instability of mood and situational factors, suicidal ideation/intent must be reevaluated at follow-up appointments.

■ MEDICAL
- Tricyclic antidepressants (TCAs) have been replaced by selective serotonin reuptake inhibitors (SSRIs, such as fluoxetine, sertraline, paroxetine, or fluvoxamine).
  1. The former demonstrated no added benefit over placebo in the treatment of depression.
  2. TCAs are highly toxic in overdose.
- Only one clinical trial of an SSRI showing effectiveness over placebo in adolescents has been published.
- If prescribed, an SSRI should be used only in combination with other effective treatments, never alone.

■ FOLLOW-UP & DISPOSITION
- Patients who have made a suicide attempt are most often hospitalized, unless their safety can be ensured at home with an "in-house hospitalization," in which they are closely monitored at all times by a responsible adult.
- Close follow-up is also needed after a suicidal gesture to assure the patient that the "cry for help" was heard.
  1. Most importantly, the patient must come to believe that "things will change" in a way that will not make suicide necessary as a means of coping or dealing with hardships.

■ PATIENT/FAMILY EDUCATION
- Two major goals include promotion of patient awareness of suicide as a public health problem and teaching that suicide is preventable.
- These goals can best be accomplished by making suicide a safe topic to talk about without normalizing it as a reasonable response to stress. Including questions about mood and coping as a part of routine comprehensive health visits fosters this approach.

■ PREVENTIVE TREATMENT
- Early identification and referral for effective treatment of mood disorder or substance use disorder is the most critical step in preventing suicide.
- Do not hesitate to assess suicidal thoughts, particularly for adolescent patients. Questioning will not create the problem, but it may be a step toward prevention, by showing an interest in the patient's well-being.
- Cooperative efforts by both the patient and a parent (preferably both parents) are beneficial in developing an effective suicide prevention plan.
- Patients and parents both benefit from a written prevention plan to take with them in the event those suicidal urges become imminent.
  1. Remember to include all relevant phone contacts with numbers included in this plan, as well as making provisions for removal of accessibility to items such as knives, guns, and medications.

■ REFERRAL INFORMATION
- Youth identified at risk for suicide are generally referred to a mental health specialist within the fields of psychiatry, psychology, and clinical social work.
- If active suicidal ideation, intent, or planning for suicide is present, a referral to a local emergency services unit for evaluation and therapeutic planning should be made without delay.
- Support services:
  1. In addition to local mental health providers and clinics, most areas have a 24-hour phone support service ("hotline") that can coordinate emergency services, transportation, or simply provide relevant referrals.

☼ PEARLS & CONSIDERATIONS

■ CLINICAL PEARLS
- Suicidal ideation and suicidal plans are the strongest predictors of suicide and can usually be easily assessed through interview with a child or adolescent.
- Adolescents are often more willing to disclose private thoughts and behaviors, such as suicidal plans, when they are interviewed separately from parents.
- Patients need to know that the disclosure of suicidal intent cannot be kept confidential if the clinician judges them to be at risk of harm to themselves or others.
  1. Patients should be included in any plan to disclose the clinician's assessment of suicidal risk to parents or other adults in authority.
- Be aware of potential bias related to mental health services and how such referrals may be perceived because a stigma is often associated with mental illness and mental health services, which can undermine this important treatment.
  1. Developing relationships with mental health providers in which the clinician has confidence facilitates success with referrals.

■ WEBSITES
- The American Academy of Child and Adolescent Psychiatry: www.aacap.org
- American Association of Suicidology: www.suicidology.org/resources.htm
- American Medical Association: www.ama-assn.org/adolhlth/
- Centers for Disease Control and Prevention: www.cdc.gov/ncipc/dvp/yvpt/suicide.htm
- Mental Health Net: http://suicide.mentalhelp.net/
- Rochford: www.rochford.org/suicide

REFERENCES
1. Asberg M: Neurotransmitters and suicidal behavior: The evidence from cerebrospinal fluid studies, *Ann NY Acad Sci* 836:158, 1997.
2. Beck AT et al: An inventory for measuring depression, *Arch Gen Psychiatry* 4:561, 1961.
3. Bell CC, Clark DC: Adolescent suicide, *Pediatr Clin North Am* 45:365, 1998.
4. Brent DA et al: Psychiatric risk factors for adolescent suicide: a case control study, *J Am Acad Child Adolesc Psychiatry* 32:521, 1993.

5. Centers for Disease Control and Prevention: Suicide among black youths, United States, 1980-1995, *MMWR Morb Mortal Wkly Rep* 47:193, 1998.

6. Emslie GJ et al: A double-blind, randomized, placebo-controlled trial of fluoxetine in children and adolescents with depression, *Arch Gen Psychiatry* 54:1031, 1997.

7. Hirschfeld RM, Russell JM: Assessment and treatment of suicidal patients, *N Engl J Med* 337:910, 1997.

8. Jellinek MS, Snyder JB: Depression and suicide in children and adolescents, *Pediatr Rev* 19:255, 1998.

9. Kovacs M: Rating scales to assess depression in school-age children, *Acta Paedopschiatrica* 46:305, 1981.

10. Pfeffer C, Normandin L, Kakuma T: Suicidal children grow up: suicidal behavior and psychiatric disorders among relatives, *J Am Acad Child Adolesc Psychiatry* 33:1087, 1994.

11. Weiss D, Coccaro EF: Neuroendocrine challenge studies of suicidal behavior, *Psychiatry Clin North Am* 20:563, 1997.

Authors: **Maria S. Ogden, Ph.D., and Richard E. Kreipe, M.D.**

BASIC INFORMATION

■ DEFINITION
Supraventricular tachycardia (SVT) is an abnormally rapid cardiac rhythm with narrow-complex (supraventricular) QRS morphology on the electrocardiogram. Rarely, wide QRS morphology occurs as a result of abnormal delayed conduction through the right or left bundle branches (supraventricular conduction with aberrancy).

■ SYNONYMS
- Reentry-type SVT
- Atrioventricular (AV) reentry tachycardia
- AV node reentry tachycardia
- Paroxysmal atrial tachycardia (now an obsolete term, unless referring to uncommon tachycardias specifically originating within atrial tissue)
- Wolff-Parkinson-White (WPW) syndrome (electrocardiographic evidence of accessory pathway when in sinus rhythm)

ICD-9CM CODE
427.0 Paroxysmal supraventricular tachycardia

■ ETIOLOGY
- There are two basic and similar mechanisms for reentry SVT:
  1. AV reentry is caused by an accessory AV conduction pathway.
     a. This pathway allows reentry of electrical wavefront back to the atrium after passing down the normal cardiac conduction tissue from atrium to ventricle.
     b. It establishes an endless loop electrical pathway.
     c. If accessory pathway conducts from the atrium to ventricle when the patient is in normal sinus rhythm, electrocardiogram (ECG) shows findings of WPW syndrome.
  2. AV node reentry tachycardia results from reentry to the atrium over a fast retrograde pathway in patients who have dual AV nodal pathways.
- Other mechanisms of narrow QRS complex tachycardia include the following:
  1. Sinus tachycardia
  2. Atrial flutter
  3. Atrial ectopic tachycardia
  4. Junctional ectopic tachycardia
  5. The latter three mechanisms much less common than reentry SVT
  6. Originate from the atrium or AV junction and do not reenter from ventricle to atrium

■ EPIDEMIOLOGY & DEMOGRAPHICS
- SVT is the most common of the important pediatric arrhythmias.
- It presents at all ages, with peaks in neonatal, school-age, and adolescent children.
- Familial occurrence is documented, but the mode of inheritance/genetic loci is not well known.
- In infants, virtually all reentry SVT is AV reentry. In adolescents, AV node reentry becomes more common.
- Most patients have structurally normal hearts, but SVT may be associated with Ebstein's anomaly of the tricuspid valve or other congenital heart diseases.
- Half of pediatric cases have their first SVT episode in the first 6 months of life. One third will have late recurrence in school-age years.

■ HISTORY
- If sustained, children or adolescents will present with continuous palpitations.
- Young infants present with congestive heart failure after several days of poor feeding.
- Nonsustained SVT causes episodic palpitations in children and adolescents.
  1. Parents may note that clothing over the chest flutters at a rate too fast to count.
  2. Rapid neck vein pulsations may be reported.
- Newborns can present with hydrops/anasarca from intrauterine heart failure.

■ PHYSICAL EXAMINATION
- Normal cardiac examination is found between episodes if no congenital heart disease exists.
- Heart sounds may be widely split if there is concomitant WPW syndrome.
- During SVT, the heart rate is from 170 to 220 beats/min in children and adolescents and from 230 to 280 beats/min in infants.
- Poor perfusion and color are seen in sustained SVT.

DIAGNOSIS

■ DIFFERENTIAL DIAGNOSIS
- Sinus tachycardia can mimic SVT with rates as fast as 260 beats/min in a febrile young infant.
- Atrial flutter with two-to-one AV conduction has a slower ventricular rate than most AV reentry SVT but may mimic classic SVT clinically and on ECG.
- Postural orthostatic tachycardia syndrome (adrenaline-mediated attacks of sinus tachycardia—"fainters who do not faint") mimics intermittent SVT in clinical history.
- Ventricular tachycardia is less common and may be misdiagnosed as SVT in children.

■ DIAGNOSTIC WORKUP
- An ECG obtained during sustained SVT shows narrow-complex tachycardia without P waves preceding QRS.
  1. Subtle retrograde P waves are usually discernible in the ST segment following the QRS in AV reentry type.
- If palpitations are episodic, a 30-day event recorder is preferable over 24-hour ambulatory (Holter) monitoring.
- The ECG should be inspected for short PR intervals and delta waves indicating WPW syndrome.
  1. This is present only when in sinus rhythm and only in patients with an accessory pathway that conducts impulses from atrium to ventricle.
- Pacing studies (programmed electrical stimulation) occasionally may be needed to secure the diagnosis. Such studies are done usually at the time of catheter ablation treatment (see following section).

THERAPY

■ NONPHARMACOLOGIC
- For sustained SVT, convert to sinus rhythm by blocking conduction in the AV node.
  1. Ice/water bag held on infant's face for 5 to 10 seconds with ECG monitoring
  2. Valsalva maneuver or carotid sinus massage in older children

■ MEDICAL
- If nonpharmacologic methods do not convert SVT to sinus rhythm, the following may be tried:
  1. Adenosine may be given at 0.1 to 0.2 mg/kg by rapid intravenous (IV) push.
  2. *Never* use IV verapamil in infants because it may cause cardiac arrest/shock.
  3. DC synchronized cardioversion may be used if patient has severe hemodynamic compromise.
- For prevention of SVT, digoxin or β-blocker drugs may be used.
  1. In infants
     a. Digoxin
     b. Propranolol if not well con-

trolled, with digoxin as first-line therapy
2. In older children
   a. Digoxin should *not* be used in older children with WPW syndrome.
   b. Atenolol is the most commonly used β-blocker.
   c. Slow-release verapamil is also useful.
3. For refractory cases, treatment with sotalol, flecainide, amiodarone, or other drugs under guidance of pediatric cardiologist

■ SURGICAL
- Invasive catheter ablation of the accessory pathway using radiofrequency energy is curative.
  1. Consider for refractory childhood SVT cases.
  2. Consider for adolescents, with or without WPW, who do not desire drug therapy.

■ FOLLOW-UP & DISPOSITION
- Infants often do not have recurrences after the first year.
- Later recurrences are more likely if the ECG shows a WPW pattern.
- Puberty is associated with recurrence as well as first-time presentation.
- Pregnancy is associated with increased risk of recurrence or initial presentation.
- Yearly ECG may show resolution of WPW pattern in some patients or development of WPW pattern in some

patients without previous WPW pattern.

■ PATIENT/FAMILY EDUCATION
- Parents of infants may be taught to auscultate the heart rate daily to detect sustained SVT recurrence during the first year of life.
- Older children and adolescents should be taught to perform the Valsalva maneuver while supine if sustained SVT occurs.

■ REFERRAL INFORMATION
Most SVT patients require pediatric cardiology consultation.

☼ PEARLS & CONSIDERATIONS

■ CLINICAL PEARLS
- Always obtain a hard-copy ECG while converting SVT with adenosine; this may elucidate the mechanism of the SVT.
- DC cardioversion should be available when using adenosine.
  1. Rare incidence of adenosine-related atrial fibrillation with rapid ventricular response if WPW syndrome is present
- WPW pattern on ECG indicates an accessory pathway that is able to conduct antegrade as well as retrograde.
  1. Rarely, atrial fibrillation develops

with extremely rapid ventricular response rate and sudden death.
  2. This can be a first presentation of WPW in adolescents.
- In adolescents with WPW, the risk of unexpected sudden death needs to be discussed versus risks of invasive catheter studies and/or curative radiofrequency ablation by an electrophysiologist.
- Infants often have poor pulses and color but may convert with ice bag maneuver and not require DC cardioversion.

■ WEBSITE
The Child's Doctor: www.childsdoc.org/fall98/st/svt.asp; current concepts and treatment of supraventricular tachycardia in children

REFERENCES
1. Dorostkar PC, Dick M II: Current management of supraventricular tachycardia in children, *Heart Dis Stroke* 3:395, 1994.
2. Jaeggi E et al: Adenosine-induced atrial pro-arrhythmia in children, *Can J Cardiol* 15:169, 1999.
3. Perry JC, Garson A Jr: Supraventricular tachycardia due to Wolff Parkinson White syndrome in children: early disappearance and late recurrence, *J Am Coll Cardiol* 16:1215, 1990.
Author: **David Hannon, M.D.**

BASIC INFORMATION

■ **DEFINITION**
Neurally mediated syncope is a sudden transient loss of postural tone and consciousness with spontaneous recovery.

■ **SYNONYMS**
- Syncope
- Fainting
- Vasovagal syncope
- Vasodepressor syncope
- Neurocardiogenic syncope

ICD-9CM CODE
780.2 Syncope and collapse

■ **ETIOLOGY**
- There is an excess of very rapid development of venous pooling in the lower extremities in association with discordant baroreceptor function and altered peripheral vascular receptor sensitivity.
- Paradoxical cerebral vasoconstriction may also play a role.

■ **EPIDEMIOLOGY & DEMOGRAPHICS**
- Syncope is common, affecting up to 15% of adolescents.
- The male:female ratio is 1:1.
- Mean age at presentation is 15 years.
- Gravitational stress is the most common precipitant.
- Minor injuries are common (25%); serious injuries occur in 1% to 2%.
- If recurrent, may have a major effect on lifestyle and/or quality of life.
- Usually there is a transient predisposition for syncope.

■ **HISTORY**
- Prodrome present in all but 1% to 2%
- Prodromal symptoms
  1. Light-headedness: 89%
  2. Visual disturbances: 71%
  3. Sensation of warmth: 39%
  4. Nausea: 35%
  5. Diaphoresis: 33%
  6. Altered hearing: 25%
  7. Sharp frontal headache: 15%
  8. Mild tachycardia: 13%
- During syncope
  1. Brief tonic-clonic activity in 6%
  2. Urinary incontinence in 2%
- May occur while standing, sitting, walking, and occasionally during exercise
- Low salt intake in 70%
- Other settings—chronic fatigue syndrome, dieting
- Family history of syncope in 20% to 30%

■ **PHYSICAL EXAMINATION**
- Examination is usually normal.
- Orthostasis may be found at the time of syncope.

 DIAGNOSIS

■ **DIFFERENTIAL DIAGNOSIS**
- Cardiovascular: arrhythmic, hemodynamic, aortic stenosis, atrial myoma
- Hypovolemia, anemia
- Seizures
- Medications or street drugs (e.g., alcohol, cocaine)
- Metabolic disorders (e.g., hypoglycemia, hypoxia)
- Psychogenic
- Pregnancy

■ **DIAGNOSTIC WORKUP**
- Electrocardiogram to rule out the following:
  1. Long QT
  2. Ventricular hypertrophy
  3. Wolff-Parkinson-White syndrome (preexcitation)
- Electrolytes: low yield unless dehydration is suspected by history or examination
- Blood glucose: low yield, usually long prodrome and long postevent confusion
- Electroencephalogram: usually not necessary; abrupt return to an alert and oriented state after syncope favors a neurally mediated event
- Echocardiogram: only if heart disease is suspected
- Cranial computed tomography, magnetic resonance imaging/angiography: not necessary unless focal neurological signs are present
- Consideration of drug screen, pregnancy test

 THERAPY

■ **NONPHARMACOLOGIC**
- Leg exercises to increase muscular, vascular tone
- Tight stockings (although compliance is an issue)
- Information to assist understanding of pathophysiology
- Lying down at the onset of a prodrome
- Biofeedback if threat-induced syncope

■ **MEDICAL**
- Sodium chloride tablets beginning with 1 g/day with food

- Addition of florinef 0.1 mg daily (check blood pressure weekly for 4 weeks)
- β-Blockers, but review first with cardiologist
- Midodrine, a peripheral α-adrenergic agonist
- Pseudoephedrine, Ritalin
- Serotonin reuptake inhibitors

■ **SURGICAL**
Very rarely, dual-chamber, rate-responsive cardiac pacing is performed.

■ **FOLLOW-UP & DISPOSITION**
- Treatment can be discontinued in 80% to 85% of patients after 12 to 18 months.
- Approximately 15% to 20% require longer intervention.
- The prognosis is usually excellent.

■ **PATIENT/FAMILY EDUCATION**
- Lie down with onset of prodromal symptoms.
- Drink an electrolyte-containing fluid, not water, during exercise, especially in a hot environment.

■ **PREVENTIVE TREATMENT**
See "Patient/Family Education."

■ **REFERRAL INFORMATION**
Cardiology referral is indicated for the following conditions:
- Syncope with exertion
- Any suggestion of heart disease
- Abnormal electrocardiogram
- Adverse family history (e.g., premature sudden cardiac death)
- Palpitations more than a mild tachycardia
- Presyncope or syncope while driving
- No prodrome
- Important injury
- Failure of conservative medical management

 PEARLS & CONSIDERATIONS

■ **CLINICAL PEARLS**
- The history is the single most important part of the workup.
- An electrocardiogram should be obtained, but other laboratory tests are usually not warranted unless drug abuse, dehydration, cardiovascular abnormalities, or neurologic problems are suspected.
- If salt tablets and/or florinef are prescribed, it is not necessary to advise patient to drink more fluids; this will naturally occur with an augmentation of sodium intake.

■ **WEBSITES**
- National Dysautonomia Research Foundation: www.ndrf.org
- The Sudden Arrhythmia Death Syndromes Foundation: www.sads.org

REFERENCES

1. Benditt DG et al: Tilt table testing for assessing syncope, *J Am Coll Cardiol* 28:263, 1998.
2. Calkins H et al: The value of the clinical history in the differentiation of syncope due to ventricular tachycardia, atrioventricular block, and neurocardiogenic syncope, *Am J Med* 98:365, 1995.
3. Grubb BP, Olshansky B: *Syncope: mechanisms and management,* Armonk, NY, 1998, Futura Publishing.

Author: **J. Peter Harris, M.D.**

II

BASIC INFORMATION

■ DEFINITION
The syndrome of inappropriate anti-diuretic hormone secretion (SIADH) comprises the finding of hyponatremia and hypoosmolality combined with a decreased amount of inappropriately concentrated urine. Patients with SIADH are euvolemic. SIADH is associated with a variety of systemic diseases and is a diagnosis of exclusion.

ICD-9CM CODE
253.6 Other disorders of
  neurohypophysis

■ ETIOLOGY
- There is no clear unifying cause or pathophysiology.
- Most patients appear to have disordered regulation of vasopressin, the human antidiuretic hormone (ADH), in response to hypoosmolality.
  1. ADH release is not suppressed when it should be (i.e., in the presence of hyponatremia).
  2. Excess ADH leads to retention of free water by the kidney. Subsequent expansion of the intravascular space leads to hyponatremia.
- Many conditions are associated with the development of SIADH, but most fall into three general categories: (1) central nervous system (CNS) disease (e.g., tumor, infection, past surgery, trauma), (2) pulmonary disorders (e.g., adult respiratory distress, infection, cancer), and (3) tumors.
- Less common forms involve the ectopic release of an ADH-like substance, most often from pulmonary tumors.

■ EPIDEMIOLOGY & DEMOGRAPHICS
- Hyponatremia is the most common electrolyte disorder seen in clinical medicine.
- SIADH is the most common cause of hyponatremia in hospitalized patients.
- Menstruating women may be more susceptible to long-term neurologic complications from hyponatremia in general. The exact reason for this association is not clear.

■ HISTORY & PHYSICAL EXAMINATION
- The hyponatremia of SIADH is usually asymptomatic.
- Signs and symptoms can include nausea, cramps, lethargy, disorientation, agitation, seizures, and coma.
- Neurologic signs and symptoms are most likely related to cerebral edema. The blood-brain barrier is permeable to water, and a gradient is set up because of the peripheral hypotonicity.

- Symptoms occur most often when sodium is less than 120 mEq/L or when a drop in sodium develops rapidly.
- The most prominent findings may be those of the underlying disease associated with SIADH.

DIAGNOSIS

■ DIFFERENTIAL DIAGNOSIS (EUVOLEMIC HYPONATREMIA)
- Glucocorticoid deficiency
- Hypothyroidism
- Cerebral salt wasting (CSW; although these patients are often volume depleted)
- Presence of drugs that cause release of ADH or potentiate its action
- Pseudohyponatremia (caused by an idiosyncrasy in assay in hyperglycemic or hyperlipidemic patients)

■ DIAGNOSTIC WORKUP
The diagnosis of SIADH should be considered in a stepwise approach:
- Establish hyponatremia (sodium less than 130 mEq/L).
- Establish that the patient is neither volume depleted nor volume overloaded.
  1. The differential diagnosis of the dehydrated or edematous patient with hyponatremia is different and does not include SIADH.
- Consider the possibility of other causes (see "Differential Diagnosis"). These need not be ruled out in every patient but should be contemplated if there is no underlying process typically associated with SIADH.
- Evaluate serum and urine sodium and osmolality in the context of urine output.
  1. Urine output should be reduced significantly in SIADH.
  2. The finding of increased urine sodium (more than 20 mEq/L) and osmolality in the setting of decreased serum sodium and osmolality strongly suggests SIADH.
  3. In the head-injured patient, this combination in the context of normal or increased urine output suggests CSW syndrome.
    a. These patients are often volume depleted.
    b. It is important to distinguish SIADH from CSW because therapies differ.

THERAPY

The treatment of SIADH is supportive.
- Fluid restriction: Fluids should be reduced to two-thirds maintenance.
- Treat the underlying disease process.
- Only in the presence of seizures or

rapidly evolving neurologic signs should administration of saline be considered.
- Care should be taken to continue to evaluate serum sodium.
  1. SIADH can resolve spontaneously without warning or obvious clinical findings.
  2. In lesions of the CNS, it can be followed by diabetes insipidus.

PEARLS & CONSIDERATIONS

■ CLINICAL PEARLS
- Care should be taken in making the diagnosis of SIADH in the presence of diuretic therapy.
- In SIADH, serum sodium will not continue to fall indefinitely because of a decline in the renal effect of ADH over time. The reason for this is unclear.
- Most of the drugs associated with SIADH are not commonly used in pediatrics. Notable exceptions are the antineoplastic drugs vincristine and cyclophosphamide. The latter is particularly worrisome in that its administration is often accompanied by vigorous hydration to avert renal complications.
- The hyponatremia of SIADH generally occurs slowly and therefore is associated with fewer symptoms and complications than other forms of hyponatremia.
- Especially in the setting of head trauma, the clinical picture is often inconsistent and changes over time. The relationship between serum and urine (sodium and osmolality) in the context of urine output and fluid intake should be continually reassessed. A broad differential diagnosis should continue to be kept in mind.

■ WEBSITE
Merck: www.merck.com/pubs/manual/section2/chapter12/12b.htm

REFERENCES
1. Ganong CA, Kappy MS: Cerebral salt wasting in children: the need for recognition and treatment, *Am J Dis Child* 147:167, 1993.
2. Harrigan MR: Cerebral salt wasting syndrome: a review, *Neurosurgery* 38:152, 1996.
3. Rogers MC, Helfaer MA (eds): *Case studies in pediatric intensive care*, Baltimore, 1993, Williams & Wilkins.
4. Schrier RW (ed): *Renal and electrolyte disorders*, ed 5, Philadelphia, 1997, Lippincott-Raven.
5. Todres ID, Fugate JH (eds): *Critical care of infants and children*, Boston, 1996, Little, Brown.
Author: **Jonathan P. Wood, M.D.**

BASIC INFORMATION

■ DEFINITION
Syphilis is a multisystem sexually transmitted disease (STD) that can be congenital or acquired.

■ SYNONYM
Venereal syphilis

ICD-9CM CODE
097.9 Syphilis, unspecified

■ ETIOLOGY
Syphilis is caused by *Treponema pallidum,* a thin, motile spirochete that cannot be cultivated in vitro.

■ EPIDEMIOLOGY & DEMOGRAPHICS
- Syphilis is acquired by direct sexual contact with ulcerative lesions of skin or mucous membranes (occasionally by other forms of close contact).
- It can be transmitted transplacentally from a woman with any stage of disease; transmission reaches almost 100% in secondary syphilis.
- In the pediatric population, it is most common among the adolescent age group. Up to 15% of adolescents and adults with syphilis are coinfected with human immunodeficiency virus (HIV).
- The incubation period for acquired primary syphilis is about 3 weeks, with a range from 10 to 90 days.
- Primary syphilis occurs in 30% of exposures.

■ HISTORY
- Painless genital ulcer
- Rash
- Sexual contact with someone with syphilis
- History of prior STD
- HIV testing

■ PHYSICAL EXAMINATION
- Primary
  1. Timing: 1 to 4 weeks after infection
  2. Ulcer or chancre at the infection site with raised indurated edge
     a. Painless, most commonly on the genitalia
  3. Painless localized lymphadenopathy
- Secondary
  1. Timing: 6 to 12 weeks after infection
  2. No chancre
  3. Rash: salmon pink macules 5 to 10 mm in size that start on the trunk and spread to most of the body, including palms and soles
  4. Mucocutaneous lesions
     a. Approximately 10% get white or gray patches on the mucous membranes.
     b. About 10% get *Condyloma lata*—raised, enlarged, painless papules in warm, moist areas such as vulva, anus, axilla, and scrotum.
  5. Generalized lymphadenopathy in 85%
- Tertiary
  1. Gummatous disease of skin, bone, and other organs occurs rarely.
  2. Approximately 10% of patients develop cardiovascular disease (e.g., aortic aneurysm, aortic insufficiency, coronary artery disease)
  3. Neurosyphilis: Involvement can be meningeal, obstructive hydrocephalus, or meningovascular.
  4. The PARESIS mnemonic stands for *p*ersonality, *a*ffect, *r*eflexes (hyperactive), *e*ye (Argyll-Robertson pupils), *s*ensorium, *i*ntellect (diminished), and *s*peech problems.
- Latent
  1. Asymptomatic syphilis, but seropositive
  2. Early latent syphilis acquired within past 1 year
  3. Late latent syphilis: duration unknown
- Congenital
  1. Symptoms range from asymptomatic to stillbirth.
  2. Manifestations include the following:
     a. Hepatosplenomegaly
     b. Hemolytic anemia
     c. Osteochondritis
     d. Thrombocytopenia
  3. Early-onset disease: Onset occurs before 2 years of age.
  4. Late-onset disease: This is seen in patients older than 2 years of age.

🔬 DIAGNOSIS

■ DIFFERENTIAL DIAGNOSIS
- Other causes of genital ulcer disease
  1. Herpes simplex
  2. *Haemophilus ducreyi* (chancroid)
  3. *Chlamydia trachomatis* (lymphogranuloma venereum)
  4. *Calymmatobacterium granulomatis* (granuloma inguinale)
- Rash on palms and soles
  1. Enteroviruses
  2. Rocky Mountain spotted fever
  3. *Neisseria meningitidis*
- Bone lesions
  1. Osteomyelitis
  2. Rickets from vitamin D deficiency
- Disseminated infection (i.e., fungal)

■ DIAGNOSTIC WORKUP
- Definitive diagnosis is determined as follows:
  1. Presence of spirochetes by microscopic dark-field examination or direct fluorescent antibody tests of lesion exudate or tissue are definitive for diagnosing early syphilis.
  2. Serologic testing is also done because false-negative microscopic results occur.
- Presumptive diagnosis is possible using two types of serologic tests:
  1. Nontreponemal tests
     a. These test include the VDRL (Venereal Disease Research Laboratory) slide test, the rapid plasma reagin test, and the automatic reagin test.
     b. These tests correlate with disease activity; results are reported quantitatively.
     c. A fourfold change is considered necessary to demonstrate a clinically significant difference (e.g., from 1:8 to 1:32).
     d. Quantitative nontreponemal tests will eventually become nonreactive after treatment.
  2. Treponemal tests (fluorescent treponemal antibody absorbed and microhemagglutination assay for antibody to *T. pallidum*)
     a. Most patients with reactive treponemal tests have reactive tests forever. Approximately 15% to 25% of patients treated during primary syphilis revert to nonreactive status after 2 to 3 years.
     b. Treponemal tests are not 100% specific for syphilis.
        (1) False-positive reactions occur in other spirochetal diseases, such as yaws, pinta, leptospirosis, ratbite fever, and Lyme disease.
        (2) The nontreponemal tests can be used to distinguish Lyme disease from syphilis. The VDRL is nonreactive in Lyme disease.
     c. In some patients, nontreponemal antibodies can persist at a low titer for a long period. These individuals are referred to as *serofast.*
- Serology
  1. Sequential serology should be performed by the same method and laboratory to gauge treatment response.
  2. HIV-infected patients can have abnormal serologic tests, and biopsy or direct microscopy is a useful addition to serology for diagnosis.
  3. Neurosyphilis is diagnosed by the combination of reactive serologic tests, cerebrospinal fluid (CSF) abnormalities (white blood cell count [WBC] or protein), or a reactive CSF-VDRL with or without clinical manifestations. CSF WBC is usually higher than 5 WBCs/mm^3. A negative CSF-VDRL does not exclude a diagnosis of

neurosyphilis, and a positive CSF-VDRL may be present in an uninfected newborn with a transplacentally acquired, high-serum VDRL titer.

4. All women should be tested for syphilis during pregnancy.
5. Maternal serology should be repeated at the time of delivery.
6. Infants should be evaluated for syphilis if they meet the following criteria:
   a. Mother has syphilis or was inadequately treated (e.g., treatment with a nonpenicillin regimen).
   b. Mother was treated within 1 month of delivery.
   c. Mother's serology has not made the expected fourfold decrease in titer to assess response to treatment.
7. Infant evaluation includes the following:
   a. Physical examination
   b. Quantitative nontreponemal serologic test for syphilis on infant's sera
   c. Antitreponemal immunoglobulin M (IgM)
   d. CSF-VDRL, cell count, protein concentration
   e. Long-bone radiographs
   f. Other tests as indicated: complete blood count, chest radiograph, liver function tests

🏥 THERAPY

■ MEDICAL
- Parenteral penicillin G is the drug of choice for treatment of syphilis at any stage.
- Recommendations for penicillin G and duration of therapy vary depending on the stage; consult current references.
- Parenteral penicillin G is the only documented effective therapy for patients with congenital syphilis, neurosyphilis, and syphilis during

pregnancy, and it is highly recommended for HIV-infected patients.

■ FOLLOW-UP & DISPOSITION
- Congenital syphilis
  1. Careful follow-up examinations are recommended at 1, 2, 4, 6, and 12 months of age.
  2. Serologic nontreponemal tests should be conducted at 3, 6, and 12 months of age or until they become nonreactive.
  3. Infants treated for congenital neurosyphilis should have repeat CSF evaluations at 6-month intervals until the CSF examination is normal.
- Early syphilis
  1. Treated pregnant women require monthly nontreponemal serologic tests for the remainder of their pregnancy.
  2. Other patients should be retested at 3, 6, and 12 months after the end of treatment.
- Latent syphilis
  1. Patients with latent syphilis should have repeat testing 24 months after treatment.
- Re-treatment is indicated if the following conditions are met:
  1. The clinical illness persists or recurs.
  2. A lasting, fourfold increase in titer of nontreponemal test occurs or, in a pregnant woman, if it occurs.
  3. A fourfold decrease in titer of nontreponemal test fails to occur in 1 year; in pregnant women with primary or secondary syphilis, it fails to decrease fourfold in 3 months; or with latent syphilis, it fails to decrease fourfold in 6 months.
- Patients with syphilis should be tested for HIV infection and other STDs.

■ PATIENT/FAMILY EDUCATION
- Education about STDs, treatment of sexual contacts, and reporting each case to the local health department are necessary.

- All recent sexual contacts should be identified.

■ REFERRAL INFORMATION
Consultation with the local health department and a pediatric infectious disease specialist can be useful.

⚙ PEARLS & CONSIDERATIONS

■ CLINICAL PEARLS
- Syphilis should be considered in the differential diagnosis of unusual rashes and multisystem disease.
- Sexually active teenagers should be screened for syphilis, especially in the presence of another STD or if they have had more than one sexual partner in the last 6 months.

■ WEBSITES
- American Social Health Association: www.iwannaknow.org
- Centers for Disease Control and Prevention: www.cdc.gov/nchstp/dstd/std98tg.htm
- The Henry J. Kaiser Family Foundation: www.itsyoursexlife.com

■ SUPPORT GROUP
National STD Hotline: 800-227-8922

REFERENCES
1. American Academy of Pediatrics: Syphilis. In Pickering LK (ed): *2000 Red Book: report of the Committee on Infectious Diseases,* ed 25, Elk Grove Village, Ill, 2000, American Academy of Pediatrics.
2. Centers for Disease Control and Prevention: *1998 guidelines for treatment of sexually transmitted disease,* www.cdc.gov.
3. Coles FB, Hipp SS: Syphilis among adolescents: the hidden epidemic, *Contemp Pediatr* 13:47, 1996.
4. Sung L, MacDonald NE: Syphilis: a pediatric perspective, *Pediatr Rev* 19:17, 1998.

Author: **Cynthia Christy, M.D.**

BASIC INFORMATION

■ DEFINITION

Systemic lupus erythematosus (SLE) is a complex autoimmune disorder that results from widespread immune complex deposition and secondary tissue injury. As such, it is characterized by the presence of antinuclear antibodies (ANAs) and multiple organ system involvement. Any organ system may be affected by SLE, but the skin, joints, and kidneys are most commonly involved.

■ SYNONYMS

- Lupus
- SLE

ICD-9CM CODE

710.0 Systemic lupus erythematosus

■ ETIOLOGY

- The cause of SLE is unknown.
- It occurs with increased frequency in first-degree family members of affected individuals and is thought to have a genetic component, but it often occurs without any family history of disease.
- Genetic absence of immunoglobulin A (IgA) and absent C4 complement both occur more often than expected among children with SLE.
- It is hypothesized that there is an immunoregulatory defect, which allows degeneration of a normal immune response into polyclonal B-cell activation.
  1. This results in production of antibodies to a wide variety of antigens unrelated to the initial immune response.
  2. These antibodies lead to immune complex deposition and tissue damage.
  3. The organ system involvement in a given individual is determined by the combination of his or her genetic background and the antigens his or her immune system has previously been exposed to.

■ EPIDEMIOLOGY & DEMOGRAPHICS

- The frequency of SLE varies by age, race, and sex.
- It most commonly affects females between the ages of 15 and 25 years.
  1. Incidence is as high as 30 per 100,000 in Asian teens.
  2. Incidence is estimated at 4 per 100,000 in Caucasians.
  3. Hispanic and African-American girls have intermediate incidences.
  4. Older and younger individuals and males are also affected.
     a. The incidence in males is roughly one fourth that for girls of the same race.

- Positive tests for ANA are found in approximately one third of first-degree relatives.
- Actual disease occurs in only about 1 in 50 first-degree relatives.

■ HISTORY

- Fever, malaise, and weight loss are the most common presenting findings.
  1. In teenagers who have unintentional weight loss, SLE should be included in the differential diagnosis.
- Less commonly, SLE may have an explosive onset, presenting with the following:
  1. Seizures and diffuse neurologic symptoms
  2. Nephritis or nephrotic syndrome
  3. Arthritis
  4. Polyserositis
  5. Any combination of above systems

■ PHYSICAL EXAMINATION

- Because SLE involves multiple organ systems, one must carefully evaluate every organ system.
- General: Children with SLE are often chronically ill and withdrawn appearing.
  1. They may be depressed.
  2. They may have undiagnosed arthritis.
  3. They often "don't want to be touched."
  4. Hypertension may be present if there is renal involvement.
- Skin: Most patients with SLE have a mild, nonspecific facial rash.
  1. One in three children have a recognized malar rash with a butterfly distribution.
  2. Bruises may be present if there is thrombocytopenia or abnormal clotting secondary to the lupus anticoagulant.
- Alopecia is a common finding, but it may be present with any chronic illness.
- Ophthalmologic findings are uncommon.
  1. If central nervous system vasculitis is present, "cotton-wool exudates" or other evidence of vasculitis may be found on funduscopic examination.
- The hard palate often has areas of irritation and redness.
  1. Helpful when the family dismisses the facial rash as being caused by cosmetics or other topical agents
- Chest and cardiac examination may be normal.
  1. SLE is a polyserositis, and the patient may have physical examination findings of pleural or pericardial effusions.
  2. Be suspicious if the patient is tachypneic.

- Examine the abdomen.
  1. Hepatosplenomegaly may be present in advanced cases.
  2. Children may have diffuse nonfocal tenderness secondary to polyserositis.
- Musculoskeletal system: Most children with active SLE have mild arthritis but may not be aware of it.
  1. Tenderness when you squeeze their hands or feet
  2. Knee effusions
- Pitting edema suggests nephrotic syndrome.

🔬 DIAGNOSIS

■ DIFFERENTIAL DIAGNOSIS

- Many rheumatic diseases and some infections may be associated with ANA.
  1. Do not accept the diagnosis of SLE based on this finding alone.
  2. However, ANA-negative SLE is extremely rare and most often an incorrect diagnosis.
- Mixed connective tissue disease is a variant of SLE that does not need to be distinguished by the nonspecialist.
- Other rheumatic diseases such as dermatomyositis, Wegener's granulomatosus, pauci-immune glomerulonephritis, and juvenile rheumatoid arthritis all occur in childhood, may have multiple system involvement, and may be associated with a positive ANA.
  1. Patients with these diseases should be referred to a pediatric rheumatologist for differentiation and care.
- Tuberculosis, malaria, subacute bacterial endocarditis, and other infections may both mimic SLE and coexist with it.
  1. A thorough evaluation to eliminate infectious problems is essential.

■ DIAGNOSTIC WORKUP

- The diagnosis of SLE is based on the presence of ANAs and multiple organ system involvement, with the exclusion of other recognized entities.
  1. SLE is often (two thirds of cases) associated with significant hypocomplementemia and antibodies to double-stranded DNA.
  2. These findings are rare in most of the other diseases considered.
- Most patients with SLE have anemia with relative or actual leukopenia and thrombocytopenia.
  1. Most chronic infections are associated with anemia, leukocytosis, and thrombocytosis.
  2. If anemic with a normal or elevated mean corpuscular volume, check for hemolysis.

- Routine clotting studies should be performed to make sure there is no evidence of a circulating anticoagulant.
    1. Both prolonged and shortened clotting times are abnormal and worrisome.
    2. Teenage girls with SLE may present with menorrhagia.
    3. Some children with SLE will have anticardiolipin antibodies.
        a. These are associated with an increased risk of stroke and thrombosis.
- Do a urinalysis to look for hematuria, pyuria, and proteinuria.
- Abnormal electrolytes or renal function studies may indicate significant nephritis or nephrotic syndrome.
- Children with SLE are often hypoalbuminemic because of chronic illness or renal loss.
    1. Total protein may be elevated secondary to hypergammaglobulinemia.
- Mild liver enzyme elevations may be caused by nonspecific liver involvement, but it may also result from increased hemolysis.
    1. If the bilirubin or aspartate aminotransferase is significantly elevated, consider hemolytic anemia.
- Specialized tests such as antibodies to Ro, La, Sm, and RNP are often helpful in distinguishing subsets of SLE.

℞ THERAPY

■ MEDICAL
- Therapy for SLE depends on the severity of the disease.
    1. Mild disease may be treated with antimalarials (e.g., hydroxychloroquine) and nonsteroidal antiinflammatory drugs.
    2. Corticosteroids are often required.
- Because of the substantial side effects associated with chronic corticosteroid use, every effort should be made to minimize the corticosteroid dosage.
- For children with severe disease, the addition of immunosuppressive drugs such as cyclophosphamide or azathioprine is required.
    1. These drugs have potentially life-threatening toxicities.

---

    2. Choice of appropriate drug, dose, and route of administration should be left to experienced physicians.
- SLE cannot be cured, and most children with significant disease require chronic use of at least low-dose corticosteroids.

■ FOLLOW-UP & DISPOSITION
- Children with SLE require chronic follow-up with an experienced pediatric rheumatologist indefinitely.
    1. With treatment, most children have a satisfactory course.
    2. Severe disease, especially with central nervous system involvement or renal involvement, may be fatal.
    3. Intercurrent infections are also a major problem for children with active disease.
- The course of the disease is unpredictable, and children who have been well for extended periods may still suddenly worsen dramatically.

■ PATIENT/FAMILY EDUCATION
- Education plays a major role in determining the outcome for children with SLE.
    1. Most of the drugs are associated with significant side effects and must be monitored carefully.
    2. Parents and children (as age appropriate) should understand why they are taking the medications and what side effects to look for.
- SLE is a chronic illness requiring children to take medications that may negatively alter their physical appearance and sense of well-being.
    1. Episodes of resistance and noncompliance should be expected.
    2. Because failure to take medications (especially corticosteroids) can be fatal, anticipate these problems and educate families accordingly.
- The risk of a second affected child in a family is small, but siblings are occasionally affected.
    1. Ill siblings should be evaluated, but well siblings do not require routine testing.
    2. One in three siblings will be ANA positive, but only 1 in 50 will ever be affected.

- Children with SLE should be encouraged to live normal, healthy lives.
    1. Most will go on to productive adulthood.
    2. As women reach reproductive age, they should be counseled about the risks of spontaneous abortion, worsening of SLE during and after pregnancy, and neonatal lupus.

■ REFERRAL INFORMATION
Most children with SLE are cared for by pediatric rheumatologists, nephrologists, or hematologists as appropriate to their disease manifestations and the availability of subspecialists in their community.

☼ PEARLS & CONSIDERATIONS

■ CLINICAL PEARLS
- Always remember SLE in the evaluation of a child of any age who is "failing to thrive," gaining weight poorly, or losing weight inappropriately.
- Chronic illness usually produces leukocytosis and thrombocytosis. If there is leukopenia or thrombocytopenia, there is either increased destruction (e.g., SLE, infection) or decreased production (e.g., marrow infiltrative disease such as leukemia).

■ WEBSITE
The Lupus Foundation: www.lupus.org

■ SUPPORT GROUPS
- The Lupus Foundation of America has offices in most major cities and provides help and support for children with SLE and their families.
- The Arthritis Foundation also has offices in most major cities and has pamphlets and informational materials available upon request.

REFERENCES
1. Lehman TJ: A practical guide to systemic lupus erythematosus, *Pediatr Clin North Am* 42:1223, 1995.
2. Lehman TJ: Systemic lupus erythematosus in childhood and adolescence. In Wallace DJ, Hahn B (eds): *Lupus erythematosus*, ed 5, Philadelphia, 1997, Lea & Febiger.
Author: **Thomas J.A. Lehman, M.D.**

BASIC INFORMATION

■ DEFINITION
Testicular torsion is twisting of the spermatic cord and testis that results in venous obstruction, progressive edema, arterial compromise, and eventually, testicular infarction.

■ SYNONYM
Spermatic cord torsion

■ ICD-9CM CODE
608.2 Testicular torsion

■ ETIOLOGY
- High attachment of the tunica vaginalis to the spermatic cord allows the testis and epididymis to hang freely in the scrotum.
- The lack of fixation allows the testis to have a more transverse lie and hang like a bell clapper; this transverse lie allows the testis to twist freely on its spermatic cord axis.
- Oblique insertion of cremasteric fibers on the spermatic cord may contribute to twist.

■ EPIDEMIOLOGY & DEMOGRAPHICS
- Occurs in 1 in 400 males younger than 25 years of age
- May occur at any age
- Biphasic peak incidence
  1. Neonate (often during late fetal development)
  2. Adolescence

■ HISTORY
- Acute onset of pain, often with nausea, vomiting, and exquisite testicular tenderness, is noted.
- Pain may be referred to the ipsilateral inguinal canal or abdomen.
- Often, patients have had similar episodes that resolved after a short period.
- A history of trauma does not rule out testicular torsion.
- Lack of severe pain does not rule out testicular torsion.

■ PHYSICAL EXAMINATION
- Test the cremasteric reflex first.
  1. Absent cremasteric reflex is consistent with torsion but not specific.
- Examine in both erect and supine positions.
- Examine the involved testis last.
- Elevated, often swollen, tender testis with a firmer consistency on the side of the torsion is seen.
- The testis may appear to be horizontal.
- Contralateral testis may have a transverse lie.

DIAGNOSIS

■ DIFFERENTIAL DIAGNOSIS
- Torsion of a testicular or epididymal appendage
- Epididymitis
- Orchitis
- Testicular neoplasm with or without hemorrhage
- Testicular abscess
- Traumatic hydrocele/hematocele
- Henoch-Schönlein purpura
- Lymphedema
- Scrotal skin inflammation
  1. Cellulitis
  2. Infected sebaceous cyst
- Incarcerated inguinal hernia
- Other intraperitoneal process manifesting in scrotum (e.g., meconium scrotitis)

■ DIAGNOSTIC WORKUP
- Surgical exploration should be carried out immediately if acute torsion cannot be ruled out clinically.
- Radiographic studies are best used to confirm torsion in a late presentation or to confirm absence of torsion.
- Color Doppler ultrasonography:
  1. Demonstrates diminished or absent blood flow to the affected testis and normal blood flow to the unaffected testis
     a. Sensitivity of 80% to 100% and specificity of 97% to 100%
  2. Operator dependent
  3. Imaging study of choice
- Scintigraphy may be performed.
  1. Scintigraphy demonstrates little or no blood flow to the affected testis and normal blood flow to the unaffected testis.
  2. This test is most helpful in "missed" or nonsalvageable torsion.
  3. It has a sensitivity of 80% to 100% and a specificity of 89% to 100%.
  4. In many centers the isotope must be prepared and is thus not readily available, causing a significant delay in diagnosis.
  5. This test does not provide anatomic data.

THERAPY

■ NONPHARMACOLOGIC
- Manual detorsion
  1. Allows for relief of symptoms
  2. Should be followed by surgical fixation because detorsion may be incomplete
  3. Recurrence common without surgical correction
  4. Procedure to untwist (detorse) testes
     a. Two thirds of torsed testes occur by medial rotation so need to untwist as if "opening a book."
     b. From foot of patient, place thumb behind and fingers on ventral surface of scrotum/testis and "open" or turn hand and testis laterally (outward).
     c. Remember, however, that in one third of cases, need to twist medially because torsion occurs by lateral rotation.

■ SURGICAL
- Surgical exploration and correction are mandatory, even when manual detorsion seems to relieve vascular compromise.
  1. Patients operated on within 3 hours have a near 100% salvage rate
     a. Salvage depends on duration, degree, and tightness of torsion.
     b. *Salvage* is defined as lack of testicular atrophy.
  2. The salvage rate drops to 92% by 6 hours and 62% at 6 to 12 hours
- Both testes should be explored and pexed, not just the torsed side.

■ FOLLOW-UP & DISPOSITION
- The infertility risk in patients with prior testicular torsion is unknown, but it is likely increased.
  1. If testis infarcts and dies but is left in scrotum, infertility is high even if other testis is fine.
  2. If one testis infarcts and dies and is removed and the other testis is normal, normal fertility is expected.
- All patients should have long-term follow-up with urologist to assess testicular atrophy.

■ REFERRAL INFORMATION
All patients with suspected testicular torsion should be referred to an urologist.

☼ PEARLS & CONSIDERATIONS

■ CLINICAL PEARLS

- Any acute scrotal pain or swelling should be considered testicular torsion until ruled out.
- The window of opportunity for testicular salvage is within the first 6 to 12 hours after the onset of symptoms.

REFERENCES

1. Hawtrey CE: Assessment of acute scrotal symptoms and findings: a clinician's dilemma, *Urol Clin North Am* 25: 715, 1998.
2. Hulbert WC, Rabinowitz R: Diagnosing testicular torsion with Doppler US, *Contemp Urol* 7:40, 1995.
3. Lerner RM et al: Testicular imaging, *Curr Opin Radiol* 3:694, 1991.
4. Rabinowitz R, Hulbert WC: Acute scrotal swelling, *Urol Clin North Am* 22: 101, 1995.

Authors: **Stephanie Sansoni, M.D., William C. Hulbert, M.D., Robert Mevorach, M.D., and Ronald Rabinowitz, M.D.**

BASIC INFORMATION

■ DEFINITION
Tetany is a state of hyperexcitability of the central and peripheral nervous systems, which results from abnormally reduced concentrations of ions (Ca^{2+}, Mg^{2+}, or H^+ [alkalosis]) in the fluid bathing nerve cells.

■ ICD-9CM CODE
781.7 Tetany

■ ETIOLOGY
- Hypocalcemia
- Vitamin D deficiency (deficient absorption of both vitamin D and calcium)
- Hypomagnesemia
  1. Occurs in various clinical states, including malabsorption syndrome (chronic diarrhea or vomiting, celiac disease), hypoparathyroidism, diuretic therapy, renal tubular acidosis, hyperaldosteronism, and prolonged intravenous fluid therapy with magnesium-free fluids
- Hyperventilation of psychogenic origin

■ EPIDEMIOLOGY & DEMOGRAPHICS
Tetany of vitamin D deficiency is rare today and usually occurs at 3 to 6 month of age; it can occur within the first week of life in infants born to vitamin D–deficient mothers.

■ HISTORY
- Manifest tetany: spontaneous clinical manifestations
  1. Classic signs of peripheral hyperexcitability of motor nerve: spasm of the muscles of the wrists and ankles (carpopedal spasm) and of the vocal cords (laryngospasm)
  2. Sensory manifestations: paresthesia, numbness and tingling of the hands and feet
  3. Motor excitability of the central nervous system: brief, recurrent convulsions; usually generalized but may be localized to one side of the body
- Latent tetany: clinical signs not evident but can be elicited after stimulation
- Alkalotic tetany: induced through spontaneous overventilation, producing respiratory alkalosis

■ PHYSICAL EXAMINATION
- Tests for the hyperexcitability of peripheral motor nerves: Trousseau sign, Chvostek sign, Peroneal sign
  1. Ischemia or mechanical or electrical stimulation of motor nerves may produce the motor response characteristic of tetany.
     a. Trousseau sign: induced carpopedal spasm through production of ischemia of the motor nerves by reducing the arterial blood supply with a tourniquet
     b. Chvostek sign: facial nerve stimulation by tapping results in contraction of the orbicularis oris with a twitch of the upper lip or entire mouth
     c. Peroneal sign: dorsiflexion and abduction of foot by tapping the peroneal nerve

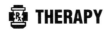

DIAGNOSIS

Diagnosis is made with a result of low serum ionized calcium or magnesium level and clinical signs of tetany.

■ DIAGNOSTIC WORKUP
- Ionized calcium concentration less than 3.0 mg/dl
- Total magnesium less than 1.0 mg/dl
- Prolonged corrected QT (QTc) interval (greater than 0.4 in infants) for a given heart rate on the electrocardiogram

THERAPY

■ MEDICAL
- Tetany of vitamin D deficiency: Give oral calcium lactate of 10 to 12 g/day in four to six doses for 10 days, or if severe, calcium gluconate (1 to 2 ml of a 10% solution per kg, intravenous infusion over 10 minutes).
- Sodium phenobarbital may be given intramuscularly when intravenous calcium gluconate does not quickly control the attacks.

■ FOLLOW-UP & DISPOSITION
See "Therapy."

PEARLS & CONSIDERATIONS

■ CLINICAL PEARLS
Tetany is still occasionally associated with cow's milk–derived formulas (related to phosphorus content greater than in human milk).

REFERENCE
1. Koo WWK, Tsang RC: Building better bones: calcium, magnesium, phosphorus, and vitamin D. In Tsang RC et al (eds): *Nutrition during infancy: principles and practice,* ed 2, Cincinnati, 1997, Digital Educational Publishing.
Authors: **Ran Namgung, M.D., Ph.D., and Reginald Tsang, M.B.B.C.**

■ DEFINITION

Tetralogy of Fallot (TOF) is a form of congenital heart disease characterized by a ventricular septal defect (VSD), an overriding aorta, right ventricular outflow tract obstruction (RVOTO), and right ventricular hypertrophy.

■ SYNONYMS

- Fallot's tetralogy
- TET
- TOF

ICD-9CM CODE

745.2 Tetralogy of Fallot

■ ETIOLOGY

- The cause is presumably heterogeneous but may depend on the interaction between genetic predisposition and environmental factors.
- Microdeletions of chromosome region 22q11 are often found in patients with TOF who have craniofacial anomalies. Deletions are also found in patients without phenotypic abnormalities.

■ EPIDEMIOLOGY & DEMOGRAPHICS

- TOF is the most common of the cyanotic congenital heart diseases, accounting for about 10% of children with congenital heart disease.
- The prevalence is 3.53 per 10,000 live births.
- There is a slight predominance of males.

■ HISTORY

- Clinical finding depends on the severity of the RVOTO.
- If the RVOTO is severe, pulmonary blood flow is limited and the infant usually presents in the neonatal period with cyanosis and a murmur.
- In patients with less severe RVOTO, the pulmonary blood flow may be enough that diagnosis is delayed for years.
- Occasionally, patients present with intense cyanosis, a tetralogy or TET spell, as a result of an acute increase in the RVOTO.

■ PHYSICAL EXAMINATION

- Examination findings depend on the severity of the RVOTO.
- With moderate to severe RVOTO, the patient will have cyanosis, normal precordial activity, a normal first heart sound, a single second heart sound, and an ejection quality murmur at the upper left sternal border.
- With mild RVOTO, the patient may have minimal cyanosis, increased precordial activity, and a flow murmur at the upper left sternal border.

⚗ DIAGNOSIS

■ DIAGNOSTIC WORKUP

- Diagnosis is usually made by echocardiography.
- This condition may be suspected in an infant with cyanosis and a murmur at the upper left sternal border.
- Key echocardiographic features are the severity of the RVOTO, the pulmonary artery size, and the coronary artery anatomy.
- Cardiac catheterization may be necessary to make an accurate preoperative diagnosis.
- Chest radiography may show a small main pulmonary artery segment, decreased pulmonary vascular markings, and an upturned cardiac apex. These abnormalities give the appearance of a "boot-shaped heart."

℞ THERAPY

■ NONPHARMACOLOGIC

- The definitive therapy for patients with TOF is surgical, but there are situations when palliative therapies are needed.
- During a tetralogy spell, pushing the knees to the chest will increase systemic vascular resistance and increase pulmonary blood flow.

■ MEDICAL

- Options for acute management of hypercyanotic (tetralogy, "TET") spells include the following:
  1. Oxygen administration
  2. Intravenous morphine
  3. Volume expansion
  4. General anesthesia
- Patients with a history of tetralogy spells who cannot be operated on in a timely fashion may benefit from beta blocker therapy.

■ SURGICAL

- The ventricular septal defect is closed, and the right ventricular outflow tract is opened.
- The timing of surgery depends on the severity of the RVOTO and the protocols of the operating center.
- Operative mortality should be less than 5%.
- In patients with very small pulmonary arteries, palliation with an aorta pulmonary shunt may be necessary to improve pulmonary blood flow and increase pulmonary artery size.
- Balloon dilation of the pulmonary valve has been used to increase pulmonary blood flow and encourage pulmonary artery growth.

■ FOLLOW-UP & DISPOSITION

- General pediatric care, including immunizations, should occur.
- Antibiotics should be given at times of endocarditis risk.
- Follow-up after repair of TOF by a cardiologist is lifelong to look for the following:
  1. Development of arrhythmias
  2. Right ventricular dysfunction
  3. Need for additional surgical intervention

■ PREVENTIVE TREATMENT

Intrauterine diagnosis is possible.

■ REFERRAL INFORMATION

All patients with TOF should be referred to a pediatric cardiologist for management and decisions about the timing of surgical intervention with the pediatric cardiothoracic surgeon.

☼ PEARLS & CONSIDERATIONS

■ CLINICAL PEARLS

- Patients with TOF and good pulmonary arteries should do very well, with low operative mortality.
- If the pulmonary arteries are small, the outlook is not as optimistic.
- Consider whether the child might have endocarditis before antibiotic administration. If endocarditis is a possibility, obtain a blood culture before starting antibiotics.

■ WEBSITES

- For parents: Congenital heart disease main page: www.tmc.edu/thi/congenit.html
- For physicians interested in congenital heart disease: NeoSoft Inc.: www.neosoft.com/~rlpierce/tof.htm

REFERENCES

1. Kirklin JW et al: Morphologic and surgical determinants of outcome events after repair of tetralogy of Fallot and pulmonary stenosis, *J Thorac Cardiovasc Surg* 103:706, 1992.
2. Momma K et al: Tetralogy of Fallot associated with chromosome 22q11 deletion, *Am J Cardiol* 76:618, 1995.
3. Zuberbuhler JR: Tetralogy of Fallot. In Moss AJ, Adams FH (eds): *Heart disease in infants, children and adolescents*, ed 5, Baltimore, 1995, Williams & Wilkins.

Author: **Michael E. McConnell, M.D.**

BASIC INFORMATION

■ DEFINITION
Thalassemia is a heterogeneous group of autosomal recessive genetic disorders characterized by decreased or absent synthesis of globin chains leading to anemia and microcytosis. Clinically, there are two major forms: α-thalassemia and β-thalassemia.

■ SYNONYMS
- Defects in the two β-globin genes and four α-globin genes have distinct names.
- β-Thalassemias:
  1. β/β   Normal
  2. β/-   β-Thalassemia trait, β-thalassemia minor
  3. -/-   β-Thalassemia major, Cooley's anemia, Mediterranean anemia
- α-Thalassemias:
  1. αα/αα   Normal
  2. αα/α-   Silent α-thalassemia
  3. αα/-- or α-/α-   α-Thalassemia trait
  4. α-/--   Hb H disease
  5. --/--   Hydrops fetalis (incompatible with extrauterine life)
- Barts hemoglobin- excess (4) γ-chains can be seen at birth, in various amounts, in all α-thalassemia disorders.

ICD-9CM CODE
282.4 Thalassemia

■ ETIOLOGY
Several hundred different genetic defects have been described that affect the structure or regulation of globin genes.

■ EPIDEMIOLOGY & DEMOGRAPHICS
- Found in regions of the world endemic for malaria
- β-Thalassemia: highest incidence in the Mediterranean basin
- α-Thalassemia: highest incidence in Southeast Asia, particularly Laos and Thailand
- African Americans: 2% to 3% have α-thalassemia trait

■ HISTORY
- Ethnicity (see "Epidemiology & Demographics"), family history of anemias, and transfusion dependence may be reported.
- Children with β-thalassemia major present with severe anemia at 1 to 2 years of age.
- Children with hydrops fetalis die in utero by 30 weeks' gestation.

■ PHYSICAL EXAMINATION
Children with severe thalassemia syndromes (β-thalassemia major, Hb H disease) have pallor and hepatosplenomegaly.

DIAGNOSIS

■ DIFFERENTIAL DIAGNOSIS
- Diseases that cause microcytic anemia, including iron deficiency, lead poisoning, sideroblastic anemia, and Hb E disease
- Iron deficiency, the most common confounding diagnosis

■ DIAGNOSTIC WORKUP
Includes complete blood count (CBC), smear, and Hb electrophoresis
- CBC
  1. Anemia (e.g., Hb 10 to 11 g/dl in β-thalassemia trait)
  2. Microcytosis (e.g., mean corpuscular volume [MCV] in high 60s in β-thalassemia trait)
  3. Mentzer index (MCV/red blood cell [RBC]) can be less than 11.5 in β-thalassemia trait and greater than 13.5 in iron deficiency
  4. Red cell distribution width (RDW) elevated in iron deficiency and Hb H disease but not in β-thalassemia trait
- Peripheral blood smear reveals microcytosis and hypochromia
- Hemoglobin electrophoresis
  1. β-Thalassemia trait: elevated HbA2 (greater than 3.5%)
  2. α-Thalassemia
     a. Hb Barts (excess γ-globin chains) at birth
     b. Hb H (excess β-globin chains) in older children

THERAPY

■ NONPHARMACOLOGIC
- For mild anemia, no therapy is warranted.
- Screen for concomitant iron deficiency.

■ MEDICAL
- Children with β-thalassemia major require regular RBC transfusions.
- Iron chelation with subcutaneous Desferal (deferoxamine) 5 to 7 days/wk is needed for iron overload.
- Oral chelators are under clinical investigation.
- Bone marrow transplantation can be curative.

■ SURGICAL
Splenectomy for hypersplenism causing an increased requirement for RBC transfusions in β-thalassemia major

■ PATIENT/FAMILY EDUCATION
- Genetic counseling is important. Risk of affected fetuses when both parents have β-thalassemia trait is 1 in 4 (autosomal recessive inheritance).
- Chronic transfusion therapy leads to iron overload and eventual death secondary to heart failure or cirrhosis.

■ PREVENTIVE TREATMENT
- Screen family members of affected individuals.
- Provide patient education.
- Prenatal diagnosis of thalassemia syndromes is available in the United States and in European countries where thalassemia is prevalent.

■ REFERRAL INFORMATION
Diagnosis and care of children with severe thalassemia syndromes is best performed by pediatric hematologists.

PEARLS & CONSIDERATIONS

■ CLINICAL PEARLS
- Hb Barts and Hb H indicate α-thalassemia and are both "fast-moving" hemoglobins.
- Clinical severity of thalassemia syndromes can be affected by the inheritance of glucose-6-phosphate dehydrogenase (G6PD) deficiency or abnormal hemoglobins (e.g., Hb E, Hb S)
  1. G6PD deficiency can make the hemolysis worse.
  2. Sickle/β-thalassemia is clinically quite similar to homozygous hemoglobin SS (sickle cell) disease and hemoglobin SC (sickle C) disease.
- The lack of the αα/-- genotype makes the prevalence of Hb H disease and hydrops fetalis extremely rare in Mediterranean and African-American populations.

■ WEBSITE
Cooley's Anemia Foundation: www.thalassemia.org

■ SUPPORT GROUPS
- Cooley's Anemia Foundation (129-09 26th Ave., Flushing, NY 11354; 800-522-7222) is a national nonprofit organization dedicated to serving patients with all forms of thalassemia.

II

- Thalassemia Action Group (129-09 26th Avenue, Flushing, NY 11354; 718-321-2873) is a support group for patients with thalassemia syndromes.
- The Ahepa Cooley's Anemia Foundation (1909 Q Street N. West, Washington, DC 20009; 202-232-6300).

REFERENCES

1. Higgs DR: α-Thalassemia, *Clin Hematol* 6:117, 1993.
2. Olivieri NF: The β-thalassemias, *N Engl J Med* 341:99, 1999.
3. The thalassemias. In Nathan DG, Orkin SH, Oski FA: *Nathan and Oski's hematology of infancy and childhood,* ed 5, Philadelphia, 1998, WB Saunders.

Author: **James Palis, M.D.**

BASIC INFORMATION

■ DEFINITION
Superficial thrombophlebitis is a thrombosis of a superficial vein with accompanying inflammatory reaction.

■ SYNONYM
Phlebitis

ICD-9CM CODE
451.89 Thrombophlebitis

■ ETIOLOGY
• Contributing factors are the three elements of Virchow's triad (intimal damage, stasis, and hypercoagulability).
• Thrombophlebitis almost always occurs in varicose veins of the leg as a result of stasis of blood.
• Occasionally, local trauma (e.g., intravenous catheters) may play a role, especially if the affected vein is normal.

■ EPIDEMIOLOGY
Almost solely a disease of adults with lower extremity varicose veins

■ HISTORY
• There is a subacute onset of pain, warmth, erythema, and swelling along the course of a superficial vein.
• Search for underlying trauma to the area, including venipuncture and intravenous catheters.
• It is important to distinguish whether the affected vein was normal before its involvement.

■ PHYSICAL EXAMINATION
• There will be pain and tenderness along the course of the vein, which may also be palpated as a tender cord or knot.
• There is often an inflammatory erythema locally.
• Occasionally, fever is present.

DIAGNOSIS

■ DIFFERENTIAL DIAGNOSIS
• Concomitant deep venous thrombosis occurs in approximately 5% of patients, so it is important to evaluate the patient for this disorder (see the section "Deep Venous Thrombosis").
• Cellulitis, calciphylaxis, and lymphangitis can mimic this disorder.

THERAPY

■ NONPHARMACOLOGIC
Warm compresses and elevation of the affected limb are mainstays of treatment.

■ MEDICAL
Nonsteroidal antiinflammatory medications such as ibuprofen or indomethacin relieve the local pain and inflammation. There is no role for anticoagulants or antibiotics.

■ FOLLOW-UP & DISPOSITION
• Resolution usually occurs within 1 to 2 weeks from the conservative measures outlined.
• The patient should be monitored for the development of deep venous thrombosis.

■ PATIENT/FAMILY EDUCATION
Elevation of the affected limb and mobilization are important to prevent the development of deep venous thrombosis.

■ PREVENTIVE TREATMENT
Elevation of the legs and simple compression stockings to decrease dependent edema and varicose veins of the legs can be helpful.

■ REFERRAL INFORMATION
This disorder can easily be diagnosed and treated by a primary care physician.

PEARLS & CONSIDERATIONS

■ CLINICAL PEARLS
• Medications most commonly associated with chemical phlebitis are nafcillin, diazepam, pentobarbital, and contrast media.
• Superficial thrombophlebitis that occurs in several distinct areas over a short period is termed *migratory superficial phlebitis*. It may signal an underlying malignancy, especially pancreatic or gastric cancer.

REFERENCES
1. Bounameaux H, Reber-Wasem M-A: Superficial thrombophlebitis and deep vein thrombosis, *Arch Intern Med* 157: 1822, 1997.
2. Goroll AH: *Primary care medicine,* ed 3, Philadelphia, 1995, JB Lippincott.
3. Messmore HL et al: Acute venous thrombosis, *Postgrad Med* 89:73, 1991.
Author: **Brett Robbins, M.D.**

II

BASIC INFORMATION

■ DEFINITION
Tinea capitis is a fungal infection of the scalp, hair shaft, and pilosebaceous apparatus.

■ SYNONYM
Ringworm of the scalp

ICD-9CM CODE
110.0 Tinea capitis

■ ETIOLOGY
- *Trichophyton tonsurans* causes the vast majority (95%) of cases in North and South America.
- The second most common cause in the United States is *Microsporum canis,* which is zoophilic and can be acquired by contact with infected animals such as pet cats and dogs.
  1. In some areas of the United States, specifically Arizona, *M. canis* is the most common cause.
  2. It is the most common cause worldwide.
- Other dermatophytes such as *M. audouinii, M. gypseum, T. mentagrophytes, T. violaceum, T. schoenleinii, T. verrucosum,* and *T. rubrum* also cause tinea capitis.

■ EPIDEMIOLOGY & DEMOGRAPHICS
- Tinea capitis is the most common dermatophytosis of childhood.
- It generally is a disease of prepubertal children between 2 and 10 years of age.
  1. Rarely affects infants
  2. Rarely occurs in postpubertal individuals
- Spread of infection has been demonstrated in households.
- Outbreaks have been reported in schools and child care centers.
- The incidence in the United States is increasing.
- This condition is much more common in African Americans.
- Asymptomatic carriage may be an important reservoir for infection.

■ HISTORY
- Usually, a caretaker notices hair or scalp changes such as patchy hair loss, scaly scalp, or pustular lesions.
- Child or parents may first notice enlarged occipital lymph nodes.

■ PHYSICAL EXAMINATION
- Scalp scaling is present.
- Infected areas are round or oval, sometimes irregular.
  1. Individual patches are 1 to 6 cm in diameter.
  2. Multiple patches are common.
- There may be coalescence of lesions, with formation of gyrate patterns.

- Broken-off hairs, 1 to 3 mm above the scalp, may be seen.
- Partial alopecia may occur.
- This condition may cause associated pustulation, suppuration, or kerion formation (see the following discussion).
- Lymphadenopathy, usually occipital and posterior cervical, may be very prominent, even with mild scalp disease.
- "Black dot" ringworm is a form characterized by multiple, small, circular patches of alopecia.
  1. The hairs are broken off at the surface of the scalp, resulting in a dot appearance; darker hairs are seen on lighter skin surfaces.
- A kerion is a sharply demarcated, inflammatory, indurated, boggy granulomatous tumefaction.
  1. It is usually not painful.
  2. The onset of kerion is acute, and it can become large; however, usually, only one area is involved.

DIAGNOSIS

■ DIFFERENTIAL DIAGNOSIS
- Seborrheic dermatitis
- Atopic dermatitis
- Psoriasis
- Alopecia areata
- Traumatic alopecia: trichotillomania, traction alopecia
- Pseudopelade
- Folliculitis decalvans
- Impetigo
- Lesions of systemic lupus erythematosus (discoid lupus)
- Syphilis
- Histiocytosis
- Scleroderma

■ DIAGNOSTIC WORKUP
- The clinical presentation is fairly distinctive, but other diagnoses can mimic tinea capitis and confirmation of the diagnosis is generally advised.
- KOH preparations can be useful for immediate confirmation of infection, but sensitivity and specificity depend on the experience of the individual performing the test and the morphology of the lesion scraped.
  1. Many false-negative and false-positive results occur.
  2. Culture is recommended.
- To obtain a fungal culture, rub several areas of the scalp with a clean disposable toothbrush or sterile cotton swab, and inoculate onto an antibiotic-enriched mycologic media.
- Wood's lamp examination is generally not helpful because *T. tonsurans* and *T. violaceum* do not fluoresce.
  1. Hairs infected by *M. audouinii* and *M. canis* produce a brilliant green fluorescence.

2. Those infected by *T. schoenleinii* produce a pale green fluorescence.

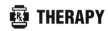

THERAPY

■ MEDICAL
- Systemic antifungal therapy is always required because topical therapies do not penetrate deeply enough into the hair follicle to adequately eradicate infection.
- Griseofulvin has been the standard therapy since 1958.
  1. The starting dose of the standard micronized griseofulvin is 20 mg/kg/day, given once a day, for 6 to 8 weeks.
  2. This dosage is higher than that recommended in several standard references.
  3. It is absorbed more rapidly when ingested along with a fatty foods.
  4. An ultramicronized griseofulvin dispersed in polyethylene glycol has twice the bioavailability, so it has allowed the dosage to be cut to half of the micronized form.
- In cases in which griseofulvin is not tolerated or is ineffective, there are some recently available alternatives; these agents cannot be recommended as first-line therapy until further comparison studies are done and more is known about safety in children.
  1. Itraconazole 5 mg/kg/day given once a day with food for 4 weeks
  2. Fluconazole 6 mg/kg/day for 3 to 4 weeks
  3. Terbinafine: not yet approved by the U.S. Food and Drug Administration for children.
     a. Effective and safe in studies so far at a dosage of 3 to 6 mg/kg/day for 2 to 4 weeks
     b. Currently only available in a pill form
     c. May not be efficacious for *M. canis* infection
- Use of adjunctive sporicidal topical agents, such as selenium sulfide 1% or 2.5% shampoo twice weekly, will limit the spread of infectious spores and may improve appearance.
- Appropriate therapy of kerion is controversial:
  1. Oral prednisone, 1 mg/kg/day for 10 days or more, may be helpful in patients with severe kerion.
     a. Increases patient comfort
     b. May prevent scarring alopecia
  2. Generally, despite the puslike appearance, antibiotics are not necessary.
     a. May use oral antistaphylococcal drug if severe with tenderness, if multiple pustules or abscesses, or if other areas of scalp show clear evidence of impetigo or pyoderma

3. Incision and drainage are not indicated because loculations are small and septa thick.

■ FOLLOW-UP & DISPOSITION
• Check the patient taking griseofulvin after 4 weeks of therapy to determine effectiveness and to decide length of therapy.
   1. If there are no signs of disease (the scalp is totally normal), continue therapy for 2 more weeks for a total of 6 weeks.
   2. If there are still signs of disease, check the dosage, review instructions and compliance, treat for 4 more weeks, and reevaluate at that time.

■ PATIENT/FAMILY EDUCATION
• *Stress the need for the prolonged (6 to 8 weeks) course of therapy.*
• Advise that the griseofulvin be taken with fatty foods (e.g., milk or ice cream).

■ PREVENTIVE TREATMENT
Avoid sharing of combs, pillows, and head gear because the organisms can be cultured from various fomites.

■ WHEN TO REFER TO A DERMATOLOGIST
• Treatment failure with griseofulvin
• Diagnosis in doubt

☼ PEARLS & CONSIDERATIONS

■ CLINICAL PEARLS
• Widespread tinea corporis, particularly when it is on the face, neck, or upper chest, can be a sign of occult scalp tinea infection or asymptomatic carriage (Cuetara).
• Although kerions often heal with treatment of the underlying fungus only, scarring alopecia is a possible complication if the inflammation is severe and diagnosis is delayed.
• Although ketoconazole is used occasionally in pediatrics, it is not recommended for treatment of this infection.
   1. Because of the risk of hepatotoxicity, the expense of the drug, the lack of superiority to griseofulvin in controlled studies, and the emergence of other more promising antifungal agents, oral ketoconazole is not a good therapy choice for tinea capitis.
• When using selenium sulfide shampoo as adjunctive treatment of tinea capitis, there is no difference between the 2.5% and 1% preparations in time required to produce a negative surface culture. The 1% is less expensive.

REFERENCES
1. Feigin RD, Cherry JD (eds): *Textbook of pediatric infectious diseases,* ed 4, Philadelphia, 1998, WB Saunders.
2. Howard RM, Friedin IJ: Dermatophyte infections in children. In Aronoff SC (ed): *Advances in pediatric infectious diseases,* vol 14, St Louis, 1999, Mosby.
3. Hurwitz S: *Clinical pediatric dermatology,* ed 2, Philadelphia, 1993, WB Saunders.
4. Lobato MN, Vugia DJ: Tinea capitis in California: a population-based study of a growing epidemic, *Pediatrics* 99: April, 1997.
5. Weston WL, Lane AT, Morelli JG: *Color textbook of pediatric dermatology,* ed 2, St Louis, 1996, Mosby.
Author: **Larry Denk, M.D.**

II

BASIC INFORMATION

■ DEFINITION
Tinea corporis is a superficial dermatophyte fungal infection of the glabrous skin. Several areas of the body are excluded in the definition and have other names, such as the scalp (tinea capitis), bearded areas (tinea barbae), the groin (tinea cruris), hands (tinea manuum), feet (tinea pedis), and nails (onychomycosis).

■ SYNONYMS
- Ringworm
- Body ringworm

ICD-9CM CODE
110.5 Tinea corporis

■ ETIOLOGY
- The species of dermatophyte causing tinea corporis depends on the source of the infection.
- *Trichophyton rubrum* is the most common cause worldwide, probably because it spreads from the feet of those with tinea pedis.
- In areas where tinea capitis is endemic, tinea corporis is more commonly caused by *Trichophyton tonsurans,* the most common cause of tinea capitis.
- *Microsporum canis* is the usual cause if the spread is from a pet.
- Other causative dermatophytes include *M. audouinii, T. mentagrophytes, T. verrucosum,* and *Epidermophyton floccosum.*

■ EPIDEMIOLOGY & DEMOGRAPHICS
- Tinea corporis is often acquired by close person-to-person contact, as occurs in a household, day care, or school.
    1. The index case may have tinea corporis, capitis, or pedis.
- Contact with domestic animals, particularly young kittens and puppies, is a common cause.
- There have been several reports of epidemics among high school wrestlers (tinea gladiatorum).
- Individuals with certain immunologic abnormalities, such as atopic dermatitis, presumably caused by a decreased cell-mediated delayed sensitivity and an increase in humoral (IgE) response, are particularly prone to chronic and recurrent dermatophyte infections.

■ HISTORY
- Usually a round lesion that may be noted to be expanding is discovered by a caretaker or the patient
- May be mildly pruritic
- No associated systemic symptoms

■ PHYSICAL EXAMINATION
- The classic lesion is annular, oval, or circinate.
    1. It is minimally inflamed, with a sharply defined papulovesicular border, and often some central clearing.
- The lesions typically begin as red papules or pustules that rupture and evolve to form papulosquamous lesions.
- These lesions then spread out from the periphery as new vesicles form and begin to clear centrally.
- Over a period of weeks, the patches may expand up to 5 cm in diameter.
- The pattern can vary and may mimic a wide variety of conditions.
    1. Lesions may be eczematous, vesicular, pustular, and less often, granulomatous.
- Sites of predilection include the nonhairy areas of the face, the trunk, and limbs.
- Lesions are usually solitary but can be multiple.
- Inappropriate treatment with topical steroids will decrease the inflammation, and hence alter the clinical appearance while the infection persists, a condition referred to as *tinea incognito.*
- An uncommon but distinctive variant of tinea is a deeper granulomatous folliculitis and perifolliculitis disorder (Majocchi's granuloma).
    1. Usually occurs on one lower leg or dorsum of a foot
    2. Nodular lesions: sometimes several in one area
    3. Often occurs on the legs of girls who shave their legs closely and get an infected ingrown hair
    4. Caused by *T. rubrum* or *T. mentagrophytes*
        a. The primary focus is a diffuse *T. rubrum* infection of the foot.

🔬 DIAGNOSIS

■ DIFFERENTIAL DIAGNOSIS
- Nummular eczema
- Psoriasis
- The Herald patch of pityriasis rosea
- Contact dermatitis
- Tinea versicolor
- Seborrheic dermatitis
- Erythema chronicum migrans
- Granuloma annulare
- Erythema multiforme
- Erythema annulare centrifugum
- Fixed drug eruptions
- Syphilis
- Systemic lupus erythematosus
- Vitiligo
- Candidiasis
- Erythrasma
- Sarcoidosis

■ DIAGNOSTIC WORKUP
- Diagnosis is usually made on clinical grounds.
- Confirm by KOH microscopic wet-mount examination.
    1. Obtain a large amount of fine scale by gentle scraping of the edge of a lesion with the belly of a No. 15-blade scalpel or the edge of a glass slide.
    2. Mount onto the center of the slide, add 1 or 2 drops of 20% KOH, apply a coverslip (gently press down with the eraser end of a pencil to crush the scales), and examine under low power.
        a. True hyphae are seen as long, branching, often septate rods of uniform width that cross the borders of epidermal cells.
        b. Cotton fibers, cell borders, or other artifacts may be misinterpreted as positive findings.
- Obtain a fungal culture of skin lesions if direct microscopy is negative and clinical suspicion is high.
- Wood's light examination is not helpful in the diagnosis of suspected lesions on glabrous skin unless the lanugo hairs are infected.

💊 THERAPY

■ MEDICAL
- Topical therapy is adequate for most cases of tinea corporis.
    1. Apply to lesions twice daily for at least 4 weeks. There are many choices:
        a. An imidazole cream such as miconazole (Micatin, Monistat-Derm) or clotrimazole (Lotrimin, Mycelex) is usually recommended because both are inexpensive, available over the counter, and relatively free of side effects.
        b. Other available imidazole creams include ketoconazole (Nizoral), econazole (Spectazole), sulconazole (Exelderm), and oxiconazole (Oxistat).
- Although clearing and relief from any associated pruritus is often seen within the first 7 to 10 days after initiation of therapy, topical treatment with the imidazoles should continue for a minimum of 2 to 3 weeks after the affected area is clinically clear.
- If therapy with any of the aforementioned agents fail, clinicians should prescribe terbinafine 1% cream (Lamisil)—a fungicidal allylamine derivative.
    1. Terbinafine (Lamisil) is also given twice daily but for a shorter time—only until clinical signs and symptoms are significantly improved (usually 1 to 2 weeks).

2. Terbinafine does not cover *M. canis*.
- Topical corticosteroids are generally unnecessary. However, a *mild* steroid cream may be used twice daily for a few days for relief in those with pruritus or severe inflammation.
  1. Combination antifungal and steroid creams are *not* indicated.
     a. The duration of steroid application should be brief.
     b. Antifungal application is prolonged.
- Some cases of tinea corporis require systemic therapy: patients with widespread or deep-seated follicular lesions (Majocchi's granuloma), those with associated tinea capitis, and immunocompromised hosts.
  1. Griseofulvin 20 mg/kg/day given once a day with fatty foods for 3 weeks is usually adequate. If there is associated tinea capitis, continue the same dose for 6 to 8 weeks (see the section "Tinea Capitis" for discussion).
  2. Itraconazole is also very effective for systemic treatment of tinea corporis and cruris.

■ FOLLOW-UP & DISPOSITION

Recheck in 2 weeks to ensure that the area is improving. If no response has occurred, either the diagnosis is incorrect or a resistant dermatophyte has been encountered.

■ PATIENT/FAMILY EDUCATION
- Emphasize the generally benign and common nature of the infection, but also explain the need for prolonged therapy to cure the infection.
- It is mildly contagious.
- Instruct the patient or caregiver to apply topical agent to the entire lesion plus about a 1 cm border beyond it.

■ PREVENTIVE TREATMENT
- Minimize spread to close contacts by frequent handwashing, adequate treatment of the index case, and not allowing the sharing of clothes. Also keep the lesion covered between medication application until it shows signs of improvement.
- Have any family pet with tinea treated.

■ WHEN TO REFER TO A DERMATOLOGIST
Resistant cases or when the diagnosis is unclear

۞ PEARLS & CONSIDERATIONS

■ CLINICAL PEARLS
- The term *fungus infection* incorporates disorders caused by both tinea (dermatophyte) and yeasts (e.g., *Candida*). They are not synonymous and often have differing response to therapy.
  1. Topical nystatin is effective against candidal infection but in-

effective in the treatment of tinea (dermatophyte) infection.
2. Tolnaftate (Tinactin) and undecylenic acid (Gordochom) are beneficial in the management of dermatophytoses such as tinea pedis, tinea cruris, and tinea corporis, but they are ineffective against disorders resulting from candidal infection.
3. Many agents treat both types of infection. These include ciclopirox (Loprox), clotrimazole (Lotrimin), econazole (Spectazole), ketoconazole (Nizoral), miconazole (Micatin, Monistat-Derm), oxiconazole (Oxistat), sulconazole (Exelderm)

REFERENCES
1. Bakos L et al: Open clinical study of the efficacy and safety of terbinafine cream 1% in children with tinea corporis and tinea cruris, *Pediatr Infect Dis J* 16:545, 1997.
2. Feigin RD, Cherry JD (eds): *Textbook of pediatric infectious diseases*, ed 4, Philadelphia, 1998, WB Saunders.
3. Howard RM, Frieden IJ: Dermatophyte infections in children. In Aronoff SC (ed): *Advances in pediatric infectious diseases*, vol 14, St Louis, 1999, Mosby.
4. Hurwitz S: *Clinical pediatric dermatology*, ed 2, Philadelphia, 1993, WB Saunders.
5. Weston WL, Lane AT, Morelli JG: *Color textbook of pediatric dermatology*, ed 2, St Louis, 1996, Mosby.
Author: **Larry Denk, M.D.**

II

BASIC INFORMATION

■ DEFINITION
Tinea cruris is an extremely common superficial dermatophyte fungal infection of the groin and upper thighs.

■ SYNONYMS
• Jock itch
• Ringworm

ICD-9CM CODE
110.3 Tinea cruris

■ ETIOLOGY
• *Trichophyton rubrum, Trichophyton mentagrophytes, Epidermophyton floccosum*

■ EPIDEMIOLOGY & DEMOGRAPHICS
• Occurs primarily in adolescent and adult males
• More common and more symptomatic in hot, humid weather
• More common in obese individuals
• More common in athletes because of sweating and chafing in the region
• Commonly seen in association with tinea pedis

■ HISTORY
• Usually, the eruption is noticed by the individual or an intimate partner.
• Itching or burning sensation may be severe.
• Vigorous physical activity, chafing, and wearing of tight-fitting clothing such as athletic supporters, jockey shorts, wet bathing suits, panty hose, or tight-fitting slacks may contribute to the development of tinea cruris.

■ PHYSICAL EXAMINATION
• Erythematous, scaly, sharply demarcated rash is seen in the groin area, possibly with some central clearing.
• The eruption is usually bilaterally symmetric on the upper inner thighs and intertriginous folds of the groin area in a half-moon shape.
  1. Occasionally extends to the perianal regions, buttocks, and abdomen
• Occasionally, a vesiculopustular border may be present.
• The scrotum or labia are often spared or more mildly involved.
  1. By comparison, *Candida* infection of the area will usually involve scrotum or labia.
• May see excoriation as a consequence of patient scratching.

DIAGNOSIS

■ DIFFERENTIAL DIAGNOSIS
• *Candida albicans* infection
• Intertrigo
• Seborrheic dermatitis
• Psoriasis
• Primary irritant or allergic contact dermatitis
  1. Diaper dermatitis in infants
  2. Medication application
• Erythrasma
• Tinea versicolor
• Erysipelas or perianal strep infection

■ DIAGNOSTIC WORKUP
• Diagnosis is based on clinical presentation.
• Wood's light examination is negative. This helps differentiate from erythrasma, which has a coral-red fluorescence.
• The diagnosis can be confirmed by KOH microscopic examination of cutaneous scrapings.
• Fungal culture generally is not necessary.

THERAPY

■ NONPHARMACOLOGIC
• Reduction of excessive chafing and irritation by wearing loose-fitting cotton underclothing.
• Weight loss in the obese patient.

■ MEDICAL
• The treatment of tinea cruris consists of topical therapy, as described in the section "Tinea Corporis," for 3 to 4 weeks.
• Friction and perspiration should be reduced in the area by use of a bland absorbent powder such as Zea-Sorb-AF Medicated Powder (Stiefel).
• Oral therapy may be indicated for lesions that are resistant or recur frequently and can be treated with oral griseofulvin or itraconazole as described under tinea corporis.

■ FOLLOW-UP & DISPOSITION
Recheck in 2 weeks

■ PATIENT/FAMILY EDUCATION
• Offer reassurance regarding the generally benign and common nature of the disorder.
• Advise that recurrences are common.

■ PREVENTIVE TREATMENT
• Improve hygiene, including bath or shower followed by thorough drying of the groin area after athletic activity (including swimming) or any activity that causes sweating.
• Avoid prolonged exposure of the groin to tight-fitting, wet, or sweaty clothes.

■ WHEN TO REFER TO A DERMATOLOGIST
Resistant cases or if the diagnosis is in doubt

PEARLS & CONSIDERATIONS

■ CLINICAL PEARLS
• The term *fungus infection* incorporates disorders caused by both tinea (dermatophyte) and yeasts (e.g., *Candida*).
  1. These conditions are not synonymous, and they have different responses to therapy.
    a. Topical nystatin (Mycostatin) is effective against candidal infection but ineffective in the treatment of tinea (dermatophyte) infection.
    b. Tolnaftate (Tinactin) and undecylenic acid (Gordochom) are beneficial in the management of dermatophytoses (tinea pedis, tinea cruris, and tinea corporis) but are ineffective against candidal infection.
  2. Many agents treat both types of infection. These include ciclopirox (Loprox), clotrimazole (Lotrimin), econazole (Spectazole), ketoconazole (Nizoral), miconazole (Micatin, Monistat-Derm), oxiconazole (Oxistat), and sulconazole (Exelderm).
• Erythrasma is a fairly common chronic superficial dermatosis of the crural area caused by *Corynebacterium minutissimum*.
  1. The treatment of choice is oral erythromycin.
  2. Erythrasma can coexist with a dermatophyte infection.

REFERENCES
1. Bakos L et al: Open clinical study of the efficacy and safety of terbinafine cream 1% in children with tinea corporis and tinea cruris, *Pediatr Infect Dis J* 16:545, 1997.
2. Feigin RD, Cherry JD: *Textbook of pediatric infectious diseases*, ed 4, Philadelphia, 1998, WB Saunders.
3. Howard RM, Frieden IJ: Dermatophyte infections in children. In Aronoff SC (ed): *Advances in pediatric infectious diseases*, vol 14, St Louis, 1999, Mosby.
4. Hurwitz S: *Clinical pediatric dermatology*, ed 2, Philadelphia, 1993, WB Saunders.
5. Weston WL, Lane AT, Morelli JG: *Color textbook of pediatric dermatology*, ed 2, St Louis, 1996, Mosby.
Author: **Larry Denk, M.D.**

BASIC INFORMATION

DEFINITION

Tinea versicolor is a superficial fungal infection of the skin caused by the yeast *Malassezia furfur*.

SYNONYM

Pityriasis versicolor

ICD-9CM CODE

111.0 Tinea versicolor

ETIOLOGY

- The infection is caused by proliferation of *Malassezia furfur*—a lipophilic yeast that is a normal inhabitant of the skin flora.
- Under certain predisposing conditions, the yeast form undergoes a dynamic change to a pathogenic mycelial form associated with clinical disease.
- The nomenclature of these yeasts is confusing.
  1. *Pityrosporum ovale* and *Pityrosporum obiculare* were used to distinguish *Malassezia furfur* with an oval or round shape, respectively.
  2. Occasionally, the term *Pityrosporum* is used instead of *Malassezia*.

EPIDEMIOLOGY & DEMOGRAPHICS

- Worldwide distribution; more common in humid and tropical climates
- Increased incidence in adolescence and young adulthood
- More commonly recognized in the summer
  1. Hypopigmented lesions become more evident when the normal skin is darkened by sun and the lesions fail to tan
- Factors that seem to favor the overgrowth of *Malassezia*: pregnancy, malnutrition, immunosuppression, oral contraceptives, and excess heat and humidity

HISTORY

- Hypopigmented lesions
  1. Can be red or hyperpigmented
- Usually on chest and trunk, neck, and upper arms
- Insidious onset
- Generally asymptomatic
  1. Some patients complain of mild pruritus.

PHYSICAL EXAMINATION

- Multiple oval, macular, and patchy lesions with fine scales are seen.
- Lesions may be hypopigmented or hyperpigmented (fawn-colored or brown), depending on the patient's complexion and exposure to sunlight.
- Occasionally, lesions are salmon pink or reddish.
- The lesions are usually distributed over the upper portions of the trunk (most common), neck, proximal arms, and occasionally, the face or other areas.
- Facial lesions are more common in children (forehead is most common facial site).
- Lesions may coalesce to involve a large contiguous area.
- Lesions can become lighter than the surrounding skin in summer and relatively darker during winter.
- Infections caused by *M. furfur* may present with follicular papules or pustules involving the same areas.

DIAGNOSIS

DIFFERENTIAL DIAGNOSIS

- Pityriasis alba
- Postinflammatory hypopigmentation
- Vitiligo
- Pityriasis rosea
- Seborrheic dermatitis
- Secondary syphilis
- Melasma (formerly referred to as *chloasma*)

DIAGNOSTIC WORKUP

- The eruption is usually distinctive, and the diagnosis can often be made on clinical grounds.
- Tinea versicolor demonstrates a green-yellow, coppery-orange, bronze, or blue-white fluorescence under Wood's light.
- The diagnosis can be confirmed by potassium hydroxide wet mounts of cutaneous scrapings.
  1. Hyphae and budding spores in grapelike clusters under microscope (spaghetti and meatballs)
- Fungal cultures are unsatisfactory because the organism is difficult to grow on culture media.

THERAPY

MEDICAL

- Tinea versicolor generally responds to a variety of topical preparations:
  1. Selenium sulfide 2.5% shampoo (Selsun, Exsel) is a convenient, inexpensive, rapid, and highly effective mode of therapy.
     a. Apply a thin layer to the entire affected area overnight once a week for 4 weeks, followed by once a month for 3 months (in an effort to help prevent recurrences).
     b. The preparation is washed off in the morning by bath or shower, at which time all night clothes, bedding, and undergarments should be changed.
  2. For the unusual patient who experiences irritation from the overnight application, an alternative is to apply the same 2.5% selenium sulfide for only 10 to 30 minutes nightly for 2 weeks.
  3. Ketoconazole 2% shampoo applied to affected areas for 10 minutes for 3 consecutive days is an alternative.
  4. Topical antifungal medications (e.g., miconazole, ciclopirox, clotrimazole) are effective but more expensive because of large surface area.
- Oral treatment is reserved for individuals with resistant or recurrent cases. Effective agents include the following:
  1. Ketoconazole 200 mg/day for 5 days
  2. Fluconazole 400 mg as a single dose
  3. Itraconazole 200 mg/day for 5 to 7 days

FOLLOW-UP & DISPOSITION

- The prognosis is good, with death of the fungus usually occurring within 3 to 4 weeks of treatment.
- Recurrences are common, especially during the hot and humid months.

PATIENT/FAMILY EDUCATION

- Patients should be informed that the hypopigmented areas will not disappear immediately after therapy.
  1. It may take several months to return to normal pigmentation, even after eradication of the fungus
- Recurrences are very common.

PREVENTIVE TREATMENT

- Tinea versicolor is mildly contagious, so measures should be taken to prevent spread to family members and close contacts.
  1. Because it is a normal inhabitant of skin, those who are at risk for pathogenic mycelial form may have no known contact.
- Some experts advise monthly application of the 2.5% selenium sulfide shampoo to prevent recurrence.

WHEN TO REFER TO A DERMATOLOGIST

Resistant cases or if the diagnosis is uncertain

PEARLS & CONSIDERATIONS

■ **CLINICAL PEARLS**
- *Malassezia (Pityrosporum)* species have also been associated with seborrheic dermatitis, folliculitis, and steroid acne.
- Patients with tinea versicolor occasionally have concomitant folliculitis, seborrheic dermatitis, and acne vulgaris.

REFERENCES
1. Assaf RR, Weil ML: The superficial mycoses, *Dermatol Clin* 14:57, 1996.
2. Feigin RD, Cherry JD: *Textbook of pediatric infectious diseases,* ed 4, Philadelphia, 1998, WB Saunders.
3. Hurwitz S: *Clinical pediatric dermatology,* ed 2, Philadelphia, 1993, WB Saunders.
4. Weston WL, Lane AT, Morelli JG: *Color textbook of pediatric dermatology,* ed 2, St Louis, 1996, Mosby.

Author: **Larry Denk, M.D.**

BASIC INFORMATION

■ DEFINITION
Toddler's diarrhea is a common benign diarrheal disorder that presents in the toddler with three to six large, loose, watery stools per day for more than 3 weeks, but without evidence of systemic illness, failure to thrive, or other gastrointestinal (GI) disorder. Diarrhea should be present at least 3 weeks (preferably 4 weeks) to be considered "chronic" and may be episodic rather than continuous.

■ SYNONYMS
- Chronic nonspecific diarrhea (CNSD)
- Irritable colon of childhood
- Sloppy stool syndrome

ICD-9CM CODE
787.91 Diarrhea

■ ETIOLOGY
- Toddler's diarrhea is a multifactorial problem. The following are contributing factors:
  1. Excessive fluid intake
  2. Disordered intestinal motility—resulting in rapid transit time
  3. Carbohydrate malabsorption from excessive fruit and fruit juice consumption
  4. Sorbitol
  5. Fructose—when the concentration exceeds glucose concentration
  6. Dietary fat restriction
  7. Elevated colonic bile salts concentration

■ EPIDEMIOLOGY & DEMOGRAPHICS
- Toddler's diarrhea is thought to be common, but the exact prevalence is unknown.
- This is the most common type of chronic diarrhea referred to a pediatric gastroenterologist.
- Typical age is 12 to 36 months; it may begin as early as 6 months and continue up to 5 years of age.
- Symptoms resolve in 90% of children by 40 months of age.
- This is possibly a variant of irritable bowel syndrome.

■ HISTORY
- When considering the large differential diagnosis of chronic diarrhea, a thorough history must include the following:
  1. Recent travel, drinking water sources, antecedent illness, infectious contacts, day care, new foods
  2. Use of antibiotics, laxatives, prescribed or over-the-counter drugs that may contain sorbitol, home remedies, alternative therapies
  3. Family history of GI diseases.

4. An accurate description of the stool appearance and pattern
5. Dietary history to ascertain total calories and fat consumed daily, quantities of milk and juice consumed daily, and any trials of elimination diets or currently eliminated foods
   a. It is possible for a child to have toddler's diarrhea and have poor weight gain merely because he or she was placed on a hypocaloric diet by the caretakers in an attempt to control the diarrhea.
   b. History of onset or change in bowel habits—essential because several diseases with diarrhea present before 3 months of age, including the following:
      (1) Congenital microvillous atrophy
      (2) Disaccharidase abnormalities
      (3) Milk and soy allergies
- Specifically, with toddler's diarrhea, the history will reveal the following:
  1. Onset is at 6 months or later.
  2. No stools occur overnight.
  3. Stooling is most common in the morning.
  4. There may be oscillation between normal and watery stools.
  5. Stools are sloppy—generally watery but occasionally with mucus.
  6. Stools often contain recognizable undigested food particles.
  7. There is no associated nausea, vomiting, abdominal pain, flatulence, blood in the stool, fevers, weakness, decreased activity, anorexia, dermatologic problems, weight loss, poor growth, or other symptoms of systemic disease.
  8. Although there may have been an antecedent illness, children with toddler's diarrhea exhibit no evidence of current enteric infection or malabsorption.
     a. They continue to show normal growth and development unless caloric intake has been inadequate.

■ PHYSICAL EXAMINATION
- The physical examination and growth parameters should be entirely normal with toddler's diarrhea. If not, different diagnoses need to be pursued.
- The single most important aspect of the physical examination is accurate measurement and plots of weight, height, and head circumference. Serial plots are needed.
- Abdominal and rectal examinations are entirely normal.
- Look for signs of dehydration—none are present in toddler's diarrhea.
- Check for evidence of malnutrition or malabsorption—none of the fol-

lowing are present in toddler's diarrhea:
1. Lack of subcutaneous fat
2. Eczematous rash of essential fatty acid deficiency and zinc deficiency
3. Glossitis
4. Easy bruising
5. Skin, hair, or nail abnormalities
6. Tired or ill appearing
7. Decreased reflexes
- Examine the perianal area—there may be evidence of irritation from toddler's diarrhea, but true perianal disease, abscesses, fistulas, or rectal prolapse would indicate other diseases.

🔬 DIAGNOSIS

■ DIFFERENTIAL DIAGNOSIS
- Enteric infection
  1. Parasite
  2. Protracted viral gastroenteritis (several viruses can rarely promote chronic diarrhea)
  3. Rare for any bacterial infection to be chronic but has been reported (usually in younger infants with *Salmonella, Yersinia, Campylobacter, Aeromonas,* and *Plesiomonas*)
- Intestinal malabsorption
  1. Postviral enteritis (caused by flattened villi after an infection with rotavirus, adenovirus, astrovirus, or coronavirus)
  2. Inflammatory bowel disease
  3. Celiac disease
- Congenital diarrhea
  1. Disaccharidase deficiency (e.g., lactase, sucrase-isomaltase)
  2. Congenital microvillous atrophy (microvillus inclusion disease)
  3. Hollow visceral myopathy
- Protein intolerance: usually unknown mechanism (e.g., animal proteins, soy proteins)
- Food allergy: will usually have other GI symptoms. such as oral pruritus, vomiting, and abdominal pain, in addition to diarrhea; may also have systemic symptoms such as skin rash, bronchospasm, or anaphylaxis
- Lactose intolerance
  1. Primary acquired (late onset): lactase levels decrease through late childhood
  2. Secondary acquired: caused by mucosal injury
  3. Congenital: mentioned earlier under congenital diarrhea (exceedingly rare)
- Medication induced
- Encopresis
- Immune system disorders: eosinophilic enteritis, acquired immunodeficiency syndrome, immunoglobulin A (IgA) deficiency, autoimmune enteropathy

II

- Acrodermatitis enteropathica (zinc deficiency)
- Anatomic abnormalities: short intestine, malrotation
- Fat malabsorption: cystic fibrosis, Schwachman-Diamond syndrome, pancreatitis
- Endocrine disorders: hyperthyroidism, diabetes
- Hormone-secreting tumors
  1. APUDomas: These tumors originate in the APUD cells (amine precursor uptake and decarboxylation of amino acids) of the gastroenteropancreatic endocrine system.
  2. Cell origin is adrenal or extraadrenal neurogenic sites.
- Hirschsprung's disease
- Vasculitis: hemolytic uremic syndrome, Henoch-Schönlein purpura
- Pseudoobstruction
- Appendicitis
- Munchausen syndrome by proxy

■ DIAGNOSTIC WORKUP
- A fresh stool sample may be the only body fluid needed and can be examined.
  1. pH, reducing substances, neutral fat, occult blood
  2. Ova and parasites, *Giardia* antigen
  3. Leukocytes, eosinophils
  4. *Clostridium difficile* toxin
- All of these stool studies are generally normal in toddler's diarrhea.
  1. Occult blood could be present if there is a perianal rash or excoriation from the frequent stools.
- Other laboratory tests should be done only if indicated because of an abnormality of certain of the fresh stool sample studies or because a different diagnosis is suspected based on history or physical examination.

℞ THERAPY

■ NONPHARMACOLOGIC
- Provide parental reassurance.
- Reduce juice consumption.
- Eliminate soda and nonjuice sweet drinks.
- Normalize fluid consumption (to about 100 ml/kg/day).

- Reduce dietary sorbitol and free fructose.
- Normalize diet (especially fats) if parents are restricting.
- Increase dietary fat content to 35% to 40% of total calories (usually more than 4 g/kg/day).
- Increase dietary fiber.

■ MEDICAL
- Usually, no medical treatment is needed; try to resist the temptation or parental pressure to use medication.
- Green stools may contain abnormally high quantities of bile acid.
  1. Treatment with the bile salt-binding medications cholestyramine and bismuth subsalicylate has reduced stool frequency and water content in some of these patients.
- Psyllium (2-3 g twice daily for 2 weeks) or Citrucel (1 to 2 tsp/day) may offer some cohesiveness to stools.
- Metronidazole will help the patient with undetected *Giardia*.
- One study suggests that ingestion of yeast can benefit some patients with toddler's diarrhea by altering the intestinal microflora and thereby decreasing the chance of bacterial overgrowth.
- Do not prescribe antispasmodic agents or antidiarrheal agents (e.g., loperamide) because these are not helpful.

■ FOLLOW-UP & DISPOSITION
- Although an extensive workup is not necessary, these children should be followed closely, at least three times a year.
- If any additional signs or symptoms of GI disease occur or if the child has poor weight gain or weight loss, further evaluation will be necessary.

■ PATIENT/FAMILY EDUCATION
- Explain the common nature and cause.
- Show parents the child's normal growth parameters.
- Give a list of fruits (and juices) that are low in sorbitol and low in free fructose (equal concentrations of

fructose and glucose or more glucose).
  1. Several fruits (and juices) have no sorbitol and also have a favorable fructose:glucose ratio. Several examples include the following:
     a. Citrus fruits
     b. Cranberries
     c. Grapes
     d. Pineapples
     e. Raspberries
     f. Blackberries
     g. Strawberries

■ PREVENTIVE TREATMENT
As under "Nonpharmacologic."

⚙ PEARLS & CONSIDERATIONS

■ CLINICAL PEARLS
- Normally, postprandial activity interrupts and replaces the migrating motor complex (MMC) the moment food enters the digestive system, slowing the transit of food through the intestine and allowing more time for the absorption of fluid, electrolytes, and nutrients. In children with toddler's diarrhea, food may fail to interrupt MMC activity, perhaps because of delayed gut motor development.
- Excess bile salts can enter the colon from rapid transit time and are thought to contribute to diarrhea because bacterial degradation of the salts produces bile acids and hydroxylated fatty acids, which may act as secretogogues in the colon.

REFERENCES
1. Judd RH: Chronic nonspecific diarrhea, *Pediatr Rev* 17:379, 1996.
2. Liacouras CA, Baldassano RN: Is it toddler's diarrhea? *Contemp Pediatr* 15: 131, 1998.
3. Wyllie R, Hyams JS: *Pediatric gastrointestinal disease: pathophysiology, diagnosis, management,* ed 2, Philadelphia, 1999, WB Saunders.
Author: **Larry Denk, M.D.**

BASIC INFORMATION

■ DEFINITION

Totticollis is unilateral contraction of the cervical or sternocleidomastoid (SCM) muscles resulting in rotation of the head and neck with associated head tilt; it may be congenital or acquired.

■ SYNONYM

Wry neck

ICD-9CM CODES

723.5 Intermittent or spastic
754.1 Congenital
767.8 Due to birth injury

Congenital Torticollis
■ ETIOLOGY

- May be secondary to mechanical constraint in utero or, less often, birth trauma
- Related most commonly to neuro-muscular abnormality with fibrotic shortening of the SCM
- Less commonly related to underlying bony anomalies (of the atlas, odon-toid, or atlantoaxial articulation), skin web (pterygium colli), central nervous system disorder (e.g., involv-ing cranial nerve XI at origin in cer-vical spinal cord or exit from base of skull)

■ EPIDEMIOLOGY & DEMOGRAPHICS

- Occurs in 0.4% of live births
- Males more frequently affected than females

■ HISTORY

- Infant prefers to keep head turned to one side.
- This condition is often unnoticed at birth. It is usually detected within the first month of life.
- The patient may have a birth history remarkable for breech presentation, forceps delivery, or orthopedic disor-ders (associated metatarsus adductus, congenital hip dysplasia, and talipes equinovarus may occur in up to 20% of cases).

■ PHYSICAL EXAMINATION

- Tight SCM muscle, often with palpa-ble, hard, olivelike mass in the mid-section of the cervical muscle, is noted.
  1. Palpable between ages 4 and 6 weeks
  2. Typically regresses by 4 to 6 months, leaving only contracture and fibrotic thickening of the in-volved muscle
- Head tilt in the direction of the muscle involved with chin turned away from the contracted side is seen.

- Later findings include facial asymme-try and plagiocephaly (flattening on affected side).
- Assess for other orthopedic abnor-malities that may be associated with torticollis (e.g., congenital hip dysplasia).
- Assess for associated ophthalmologic or neurologic abnormalities.

⚕ DIAGNOSIS

■ DIFFERENTIAL DIAGNOSIS

- Other causes of neck masses in region of the SCM muscle
  1. Cystic hygroma
  2. Branchial cleft cyst
- Underlying vertebral or neurologic abnormalities
  1. Vertebral dislocation
  2. Klippel-Feil syndrome with failure of normal vertebral segmentation of the cervical spine
  3. Sprengel's deformity with congen-ital elevation of the scapula

■ DIAGNOSTIC WORKUP

- Most patients require only a careful physical examination.
- When a cervical muscle mass is not palpable or torticollis is not respond-ing to therapy, plain films of the neck should be obtained to look for cervical bony abnormalities (e.g., hemivertebrae). Magnetic resonance imaging (MRI) should be done for patients with complicated cervical anomalies.
- In cases of plagiocephaly without obvious torticollis, need to evaluate for craniosynostosis.

℞ THERAPY

■ NONPHARMACOLOGIC

- Passive stretching involves lateral flexion of the head to the side oppo-site the torticollis and rotation of the chin to the affected side; supervision by a physical therapist is helpful.
- The infant should be placed in rela-tion to objects of interest so that active head turning to the unaffected side is encouraged.
- In certain cases with significant sec-ondary plagiocephaly, treatment with a fitted plastic helmet may remediate the plagiocephaly.

■ SURGICAL

- Most cases resolve by 1 year of age.
- Surgical referral is indicated if not resolved by 1 year for potential lengthening of the SCM muscle.

■ PATIENT/FAMILY EDUCATION

- See nonpharmacologic therapy for stretching exercises and infant positioning.
- Resolution of torticollis before 1 year of age can lead to a resolution of facial asymmetry.

■ REFERRAL INFORMATION

Refer patients with any of the following:
- Failure to improve after 2 to 3 months of conservative treatment
- Presence of anomalies of the skull or cervical spine
- Abnormal neurologic or ophthalmo-logic examinations
- Failure to resolve by 1 year of age

Acquired Torticollis
■ ETIOLOGY

Acute and short term
- Secondary to an acute process result-ing in spasm of the SCM muscle
  1. Most cases are related to ligamen-tous or muscular injuries with sudden onset following minor injury, strenuous activity, or sudden position change.
  2. Inflammatory or infectious causes include tonsillitis, cervi-cal adenitis, or retropharyngeal abscess causing cervical node enlargement.
  3. Atlantoaxial rotational subluxa-tion can occur secondary to trauma or in children with under-lying conditions that predispose to atlantoaxial instability (e.g., trisomy 21, bone dysplasia, Morquio syndrome).
- Reversible torticollis (apparent torti-collis without SCM muscle shortening)
  1. Idiosyncratic response to phe-nothiazines, metoclopramide, or haloperidol
  2. Paroxysmal torticollis of infancy
    a. Rare
    b. Associated with vestibular dysfunction
    c. Presents at age 2 to 8 months with associated distress, pallor, possible eye rolling/deviation, and ataxia
  3. Sandifer syndrome with arching and posturing secondary to gas-troesophageal reflux
- Pseudotorticollis
  1. Secondary to abducens or other oculomotor palsies, spasmus nutans, or congenital nystagmus; is a mechanical compensation that allows for one visual image
- Progressive torticollis
  1. Infratentorial tumor
  2. Structural lesions: colloid cyst of the third ventricle and syringomyelia

II

3. Sarcoma with invasion and entrapment of cranial nerves
4. Basal ganglia dysfunction or destruction (e.g., Wilson disease with destruction secondary to copper deposition)
5. Myositis of the sternocleidomastoid muscle

■ HISTORY

- Assess for history of trauma, recent or concurrent illness, and drug exposure.
- Inquire regarding any associated neurologic symptoms such as dizziness, unsteadiness, or abnormal eye movements.

■ PHYSICAL EXAMINATION

- Tight SCM muscle with head tilt in the direction of the muscle involved with chin turned away from the contracted side is noted.
- Assess for associated infection and lymphadenopathy.
- In the absence of obvious infection, careful neurologic and ophthalmologic examinations are essential.

⚕ DIAGNOSIS

■ DIFFERENTIAL DIAGNOSIS

See preceding "Etiology."

■ DIAGNOSTIC WORKUP

Acute and short term
- A careful physical examination and history will dictate further workup.
  1. Cervical spine films or imaging

studies may be required in cases of trauma
  2. Barium swallow and/or pH probe in cases of suspected gastroesophageal reflux (Sandifer syndrome)
- Computed tomography of the neck may be useful if a retropharyngeal abscess is suspected.

Progressive torticollis
- MRI and radiographic imaging of the head and neck
- Slit-lamp examination for Kayser-Fleischer corneal ring; serum tests to assess for Wilson disease
- Creatinine phosphokinase to rule out myopathy

℞ THERAPY

■ NONPHARMACOLOGIC

- In cases with torticollis secondary to muscle spasm, strain, or intervertebral disc calcification, use local heat, analgesics, and muscle relaxants.
- Appropriately treat the underlying cause (e.g., systemic antibiotics for infection).

■ SURGICAL

Patients with atlantoaxial subluxation require referral to an orthopedic or neurologic surgeon.

■ REFERRAL INFORMATION

Refer patients with any of the following:
- Presence of anomalies of the skull or cervical spine

- Progressive torticollis or failure to respond to conventional therapy
- Abnormal neurologic or ophthalmologic examinations

☼ PEARLS & CONSIDERATIONS

■ CLINICAL PEARLS

- Head tilt toward the muscle involved with the chin turned to the opposite side is seen.
- In congenital torticollis, early detection and treatment with stretching exercises can promote resolution of craniofacial abnormalities.
- A careful history and clinical examination focusing on the neck and neurologic and ophthalmologic examinations should sort out the many causes and allow appropriate diagnosis and management.

REFERENCES

1. Braun MA: Torticollis. In Dershewitz RA (ed): *Ambulatory pediatric care*, ed 3, Philadelphia, 1999, Lippincott Williams & Wilkins.
2. Snider RK (ed): *Essentials of musculoskeletal care*, Rosemont, Ill, 1997, American Academy of Orthopedic Surgeons and the American Academy of Pediatrics.
3. Rosenstein BJ: Torticollis. In Hoekelman RA (ed): *Primary pediatric care*, ed 4, St Louis, 2001, Mosby.

Author: **Laura Jean Shipley, M.D.**

BASIC INFORMATION

■ DEFINITION

Tourette's syndrome (TS) is a chronic neuropsychiatric condition with onset in childhood. It is characterized by motor and vocal tics that wax and wane in severity and persist longer than 1 year. In addition, affected individuals often have behavioral characteristics that include features of obsessive-compulsive disorder and/or of attention deficit/hyperactivity disorder (AD/HD).

■ SYNONYM

Tic disorder

ICD-9CM CODE

307.23 Tourette's syndrome

■ ETIOLOGY

- Genetic factors play a prominent role in vulnerability in majority of individuals.
- Nongenetic factors may determine the clinical phenotype (e.g., chronic motor tics, TS, obsessive-compulsive features). Prenatal and postnatal factors are included.
- The specific neuropathology is not yet clear. It seems to involve the basal ganglia and, possibly, cortico-striatothalamocortical circuitry.
- A minority of individuals do not have a genetic etiology. Symptoms may result from trauma, toxins, and possibly postinfectious autoimmune mechanisms (PANDAS—pediatric autoimmune neuropsychiatric disorders associated with streptococcal infection).

■ EPIDEMIOLOGY & DEMOGRAPHICS

- TS may occur in up to 1 to 8 cases per 1000 boys and 0.1 to 4 cases per 1000 girls.
- Motor tics occur at some time in 5% to 15% of school-age children.

■ HISTORY

- DSM-IV criteria are as follows:
  1. Both multiple motor and one or more vocal tics have been present, not necessarily simultaneously, during the illness.
  2. Tics occur many times a day, nearly every day, or intermittently throughout a period of more than 1 year. During this period, there has never been a tic-free period of more than 3 consecutive months.
  3. The disturbance causes marked distress or significant impairment in social, occupational, or other important areas of functioning.
  4. The onset is before age 18 years.
  5. The disturbance is not caused by the effects of a substance or a general medical condition.

- Symptoms of AD/HD may precede any tics.
- More than 50% of patients have associated features of AD/HD.
- The onset of simple motor tics, initially involving the head and neck, occurs during the first decade of life, with the median onset at 5 to 6 years.
- The type of tics varies over time; frequency and severity wax and wane.
- Complex motor tics, involving combinations of muscle groups, also change over time.
- Vocal tics usually follow motor tics by 1 to 2 years. Throat clearing and involuntary sounds are the most common vocal tics. The most severe form is coprolalia.
- Worst tic severity usually occurs between 7 and 15 years.
- As many as 80% of patients have some obsessive-compulsive features, with 30% having obsessive-compulsive disorder.
- Family history of tics and obsessive-compulsive features is common.
- If there is very sudden onset or marked and sudden increase in severity, question about recent infectious illness and consider getting ASO and anti-DNAase B titers.

■ PHYSICAL EXAMINATION

- The neurologic examination is remarkable for tics.
  1. Simple motor tics: sudden, brief, meaningless movements such as eye blinking, eye movements, grimacing, head jerks, arm jerks, tooth clicking, finger movements, and kicks
  2. Complex motor tics: slower, longer, more purposeful movements such as sustained looks, facial gestures, biting, touching objects or self, gestures with hands, gyrating and bending, and copropraxia (obscene gestures)
  3. Simple phonic (vocal) tics: sudden, meaningless sounds or noises such as throat clearing, barking, coughing, spitting, clacking, hissing, and many other sounds
  4. Complex phonic tics: sudden, more meaningful utterances such as syllables, words, phrases, or statements; may have echo phenomenon and coprolalia

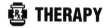 **DIAGNOSIS**

■ DIFFERENTIAL DIAGNOSIS

- Transient motor tic disorder
- Chronic motor tic disorder
- AD/HD (can be comorbid)
- Obsessive-compulsive disorder (can be comorbid)

- Continuous movement disorders: athetosis, chorea, tremor, myoclonus, dystonia, dyskinesia, and akathisia
- Paroxysmal movement disorders: paroxysmal ataxia, paroxysmal tremor, and stereotypies
- Wilson disease
- PANDAS

■ DIAGNOSTIC WORKUP

- History, including careful family history
- Careful physical examination and neurologic examination
- Electroencephalogram only if strong suspicion of seizure disorder
- Streptozyme and DNAase B if very abrupt onset or very abrupt exacerbation of symptoms
- Neuroimaging only if presentation is atypical or symptoms are very severe
- Careful psychiatric history for comorbid disorders

℞ THERAPY

■ NONPHARMACOLOGIC

- Education of patient, family, and school personnel about TS and its manifestations
- Specific educational modifications, especially during times of increased tic severity
- Cognitive-behavioral therapy may be helpful for obsessive-compulsive disorder symptoms
- Supportive psychotherapy as indicated

■ MEDICAL

- In this complex condition, it is important to clarify the target symptom for pharmacologic intervention and to watch carefully for potential exacerbation of other symptoms.
- Treatment is indicated only if symptoms are significantly interfering with the patient's functional status.
- Because of the complexity of symptoms and the frequent need for combinations of pharmacologic agents, medication is often managed by a child neurologist or developmental pediatrician.

■ MEDICAL INTERVENTIONS FOR TICS

- α-Adrenergic receptor agonists (e.g., clonidine, guanfacine [Tenex])
- Typical neuroleptics (e.g., haloperidol, pimozide)
- Atypical neuroleptics (e.g., risperidone, clozapine)

■ MEDICAL INTERVENTIONS FOR OBSESSIVE-COMPULSIVE SYMPTOMS

See the section "Obsessive-Compulsive Disorder."

II

■ MEDICAL INTERVENTION FOR AD/HD SYMPTOMS

See the section "Attention Deficit/Hyperactivity Disorder."

■ FOLLOW-UP & DISPOSITION

- A multidisciplinary team, including child neurologist or developmental pediatrician, psychologist, and educational specialist, is most effective at case management.
- Alternatively, referral to child neurologist or developmental pediatrician with expertise in TS is recommended.
- Collaboration between provider, school, and family is essential.
- Waxing and waning symptoms may necessitate frequent medication changes.
- It is important to watch for signs of increasing depression or anxiety.

■ PATIENT/FAMILY EDUCATION

- Most patients do not progress to severe forms depicted by media.
- Waxing and waning severity of symptoms is to be expected.
- The child may need specific educational accommodations.
- Parents serve a very important advocacy role.
- Associated learning disabilities are common.
- Local support groups are extremely helpful for family and patients.

- Symptoms usually peak during early adolescence, and then tend to diminish and stabilize.

■ REFERRAL INFORMATION

- Multidisciplinary team with expertise in TS
- Child neurologist
- Developmental pediatrician
- Psychologist to work on behavior management strategies and cognitive strategies and to help with depression as necessary

☼ PEARLS & CONSIDERATIONS

■ CLINICAL PEARLS

- Tics are extremely common during childhood. It is important that the child meet the full diagnostic criteria before making the diagnosis of TS.
- It is often extremely difficult, sometimes impossible, to distinguish between complex tics and compulsions.
- Complex tics, such as touching and eye rolling, are often interpreted as intentional oppositional behavior. It is important to help school personnel understand the nature of the tics.
- Watch for ongoing studies about PANDAS.

■ WEBSITE

Tourette Syndrome Association: National organization for education and information: http://tsa.mgh.harvard.edu

■ SUPPORT GROUPS

- Information about local support groups is available by contacting the national Tourette Syndrome Association.
- Local neurologists, child development centers, and school social workers may know of other local groups.

REFERENCES

1. Bagheri MM: Recognition and management of Tourette's syndrome and tic disorders, *Am Fam Physician* 59: 2263, 1999.
2. Bruun RD: The course and prognosis of Tourette syndrome, *Neurol Clin* 15: 291, 1997.
3. Kurlan R: Tourette's syndrome and "PANDAS": will the relation bear out? *Neurology* 50:1530, 1998.
4. Leckman JF et al: Tic disorders, *Psychiatric Clin North Am* 20:839, 1997.

Author: **Ellen Gellerstedt, M.D.**

BASIC INFORMATION

■ DEFINITION
- Streptococcal toxic shock syndrome (TSS) case definition:
  1. Isolation of group A streptococcus (groups B, C, F, and G also reported) from sterile site (if from nonsterile site, a probable case)
  2. Hypotension: systolic blood pressure 90 mm Hg or lower in adults, less than the 5th percentile for age in children
  3. Organ system involvement, including at least *two* of the following:
     a. Renal: creatinine level elevated twice the upper limit of normal for age (twice the baseline if preexisting elevation), or 2 mg/dl or more
     b. Hematologic: platelets 100,000/mm^3 or less or disseminated intravascular coagulation based on prolonged clotting time, low fibrinogen, and presence of fibrin degradation products
     c. Hepatic: transaminase or bilirubin levels twice the upper limits of normal or twice the baseline if underlying liver disease
     d. Respiratory: acute respiratory distress syndrome (ARDS), acute pulmonary edema, or pleural effusion with hypoalbuminemia
     e. Integument: generalized erythematous macular rash; may desquamate
     f. Integument: tissue necrosis, including necrotizing fasciitis, myositis, or gangrene
- Staphylococcal TSS case definition:
  1. Temperature 38.9° C (102.0° F) or higher
  2. Diffuse erythroderma or polymorphic maculopapular rash
  3. Desquamation of the palms and soles 1 to 2 weeks after syndrome onset
  4. Hypotension: systolic blood pressure less than 90 mm Hg or less than the 5th percentile in children, *or* drop in systolic blood pressure 10 mm Hg or more from lying to sitting position, *or* orthostatic syncope
  5. Involvement of *three* or more of the following organ systems:
     a. Gastrointestinal: vomiting or diarrhea at onset
     b. Musculoskeletal: myalgias or creatinine phosphokinase (CPK) greater than twice the upper limits of normal or higher

  c. Mucous membrane hyperemia: conjunctival, oropharyngeal, or vaginal
  d. Renal: blood urea nitrogen (BUN) or creatinine level greater than twice the upper limit of normal, *or* pyuria 5 or more white blood cells per high-power field without evidence of a urinary tract infection
  e. Hepatic: transaminase or bilirubin levels twice the upper limits of normal
  f. Hematologic: platelets 100,000/mm^3 or less
  g. Central nervous system: disorientation or altered consciousness without focal signs (in the absence of fever or hypotension).
  h. Cardiopulmonary: ARDS, pulmonary edema, new-onset second- or third-degree atrioventricular block, evidence of myocarditis
  6. Negative cultures (throat, cerebrospinal fluid [CSF], urine), except positive blood culture for *Staphylococcus aureus*
  7. Negative serologies for Rocky Mountain spotted fever, leptospirosis, and rubeola

ICD-9CM CODES
040.89 Toxic shock
041.11 *S. aureus*
041.19 *Staphylococcus,* other
041.00 *Streptococcus*

■ ETIOLOGY
This is a systemic inflammatory response syndrome resulting from toxin-mediated effects on the immune system. It requires a conducive environment for toxin production, a susceptible host, and specific toxin-producing strains of certain microbes. Staphylococcal toxins TSST-1, enterotoxins B and C, or streptococcal pyrogenic exotoxins A and B probably act as "superantigens" to suppress certain protective cellular immune responses and to enhance production of cytokines and tumor necrosis factor. This inflammatory cascade bypasses conventional immune activation sequences.

■ EPIDEMIOLOGY & DEMOGRAPHICS
- Streptococcal TSS has a moderately high incidence at 0 to 4 years, is low in school-age children, with increased risk with advancing age beyond young adult. Males may be predominately affected.
- Staphylococcal TSS has no age or sex predominance.
- Healthy individuals with normal immune systems are usually affected.

- Patients probably lack immunity to virulence factors *and* have predisposing conditions.
- Secondary cases are extremely rare.

■ HISTORY
- Streptococcal TSS often begins with severe, localized pain at the infection site, but may begin with influenza-like symptoms.
  1. Altered mental status is present in most patients.
  2. Invasive infection is almost invariably present, although symptoms of pneumonia, sinus infections, or pharyngitis may be noted.
- Staphylococcal TSS begins with nonspecific constitutional symptoms for 2 to 3 days; fever follows, and diarrhea and orthostasis may develop early.
  1. Menstrual staphylococcal TSS now represents a minority of TSS cases, almost exclusively with tampon use. However, it has occurred with contraceptive sponge or intrauterine device use.
  2. Nonmenstrual TSS can occur in association with focal tissue infections (e.g., impetigo, abscess, varicella lesions), pneumonia, sinusitis, osteomyelitis, septic arthritis, burns, empyema, and nasal packing, as well as in the postpartum (endometriosis/mastitis) and postoperative settings.

■ PHYSICAL EXAMINATION
- TSS generally presents with fever, tachycardia, tachypnea, and hypotension.
- Generalized erythema (less commonly patchy) is common with the staphylococcal form; it is more rare with the streptococcal form. It involves the palms and soles and may have flexor accentuation.
- Mucosal hyperemia, conjunctival hemorrhages, "strawberry tongue," and aphthous ulcers are more common in the staphylococcal form.
- Bullae are more common with the streptococcal form.
- Later evidence of anasarca from interstitial fluid losses is possible.
- Streptococcal disease usually occurs in association with invasive infection, especially necrotizing fasciitis (up to 70% of cases). Less common sources include septic arthritis, pneumonia, peritonitis, sinusitis, epiglottis, meningitis, cellulitis (especially with varicella), and pharyngitis (rare).
- Staphylococcal disease infection site findings are generally unimpressive but may include tissue infections, pneumonia, sinus tenderness, joint or bony findings, or incisional infection.

II

🔬 DIAGNOSIS

■ DIFFERENTIAL DIAGNOSIS
- Acute rheumatic fever
- Disseminated Epstein-Barr virus or fungal infection
- Gram-negative sepsis
- Heat stroke
- Kawasaki disease
- Legionnaire's disease
- Leptospirosis
- Lyme disease
- Meningococcemia
- Recalcitrant erythematous desquamating disorder (acquired immunodeficiency syndrome associated)
- Rocky Mountain spotted fever
- Scarlet fever and other exanthems
- Staphylococcal scalded skin syndrome
- Stevens-Johnson syndrome
- Systemic juvenile rheumatoid arthritis
- Systemic lupus erythematosus
- Toxoplasmosis
- Typhus

■ DIAGNOSTIC WORKUP
Laboratory tests include the following:
- Electrolytes, calcium, creatine, and BUN
- Complete blood count and coagulation studies
- Blood and urine cultures; consider CSF studies
- CPK
- Urinalysis
- Liver function tests, pancreatic function test(s)
- Chest radiograph and oxygen saturation; consider arterial blood gases
- Electrocardiogram; consider creatine kinase-muscle/brain (CK-MB) and/or troponin testing; consider echo for hemodynamically unstable patient

Expected results are as follows:
- See organ system information under case definitions.
- Frequent metabolic acidosis secondary to poor perfusion can occur.
- Leukocytosis with prominent left shift is expected and anemia often seen.
- Coagulation studies are abnormal in 40% of patients.
- Hypokalemia and hypocalcemia are common; hyponatremia is less common.
- Hypoalbuminemia is common.
- Bacteremia is seen in most streptococcal cases but is rare in staphylococcal TSS.

℞ THERAPY

■ NONPHARMACOLOGIC
- Provide supplemental oxygen at high concentrations; consider intubation based on clinical condition.
- Provide aggressive fluid resuscitation with normal saline (may consider colloid preparations in the later stages).
- Consider central access and hemodynamic monitoring to guide further resuscitation.
- The patient may require correction of coagulopathy with fresh frozen plasma, platelets, or cryoprecipitate.
- Anemia may require transfusion of packed red blood cells.
- Correct electrolyte abnormalities as needed.

■ MEDICAL
- For streptococcal cases:
  1. Clindamycin with or without penicillin G may be administered intravenously.
  2. Intravenous immune gammaglobulin (IVIg) may result in dramatic improvement (0.5 g/kg).
- For staphylococcal cases:
  1. Clindamycin is given intravenously; add vancomycin, first-generation cephalosporin, or antistaphylococcal penicillin (e.g., nafcillin); antistaphylococcal β-lactam antibiotics *may* enhance toxin production.
  2. IVIg (0.5 g/kg) may be given.
  3. Steroids have been recommended for refractory cases, but evidence to support their use is lacking.
- Consider vasopressors for shock refractory to fluid resuscitation. Dopamine may be supplemented with norepinephrine if needed.
- Ceftriaxone may need to be added to cover for meningitis (until definite diagnosis made) or doxycycline for Rocky Mountain spotted fever and leptospirosis.
- Consider sodium bicarbonate if the patient is severely acidotic (pH less than 7.1) and has a worsening acid-base status despite appropriate fluid resuscitation and ventilatory correction.
- Consider acetaminophen for antipyresis. Nonsteroidal medications are relatively contraindicated.

■ SURGICAL
Streptococcal forms may require surgical debridement, fasciotomy, laparotomy, hysterectomy, or amputation, depending on site of origin and degree of necrosis.

■ FOLLOW-UP & DISPOSITION
All patients with suspected TSS should be admitted to an intensive care unit.

■ PATIENT/FAMILY EDUCATION
Completion of a full 10-day course of antibiotics helps reduce the rate of relapse (30% to 40% of inadequately treated staphylococcal TSS cases relapse).

■ PREVENTIVE TREATMENT
Few preventive measures are available. Avoidance of tampon use, a reduction in the duration of nasal packing to a few days (possibly with use of antibiotic prophylaxis), and appropriate treatment of wounds and burns may reduce chances of TSS.

■ REFERRAL INFORMATION
Early consultation with pediatric intensivist is recommended. Surgical consultation may be necessary for streptococcal-associated tissue necrosis.

💡 PEARLS & CONSIDERATIONS

■ CLINICAL PEARLS
- Few signs of infection are present at the originating site of staphylococcal TSS; significant findings are usually present at the infected site of streptococcal TSS.
- Streptococcal TSS may present with early-onset shock and organ failure without typical rash.
- Mortality is much higher in streptococcal (30% to 70%) than staphylococcal (less than 3% menstrual, 6% to 9% nonmenstrual) TSS.
- Renal dysfunction *precedes* shock in TSS.
- Most patients improve significantly within 48 to 72 hours with treatment. Evidence of ARDS or refractory hypotension is a poor prognostic indicator.

REFERENCES
1. Centers for Disease Control and Prevention: Toxic shock syndrome—United States, 1970-1982, *MMWR Morb Mortal Wkly Rep* 31:201, 1982.
2. Eriksson BG et al: Epidemiological and clinical aspects of invasive group A streptococcal infections and the streptococcal toxic shock syndrome, *Clin Infect Dis* 27:1428, 1998.
3. Manders SM: Toxin-mediated streptococcal and staphylococcal disease, *J Am Acad Derm* 39:383, 1998.
4. Stevens DL: The toxic shock syndromes, *Infect Dis Clin North Am* 10:727, 1996.
5. The working group on severe streptococcal infections: Defining the group A streptococcal toxic shock syndrome: rationale and consensus definition, *JAMA* 269:390, 1993.
Authors: **John L. Hick, M.D.,** and **Karen L. Resch, M.D.**

BASIC INFORMATION

■ DEFINITION
Toxoplasmosis is a parasitic infection caused by the single-celled organism *Toxoplasma gondii*. Normally asymptomatic, it may produce severe ocular and central nervous system sequelae in immunocompromised hosts (e.g., patients with human immunodeficiency virus [HIV], transplant and chemotherapy recipients) or transplacentally infected infants.

■ SYNONYMS
- Toxo
- Toxoplasma

ICD-9CM CODE
130.0-130.9 Toxoplasmosis

■ ETIOLOGY
- *T. gondii* is a protozoan parasite. Although cat species are the definitive host, it may encyst in the tissue of virtually all mammals.
- Infection is generally via oral or parenteral routes, specifically from the following:
  1. Oocysts in cat feces contaminating either a litter box or garden soil
  2. Eating or improperly handling raw meat, especially lamb, pork, or venison
  3. Maternal-fetal transmission from a recently infected (or immunocompromised) mother
  4. Rarely blood or organ donation

■ EPIDEMIOLOGY & DEMOGRAPHICS
- Toxoplasmosis is ubiquitous, occurring worldwide. More than 60 million persons in the United States are infected.
- The incidence of congenital infection is estimated as 1 per 1000 to 1 per 10,000 live births.
- The risk of transplacental transmission is highest in third trimester; the risk of severe sequelae is highest if infection occurs in the first trimester.
- The incubation period is 4 to 21 days, averaging 7 days.
- Reactivation of latent infection may occur in immunocompromised hosts.

■ HISTORY
- Infection acquired after birth is usually asymptomatic but may cause generalized self-limiting flulike symptoms (e.g., malaise, muscle aches, lymphadenopathy).
- Congenital infection is asymptomatic at birth in 70% to 90% of cases.
- There is often a maternal history of cat exposure (e.g., cat box, gardening) or eating undercooked meat.

- Symptoms at birth may include the following:
  1. Maculopapular rash
  2. Microcephaly
  3. Intrauterine growth retardation
  4. Jaundice
  5. Seizures
- Late manifestations of congenital infection include the following:
  1. Visual impairment (very common)
  2. Developmental delay
  3. Spasticity
  4. Hydrocephalus
  5. Seizures
  6. Learning disabilities
- Rare manifestations include the following:
  1. Pneumonitis
  2. Myocarditis
  3. Pericarditis

■ PHYSICAL EXAMINATION
- Chorioretinitis, decreased visual acuity
- Cervical (or generalized) lymphadenopathy
- Hepatomegaly and/or splenomegaly
- Microcephaly or macrocephaly
- Hyperreflexia
- Increased tone

DIAGNOSIS

■ DIFFERENTIAL DIAGNOSIS
- Other (S)TORCH (syphilis, toxoplasmosis, other, rubella, cytomegalovirus, herpes simplex) infections, especially syphilis and cytomegalovirus
- Neonatal sepsis or aseptic meningitis
- Other lymphadenopathic disease (e.g., lymphoma, infectious mononucleosis)
- Other hemolytic disease (e.g., erythroblastosis fetalis)
- Other ocular disease (e.g., idiopathic chorioretinitis, colobomatous defect, intraocular hemorrhage, retinoblastoma, glioma)

■ DIAGNOSTIC WORKUP
- Signs and symptoms of infection can be protean and nonspecific.
- Workup includes serology, imaging studies, and ophthalmologic examination for diagnosis.
- Maternal infection:
  1. Serology: simultaneously assay IgG and either IgM or IgA
- Fetal infection:
  1. Polymerase chain reaction (PCR) or antigen detection on amniotic fluid
     a. Very sensitive at 18 weeks' gestation
  2. Parasite isolation from amniotic fluid or blood cells (mouse inoculation)

  3. Serology: enzyme immunoassay for IgM or IgA
  4. Radiology: serial cranial ultrasound for dilated lateral ventricles
- Neonatal infection:
  1. Serology: sequential IgG, double-sandwich IgM or IgA
  2. Radiology: computed tomography scan of the head for intracranial calcifications or hydrocephalus
  3. Parasite isolation from cord, placenta, or peripheral blood (mouse inoculation)
  4. PCR on buffy coat or cerebrospinal fluid (CSF) pellet
  5. Ophthalmology: funduscopic examination for necrotizing retinitis ("cotton-wool" patches or punched-out pigmented lesions)
- HIV-positive patients:
  1. Serology: IgG
  2. Ophthalmology: funduscopic examination for necrotizing retinitis ("cotton-wool" patches or punched-out pigmented lesions)
  3. PCR or antigen detection from blood (buffy coat), biopsy tissue, or CSF pellet

THERAPY

- Asymptomatic immunocompetent adults and children 5 years of age or older do not require treatment.
  1. Women infected with *T. gondii* 6 months before pregnancy do not require treatment during pregnancy.
- Pregnant women require treatment if they:
  1. Have recently become infected with *T. gondii*
  2. Are immunocompromised (i.e., HIV positive) and *T. gondii* infected
- All infections in neonates and immunocompromised individuals should be treated.

■ MEDICAL
- Prenatal
  1. First trimester: spiramycin (available only from the U.S. Food and Drug Administration)
  2. After 17 weeks' gestation: pyrimethamine/sulfadiazine and calcium leucovorin
- Neonatal/congenital
  1. Pyrimethamine/sulfadiazine plus calcium leucovorin for at least 1 year
- HIV positive/immunosuppressed
  1. Pyrimethamine/sulfadiazine plus calcium leucovorin is given for active infection.
  2. Trimethoprim/sulfamethoxazole is used for prophylaxis of inactive infections.
  3. Clindamycin may be substituted

for sulfadiazine in sulfa-sensitive individuals.
4. *Note:* Zidovudine (AZT, Retrovir) may compromise the efficacy of pyrimethamine/sulfadiazine treatment.
- Isolated chorioretinitis
  1. Pyrimethamine/sulfadiazine plus calcium leucovorin is given for 1 month.
  2. If infection involves macula or optic nerve head, steroids may be added.

■ SURGICAL
If chorioretinitis does not respond to systemic antimicrobials (with or without steroids), photocoagulation may be indicated, and rarely, vitrectomy or lens removal.

■ FOLLOW-UP & DISPOSITION
- All patients taking pyrimethamine require a complete blood count with platelets checked biweekly for signs of marrow suppression.

- Congenital infections require close ophthalmology, audiology, and neurology follow-up, as well as serial brain imaging for signs of obstructing hydrocephalus.

■ PREVENTIVE TREATMENT
- This consists primarily of patient education.
- Pregnant, prepregnant, and immunocompromised individuals should do the following:
  1. Avoid handling cat litter boxes, sand, or garden soil.
  2. Avoid handling or eating raw and undercooked meat.
  3. If performing these high-risk activities, always wear gloves and wash hands thoroughly with soap and water afterward.
  4. Keep cats indoors, and feed them only dry or canned/prepared foods.

■ REFERRAL INFORMATION
- Referral to an infectious disease specialist is needed.

- Congenital infections also require close ophthalmology, audiology, and neurology follow-up.
  1. These children will often need special services for developmental delays.

☼ PEARLS & CONSIDERATIONS

■ WEBSITE
Centers for Disease Control and Prevention: www.cdc.gov; keyword search: toxoplasmosis

REFERENCES
1. Behrman RE, Klegman R, Jenson HB: *Nelson textbook of pediatrics,* ed 16, Philadelphia, 2000, Saunders.
2. Gilbert DN et al: *The Sanford guide to antimicrobial therapy,* ed 31, Hyde Park, Vt, 2001, Antimicrobial Therapy, Inc.
Author: **D. Steven Fox, M.D.**

BASIC INFORMATION

■ DEFINITION
Tracheomalacia/laryngomalacia is a disorder of the trachea or larynx that causes it to be abnormally collapsible as a result of the loss of structural integrity. In tracheomalacia, there is a softening of the tracheal rings, making them unable to maintain airway patency, particularly during expiration. More commonly encountered, laryngomalacia is caused by softness of laryngeal structures and is more likely to cause inspiratory symptoms. These conditions are closely related to the less commonly encountered tracheobronchomalacia and bronchomalacia.

ICD-9CM CODES
519.1 Unspecified
748.3 Congenital

■ ETIOLOGY
- A congenital process of uncertain origin that results in diffuse softness of the upper airway system, *or*
- A congenital process brought about by abnormal development of the embryonic foregut and vasculature, which results in a localized weakening of the tracheal rings, *or*
- A weakness brought about by an impinging structure such as a vascular ring, tracheoesophageal fistula, atretic esophagus, or tracheostomy tube

■ EPIDEMIOLOGY & DEMOGRAPHICS
- The two most common causes of stridor in infants
- Difficult to assess incidence because of the spectrum of disease
- Twice as common in males
- Presentation generally between birth and 2 months

■ HISTORY
- Usually begins within first few days of life, rarely as late as 3 months
- Symptoms worst with upper respiratory infections, exertion, or supine position
- Better with prone sleeping position
- Often associated with wheezing, dyspnea, hoarseness, aphonia, or chronic cough
- In severe cases, poor weight gain may be present

■ PHYSICAL EXAMINATION
- Coarse wheezing worse on expiration in tracheomalacia; worse on inspiration in laryngomalacia
- Stridor
- Prolonged expiratory phase
- Croupy cough
- In severe cases, chest retractions (possibly even causing chest wall deformity)

- Apnea, bradycardia, cyanosis ("dying spell") with feeding
  1. Seen in those with esophageal anomaly repair(s) who have persistent tracheomalacia

DIAGNOSIS

■ DIFFERENTIAL DIAGNOSIS
- Tracheobronchomalacia, bronchomalacia
- Tracheoesophageal fistula
- Vascular ring
- Esophageal atresia
- Laryngeal cartilaginous or vocal cord anomalies
- Neonatal tetany
- Dysfunctional suck or swallow
- Laryngeal edema secondary to trauma or aspiration
- Severe generalized laryngeal/tracheal chondromalacia (e.g., Ehlers-Danlos syndrome)
- Intraluminal or laryngeal webs
- Airway tumor
- Macroglossia
- Mandibular hypoplasia syndromes (e.g., Pierre-Robin syndrome)
- Branchial cleft cyst, thyroglossal duct remnant, mucous retention cyst
- Congenital goiter
- Lymphoma
- Bifid epiglottis
- Epiglottic or laryngeal atresia
- Laryngocele
- Laryngeal cysts
- Laryngotracheoesophageal cleft

■ DIAGNOSTIC WORKUP
- Presumptively by history and physical examination
- Chest radiograph to exclude some vascular anomalies
- Direct laryngoscopy to reveal laryngomalacia
- Bronchoscopy to reveal severity and extent of weakness in tracheomalacia may be needed
- Echocardiography and computed tomography (CT) for severe cases
- In rare cases, angiography, fluoroscopy, or cine CT to elucidate certain vascular or dynamic abnormalities

THERAPY

■ NONPHARMACOLOGIC
- Reassure that most cases become clinically insignificant by 18 months.
- Most patients require no therapy other than monitoring of growth and development.
- May need a prone sleeping positioning.
- Instruct on upright awake positioning.
- Encourage slow, careful feedings.

■ SURGICAL
- Correction of the underlying vascular anomaly or other provoking structural defect
- Rarely, nasotracheal intubation or tracheostomy

■ FOLLOW-UP & DISPOSITION
Verification of resolution by clinical examination

■ PATIENT/FAMILY EDUCATION
- Nearly all cases require no surgical intervention and spontaneously resolve.
- Most important parameters to monitor are respiratory status, feeding, and growth.

■ REFERRAL INFORMATION
Depending on the cause, involvement of a radiologist, otolaryngologist, or cardiothoracic surgeon may be warranted.

PEARLS & CONSIDERATIONS

■ CLINICAL PEARLS
- Most patients have a congenital form, which nearly always resolves by 18 months, although some predisposition to airway illnesses (e.g., croup) may persist for years.
- Presence of expiratory symptoms helps differentiate tracheomalacia from laryngomalacia, which is usually inspiratory.

■ WEBSITES
- Pediatric Database (PEDBASE): www.icondata.com/health/pedbase/files/tracheom
- Virtual Hospital: Electric Airway—Upper Airway Problems in Children: www.vh.org/Providers/ElectricAirway/Text/TracheoLaryngo.html

REFERENCES
1. Behrman RE, Kliegman R, Jenson HB: *Nelson textbook of pediatrics,* ed 16, Philadelphia, 2000, WB Saunders.
2. Gandy: Pediatric Database. Available at wwww.icondata.com/health/pedbase/files/tracheom
3. Hathaway WE (ed): *Current pediatric diagnosis and treatment,* ed, 15, New York, 2000, McGraw-Hill.
4. Myer CM, Cotton RT: A practical approach to: pediatric otolaryngology, St Louis, 1988, Mosby.
5. Santer, D'Allessandro: Virtual Hospital: Electric airway: upper respiratory problems in children. Available at www.vh.org/Providers/ElectricAirway/Text/TracheoLaryngo.html
6. Zalzal GH: Stridor and airway compromise, *Pediatr Clin North Am* 36:1394, 1989.

Author: **Chris Bolling, M.D.**

II

BASIC INFORMATION

■ DEFINITION

Transfusion reactions include urticaria, fevers, and/or hemolysis caused by antibodies in the recipient directed against components of the transfused product, including antigens on the red cells themselves, plasma proteins, or antigens on contaminating white cells or platelets.

■ SYNONYMS

- Urticarial reactions
- Febrile nonhemolytic reactions
- Acute hemolytic reactions
- Delayed hemolytic reactions
- Transfusion-related acute lung injury

ICD-9CM CODE
999.8 Transfusion reaction

■ ETIOLOGY

- Febrile nonhemolytic reactions are caused by antibodies in the recipient directed against donor plasma proteins or antigens on contaminating white cells or platelets.
- Urticarial reactions are thought to be caused by recipient allergies to donor plasma proteins.
- Delayed hemolytic reactions are caused by antibodies to minor group red cell antigens not detected by routine screening. The reticuloendothelial system clears antibody-coated red cells, producing a slow, extravascular hemolysis.
- Transfusion-related acute lung injury is caused by activation of endogenous neutrophils with subsequent damage to pulmonary capillary endothelium, leading to acute respiratory distress syndrome.
- Acute hemolytic reactions are caused by antibodies in the recipient directed against ABO group antigens present on transfused red blood cells. These isohemagglutinins bind to the transfused red cells, activate complement, and cause brisk intravascular hemolysis.

■ EPIDEMIOLOGY & DEMOGRAPHICS

- Febrile nonhemolytic reactions occur as often as 1 in 100 units of red cells transfused.
- Urticarial reactions occur in 1 in 1000 units of red cells transfused.
- Delayed hemolytic reactions occur in 1 in 1000 units of red cells transfused.
- Transfusion-related acute lung injury has an estimated frequency of 1 in 10,000 units of red cells transfused, and it is more likely to occur in the setting of sepsis.
- Acute hemolytic reactions occur 1 in 250,000 to 1 in 1,000,000 units of

red cells transfused and are usually caused by administrative/clerical errors (i.e., misidentification of the blood sample tested or misidentification of the recipient receiving the transfusion).

■ HISTORY

- Febrile nonhemolytic reactions can be associated with shortness of breath and back, chest, or neck pain.
- Urticarial reactions can occur on a first transfusion and cause pruritus.
- Delayed hemolytic transfusion reactions occur 3 to 14 days after a transfusion.
- Transfusion-related acute lung injury causes dyspnea within 4 hours of a transfusion.
- Acute hemolytic reactions occur early in the course of the transfusion, with chills, chest pain, and nausea being common symptoms.

■ PHYSICAL EXAMINATION

- Febrile nonhemolytic reactions cause fevers that may be associated with tachypnea and hypertension.
- Urticarial reactions cause hives.
- Delayed hemolytic reactions are characterized by fever, jaundice, and hemoglobinuria.
- Transfusion-related acute lung injury is characterized by hypoxia and respiratory distress.
- Acute hemolytic reactions cause fever, flank pain, dyspnea, tachycardia, hematuria, and hypotension, potentially leading to shock and death.

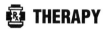 **DIAGNOSIS**

■ DIFFERENTIAL DIAGNOSIS

The onset of fever in the setting of a red cell transfusion may be caused by the following:

- Acute nonhemolytic reactions (clinically benign)
- Acute hemolytic reactions (potentially life-threatening)
- A coincident febrile illness
- Bacterial contamination of the transfused product

■ DIAGNOSTIC WORKUP

- With the guidance of the blood bank, the workup should include the following:
  1. A Coombs' test to look for red cell antibodies
  2. Measurement of hemoglobinemia on pretransfusion and posttransfusion blood samples to look for evidence of ongoing hemolysis
- Measure hemoglobinuria on a urine sample as evidence of acute hemolysis. A negative workup rules out an acute hemolytic transfusion reaction.

- Delayed hemolytic transfusion reactions cause anemia (complete blood count) and increase in indirect bilirubin but no hemoglobinemia.

■ THERAPY

■ NONPHARMACOLOGIC

- *Febrile nonhemolytic reactions:* Stop the transfusion and assess for evidence of hemolysis. It is usually possible to complete the transfusion.
- *Urticarial reactions:* Stop the transfusion temporarily. If the urticaria improves within 30 minutes, resume the transfusion.
- *Delayed hemolytic reactions:* Treat the anemia with transfusion therapy.
- *Transfusion-related acute lung injury:* Provide supportive care, including ventilatory support as needed.
- *Acute hemolytic reactions:* Stop the transfusion immediately. Maintain veinous access and hydrate to maintain urine output and minimize the risk of renal failure.

■ MEDICAL

- Febrile nonhemolytic reactions can be treated with antipyretics such as Tylenol.
- Urticarial reactions are treated with antihistamines, such as intravenous diphenhydramine. Steroids (1 to 2 mg/kg methylprednisolone) may be necessary for severe reactions.
- Acute hemolytic transfusion reactions may require furosemide, mannitol, or a renal dose dopamine to maintain urine output.

■ FOLLOW-UP & DISPOSITION

- *Urticarial reactions:* Monitor carefully for evidence of anaphylaxis, including laryngeal edema, bronchospasm, or vascular collapse.
- *Delayed hemolytic reactions:* Treat the anemia that develops.
- *Transfusion-related acute lung injury:* Admit to hospital for supportive care.
- *Acute hemolytic reactions:* Admit to the hospital to monitor intake and output and renal function.

■ PATIENT/FAMILY EDUCATION

- Obtain informed consent before any transfusion.
- Make the patient aware of the potential of a delayed transfusion reaction, which can cause anemia and jaundice.

■ PREVENTIVE TREATMENT

- *Febrile nonhemolytic reactions:* Deplete contaminating white cells by filtration of the red cells.
  1. Pretreat the patient with antipyretics.

2. *Repeat delayed hemolytic reactions:* Perform detailed blood typing to exclude red cell units that express offending minor group antigens.

3. *Acute hemolytic transfusion reactions:* Increase vigilance regarding the identification of patients and units of blood to reduce administrative/clerical errors.

■ REFERRAL INFORMATION
- The blood bank should be notified immediately of any transfusion reactions.

- Chronic transfusion therapy of patients with thalassemia major or sickle cell disease should be managed by pediatric hematologists.

 PEARLS & CONSIDERATIONS

■ CLINICAL PEARLS
Patients with sickle cell disease who are on chronic transfusion programs are at increased risk of developing antibodies to minor group antigens that can cause delayed hemolytic transfusion reactions.

REFERENCES
1. Goodnough LT et al: Transfusion medicine, *N Engl J Med* 340:438, 1999.
2. Sloop GD, Friedberg RC: Complications of blood transfusion: how to recognize and respond to noninfectious reactions, *Postgrad Med* 98:159, 1995.
Author: **James Palis, M.D.**

II

BASIC INFORMATION

■ DEFINITION
Transient synovitis of the hip is a non-specific, self-limited inflammation of synovial membrane of the hip joint.

■ SYNONYMS
- Transitory synovitis
- Transitory coxitis
- Reactive synovitis
- Acute transient epiphysitis
- Coxitis fugax
- Coxitis serosa
- Phantom hip
- Toxic synovitis
- Observation hip
- Irritable hip
- Intermittent hydrarthrosis

ICD-9CM CODE
719.25 Transient synovitis of the hip

■ ETIOLOGY
- No definitive cause known
- Hypotheses include association with the following:
  1. Active or recent infection
  2. Allergic hypersensitivity
  3. Preceding trauma

■ EPIDEMIOLOGY & DEMOGRAPHICS
- Most common cause of hip pain in children age 3 to 10 years old
- Average age of onset is 6 years; can occur in infancy through adolescence
- No seasonal preference
- Right and left hip involvement essentially equal
- Usually unilateral (less than 5% bilateral)
- Male:female ratio of 2:1
- Much lower incidence in African Americans

■ HISTORY
- The presenting complaint is acute onset of unilateral hip pain in an otherwise healthy child.
- Pain typically occurs in the groin or hip area or is referred to the anterior thigh or knee.
- Associated limp, antalgic gait, or refusal to bear weight may be seen.
- Approximately 50% of patients present after 1 to 3 days of symptoms.

■ PHYSICAL EXAMINATION
- Affected extremity held in flexed and externally rotated position
- Restricted range of motion at the hip, especially with abduction and internal rotation
- Temperature rarely exceeds 38° C (100.4° F)

DIAGNOSIS

■ DIFFERENTIAL DIAGNOSIS
- Septic arthritis
- Osteomyelitis of pelvis or femur
- Juvenile rheumatoid arthritis
- Legg-Calvé-Perthes (LCP) disease
- Acute rheumatic fever
- Tuberculous arthritis
- Tumor
- Slipped capital femoral epiphysis (SCFE)

■ DIAGNOSTIC WORKUP
- Complete blood count with differential (usually less than 13,000/mm^3 and may be elevated in septic arthritis)
- Erythrocyte sedimentation rate (ESR) (usually less than 20 mm/hr)
- Anteroposterior and frog-leg radiographs of pelvis (usually normal; rule out LCP disease and SCFE)
- Ultrasound of hip joint
  1. Not routinely required
  2. May be used to monitor resolution of effusion or in conjunction with needle aspiration of the joint
- Joint aspiration if septic arthritis is suspected
  1. More than 90% polymorphonuclear leukocytes in septic arthritis
- Purified protein derivative if tuberculous arthritis is suspected
- Blood culture if septic arthritis or osteomyelitis is suspected

THERAPY

■ NONPHARMACOLOGIC
- Bed rest
  1. Non–weight bearing until pain resolves and full joint motion returns
  2. Usually 3 to 7 days
- Abstinence from strenuous activities involving the hip additional 7 to 10 days after regain full range of motion

■ MEDICAL
- Nonsteroidal antiinflammatory agents may be given for pain relief.
- Avoid use of aspirin because of association with Reye syndrome.

- Antibiotics and steroids are not routinely recommended.

■ SURGICAL
- Routine joint aspiration is not recommended.
- Joint aspiration is done to rule out other causes of hip pain in questionable cases.

■ FOLLOW-UP & DISPOSITION
- If pain and/or limp persists for more than 10 days, reevaluate.
- Check temperature regularly to monitor for fever.
- Some recommend reevaluating at 14 days to detect recurrence before allowing resumption of full activity.
- Some recommend repeat radiographs at 2 and 4 to 6 months to detect LCP disease.

■ PATIENT/FAMILY EDUCATION
- Noncompliance with regimen is associated with longer duration of symptoms and increased risk for recurrence.
- Twenty-one-year follow up in some studies has shown radiologic changes not associated with functional limitations.

PEARLS & CONSIDERATIONS

■ CLINICAL PEARLS
- Suspect septic arthritis if have severe pain or spasm with movement of the hip, tenderness on palpation, temperature greater than 38° C (100.4° F), or ESR greater than 20 mm/hr.
- Using criteria of ESR greater than 20 mm/hr and/or temperature greater than 37.5° C (99.5° F) identified 97% of all cases of septic arthritis of the hip.
- An association between the development of LCP disease and transient synovitis has been reported (range of 0% to 17% with average of 1.5%).

REFERENCES
1. Hart JJ: Transient synovitis of the hip in children, *Am Fam Physician* 54:1587, 1996.
2. Morrissy RT, Weinstein SL: *Lovell and Winter's pediatric orthopaedics*, ed 4, Philadelphia, 1996, Lippincott-Raven.
3. Tachdjian MO: *Pediatric orthopedics*, ed 2, Philadelphia, 1990, WB Saunders.
Author: **Indra Kancitis, M.D.**

BASIC INFORMATION

DEFINITION
Transposition of the great arteries (TGA) is discordant ventriculoarterial connection wherein the aorta originates from the right ventricle and the pulmonary artery arises from the left ventricle, resulting in systemic and pulmonary circulations in parallel rather than in series.

SYNONYMS
- Transposition of the great vessels (TGV)
- Complete transposition
- D-transposition

ICD-9CM CODE
745.1 Transposition of the great arteries

ETIOLOGY
An abnormality of conotruncal development related to differential conal absorption and abnormal aortopulmonary septation

EPIDEMIOLOGY & DEMOGRAPHICS
- The incidence is 3 per 10,000 live births; it occurs in 2.5% to 5.0% of infants born with congenital heart disease.
- There is a sporadic, nonfamilial occurrence, but the male:female ratio is 2:1.
- This is the most common type of cyanotic cardiac malformation in the first month of life.
- A patent foramen ovale, atrial defect, ventricular defect, or patent ductus arteriosus (PDA) is essential for early survival.
- Mortality is greater than 90% by 1 year in untreated patients.
- In simple transposition, there is a patent foramen and a PDA, which subsequently close.
- Associated defects include the following:
  1. Ventricular septal defect (VSD): 20%
  2. Large atrial septal defect: 10%
  3. VSD and pulmonary stenosis: 5%
- Extracardiac malformations are uncommon and usually minor.

HISTORY
- Generally no interference with fetal well-being
- Cyanosis: may be mild initially but rapidly progresses
- Tachypnea and exertional dyspnea

PHYSICAL EXAMINATION
- Cyanosis
- Tachypnea with or without dyspnea
- Single or narrowly split, accentuated second heart sound
- Usually no murmur unless pulmonary stenosis is present
- Otherwise normal but if a large VSD is a complicating lesion, mild cyanosis with congestive heart failure developing at 2 to 6 weeks dominates the clinical picture

DIAGNOSIS

DIFFERENTIAL DIAGNOSIS
- Cyanotic malformations of the heart with increased pulmonary blood flow, but in other lesions, in general, the greater the amount of pulmonary blood flow, the higher the saturation
- Pulmonary hypertension of the newborn

DIAGNOSTIC WORKUP
- Electrocardiogram reveals normal right ventricular dominance in neonates.
- Chest radiograph reveals an abnormal silhouette.
  1. Egg-on-side
  2. Narrow pedicle
  3. No visible conus
  4. Increased pulmonary blood flow
  5. Mild cardiomegaly
- Blood gases reveal hypoxemia and a low-normal carbon dioxide tension (e.g., 32 to 35 mm Hg).
- Echocardiography reveals the following:
  1. Side-by-side great vessels
  2. Anterior aorta arises from right ventricle
  3. Posterior pulmonary artery from left ventricle
  4. Size, patency of fossa ovalis, ductus
  5. Associated lesions: VSD, pulmonary valve stenosis (PS)
  6. Distribution of coronary arteries
- Catheterization/angiography is done if questions persist about the coronary artery distribution or pattern or associated anomalies.

THERAPY

MEDICAL & SURGICAL
- Prostaglandin E_1 infusion to maintain ductal patency
- Balloon atrial septostomy if a very restrictive atrial communication is present
- Early arterial switch procedure (great arteries and coronary arteries) within the first 2 weeks of life
- Rarely, an atrial switch procedure (Mustard or Senning operation) because of a coronary artery pattern precluding coronary transfer

FOLLOW-UP & DISPOSITION
- Lifelong follow-up by a cardiologist is necessary, as is infective endocarditis prophylaxis.
- Short- and long-term survival after arterial switch procedure should now be 95% or more.
- Postarterial switch problems are unusual.
- If an atrial switch procedure has been performed, there is a substantial risk of the development of atypical atrial flutter and other atrial arrhythmias, sudden death, and right or systemic ventricular failure with a cumulative survival rate of 80% at 20 years of follow-up.

PATIENT/FAMILY EDUCATION
- The risk of recurrence is very low.
- Intelligence after an early arterial switch should be in the normal range.
- Malformation will preclude some competitive sports as the child grows.

REFERRAL INFORMATION
All patients with suspected TGA should be referred immediately to a pediatric cardiologist.

PEARLS & CONSIDERATIONS

CLINICAL PEARLS
- Suspect TGA in an infant with deep cyanosis, increased pulmonary blood flow, and an unusual cardiac silhouette.
- Arterial saturation is related to the size of the atrial communication and the amount of pulmonary blood flow.

SUPPORT GROUPS
Local Helping Hearts or related parental organizations provide both support and information.

REFERENCES
1. Helbing WA et al: Long-term results of atrial correction for transposition of the great arteries, *J Thor Cardiovasc Surg* 108:363, 1994.
2. Karl TR, Cochrane A, Brizard CPR: Arterial switch operation, *Tex Heart Inst J* 24:322, 1997.
3. Kirklin JW et al: Clinical outcomes after the arterial switch operation for transposition, *Circulation* 86:1501, 1992.
4. Rigby ML, Chan K-Y: The diagnostic evaluation of patient with complete transposition, *Cardiol Young* 1:26, 1991.

Author: **J. Peter Harris, M.D.**

BASIC INFORMATION

■ DEFINITION
Trichomoniasis is an infection of the genitourinary system (vagina, urethra, and periurethral glands) with the flagellated protozoa *Trichomonas vaginalis*.

■ SYNONYM
Trich

ICD-9CM CODES
131.01 Vagina, vulva, or vulvovaginal
131.02 Urethra

■ ETIOLOGY
- Sexually transmitted infection from the protozoa *T. vaginalis*
- Also evidence showing nonsexually transmitted infections can occur with trichomonads surviving in wet sponges or towels for up to 1.5 hours.

■ EPIDEMIOLOGY & DEMOGRAPHICS
- Prevalence in teenagers varies from 8% to 34%.
- Peak prevalence rates are between 16 and 35 years of age.
- Onset of symptoms varies from several days to weeks.

■ HISTORY
- Perineal pruritus (60% to 75%)
- Bothersome and irritating vaginal discharge (50%)
- Dysuria (20%)
- Dyspareunia
- Asymptomatic (up to 25% of females and 90% of males)

■ PHYSICAL EXAMINATION
- Frothy gray, green, or yellow vaginal discharge of varying consistency (pH greater than 4.5)
- Diffuse vulvitis
- Colpitis macularis or "strawberry spots"—petechiae on the cervix (not always present)

DIAGNOSIS

■ DIFFERENTIAL DIAGNOSIS
- Nonspecific vaginitis
- *Candida vaginitis*
- Bacterial vaginosis
- *Chlamydia cervicitis*
- Gonococcal cervicitis
- Nongonococcal urethritis

■ DIAGNOSTIC WORKUP
- Culture methods (gold standard): sensitivity 86% to 97%
- Wet-mount microscopy: sensitivity approximately 45% to 60%
- In-pouch TV culture system: sensitivity 81%
- Pap smear: sensitivity approximately 56% to 78% (unreliable because of high false-positive rate).
- Also available: enzyme immunoassay and immunofluorescence methods

THERAPY

■ MEDICAL
- First-line therapy: metronidazole 2 g orally for one dose
  1. Avoid in first trimester; pregnancy category B
  2. Approximate 90% cure rate
- Alternative therapy: metronidazole vaginal gel one applicator intravaginally twice daily for 5 days
  1. Avoid in the first trimester
  2. Approximate 50% cure rate
- Alternative therapy: metronidazole 500 mg orally twice daily for 7 days
  1. Avoid in first trimester
  2. Approximate 90% cure rate
- In pregnancy: clotrimazole 100 mg vaginal tabs at bedtime every day for 2 weeks
  1. If infection continues, re-treat after first trimester with metronidazole 7-day course (lower blood levels than 2-g dose).
  2. If untreated in pregnancy, ongoing infection is associated with premature rupture of membranes, postpartum endometritis, and prematurity.
- For treatment failure: metronidazole 2 g/day orally for 5 days
- For trichomoniasis resistant to metronidazole: tinidazole (a 5-nitroimidazole) or topical paromomycin

■ FOLLOW-UP & DISPOSITION
Most guidelines recommend no follow-up visit unless patients remain or become symptomatic.

■ PATIENT/FAMILY EDUCATION
- Sexual contacts also must be treated (metronidazole 2 g orally in a single dose).
- While taking metronidazole, patients must not drink alcohol, which could result in a disulfiram-like reaction (abdominal cramping, nausea, vomiting).

■ PREVENTIVE TREATMENT
"Safe sex" practices, including abstinence from sex and condom use with sexual contact to prevent contracting sexually transmitted diseases

■ REFERRAL INFORMATION
Consider referrals for patients with infections refractory to standard treatments and infections causing complications (especially in the prenatal patient).

PEARLS & CONSIDERATIONS

■ CLINICAL PEARLS
- There is an increased risk for human immunodeficiency virus transmission with preexisting trichomoniasis infection.
- Remember to check for other sexually transmitted diseases because the prevalence will be higher in someone who has one sexually transmitted disease.

■ WEBSITES
- Centers for Disease Control and Prevention, Division of Parasitic Diseases: www.dpd.cdc.gov/dpdx/html/trichomoniasis.htm
- STD Services: www.stdservices.on.net/std/trichomoniasis/facts09.htm
- Support-Group.com: www.support-group.com/

REFERENCES
1. Emans SJ: Vulvovaginal complaints in the adolescent. In Emans SJ, Laufer MR, Goldstein DP (eds): *Pediatric and adolescent gynecology*, ed 4, Philadelphia, 1998, Lippincott Williams & Wilkins.
2. Gülmezoglu AM: Interventions for treating trichomoniasis in women (Cochrane review), *Cochrane Database Syst Rev* Issue 1, 1999.
3. Ohlemeyer et al. Diagnosis of *Trichomonas vaginalis* in adolescent females: InPouch TV culture versus wet-mount microscopy, *J Adolesc Health* 22:205, 1998.
4. Sobel J: Current concepts: vaginitis, *N Engl J Med* 337:1896, 1997.
5. Vaginitis and cervicitis. In Neinstein LS (ed): *Adolescent health care*, Baltimore, 1996, Williams & Wilkins.
Author: **Susan Birndorf, D.O.**

BASIC INFORMATION

■ DEFINITION

Tuberculosis (TB) is a chronic systemic bacterial infection that may involve the lungs, meninges, bones, joints, kidneys, and skin.

- *TB exposure:* an asymptomatic individual with a negative TB skin test, normal physical examination, and normal chest radiograph who has had recent contact with a patient with suspected or confirmed TB
- *TB infection:* an asymptomatic individual with a positive TB skin test, a normal physical examination, and a normal chest radiograph
- *TB disease:* a symptomatic patient with definitive evidence (usually radiographic) of TB
  1. In young children, the distinction between infection and disease often may be unclear, and children with TB disease may be asymptomatic.

ICD-9CM CODES
010.9 Primary tuberculosis
011.9 Pulmonary tuberculosis
771.2 Congenital tuberculosis

■ ETIOLOGY

Mycobacterium tuberculosis is the acid-fast bacterium that resists acid discoloration following staining with aniline dyes. In developing countries, *Mycobacterium bovis,* acquired from contaminated milk, causes both pulmonary and gastrointestinal disease. There have been rare cases of *M. bovis* disease in the United States and Canada.

■ EPIDEMIOLOGY & DEMOGRAPHICS

- Congenital TB is acquired via transplacental spread from an infected mother or by the aspiration or swallowing of infected amniotic fluid.
- Most pediatric infections are acquired from household contacts via the inhalation of droplets containing the tubercle bacilli.
- Crowded living conditions, poverty, poor nutrition, and human immunodeficiency virus (HIV) infection are predisposing factors.
- The incubation period from acquisition of bacilli to a positive TB skin test is 2 to 12 weeks (median, 3 to 4 weeks). The highest risk for developing disease is within 6 months of infection.

■ HISTORY

- History of household exposure to an individual with active pulmonary TB
- History of a positive tuberculin skin test
- Unlike adults, most young children with pulmonary TB do not have a history of fever, weight loss, and malaise.

■ PHYSICAL EXAMINATION

- The following features may be present with advanced TB:
  1. Chest: wheezing, rhonchi, and crackles on auscultation
  2. Abdomen: hepatosplenomegaly
  3. Skin: newborns with congenital tuberculosis may have erythematous papules with necrotic or crusted centers known as *tuberculids*
  4. Bones and joints: tenderness to palpation and motion and limitation of motion

DIAGNOSIS

■ DIFFERENTIAL DIAGNOSIS

- Sarcoidosis
- Nontuberculous mycobacterial disease
- Bacterial infection
- Fungal infections (e.g., histoplasmosis, coccidioidomycosis)

■ DIAGNOSTIC WORKUP

- The Mantoux skin test (5 TU of purified protein derivative [PPD] injected intradermally) is the most important initial step in the diagnosis of TB.
- Definition of a positive test as per the American Academy of Pediatrics is as follows:
  1. Induration 5 mm or greater
     a. Children with history of close contact with a known or suspected case of TB
     b. Clinical and/or radiographic evidence of disease
     c. Children with HIV and those with immunosuppressive conditions or those receiving immunosuppressive therapy
  2. Induration 10 mm or greater
     a. Children 4 years of age or younger
     b. History of increased environmental exposure to TB, such as frequent exposure to people at high risk for TB, including HIV-infected individuals and institutionalized people
     c. History of travel to high-prevalence regions of the world or emigration from areas where TB is endemic
  3. Induration 15 mm or greater
     a. Asymptomatic children 4 years of age or older with no risk factors
- Radiographic diagnosis requires multiple chest radiographs, including anterior and posterior, lateral, and oblique views.

- Radiographic features of pulmonary TB include the following:
  1. Hilar adenopathy
  2. Infiltrates
  3. Miliary spread of disease
  4. Cavitations
  5. Calcifications
  6. Pleural effusion
- A computed tomography scan of the chest may be helpful.
- Laboratory diagnosis requires samples of gastric lavage fluid (first morning for 3 days) and/or samples of pulmonary secretions obtained on bronchoscopy to be sent for acid-fast staining and culture for *M. tuberculosis*. Some older children and adolescents may be able to produce sputum for testing.

THERAPY

■ NONPHARMACOLOGIC

The child with a positive TB skin test must be removed from the TB contact individual as soon as possible.

■ MEDICAL

- Therapy for TB exposure:
  1. Following household exposure within 3 months to active TB, the child younger than 4 years of age should receive at least 3 months of isoniazid (INH), if the initial skin test is negative. The child should then be skin tested again and treated accordingly.
  2. Other candidates for preventive therapy if the TB skin test is negative include recent contacts, household contacts, and anergic individuals.
- Therapy for TB infection:
  1. Infants and children with a history of a positive TB skin test should be started on INH alone, unless there is a history of prior antituberculosis therapy or drug resistance is suspected.
  2. INH should be continued for at least 6 to 9 months and at least 12 months in HIV-infected individuals.
- Therapy for TB disease:
  1. A 6-month course of INH, rifampin, and pyrazinamide is given for the first 2 months and INH and rifampin for the next 4 months.
  2. If drug resistance is suspected, a fourth drug, ethambutol or streptomycin, should be added.
  3. With concomitant HIV infection, treat with INH and rifampin for at least 12 months.

■ SURGICAL

Surgical resection of an involved lobe is occasionally indicated in chronic advanced pulmonary disease.

■ PREVENTIVE TREATMENT

- Isolation of adults with active disease
- INH treatment of children with household contacts
- Bacille Calmette-Guérin vaccine
  1. Currently recommended in the United States only for those unusual situations in which a child is exposed continually to a person with untreated or drug-resistant disease and the child cannot be removed from the exposure

☼ PEARLS & CONSIDERATIONS

■ CLINICAL PEARLS

- The TB skin test is often underread.
- Confirmed and suspected cases of TB must be reported to the local health department in all states.
- Chemotherapy, in cases of active TB disease, should be undertaken with the help and consultation of specialists in pediatric pulmonology and pediatric infectious disease.
- For directly observed therapy, it is recommended that a trained third party (not a relative or friend) be present to document the ingestion of each dose of oral medication.
- All individuals with TB should be tested for HIV.
- A negative TB skin test never excludes TB infection or disease.

REFERENCES

1. American Academy of Pediatrics: Tuberculosis. In Pickering LK (ed): *2000 Red Book: report of the Committee on Infectious Diseases,* ed 25, Elk Grove Village, Ill, 2000, American Academy of Pediatrics.
2. Inselman LS, Kendig EL Jr: Tuberculosis. In Chernick V, Boat TF (eds): *Kendig's disorders of the respiratory tract in children,* ed 6, Philadelphia, 1998, WB Saunders.
3. Kendig EL Jr et al: Underreading of the tuberculin skin test reaction, *Chest* 113:1175, 1998.

Authors: **James W. Kendig, M.D., Laura S. Inselman, M.D., and Edwin L. Kendig, Jr., M.D.**

BASIC INFORMATION

■ DEFINTION
Tuberous sclerosis (TS) is a neurocutaneous syndrome inherited in an autosomal dominant fashion. It is characterized by skin lesions (angiofibromas, hypopigmented macules) and tumors (hamartomas) of the nervous system (cortical tubers, subependymal nodules, giant cell astrocytomas). Kidney cysts and tumors (angiomyolipomas), cardiac tumors (rhabdomyomas), pulmonary cystic and fibrotic disease, and rectal polyps may also be seen.

■ SYNONYMS
• Bourneville's disease
• Epiloia

ICD-9CM CODE
759.5 Tuberous sclerosis

■ ETIOLOGY
• Two clearly identified genetic loci at 9q34 and 16p13
• Hypothesized that gene products may function as tumor suppressors
• Also hypothesized that tumors seen in TS may require the dysfunction of at least two genes—similar to the "two-hit" mutations responsible for retinoblastoma
  1. It is possible that genetic transmission provides the miscoding in one gene with spontaneous mutation supplying the other.

■ EPIDEMIOLOGY & DEMOGRAPHICS
• The second most common neurocutaneous syndrome seen in children (after neurofibromatosis)
• Prevalence of about 10 cases per 100,000 individuals
• Autosomal dominant inheritance but 50% to 70% of cases represent new mutations

■ HISTORY
• Seizures, especially infantile spasms
• Developmental delay/mental retardation
• Unusual skin lesions

■ PHYSICAL EXAMINATION
• Skin lesions
  1. Ash leaf spots: hypopigmented macules, often elliptical in shape
  2. Multiple café-au-lait spots in many patients as well
  3. Adenoma sebaceum: facial angiofibromas less than 0.5 cm in diameter, pink to red in color, seen in bilaterally symmetric distribution on the face around the nose and cheeks
  4. Shagreen patch: large patch of fused fibromas on the trunk in approximately 25% of patients with TS

  5. Ungual fibromas: fleshy growths along the nailbed
  6. Polygonal hypopigmented macules ("thumbprints"): most common but least specific skin lesions
  7. Confetti-type hypopigmented macules pathognomonic for TS
• *Note:* Visualization of all hypopigmented skin lesions is enhanced by ultraviolet/Wood's lamp illumination
• Teeth: characteristic diffuse small pits in the enamel
• Eye
  1. Hypopigmented areas in the iris occasionally seen
  2. Whitish yellow choroidal hamartomas around the optic nerve head on funduscopic examination
• Heart: symptoms of congestive heart failure possible (rare)
• Kidney: hypertension or hematuria (rare)
• Lungs: difficulty breathing, rales (rare)

DIAGNOSIS

■ DIFFERENTIAL DIAGNOSIS
• Neurofibromatosis
• Incontinentia pigmenti
• Linear sebaceous nevus syndrome
• Neurocutaneous melanosis

■ DIAGNOSTIC WORKUP
• Made on clinical grounds on the basis of characteristic distinctive malformations such as the following:
  1. Central nervous system and retinal hamartomas
  2. Skin angiofibromas
  3. Multiple less specific lesions as described previously

THERAPY

There is no specific or curative treatment for TS.

■ NONPHARMACOLOGIC
Educational and behavioral therapies are important in the management of developmental delays and mental retardation.

■ MEDICAL
Medical treatment of seizures and other complications is the same as if TS were not present.

■ SURGICAL
Surgical treatment is usually not undertaken until symptoms from a growing tumor appear.

■ FOLLOW-UP & DISPOSITION
• Periodic imaging of affected organs is necessary, especially imaging of the brain and kidneys.

• Many experts recommend magnetic resonance imaging of the head and renal ultrasound or a computed tomography scan every 1 to 2 years.
• Periodic echocardiography is also recommended.
• Developmental status and school performance should be followed closely.

■ PATIENT/FAMILY EDUCATION
• The risk of a child having TS if one parent is affected is 50%.
• Generally, the severity of various symptoms changes little over the years. If a child is mildly affected, the child is likely to remain mildly affected as he or she matures.
• Periodic screening may be necessary, as described previously.
• Parents should be educated regarding the common manifestations of TS.

■ REFERRAL INFORMATION
Most children with TS are referred to a neurologist. Other subspecialty referrals, including cardiology, nephrology, dermatology, and neurosurgery, may be warranted.

⚙ PEARLS & CONSIDERATIONS

■ CLINICAL PEARLS
• About 25% of children with infantile spasms have TS.
• The eye findings, although helpful diagnostically, are not symptomatic.
• Dental pitting is seen in virtually all patients by the time they reach adulthood.

■ WEBSITE
National Tuberous Sclerosis Association (NTSA): www.ntsa.org

■ SUPPORT GROUPS
• The National Tuberous Sclerosis Association has a support group. Information can be obtained from the preceding web address.
• There is a TS chat group available by sending an email message to tsctalk-requests@pebbs.com.
• Many cities and state regions have their own TS support groups. Neurologists often are aware of the support groups in the local area.

REFERENCES
1. Gomez MR: *Tuberous sclerosis: neurologic and psychiatric features,* ed 2, New York, 1988. Raven Press.
2. Online Mendelian Inheritance in Man (OMIM) at website www3.ncbi.nlm.nih.gov/omim/ (search "tuberous sclerosis"; this reference is updated several times per year).
Author: Jeffrey Kaczorowski, M.D.

II

BASIC INFORMATION

■ DEFINITION

Turner syndrome is a chromosomal condition in females in which the complete or partial absence of a second normal X chromosome results in short stature and ovarian failure.

■ SYNONYMS

- Ulrich-Turner syndrome
- XO genotype

ICD-9CM CODE

758.6 Turner syndrome

■ ETIOLOGY

- With conventional chromosomal studies, about 50% of Turner syndrome patients show a 45,X pattern
- Mosaicism of 45,X with other cell lines such as 46,XX, 46,XY, or 47,XXX are common.
- Structural abnormality of an X chromosome (deletions, rings, or translocations), either isolated or mosaic with a 45,X or 46,XX cell line, are also seen.
- With modern cytogenetic techniques, mosaicism is increasingly being detected
- The short stature in Turner syndrome appears to be caused by the absence of one copy of the SHOX gene, which is located on the short arm of the X chromosome

■ EPIDEMIOLOGY & DEMOGRAPHICS

- The incidence is 1 in 1500 to 1 in 2500 liveborn females among all racial groups.
- It affects approximately 3% of all females conceived, with only about 1% of these conspectuses surviving to term.

■ HISTORY

- Mild intrauterine growth retardation is followed by normal height increase from birth until approximately 3 years.
  1. After age 3, there is a progressive decrease in growth velocity until 14 years of age.
  2. Adolescent growth is prolonged because of delayed epiphyseal fusion. The final expected height typically falls between 142 and 146.8 cm (46 to 48 inches).
- Primary amenorrhea and infertility may occur.
- Prenatal diagnosis of Turner syndrome is becoming more common with increasing prenatal testing in advanced maternal age.
  1. Turner syndrome is not associated with advanced maternal age per se.

■ PHYSICAL EXAMINATION

- All ages
  1. Triangular faces
  2. Ptosis, strabismus
  3. Posteriorly rotated ears
  4. Short stature
  5. Shield chest, increased internipple distance
  6. Short fourth metacarpal
  7. Madelung deformity of the radius: cubitus valgus (increased carrying angle at the elbows)
  8. Nail dysplasia
- Newborn period
  1. Congenital lymphedema: puffy hands and feet, webbed neck
  2. Low posterior hairline
- Infancy
  1. Heart murmur
  2. Decreased peripheral pulses and capillary refill
- Childhood
  1. Short stature
  2. Hypertension
- Adolescence
  1. Delayed or absence of puberty
  2. Pigmented nevi

DIAGNOSIS

■ DIFFERENTIAL DIAGNOSIS

- Noonan syndrome affects both males and females and consists of Turner-like physical features, predominantly right-sided cardiac defects (e.g., pulmonic stenosis, asymmetric hypertrophy of the septum), and generally more significant developmental disabilities.
- Pure gonadal dysgenesis consists of a group of mendelian disorders in which affected individuals are phenotypically female but may have 46,XX or 46,XY chromosomal pattern.
- Mixed gonadal dysgenesis is associated with the presence of a testis on one side and a streak gonad on the contralateral side. Most patients with this disorder have a 45,X/46,XY chromosomal pattern.
- An isolated SHOX gene defect results in short stature and the skeletal manifestation of Turner syndrome, but it is not associated with primary amenorrhea or lymphedema.

■ DIAGNOSTIC WORKUP

- Routine chromosome study
  1. Occasionally, fluorescence in situ hybridization or other DNA-based methods may be used to define more complex alterations.
- Cardiac evaluation, often including echocardiography
  1. Aortic coarctation: approximately 20%
  2. Bicuspid aortic valve: approximately 50%

- Endocrine evaluation
  1. Primary hypothyroidism (10% to 30%), thyroiditis
  2. Glucose intolerance
  3. Delayed puberty and primary amenorrhea
- Renal ultrasound for anomalies
  1. Horseshoe kidney
  2. Ectopic kidneys
  3. Double collecting system
- Prenatal diagnosis
  1. Aided by ultrasound
     a. Thickened nuchal folds
     b. Cystic hygroma
     c. Renal anomalies
     d. Cardiac anomalies
  2. Definitive diagnosis done by chromosomal analysis on chorionic villus or amniocytes

THERAPY

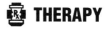

■ NONPHARMACOLOGIC

Support stocking for lymphedema

■ MEDICAL

- Growth hormone replacement therapy (usually with a weak anabolic agent such as oxandrolone) beginning between 2 to 5 years of age, until bone age exceeds 15 years
- Estrogen replacement beginning in adolescent years to promote the development of secondary sexual characteristics
- Thyroid replacement as needed

■ SURGICAL

- Repair of aortic coarctation if needed
- Ophthalmologic intervention for ptosis and strabismus if needed
- Plastic surgery
  1. Some families have elected to have plastic surgery to correct dysmorphic features.
- Myringotomy tube placement if needed

■ FOLLOW-UP & DISPOSITION

- Blood pressure monitoring
- Annual monitoring of thyroid function and glucose tolerance
- Monitoring of luteinizing hormone and follicle-stimulating hormone during adolescent years
- Annual check for scoliosis
- Hearing evaluation
- Monitoring for lymphedema, which may persist for months and even recur
- Monitoring for gastrointestinal bleeding resulting from mesenteric vascular abnormalities or inflammatory bowel disease
- Dietary management, exercise, and weight control
- Screen for learning disability, especially for deficits in attention, mathe-

matical and visuospatial organization skills

- Psychologic support for patient and family as needed
- Cardiac, otolaryngologic, ophthalmologic follow-up as needed

■ PATIENT/FAMILY EDUCATION

- For teenagers, sex education counseling should be done to emphasize that primary amenorrhea is not enough reason not to practice "safe sex."
- For late teens and young adults, counseling about modern reproductive technologies such as egg donation program should be done.
- Intelligence is usually normal except in patients with unusual chromosomal variants, such as a ring X chromosome.

■ PREVENTIVE TREATMENT

- Prophylactic antibiotics before dental procedure for patients with cardiac anomalies
- Aggressive treatment of middle ear disease to prevent conductive hearing loss

■ REFERRAL INFORMATION

- Cardiology
- Endocrine

- Genetics
- Developmental intervention as needed
- Nephrology, otolaryngology, ophthalmology, dermatology, plastic surgery as needed

☼ PEARLS & CONSIDERATIONS

■ CLINICAL PEARLS

- Because of the consistent presence of short stature and the variability of the other findings, which often manifest only during certain age windows, any girl with unexplained short stature should be evaluated for Turner syndrome by chromosome analysis.
- Approximately 10% of patients with Turner syndrome go through puberty spontaneously. The presence of pubic and axillary hair does not rule out primary ovarian failure.
- In prepubertal girls, the position of nipples lateral to the midclavicular line usually indicates increased internipple distance.
- When Turner syndrome is diagnosed, cytogenetic results should be evaluated carefully for the presence of a covert Y chromosome. DNA-

based studies may be needed for this purpose. The presence of a Y chromosome increases the risk for gonadoblastoma and dysgerminoma to 15% to 25%, necessitating prophylactic gonadectomy.

- Cheek-swab and Barr-body analysis are not acceptable for the diagnosis of Turner syndrome
- There is a tendency for keloid formation in patients with Turner syndrome, which should be taken into account when plastic surgery or removal of pigmented nevi are considered.

■ WEBSITE

Turner Syndrome Society: www.turner-syndrome-us.org/

REFERENCES

1. American Academy of Pediatrics Committee on Genetics: Health supervision for children with Turner syndrome, *Pediatrics* 96:1166, 1995.
2. Rosenfeld RG: Turner syndrome: a guide for physicians, 1992, The Turner Syndrome Society, Genetic Mason Medical Communications, Inc.
3. Saenger P: Turner's syndrome, *N Engl J Med* 335:1649, 1996.

Author: **Chin-To Fong, M.D.**

BASIC INFORMATION

■ DEFINITION
Ureteropelvic junction obstruction (UPJO) is a congenital resistance to the transport of urine from the renal pelvis into the proximal ureter.

■ SYNONYM
Ureteral valves—upper

ICD-9CM CODE
753.21 Congenital obstruction of ureteropelvic junction

■ ETIOLOGY
- The ureteropelvic junction (UPJ) is a normal site of relative narrowing of the urinary collecting system.
  1. UPJOs are partial blockages that commonly result in some degree of hydronephrosis.
  2. This hydronephrosis, in turn, may pose a risk to ultimate renal function.
  3. Obstructions are dynamic and may regress, progress, or remain unchanged over time.
  4. UPJOs may lie on a pathophysiologic continuum from the functionally irrelevant extrarenal pelvis, to the uniformly nonfunctioning multicystic dysplastic kidney (MCDK).
- Specific causes include the following:
  1. Intrinsic narrowing: 75%
     a. Aperistalsis
     b. Smooth muscle deficiency
  2. Ureterovascular tangles: 15%
  3. High, abnormal ureteral insertion: 7%
  4. Periureteral fibrosis: 3%
  5. Ureteral valve: rare

■ EPIDEMIOLOGY & DEMOGRAPHICS
- Prenatal ultrasound diagnosis of hydronephrosis occurs in 1% of all births.
  1. Approximately 50% of these patients have hydronephrosis at their postnatal examination.
- UPJO
  1. Incidence is 1 per 20,000: sporadic, but familial tendency.
  2. Male:female ratio is 2:1 to 4:1.
  3. There is a 15% to 40% incidence with horseshoe ectopic kidney.
  4. One third of patients with UPJO have the abnormality bilaterally.
     a. Degree of obstruction varies between kidneys
  5. Approximately 10% are associated with vesicoureteral reflux.

■ HISTORY
- Prenatal hydronephrosis
- Younger than 18 months old
  1. Visible abdominal mass
  2. Failure to thrive

3. Fever
4. Emesis
5. History of urinary tract infection
6. History of renal calculi
7. Hematuria
- Abdominal pain

■ PHYSICAL EXAMINATION
- Palpable abdominal mass (may transilluminate)
- Hypertension uncommon (0.1%)

🔬 DIAGNOSIS

■ DIFFERENTIAL DIAGNOSIS
- Prenatal hydronephrosis
  1. MCDK
  2. Vesicoureteral reflux
  3. Ureterovesical junction obstruction
  4. Megacalycosis
  5. Multiple renal cysts
- Abdominal mass
  1. MCDK
  2. Congenital mesoblastic nephroma
  3. Wilms' tumor
  4. Neuroblastoma

■ DIAGNOSTIC WORKUP
- Prenatally detected
  1. Serum creatinine after 5 days to reflect baby's renal status
- Ultrasound—renal and bladder
  1. Hydronephrosis without ureterectasis should be present.
  2. Assess for duplication anomaly (lower-pole UPJO is more common), parenchymal thickness, and presence of corticomedullary differentiation.
  3. Hydronephrosis is graded from 0 to 4 using the Society for Fetal Urology (SFU) scale (see "Websites").
  4. Early ultrasound, within first few days of life, may underestimate grading because of the relative decrease in urine output in the newborn.
  5. Solid masses should be defined by this study.
- Nuclear medicine scanning
  1. Radionuclide scans are used to assess relative function and drainage of the kidneys.
  2. ^{99}Tc-DTPA is filtered and therefore is used to calculate the glomerular filtration rate (relative function is calculated from this data).
     a. Administration of furosemide (Lasix) at a fixed time after administration, or at maximal filling of the renal pelvis, can aid in diagnosing abnormal drainage.
     b. Drainage or washout of radionuclide from the affected kidney is expected to be delayed.

c. Arbitrary categories of the T½ for the ^{99}Tc-DTPA studies are as follows:
     (1) Normal: less than 10 minutes
     (2) Equivocal: 10 to 20 minutes
     (3) Obstructed: more than 20 minutes
  d. The definition of T½ varies between centers.
  e. Patient variables (hydration; age; response, dose, and timing of furosemide) create a barrier for uniformity in these studies.
  3. "Well-tempered renogram" has been advocated by the SFU to provide some standardization and thus the ability to compare outcomes for advocated treatments (see website for reference and protocol).
  4. MAG-3 is cleared primarily by tubular secretion, with a small component filtered.
     a. This can be used to estimate renal plasma flow (relative function is calculated).
     b. Furosemide administration is used to assess poor drainage.
     c. Define areas of parenchymal loss.
  5. ^{99}Tc-DMSA and glucoheptonate bind to proximal tubular cells.
     a. Assess relative functional parenchyma.
     b. Furosemide administration is used to assess drainage.
     c. Define areas of parenchymal loss.
- Voiding cystourethrogram
  1. There was a reported 10% incidence of vesicoureteral reflux in UPJO series.
- Whitaker tests
  1. Antegrade pressure and flow studies originally described for use in adults
  2. Involve invasive, nonphysiologic infusions without standardization and are of anecdotal utility only

💊 THERAPY

■ NONPHARMACOLOGIC
- Observe the patient.
- Most cases of hydronephrosis, from prenatally detected UPJO, resolve upon continued follow-up postnatally.
- Some authors have advocated "aggressive observation" of all UPJOs.
  1. Only 1 in 4 cases require surgery; requisite events include the following:
     a. Symptoms
     b. Gross loss of function
     c. Urinary tract infections
  2. Optimal observation should not allow a 10% rate of renal injury to be incurred.

3. Application of this approach should be with care, in the well-counseled family.

MEDICAL
- Antibiotics
  1. One in three children with UPJO will have an associated urinary tract infection at some point in his or her care.
  2. Because the adverse effect of low-dose antibiotic prophylaxis is minimal, routine use of amoxicillin in neonates and nitrofurantoin or trimethoprim-sulfamethoxazole in infants is reasonable.
  3. Use of antibiotics in older children is best guided by cultures and manner of presentation.

SURGICAL
- Pyeloplasty
  1. The surgical principal is removal or bypass of the site of blockage.
  2. Drains, splints, nephrostomy tubes (direct catheter drainage of the affected renal pelvis), and timing of repair are a matter of surgeon preference.
  3. There is no clearly defined effect on long-term outcomes.
  4. This procedure is successful in more than 90% of patients treated.
- Endopyelotomy
  1. An incision is made at the site of blockage as visually defined through an endoscope or under fluoroscopy.

2. The instrument for incision may be inserted retrograde via the urethra/bladder/ureter or via a direct puncture into the renal pelvis through the kidney.
3. This procedure is successful in less than 80% of patients treated.
4. In cases of failed initial pyeloplasty, endopyelotomy is the procedure of choice and carries a success of up to 91%.

FOLLOW-UP & DISPOSITION
- Follow-up is dictated by therapy.
- One of three functionally unobstructed kidneys will show persistent hydronephrosis.
- Long-term follow-up is mandatory in all children with UPJO, regardless of grade, to ensure renal preservation and no increase in obstruction.

PATIENT/FAMILY EDUCATION
- The goal of therapy is to ensure optimal function of the involved kidney.
- The grade of hydronephrosis does not correlate to degree of obstruction.

REFERRAL INFORMATION
- Prenatal consultation with the pediatric urologist is highly encouraged.
- All patients with prenatal hydronephrosis should be evaluated by a pediatric urologist and those with bilateral findings (or UPJO in solitary kidneys) should be seen within 48 hours of birth.

☼ PEARLS & CONSIDERATIONS

CLINICAL PEARLS
- Approximately 33% of patients with kidneys with more than 12 mm of maximal renal pelvis diameter after 24 weeks' gestational age require eventual pyeloplasty.
- Hematuria following minor trauma should bring UPJO into the differential.
- Abdominal pain with UPJO is localized to the kidney whether in an orthotopic or ectopic location.
- Renal dysplasia may be noted on ultrasound as small cysts or echogenic foci within the parenchyma. This may influence therapeutic decisions.

WEBSITES
- Society for Fetal Urology: www.fetalurology.org
- Society of Pediatric Urology: www.spu.org

REFERENCES
1. Koff SA, Campbell KD: Non-operative management of unilateral neonatal hydronephrosis, *J Urol* 25:1, 1992.
2. Park JM, Bloom DA: The pathophysiology of UPJ obstruction: current concepts, *Urol Clin North Am* 25:2, 1998.
Authors: **Robert A. Mevorach, M.D., William C. Hulbert, M.D., and Ronald Rabinowitz, M.D.**

BASIC INFORMATION

■ DEFINITION
Urethritis is inflammation of the urethra as a result of any of a variety of infectious and noninfectious causes.

■ SYNONYMS
- Urethral inflammation
- Urethral irritation

ICD-9CM CODES
098.0 Gonococcal infection, acute, of lower genitourinary tract
098.2 Gonococcal infection, chronic, of lower genitourinary tract
099.40 Nongonococcal
099.3 Reiter's disease
099.41 Chlamydial
099.49 Specified organism

■ ETIOLOGY
- Infectious: local invasion of infectious (gonococcal or nongonococcal) organism into urethral lining cells with subsequent host inflammatory response
  1. Gonococcal urethritis is caused by *Neisseria gonorrhoeae*.
  2. Nongonococcal urethritis (NGU) is most commonly caused by *Chlamydia trachomatis;* less commonly it is caused by *Ureaplasma urealyticum*.
  3. Approximately 20% to 30% of NGU cases are caused by organisms such as *Haemophilus* species, *Bacteroides* or other anaerobes, genital mycoplasmas, *Candida albicans, Trichomonas vaginalis,* herpes simplex virus, human papillomavirus, or pinworm infestation.
     a. Genital infection with these organisms most commonly presents as urethritis in males and cervicitis in females.
- Noninfectious: physical (e.g., noncotton underwear in young girls, sexual abuse), or chemical (e.g., bubble bath, soaps, lotions, powders) irritation

■ EPIDEMIOLOGY & DEMOGRAPHICS
- Urethritis is most common in the older and sexually active male; only occasionally is it seen in the prepubertal child.
- Gonococcal urethritis is the most commonly reported sexually transmitted disease in the United States, accounting for 35% of adolescent males and men evaluated for urethritis.
- The incidence of gonococcal urethritis is decreasing, but the incidence of NGU is increasing.

■ HISTORY
- Adolescents and older children: dysuria, itching, and discharge
- Sexual activity
- Young children and infants: crying concomitant with voiding, urinary retention
- Use of bubble bath, irritating soaps or lotions, noncotton underwear, sexual abuse, poor hygiene in younger child

■ PHYSICAL EXAMINATION
- It is often difficult to differentiate gonococcal from nongonococcal urethritis based on symptoms and signs alone.
- Penile/urethral discharge, which is often purulent, mucoid, and yellow-green, is easily expressed; discharge may also be scant and clear.
- Erythematous, edematous urethral and periurethral tissues may be noted.

🔬 DIAGNOSIS

■ DIFFERENTIAL DIAGNOSIS
- Meatitis
- Balanitis
- Vaginitis
- Cervicitis

■ DIAGNOSTIC WORKUP
- Document the presence of urethritis with any of the following:
  1. Mucopurulent or purulent discharge in males
  2. Five or more leukocytes per oil immersion field on a Gram-stained smear of urethral secretions
  3. Intracellular (within polymorphonuclear leukocytes) gram-negative diplococci in a Gram-stained urethral discharge specimen for gonorrhea
  4. Ten or more white blood cells (WBCs) per high-power field in the sediment of a first-void, early-morning urine specimen
- Newer DNA amplification assays (polymerase chain reaction [PCR] and ligase chain reaction) for *N. gonorrhoeae* and *C. trachomatis* are largely replacing traditional cultures because of their greater sensitivity and ease and convenience of patient sample collection.
- For males with urethritis who have a purulent discharge:
  1. Perform Gram stain on urethral discharge.
  2. Send swab of discharge for PCR test for *N. gonorrhoeae* and *C. trachomatis*.
  3. Treat for infection with both *N. gonorrhoeae* and *C. trachomatis*.

- For males with urethritis but no discharge:
  1. Send first 15 ml of a first-voided urine for PCR test for *N. gonorrhoeae* and *C. trachomatis*.
  2. Send urine for urinalysis and urine culture.
  3. Defer therapy until test results for *N. gonorrhoeae* and *C. trachomatis* are available, except in patients unlikely to return for follow-up evaluation, in which case treatment should be given for both gonorrheal and chlamydial infection.
- If opted for, culture *N. gonorrhoeae* on Thayer-Martin medium/chocolate agar:
  1. Males: Proper culture is obtained by inserting a small, noncotton swab 2 to 3 cm into the urethra and plating the specimen immediately onto appropriate culture media.
  2. Females: Proper culture is obtained by first wiping the exocervix and then placing a noncotton swab into the cervical os and rotating the swab several times; the specimen is then immediately plated onto appropriate culture media.
- *C. trachomatis* culture: The swab is placed into *Chlamydia* transport media.
- Viral culture should be done for herpes simplex when suspected.

💊 THERAPY

■ MEDICAL
- Patients infected with *N. gonorrhoeae* are often coinfected with *C. trachomatis* and are most often treated for both organisms presumptively, especially when follow-up cannot be ensured.
- In populations in which coinfection rates are low, patients may be treated for gonorrhea and tested for *Chlamydia* if follow-up is ensured.
- Recommended regimens for the treatment of gonococcal urethritis are as follows:
  1. Cefixime 400 mg orally in a single dose, *or*
  2. Ceftriaxone 125 mg intramuscularly in a single dose, *or*
  3. Ciprofloxacin 500 mg orally in a single dose, *or*
  4. Ofloxacin 400 mg orally in a single dose, *plus*
  5. Azithromycin 1 g orally in a single dose, *or*
  6. Doxycycline 100 mg orally twice a day for 7 days

- Recommended regimens for the treatment of NGU are as follows:
  1. Azithromycin 1 g orally in a single dose, *or*
  2. Doxycycline 100 mg orally twice a day for 7 days
- Alternative regimens include the following:
  1. Erythromycin base 500 mg orally four times a day for 7 days, *or*
  2. Erythromycin ethylsuccinate 800 mg orally four times a day for 7 days, *or*
  3. Ofloxacin 300 mg orally twice a day for 7 days
- If only erythromycin can be used and a patient cannot tolerate high-dose erythromycin, one of the following regimens can be used:
  1. Erythromycin base 250 mg orally four times a day for 14 days, *or*
  2. Erythromycin ethylsuccinate 400 mg orally four times a day for 14 days
- Recommended regimens for the treatment of recurrent or persistent urethritis are as follows*:
  1. Metronidazole 2 g orally in a single dose, *plus*
  2. Erythromycin base 500 mg orally four times a day for 7 days, *or*
  3. Erythromycin ethylsuccinate 800 mg orally four times a day for 7 days
- Recommended regimens for the treatment of chlamydial infection in adolescents are as follows:
  1. Azithromycin 1 g orally in a single dose, *or*
  2. Doxycycline 100 mg orally twice a day for 7 days
- Alternative regimens include the following:
  1. Erythromycin base 500 mg orally four times a day for 7 days, *or*

2. Erythromycin ethylsuccinate 800 mg orally four times a day for 7 days, *or*
3. Ofloxacin 300 mg orally twice a day for 7 days
- Recommended regimens for the treatment of chlamydial infection in children are as follows:
- Children who weigh less than 45 kg:
  1. Erythromycin base 50 mg/kg/day orally divided four times daily for 10 to 14 days*
  2. Children who weigh more than 45 kg but who are younger than 8 years of age:
     a. Azithromycin 1 g orally in a single dose
  3. Children older than 8 years of age:
     a. Azithromycin 1 g orally in a single dose, *or*
     b. Doxycycline 100 mg orally twice a day for 7 days

■ PATIENT/FAMILY EDUCATION & PREVENTIVE TREATMENT
- Counsel patients that sexual activity is the most common mode of transmission.
- Each and every sexual contact of an infected individual needs to be evaluated and treated.
- Preventive measures that are most successful include abstinence, use of condoms, and good hygiene.

■ REFERRAL INFORMATION
- Adolescent medicine specialist, especially in complicated cases
- Child protective services (social services) evaluation for possibility of sexual abuse in young children found to be infected with *N. gonorrhoeae* or *C. trachomatis*

✵ PEARLS & CONSIDERATIONS

■ CLINICAL PEARLS
- Most individuals with NGU are asymptomatic.
- Potential complications arising from urethritis may include epididymitis and Reiter's syndrome in males and pelvic inflammatory disease and infertility in females.

■ WEBSITES
- Journal of the American Medical Association: Sexually Transmitted Disease Information Center: www.ama-assn.org/special/std/treatmnt/guide/stdg3443.htm
- Centers for Disease Control and Prevention: Sexually Transmitted Diseases Website: http://www.cdc.gov/od/owh/whstd.htm

REFERENCES
1. Centers for Disease Control and Prevention: 1998 guidelines for treatment of sexually transmitted diseases, *MMWR Morb Mortal Wkly Rep* 47(No. RR-1):49, 1998.
2. Gaydos CA et al: Molecular amplification assays to detect chlamydial infections in urine specimens from high school female students and to monitor the persistence of chlamydial DNA after therapy, *J Infect Dis* 177:417, 1998.
3. Oh MK et al: High prevalence of *Chlamydia trachomatis* infections in adolescent females not having pelvic examinations: utility of PCR-based urine screening in an urban adolescent clinic setting, *J Adolesc Health* 21:80, 1997.

Author: **Chris Nelson, M.D.**

---

*Assumes compliance with initial treatment regimen and no reexposure to infected individuals; wet-mount examination and urethral swab culture for *T. vaginalis* should be performed.

---

*The effectiveness of treatment with erythromycin is approximately 80%; a second course of therapy may be required.

BASIC INFORMATION

■ DEFINITION

Infection of the bladder or lower urinary tract is called *cystitis;* infection of the kidney or upper urinary tract is termed *acute pyelonephritis.*

■ SYNONYMS

- Kidney infection
- Bladder infection
- Cystitis

ICD-9CM CODES

599.0   Urinary tract infection, site not specific
590.10 Acute pyelonephritis
595.0   Acute cystitis

■ ETIOLOGY

- Organisms: *Escherichia coli* is responsible for 85% of cases; other gram-negative bacteria include *Klebsiella pneumoniae, Proteus* species, *Pseudomonas aeruginosa,* and *Enterobacter* species. Gram-positive organisms (less common) include enterococci, staphylococci, and group B streptococci.
- Mechanisms: Ascending infection or hematogenous dissemination (neonates) are possible.
- Predisposing risk factors include vesicoureteral reflux (VUR), congenital renal anomalies (e.g., hydronephrosis, posterior urethral valves), neurologic abnormalities (e.g., dysfunctional voiding, neurogenic bladder), uncircumcised boys, infant girls, constipation, indwelling catheters, and sexual activity.

■ EPIDEMIOLOGY & DEMOGRAPHICS

- Urinary tract infection (UTI) is the most common serious bacterial infection in febrile infants.
- Overall, there is a 5% prevalence in febrile infants.
- Prevalence is high in young children when no apparent source of fever is identified.
- High prevalence (17%) is seen in Caucasian girls with temperatures greater than 39° C.
- Uncircumcised boys have a tenfold higher risk than circumcised boys.
- Male infants younger than 2 months of age are more likely to develop a UTI than girls of the same age.
- In children 2 months to 2 years, girls have a 2.3-fold higher risk than boys.

■ HISTORY

- Wide range of symptoms, nonspecific symptoms more likely in neonates and infants

- Cystitis
  1. Specific: frequency, urgency, dysuria
  2. Nonspecific: irritability, fever
- Pyelonephritis
  1. Specific: flank pain
  2. Nonspecific: fever, rigors, poor feeding, vomiting, failure to thrive

■ PHYSICAL EXAMINATION

- Varies from normal to toxic appearance
- Fever, signs of sepsis (e.g., hypotension, tachycardia, lethargy, hyperpnea, tachypnea), jaundice (neonate), costovertebral angle tenderness, abdominal tenderness

🔬 DIAGNOSIS

■ DIFFERENTIAL DIAGNOSIS

- Occult bacteremia
- Sepsis
- Metabolic disease
- Other abdominal and retroperitoneal disease (e.g., acute gastroenteritis, appendicitis, pelvic inflammatory disease, vaginitis, cervicitis).

■ DIAGNOSTIC WORKUP

Methods of urine collection include the following:
- Infants and children with no bladder control: catheterized urine or suprapubic aspiration
- Older children: midstream, clean-catch specimen
Laboratory evaluation includes the following:
- Urinalysis (UA)
  1. "Enhanced" UA, preferred method (see box on the following page)
     a. Pyuria: more than 10 white blood cells (WBCs)/mm^3 (uncentrifuged urine)
     b. Bacteriuria: any bacteria/any of 10 oil immersion fields (Gram-stained smear)
  2. Standard UA
     a. Pyuria: more than 5 WBCs/high-power field (centrifuged urine)
     b. Bacteriuria: any bacteria/high-power field (unstained)
  3. Urine dipstick for leukocyte esterase and nitrite, poor sensitivity for detecting UTI
- Urine culture
  1. Urine culture may be eliminated in a child with a negative enhanced UA.
  2. Obtain urine culture in a child with the following:
     a. Previous history of UTI
     b. Anomalies of the urinary tract
     c. Planned treatment with antimicrobials.

  3. Urine culture is considered positive if the following criteria are met:
     a. Suprapubic specimen: any bacterial growth
     b. Catheterized specimen: more than 50,000 colony-forming units (CFU)/ml, single pathogen
     c. Midstream specimen: more than 100,000 CFU/ml, single pathogen
Radiologic evaluation includes the following:
- Radiologic evaluation should be performed in the following cases:
  1. Acute pyelonephritis
  2. First UTI in boy, any age
  3. First UTI in girl younger than 3 years of age
  4. Second UTI in girl 3 years or older
  5. First UTI in child of any age with family history of UTIs, urinary tract abnormalities, voiding abnormalities, hypertension, or poor growth
- Renal ultrasound (US) is used to identify gross anatomic abnormalities. Because of the widespread use of prenatal US, it may be redundant if known to have a normal, late prenatal US. Obtain US in patients with poor clinical response within 48 hours of antimicrobial therapy.
- Voiding cystourethrogram (VCUG) is used to identify VUR. Perform immediately after therapy, thus eliminating the need for prophylaxis. If unable to schedule immediately after therapy, keep patient on antimicrobial prophylaxis until VCUG can be done.
- ^{99m}Tc-dimercaptosuccinic acid (DMSA) or ^{99m}Tc-glucoheptonate is used to identify acute pyelonephritis and renal scars. It is of limited value during acute pyelonephritis. It is useful to detect renal scars if performed at least 5 months after infection.
- Intravenous pyelography is no longer used routinely. It has been replaced by renal US because of its noninvasiveness and comparable accuracy.

💊 THERAPY

Pyelonephritis
- Oral therapy
  1. Cefixime (double dose on day 1) is the only oral antimicrobial evaluated in a randomized, controlled trial for UTI in young children with fever.
  2. Other possible antimicrobials include second- and third-generation cephalosporins or amoxicillin-clavulanate potassium.

3. Resistance rates of *Escherichia coli* to amoxicillin and trimethoprim-sulfamethoxazole (TMP-SMX) are 50% and 18%, respectively.
4. Duration of treatment is 10 to 14 days.

- Parenteral therapy (if toxic appearing or unable to tolerate an oral antimicrobial)
  1. Second-generation (cefuroxime) or third-generation (cefotaxime, ceftriaxone) cephalosporin, ampicillin-sulbactam, or gentamicin may be used.
  2. Switch to oral medications when patient becomes afebrile. Continue oral treatment to complete 10- to 14-day course.

Cystitis
- Oral
- Second or third-generation cephalosporins, amoxicillin-clavulanate potassium, trimethoprim-sulfamethoxazole

Other Therapeutic Considerations
- Dysfunctional voiding: liberal intake of fluids, frequent voiding (every 1 to 2 hours)
- Management of constipation

■ FOLLOW-UP & DISPOSITION
- Repeat urine culture within 48 to 72 hours if the clinical response is poor. Routine "test of cure" is generally not necessary.
- If VUR is detected, need prophylaxis with nitrofurantoin (1 to –2 mg/kg/day) or TMP-SMX (2 mg/kg/day) for 1 year. Perform a radionuclide cystogram at 1 year to determine the need for continued prophylaxis.
- If the patient has recurrent UTI (more than two in 6 months or more than three in 1 year) but no VUR,

may still consider prophylaxis for 6 months, as just stated.

■ PATIENT/FAMILY EDUCATION
- In young girls: cleaning front to back, frequent diaper changes, avoiding bubble baths
- Cranberry juice
- Need for evaluation of fever in patients with history of UTI or with underlying anomalies of the urinary tract

■ PREVENTIVE TREATMENT
See "Follow-Up & Disposition."

■ REFERRAL INFORMATION
Refer to a urologist if grade III or higher VUR or recurrence of UTI to assess for surgical repair and ureteral reimplantation.

☼ PEARLS & CONSIDERATIONS

■ CLINICAL PEARLS
The "enhanced" UA may become the preferred method for UA.

■ WEBSITES
- National Institute of Diabetes & Digestive & Kidney Diseases: www.niddk.nih.gov/health/urolog/pubs/utichild/utichild.htm
- Johns Hopkins: www.med.jhu.edu

REFERENCES
1. American Academy of Pediatrics: Practice guideline: the diagnosis, treatment, and evaluation of the initial urinary tract infection in febrile infants and young children, *Pediatrics* 103:843, 1999.
2. Batisky D: Pediatric urinary tract infections, *Pediatr Ann* 25:269, 1996.
3. Crain EF, Gershel JC: Urinary tract infection in febrile infants younger than 8 weeks of age, *Pediatrics* 86:363, 1990.
4. Hoberman A, Wald ER: UTI in young children: new light on old questions, *Contemp Pediatr* 14:140, 1997.
5. Hobertman A et al: Oral versus initial intravenous therapy for urinary tract infections in young febrile children, *Pediatrics* 104:79, 1999.
6. Rushton GH: Urinary tract infections in children: epidemiology, evaluation and management, *Pediatr Clin North Am* 44:1133, 1997.
Authors: **Rosemary Amofah Dayie, M.D., and Alejandro Hoberman, M.D.**

The Enhanced Urinalysis
The enhanced urinalysis is performed on a specimen of uncentrifuged urine. The urine is drawn into a Neubauer hemocytometer by capillary action. White blood cells (WBCs) are counted on one side of the chamber and multiplied by 1.1 to obtain a total cell count per cubic millimeter. *Pyuria* is at least 10 WBCs per cubic millimeter. Smears are prepared by using 2 drops of uncentrifuged urine on a sterile slide within a standardized marked area of 1.5-cm diameter, air-dried, and Gram-stained. *Bacteremia* is any bacteria per 10 oil immersion fields. The positive predictive value of both pyuria and bacteremia is 93.1%.

II

BASIC INFORMATION

DEFINITION
Urolithiasis is an abnormal development of calculi, or stones, in the urinary tract.

SYNONYMS
- Nephrolithiasis
- Renal stone disease
- Kidney stone
- Urinary calculi

ICD-9CM CODE
592.9 Urinary calculus, unspecified

ETIOLOGY
- Metabolic conditions, the most common cause, involve concentration of precipitating substances in the urine, which form stones.
- Urinary tract anomalies and infections are also a common cause in children.
  1. Calcium stones are the most common type, either calcium oxalate or calcium phosphate.
     a. Hypercalciuria can occur with or without hypercalcemia.
     b. Diet-dependent hypercalciuria is more common in adults.
     c. Hyperoxaluria, either primary or secondary, may occur.
     d. Hypocitraturia is a condition with decreased levels of stone inhibitor.
  2. Struvite stones are associated with urinary tract infections.
     a. Only occur with urease-producing bacteria
        (1) Gram-negative rods include *Proteus, Providencia, Klebsiella, Pseudomonas,* and *Serratia.*
        (2) Other organisms include *Streptococcus* and *Mycoplasma.*
     b. Composed of magnesium ammonium phosphate
     c. Precipitate at pH greater than 6.8
  3. Uric acid stones are a third type of renal stone.
     a. Hyperuricosuria with or without hyperuricemia
     b. Precipitate at pH less than 5.8
  4. Cystine stones are usually associated with cystinuria.
     a. Cystinuria: an autosomal recessive trait
     b. Precipitate at pH less than 7.0
  5. Rare stones include xanthine, orotic acid, and dihydroxyadenine.

EPIDEMIOLOGY & DEMOGRAPHICS
- The incidence is 1 in 1000 to 1 in 7600 pediatric hospital admissions in the United States.
- Boys and girls are affected equally, unlike adults.

- Greater risk is seen in southern California and southeastern states.
- Caucasian children are more at risk than African-American children.
- In developed countries, most stones are in the upper urinary tract.
- Bladder stones are endemic in Africa and Asia.

HISTORY
- Children do not usually present with the classic symptoms of renal colic.
- Pain can be abdominal, flank, or pelvic.
- Gross (or microscopic) hematuria is often present.
- Symptoms of urinary tract infection (UTI) are noted almost half the time:
  1. Fever
  2. Dysuria
  3. Urgency
  4. Frequency
- Obstructive symptoms are less common:
  1. Urinary retention
  2. Anuria
  3. Nausea
  4. Vomiting
- Colicky or persistent abdominal pain may be described along the entire length of the ureter from the flank and lateral abdominal walls to the lower abdomen, pelvis, and groin.
- Family, medication, and dietary histories are important to assess risk.

PHYSICAL EXAMINATION
- It is important to determine signs of congenital or anatomic abnormalities and systemic disorders.
- Blood pressure, height, and weight can provide clues about systemic disease or chronic renal failure.
- Findings consistent with stones include abdominal and flank tenderness.
- Plain films together with ultrasound are gaining acceptance as the initial tests.

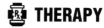 **DIAGNOSIS**

DIFFERENTIAL DIAGNOSIS
- Other renal disease such as pyelonephritis or obstruction (e.g., ureteropelvic or vesicoureteral stenosis)
- Gastrointestinal disease such as appendicitis, volvulus, intussusception, or gastroenterocolitis
- Genital tract disease such as ovarian or testicular torsion or pelvic inflammatory disease

DIAGNOSTIC WORKUP
- Radiologic
  1. Ultrasound with plain films are the most reliable initial tests.
  2. Intravenous urography is more invasive and less sensitive in children.

  3. Most stones can be seen on plain abdominal radiographs.
     a. Cystine stones are weakly radiopaque.
     b. Uric acid stones are radiolucent.
- Urine studies
  1. Urinalysis should be done to assess pH, pyuria, bacteriuria, and crystals.
  2. Urine culture should be done when UTI is suspected.
  3. A 24-hour urine sample can be analyzed for calcium, uric acid, phosphorus, citrate, sodium, cystine, and creatinine concentrations.
     a. Normal 24-hour urine calcium excretion is less than 4 mg/kg/day.
  4. Spot urinary solute:creatinine ratios are easier to obtain but are less reliable.
     a. Normal infant value for calcium:creatinine ratio is less than 0.42.
     b. Normal child value for calcium:creatinine ratio is less than 0.21.
- Blood work: should include complete blood count, blood urea nitrogen, creatinine, calcium, phosphorus, uric acid, and electrolytes
  1. Consider parathyroid hormone level if serum or urine calcium is high.

THERAPY

MEDICAL
For management of acute symptoms:
- Pain relief
- Oral or parenteral hydration, 1.5 to 2 times maintenance
- Treatment of concomitant UTI

SURGICAL
- Indications for surgical stone removal include intractable pain, persistent obstruction, and persistent UTI.
- Shock-wave lithotripsy, percutaneous techniques, and endourologic treatments are replacing open stone surgery.
- Congenital anomalies in young children may necessitate open surgical repair.

PREVENTIVE TREATMENT
- High fluid intake to keep urine volume high and specific gravity low
- If a child has hypercalciuria:
  1. Low-sodium diet
  2. Low-oxalate diet
  3. Hydrochlorothiazide (1 to 2 mg/kg/day)

4. Potassium citrate (1 to 4 mg/kg/day) in cases of hypocitraturia or renal acidosis contributing to calcium stone formation
- If a child has cystinuria:
  1. Low-sodium diet
  2. Potassium citrate
  3. Chelating agents: considered with recurrent stones
- If a child has hyperuricosuria:
  1. Potassium citrate
  2. Allopurinol (10 mg/kg/day)

■ **REFERRAL INFORMATION**
- Pediatric urologist for congenital anomalies and surgical management
- Pediatric nephrologist for medical management of metabolic conditions

☼ PEARLS & CONSIDERATIONS

■ **WEBSITE**
National Institute of Diabetes & Digestive & Kidney Diseases: www.niddk.nih.gov

REFERENCES

1. Cohen TD et al: Pediatric urolithiasis: medical and surgical management, *Urology* 47:292, 1996.
2. Drach GW: Metabolic evaluation of pediatric patients with stones, *Urol Clin North Am* 22:95, 1995.
3. Santos-Victoriano M, Brouhard BH, Cunningham RJ III: Renal stone disease in children, *Clin Pediatr* 37:583, 1998.
4. Stapleton FB: Clinical approach to children with urolithiasis, *Semin Nephrol* 16:389, 1996.

Author: **Edgard A. Segura, M.D.**

II

BASIC INFORMATION

■ DEFINITION
Urticaria is a rash characterized by the appearance of pruritic, erythematous, cutaneous elevations that blanch with pressure.

■ SYNONYMS
- Hives
- Welts

ICD-9CM CODES
708.9 Unspecified urticaria
708.8 Chronic urticaria
995.1 Urticaria with angioneurotic edema

■ ETIOLOGY
- Urticaria results from the release of a variety of vasoactive mediators that arise from the immune (e.g., immunoglobulin E [IgE]) or nonimmune (e.g., physical stimuli) activation of cells (e.g., mast cells—histamine, prostaglandin D_2, leukotrienes C and D, platelet-activating factor) or enzymatic pathways (e.g., complement system or Hageman factor–dependent pathway).
- Biopsy of an urticarial lesion reveals dilation of small venules and capillaries located in the superficial dermis with widening of the dermal papillae, flattening of the rete pegs, and swelling of collagen fibers.
- Angioedema (swelling), which often occurs with urticaria, occurs in deeper skin layers.
- Urticaria/angioedema can be triggered by multiple causes, including exogenous factors (e.g., foods, drugs, contactants) or endogenous disease states with allergic, inflammatory, or infectious mechanisms.
- In chronic urticaria, an underlying cause often is not found.

■ EPIDEMIOLOGY & DEMOGRAPHICS
- Acute urticaria is common, affecting as many as 10% to 20% of the population at some time in their life.
- When the duration of urticaria exceeds 6 weeks, it is designated as *chronic*.
- Acute urticaria is more common in children and young adults, whereas the peak incidence of chronic urticaria is during the third and fourth decades of life.

■ HISTORY
- A thorough, detailed history is essential to accurately diagnose the underlying cause of urticaria.
- Information should include the following:
  1. Onset, duration, distribution, pattern (e.g., relationship to food or drug ingestion) of lesions

2. Physical exposures (e.g., cold, pressure, heat, exercise, vibrations, sunlight, water)
3. Associated symptoms (e.g., fever, joint pain, gastrointestinal symptoms)
4. History of atopy (e.g., allergic rhinitis or asthma)
5. Environmental (especially pets) exposures
6. Current medications (e.g., prescription and over-the-counter medications such as nonsteroidal antiinflammatory drugs or herbal remedies)
7. Menstrual cycle and oral contraceptive pill use in females
8. Travel history
9. Family history of hives (e.g., Muckle-Wells syndrome) or angioedema (hereditary angioneurotic edema)

■ PHYSICAL EXAMINATION
- A thorough examination is required to exclude an underlying systemic condition.
- The size and pattern of urticarial lesions can vary greatly. If individual lesions persist longer than 24 hours, other diagnoses should be considered.
- Lesions are anywhere from several millimeters to 10 to 20 cm, but in general, they are 2 to 8 cm.
- Lesions may present anywhere on the body.
- They are palpable, pink, and blanch.
- They may last minutes to hours.
- Lesions are very pruritic.
- They do not leave scars.
- Lesions may coalesce and look serpiginous or serpentarial.

DIAGNOSIS

■ DIFFERENTIAL DIAGNOSIS
- Urticarial vasculitis has a characteristic residual pigmentation; palpable purpura and petechiae; arthralgias and myalgias; and palm, sole, and extremity predilection.
- Erythema multiforme can also resemble acute urticaria but usually has target lesions that are slightly raised, not necessarily pruritic, and often found on the extremities.

■ DIAGNOSTIC WORKUP
- Acute urticaria is generally a straightforward diagnosis based on the history (e.g., temporal relationship to food or drug ingestion) and physical examination.
- The cause of chronic urticaria is often unknown despite an in-depth evaluation. Fortunately, idiopathic chronic urticaria is usually self-limited and benign. Recurrences are common.

1. The extent of the laboratory evaluation for chronic urticaria depends on the history.
2. Commonly obtained tests (especially if vasculitis suspected) include the following:
   a. Complete blood count and differential
   b. Erythrocyte sedimentation rate
   c. Antinuclear antibody
   d. Urinalysis
   e. Complement studies
   f. Antithyroid antibody
   g. Skin biopsy

THERAPY

■ NONPHARMACOLOGIC
If identified, any inciting agent (e.g., drug, food, or physical factor such as sunlight, cold, heat, pressure) should be avoided.

■ MEDICAL
- Oral antihistamines remain the first-line drugs of choice.
- Sedating antihistamines (diphenhydramine or hydroxyzine) effectively control itching and the number and size of lesions. However, their use (especially chronic) is limited by undesirable side effects (sedation or paradoxical activity).
- Nonsedating antihistamines can help suppress chronic idiopathic urticaria. The loratadine (Claritin) dosage is 10 mg/day in children older than 6 years of age.
- Fexofenadine, a nonsedating antihistamine, is not currently approved for urticaria but is approved in children 12 years and older with allergic rhinitis.
- A "low-sedating" antihistamine like cetirizine (Zyrtec) is recommended for chronic idiopathic urticaria in children 2 years old and older.
  1. Initial dosages: age 2 to 5 years: 2.5 mg/day; age 6 to 11 years: 5 to 10 mg/day; age 12 years and older: 10 mg/day
- H_2 antagonists (e.g., cimetidine, ranitidine) have been used with H_1 antihistamines in some adults to help relieve pruritus and wheal formation.
- Epinephrine by injection can provide short-lived relief in patients with severe urticaria or angioedema.
- Mast-cell stabilizers (e.g., nedocromil or cromolyn) are not effective agents for urticaria.
- Oral corticosteroids are effective antiinflammatory agents that can provide short-term relief for acute flares of urticaria (e.g., food- or drug-induced, delayed pressure urticaria).
  1. Long-term side effects limit the usefulness of corticosteroids in chronic urticaria.
  2. Patients with urticarial vasculitis

may require high dosages of corticosteroids, and relapses can occur when the corticosteroids are tapered.
- Leukotriene antagonists have shown efficacy in chronic urticaria.

■ PATIENT/FAMILY EDUCATION
- Education of parents and patients about symptoms and triggers of urticaria
- Appropriate use of medications, especially extended administration of antihistamines for adequate control of chronic urticaria

■ REFERRAL INFORMATION
Consider referral to an allergist or dermatologist for patients with prolonged manifestations of urticaria or angioedema that impair functioning or quality of life and require more extensive evaluation (e.g., skin biopsy to exclude the diagnosis of vasculitis).

○ PEARLS & CONSIDERATIONS

■ CLINICAL PEARLS
- Dermographism ("write on skin"), a physical urticaria affecting 2% to 5% of the population, occurs within 2 to 5 minutes of gently stroking the skin with a tongue blade or fingernail. Systemic symptoms are absent.
- Dermagraphism can follow an acute viral infection or drug reaction; it is commonly seen in patients with chronic urticaria.

■ WEBSITES
- American Academy of Allergy, Asthma, and Immunology: www.aaai.org
- American College of Allergy, Asthma, and Immunology: www.acaai.org

REFERENCES
1. Kaplan AP: Urticaria and angioedema. In Middleton E et al (eds): *Allergy: principles and practice,* St Louis, 1998, Mosby.
2. Zacharisen MC: Pediatric urticaria and angioedema, *Immunol Allergy Clin North Am* 19:363, 1999.

Author: **Thomas J. Fischer, M.D.**

II

BASIC INFORMATION

■ DEFINITION
- Uveitis is inflammation of the uveal tract.
- It is further differentiated by anatomic site (e.g., iritis, cyclitis, vitreitis) or linearly along the axis of the eye (anterior, intermediate, or posterior).
- Uveitis may be acute or chronic.

ICD-9CM CODES
364.00 Iritis, acute, unspecified
364.11 Iritis, chronic, other disease

■ ETIOLOGY
- Anterior: in pediatric age group, often traumatic
  1. Infectious diseases such as herpes simplex, herpes zoster, Lyme disease
  2. Rheumatologic disorders such as juvenile arthritis, Crohn's disease
  3. Vasculitis such as Kawasaki disease
- Intermediate
  1. Pars planitis (inflammation of the pars plana, a part of the uveal tract)
- Posterior
  1. Infectious diseases such as toxoplasmosis, toxocara, human immunodeficiency virus
  2. Neoplastic disorders such as retinoblastoma, lymphoma
  3. Rheumatologic disorders such as sarcoidosis

■ EPIDEMIOLOGY & DEMOGRAPHICS
- Approximately 5% of all uveitis cases are pediatric.
- About 50% of pediatric uveitis cases are posterior, most commonly toxoplasmosis.
- No cause is found in 50% of pediatric anterior uveitis cases.
- About 25% of pediatric uveitis is intermediate.

■ HISTORY
- Anterior: unilateral or bilateral red eye, light sensitivity, pain, headache, tearing but usually no discharge
- Intermediate: gradual onset, bilateral, decreased vision, floaters
- Posterior: unilateral or bilateral, decreased vision, floaters, distorted vision

■ PHYSICAL EXAMINATION
- Anterior
  1. Conjunctival injection, especially encircling the limbus
  2. Mid-dilated pupil and occasionally an irregular pupil because of scarring of the iris to the anterior surface of lens
  3. Anterior segment cells and occasionally corneal edema
- Intermediate
  1. Classic finding is "snowbanking" (a collection of cells in the vitreous at the pars plana seen by indirect ophthalmoscopy).
- Posterior
  1. Usually unilateral findings
  2. White cells in the vitreous and inflammatory cells lining retinal vasculature seen by ophthalmoscopy

DIAGNOSIS

■ DIFFERENTIAL DIAGNOSIS
- Diagnosis based on the physical examination and differentiated on the basis of location of inflammation
- Anterior uveitis differential and workup
  1. May defer workup in first case of anterior uveitis, especially if trauma is involved
  2. Juvenile arthritis: systemic examination and antinuclear antibodies
  3. Trauma
  4. Herpes simplex or zoster
  5. Lyme disease: serology
  6. Unknown: 50% of cases

- Intermediate uveitis: differential and workup
  1. Unknown
  2. Sarcoid
  3. Lyme disease
- Posterior uveitis: differential and workup
  1. Toxoplasmosis: toxoplasmosis IgG and IgM titers
  2. Ocular histoplasmosis: diagnosis on basis of history and ophthalmic examination
  3. Toxocariasis: may have increased eosinophils, enzyme-linked immunosorbent assay

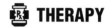

THERAPY

■ MEDICAL
- Topical steroids and cycloplegia may be given under the supervision of an ophthalmologist.
- Occasionally, systemic steroids or other antimicrobials will be necessary.

■ SURGICAL
Rarely, in some cases of posterior uveitis, photocoagulation or surgery may be required.

■ FOLLOW-UP & DISPOSITION
- Children at risk for uveitis should be referred to an ophthalmologist.
- A patient with persistent red eye, photophobia, or decreased vision should be referred to an ophthalmologist.
- Uveitis should be treated by an ophthalmologist.

REFERENCES
1. Giles CL: Uveitis in children. In Nelson LB, Calhoun JH, Harley R (eds): *Pediatric ophthalmology,* ed 3, Philadelphia, 1991, WB Saunders.
2. Uveitis in the pediatric age group. In *Basic and clinical science course,* San Francisco, 1998-1999, American Academy of Ophthalmology.
Author: **Anna F. Fakadej, M.D., F.A.A.O.**

BASIC INFORMATION

DEFINITION
Vaginitis is inflammation of the vaginal mucosa.

ICD-9CM CODES
616.10 Acute, chronic, nonspecific
616.10 Bacterial
112.1 Candidal
131.01 Trichomonal

ETIOLOGY
- Prepubertal cases are most commonly caused by the following:
  1. Group A β-hemolytic streptococci
  2. Coagulase-positive *Staphylococcus*
  3. *Shigella*
  4. Other coliform bacteria from fecal contamination (*Haemophilus influenzae* controversial)
- Adolescent cases are most commonly caused by the following:
  1. *Candida albicans* (vulvovaginal candidiasis [VVC])
  2. Replacement of normal vaginal H_2O_2-producing *Lactobacillus* species with anaerobic bacteria, *Gardnerella vaginalis* (bacterial vaginosis [BV]), and *Mycoplasma hominis*
  3. *Trichomonas vaginalis* (trichomoniasis)

EPIDEMIOLOGY & DEMOGRAPHICS
- In prepubertal children:
  1. Uncommon
  2. Predisposed by intravaginal foreign body, pinworm infection, or poor perineal hygiene
  3. Consider sexual abuse
- In adolescents:
  1. Common reason for adolescent reproductive health visit
- VVC, BV, and trichomoniasis are often asymptomatic and do not result in clinical syndromes.
- BV is more common among females who are sexually active, although classification as a sexually transmitted disease is debatable.
- Recurrence of BV and VVC is not prevented by treating male sex partners.
- Complications include the following:
  1. BV: pelvic inflammatory disease with gonorrhea/*Chlamydia* coinfection (see the section "Pelvic Inflammatory Disease")
  2. BV and trichomoniasis:
     a. Increased risk of human immunodeficiency virus (HIV) transmission and infection
     b. Perinatal complications
  3. VVC: chronic or recurrent infection

HISTORY
- Vaginal discharge
- Vaginal or vulvar vaginal pruritus
- Vaginal odor

PHYSICAL EXAMINATION
- Vaginal discharge
  1. VVC: thick, white, "cottage cheese" appearance
  2. BV: fishy vaginal odor
  3. Trichomoniasis: yellow-green to gray frothy vaginal discharge
- Evidence of pruritus: excoriation of vaginal mucosa
- Vaginal irritation
  1. Erythema and edema
  2. Trichomoniasis: "strawberry"-appearing cervix because of punctate hemorrhages

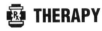 **DIAGNOSIS**

DIFFERENTIAL DIAGNOSIS
- Cervicitis
- Foreign body (i.e., tampon)
- Allergic or chemical reaction to soaps, detergent, and so forth.
- Physiologic vaginal discharge

DIAGNOSTIC WORKUP
- VVC: visualization of pseudohyphae or yeasts on microscopy
  1. Microscopy: 10% KOH on wet-mount preparations improves visualization.
  2. Culture is not routinely recommended because it leads to overdiagnosis.
- BV: clinical or Gram stain criteria
  1. Clinical criteria: three of the following four required:
     a. Homogeneous gray-white discharge that smoothly coats the vaginal walls
     b. Microscopic examination of vaginal fluid saline preparation
        (1) More than 20% of vaginal squamous epithelial cells identified as clue cells (squamous epithelial cells covered with adherent bacteria)
        (2) White blood cells on microscopy not consistent with BV; coinfection probable
     c. Vaginal fluid pH greater than 4.5
     d. Whiff test: addition of 10% KOH to vaginal discharge eliciting a fishy odor
  2. Gram stain criteria: shift in vaginal flora to predominance of BV-associated bacterial morphotypes with clinical correlation
     a. Shift in vaginal flora from predominance of lactobacilli to predominance of *Gardnerella* and anaerobic bacterial morphotypes

- Trichomoniasis: trichomonads visualized in culture or under microscopic examination
  1. Microscopic examination
     a. A saline preparation of the vaginal discharge
     b. Medium (×400) magnification
  2. Culture
     a. Diamond's medium
     b. InPouch TV system (BioMed Diagnostics, San Jose, California)
- Affirm VPII (Becton Dickinson, Franklin Lakes, New Jersey) DNA probe for VVC, BV and trichomoniasis diagnosis
  1. Superior sensitivity to wet mount
  2. Correlation with clinical symptoms and vaginal pH greater than 4.5 for improved specificity
- Prepubertal vaginitis: culture of discharge

THERAPY

CENTERS FOR DISEASE CONTROL AND PREVENTION RECOMMENDED REGIMENS
- VVC (one of the following):
  1. Azole intravaginal creams and suppositories, such as clotrimazole, terconazole, or butoconazole, for 3 to 7 days (most over-the-counter preparations)
  2. Fluconazole 150 mg orally in a single dose
- BV (for symptomatic cases only):
  1. Recommended regimens (one of the following):
     a. Metronidazole 500 mg orally twice a day for 7 days
     b. Clindamycin cream 2%, one full applicator (5 g) intravaginally at bedtime for 7 days
     c. Metronidazole gel 0.75%, one full applicator (5 g) intravaginally twice a day for 5 days
  2. Alternative regimens (one of the following):
     a. Metronidazole 2 g orally in a single dose
     b. Clindamycin 300 mg orally twice a day for 7 days
- Trichomoniasis: metronidazole 2 g orally in a single dose
- Prepubertal vaginitis: broad-spectrum antibiotic, such as amoxicillin or cephalosporins, that covers group A β-homolytic streptococci and gram-negative bacteria

FOLLOW-UP & DISPOSITION
Not necessary if patient is asymptomatic after treatment

MANAGEMENT OF SEX PARTNERS
Routine treatment of sex partners is recommended for trichomoniasis but not for VVC or BV.

II

☼ PEARLS & CONSIDERATIONS

■ CLINICAL PEARLS
- Pregnancy
  1. BV is associated with adverse pregnancy outcomes for the mother and newborn.
  2. Recommended BV treatment regimen is metronidazole 250 mg three times a day for 7 days.
  3. Metronidazole was not found to be teratogenic in recent meta-analysis.
  4. Oral fluconazole and clindamycin vaginal cream are contraindicated during pregnancy.
- HIV-infected females receive same vaginitis treatments
- Recurrent VVC (RVVC): more than four episodes of symptomatic VVC in 1 year
  1. Initial treatment for 10 to 14 days, immediately followed by maintenance therapy for at least 6 months
  2. RVVC frequency reduced by ketoconazole 100 mg orally per day for more than 6 months

- Sexual abuse: a consideration in prepubertal vaginitis

■ WEBSITES & SUPPORT GROUPS
Health care provider information
- Centers for Disease Control and Prevention, Division of STD Prevention: www.cdc.gov/nchstp/dstd/dstdp.html

Patient information
- Adolescent-appropriate STD information websites:
  1. www/owammaknow.org
  2. www.itsyoursexlife.com
  3. American Social Health Association (ASHA) for patient information brochures, STD Hotline telephone number, online STD information; 800-783-9877; www.ashastd.org
  4. ETR Associates for patient information brochures; 831-438-4060; www.etr.org
  5. Adolescent appropriate STD information hotlines: National STD Hotline: 800-227-8922

REFERENCES
1. Burtin P et al: Safety of metronidazole in pregnancy: a meta-analysis, *Am J Obstet Gynecol* 172:525, 1995.
2. Centers for Disease Control and Prevention: 1998 guidelines for treatment of sexually transmitted diseases, *MMWR Morb Mortal Wkly Rep* 47(No. RR-14), 1998.
3. Holmes KK, Stamm WE: Lower genital tract infections in women. In Homes KK et al (eds): *Sexually transmitted diseases,* ed 3, New York, 1999, McGraw-Hill.
4. Sanfilippo JS: Vulvovaginitis. In Behrman RE, Kliegman RM, Arvin AM (eds): *Nelson textbook of pediatrics,* ed 15, Philadelphia, 1996, WB Saunders.
5. Schwebke JR: Vaginal infections. In Goldman MB, Hatch MC (eds): *Women and health,* San Diego, 1999, Academic Press.
Authors: **Gale R. Burstein, M.D., M.P.H., and Sheryl A. Ryan, M.D.**

BASIC INFORMATION

■ DEFINITION
A defect in one of the four components of the ventricular septum—perimembranous, inlet, trabecular, or outlet septum—allowing communication between the left and right ventricles is called a *ventricular septal defect* (VSD).

■ SYNONYMS
- VSD
- Perimembranous VSD
- Muscular VSD

ICD-9CM CODE
745.4 Ventricular septal defect

■ ETIOLOGY
Failure of fusion of the muscular (trabecular), inflow (inlet), and outflow (conus or outlet) septa; deficient extracellular matrix formation, and excessive cell death

■ EPIDEMIOLOGY & DEMOGRAPHICS
- VSD is the most common congenital cardiac malformation.
- Incidence is 2 to 5 per 1000 live births (isolated VSDs).
- It is often an integral part of complex congenital heart lesions.
- Perimembranous defects account for 75% to 80%, and muscular defects account for 20% to 25%.
- VSD is slightly more common in females.
- It is the most common cardiac defect in patients with genetic trisomies.
- Small defects have a high rate of spontaneous closure.
- More than half of large defects decrease in size.

■ HISTORY
The clinical history and pathophysiology are determined by the size of the defect and the level of pulmonary vascular resistance.
- Patients with small defects are usually asymptomatic.
- Congestive heart failure may develop in patients with moderate-sized to large defects at 2 to 12 weeks of age.
- Moderate to large defects are often associated with a decrease in lung compliance and a secondary severe and prolonged course with viral lower respiratory tract infections.
- Patients usually come to attention because of a murmur, often earlier with smaller defects.
- Approximately 80% of small defects close spontaneously during the first year of life.

■ PHYSICAL EXAMINATION
- Small defects
  1. Growth and development are normal.
  2. A grade IV to V/VI harsh pansystolic murmur of even amplitude (regurgitant murmur) is heard at the lower left sternal border (LLSB).
  3. Pulmonary closure sound is normal.
  4. No diastolic murmur is present.
  5. Infants with tiny muscular defects often have a short, high-pitched, soft murmur cut off in midsystole as a result of late systolic closure from muscular contraction of the septum.
- Moderate-sized defects
  1. Height is preserved, but weight may be decreased.
  2. Precordial activity is increased.
  3. A grade III to IV regurgitant murmur is heard at the LLSB.
  4. Apical middiastolic murmur is present.
  5. Pulmonary closure sound may be accentuated.
  6. Signs of congestive heart failure, such as tachycardia, tachypnea, hepatomegaly, diaphoresis, or diminished pulses, may develop.
- Large defects
  1. Weight or weight and height may be decreased.
  2. Precordial activity is increased.
  3. Soft systolic ejection murmur is heard at the upper left sternal border as a result of relative pulmonary stenosis; no murmur arises from the VSD because the ventricular pressures are equal.
  4. A single loud second heart sound resulting from an early and accentuated pulmonary closure sound may be noted.
  5. Apical middiastolic murmur is present.
  6. Congestive heart failure is common.

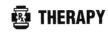 **DIAGNOSIS**

■ DIFFERENTIAL DIAGNOSIS
- Atrioventricular septal or canal defects
- Mitral regurgitation
- Tricuspid regurgitation

■ DIAGNOSTIC WORKUP
- Electrocardiogram
  1. Normal with small defects
  2. Left ventricular hypertrophy or left and right ventricular hypertrophy
  3. Left atrial enlargement
- Chest roentgenogram
  1. Normal with small defects
  2. Cardiomegaly
  3. Increased pulmonary blood flow
  4. Left atrial enlargement
- Echocardiogram
  1. Location and size of defect
  2. Pressure gradient across defect
  3. Direction of flow across defect
  4. Size of chambers, great vessels
  5. Associated anomalies
- Catheterization/angiography
  1. Usually not necessary unless atypical features are present or for further delineation of associated malformations

THERAPY

■ NONPHARMACOLOGIC
Provision of adequate caloric intake

■ MEDICAL
- Infective endocarditis prophylaxis for all patients (see "Endocarditis Prophylaxis," Part III)
- Digoxin, furosemide (Lasix), or other diuretic therapy; afterload reduction with an angiotensin-converting enzyme inhibitor for patients with congestive heart failure

■ SURGICAL
- Patch closure of a ventricular defect is indicated in the following cases:
  1. Persistent congestive heart failure with failure to thrive despite maximal medical management
  2. Development of right ventricular outflow tract obstruction (tetralogy physiology)
  3. Development of a rising pulmonary vascular or arteriolar resistance
  4. Development of aortic insufficiency
  5. Recurrent endocarditis
  6. Persistence of a moderate to large left-to-right shunt after 2 years of age
- Surgical morbidity and mortality should be less than 5%.

■ FOLLOW-UP & DISPOSITION
- Patients with small defects should be followed until spontaneous closure is documented, usually by auscultation.
- If a moderate or large left-to-right shunt is present, long-term follow-up is necessary.
- After surgical closure, long-term follow-up is also indicated because of small residual ventricular defects and late arrhythmias, including complete heart block and ventricular arrhythmias.

■ PATIENT/FAMILY EDUCATION
- In general, the prognosis for small defects, small to moderate-sized defects, and surgically closed ventricular defects is excellent.

II

- The risk of recurrence among siblings is less than 4%, unless a microdeletion of chromosome 22 is present.

■ REFERRAL INFORMATION
All patients with VSD should have an initial consultation with a pediatric cardiologist.

☼ PEARLS & CONSIDERATIONS

■ CLINICAL PEARLS
- Neonates and young infants with large ventricular defects and equalization of ventricular pressures may not have a murmur.

- Nevertheless, if a single loud second heart sound, peaceful tachypnea, and increased precordial activity are present, a congenital cardiac malformation should be suspected.
- Defects in the outlet septum and large muscular defects are unlikely to become smaller or close spontaneously.

■ SUPPORT GROUPS
Local Helping Hearts or related parental organizations are available to provide support and information.

REFERENCES
1. Anderson RH, Lenox CC, Zuberbuhler JR: Mechanisms of closure of perimembranous ventricular septal defects, *Am J Cardiol* 52:341, 1983.
2. Graham TP, Gutgesell HP: Ventricular septal defect. In Emmanouillides GC et al (eds): *Heart disease in infants, children, and adolescents,* Baltimore, 1995, Williams & Wilkins.
3. Kidd L et al: Second natural history study of congenital heart defects: results of treatment of patients with ventricular septal defects, *Circulation* Suppl I:I38, 1993.

Author: **J. Peter Harris, M.D.**

BASIC INFORMATION

■ DEFINITION
Vesicoureteral reflux (VUR) is the retrograde flow of urine from the bladder into the ureter.

ICD-9CM CODES
593.70 Vesicoureteral reflux
593.71 With reflux nephropathy, unilateral
593.72 With reflux nephropathy, bilateral

■ ETIOLOGY
- Abnormal ureteral orifice or an abnormal submucosal ureteral tunnel prevents the normal valvelike effect of the bladder smooth muscle, allowing retrograde flow of urine.
- VUR may be primary or secondary.
- The primary form of VUR is a congenital condition with isolated abnormality of the ureteral orifice.
- Primary VUR is an autosomal dominant disease.
- The secondary forms of VUR may also be congenital, but they occur in association with other congenital renal abnormalities, such as posterior urethral valves or renal dysplasia

■ EPIDEMIOLOGY & DEMOGRAPHICS
- It is estimated that the gene frequency for VUR is 1 in 600.
- Incidence of primary VUR in the general population is between 0.1% and 1.0%.
- Incidence in children is higher than in adults, ranging from 12% to 50%.
- The girl:boy ratio is approximately 5:1.
- VUR is more common in Caucasians than in African Americans.
- There is an increased incidence in patients with other forms of congenital renal disease or genetic syndromes.

■ HISTORY
- Hydronephrosis on antenatal ultrasound (approximately 20% of fetal hydronephrosis)
- Urinary tract infection (UTI) (20% to 40% of children with UTI have VUR)
- Family history (50% if parent, 30% if sibling)
- Gross hematuria (as a result of distended urinary mucosa)
- If missed in early childhood, may present with hypertension or renal failure

■ PHYSICAL EXAMINATION
In severe reflux, the patient may have an abdominal mass secondary to the massive dilation of the ureter.

DIAGNOSIS

■ DIFFERENTIAL DIAGNOSIS
Diagnosis is made by radiologic evaluation with little else on differential.

■ DIAGNOSTIC WORKUP
- Ultrasound is inadequate because even high-grade reflux may not show hydronephrosis.
- Voiding cystourethrogram (VCUG) is the radiographic test needed for diagnosis.
- Two types of VCUG are available: fluoroscopic and isotope.
- In fluoroscopic VCUG, radiopaque contrast is instilled into the bladder and imaging is done by fluoroscopy with intermittent radiographs.
  1. Gives detailed anatomic picture of the bladder and urethral anatomy
  2. Allows for precise grading of VUR severity
  3. Relatively high gonadal radiation
  4. Most appropriate initial test for the evaluation of a child suspected of having VUR
- In isotope VCUG, a radioisotope is placed in the bladder with continuous monitoring of the bladder and ureters via an isotope emission camera.
  1. Decreased gonadal radiation (only 1% the radiation exposure of fluoroscopic VCUG)
  2. Good for follow-up and screening examination
- VUR is graded according to severity.
  1. Grade I: retrograde flow of urine into a nondilated ureter only
  2. Grade II: filling of a nondilated ureter and a nondilated renal pelvis
  3. Grade III: filling of a dilated renal pelvis with sharp renal fornices
  4. Grade IV: filling of a dilated renal pelvis with blunted renal fornices
  5. Grade V: filling of massively dilated renal pelvis and ureter
- Evaluate for any associated voiding dysfunction (e.g., dribbling, urgency, incontinence).

THERAPY

All modes of therapy are directed toward decreasing the incidence of UTI.

■ NONPHARMACOLOGIC
- Meticulous perineal hygiene
- Avoidance of chemical irritants such as bubble bath
- Aggressive treatment of constipation

- Avoidance of dietary bladder irritants: caffeinated substances, carbonated beverages, chocolate, and citrus

■ MEDICAL
- Found to be equivalent to surgical correction
- Prophylactic antibiotic suppression of UTI
  1. For children older than 2 months of age:
     a. Trimethoprin-sulfamethoxazole 2 to 4 mg/kg/day of trimethoprim
     b. Nitrofurantoin 1 to 2 mg/kg/day
  2. For children younger than 2 months of age:
     a. Amoxicillin 10 to 15 mg/kg/day
     b. Cefazolin 20 to 30 mg/kg/day
  3. Prophylactic antibiotics are continued until VUR is outgrown.
  4. In some children, alternative drug therapy, twice-daily dosage, or two-drug therapy is needed.

■ SURGICAL
- The ureter is reimplanted in the bladder through a mucosal tunnel, recreating a normal ureteral insertion.
- Surgery is indicated in children who fail to outgrow their VUR, those with severe reflux, or those who have recurrent UTI with progressive renal damage.
- It may also be needed in patients with associated renal anomalies.

■ FOLLOW-UP & DISPOSITION
- Approximately 10% to 15% of cases resolve spontaneously each year.
- Up to 80% of low-grade (grades I and II) and 40% of high-grade VUR resolve without surgery.
- In children older than 5 years of age, the probability of high-grade reflux spontaneously resolving is low.
- Children should receive follow-up VCUG, preferably isotope, every 6 to 12 months until VUR is resolved.

■ PATIENT/FAMILY EDUCATION
- The risk of a child having VUR if one parent is affected is 50%.
- The risk of a child having VUR if a sibling is affected is 30%.
- The long-term morbidity from VUR is primarily caused by recurrent UTI.

■ PREVENTIVE TREATMENT
There is no known way to prevent VUR, but early identification of patients with VUR and the prevention of recurrent UTI decreases incidence of reflux nephropathy, the primary morbidity of VUR.

II

■ REFERRAL INFORMATION

- Referrals should be made to a pediatric urologist or pediatric nephrologist, especially with any of the following:
  1. Children with grade III or higher VUR
  2. Children with associated renal anomalies
  3. Children with hypertension or abnormal renal function
  4. Children with VUR and recurrent UTI despite antibiotic prophylaxis
  5. Children with voiding dysfunction: urinary urgency, incontinence, dribbling

☼ PEARLS & CONSIDERATIONS

■ CLINICAL PEARLS

Older siblings (older than 5 years of age) of children with VUR who have no history of UTI can be screened with a renal ultrasound and, if abnormal, a VCUG.

■ WEBSITES

Description of VUR and clinical course
- Johns Hopkins: www.med.jhu.edu/pediurol/pediatric/access/vur.html
- National Institute of Diabetes & Digestive & Kidney Diseases: www.niddk.nih.gov/health/kidney/summary/vesico/vesico.htm

Description of VCUG and suggestions on preparing a child for the test

- Children's Hospital Boston: http://web1.tch.harvard.edu/urology/testing.html

REFERENCES

1. Elder JS et al: Pediatric vesicoureteral reflux guidelines panel summary report on the management of primary vesicoureteral reflux in children, *J Urol* 157:1846, 1997.
2. Sheldon CA, Wacksman J: Vesicoureteral reflux, *Pediatr Rev* 16:22, 1995.
3. Smellie JM et al: Five-year study of medical or surgical treatment in children with severe reflux: radiological renal findings, *Pediatr Nephrol* 6:223, 1992.

Author: **Melissa Gregory, M.D.**

BASIC INFORMATION

■ DEFINITION

Malrotation is an abnormal rotation of the intestines as they return from the umbilical cord to the abdomen during early fetal life. The abnormal position and lack of fixation within the abdomen predisposes the infant to volvulus, abnormal twisting of the intestine and obstruction, often with secondary ischemia and infarction.

■ SYNONYMS

- Nonrotation
- Midgut volvulus

ICD-9CM CODES

560.2 Volvulus
751.4 Malrotation of the intestine
751.5 Congenital

■ ETIOLOGY

- Normal rotation of the intestine occurs within the first 3 months of fetal life.
  1. The "midgut" lengthens and extends outside the abdominal cavity.
  2. As the gut returns to the abdominal cavity, it rotates 270 degrees and is fixed to the retroperitoneum.
     a. Duodenum behind the superior mesenteric vessels
     b. Normal ligament of Treitz
     c. Attachment of cecum in the right lower quadrant
- Failure of the intestine to return to the abdominal cavity, rotate, and become correctly fixed in the retroperitoneum results in a variety of rotational anomalies.
- Abortive attempts to form the normal retroperitoneal fixation result in Ladd's bands.
  1. Fibrous bands of connective tissue
  2. Can lead to obstruction secondary to intestinal compression or luminal kinking
- Most common and dangerous anomaly of rotation is "nonrotation."
  1. Midgut does not rotate or fix.
  2. The result is that the duodenum descends along the right paravertebral gutter.
  3. The proximal colon ascends parallel to the duodenum.
  4. Both intestinal structures are enclosed in a common serosal sheath and contain the superior mesenteric artery and vein.
  5. This anatomic arrangement is particularly prone to twisting along the vascular axis, creating an intestinal volvulus.
  6. Further twisting of the intestine results in venous followed by arterial obstruction, leading to intestinal ischemia and necrosis.

- Other rare rotational anomalies include the following:
  1. Nonrotation of the duodenum with normal colonic rotation
     a. Also prone to volvulus
  2. Reversed rotation of the duodenum and colon, leading to transverse colonic obstruction
  3. Reversed rotation, paraduodenal hernias, and anomalies of attachment of the normally rotated intestine.

■ EPIDEMIOLOGY & DEMOGRAPHICS

- Of the patients who present with the syndrome of intestinal volvulus, 75% do so within the first month of life.
- There is no known ethnic, racial, or gender associations.
- This condition almost never predates delivery.

■ HISTORY

- Bilious vomiting
  1. Because of obstruction of distal duodenal/jejunal segment
- Lethargy or irritability
- Blood-tinged mucus or stool: may be passed
- Older child
  1. Recurrent abdominal pain
  2. Failure to thrive

■ PHYSICAL EXAMINATION

- Ill-appearing or toxic infant
  1. This is the only reliable and consistent sign.
- Fever: not always present, not reliable
- Tachycardia and tachypnea common
- Grunting
- Hypotension
- Distended abdomen or vague abdominal fullness

DIAGNOSIS

■ DIFFERENTIAL DIAGNOSIS

- Necrotizing enterocolitis (NEC)
- Stenosis or stricture, especially following NEC
- Duplication
- Toxic megacolon
- Sepsis

■ DIAGNOSTIC WORKUP

- Upper gastrointestinal series (UGI) is the study of choice.
  1. Radiographic confirmation demonstrates inappropriate position of the ligament of Treitz and abnormal colonic rotation.
  2. Anomalous Ladd's bands and partial obstruction will also be confirmed in an older child.
- Plain abdominal radiographs are not diagnostic and are often normal at initial presentation.

- Although barium enema can demonstrate the colonic nonrotation and confirm volvulus, diagnostic accuracy is not as high as with a UGI series.

THERAPY

■ SURGICAL

- Malrotation with volvulus is a surgical emergency.
- Surgical correction is the only therapy.
- Operative treatment includes counterclockwise rotation of the volvulus to restore normal perfusion.
- Abnormal Ladd's bands are divided to free the duodenal lumen from extrinsic compression.
- If significant ischemic damage has occurred to the midgut, appropriate resection decisions may need to await a second-look laparotomy 18 to 24 hours after correction of the volvulus and reestablishment of vascular perfusion to the intestine.
- In cases in which significant irreversible ischemic damage has occurred, enterectomy will be needed.
- When anomalies of intestinal rotation are recognized during the evaluation of recurrent abdominal pain or failure to thrive, operative correction is indicated.
  1. Most cases do not have vascular compromise, but a limited volvulus with nonocclusive kinking of the mesenteric pedicle is common.
  2. Operative separation of the mesenteric pedicle and division of any obstructing Ladd's bands are both required.
  3. Improved lymphatic and venous flow within the unobstructed mesentery and correction of partial intestinal obstruction often result in significant clinical improvement.
- Appendectomy is usually done because the cecum is not in the right lower quadrant; this prevents later diagnostic confusion.

■ FOLLOW-UP & DISPOSITION

- Symptomatic only
- Recurrence in 3%, most commonly in the early postoperative period

■ REFERRAL INFORMATION

- Emergency pediatric surgical consultation is mandatory in an infant with bilious vomiting.
- Nonemergent consultation with a pediatric surgeon is appropriate for older infants or children with failure to thrive.

II

☼ PEARLS & CONSIDERATIONS

■ CLINICAL PEARLS

• Bilious vomiting in an infant is a surgical emergency until proven otherwise.

1. Although there are many causes of bilious vomiting in infancy, no condition can result in irreversible damage in such a short time as malrotation with volvulus.
2. Evaluation and treatment must proceed with haste.

■ WEBSITE

University of Hawaii: www2.hawaii. edu/medicine/pediatrics/pemxray/ v2c08.html
Authors: **Mark Arkovitz, M.D., and Frederick Ryckman, M.D.**

BASIC INFORMATION

■ DEFINITION
- Von Willebrand disease is an absolute or functional deficiency of the von Willebrand factor (vWf) protein. This protein plays a key role in hemostasis in localizing platelets to the site of bleeding. vWf also "protects" coagulant protein factor VIII from proteolytic cleavage.
- The clinical consequence of vWf deficiency is excessive bleeding at mucous and cutaneous surfaces ("mucocutaneous" bleeding).
- This is the most common of all congenital bleeding disorders but is typically mild.

■ SYNONYM
Pseudohemophilia

ICD-9CM CODE
286.4 von Willebrand disease

■ ETIOLOGY
- Congenital disorder caused by a mutation in the gene on chromosome 12 that codes for vWf
- Rarely an acquired autoantibody in the setting of hypothyroidism
  1. Autoimmune disorder
  2. Malignancy

■ EPIDEMIOLOGY & DEMOGRAPHICS
- Prevalence is 0.8% to 1.2% based on two large-scale epidemiologic studies done in Virginia and Vincenza, Italy.
- In addition, patients with type O blood (approximately 45% of the general population) have vWf levels 60% to 70% lower than levels in patients with non–type O blood.
  1. They do not necessarily have a mutation in the vWf gene.
  2. These patients may be at increased risk of bleeding.

■ HISTORY
- Mucocutaneous bleeding is the hallmark symptom.
- Frequent epistaxis occurs through childhood and often necessitates packing or cauterization before the diagnosis is made.
- Gum bleeding, especially upon eruption of new teeth and with flossing, is common.
- Excessive bleeding is seen with wisdom tooth extractions.
- Rectal bleeding may be more pronounced from hemorrhoids.
- These patients bruise easily.
  1. A bruise in a child greater than the circumference of the palm of his or her hand may signify von Willebrand disease.
- Menorrhagia: Females with von Willebrand disease have a far greater tendency to present with heavy bleeding from monthly menstruation and after childbirth.
  1. Perceived heavy menses typically from onset of menarche
  2. Two pads or a tampon with a pad used
  3. Change tampon and/or pad every 30 to 120 minutes on the heaviest day
  4. Stain through underclothes
  5. Iron deficient
  6. High risk of undergoing dilation and curettage and/or hysterectomy for control of menorrhagia
  7. Approximate 5% to 10% risk of necessitating red blood cell transfusions postpartum

■ PHYSICAL EXAMINATION
- Fresh or crusted bloody discharge may be noted at the nares and gum line.
- Ecchymoses, typically 1 to 2 inches in diameter, are present in dependent lower extremities.
- Approximately 5% of patients with von Willebrand disease have telangiectasias.

DIAGNOSIS

■ DIFFERENTIAL DIAGNOSIS
- Mild hemophilia A
- Congenital platelet disorders: Bernard Soulier, Hermansky-Pudlak
- Acquired platelet disorders: aspirin-induced platelet dysfunction, uremia

■ DIAGNOSTIC WORKUP
- Workup is predicated first on the presence of mucocutaneous bleeding symptoms.
- Initial laboratory diagnosis is based on a constellation of tests:
  1. Subnormal vWf antigen and/or vWf activity ("Ristocetin cofactor test")
  2. Bleeding time prolonged in 50% of patients
  3. Factor VIII activity subnormal in approximately 40% of patients
- Laboratory testing should entail the following tests for purposes of classifying von Willebrand disease:
  1. Protein electrophoresis of vWf multimer pattern
  2. Normal pattern
     a. Type 1 is associated with a vWf level normally less than 10% to 50% of normal.
     b. Approximately 80% to 85% of patients have type 1 von Willebrand disease.
     c. Type 3 is associated with vWf levels less than 5% normal.
     d. Type 3 is also associated with a normal pattern and is seen in approximately 5% of patients with von Willebrand disease.
  3. Abnormal pattern
     a. Approximately 10% to 15% of patients with von Willebrand disease have type 2 disease.
     b. Usually, type 2 patients have more severe bleeding than type 1 patients.
     c. Type 2 patients do not respond to DDAVP like type 1 patients.
  4. Ristocetin-induced platelet aggregation
     a. Decreased pattern: consistent with type 2A or 2M
     b. Increased pattern: consistent with type 2B (which is often associated with thrombocytopenia, 50 to 150,000/μl range)

THERAPY

■ MEDICAL
- Based on severity of bleeding and von Willebrand disease type
- Type 1 von Willebrand disease: intravenous or intranasal desmopressin
  1. Desmopressin is approximately 80% to 85% effective in patients with type 1 von Willebrand disease.
  2. Before DDAVP use, a trial should be done to document at least a twofold rise in the vWf levels.
  3. Dosing is based on weight:
     a. Less than 50 kg: 1 puff
     b. More than 50 kg: 2 puffs
  4. In general, for any of the situations that follow, administration of DDAVP should not exceed more than 3 consecutive days.
     a. Tachyphylaxis can develop.
     b. Hyponatremia can develop.
     c. Fluid intake should be less than 5 glasses a day while using DDAVP.
  5. Intranasal DDAVP (Stimate) may be used for the following:
     a. Active bleeding
        (1) Epistaxis
        (2) Menorrhagia: daily for 3 days; oral contraceptive approximately 50% effective
        (3) Minor laceration: every 12 to 24 hours for 2 to 3 days
     b. Prophylaxis for bleeding
        (1) Before dental work (e.g., wisdom tooth extraction)
        (2) Before minor surgical procedures
  6. Intravenous DDAVP is indicated for the following:
     a. Active bleeding: major laceration
     b. Prophylaxis: major surgical procedure, including the following:
        (1) Tonsillectomy
        (2) Abdominal surgery

II

- Types 2 and 3: infusion of vWf-containing plasma-derived factor VIII concentrates

■ FOLLOW-UP & DISPOSITION
- Yearly inventory of mucocutaneous bleeding
- Communication with surgeon, dentist, and gynecologist before any surgical intervention.

■ PATIENT/FAMILY EDUCATION
- Major head trauma necessitates immediate evaluation, but unlike hemophilia, intracranial hemorrhage is exceedingly rare.
- Avoid intramuscular injections.
- Try topical thrombin and a pressure bandage for minor lacerations.
- Oral epsilon-amino caproic acid (Amicar) can be an adjunct for epistaxis, dental-related procedures, and menorrhagia.
- Intranasal DDAVP should be self-administered before high-risk bleeding situations (e.g., onset of menses, dental work, horseback riding)
- Other than football and hockey, there should be no major restrictions for physical education.

■ REFERRAL INFORMATION
- An evaluation by a hematologist with on-site laboratory analysis and interpretation for von Willebrand disease is appropriate.
- A trial of intranasal desmopressin should be planned and carried out by a hematologist.

☼ PEARLS & CONSIDERATIONS

■ CLINICAL PEARLS
- Von Willebrand disease is a far more common cause of bleeding than hemophilia.
- Relatively common situations such as epistaxis or menorrhagia warrant testing for von Willebrand disease, particularly if the patient has a family history of bleeding.
- One third of patients are index cases.
- Intranasal DDAVP can help restore those patients to a normal lifestyle.

■ WEBSITES
- Mary M. Gooley Hemophilia Center of Rochester, NY: www.hemocenter.org

- National Hemophilia Foundation: www.hemophilia.org
- World Federation of Hematology: www.wfh.org

■ SUPPORT GROUPS
- National Hemophilia Foundation, 116 West 32nd Street, 11th Floor, New York, NY 10001; 212-328-3700, fax: 212-328-3777; email: info@hemophilia.org
- World Federation of Hemophilia

REFERENCES
1. Claessens EA, Cowell CA: Acute adolescent menorrhagia, *Am J Obstet Gynecol* 139:277, 1981.
2. Kouides PA: Females with von Willebrand disease: 72 years as the silent majority, *Haemophilia* 4:665, 1998.
3. Mannucci PM: Desmopressin (DDAVP) in the treatment of bleeding disorders: the first 20 years, *Blood* 90:2515, 1997.
4. Werner EJ: Von Willebrand disease in children and adolescents, *Pediatr Clin North Am* 43:683, 1996.
Author: **Peter A. Kouides, M.D.**

BASIC INFORMATION

■ DEFINITION
Human papillomavirus (HPV) infection of the skin or mucous membranes may present as common warts (verruca vulgaris), genital warts (condylomata acuminata), plantar warts (verruca plantaris), or flat warts (verruca plana).

ICD-9CM CODES
078.10 Viral warts
078.19 Genital warts

■ ETIOLOGY
- Papillomaviruses are part of family Papovaviridae, a double-stranded DNA virus.
- More than 80 HPV types have been identified.
- Warts on the fingers, hands, and knees are usually caused by HPV-2 but may also be caused by HPV types 1, 3, 5, 7, 10, 26 to 29, and 41.
- Plantar warts are mainly caused by HPV types 1, 2, and 4.
- Flat warts are caused by HPV types 3 and 10.

■ EPIDEMIOLOGY & DEMOGRAPHICS
- Infection originates from a person who harbors HPV.
- Peak age affected is 12 to 16 years; it affects 10% of children.
- Defective cell-mediated immunity is a risk factor for infection.
- Some warts regress and recur after a period of latency.
- HPV-16 and HPV-18 are the most common types to progress to anogenital cancer.
- Approximately 30% of warts disappear within 6 months, and two thirds resolve within 2 years.

■ HISTORY
- Family members may be affected with warts.
- Genital warts may occur as a sign of sexual abuse, and a thorough history and physical examination must be taken to confirm whether this is the case.
- Vertical transmission from an infected mother to offspring is a source of anogenital warts in infants.

■ PHYSICAL EXAMINATION
- Common warts often appear on the dorsal side of hands as skin-colored rough keratotic papules studded with black dots.
  1. Gentle scraping reveals small capillaries (black dots).
- Plantar warts are thickened, yellow plaques on the soles, especially over pressure sites (e.g., heels, metatarsal heads) and are often painful.
- Flat warts are tan, smooth papules often found on the face and dorsum of hands.
- Genital warts are soft, flesh-colored papules that occur on the genitalia and buttocks; they may progress to large, cauliflower-like growths.

DIAGNOSIS

■ DIFFERENTIAL DIAGNOSIS
- Molluscum contagiosum
- Seborrheic keratoses
- Callus
- Corn (keratosis)
- Lichen planus
- Skin tags

■ DIAGNOSTIC WORKUP
- Diagnosis usually is made by clinical appearance.
- Serotyping of HPV is not routinely done in clinical practice.
- Surgical removal could be considered to confirm the diagnosis by histopathology.
- Evaluate for possible sexual abuse when a child presents with genital warts.

THERAPY

■ NONPHARMACOLOGIC
- Warts can be observed for spontaneous resolution.
- Adhesion therapy (occlusive tape) applied continuously can be effective.
- Hypnosis can cause resolution.

■ MEDICAL
- Cytodestructive
  1. Acids
     a. Salicylic acid is available over-the-counter.
     b. Bichloracetic and trichloroacetic acid may cause ulceration; avoid use on normal skin.
     c. Cantharidin (extract from blister beetle) may cause severe blisters and must be applied carefully.
  2. Cryotherapy
     a. Cryotherapy is the freezing of a wart with liquid nitrogen or dry ice
     b. This can be painful and requires repeated office visits every 2 to 3 weeks.
- Chemotherapeutic
  1. Intralesional bleomycin, for severe recalcitrant warts, can cause ulceration.
  2. 5-Fluorouracil cream can be used for genital warts; it is a teratogen and causes significant inflammation.
  3. Podophyllin and podophyllotoxin are effective for genital warts and are available by prescription for home application.
  4. Topical retinoic acid can be used for flat warts; it is moderately successful and mildly irritating.
  5. Cimetidine, high-dose (30 to 40 mg/kg/day), has been shown in several studies to improve or clear warts after 2 to 3 months of therapy.
- Antiviral/immunomodulatory
  1. Interferon: given subcutaneously, very expensive, causes flulike side effects
  2. Imiquimod: topical immunomodulator, causes local skin irritation
  3. Cidofovir and HPV vaccines: efficacy not yet proven but experimental reports are encouraging

■ SURGICAL
- Cold-knife surgery and electrosurgery can be performed under local anesthesia; risks are pain and recurrences (25% to 30%).
- Laser surgery destroys the HPV by absorbing laser light in the cells causing vaporization. Laser surgery has advantages of less postoperative pain and less bleeding, but it is limited by cost, prolonged healing time, scarring, and risk of recurrence (5% to 10%).

■ FOLLOW-UP & DISPOSITION
Warts may need to be treated multiple times at 1- to 2-week intervals until resolution.

■ PATIENT/FAMILY EDUCATION
- Make patient aware of risks associated with treatments (e.g., slow response, possible scars, pain).
- Make patient aware of risk of recurrence.

■ PREVENTIVE TREATMENT
- Patient should avoid picking at or chewing warts (promotes spread).
- It may be helpful to change socks when feet are damp or sweaty because dampness may promote spread.

■ REFERRAL INFORMATION
Referral to dermatologist is appropriate when warts are painful, bleeding, spreading, a cosmetic concern (face, hands), or not responding to first-line therapy (e.g., salicylic acid).

PEARLS & CONSIDERATIONS

■ CLINICAL PEARLS

It is important not to make the treatment worse than the disease; if treatments become painful or traumatic, it is reasonable to choose alternative therapy (e.g., observation, salicylic acid).

REFERENCES

1. Baker G, Tyring S: Therapeutic approaches to papillomavirus infections, *Dermatol Clin* 15:331, 1997.
2. Ordovknanian E, Lane A: Warts and molluscum contagiosum, *Postgrad Med* 101:223, 1997.
3. Severson J, Tyrin S: Viral disease update, *Curr Prob Dermatol* 11:37, 1999.
4. Siegfried E: Warts on children: an approach to therapy, *Pediatr Ann* 25:79, 1996.

Author: **Allison L. Holm, M.D.**

BASIC INFORMATION

DEFINITION
Wilms' tumor is a malignant neoplasm of the kidney, derived from primitive metanephric blastema.

SYNONYM
Nephroblastoma

ICD-9CM CODE
189.0 Malignant neoplasm of kidney, except pelvis

ETIOLOGY
- There are no identified environmental risk factors.
- Approximately 1% to 2% of patients have relatives with Wilms' tumor.
  1. An estimated 15% to 20% of patients have Wilms' tumor that is hereditary in nature, but penetrance is incomplete.
- A minority of patients with Wilms' tumor have other anomalies and syndromes associated with the development of Wilms' tumor, including the following:
  1. Aniridia, genitourinary malformations, or a syndrome with those abnormalities, and mental retardation
  2. Hemihypertrophy as an isolated finding or Beckwith-Wiedemann syndrome
  3. Denys-Drash syndrome
  4. Trisomy 18
- Potential "Wilms' tumor complex" is in the region of chromosome 11p, which may be involved in both sporadic and heritable forms of Wilms' tumor.
- Unidentified gene defects on chromosomes 1 and 16 may also be involved in the development of some cases of Wilms' tumor.

EPIDEMIOLOGY & DEMOGRAPHICS
- Approximately 5% to 6% of pediatric cancers
- Incidence approximately 8 cases per 1 million per year in children younger than 15 years of age
- Total incidence approximately 400 to 500 cases per year in the United States
- Incidence in females slightly higher than in males, especially for bilateral disease
- Highest incidence in African Americans, followed by Caucasians and then Asian Americans
- Approximately 75% of patients diagnosed before 5 years of age; 90% before 7 years of age

HISTORY
- Asymptomatic abdominal fullness or mass
- Abdominal pain
- Hematuria
- Fever
- Presentation with rapid abdominal enlargement and anemia: may be related to hemorrhage in tumor

PHYSICAL EXAMINATION
- Abdominal mass is usually palpable; it may be difficult to differentiate from hepatomegaly, splenomegaly, or other tumor by physical examination.
- Hypertension is present.
- Examination should include assessment for any associated physical anomalies, including aniridia, hemihypertrophy, or genitourinary abnormalities.

DIAGNOSIS

DIFFERENTIAL DIAGNOSIS
- Other kidney tumors, including clear cell sarcoma, rhabdoid tumor of the kidney
- Benign renal masses, including mesoblastic nephroma (especially in children younger than 1 year of age)
- Renal cysts
- Other abdominal tumors, including neuroblastoma, lymphoma, hepatoblastoma, rhabdomyosarcoma

DIAGNOSTIC WORKUP
- Abdominal ultrasound, including Doppler to evaluate inferior vena cava involvement
- Computed tomogram (CT) of the abdomen and pelvis
- Chest roentgenogram
- CT of the chest
- No diagnostic laboratory tests, but complete blood count, chemistries (including renal and liver function tests), and urinalysis important components of complete baseline evaluation

PATHOLOGY
- Favorable histology (FH): absence of anaplasia
- Unfavorable histology (UH): presence of anaplasia, defined by gigantic polypoid nuclei within the tumor sample.
  1. Anaplasia may be focal or diffuse.

STAGING
- Stage I: Tumor is limited to the kidney and completely resected. No tumor rupture, and vessels of the renal sinus are not involved.
- Stage II: Tumor extends beyond the kidney but is completely resected.

Tumor may have been biopsied or local tumor spillage may have occurred, but it was confined to the flank.
- Stage III: Residual nonhematogenous tumor, including any unresectable tumor, is present but confined to the abdomen.
- Stage IV: Hematogenous metastases (i.e., lung, liver, or bone) or involved lymph nodes outside the abdomen are present.
  1. The lung is the most common site of metastases and the only site in approximately 80% of patients with metastatic disease.
  2. Liver involvement, with or without lung metastases, is present in 15% of patients.
- Stage V: Bilateral renal involvement is seen at diagnosis. Each side is then staged separately.

THERAPY

MEDICAL
- Chemotherapy and radiation therapy depend on the stage and histology.
  1. Current chemotherapy regimens include vincristine and dactinomycin for stage I and II FH and stage I UH.
  2. Doxorubicin is added for stage II, III, and IV focal anaplasia and stage III and IV FH.
  3. Stage II, III, and IV diffuse anaplasia is treated with vincristine, doxorubicin, cyclophosphamide, and etoposide.
- Therapy for bilateral tumors is individualized with the goal of sparing adequate renal parenchyma for normal renal function.
- Chemotherapy is generally administered in the outpatient setting.
- Duration of treatment is 18 to 24 weeks.
- Radiation therapy is indicated for stages II, III, and IV UH, and stages III and IV FH.
- Radiation therapy may be considered for pulmonary metastases visible on chest roentgenogram or for pulmonary nodules visible on CT only that are unresponsive to chemotherapy.

SURGICAL
Radical nephrectomy with examination of the contralateral kidney if tumor is deemed resectable; biopsy only if tumor is unresectable

PROGNOSIS
- Current studies demonstrate an approximate 90% to 95% 5-year survival for Wilms' tumor patients as a group.
- Relapses beyond 5 years are rare.

- Prognosis after relapse is worse for patients who received doxorubicin or radiation therapy as part of their initial therapy.

■ **FOLLOW-UP & DISPOSITION**
- Serial abdominal ultrasounds or CT scans, and chest roentgenograms (timing dependent on stage) are appropriate.
- Late effects of chemotherapy are limited but may include cardio-myopathy in patients receiving doxorubicin and renal tubular dysfunction in patients receiving cyclophosphamide.
- Late effects of radiation may include hypoplasia and potential reproductive difficulties in females, including pregnancy loss and premature delivery. There is a smaller risk of ovarian failure, pulmonary fibrosis, and second malignancies.
- Some restrictions may be recommended to single-kidney status, and renal function should be monitored.

■ **PATIENT/FAMILY EDUCATION**
- Most cases are sporadic, but bilateral, multicentric disease or disease diagnosed at younger ages is more likely to be heritable.
- Multimodal approach to therapy, including surgery, chemotherapy, and radiation therapy if necessary, has re-sulted in excellent cure rates for all stages of disease, including meta-static disease.

■ **REFERRAL INFORMATION**
- All patients should be referred to pediatric oncologists and treated on National Wilms' Tumor Study protocols as appropriate.
- A pediatric surgeon or pediatric urologist with experience in oncologic surgery should perform nephrectomy.

☼ PEARLS & CONSIDERATIONS

■ **CLINICAL PEARLS**
- Many patients with Wilms' tumor will have their mass detected by a family member.
- Although only a small number of patients will be diagnosed after hypertension is detected on routine examination, it is another reason to measure blood pressure during well-child visits.

■ **WEBSITES**
- American Cancer Society: www.cancer.org
- National Cancer Institute: www.nci.nih.gov
- OncoLink: www.oncolink.com

■ **SUPPORT GROUPS**
- Pediatric oncologists can refer patients and parents to local or national support organizations for children with cancer and their families.
- National organizations include the American Cancer Society and Candlelighters.

REFERENCES

1. Crist WM, Kun LE: Common solid tumors of childhood, *N Engl J Med* 324:461, 1991.
2. Green DM et al: Wilms' tumor. In Pizzo PA, Poplack DG (eds): *Principles and practice of pediatric oncology*, ed 3, Philadelphia, 1997, JB Lippincott.
3. Halperin EC et al: Wilms' tumor. In Halperin EC et al (eds): *Pediatric radiation oncology*, ed 3, Philadelphia, 1999, Lippincott Williams & Wilkins.
4. Kobrinsky NL et al: Wilms' tumor, *Hematol Oncol Ann* 1:173, 1993.
5. Personal communication. National Wilms' Tumor Study Group. Green D, Chairman, National Wilms' Tumor Study-5: Therapeutic Trial and Biology Study. Approved CTEP, NCI. Pediatric Oncology Group #9440, opened July, 1995.

Author: **Andrea S. Hinkle, M.D.**

BASIC INFORMATION

■ DEFINITION
Wilson disease is an autosomal recessive disorder of copper metabolism characterized by degenerative changes in the brain, liver disease, Kayser-Fleischer rings in the cornea, and sometimes hemolysis.

■ SYNONYM
Hepatolenticular degeneration

ICD-9CM CODE
275.1 Disorders of copper metabolism

■ ETIOLOGY
- Mutations occur in the ATPB7 gene located at chromosome 13 at q14.3-q21.1.
- Gene encodes a P-type ATPase that plays a role in copper transport.
- Defective mobilization of copper from lysosomes in liver cells for excretion into bile leads to accumulation of copper in the liver.
- Copper is a potent inhibitor of enzymatic processes.
- When the liver's capacity for storing copper is exceeded, copper then escapes the liver and causes damage to other organs, including the brain, kidneys, and eyes.

■ EPIDEMIOLOGY & DEMOGRAPHICS
- Estimated prevalence is 1 in 200,000 children.
- Symptoms are rarely present before age 5 years.
- Patients younger than 20 years of age tend to present with hepatic manifestations, sometimes with a brisk hemolytic anemia.
- Older individuals tend to have more neurologic and psychiatric manifestations.
- This disease is autosomal recessive.
- Markers close to the Wilson disease gene allow presymptomatic diagnosis in siblings.

■ HISTORY
- Abdominal mass or distention from asymptomatic hepatomegaly
- Jaundice, nausea, vomiting, and right upper quadrant pain associated with acute hepatitis
- Jaundice, edema, malaise, and pallor associated with hepatic failure and hemolytic anemia
- Esophageal bleeding and ascites from portal hypertension
- Neurologic manifestations, particularly those of a movement disorder, such as resting and intention tremors, spasticity, rigidity, chorea, dysphagia, and dysarthria
- Psychiatric disturbances, including syndromes indistinguishable from schizophrenia, manic-depressive disorder, and classic neuroses, as well as more bizarre behavioral disturbances
- Deterioration in school performance, marked behavioral changes

■ PHYSICAL EXAMINATION
- Hepatomegaly or hepatosplenomegaly
- Right upper quadrant tenderness
- Ascites
- Edema
- Jaundice
- Pallor associated with hemolytic anemia
- Tremor, spasticity, rigidity, chorea, dysphagia, and dysarthria
- Bizarre behavior
- Progressive renal failure, manifestations of Fanconi's syndrome present on urinalysis
- Kayser-Fleischer rings in the cornea (slit-lamp examination is most often required, although detection is occasionally possible on routine examination)
- Rare: arthritis, endocrinopathies

🔬 DIAGNOSIS

■ DIFFERENTIAL DIAGNOSIS
- Acute viral hepatitis
- Chronic hepatitis
- α_1-Antitrypsin deficiency
- Porphyria
- Hepatic copper overload syndrome
- Indian childhood cirrhosis
- Copper poisoning

■ DIAGNOSTIC WORKUP
- The diagnosis is fairly straightforward, *as long as it is suspected.*
- The best screening test is to measure serum ceruloplasmin.
  1. Most patients have a serum ceruloplasmin level that is decreased: less than 20 mg/dl.
- An ophthalmologic examination should be done to look for Kayser-Fleischer rings.
- Consider measuring urinary copper excretion.
- Liver biopsy should also be considered.
  1. Hepatic copper concentration is the gold standard in diagnosing Wilson disease.

💊 THERAPY

■ NONPHARMACOLOGIC
- Restrict copper intake (avoid shellfish, nuts, chocolate, liver, and other foods high in copper).
- If the copper content of local water is high, it may be necessary to demineralize the water.

■ MEDICAL
- Administer copper-chelating agents: currently oral penicillamine.
- Because penicillamine is a vitamin B_6 antimetabolite, additional amounts of B_6 are necessary.
- For patients who do not tolerate penicillamine because of hypersensitivity reactions, triethylene tetramine dihydrochloride (Trien) can be used.
- Zinc acetate may be helpful to block absorption of copper in the intestinal tract; at least one study has demonstrated efficacy of zinc as a sole therapy for adults with Wilson disease.

■ SURGICAL
Liver transplantation may be undertaken for patients with fulminant hepatic disease or cirrhosis.

■ PROGNOSIS
- Wilson disease is fatal if untreated.
- The prognosis for patients receiving medical therapy depends on the progression of disease at the initiation of treatment and individual variation.
- Once initiated, therapy must be maintained for life.

■ PATIENT/FAMILY EDUCATION
- Most people with Wilson disease do not have any family history of the disease.
- The chance of a sibling of a child with Wilson disease being affected is 25%.
- There is no simple genetic test for Wilson disease, but within individual families, genetic testing is usually possible.
- Early treatment is important to prevent progression of the disease; once treatment is initiated, it is lifelong.

■ REFERRAL INFORMATION
- Children with Wilson disease should be referred to a pediatric gastroenterologist specializing in this disorder.
- Consultations with pediatric neurology and hematology may also be warranted.

💡 PEARLS & CONSIDERATIONS

■ CLINICAL PEARLS
- Wilson disease should be considered in any child with an unexplained neurologic or psychiatric problem and evidence of elevated liver transaminases, hepatitis, or hepatomegaly.
- All patients with neurologic or psychiatric disturbance have Kayser-Fleischer rings; however, Kayser-

Fleisher rings may be absent in the young patient with only liver disease.

• Unexplained hemolysis should always be regarded as a possible sign of Wilson disease.

■ **WEBSITE**

Wilson's Disease Association International: www.wilsonsdisease.org

■ **SUPPORT GROUPS**

• The Wilson's Disease Association has a support group. Information can be obtained at www.wilsonsdisease.org
• American Liver Foundation, 1425 Pompton Avenue, Cedar Grove, NJ 07009, 800-465-4837
• National Organization for Rare Disorders Inc., P.O. Box 8923, New Fairfield, CT 06812, 800-999-6673

REFERENCES

1. Brewer GJ et al: Treatment of Wilson's disease with zinc. XV. Long-term follow-up studies, *J Clin Lab Med* 132: 264, 1998.
2. Dobyns WB, Goldstein NP, Gordon H: Clinical spectrum of Wilson's disease (hepatolenticular degeneration), *Mayo Clin Proc* 54:35, 1979.
3. Online Mendelian Inheritance in Man (OMIM) at website: www3.ncbi.nlm. nih.gov/omim/ (search "Wilson disease"—this reference is updated several times per year).

Author: **Jeffrey Kaczorowski, M.D.**

BASIC INFORMATION

DEFINITION
Infection caused by *Yersinia enterocolitica* (and less commonly, by the closely related species *Y. pseudotuberculosis*) is an increasingly recognized zoonosis causing food poisoning and mesenteric lymphadenitis. A separate species *(Y. pestis)* is responsible for the distinctly different disease plague.

SYNONYMS
• Nonplague yersiniosis
• Bacterial enterocolitis

ICD-9CM CODE
027.8 *Y. enterocolitica,* other bacterial zoonoses

ETIOLOGY
• *Y. enterocolitica* is a gram-negative, rod-shaped aerobic bacterium.
• Serotypes O:3, O:8, and O:9 predominate in human disease.
• Both iron overload states and iron chelation therapy with deferoxamine enhance the virulence of *Y. enterocolitica.*

EPIDEMIOLOGY & DEMOGRAPHICS
• *Y. enterocolitica* is widespread in nature. The most common reservoir is the pig; sheep, cattle, horses, rodents, and household pets can also serve as reservoirs.
• This infection is more common in temperate areas (Northern Europe, Canada, United States) than in tropical areas.
• This is the fifth most common bacterial cause of foodborne illness in the United States (following *Campylobacter, Salmonella, Shigella, Escherichia coli* O157:H7).
• Modes of transmission include the following:
  1. Contaminated food or milk
  2. Rarely person-to-person (fecal-oral spread)
  3. Rarely transfusion-related from contaminated blood products
  4. Organisms persisting and growing in refrigerated stored food and banked blood
• The most common foods associated with transmission are pork and dairy products.
• Risk groups include the following:
  1. Children exposed to contaminated food (especially undercooked pork)
  2. Patients with iron overload states (e.g., hemochromatosis, thalassemia, renal failure with transfusion therapy)
  3. Patients receiving iron chelation therapy with deferoxamine
• Geographically neighboring farming communities of Belgium and France have very different rates of yersiniosis because of cultural and regulatory differences in food handling.

PREDOMINANT CLINICAL SYNDROMES
• Gastroenteritis
  1. Enterocolitic diarrhea, with fever, abdominal pain, mucus- and blood-containing stools, and sometimes with vomiting, occurs.
  2. Incubation period is 3 to 7 days.
  3. Symptoms persist for 1 to 3 weeks.
  4. Gastroenteritis predominantly occurs in children younger than 5 years of age.
• Mesenteric lymphadenitis/ pseudoappendicitis
  1. Mimics acute appendicitis with fever, right lower quadrant pain, leukocytosis, but not diarrhea
  2. Predominantly seen in children older than 6 to 10 years of age
  3. Often misdiagnosed, resulting in laparotomy
• Extraintestinal infection
  1. Bacteremia may occur with or without diarrhea and may lead to metastatic lesions such as lymphadenitis, pharyngitis, osteomyelitis, septic arthritis, meningitis, peritonitis, and hepatic or splenic abscesses.
  2. Invasive disease is more common after transfusions and in patients receiving iron overload or chelation therapy.
  3. Mortality can approach 50%.
• Immunologic sequelae
  1. Reactive arthritis, erythema nodosum, and Reiter's syndrome may occur.
  2. Adults with the HLA-B27 genotype are especially at risk.

HISTORY
• Risk factor discussed earlier
• Ingestion of food associated with transmission in preceding 2 weeks
• Contact with preparers of high-risk food such as pork chitterlings

PHYSICAL EXAMINATION
Depends on clinical syndrome (see previous discussion)

DIAGNOSIS

DIFFERENTIAL DIAGNOSIS
• Colitis
  1. *Shigella*
  2. *Salmonella*
  3. *Campylobacter enteritis*
• Mesenteric adenitis
  1. Appendicitis
  2. Crohn's disease
  3. Terminal ileitis
• Bacteremia with extraintestinal manifestations
  1. Lymphadenitis
  2. Peritonitis
  3. Hepatic and splenic abscesses
  4. Septic arthritis

DIAGNOSTIC WORKUP
• Bacterial cultures of blood and stool should be obtained.
  1. Stool cultures require special media and selection techniques.
  2. Laboratory should be alerted to isolate *Yersinia.*
• Abdominal computed tomography scan may help differentiate appendicitis from mesenteric adenitis.

THERAPY

NONPHARMACOLOGIC
• Supportive therapy is provided for diarrhea, fever, and pain.
• Uncomplicated cases of enterocolitis and mesenteric adenitis in older children may not require antibiotic therapy.

MEDICAL
• Antibiotic therapy is indicated for bacteremia, systemic focal infections, infections in immunocompromised hosts, and severe cases of mesenteric adenitis.
• Most *Y. enterocolitica* isolates are susceptible to trimethoprim-sulfamethoxazole, aminoglycosides, third-generation cephalosporins, and fluoroquinolones.

PREVENTIVE TREATMENT & PATIENT/FAMILY EDUCATION
• Do not let children handle raw pork products (e.g., chitterlings).
• Thoroughly cook all pork products.
• Keep uncooked pork products separate from other foods.
• Wash hands, knives, and cutting boards after handling uncooked pork products.
• Avoid raw or unpasteurized milk.

PEARLS & CONSIDERATIONS

CLINICAL PEARLS
• Recent outbreaks of *Y. enterocolitica* febrile gastroenteritis have occurred in urban African-American children after Thanksgiving, Christmas, and New Year's holiday gatherings.
  1. Pork chitterlings (intestines), often prepared at such times, have been implicated as the vehicle of spread of infection.
  2. Most children did not have direct contact with raw chitterlings.
    a. Preparation of chitterlings is

labor intensive and time-consuming.
  b. Presumably food-handling adults infect the children.

■ **WEBSITE**

Centers for Disease Control and Prevention: www.cdc.gov/health/diseases.htm

REFERENCES

1. Butler T: *Yersinia* species, including plague. In Mandell GL, Bennett JE, Dolin R (eds): *Mandell, Douglas, and Bennett's principles and practice of infectious diseases,* ed 5, Philadelphia, 2000, Churchill Livingstone.
2. Lee LA et al: *Yersinia enterocolitica* O3: an emerging cause of pediatric gastroenteritis in the United States, *J Infect Dis* 27:59, 1991.
3. Smego RA, Frean J, Koornhof HJ: Yersiniosis I: microbiological and clinicoepidemiological aspects of plague and non-plague *Yersinia* infections, *Eur J Clin Microbiol Infect Dis* 18:1, 1999.
4. Verhaegen J et al: Surveillance of human *Yersinia enterocolitica* infections in Belgium: 1967-1996, *Clin Infect Dis* 27:59, 1998.
5. Woods CR: Other *Yersinia* species. In Feigin RD, Cherry JD (eds): *Textbook of pediatric infectious diseases,* ed 4, Philadelphia, 1998, WB Saunders.

Author: **Geoffrey A. Weinberg, M.D.**

PART III

Charts, Formulas, and Tests

Section 1
GROWTH

■ WEIGHT-FOR-AGE PERCENTILES

■ LENGTH-FOR-AGE PERCENTILES

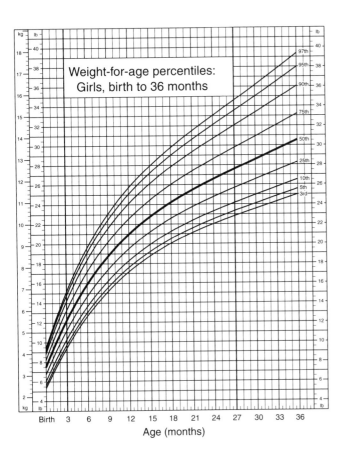

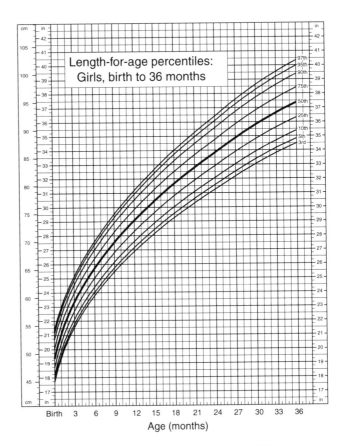

Fig. 3-1 Weight-for-age percentiles, girls, birth to 36 months, CDC growth charts: United States. (Developed by the National Center for Health Statistics in collaboration with the National Center for Chronic Disease Prevention and Health Promotion, 2000.)

Fig. 3-2 Length-for-age percentiles, girls, birth to 36 months, CDC growth charts: United States. (Developed by the National Center for Health Statistics in collaboration with the National Center for Chronic Disease Prevention and Health Promotion, 2000.)

III

■ HEAD CIRCUMFERENCE-FOR-AGE PERCENTILES ■ WEIGHT-FOR-LENGTH PERCENTILES

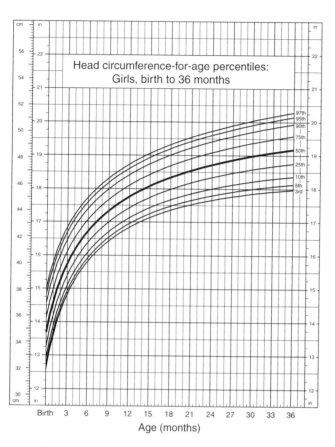

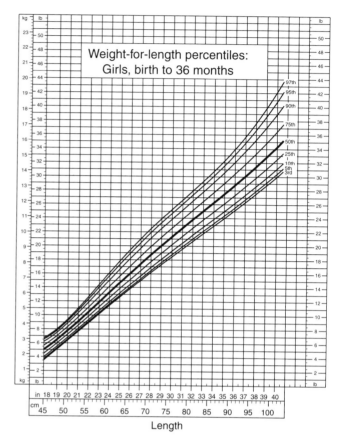

Fig. 3-3 **Head circumference-for-age percentiles, girls, birth to 36 months, CDC growth charts: United States.** (Developed by the National Center for Health Statistics in collaboration with the National Center for Chronic Disease Prevention and Health Promotion, 2000.)

Fig. 3-4 **Weight-for-length percentiles, girls, birth to 36 month, CDC growth charts: United States.** (Developed by the National Center for Health Statistics in collaboration with the National Center for Chronic Disease Prevention and Health Promotion, 2000.)

■ WEIGHT-FOR-AGE PERCENTILES

■ LENGTH-FOR-AGE PERCENTILES

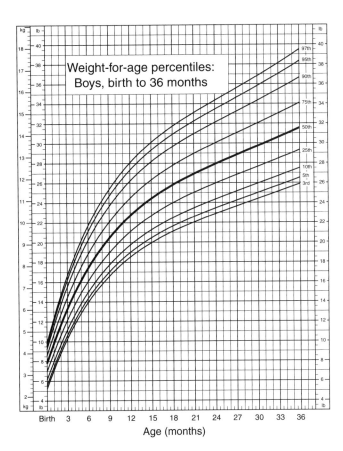

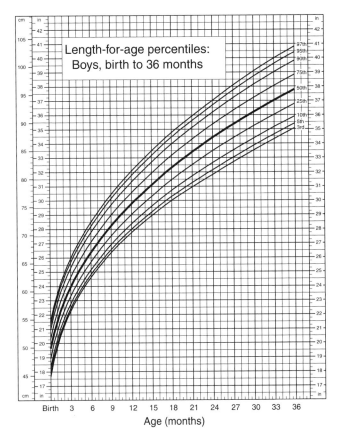

Fig. 3-5   Weight-for-age percentiles, boys, birth to 36 months, CDC growth charts: United States. (Developed by the National Center for Health Statistics in collaboration with the National Center for Chronic Disease Prevention and Health Promotion, 2000.)

Fig. 3-6   Length-for-age percentiles, boys, birth to 36 months, CDC growth charts: United States. (Developed by the National Center for Health Statistics in collaboration with the National Center for Chronic Disease Prevention and Health Promotion, 2000.)

III

■ HEAD CIRCUMFERENCE-FOR-AGE PERCENTILES

■ WEIGHT-FOR-LENGTH PERCENTILES

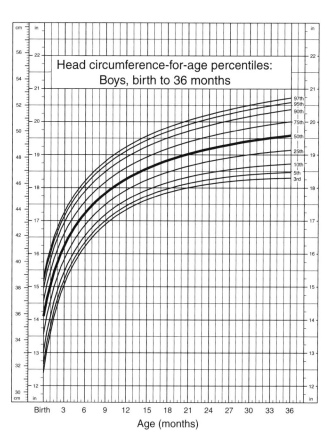

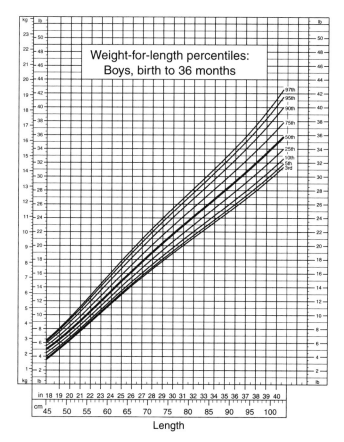

Fig. 3-7 Head circumference-for-age percentiles, boys, birth to 36 months, CDC growth charts: United States. (Developed by the National Center for Health Statistics in collaboration with the National Center for Chronic Disease Prevention and Health Promotion, 2000.)

Fig. 3-8 Weight-for-length percentiles, boys, birth to 36 months, CDC growth charts: United States. (Developed by the National Center for Health Statistics in collaboration with the National Center for Chronic Disease Prevention and Health Promotion, 2000.)

■ **WEIGHT-FOR-AGE PERCENTILES**

■ **STATURE-FOR-AGE PERCENTILES**

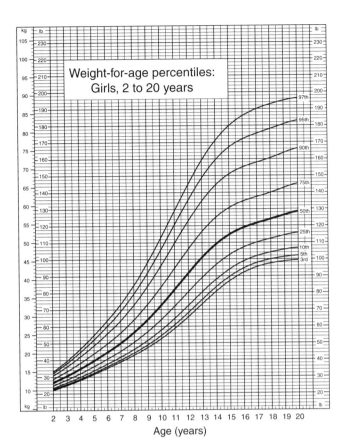

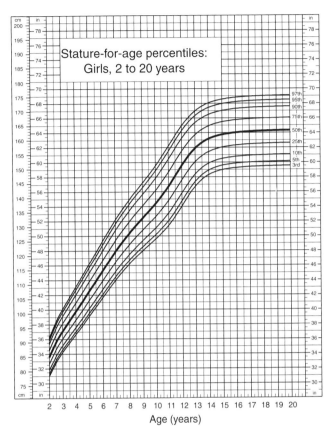

Fig. 3-9   Weight-for-age percentiles, girls, 2 to 20 years, CDC growth charts: United States. (Developed by the National Center for Health Statistics in collaboration with the National Center for Chronic Disease Prevention and Health Promotion, 2000.)

Fig. 3-10   Stature-for-age percentiles, girls 2 to 20 years, CDC growth charts: United States. (Developed by the National Center for Health Statistics in collaboration with the National Center for Chronic Disease Prevention and Health Promotion, 2000.)

■ WEIGHT-FOR-STATURE PERCENTILES

■ BODY MASS INDEX-FOR-AGE PERCENTILES

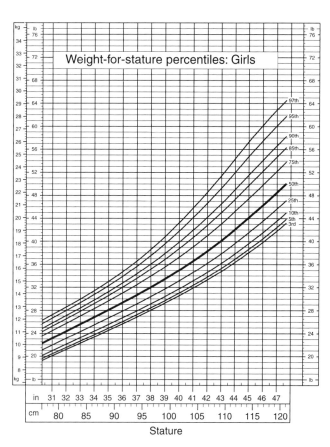

Fig. 3-11   Weight-for-stature percentiles, girls, CDC growth charts: United States. (Developed by the National Center for Health Statistics in collaboration with the National Center for Chronic Disease Prevention and Health Promotion, 2000.)

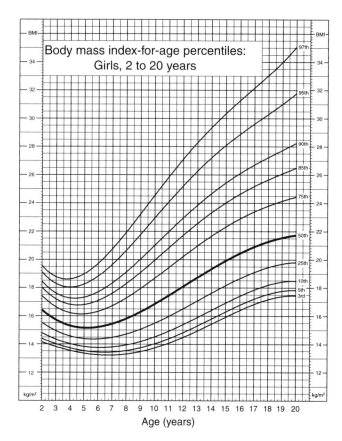

Fig. 3-12   Body mass index-for-age percentiles, girls, 2 to 20 years, CDC growth charts: United States. (Developed by the National Center for Health Statistics in collaboration with the National Center for Chronic Disease Prevention and Health Promotion, 2000.)

■ WEIGHT-FOR-AGE PERCENTILES

■ STATURE-FOR-AGE PERCENTILES

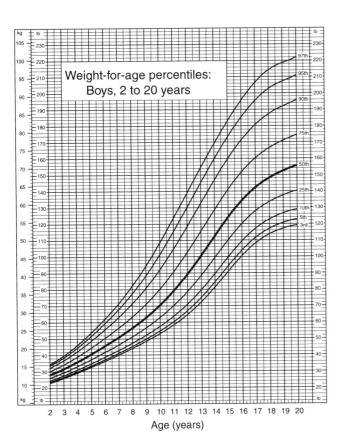

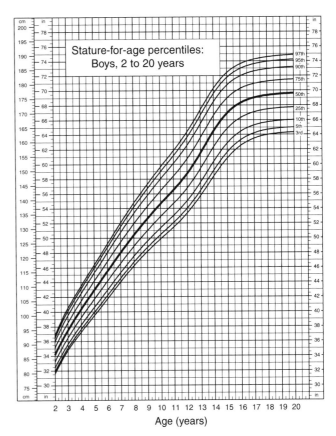

Fig. 3-13 Weight-for-age percentiles, boys, 2 to 20 years, CDC growth charts: United States. (Developed by the National Center for Health Statistics in collaboration with the National Center for Chronic Disease Prevention and Health Promotion, 2000.)

Fig. 3-14 Stature-for-age percentiles, boys, 2 to 20 years, CDC growth charts: United States. (Developed by the National Center for Health Statistics in collaboration with the National Center for Chronic Disease Prevention and Health Promotion, 2000.)

III

■ WEIGHT-FOR-STATURE PERCENTILES

■ BODY MASS INDEX-FOR-AGE PERCENTILES

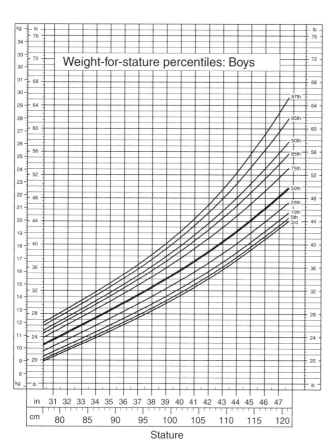

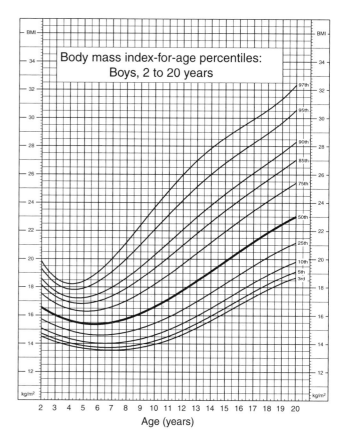

Fig. 3-15   Weight-for-stature percentiles, boys, CDC growth charts: United States. (Developed by the National Center for Health Statistics in collaboration with the National Center for Chronic Disease Prevention and Health Promotion, 2000.)

Fig. 3-16   Body mass index-for-age percentiles, boys, 2 to 20 years, CDC growth charts: United States. (Developed by the National Center for Health Statistics in collaboration with the National Center for Chronic Disease Prevention and Health Promotion, 2000.)

■ HEAD CIRCUMFERENCE

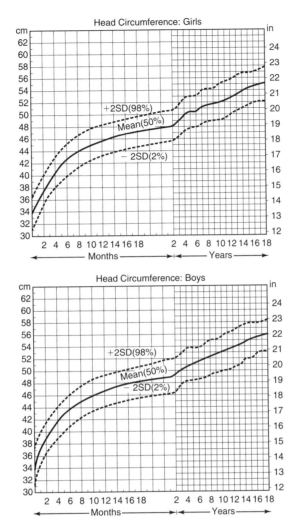

Fig. 3-17   Head circumference for boys and girls 2 to 18 years. (Modified from Niehaus G: *J Pediatr* 41:106, 1968. In Siberry GK, Iannone R [eds]: *The Harriet Lane handbook: a manual for pediatric house officers,* ed 15, St Louis, 2000, Mosby.)

■ **LENGTH, WEIGHT, & HEAD CIRCUMFERENCE**

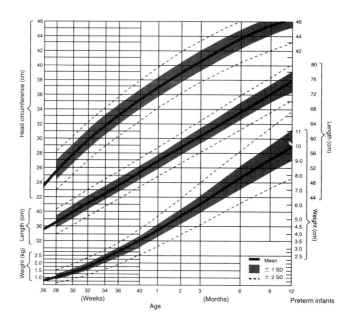

Fig. 3-18   Length, weight, and head circumference for preterm infants. (Modified from Babson SG, Benda GI: *J Pediatr* 89:815, 1976. In Siberry GK, Iannone R [eds]: *The Harriet Lane handbook: a manual for pediatric house officers,* ed 15, St Louis, 2000, Mosby.)

■ **HEIGHT FOR GIRLS 2 TO 18 YEARS**

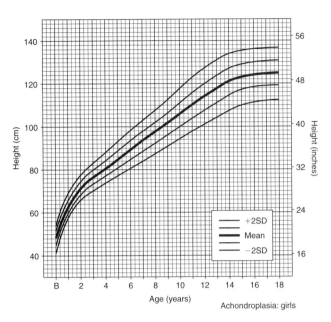

Fig. 3-19   Height for girls with achondroplasia, from birth to 18 years. (From Horton WA et al: *J Pediatr* 93:435, 1978. In Siberry GK, Iannone R [eds]: *The Harriet Lane handbook: a manual for pediatric house officers,* ed 15, St Louis, 2000, Mosby.)

■ **HEAD CIRCUMFERENCE FOR GIRLS 2 TO 18 YEARS**

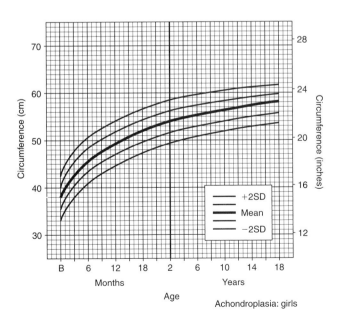

Fig. 3-20   Head circumference for girls with achondroplasia, from birth to 18 years. (From Horton WA et al: *J Pediatr* 93:435, 1978. In Siberry GK, Iannone R [eds]: *The Harriet Lane handbook: a manual for pediatric house officers,* ed 15, St Louis, 2000, Mosby.)

■ **HEIGHT FOR BOYS 2 TO 18 YEARS**

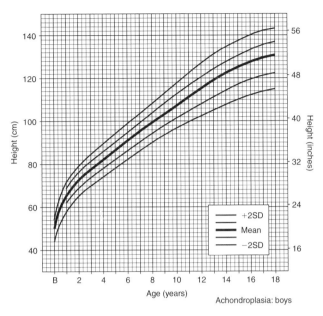

Fig. 3-21   Height for boys with achondroplasia, from birth to 18 years. (From Horton WA et al: *J Pediatr* 93:435, 1978. In Siberry GK, Iannone R [eds]: *The Harriet Lane handbook: a manual for pediatric house officers,* ed 15, St Louis, 2000, Mosby.)

■ **HEAD CIRCUMFERENCE FOR BOYS 2 TO 18 YEARS**

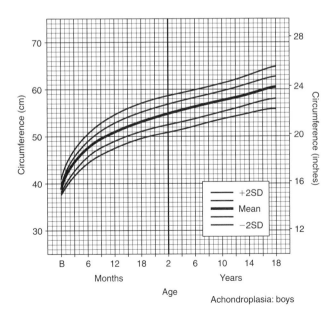

Fig. 3-22   Head circumference for boys with achondroplasia, from birth to 18 years. (From Horton WA et al: *J Pediatr* 93:435, 1978. In Siberry GK, Iannone R [eds]: *The Harriet Lane handbook: a manual for pediatric house officers,* ed 15, St Louis, 2000, Mosby.)

III

■ **LENGTH & WEIGHT**
FOR GIRLS 0 TO 36 MONTHS

■ **HEAD CIRCUMFERENCE**
FOR GIRLS 0 TO 36 MONTHS

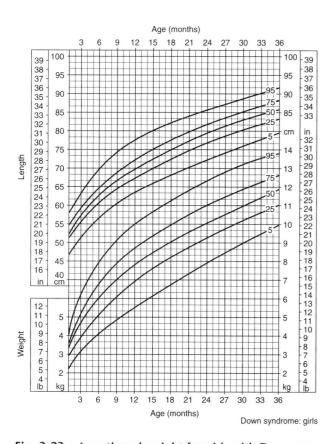

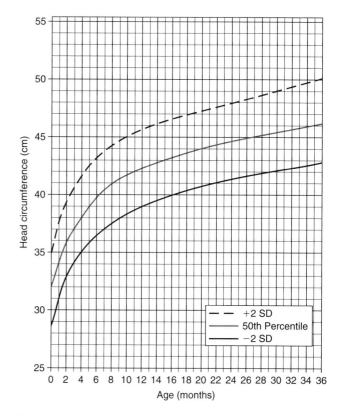

Fig. 3-23   Length and weight for girls with Down syndrome, from birth to 36 months. (Modified from Cronk C et al: *Pediatrics* 81:102, 1988. In Siberry GK, Iannone R [eds]: *The Harriet Lane handbook: a manual for pediatric house officers,* ed 15, St Louis, 2000, Mosby.)

Fig. 3-24   Head circumference for girls (0 to 3) with Down syndrome.

■ **LENGTH & WEIGHT FOR BOYS 0 TO 36 MONTHS**

■ **HEAD CIRCUMFERENCE FOR BOYS 0 TO 36 MONTHS**

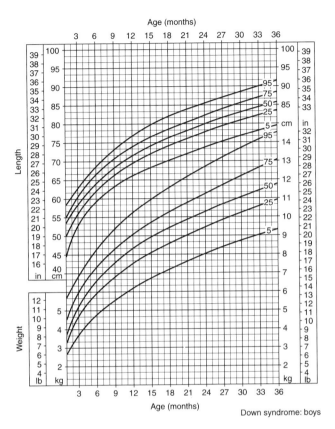

Fig. 3-25 **Length and weight for boys with Down syndrome, from birth to 36 months.** (Modified from Cronk C et al: *Pediatrics* 81:102, 1988. In Siberry GK, Iannone R [eds]: *The Harriet Lane handbook: a manual for pediatric house officers,* ed 15, St Louis, 2000, Mosby.)

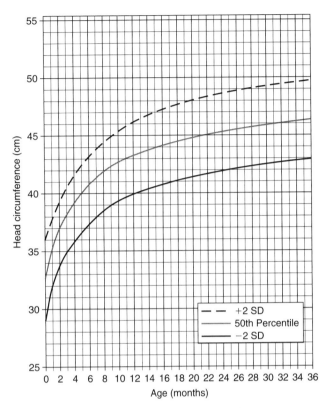

Fig. 3-26 **Head circumference for boys (0 to 3) with Down syndrome.**

■ STATURE & WEIGHT FOR GIRLS 2 TO 18 YEARS   ■ STATURE & WEIGHT FOR BOYS 2 TO 18 YEARS

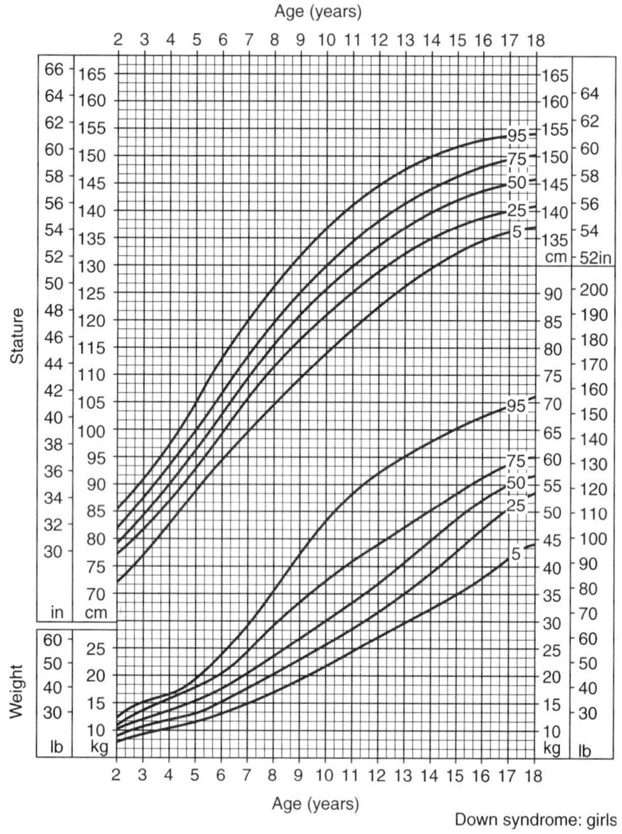

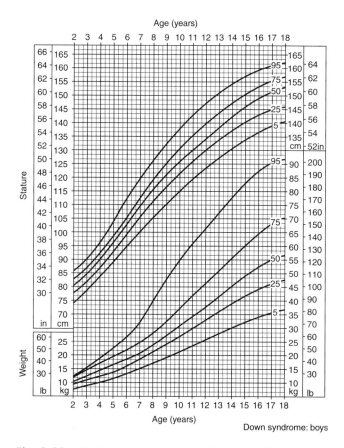

Fig. 3-27   Stature and weight for girls with Down syndrome 2 to 18 years. (Modified from Cronk C et al: *Pediatrics* 81:102, 1988. In Siberry GK, Iannone R [eds]: *The Harriet Lane handbook: a manual for pediatric house officers,* ed 15, St Louis, 2000, Mosby.)

Fig. 3-28   Stature and weight for boys with Down syndrome 2 to 18 years. (Modified from Cronk C et al: *Pediatrics* 81:102, 1988. In Siberry GK, Iannone R [eds]: *The Harriet Lane handbook: a manual for pediatric house officers,* ed 15, St Louis, 2000, Mosby.)

■ **PHYSICAL GROWTH (HEIGHT)**
FOR GIRLS 2 TO 18 YEARS

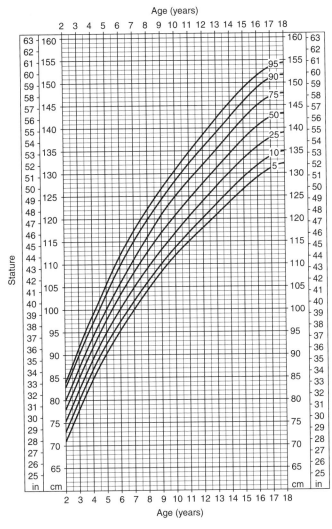

Fig. 3-29   Stature for girls with Turner syndrome 2 to 18 years. (From Lyon AJ, Preece MA, Grant DB: *Arch Dis Child* 60:932, 1985. Courtesy Greentech, Inc., 1987. In Siberry GK, Iannone R [eds]: *The Harriet Lane handbook: a manual for pediatric house officers,* ed 15, St Louis, 2000, Mosby.)

Section 2
DEVELOPMENT

TABLE 3-1 Developmental Milestones

AGE	GROSS MOTOR	VISUAL-MOTOR/ PROBLEM-SOLVING	LANGUAGE	SOCIAL/ADAPTIVE	SPECIFIC GUIDANCE ISSUES
1 mo	Raises head slightly from prone, makes crawling movements	Birth: visually fixes 1 mo: has tight grasp, follows to midline	Alerts to sound	Regards face	Car seats, fever control, thermometers, talking to baby, sleeping, stimulating mobiles
2 mo	Holds head in midline, lifts chest off table	No longer clenches fist tightly, follows object past midline	Smiles socially (after being stroked or talked to)	Recognizes parent	
3 mo	Supports on forearms in prone, holds head up steadily	Holds hands open at rest, follows in circular fashion, responds to visual threat	Coos (produces long vowel sounds in musical fashion)	Reaches for familiar people or objects, anticipates feeding	Car seats, diet, stimulating safe toys, babysitters
4 mo	Rolls front to back, supports on wrists and shifts weight	Reaches with arms in unison, brings hands to midline	Laughs, orients to voice	Enjoys looking around environment	
5 mo	Rolls back to front, sits supported	Transfers objects	Says "ah-goo," razzes, orients to bell (localizes laterally)	—	
6 mo	Sits unsupported, puts feet in mouth in supine position	Unilateral reach, uses raking grasp	Babbles	Recognizes strangers	Car seats, stair gates, electric cord and outlet covers, crawling, stranger anxiety, peek-a-boo, banging toys
7 mo	Creeps	—	Orients to bell (localized indirectly)	—	
8 mo	Comes to sit, crawls	Inspects objects	"Dada" indiscriminately	Fingerfeeds	
9 mo	Pivots when sitting, pulls to stand, cruises	Uses pincer grasp, probes with forefinger, holds bottle, throws objects	"Mama" indiscriminately, gestures, waves bye-bye, understands "no"	Starts to explore environment; plays gesture games (e.g., pat-a-cake)	Car seats, water bath safety, finger-foods, cup weaning, teeth care, first book, appropriate discipline, ipecac
10 mo	Walks when led with both hands held	—	"Dada/mama" discriminately; orients to bell (directly)	—	
11 mo	Walks when led with one hand held	—	One word other than "dada/mama," follows 1-step command with gesture	—	

From Bravo AM: Development. In Siberry GK, Iannone R (eds): *The Harriet Lane handbook: a manual for pediatric house officers,* ed 15, St Louis, 2000, Mosby. Rounded norms from Capute AJ et al: *Dev Med Child Neurol* 28:762, 1986.

TABLE 3-1 Developmental Milestones—cont'd

AGE	GROSS MOTOR	VISUAL-MOTOR/ PROBLEM-SOLVING	LANGUAGE	SOCIAL/ADAPTIVE	SPECIFIC GUIDANCE ISSUES
12 mo	Walks alone	Uses mature pincer grasp, releases voluntarily, marks paper with pencil	Uses two words other than "dada/mama," immature jargoning (runs several unintelligible words together)	Imitates actions, comes when called, cooperates with dressing	Car seats, books, water safety, burns, scalds, decreased appetite, riding toys, pull toys, temper tantrums, nightmares
13 mo	—	—	Uses three words	—	
14 mo	—	—	Follows 1-step command without gesture	—	
15 mo	Creeps up stairs, walks backwards	Scribbles in imitation, builds tower of 2 blocks in imitation	Uses 4-6 words	15-18 mo: uses spoon, uses cup independently	
17 mo	—	—	Uses 7-20 words, points to 5 body parts, uses mature jargoning (includes intelligible words in jargoning)	—	
18 mo	Runs, throws objects from standing without falling	Scribbles spontaneously, builds tower of 3 blocks, turns 2-3 pages at a time	Uses 2-word combinations	Copies parent in tasks (sweeping, dusting), plays in company of other children	
19 mo	—	—	Knows 8 body parts	—	
21 mo	Squats in play, goes up steps	Builds tower of 5 blocks	Uses 50 words, 2-word sentences	Asks to have food and to go to toilet	
24 mo	Walks up and down steps without help	Imitates stroke with pencil, builds tower of 7 blocks, turns pages one at a time, removes shoes, pants, etc.	Uses pronouns (I, you, me) inappropriately, follows 2-step commands	Parallel play	Car seats, books, playground safety, babysitter, giving up blanket, etc., appropriate discipline, learning to play with others
30 mo	Jumps with both feet off floor, throws ball overhand	Holds pencil in adult fashion, performs horizontal and vertical strokes, unbuttons	Uses pronouns appropriately, understands concept of "1," repeats 2 digits forward	Tells first and last names when asked; gets self drink without help	
3 yr	Can alternate feet when going up steps, pedals tricycle	Copies a circle, undresses completely, dresses partially, dries hands if reminded	Uses minimum 250 words, 3-word sentences; uses plurals, past tense; knows all pronouns; understands concept of "2"	Group play, shares toys, takes turns, plays well with others, knows full name, age, sex	
4 yr	Hops, skips, alternates feet going down steps	Copies a square, buttons clothing, dresses self completely, catches ball	Knows colors, says song or poem from memory, asks questions	Tells "tall tales," plays cooperatively with a group of children	Consideration should be given to discussing "private" areas and setting limits for those areas
5 yr	Skips alternating feet, jumps over low obstacles	Copies triangle, ties shoes, spreads with knife	Prints first name, asks what a word means	Plays competitive games, abides by rules, likes to help in household tasks	

From Bravo AM: Development. In Siberry GK, Iannone R (eds): *The Harriet Lane handbook: a manual for pediatric house officers,* ed 15, St Louis, 2000, Mosby. Rounded norms from Capute AJ et al: *Dev Med Child Neurol* 28:762, 1986.

TABLE 3-2 Primitive Reflexes

PRIMITIVE REFLEXES	ELICITATION	RESPONSE	TIMING
Moro reflex (MR, "embrace" response) of fingers, wrists, and elbows	Supine: sudden neck extension; allow head to fall back about 3 cm	Extension, adduction, and then abduction of UEs, with semiflexion	Present at birth, disappears by 3-6 mo
Galant reflex (GR)	Prone suspension: stroking paravertebral area from thoracic to sacral region	Produces truncal incurvature with concavity towards stimulated side	Present at birth, disappears by 2-6 mo
Asymmetric tonic neck reflex (ATNR, "fencer" response)	Supine: rotate head laterally about 45°-90°	Relative extension of limbs on chin side and flexion on occiput side	Present at birth, disappears by 4-9 mo
Symmetric tonic neck reflex (STNR, "cat" reflex)	Sitting: head extension/flexion	Extension of UEs and flexion of LEs/flexion of UEs and LE extension	Appears at 5 mo; not present in most normal children; disappears by 8-9 mo
Tonic labyrinthine supine (TLS)	Supine: extension of the neck (alters relation of labyrinths)	Tonic extension of trunk and LEs, shoulder retraction and adduction, usually with elbow flexion	Present at birth, disappears by 6-9 mo
Tonic labyrinthine prone (TLP)	Prone: flexion of the neck	Active flexion of trunk with protraction of shoulders	Present at birth, disappears by 6-9 mo
Positive support reflex (PSR)	Vertical suspension; bouncing hallucal areas on firm surface	Neonatal: momentary LE extension followed by flexion Mature: extension of LEs and support of body weight	Present a birth; disappears by 2-4 mo Appears by 6 mo
Stepping reflex (SR, walking reflex)	Vertical suspension; hallucal stimulation	Stepping gait	Disappears by 2-3 mo
Crossed extension reflex (CER)	Prone; hallucal stimulation of a LE in full extension	Initial flexion, adduction, then extension of contralateral limb	Present at birth; disappears by 2-3 mo
Plantar grasp (PG)	Stimulation of hallucal area	Plantar flexion grasp	Present at birth; disappears by 9 mo
Palmar grasp	Stimulation of palm	Palmar grasp	Present at birth; disappears by 4 mo
Lower extremity placing (LEP)	Vertical suspension; rubbing tibia or dorsum of foot against edge of tabletop	Initial flexion, then extension, the placing of LE on tabletop	Appears at 1 day
Upper extremity placing (UEP)	Rubbing lateral surface of forearm along edge of tabletop from elbow to wrist to dorsum	Flexion, extension, then placing of hand on tabletop	Appears at 3 mo
Downward thrust (DT)	Vertical suspension; thrust LEs downward	Full extension of LEs	Appears at 3 mo

From Bravo AM: Development. In Siberry GK, Iannone R (eds): *The Harriet Lane handbook: a manual for pediatric house officers,* ed 15, St Louis, 2000, Mosby.
LE, Lower extremity; *UE,* upper extremity.

TABLE 3-3 Postural Reactions

POSTURAL REACTION	AGE OF APPEARANCE	DESCRIPTION	IMPORTANCE
Head righting	6 wk-3 mo	Lifts chin from tabletop in prone position	Necessary for adequate head control and sitting
Landau response	2-3 mo	Extension of head, then trunk and legs when held prone	Early measure of developing trunk control
Derotational righting	4-5 mo	Following passive or active head turning, the body rotates to follow the direction of the head	Prerequisite to independent rolling
Anterior propping	4-5 mo	Arm extension anteriorly in supported sitting	Necessary for tripod sitting
Parachute	5-6 mo	Arm extension when falling	Facial protection when falling
Lateral propping	6-7 mo	Arm extension laterally in protective response	Allows independent sitting
Posterior propping	8-10 mo	Arm extension posteriorly	Allows pivoting in sitting

From Bravo AM: Development. In Siberry GK, Iannone R (eds): *The Harriet Lane handbook: a manual for pediatric house officers,* ed 15, St Louis, 2000, Mosby.

III

TABLE 3-4 **Chronology of Human Dentition of Primary or Deciduous and Secondary or Permanent Teeth**

	AGE AT ERUPTION		AGE AT SHEDDING	
	MAXILLARY	MANDIBULAR	MAXILLARY	MANDIBULAR
Primary Teeth				
Central incisors	6-8 mo	5-7 mo	7-8 yr	6-7 yr
Lateral incisors	8-11 mo	7-10 mo	8-9 yr	7-8 yr
Cuspids (canines)	16-20 mo	16-20 mo	11-12 yr	9-11 yr
First molars	10-16 mo	10-16 mo	10-11 yr	10-12 yr
Second molars	20-30 mo	20-30 mo	10-12 yr	11-13 yr
Secondary Teeth				
Central incisors	7-8 yr	6-7 yr		
Lateral incisors	8-9 yr	7-8 yr		
Cuspids (canines)	11-12 yr	9-11 yr		
First premolars (bicuspids)	10-11 yr	10-12 yr		
Second premolars (bicuspids)	10-12 yr	11-13 yr		
First molars	6-7 yr	6-7 yr		
Second molars	12-13 yr	12-13 yr		
Third molars	17-22 yr	17-22 yr		

From Behrman RE, Kliegman RM, Arvin AM: *Nelson textbook of pediatrics,* ed 15, Philadelphia, 1996, WB Saunders.

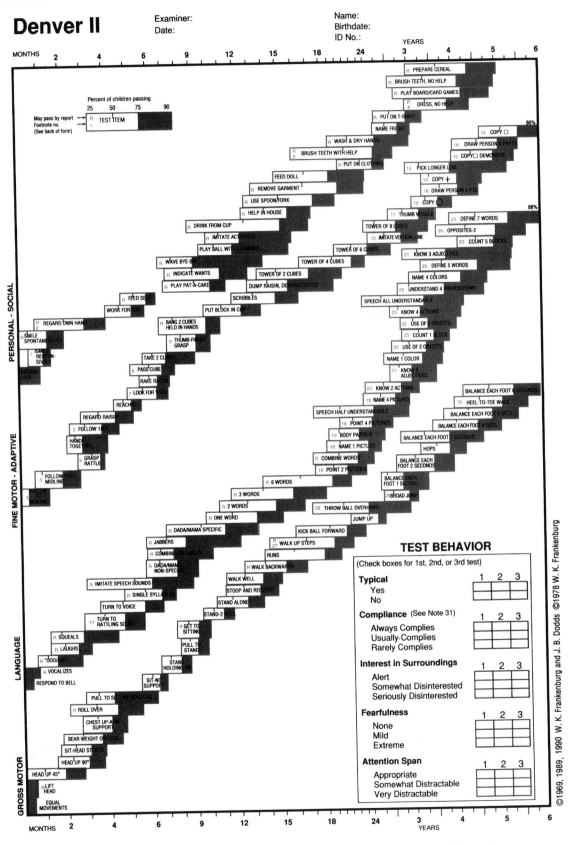

Fig. 3-30 **Denver II.** Testing kits, test forms, and reference manuals (which must be used to ensure accuracy in administration of the test) for the DDST may be ordered from Denver Developmental Material, Inc., P.O. Box 6919, Denver, CO 80206-0919. (Copyright by William K. Frankenburg and J.B. Dodds.)

DIRECTIONS FOR ADMINISTRATION

1. Try to get child to smile by smiling, talking, or waving. Do not touch him/her.
2. Child must stare at hand several seconds.
3. Parent may help guide toothbrush and put toothpaste on brush.
4. Child does not have to be able to tie shoes or button/zip in the back.
5. Move yarn slowly in an arc from one side to the other, about 8" above child's face.
6. Pass if child grasps rattle when it is touched to the backs or tips of fingers.
7. Pass if child tries to see where yarn went. Yarn should be dropped quickly from sight from tester's hand without arm movement.
8. Child must transfer cube from hand to hand without help of body, mouth, or table.
9. Pass if child picks up raisin with any part of thumb and finger.
10. Line can vary only 30 degrees or less from tester's line. /
11. Make a fist with thumb pointing upward and wiggle only the thumb. Pass if child imitates and does not move any fingers other than the thumb.

   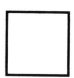

12. Pass any enclosed form. Fail continuous round motions.	13. Which line is longer? (Not bigger.) Turn paper upside down and repeat. (pass 3 of 3 or 5 of 6)	14. Pass any lines crossing near midpoint.	15. Have child copy first. If failed, demonstrate.

When giving items 12, 14, and 15, do not name the forms. Do not demonstrate 12 and 14.

16. When scoring, each pair (2 arms, 2 legs, etc.) counts as one part.
17. Place one cube in cup and shake gently near child's ear, but out of sight. Repeat for other ear.
18. Point to picture and have child name it. (No credit is given for sounds only.)
   If less than 4 pictures are named correctly, have child point to picture as each is named by tester.

 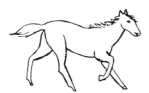 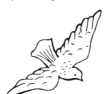 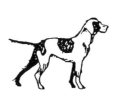 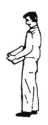

19. Using doll, tell child: Show me the nose, eyes, ears, mouth, hands, feet, tummy, hair. Pass 6 of 8.
20. Using pictures, ask child: Which one flies?... says meow?... talks?... barks?... gallops? Pass 2 of 5, 4 of 5.
21. Ask child: What do you do when you are cold?... tired?... hungry? Pass 2 of 3, 3 of 3.
22. Ask child: What do you do with a cup? What is a chair used for? What is a pencil used for? Action words must be included in answers.
23. Pass if child correctly places <u>and</u> says how many blocks are on paper. (1, 5).
24. Tell child: Put block **on** table; **under** table; **in front of** me, **behind** me. Pass 4 of 4. (Do not help child by pointing, moving head or eyes.)
25. Ask child: What is a ball?... lake?... desk?... house?... banana?... curtain?... fence?... ceiling? Pass if defined in terms of use, shape, what it is made of, or general category (such as banana is fruit, not just yellow). Pass 5 of 8, 7 of 8.
26. Ask child: If a horse is big, a mouse is __? If fire is hot, ice is __? If the sun shines during the day, the moon shines during the __? Pass 2 of 3.
27. Child may use wall or rail only, not person. May not crawl.
28. Child must throw ball overhand 3 feet to within arm's reach of tester.
29. Child must perform standing broad jump over width of test sheet (8 1/2 inches).
30. Tell child to walk forward, ⦿⟳⦿⟳⦿⟳➔ heel within 1 inch of toe. Tester may demonstrate. Child must walk 4 consecutive steps.
31. In the second year, half of normal children are noncompliant.

OBSERVATIONS:

Fig. 3-31 **Instructions for administering the DDST.** (Copyright by William K. Frankenburg and J.B. Dodds.)

■ CLAMS/CAT*

CLAMS/CAT (Capute Scales) (Table 3-5): The Capute Scales are an assessment tool that gives quantitative developmental quotients for visual-motor/problem-solving and language abilities. The CLAMS (Clinical Linguistic and Auditory Milestone Scale) was developed, standardized, and validated for assessment of language development from birth to 36 months of age. The CAT (Clinical Adaptive Test) consists of problem-solving items, for ages from birth to 36 months, adapted from standardized infant psychologic tests.

1. **Supplies:** The kit includes the following items: red ring, cup, 10 cubes, pegboard with six holes and two pegs, metal bell, crayon and paper, tissues, card with four pictures, card with six pictures, bottle and pellets, round stick, glass/Plexiglas, formboard with three shapes.
2. **Responses:** Responses to the test item are recorded as "yes" for pass and "no" for fail. A basal age is determined when all items for 2 consecutive months are scored as "yes." Items for tests at the next higher age group are administered until two consecutive levels of all "no" responses are obtained. Items marked with an asterisk must be answered or demon-strated by the child and not per report of the parent/caregiver.

3. **Scoring:** Scoring is done by calculating the basal age as the highest age group where a child accomplishes all of the test tasks correctly. The age equivalent is then determined by adding the decimal number (recorded in parentheses) next to each correctly scored item passed at age groups beyond the basal age to the basal age itself. This is done to calculate the language age equivalent and the problem-solving age equivalent. Each of these age equivalents is then divided by the child's chronologic age and multiplied by 100 to determine a developmental quotient (DQ). Again, a DQ less than 70% constitutes delay and warrants referral for evaluation to rule out MR or auditory/visual impairment. For example, a 6-month-old child who *can* orient to voice, laugh out loud, and orient toward bell laterally, but who *cannot* ah-goo or razz has a basal age (age where child accomplishes all tasks correctly) of 4 months. An additional 0.3 is added for the ability to orient toward bell laterally, as per the decimal number recorded in parentheses. Together, this gives an age-equivalent of 4.3. The DQ of this patient's linguistic and auditory skills is 4.3 (age equivalent) ÷ 6.0 (chronologic age) × 100 = 71.7.

*From Bravo AM: Development. In Siberry GK, Iannone R (eds): *The Harriet Lane handbook: a manual for pediatric house officers,* ed 15, St Louis, 2000, Mosby.

TABLE 3-5 CLAMS/CAT

AGE (mo)	CLAMS	YES	NO	CAT	YES	NO
1	1. Alerts to sound (0.5)*	—	—	1. Visually fixates momentarily upon red ring (0.5)	—	—
	2. Soothes when picked up (0.5)	—	—	2. Chin off table in prone (0.5)	—	—
2	1. Social smile (1.0)*	—	—	1. Visually follows ring horizontally and vertically (0.5)	—	—
				2. Chest off table prone (0.5)	—	—
3	1. Cooing (1.0)	—	—	1. Visually follows ring in circle (0.3)	—	—
				2. Supports on forearms in prone (0.3)	—	—
				3. Visual threat (0.3)	—	—
4	1. Orients to voice (0.5)*	—	—	1. Unfisted (0.3)	—	—
	2. Laughs aloud (0.5)	—	—	2. Manipulates fingers (0.3)	—	—
				3. Supports on wrists in prone (0.3)	—	—
5	1. Orients toward bell laterally (0.3)*	—	—	1. Pulls down rings (0.3)	—	—
	2. Ah-goo (0.3)	—	—	2. Transfers (0.3)	—	—
	3. Razzing (0.3)	—	—	3. Regards pellet (0.3)	—	—

From Bravo AM: Development. In Siberry GK, Iannone R (eds): *The Harriet Lane handbook: a manual for pediatric house officers,* ed 15, St Louis, 2000, Mosby.

Continued

TABLE 3-5 CLAMS/CAT—cont'd

AGE (mo)	CLAMS	YES	NO	CAT	YES	NO
6	1. Babbling (1.0)	—	—	1. Obtains cube (0.3) 2. Lifts cup (0.3) 3. Radial rake (0.3)	— — —	— — —
7	1. Orients toward bell (1.0)* (upwardly/ indirectly 90°)	—	—	1. Attempts pellet (0.3) 2. Pulls out peg (0.3) 3. Inspects ring (0.3)	— — —	— — —
8	1. "Dada" inappropriately (0.5) 2. "Mama" inappropriately (0.5)	— —	— —	1. Pulls out ring by string (0.3) 2. Secures pellet (0.3) 3. Inspects bell (0.3)	— — —	— — —
9	1. Orients toward bell (upward directly 180°) (0.5)* 2. Gesture language (0.5)	— —	— —	1. Three finger scissor grasp (0.3) 2. Rings bell (0.3) 3. Over the edge for toy (0.3)	— — —	— — —
10	1. Understands "no" (0.3) 2. Uses "dada" appropriately (0.3) 3. Uses "mama" appropriately (0.3)	— — —	— — —	1. Combine cube-cup (0.3) 2. Uncovers bell (0.3) 3. Fingers pegboard (0.3)	— — —	— — —
11	1. One word (other than "mama" and "dada") (1.0)	—	—	1. Mature overhand pincer movement (0.5) 2. Solves cube under cup (0.5)	— —	— —
12	1. One-step command with gesture (0.5) 2. Two-word vocabulary (0.5)	— —	— —	1. Release one cube in cup (0.5) 2. Crayon mark (0.5)	— —	— —
14	1. Three-word vocabulary (1.0) 2. Immature jargoning (1.0)	— —	— —	1. Solves glass frustration (0.6) 2. Out-in with peg (0.6) 3. Solves pellet-bottle with demonstration (0.6)	— — —	— — —
16	1. Four- to six-word vocabulary (1.0) 2. One-step command without gesture (1.0)	— —	— —	1. Solves pellet-bottle spontaneously (0.6) 2. Round block on form board (0.6) 3. Scribbles in imitation (0.6)	— — —	— — —
18	1. Mature jargoning (0.5) 2. 7-10 word vocabulary (0.5) 3. Points to one picture (0.5)* 4. Body parts (0.5)	— — — —	— — — —	1. Ten cubes in cup (0.5) 2. Solves round hole in form board reversed (0.5) 3. Spontaneous scribbling with crayon (0.5) 4. Pegboard completed spontaneously (0.5)	— — — —	— — — —
21	1. 20-word vocabulary (1.0) 2. Two-word phrases (1.0) 3. Points to two pictures (1.0)*	— — —	— — —	1. Obtains object with stick (1.0) 2. Solves square in form board (1.0) 3. Tower of three cubes (1.0)	— — —	— — —
24	1. 50-word vocabulary (1.0) 2. Two-step command (1.0) 3. Two word sentences (1.0)	— — —	— — —	1. Attempts to fold paper (0.7) 2. Horizontal four cube train (0.7) 3. Imitates stroke with pencil (0.7) 4. Completes form board (0.7)	— — — —	— — — —
30	1. Uses pronouns appropriately (1.5) 2. Concept of one (1.5)* 3. Points to seven pictures (1.5)* 4. Two digits forward (1.5)*	— — — —	— — — —	1. Horizontal-vertical stroke with pencil (1.5) 2. Form board reversed (1.5) 3. Folds paper with definite crease (1.5) 4. Train with chimney (1.5)	— — — —	— — — —
36	1. 250-word vocabulary (1.5) 2. Three-word sentence (1.5) 3. Three digits forward (1.5)* 4. Follows two prepositional commands (1.5)*	— — — —	— — — —	1. Three cube bridge (1.5) 2. Draws circle (1.5) 3. Names one color (1.5) 4. Draw-a-person with head plus one other part of body (1.5)	— — — —	— — — —

From Bravo AM: Development. In Siberry GK, Iannone R (eds): *The Harriet Lane handbook: a manual for pediatric house officers*, ed 15, St Louis, 2000, Mosby.

■ BLOCK SKILLS*

The structures should be demonstrated for the child. Figure 3-32 includes the developmental age at which each structure can usually be accomplished.

*From Siberry GK, Iannone R (eds): *The Harriet Lane handbook: a manual for pediatric house officers,* ed 15, St Louis, 2000, Mosby.

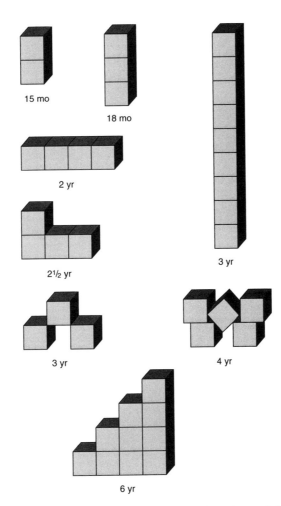

Fig. 3-32   Block skills. (From Capute AJ, Accardo PJ: *The pediatrician and the developmentally disabled child: a clinical textbook on mental retardation,* Baltimore, 1979, University Press.)

■ GESELL FIGURES* (Figure 3-33)

One should note that the examiner is not supposed to demonstrate the drawing of the figures for the patient; however, most developmentalists do demonstrate and do not feel that it makes a difference.

*From Siberry GK, Iannone R (eds): *The Harriet Lane handbook: a manual for pediatric house officers,* ed 15, St Louis, 2000, Mosby.

15 months	Imitates scribble
18 months	Scribbles spontaneously
2 years	Imitates stroke
2½ years	Differentiates horizontal and vertical stroke

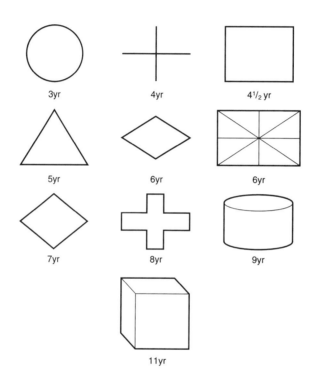

Fig. 3-33   Gesell figures. (From Illingsworth RS: *The development of the infant and young child, normal and abnormal,* ed 5, Baltimore, 1972, Williams & Wilkins; and Cattel P: *The measurement of intelligence of infants and young children,* New York, 1960, The Psychological Corporation.)

■ GOODENOUGH-HARRIS DRAW-A-PERSON TEST

a. Procedure: Give the child a pencil (preferably a no. 2 with eraser) and a sheet of blank paper. Instruct the child to "Draw a person; draw the best person you can." Supply encouragement if needed (i.e., "Draw a whole person"); however, do not suggest specific supplementation or changes.

b. Scoring: Ask the child to describe or explain the drawing to you. Give the child one point for each detail present using the guide in Table 3-6. (Maximum score = 51.)

c. Age norms (Table 3-7).

*From Straub DM: Adolescent medicine. In Siberry GK, Iannone R (eds): *The Harriet Lane handbook: a manual for pediatric house officers,* ed 15, St Louis, 2000, Mosby.

TABLE 3-6 Goodenough-Harris Scoring

General	☐ Head present ☐ Legs present ☐ Arms present	**Joints:**	☐ Elbow, shoulder, or both ☐ Knee, hip, or both
Trunk:	☐ Present ☐ Length greater than breadth ☐ Shoulders	**Proportion:**	☐ Head: 10% to 50% of trunk area ☐ Arms: Approx. same length as trunk ☐ Legs: 1-2 times trunk length; width less than trunk width ☐ Feet: 10% to 30% leg length ☐ Arms and legs in two dimensions ☐ Heel
Arms/legs:	☐ Attached to trunk ☐ At correct point		
Neck:	☐ Present ☐ Outline of neck continuous with head, trunk, or both	**Motor coordination:**	☐ Lines firm and well connected ☐ Firmly drawn with correct joining ☐ Head outline ☐ Trunk outline ☐ Outline of arms and legs ☐ Features
Face:	☐ Eyes ☐ Nose ☐ Mouth ☐ Nose and mouth in two dimensions ☐ Nostrils	**Ears:**	☐ Present ☐ Correct position and proportion
Hair:	☐ Present ☐ On more than circumference; nontransparent	**Eye detail:**	☐ Brow or lashes ☐ Pupil ☐ Proportion ☐ Glance directed front in profile drawing
Clothing:	☐ Present ☐ Two articles; nontransparent ☐ Entire drawing nontransparent (sleeves and trousers) ☐ Four articles ☐ Costume complete	**Chin:**	☐ Present; forehead ☐ Projection
		Profile:	☐ Not more than one error ☐ Correct
Fingers:	☐ Present ☐ Correct number ☐ Two dimension; length, breadth ☐ Thumb opposition ☐ Hand distinct from fingers and arm		

From Bravo AM: Development. In Siberry GK, Iannone R (eds): *The Harriet Lane handbook: a manual for pediatric house officers,* ed 15, St Louis, 2000, Mosby.

TABLE 3-7 Goodenough Age Norms

Age (yr)	3	4	5	6	7	8	9	10	11	12	13
Points	2	6	10	14	18	22	26	30	34	38	42

From Taylor E: *Psychological appraisal of children with cerebral defects,* Boston, 1961, Harvard University. Adapted from Goodenough FL: *Measurement of intelligence by drawings,* Chicago, 1926, World Book Co.

Section 3
ADOLESCENT

■ **CONTENT FOR ROUTINE ADOLESCENT HEALTH VISIT***

A. **MEDICAL HISTORY:** Immunizations, chronic illness, chronic medications (including hormonal contraception), recent dental care, hospitializations, surgeries.

B. **FAMILY HISTORY:** Psychiatric disorders, suicide, alcoholism/substance abuse.

C. **REVIEW OF SYSTEMS**
   1. **Dietary habits:** Typical foods consumed, types and frequency of meals skipped, vomiting, use of laxatives or other weight-loss methods, dietary sources of calcium
   2. **Recent weight gain or loss**

D. **PSYCHOSOCIAL/MEDICOSOCIAL HISTORY (HEADSS)**
   1. **H(ome)**
      a. Household composition.
      b. Family dynamics and relationships with adolescent.
      c. Living/sleeping arrangements.
      d. Guns in the home.
   2. **E(ducation)**
      a. School attendance/absences.
      b. Ever failed a grade(s); grades as compared to last year's?
      c. Attitude toward school.
      d. Favorite, most difficult, best subjects
      e. Special educational needs.
      f. Goals: vocational/technical school, college, career.
   3. **A(ctivities)**
      a. Physical activity, exercise, hobbies.
      b. Sports participation.
      c. Job.
      d. Weapon carrying and fighting.
   4. **D(rugs)**
      a. Cigarettes/smokeless tobacco: Age at first use, packs per day.
      b. Alcohol and/or other drugs: Use at school or parties; use by friends, self; kind (i.e., beer, wine coolers), frequency, and quantity used. If yes, CAGE: Have you ever felt the need to **C**ut down; have others **A**nnoyed you by commenting on your use; have you ever felt **G**uilty about your use; have you ever needed an **E**yeopener (alcohol first thing in morning)?
   5. **S(exuality)**
      a. Sexual feelings: Opposite or same sex.
      b. Sexual intercourse: Age at first intercourse, number of lifetime and current partners, recent change in partners.
      c. Contraception/sexually transmitted disease (STD) prevention.
      d. History of STDs.
      e. Prior pregnancies, abortions; ever fathered a child?
      f. History of/current nonconsensual intimate physical contact/sex.
   6. **S(uicide)/depression**
      a. Feelings about self: Positive and negative.
      b. History of depression or other mental health problems, prior suicidal thoughts, prior suicide attempts.
      c. Sleep problems: Difficulty getting to sleep, early waking.

E. **PHYSICAL EXAMINATION (MOST PERTINENT ASPECTS)**
   1. **Skin:** Acne (type and distribution of lesions).
   2. **Thyroid**
   3. **Spine:** Scoliosis (see p. 812 for assessment and treatment).
   4. **Breasts:** Tanner stage (Fig. 3-34 and Table 3-8), masses.
   5. **External genitalia**
      a. Pubic hair distribution: Tanner stage (Figs. 3-35 and 3-36 and Table 3-9)
      b. Testicular examination: Tanner stage (Fig. 3-36 and Table 3-10), masses.
   6. **Pelvic examination:** Sexually active, gynecologic compliant.

F. **LABORATORY TESTS**
   1. **Purified protein derivative (PPD):** If high risk.
   2. **Hemoglobin/hematocrit:** Once during puberty for boys, once after menarche for girls.
   3. **Sexually active adolescents:** Serologic tests for syphilis annually; offer HIV testing, especially if syphilis or other ulcerative genital disease.
      a. Males: First part voided urinalysis/leukocyte esterase screen with positive results confirmed by detection tests for gonorrhea and chlamydia (i.e., cultures, ligase/polymerase chain reaction).
      b. Females: Detection tests for gonorrhea

---

*From From Straub DM: Adolescent medicine. In Siberry GK, Iannone R (eds): *The Harriet Lane handbook: a manual for pediatric house officers,* ed 15, St Louis, 2000, Mosby.

and chlamydia (i.e., cultures, LCR/PCR), wet preparation, potassium hydroxide (KOH), cervical Gram stain, Papanicolaou smear, midvaginal pH.

G. IMMUNIZATIONS (see p. 822 for specifics of dosing, route, formulation, and schedules)
   1. **Tetanus and diphtheria (Td):** Booster age 11-15 years.
   2. **Measles:** Two doses of live attenuated vaccine are required after first birthday. Use measles, mumps, rubella (MMR) vaccine if not previously immunized for mumps or rubella. Assess pregnancy status, and do not administer rubella vaccine to woman anticipating pregnancy within 90 days.
   3. **Hepatitis B vaccine:** Recommended for all adolescents (three doses) if not previously vaccinated.
   4. **Varicella vaccine:** Two doses at least 1 month apart are recommended for adolescents ≥13 years old with no history of disease.

H. ANTICIPATORY GUIDANCE
   1. **Sexuality** (e.g., abstinence, STD/pregnancy prevention)
   2. **Nutrition:** Excessive/inadequate calories, balanced diet, calcium.
   3. **Coping skills/violence prevention**
   4. **Safety:** Driving/seat belts, guns, bicycle helmets.
   5. **Substance abuse prevention**

III

■ **PUBERTAL EVENTS & TANNER STAGE DIAGRAMS***

The temporal interrelationship of the biologic and psychosocial events of adolescence are illustrated in Figs. 3-34 to 3-37 and Tables 3-8 to 3-10. Age limits for the events and stages are appropriate and may differ from those used by other authors.

From Straub DM: Adolescent medicine. In Siberry GK, Iannone R (eds): *The Harriet Lane handbook: a manual for pediatric house officers*, ed 15, St Louis, 2000, Mosby.

■ **BREAST DEVELOPMENT IN FEMALES**

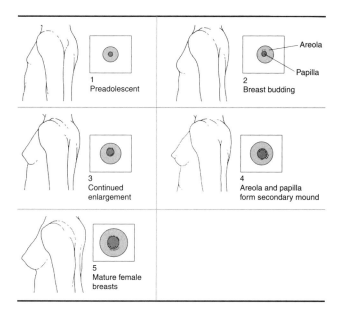

Fig. 3-34 **Tanner states of breast development in females.** (Modified from Johnson TR, Moore WM, Jefferies JE: *Children are different: development physiology*, ed 2, Columbus, Ohio, 1979, Ross Laboratories, Division of Abbott Laboratories. In Straub DM: Adolescent medicine. In Siberry GK, Iannone R [eds]: *The Harriet Lane handbook: a manual for pediatric house officers*, ed 15, St Louis, 2000, Mosby.)

TABLE 3-8 **Breast Development**

STAGE	COMMENT (MEAN AGE ± STANDARD DEVIATION)
I	Preadolescent; elevation of papilla only
II	Breast bud; elevation of breast and papilla as small mound; enlargement of areolar diameter (11.15 ± 1.10)
III	Further enlargement and elevation of breast and areola; no separation of their contours (12.15 ± 1.09)
IV	Projection of areola and papilla to form secondary mound above level of breast (13.11 ± 1.15)
V	Mature stage; projection of papilla only as a result of recession of areola to general contour of breast (15.3 ± 1.74)

Modified from Marshall WA, Tanner JM: *Arch Dis Child* 44:291, 1969; and Marshall WA, Tanner JM: *Arch Dis Child* 45:13, 1970. In Oski FA (eds): *Principles and practice of pediatrics*, Philadelphia, 1994, JB Lippincott.

■ PUBIC HAIR DEVELOPMENT IN FEMALES

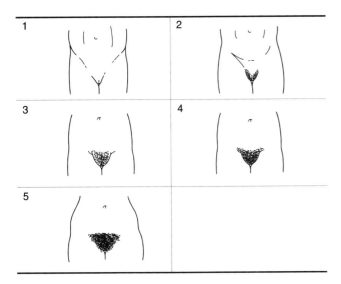

Fig. 3-35   Tanner stages of pubic hair development in females. (Modified from Neinstein LS: *Adolescent health care: a practical guide,* ed 2, Baltimore, 1991, Urban & Schwarzenberg. In Straub DM: Adolescent medicine. In Siberry GK, Iannone R [eds]: *The Harriet Lane handbook: a manual for pediatric house officers,* ed 15, St Louis, 2000, Mosby.)

■ PUBLIC HAIR & GENITAL DEVELOPMENT IN MALES

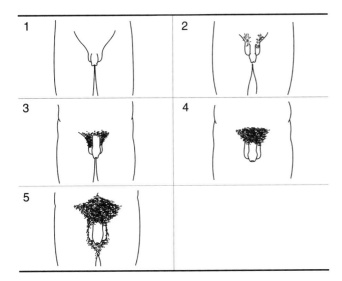

Fig. 3-36   Pubic hair and genital development in males. (Modified from Neinstein LS: *Adolescent health care: a practical guide,* ed 2, Baltimore, 1991, Urban & Schwarzenberg. In Straub DM: Adolescent medicine. In Siberry GK, Iannone R [eds]: *The Harriet Lane handbook: a manual for pediatric house officers,* ed 15, St Louis, 2000, Mosby.)

TABLE 3-9   Pubic Hair (Male and Female)

STAGE	COMMENT (MEAN AGE ± STANDARD DEVIATION)
I	Preadolescent; Vellus over pubes no further developed than that over abdominal wall (i.e., no pubic hair)
II	Sparse growth of long, slightly pigmented downy hair, straight or only slightly curled, chiefly at base of penis or along labia (male: 13.44 ± 1.09; female: 11.69 ± 1.21)
III	Considerably darker, coarser and more curled; hair spreads sparsely over junction of pubes (male: 13.9 ± 1.04; female: 12.36 ± 1.10)
IV	Hair resembles adult in type; distribution still considerably less than in adult; no spread to medial surface of thighs (male: 14.36 ± 1.08; female: 12.95 ± 1.06)
V	Adult in quantity and type with distribution of the horizontal pattern (male: 15.18 ± 1.07; female: 14.41 ± 1.12)
VI	Spread up linea alba: "Male escutcheon"

Modified from Marshall WA, Tanner JM: *Arch Dis Child* 44:291, 1969; and Marshall WA, Tanner JM: *Arch Dis Child* 45:13, 1970. In Oski FA (eds): *Principles and practice of pediatrics,* Philadelphia, 1994, JB Lippincott.

TABLE 3-10   Genital Development (Male)

STAGE	COMMENT (MEAN AGE ± STANDARD DEVIATION)
I	Preadolescent; testes, scrotum, and penis about same size and proportion as in early childhood
II	Enlargement of scrotum and testes; skin of scrotum reddens and changes in texture; little or no enlargement of penis (11.64 ± 1.07)
III	Enlargement of penis, first mainly in length; further growth of testes and scrotum (12.85 ± 1.04)
IV	Increased size of penis with growth in breadth and development of glans; further enlargement of testes and scrotum and increased darkening of scrotal skin (13.77 ± 1.02)
V	Genitalia adult in size and shape (14.92 ± 1.10)

Modified from Marshall WA, Tanner JM: *Arch Dis Child* 44:291, 1969; and Marshall WA, Tanner JM: *Arch Dis Child* 45:13, 1970. In Oski FA (eds): *Principles and practice of pediatrics,* Philadelphia, 1994, JB Lippincott.

III

■ **EARLY ADOLESCENCE THROUGH
   YOUNG ADULTS**

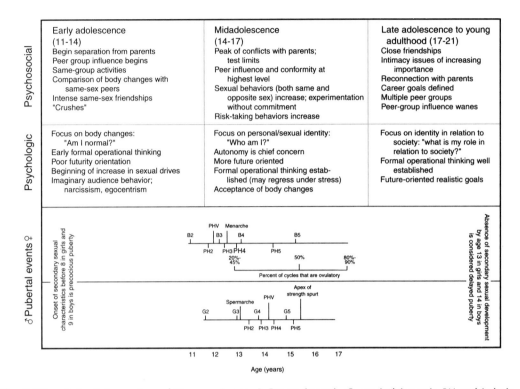

Fig. 3-37   Pubertal events and Tanner stages. *B,* Breast (stage); *G,* genital (stage); *PH,* pubic hair (stage); *PHV,* peak height velocity. (Modified from Joffe A: Adolescent medicine. In Oski FA et al [eds]: *Principles and practice of pediatrics,* Philadelphia, 1994, JB Lippincott.)

■ GIRLS 2 TO 18 YEARS

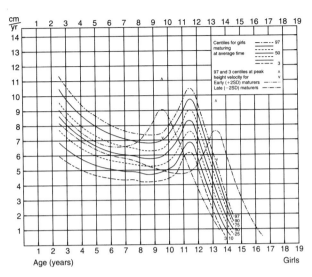

Fig. 3-38   Height velocity for girls 2 to 18 years. (Modified from Tanner JM, Davis PS: *J Pediatr* 107:317, 1985. Courtesy Castlemead Publications, 1985. Distributed by Sereno Laboratories. In Siberry GK, Iannone R [eds]: *The Harriet Lane handbook: a manual for pediatric house officers,* ed 15, St Louis, 2000, Mosby.)

■ BOYS 2 TO 18 YEARS

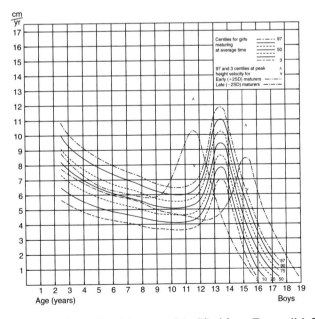

Fig. 3-39   Height velocity for boys 2 to 18 years. (Modified from Tanner JM, Davis PS: *J Pediatr* 107:317, 1985. Courtesy Castlemead Publications, 1985. Distributed by Sereno Laboratories. In Siberry GK, Iannone R [eds]: *The Harriet Lane handbook: a manual for pediatric house officers,* ed 15, St Louis, 2000, Mosby.)

■ **SCOLIOSIS***

Refer to Fig. 3-40 and see the section "Scoliosis" in Part II for routine screening for scoliosis. Many curves that are detected on screening are nonprogressive and/or too slight to be significant.

Assessment

1. **Radiographic determination of the Cobb angle** (Fig. 3-41). If clinical suspicion of significant scoliosis.
2. **Bone scan ± MRI:** If there is pain that is worse at night, progressive, well localized, or otherwise suspicious.
3. **MRI:** If presents at <10 years old or presence of "opposite" curves (left-sided thoracic, right-sided lumbar).

---

*From Straub DM: Adolescent medicine. In Siberry GK, Iannone R (eds): *The Harriet Lane handbook: a manual for pediatric house officers,* ed 15, St Louis, 2000, Mosby.

Treatment

According to the Cobb angle and skeletal maturity, which is assessed by grading the ossification of the iliac crest.

1. **Skeletally immature**
   a. <10 degrees: Single follow-up radiograph in 4-6 months to ensure no significant progression.
   b. 10-20 degrees: Radiographs every 4-6 months.
   c. 20-40 degrees: Bracing.
   d. >40 degrees: Surgical correction.
2. **Skeletally mature**
   a. <40 degrees: No further evaluation or intervention indicated.
   b. >40 degrees: Surgical correction.
3. **Orthopedic referral:** This is indicated if skeletally immature with curve >20 degrees, skeletally mature with curve >40 degrees, and/or presence of suspicious pain or neurologic symptoms.

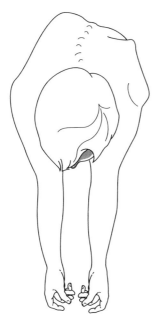

Fig. 3-40 Forward-bending test. This emphasizes any asymmetry of the paraspinous muscles and rib cage. (From Straub DM: Adolescent medicine. In Siberry GK, Iannone R [eds]: *The Harriet Lane handbook: a manual for pediatric house officers,* ed 15, St Louis, 2000, Mosby.)

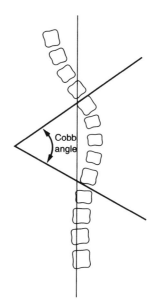

Fig. 3-41 Cobb angle. This is measured using the superior and inferior endplates of the most tilted vertebrae at the end of each curve. (From Scoliosis. In Siberry GK, Iannone R [eds]: *The Harriet Lane handbook: a manual for pediatric house officers,* ed 15, St Louis, 2000, Mosby.)

Section 4
VITAL SIGNS

TABLE 3-11 **Mean Respiratory Rates ± 1 Standard Deviation**

AGE (yr)	BOYS	GIRLS	AGE (yr)	BOYS	GIRLS
0-1	31 ± 8	30 ± 6	9-10	19 ± 2	19 ± 2
1-2	26 ± 4	27 ± 4	10-11	19 ± 2	19 ± 2
2-3	25 ± 4	25 ± 3	11-12	19 ± 3	19 ± 3
3-4	24 ± 3	24 ± 3	12-13	19 ± 3	19 ± 2
4-5	23 ± 2	22 ± 2	13-14	19 ± 2	18 ± 2
5-6	22 ± 2	21 ± 2	14-15	18 ± 2	18 ± 3
6-7	21 ± 3	21 ± 3	15-16	17 ± 3	18 ± 3
7-8	20 ± 3	20 ± 2	16-17	17 ± 2	17 ± 3
8-9	20 ± 2	20 ± 2	17-18	16 ± 3	17 ± 3

From Iliff A, Lee V: *Child Dev* 23:240, 1952. In Siberry GK, Iannone R (eds): *The Harriet Lane handbook: a manual for pediatric house officers,* ed 15, St Louis, 2000, Mosby.

III

TABLE 3-12   Age-Specific Heart Rates
              (beats/min)

AGE	2%	MEAN	98%
<1 day	93	123	154
1-2 days	91	123	159
3-6 days	91	129	166
1-3 wk	107	148	182
1-2 mo	121	149	179
3-5 mo	106	141	186
6-11 mo	109	134	169
1-2 yr	89	119	151
3-4 yr	73	108	137
5-7 yr	65	100	133
8-11 yr	62	91	130
12-15 yr	60	85	119

From Chiang LK, Dunn AE: Cardiology. In Siberry GK, Iannone R (eds): *The Harriet Lane handbook: a manual for pediatric house officers,* ed 15, St Louis, 2000, Mosby.

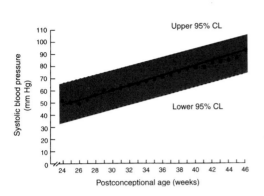

Fig. 3-42 Linear regression of mean systolic blood pressure on postconceptual age (gestational age in weeks + weeks after delivery). (From Zubrow AB et al: *J Perinatol* 15:470, 1995.)

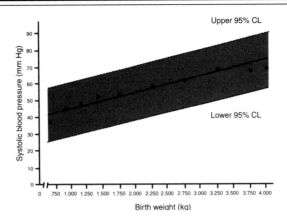

Fig. 3-43 Linear regression of mean systolic blood pressure on birth weight on day 1 of life. (From Zubrow AB et al: *J Perinatol* 15:470, 1995.)

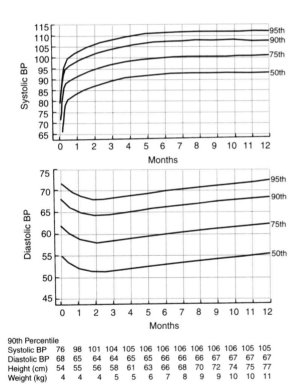

90th Percentile

Systolic BP	76	98	101	104	105	106	106	106	106	106	106	105	105
Diastolic BP	68	65	64	64	65	65	66	66	66	67	67	67	67
Height (cm)	54	55	56	58	61	63	66	68	70	72	74	75	77
Weight (kg)	4	4	4	5	5	6	7	8	9	9	10	10	11

Fig. 3-44 Age-specific percentiles of blood pressure *(BP)* measurements in girls from birth to 12 months of age; Korotkoff phase IV (K4) used for diastolic BP. (From Horan MJ: *Pediatrics* 79:1, 1987.)

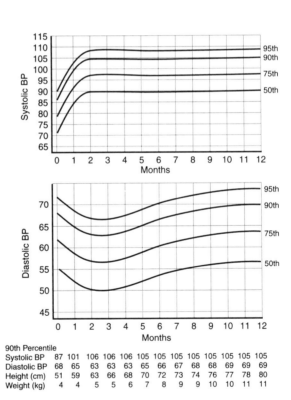

90th Percentile

Systolic BP	87	101	106	106	106	105	105	105	105	105	105	105	105
Diastolic BP	68	65	63	63	63	65	66	67	68	68	69	69	69
Height (cm)	51	59	63	66	68	70	72	73	74	76	77	78	80
Weight (kg)	4	4	5	5	6	7	8	9	9	10	10	11	11

Fig. 3-45 Age-specific percentiles of blood pressure *(BP)* measurements in boys from birth to 12 months of age; Korotkoff phase IV (K4) used for diastolic BP. (From Horan MJ: *Pediatrics* 79:1, 1987.)

III

TABLE 3-13 Blood Pressure Levels for the 90th and 95th Percentiles of Blood Pressure for *Girls* Aged 1-17 Years by Percentiles of Height

		SYSTOLIC BP (mm Hg) BY PERCENTILE OF HEIGHT							DIASTOLIC BP (DBP) (mm Hg) BY PERCENTILE OF HEIGHT						
PERCENTILES AGE (yr)	HEIGHT*→ BP†↓	5%	10%	25%	50%	75%	90%	95%	5%	10%	25%	50%	75%	90%	95%
1	90th	97	98	99	100	102	103	104	53	53	53	54	55	56	56
	95th	101	102	103	104	105	107	107	57	57	57	58	59	60	60
2	90th	99	99	100	102	103	104	105	57	57	58	58	59	60	61
	95th	102	103	104	105	107	108	109	61	61	62	62	63	64	65
3	90th	100	100	102	103	104	105	106	61	61	61	62	63	63	64
	95th	104	104	105	107	108	109	110	65	65	65	66	67	67	68
4	90th	101	102	103	104	106	107	108	63	63	64	65	65	66	67
	95th	105	106	107	108	109	111	111	67	67	68	69	69	70	71
5	90th	103	103	104	106	107	108	109	65	66	66	67	68	68	69
	95th	107	107	108	110	111	112	113	69	70	70	71	72	72	73
6	90th	104	105	106	107	109	110	111	67	67	68	69	69	70	71
	95th	108	109	110	111	112	114	114	71	71	72	73	73	74	75
7	90th	106	107	108	109	110	112	112	69	69	69	70	71	72	72
	95th	110	110	112	113	114	115	116	73	73	73	74	75	76	76
8	90th	108	109	110	111	112	113	114	70	70	71	71	72	73	74
	95th	112	112	113	115	116	117	118	74	74	75	75	76	77	78
9	90th	110	110	112	113	114	115	116	71	72	72	73	74	74	75
	95th	114	114	115	117	118	119	120	75	76	76	77	78	78	79
10	90th	112	112	114	115	116	117	118	73	73	73	74	75	76	76
	95th	116	116	117	119	120	121	122	77	77	77	78	79	80	80
11	90th	114	114	116	117	118	119	120	74	74	75	75	76	77	77
	95th	118	118	119	121	122	123	124	78	78	79	79	80	81	81
12	90th	116	116	118	119	120	121	122	75	75	76	76	77	78	78
	95th	120	120	121	123	124	125	126	79	79	80	80	81	82	82
13	90th	118	118	119	121	122	123	124	76	76	77	78	78	79	80
	95th	121	122	123	125	126	127	128	80	80	81	82	82	83	84
14	90th	119	120	121	122	124	125	126	77	77	78	79	79	80	81
	95th	123	124	125	126	128	129	130	81	81	82	83	83	84	85
15	90th	121	121	122	124	125	126	127	78	78	79	79	80	81	82
	95th	124	125	126	128	129	130	131	82	82	83	83	84	85	86
16	90th	122	122	123	125	126	127	128	79	79	79	80	81	82	82
	95th	125	126	127	128	130	131	132	83	83	83	84	85	86	86
17	90th	122	123	124	125	126	128	128	79	79	79	80	81	82	82
	95th	126	126	127	129	130	131	132	83	83	83	84	85	86	86

From Chiang LK, Dunn AE: Cardiology. In Siberry GK, Iannone R (eds): *The Harriet Lane handbook: a manual for pediatric house officers*, ed 15, St Louis, 2000, Mosby.
*Height percentile determined by standard growth curves.
†Blood pressure percentile determined by a single measurement.

TABLE 3-14 Blood Pressure Levels for the 90th and 95th Percentiles of Blood Pressure for *Boys* Aged 1-17 Years by Percentiles of Height

		SYSTOLIC BP (mm Hg) BY PERCENTILE OF HEIGHT							DIASTOLIC BP (DBP) (mm Hg) BY PERCENTILE OF HEIGHT						
PERCENTILES AGE (yr)	HEIGHT*→ BP†↓	5%	10%	25%	50%	75%	90%	95%	5%	10%	25%	50%	75%	90%	95%
1	90th	94	95	97	98	100	102	102	50	51	52	53	54	54	55
	95th	98	99	101	102	104	106	106	55	55	56	57	58	59	59
2	90th	98	99	100	102	104	105	106	55	55	56	57	58	59	59
	95th	101	102	104	106	108	109	110	59	59	60	61	62	63	63
3	90th	100	101	103	105	107	108	109	59	59	60	61	62	63	63
	95th	104	105	107	109	111	112	113	63	63	64	65	66	67	67
4	90th	102	103	105	107	109	110	111	62	62	63	64	65	66	66
	95th	106	107	109	111	113	114	115	66	67	67	68	69	70	71
5	90th	104	105	106	108	110	112	112	65	65	66	67	68	69	69
	95th	108	109	110	112	114	115	116	69	70	70	71	72	73	74
6	90th	105	106	108	110	111	113	114	67	68	69	70	70	71	72
	95th	109	110	112	114	115	117	117	72	72	73	74	75	76	76
7	90th	106	107	109	111	113	114	115	69	70	71	72	72	73	74
	95th	110	111	113	115	116	118	119	74	74	75	76	77	78	78
8	90th	107	108	110	112	114	115	116	71	71	72	73	74	75	75
	95th	111	112	114	116	118	119	120	75	76	76	77	78	79	80
9	90th	109	110	112	113	115	117	117	72	73	73	74	75	76	77
	95th	113	114	116	117	119	121	121	76	77	78	79	80	80	81
10	90th	110	112	113	115	117	118	119	73	74	74	75	76	77	78
	95th	114	115	117	119	121	122	123	77	78	79	80	80	81	82
11	90th	112	113	115	117	119	120	121	74	74	75	76	77	78	78
	95th	116	117	119	121	123	124	125	78	79	79	80	81	82	83
12	90th	115	116	117	119	121	123	123	75	75	76	77	78	78	79
	95th	119	120	121	123	125	126	127	79	79	80	81	82	83	83
13	90th	117	118	120	122	124	125	126	75	76	76	77	78	79	80
	95th	121	122	124	126	128	129	130	79	80	81	82	83	83	84
14	90th	120	121	123	125	126	128	128	76	76	77	78	79	80	80
	95th	124	125	127	128	130	132	132	80	81	81	82	83	84	85
15	90th	123	124	125	127	129	131	131	77	77	78	79	80	81	81
	95th	127	128	129	131	133	134	135	81	82	83	83	84	85	86
16	90th	125	126	128	130	132	133	134	79	79	80	81	82	82	83
	95th	129	130	132	134	136	137	138	83	83	84	85	86	87	87
17	90th	128	129	131	133	134	136	136	81	81	82	83	84	85	85
	95th	132	133	135	136	138	140	140	85	85	86	87	88	89	89

From Chiang LK, Dunn AE: Cardiology. In Siberry GK, Iannone R (eds): *The Harriet Lane handbook: a manual for pediatric house officers*, ed 15, St Louis, 2000, Mosby.
*Height percentile determined by standard growth curves.
†Blood pressure percentile determined by a single measurement.

TABLE 3-15 **Predicted Average Peak Expiratory Flow Rates for Normal Children**

HEIGHT (in)	PEFR (L/min)	HEIGHT (in)	PEFR (L/min)
43	147	56	320
44	160	57	334
45	173	58	347
46	187	59	360
47	200	60	373
48	214	61	387
49	227	62	400
50	240	63	413
51	254	64	427
52	267	65	440
53	280	66	454
54	293	67	467
55	307		

From Polger G, Promedhat V: *Pulmonary function testing in children: techniques and standards,* Philadelphia, 1971, WB Saunders. In Siberry GK, Iannone R (eds): *The Harriet Lane handbook: a manual for pediatric house officers,* ed 15, St Louis, 2000, Mosby.

Section 5
COMMONLY USED FORMULAS AND GRAPHS

BOX 3-1   Commonly Used Formulas

1. Calculation of creatinine clearance (CCr)

$$CCr = \frac{UV}{P} \times \frac{1.73}{S.A.} = ml/min/1.73 \ m^2$$

U (mg/dl) = Urine creatinine concentration
V (ml/min) = Total urine volume ÷ length of collection time
P (mg/dl) = Serum creatinine
S.A. (m^2) = Surface area

2. Alveolar-arterial oxygen gradient (Aa gradient)

$$Aa \ gradient = \left[(713)(FIo_2) - \left(\frac{Paco_2}{0.8} \right) \right] - Pao_2$$

Normal Aa gradient = 5-15 mm
FIo$_2$ = Fraction of inspired oxygen (normal = 0.21-1.0)
Paco$_2$ = Arterial carbon dioxide tension (normal = 35-45 mm Hg)
Pao$_2$ = Arterial partial pressure oxygen (normal = 70-100 mm Hg)
Differential diagnosis of Aa gradient:

ABNORMALITY	15% O$_2$	100% O$_2$
Diffusion defect	Increased gradient	Correction of gradient
Ventilation/perfusion mismatch	Increased gradient	Partial or complete correction of gradient
Right-to-left shunt (intracardiac or pulmonary)	Increased gradient	Increased gradient (no correction)

3. Anion gap (AG) $$AG = Na^+ - (Cl^- + HCO_3^-)$$

4. Fractional excretion of sodium $$FE_{Na} = \frac{U_{Na}/P_{Na}}{U_{Cr}/P_{Cr}} \times 100$$

5. Serum osmolality $$Osm = 2(Na^+ + K^+) + \frac{Glucose}{18} + \frac{BUN}{2.8}$$

6. Corrected sodium in hyperglycemic patients

$$Corrected \ Na^+ = Measured \ Na^+ + 1.6 \times \frac{Glucose - 140}{100}$$

7. Water deficit in hypernatremic patients

$$Water \ deficit \ (in \ liters) = 0.6 \times Body \ weight \ (kg) \times \left(\frac{Measured \ serum \ sodium}{Normal \ serum \ sodium} - 1 \right)$$

From Ferri FF: *Ferri's clinical advisor: instant diagnosis and management*, St Louis, 1999, Mosby.

■ NORMAL VALUES OF GFR

Age	GFR - mean (ml/min/1.73 m^2)	Range (ml/min/1.73 m^2)
Neonates <34 wk gestational age		
2-8 days	11	11-15
4-28 days	20	15-28
30-90 days	50	40-65
Neonates >34 wk gestational age		
2-8 days	39	17-60
4-28 days	47	26-68
30-90 days	58	30-86
1-6 mo	7	39-114
6-12 mo	103	49-157
12-19 mo	127	62-191
2 yr-adult	127	89-165

*From Renal function tests. In Siberry GK, Iannone R (eds): *The Harriet Lane handbook: a manual for pediatric house officers*, ed 15, St Louis, 2000, Mosby.

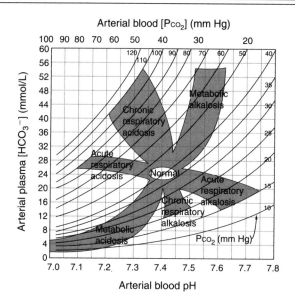

Fig. 3-46 **Acid-base nomogram.** (Modified from Brenner BN, Floyd CR Jr [eds]: *The kidney,* vol 1, Philadelphia, 1991, WB Saunders. In Siberry GK, Iannone R [eds]: *The Harriet Lane handbook: a manual for pediatric house officers,* ed 15, St Louis, 2000, Mosby.)

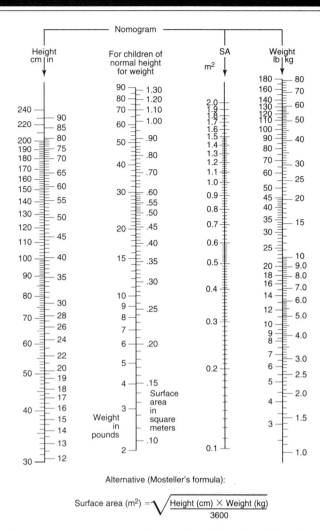

Alternative (Mosteller's formula):

$$\text{Surface area (m}^2) = \sqrt{\frac{\text{Height (cm)} \times \text{Weight (kg)}}{3600}}$$

Fig. 3-47 **Body surface area nomogram and equation.** (Data from Briars GL, Bailey BJ: *Arch Dis Child* 70:246, 1994; In Siberry GK, Iannone R [eds]: *The Harriet Lane handbook: a manual for pediatric house officers,* ed 15, St Louis, 2000, Mosby.)

III

Section 6
IMMUNIZATIONS AND INFECTIOUS DISEASES AND PREVENTION

TABLE 3-16 Childhood Immunization Schedule

Age ▶ Vaccines ▼	Birth	1 mo	2 mos	4 mos	6 mos	12 mos	15 mos	18 mos	24 mos	4-6 yrs	11-12 yrs	14-16 yrs
Hepatitis B	Hep B #1		Hep B # 2		Hep B # 3						Hep B	
Diphtheria, Tetanus, Pertussis			DTaP	DTaP	DTaP		DTaP			DTaP	Td	
H. influenzae type b			Hib	Hib	Hib	Hib						
Inactivated Polio			IPV	IPV		IPV				IPV		
Pneumococcal Conjugate			PCV	PCV	PCV	PCV						
Measles, Mumps, Rubella						MMR				MMR	MMR	
Varicella						Var					Var	
Hepatitis A										Hep A—in selected areas		

☐ Range of recommended ages for vaccination

⬭ Vaccines to be given if previously recommended doses were missed or were given earlier than the recommended minimum age.

▨ Recommended in selected states and/or regions.

From the Advisory Committee on Immunization Practices (ACIP), the American Academy of Family Physicians, and the American Academy of Pediatrics: *MMWR Morb Mortal Wkly Rep* 50:8, 2001.

■ **RELEVANT WEBSITES**
- www.immunizationinfo.org
- www.cdc.gov

TABLE 3-17 Administration of Multiple Vaccines and Immune Globulins

VACCINE COMBINATION	RECOMMENDED MINIMUM INTERVAL BETWEEN DOSES
≥2 killed vaccines	None. May be administered simultaneously or at any interval between doses. (If possible, cholera, parenteral typhoid, and plague vaccines should be given on separate occasions to avoid accentuating their side effects.)
Killed and live vaccines	None. May be administered simultaneously or at any interval between doses. (Cholera vaccine with yellow fever vaccine is the exception. These vaccines should be given separately at least 3 wk apart; otherwise the antibody response to each may be suboptimal.)
≥2 live vaccines	May be administered simultaneously. If given separately, there must be an interval at least 4 wk between them. However, OPV can be administered at any time before, with, or after an MMR or oral typhoid, if indicated.
Live vaccine and purified protein derivative (PPD)	May be administered simultaneously. If given separately, the PPD should be given 4 to 6 wk after the live vaccine.
Immune globulin and killed vaccine	None. May be administered simultaneously or at any interval between doses.
Immune globulin and live vaccine	Should not be given together. The live vaccine should be given a minimum of 2 wk before the immune globulin. If the live vaccine is to be given after the immune globulin, the minimum time that should elapse between administration is dose dependent and is outlined in Table 3-6. Of note, OPV, oral typhoid, and yellow fever are exceptions to these recommendations and can be given any time before, during, or after an immune globulin–containing product.

Modified from *MMWR* 43(RR-1):15-16, 1994.
MMR, Measles, mumps, rubella; *OPV,* oral polio vaccine.

■ WEBSITE
Centers for Disease Control and Prevention:
www.cdc.gov

III

TABLE 3-18 **Suggested Intervals between Administration of Immune Globulin Preparations for Various Indications and Vaccines Containing Live Measles Virus***

INDICATION	DOSE (INCLUDING mg IgG/kg)	TIME INTERVAL (mo) BEFORE MEASLES VACCINATION
Tetanus (TIG) prophylaxis	250 units (10 mg IgG/kg) IM	3
Hepatitis A (IG) prophylaxis		
Contact prophylaxis	0.02 ml/kg (3.3 mg IgG/kg) IM	3
International travel	0.06 ml/kg (10 mg IgG/kg) IM	3
Hepatitis B prophylaxis (HBIG)	0.06 ml/kg (10 mg IgG/kg) IM	3
Rabies immune globulin (HRIG)	20 IU/kg (22 mg IgG/kg) IM	4
Varicella prophylaxis (VZIG)	125 units/10 kg (20-40 mg IgG/kg) IM (maximum, 625 units)	5
Measles prophylaxis (IG)		
Standard (i.e., nonimmuno-compromised contact)	0.25 ml/kg (40mg IgG/kg) IM	5
Immunocompromised contact	0.50 ml/kg (80 mg IgG/kg) IM	6
Blood transfusion:		
Red blood cells (RBCs), washed	10 ml/kg (negligible IgG/kg) IV	0
RBCs, adenine-saline added	10 ml/kg (10 mg IgG/kg) IV	3
Packed RBCs (Hct 65%)†	10 ml/kg (20-60 mg IgG/kg) IV	6
Whole blood cells (Hct 35%-50%)†	10 ml/kg (80-100 mg IgG/kg) IV	6
Plasma/platelet products	10 ml/kg (160 mg IgG/kg) IV	7
Replacement therapy for immune deficiencies	300-400 mg/kg IV‡ (as IGIV)	8
Treatment of the following:		
Immune thrombocytopenic purpura§	400 mg/kg IV (as IGIV)	8
Immune thrombocytopenic purpura§	1000 mg/kg IV (as IGIV)	10
Kawasaki's disease	2 g/kg IV (as IGIV)	11

From *MMWR* 45(RR-12), 1996.

*This table is not intended for determining the correct indications and dosage for the use of immune globulin preparations. Unvaccinated persons may not be fully protected against measles during the entire suggested time interval, and additional doses of immune globulin and/or measles vaccine may be indicated after measles exposure. The concentration of measles antibody in a particular immune globulin preparation can vary by lot. The rate of antibody clearance after receipt of an immune globulin preparation also can vary. The recommended time intervals are extrapolated from an estimated half-life of 30 days for passively acquired antibody and an observed interference with the immune response to measles vaccine for 5 mo after a dose of 80 mg IgG/kg.

†Assumes a serum IgG concentration of 16 mg/ml.

‡Measles vaccination is recommended for most HIV-infected children who do not have evidence of severe immunosuppression, but it is contraindicated for patients who have congenital disorders of the immune system.

§Formerly referred to as *idiopathic thrombocytopenic purpura*.

TABLE 3-19 Recommendations for Hepatitis B Prophylaxis after Percutaneous or Permucosal Exposure to Blood

| EXPOSED PERSON | TREATMENT OF EXPOSED PERSON BASED ON STATUS OF SOURCE | | |
	HBsAg-POSITIVE SOURCE	HBsAg-NEGATIVE SOURCE	SOURCE NOT TESTED OR SOURCE UNKNOWN
Unvaccinated	One dose of HBIG*; initiate hepatitis B vaccine	Initiate hepatitis B vaccine	Initiate hepatitis B vaccine
Previously vaccinated			
Known responder	Test exposed person for anti-HBsAg† 1. If adequate, no treatment 2. If inadequate, hepatitis B vaccine booster dose	No treatment	No treatment
Known nonresponder	Two doses of HRIG or one dose of HBIG plus one dose of hepatitis B vaccine	No treatment	If known high-risk source, may treat as if source were HBsAg positive
Response unknown	Test exposed person for anti-HBsAg 1. If adequate, no treatment 2. If inadequate, one dose of HBIG plus hepatitis B vaccine booster dose	No treatment	Test exposed person for anti-HBsAg† 1. If adequate, no treatment 2. If inadequate, hepatitis B vaccine booster dose

Adapted from Recommendations of the Immunization Practices Advisory Committee (ACIP): *MMWR* 46(RR-18):22, 1997.
HBsAg, Hepatitis B surface antigen; *anti-HBsAg,* antibody to hepatitis B surface antigen; *HBIG,* hepatitis B immune globulin.
*HBIG dose, should be 0.06 ml/kg intramuscularly.
†Adequate anti-HBsAg level is ≥10 mIU.

III

TABLE 3-20 Recommended Schedule of Hepatitis B Immunoprophylaxis to Prevent Perinatal Transmission

POPULATION GROUP	VACCINE DOSE	AGE OF INFANT
Infants born to HBsAg-positive mothers	First dose	Birth (within 12 hr)
	HBIG*	Birth (within 12 hr)
	Second dose	1-2 mo
	Third dose	6 mo†
Infants born to mothers not screened for HBsAg	First dose	Birth (within 12 hr)
	HBIG†	If mother is HBsAg positive, administer 0.5 ml HBIG to infant as soon as possible, not later than 1 wk after birth
	Second dose	1-2 mo‡
	Third dose	6 mo†

Modified from Recommendations of the Immunization Practices Advisory Committee (ACIP): *MMWR* 40(RR-13):12, 1991. In Hepatitis B prophylaxis/HIV chemoprophylaxis. In Ferri FF (ed): *Ferri's clinical advisor: instant diagnosis and treatment,* St Louis, 1999, Mosby.
HBsAg, Hepatitis B surface antigen; *HBIG,* hepatitis B immune globulin.
*HBIG is given in a dose of 0.5 ml, administered intramuscularly at a site different from that used for vaccine.
†If four-dose schedule (Engerix-B) is used, the third dose is administered at 2 mo of age and the fourth dose at 12-18 mo.
‡Infants of women who are HBsAg negative can be vaccinated at 2 mo of age.

TABLE 3-21 Vaccinations for International Travel

DISEASE*	AREAS AFFECTED†	PROPHYLAXIS RECOMMENDED
Tetanus	All	All travelers: vaccine series/booster (Td) every 10 years.
Measles	All	Born after 1956: ensure immunity by antibody titer, diagnosed measles, or two doses of vaccine.
Rubella	All	All travelers: ensure immunity by antibody titer or vaccine.
Mumps	All	Born after 1956: ensure immunity by antibody titer, diagnosed mumps, or one dose of vaccine.
Poliomyelitis	Developing countries not in the western hemisphere but including Peru and Colombia and the new independent states of the former Soviet Union; tropics at risk all year; temperate zones have increased cases in summer and fall	All travelers: vaccine series/booster. IPV recommended for this dose.
Hepatitis B	5%-20% of population are carriers—Africa, Middle East except Israel, all Southeast Asia, Amazon basin, Haiti, Dominican Republic; 1%-5% of population are carriers—South Central and Southwest Asia, Israel, Japan, the Americas, Russia, eastern and southern Europe	Travelers for more than 6 mo and having close contact with the population or staying less time but having higher-risk activities (sex, close household contact, seeking dental or medical care): vaccine series.
Hepatitis A	Developing countries	Travelers to rural areas, eating and drinking in settings of poor sanitation: hepatitis A vaccine or pooled IG prophylaxis.
Influenza	Tropics throughout the year; southern hemisphere April to September	Travelers for whom vaccine is otherwise indicated: give the current vaccine and revaccinate in fall as usual.
Meningococcus*	Tanzania, Kenya, sub-Saharan Africa from Mali to Ethiopia; required for pilgrims to Mecca, Saudi Arabia, during the hajj	All travelers: vaccine.

From Noble J (ed): *Primary care medicine,* ed 2, St Louis, 1996, Mosby.

*Only yellow fever vaccine is required for entry by any country, cholera vaccine may be required by some local authorities, and meningococcus vaccine is only required for pilgrims to Mecca, Saudi Arabia, during the hajj. However, it is important to follow the recommendations for other vaccines for disease prevention. If a required vaccine is contraindicated or withheld for any reason, attempts should be made to obtain a waiver from the country's consulate or embassy.

†Because areas affected can change, and for more specific details, consult the Centers for Disease Control and Prevention's traveler's hotline or the most recent edition of *Health Information for the International Traveler.*

TABLE 3-21 Vaccinations for International Travel—cont'd

DISEASE*	AREAS AFFECTED†	PROPHYLAXIS RECOMMENDED
Rabies	Endemic dog rabies exist in parts of Mexico, El Salvador, Guatemala, Peru, Colombia, Ecuador, India, Nepal, Philippines, Sri Lanka, Thailand, Viet Nam	Travelers staying for more than 30 days or at high risk of exposure: vaccine series/booster.
Yellow fever*	North and central South America, forest-savannah zones of Africa, some countries in Africa, Asia and Middle East require travelers from endemic areas to be vaccinated	All travelers: vaccine/booster at approved Yellow Fever Vaccination Center.
Japanese encephalitis	Seasonally in most areas of Asia; in temperate zones the incidence is increased in summer and early fall; in the tropics occurs all year	Travelers to high-risk rural areas, staying outdoors or during the transmission season: vaccine series.
Cholera*	Certain undeveloped countries	If required by local authorities, one dose usually suffices. Primary series only for those living in high-risk areas under poor sanitary conditions or those with compromised gastric defense mechanisms (achlorhydria, antacid therapy or previous ulcer surgery): booster every 6 mo.
Typhoid fever	Many countries of Asia, Africa, Central and South America	Travelers with prolonged stay in rural areas with poor sanitation: vaccine series/booster.
Plague	Africa, Asia, Americas in rural mountainous or upland areas	Travelers with research or field activities that bring them in contact with rodents: vaccine series/booster. Consider taking tetracycline (500 mg qid) for chemoprophylaxis (inferred from clinical experience in treating plague).
Pneumococcus		Recommended for adults ≥65 years or older and other high-risk travelers.

III

■ **WEBSITE**

Centers for Disease Control and Prevention:
www.cdc.gov

TABLE 3-22 Cardiac Conditions Associated with Endocarditis

ENDOCARDITIS PROPHYLAXIS		
RECOMMENDED		NOT RECOMMENDED
High Risk	**Moderate Risk**	**Negligible Risk***
Prosthetic cardiac valves, including bioprosthetic and homograft valves	Most other congenital cardiac malformations (other than those in the high-risk and negligible-risk categories)	Isolated secundum atrial septal defect
Previous bacterial endocarditis	Acquired valvular dysfunction (e.g., rheumatic heart disease)	Surgical repair of atrial septal defect, ventricular septal defect, or patent ductus arteriosus (without residua and beyond 6 mo of age)
Complex cyanotic congenital heart disease (e.g., single ventricle states, transposition of the great arteries, tetralogy of Fallot)	Hypertrophic cardiomyopathy	Previous coronary artery bypass graft surgery
Surgically constructed systemic pulmonary shunts or conduits	Mitral valve prolapse with valvular regurgitation and/or thickened leaflets†	Mitral valve prolapse without valvular regurgitation†
		Physiologic, functional, or innocent heart murmurs†
		Previous Kawasaki's disease without valvular dysfunction
		Previous rheumatic fever without valvular dysfunction
		Cardiac pacemakers (intravascular and epicardial) and implanted defibrillators

From American Academy of Pediatrics: Prevention of bacterial endocarditis. In Pickering LK (ed): *2000 Red Book: report of the Committee on Infectious Diseases,* ed 25, Elk Grove Village, Ill, 2000, American Academy of Pediatrics.
*No greater risk than the general population.
†For further details, see Dajani AS et al: Prevention of bacterial endocarditis: recommendations by the American Heart Association, *JAMA* 277:1794, 1997.

TABLE 3-23 Dental Procedures and Endocarditis Prophylaxis

RECOMMENDED*	NOT RECOMMENDED
Dental extractions	Restorative dentistry† (operative and prosthodontic) with or without retraction cord‡
Periodontal procedures, including surgery, scaling and root planing, probing, and routine maintenance	Local anesthetic injections (nonintraligamentary)
Dental implant placement and reimplantation of avulsed teeth	Intracanal endodontic treatment; postplacement and buildup
Endodontic (root canal) instrumentation or surgery only beyond the apex	Placement of rubber dams
Subgingival placement of antibiotic fibers or strips	Postoperative suture removal
Initial placement of orthodontic bands but not brackets	Placement of removable prosthodontic or orthodontic appliances
Intraligamentary local anesthetic injections	Taking of oral impressions
Prophylactic cleaning of teeth or implants during which bleeding is anticipated	Fluoride treatments
	Taking of oral radiographs
	Orthodontic appliance adjustment
	Shedding of primary teeth

From American Academy of Pediatrics: Prevention of endocarditis. In Pickering LK (ed): *2000 Red Book: report of the Committee on Infectious Diseases,* ed 25, Elk Grove Village, Ill, 2000, American Academy of Pediatrics.
*Prophylaxis is recommended for patients with high- and moderate-risk cardiac conditions.
†This includes restoration of decayed teeth (filling cavities) and replacement of missing teeth.
‡Clinical judgment may indicate antibiotic use in selected circumstances that may create significant bleeding.

BOX 3-2 Other Procedures and Endocarditis Prophylaxis

Endocarditis Prophylaxis Recommended
Respiratory Tract

Tonsillectomy and/or adenoidectomy
Surgical operations that involve respiratory mucosa
Bronchoscopy with a rigid bronchoscope

Gastrointestinal Tract*

Sclerotherapy for esophageal varices
Esophageal stricture dilation
Endoscopic retrograde cholangiography* with biliary obstruction
Biliary tract surgery
Surgical operations that involve intestinal mucosa

Genitourinary Tract

Prostatic surgery
Cystoscopy
Urethral dilation

Endocarditis Prophylaxis Not Recommended
Respiratory Tract

Endotracheal intubation
Bronchoscopy with a flexible bronchoscope, with or without biopsy†
Tympanostomy tube insertion

Gastrointestinal Tract

Transesophageal echocardiography†
Endoscopy with or without gastrointestinal biopsy†

Genitourinary Tract

Vaginal hysterectomy†
Vaginal delivery†
Cesarean section
In uninfected tissue:
 Urethral catheterization
 Uterine dilation and curettage
 Therapeutic abortion
 Sterilization procedures
 Insertion or removal of intrauterine devices

Other

Cardiac catheterization, including balloon angioplasty
Implanted cardiac pacemakers, implanted defibrillators, and coronary stents
Incision or biopsy of surgically scrubbed skin
Circumcision

From Dajani AS et al: *JAMA* 277:1794, 1997.
*Prophylaxis is recommended for high-risk patients; optional for medium-risk patients.
†Prophylaxis is optional for high-risk patients.

TABLE 3-24 Prophylactic Regimens for Dental, Oral, Respiratory Tract, or Esophageal Procedures

SITUATION	AGENT	REGIMEN*
Standard general prophylaxis	Amoxicillin	Adults: 2.0 g; children: 50 mg/kg orally 1 hr before procedure
Unable to take oral medications	Ampicillin	Adults: 2.0 g IM or IV; children: 50 mg/kg IM or IV within 30 min before procedure
Allergic to penicillin	Clindamycin	Adults: 600 mg; children: 20 mg/kg orally 1 hr before procedure
	or Cephalexin† or cefadroxil†	Adults: 2.0 g; children: 50 mg/kg orally 1 hr before procedure
	or Azithromycin or clarithromycin	Adults: 500 mg; children: 15 mg/kg orally 1 hr before procedure
Allergic to penicillin and unable to take oral medications	Clindamycin *or*	Adults: 600 mg; children: 20 mg/kg IV within 30 min before procedure
	Cefazolin†	Adults 1.0 g; children: 25 mg/kg IM or IV within 30 min before procedure

From Dajani AS et al: *JAMA* 277:1794, 1997.
*Total children's dose should not exceed adult dose.
†Cephalosporins should not be used in individuals with immediate-type hypersensitivity reaction (urticaria, angioedema, or anaphylaxis) to penicillins.

TABLE 3-25 **Duration of Prophylaxis for Persons Who Have Had Rheumatic Fever: Recommendations of the American Heart Association**

CATEGORY	DURATION
Rheumatic fever without carditis	5 yr or until age 21 yr, whichever is longer
Rheumatic fever with carditis but without residual heart disease (no valvular disease*)	10 yr or well into adulthood, whichever is longer
Rheumatic fever with carditis and residual heart disease (persistent valvular disease*)	At least 10 yr since last episode and at least until age 40 yr; sometimes lifelong prophylaxis

Modified from Dajani A et al: *Pediatrics* 96:758, 1995.
*Clinical or echocardiographic evidence.

TABLE 3-26 **Chemoprophylaxis for Recurrences of Rheumatic Fever**

DRUG	DOSE	ROUTE
Benzathine penicillin G	1,200,000 U every 4 wk*	Intramuscular
OR		
Penicillin V	250 mg twice a day	Oral
OR		
Sulfadiazine or sulfisoxazole	0.5 g once a day for patients ≤27 kg (60 lb)	Oral
	1.0 g once a day for patients >27 kg (60 lb)	

For persons allergic to penicillin and sulfonamide drugs

Erythromycin	250 mg twice a day	Oral

Modified from Dajani A et al: *Pediatrics* 96:758, 1995.
*In high-risk situations, administration every 3 weeks is recommended.

TABLE 3-27 Provisional Public Health Service Recommendations for Chemoprophylaxis after Occupational Exposure to HIV, by Type of Exposure and Source Material—1998

TYPE OF EXPOSURE	SOURCE MATERIALS*	ANTIRETROVIRAL PROPHYLAXIS†	ANTIRETROVIRAL REGIMEN‡
Percutaneous	Blood		
	Highest risk	Recommend	Zidovudine plus lamivudine plus either indinavir or nelfinavir
	Increased risk	Recommend	Zidovudine plus lamivudine with or without either indinavir or nelfinavir
	No increased risk	Offer	Zidovudine plus lamivudine
	Fluid containing visible blood, other potentially infectious fluid,§ or tissue	Offer	Zidovudine plus lamivudine
	Other body fluid (e.g., urine)	Not offer	
Mucous membrane	Blood	Offer	Zidovudine plus lamivudine with or without either indinavir or nelfinavir
	Fluid containing visible blood, other potentially infectious fluid,§ or tissue	Offer	Zidovudine with or without lamivudine
	Other body fluid (e.g., urine)	Not offer	
Skin, increased risk‖	Blood	Offer	Zidovudine plus lamivudine with or without either indinavir or nelfinavir
	Fluid containing visible blood, other potentially infectious fluid,§ or tissue	Offer	Zidovudine with or without lamivudine
	Other body fluid (e.g., urine)	Not offer	

From Centers for Disease Control and Prevention: *MMWR Morb Mortal Wkly Rep* 47(RR-7):1, 1998.

AIDS, Acquired immunodeficiency syndrome; *HIV,* human immunodeficiency virus.

*Any exposure to concentrated HIV (e.g., in a research laboratory or production facility) is treated as percutaneous exposure to blood with highest risk. *Highest risk,* exposure that involves BOTH a larger volume of blood (e.g., deep injury with large diameter hollow needle previously in source patient's vein or artery, especially involving an injection of source-patient's blood) AND blood containing a high titer of HIV (e.g., source with acute retroviral illness or end-stage AIDS; viral load measurement may be considered, but its use in relation to postexposure prophylaxis has not been evaluated). *Increased risk,* EITHER exposure to a larger volume of blood OR blood with a high titer of HIV. *No increased risk,* NEITHER exposure to larger volume of blood NOR blood with a high titer of HIV (e.g., solid suture needle injury from source patient with asymptomatic HIV infection).

†*Recommend,* postexposure prophylaxis should be recommended to the exposed worker with counseling. *Offer,* postexposure prophylaxis should be offered to the exposed worker with counseling. *Not offer,* postexposure prophylaxis should not be offered because it is not an occupational exposure to HIV.

‡Regimens for adults: zidovudine, 200 mg three times a day; lamivudine, 150 mg twice a day; indinavir, 800 mg three times a day (if indinavir is not available, ritonavir, 600 mg twice a day, or saquinavir, 600 mg three times a day, may be used); nelfinavir, 750 mg three times a day. Prophylaxis is given for 4 weeks. For full prescribing information, see package inserts. Possible toxic effects from indinavir or nelfinavir may not be warranted.

§Includes semen; vaginal secretions; and cerebrospinal, synovial, pleural, peritoneal, pericardial, and amniotic fluids.

‖For skin, risk is increased for exposures involving a high titer of HIV, prolonged contact, an extensive area, or an area in which skin integrity is visibly compromised. For skin exposures without increased risk, the risk for toxic effects of the drug outweigh the benefit of postexposure prophylaxis.

■ **WEBSITE**

Centers for Disease Control and Prevention: www.cdc.gov

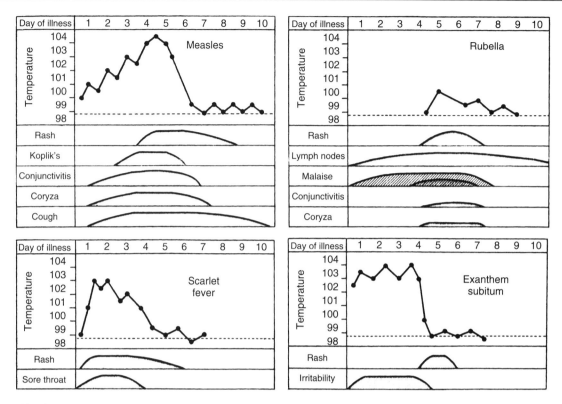

Fig. 3-48 Location of rash on days 1 and 3 of measles, rubella, and scarlet fever. (From McMillan JA, Stockman JA III, Oski FA [eds]: *The whole pediatrician catalog: a compendium of clues to the diagnosis and management,* Philadelphia, 1979, WB Saunders.)

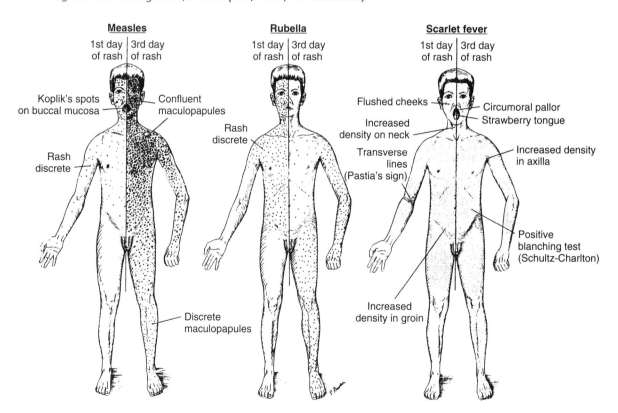

Fig. 3-49 Prevalence of signs and symptoms in chickenpox, smallpox, eczema vaccinatum or herpeticum, and rickettsialpox. (From McMillan JA, Stockman JA III, Oski FA [eds]: *The whole pediatrician catalog: a compendium of clues to the diagnosis and management,* Philadelphia, 1979, WB Saunders.)

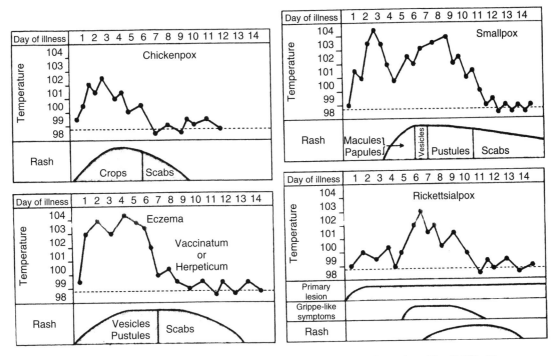

Fig. 3-50 Location and intensity of rash in chickenpox and smallpox (see Fig. 3-51). (From McMillan JA, Stockman JA III, Oski FA [eds]: *The whole pediatrician catalog: a compendium of clues to the diagnosis and management,* Philadelphia, 1979, WB Saunders.)

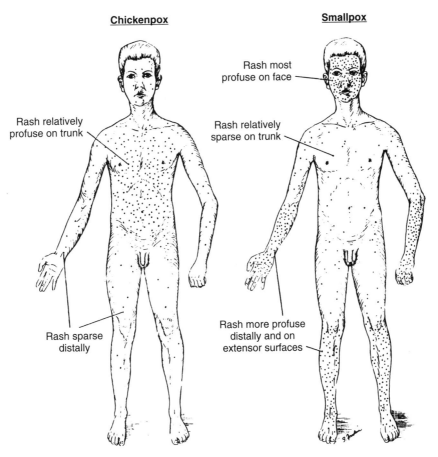

Fig. 3-51 Prevalence of signs and symptoms in measles, rubella, scarlet fever, and exanthem subitum. (From McMillan JA, Stockman JA III, Oski FA [eds]: *The whole pediatrician catalog: a compendium of clues to the diagnosis and management,* Philadelphia, 1979, WB Saunders.)

■ INTESTINAL NEMATODES

- The intestinal nematode worms are extremely common parasites of humans and other animals.
- More than 1 billion people are infected worldwide.
- Infection may cause only subtle growth and performance deficits, or it may result in severe anemia, debilitation, or even death.
- All intestinal nematodes share a roughly common life cycle.
    1. Eggs are passed in the feces of an infected host, where they ripen and/or hatch.
    2. New infection (usually) occurs when a suitable host comes in contact with fecally contaminated soil.
    3. Either eggs are swallowed or larval worms directly penetrate the host's skin.
    4. After maturation and (usually) a migration through the lungs, adult worms take up residence (and egg production) in some portion of the host gut.

Author: **D. Steven Fox, M.D.**

TABLE 3-28 Intestinal Nematodes

AGENT	CHARACTERISTICS	OCCURRENCE	LIFE CYCLE	SIGNS AND SYMPTOMS	DIAGNOSTIC PROCEDURE	TREATMENT
Whipworm: Trichuris trichiuria ICD-9CM: 127.3	Medium length (2-5 cm) Narrow anterior half, wider posterior half	Warm, moist climates worldwide	1000-10,000 eggs/female/day Eggs infectious after 2 weeks *No tissue or lung migration* Suck tissue fluids in large intestine Sexually mature in about 3 months	Malnutrition Anemia Rectal prolapse	Direct stool microscopy	Albendazole or Mebendazole
Threadworm: Strongyloides stercoralis ICD-9CM: 127.2	Tiny (2 mm)	Very moist conditions worldwide, especially tropics and subtropics	Adult males rapidly expelled from GI tract Females reproduce parthenogenically Eggs hatch in GI tract Immature larvae usually passed in feces, but may penetrate gut wall and autoinfect Can live free and reproduce in the soil Direct skin penetration with tissue/lung migration Sexually mature in 4 weeks Live in small bowel mucosa Autoinfection can continue for decades	Ground itch (mild): purulent eosinophilic rash at site of penetration Lung symptoms: cough, mild wheeze, larvae in sputum Steatorrhea (in early infection), often associated with eosinophilia Chronic intermittant diarrhea Larva currens: serpiginous wheal and flare reaction, evanescent, appears at irregular intervals Hyperinfection syndrome: eosinopenia (from steroids, lymphoma, transplant), causes disseminated disease; rapidly fatal	Stool microscopy Enterocapsule (string test) Stool culture ELISA	Albendazole or Ivermectin

Continued

ELISA, Enzyme-linked immunosorbent assay; *GI,* gastrointestinal.

III

TABLE 3-28 Intestinal Nematodes—cont'd

AGENT	CHARACTERISTICS	OCCURRENCE	LIFE CYCLE	SIGNS AND SYMPTOMS	DIAGNOSTIC PROCEDURE	TREATMENT
Pinworm: Enterobius vermicularis ICD-9CM: 127.4	Small, round white About 1 cm in length	Very cosmopolitan Very common in children worldwide	Female exits anus nocturnally, deposits eggs perianally Scratching transfers eggs to fingernails, mouth, environment Eggs infectious in 6 hours Eggs viable for 3 weeks	Rectal itching/ excoriation Rectal prolapse Vulvovaginitis	Visualizing worms perianally at night Microscopy of scotch tape applied to perianal area in am	Mebendazole or Pyrantel pamoate
Roundworm: Ascaris lumbricoides ICD-9CM: 127.0	Large, round, cream colored Up to 40 cm in length	Cosmopolitan Greater than 1 billion infected worldwide, especially children	More than 200,000 eggs/female/day Eggs infectious after 10 days Have a lung maturation phase Adults live in small intestine Egg to adult in 60-75 days	Verminous pneumonia (Loeffler's syndrome): cough, fever, wheeze, dyspnea, eosinophilia, eosinophils or worms in sputum Mechanical: obstruction, volvulus, intussus- ception, pancreatitis, obstructive jaundice, hepatic abcess, asphyxia, brain abcess Malnutrition	Worms in stool or vomitus ("He's eating earthworms!") Stool microscopy	Albendazole or Mebendazole

Hookworms: Ancylostoma duodenale and Necator americanus ICD-9CM: 126.0 and 126.1	Small (1 cm) Gaping jaws; teeth or cutting plates for mucosal penetration and blood sucking	Very widespread Tropics and subtropics	Eggs hatch in soil in 1 day; larvae infectious after 1 week. Either swallowed (*A. duodenale*) or can directly penetrate skin between toes. Migrate via lung. Sexually mature in 3-5 weeks. Prolonged prepatent phase (no egg production) exists	Ground itch: purulent eosinophilic rash at site of penetration. Lung symptoms: mild, transient cough or wheeze. Hookworm anemia: blood loss about 0.05 ml/worm/day. If adequate iron intake, then no anemia; in heavy infections, protein loss and edema also possible	Quantitative stool microscopy. Stool culture. Iron deficiency anemia in endemic area	Albendazole or Mebendazole
Larva Migrans: Toxicara canus ICD-9CM: 125.9	Dog roundworm. Only larval stage found in humans	Wherever dogs are found	Active infection mostly in puppies/pregnant dogs. Feces/Egg ingestion by humans yields prolonged (1-2 year) tissue migration. No maturation in humans	Visceral larva migrans (VLM): fever, eosinophilia, hepatomegaly, asthma (rare). Ocular VLM: retinal granulomas	Eosinophilia. Liver biopsy. Enucleation	VLM: DEC and steroids. Ocular VLM: steroids
Cutaneous Larva Migrans: Ancylostoma braziliense ICD-9CM: 126.2	Dog hookworm. Only larval stage found (subcutaneously) in humans	Wherever dogs are found, especially tropics and subtropics	Direct penetration of skin, especially feet/legs and buttocks/genitalia. Cannot penetrate through dermal layer. Wander in skin for few weeks, then die	Cutaneous larva migrans: slowly evolving, intensely puritic, excoriated tracks in skin	History and physical examination	Freeze worm heads or Topical thiabendazole or Metriphonate or Ivermectin or Albendazole

III

Section 7
NUTRITION3-29

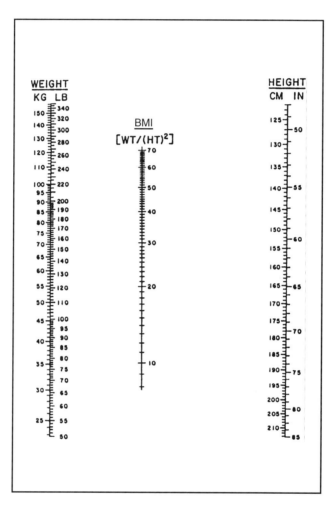

Fig. 3-52   Nomogram for body mass index *(BMI).* (From Bray GA: *Obesity in America,* NIH Publication No. 79-359, Nov 1979.)

■ **CALCULATION**

$$BMI = \frac{Weight\ (kg)}{[Height\ (m)]^2}$$

TABLE 3-29   Body Mass Index (BMI, in kg/m²) for Selected Statures and Weights

HEIGHT m (in)

WEIGHT kg (lb)	1.24 (49)	1.27 (50)	1.30 (51)	1.32 (52)	1.35 (53)	1.37 (54)	1.40 (55)	1.42 (56)	1.45 (57)	1.47 (58)	1.50 (59)	1.52 (60)	1.55 (61)	1.57 (62)	1.60 (63)	1.63 (64)	1.65 (65)	1.68 (66)	1.70 (67)	1.73 (68)	1.75 (69)	1.78 (70)	1.80 (71)	1.83 (72)	1.85 (73)	1.88 (74)	1.90 (75)	1.93 (76)
20 (45)	13	12	12	11	11	11	10	10	10	9	9	9	8	8	8	8												
23 (50)	15	14	14	13	13	12	12	11	11	11	10	10	10	9	9	9	8											
25 (55)	16	16	15	14	14	13	13	12	12	12	11	11	10	10	10	9	9	9										
27 (60)	18	17	16	16	15	14	14	13	13	13	12	12	11	11	11	10	10	10	9									
29 (65)	19	18	17	17	16	15	15	14	14	13	13	13	12	12	11	11	11	10	10	10								
32 (70)	21	20	19	18	18	17	16	16	15	15	14	14	13	13	13	12	12	11	11	11	10							
34 (75)	22	21	20	20	19	18	17	17	16	16	15	15	14	14	13	13	12	12	12	11	11	11						
36 (80)	23	22	21	21	20	19	18	18	17	17	16	16	15	15	14	14	13	13	12	12	12	11	11					
39 (85)	25	24	23	22	21	21	20	19	19	18	17	17	16	16	15	15	14	14	13	13	13	12	12	12				
41 (90)	27	25	24	24	23	22	21	20	20	19	18	18	17	17	16	15	15	15	14	14	13	13	13	12	12			
43 (95)	28	27	25	25	24	23	22	21	20	20	19	19	18	17	17	16	16	15	15	14	14	14	13	13	13	12		
45 (100)	29	28	27	26	25	24	23	22	21	21	20	19	19	18	18	17	17	16	16	15	15	14	14	13	13	13	12	
48 (105)	31	30	28	28	26	26	24	24	23	22	21	21	20	19	19	18	18	17	17	16	16	15	15	14	14	14	13	13
50 (110)	33	31	30	29	27	27	26	25	24	23	22	22	21	20	20	19	18	18	17	17	16	16	15	15	15	14	14	13
52 (115)	34	32	31	30	29	28	27	26	25	24	23	23	22	21	20	20	19	18	18	17	17	16	16	16	15	15	14	14
54 (120)	35	33	32	31	30	29	28	27	26	25	24	23	22	22	21	20	20	19	19	18	18	17	17	16	16	15	15	15
57 (125)	37	35	34	33	31	30	29	28	27	26	25	25	24	23	22	21	21	20	20	19	19	18	18	17	17	16	16	15
59 (130)	38	37	35	34	32	31	30	29	28	27	26	26	25	24	23	22	22	21	20	20	19	19	18	18	17	17	16	16
61 (135)	40	38	36	35	33	33	31	30	29	28	27	26	25	25	24	23	22	22	21	20	20	19	19	18	18	17	17	16
64 (140)	42	40	38	37	35	34	33	32	30	30	28	28	27	26	25	24	24	23	22	21	21	20	20	19	19	18	18	17
66 (145)	43	41	39	38	36	35	34	33	31	31	29	29	27	27	26	25	24	23	23	22	22	21	20	20	19	19	18	18
68 (150)	44	42	40	39	37	36	35	34	32	31	30	29	28	28	27	26	25	24	24	23	22	21	21	20	20	19	19	18
70 (155)	46	43	41	40	38	37	36	35	33	32	31	30	29	28	27	26	26	25	24	23	23	22	22	21	20	20	19	19
73 (160)	47	45	43	42	40	39	37	36	35	34	32	32	30	30	29	27	27	26	25	24	24	23	23	22	21	21	20	20
77 (170)	50	48	46	44	42	41	39	38	37	36	34	33	32	31	30	29	28	27	27	26	25	24	24	23	23	22	21	21

Continued

From Green M (ed): *Bright futures: guidelines for health supervision of infants, children, and adolescents,* 1994, National Center for Education in Maternal and Child Health.

III

TABLE 3-29 Body Mass Index (BMI, in kg/m²) for Selected Statures and Weights—cont'd

HEIGHT m (in)

WEIGHT kg (lb)	1.24 (49)	1.27 (50)	1.30 (51)	1.32 (52)	1.35 (53)	1.37 (54)	1.40 (55)	1.42 (56)	1.45 (57)	1.47 (58)	1.50 (59)	1.52 (60)	1.55 (61)	1.57 (62)	1.60 (63)	1.63 (64)	1.65 (65)	1.68 (66)	1.70 (67)	1.73 (68)	1.75 (69)	1.78 (70)	1.80 (71)	1.83 (72)	1.85 (73)	1.88 (74)	1.90 (75)	1.93 (76)
79 (175)	51	49	47	45	43	42	40	39	38	37	35	34	33	32	31	30	29	28	27	26	26	25	24	24	23	22	22	21
82 (180)		51	49	47	45	44	42	41	39	38	36	35	34	33	32	31	30	29	28	27	27	26	25	24	24	23	23	22
84 (185)			50	48	46	45	43	42	40	39	37	36	35	34	33	32	31	30	29	28	27	27	26	25	25	24	23	23
86 (190)			51	49	47	46	44	43	41	40	38	37	36	35	34	32	32	30	30	29	28	27	27	26	25	24	24	23
88 (195)				51	48	47	45	44	42	41	39	38	37	36	34	33	32	31	30	29	29	28	27	26	26	25	24	24
91 (200)					50	48	46	45	43	42	40	39	38	37	36	34	33	32	31	30	30	29	28	27	27	26	25	24
93 (205)						50	47	46	44	43	41	40	39	38	36	35	34	33	32	31	30	29	29	28	27	26	26	25
95 (210)						51	48	47	45	44	42	41	40	39	37	36	35	34	33	32	31	30	29	28	28	27	26	26
98 (215)							50	49	47	45	44	42	41	40	38	37	36	35	34	33	32	31	30	29	29	28	27	26
100 (220)								50	48	46	44	43	42	41	39	38	37	35	35	33	33	32	31	30	29	28	28	27
102 (225)								51	49	47	45	44	42	41	40	38	37	36	35	34	33	32	31	30	30	29	28	27
104 (230)									49	48	46	45	43	42	41	39	38	37	36	35	34	33	32	31	30	29	29	28
107 (235)									51	50	48	46	45	43	42	40	39	38	37	36	35	34	33	32	31	30	30	29
109 (240)										50	48	47	45	44	43	41	40	39	38	36	36	34	34	33	32	31	30	29
111 (245)											49	48	46	45	43	42	41	39	38	37	36	35	34	33	32	31	31	30
113 (250)											50	49	47	46	44	43	42	40	39	38	37	36	35	34	33	32	31	30
116 (255)												50	48	47	45	44	43	41	40	39	38	37	36	35	34	33	32	31
118 (260)													49	48	46	44	43	42	41	39	39	37	36	35	34	33	33	32
120 (265)													50	49	47	45	44	43	42	40	39	38	37	36	35	34	33	32
122 (270)													51	49	48	46	45	43	42	41	40	39	38	36	36	35	34	33
125 (275)														51	49	47	46	44	43	42	41	39	39	37	37	35	35	34
127 (280)															50	48	47	45	44	42	41	40	39	38	37	36	35	34
129 (285)															50	49	47	46	45	43	42	41	40	39	38	37	36	35
132 (290)																50	48	47	46	44	43	42	41	39	39	37	37	35
134 (295)																50	49	47	46	45	44	42	41	40	39	38	37	36
136 (300)																	50	48	47	45	44	43	42	41	40	38	38	37

From Green M (ed): *Bright futures: guidelines for health supervision of infants, children, and adolescents,* 1994, National Center for Education in Maternal and Child Health.

TABLE 3-30   **Evaluation for Obesity in Children and Adolescents in the United States Using BMI (kg/m^2)**

AGE (yr)	AT RISK OF OVERWEIGHT (85th PERCENTILE BMI)		OVERWEIGHT (95th PERCENTILE BMI)	
	MALES	FEMALES	MALES	FEMALES
5	17.2	16.9	18.3	18.5
6	17.4	17.2	19.0	19.3
7	17.8	17.9	20.0	20.4
8	18.6	18.9	21.5	21.7
9	19.7	20.1	23.1	23.0
10	20.9	21.4	24.6	24.5
11	21.9	22.6	25.7	26.1
12	22.6	23.6	26.5	27.5
13	23.2	24.4	27.1	28.6
14	23.7	24.9	27.8	29.3
15	24.5	25.2	28.7	29.6
16	25.4	25.5	29.8	29.9
17	25.9	25.9	30.1	31.3

Modified from Rosner B et al: *J Pediatr* 132:211, 1998. In Siberry GK, Iannone R (eds): *The Harriet Lane handbook: a manual for pediatric house officers,* ed 15, St Louis, 2000, Mosby.

III

TABLE 3-31 Classification of Formulas by Carbohydrate

	LACTOSE	SUCROSE AND GLUCOSE POLYMERS	GLUCOSE POLYMERS	MINIMAL CARBOHYDRATE
Common ingredient names		See glucose polymers	Glucose polymers Maltodextrins Corn syrup solids Modified tapioca starch	
Comments	Requires lactase enzyme for digestion Contraindicated in galactosemia	Requires sucrase enzyme for digestion (see also glucose polymers)	Easily digested For individuals with lactose malabsorption	For severe carbohydrate intolerance
Infants	Enfamil Enfamil 22* Enfamil AR Enfamil Premature Carnation Follow-up Carnation Good Start Neosure* Similac Similac PM 60/40 Similac Special Care	Alimentum Alsoy Isomil Isomil DF (Fiber) Portagen	Isomil SF Lactofree Neocate Nutramigen Pregestimil ProSobee Similac Lactose Free	MJ3232A RCF
Toddlers and young children	Next Step*	Compleat Pediatric† Kindercal (Fiber) Neocate One Plus Next Step Soy Nutren Junior PediaSure (also with Fiber) Peptamen Junior ProPeptide for Kids Resource Just for Kids	Vivonex Pediatric L-Emental Pediatric	
Older children and adolescents	Carnation Instant Breakfast Scandishake	All other formulas in Table 3-34	Criticare HN Deliver 2.0 Glucerna Isocal Jevity (fiber) L-Emental L-Emental Plus Peptamen PropPeptide Tolerex Vivonex TEN Vivonex Plus	

From Cox J: Nutrition. In Siberry GK, Iannone R (eds): *The Harriet Lane handbook: a manual for pediatric house officers,* ed 15, St Louis, 2000, Mosby.
*Also contains glucose polymers.
†Also contains fruit and vegetable purees.

TABLE 3-32 Classification of Formulas by Protein

	COW'S MILK	SOY	HYDROLYSATE	FREE AMINO ACIDS
Common ingredient names	Cow's milk protein Nonfat milk Demineralized whey Reduced mineral whey Sodium, calcium, magnesium caseinate Casein	Soy protein Soy protein isolate	Casein hydrolysate Hydrolyzed whey, meat, and soy	
Comments	Requires normal protein digestion and absorption	Requires normal protein digestion and absorption Not recommended for premature infants or those with cystic fibrosis	For individuals with protein allergy and/or malabsorption	For individuals with severe protein allergy and/or severe protein malabsorption
Infants	Enfamil Enfamil 22 Enfamil AR Follow-up Lactofree Neosure Portagen Enfamil Premature Similac Similac PM 60/40 Similac Special Care Similac Lactose Free	Alsoy Follow-up Soy Isomil Isomil DF ProSobee RCF	Alimentum Good Start Nutramigen Pregestimil MJ3232A	Neocate
Toddlers and young children	Compleat Pediatric* Resource Just for Kids Kindercal Next Step Nutren Junior PediaSure	Next Step Soy	Peptamen Junior Pro-Peptide for Kids	Vivonex Pediatric Neocate One Plus EleCare L-Emental Pediatric
Older children and adolescents	All other formulas in Table 3-33	Ensure† Ensure with Fiber† Isocal† Osmolite† Promote† Sustacal† Boost High-Protein† Boost with Fiber†	Criticare HN Peptamen Vital HN ProPeptide	Tolerex Vivonex TEN Vivonex Plus L-Emental L-Emental Plus

From Cox J: Nutrition. In Siberry GK, Iannone R (eds): *The Harriet Lane handbook: a manual for pediatric house officers,* ed 15, St Louis, 2000, Mosby.
*Blenderized protein diet of meat, vegetables, and fruit.
†Also contains cow's milk.

TABLE 3-33   **Classification of Formulas by Fat**

	LONG-CHAIN TRIGLYCERIDES		MEDIUM-CHAIN AND LONG-CHAIN TRIGLYCERIDES
Common ingredient names	Safflower oil Soy oil Palm olein Coconut oil	Sunflower oil Corn oil Canola oil Butterfat	Medium-chain triglycerides (MCT oil) Fractioned coconut oil
Comments	Requires normal fat digestion and absorption		For individuals with fat malabsorption Bile digestion not required Absorbed directly into portal circulation
Infants	Alsoy Enfamil Enfamil AR Carnation Follow-up Carnation Follow-up Soy Carnation Good Start	Isomil (all) Lactofree Neocate Nutramigen ProSobee RCF Similac Similac PM 60/40 Similac Lactose Free	Alimentum Enfamil Premature Enfamil 22 Pregestimil Portagen Neosure Similac Special Care
Toddlers and young children	Next Step Compleat Pediatric Toddler's Best		Resource Just For Kids Kindercal Neocate One Plus Nutren Junior PediaSure L-Emental Pediatric Peptamen Junior Vivonex Pediatric
Older children and adolescents	Carnation Instant Breakfast Ensure Ensure with Fiber Ensure Plus Glucerna	Nepro Pulmocare Scandishake Suplena Boost Plus Boost High-Protein Boost with Fiber	Deliver 2.0 Isocal Jevity Lipisorb Nutren 2.0 Nutrivent Osmolite Promote Respalor Traumacal Ultracal

From Cox J: Nutrition. In Siberry GK, Iannone R (eds): *The Harriet Lane handbook: a manual for pediatric house officers,* ed 15, St Louis, 2000, Mosby.

TABLE 3-34   Infant Formula Analysis (Per Liter)

FORMULA	kcal/ml (kcal/oz)	PROTEIN g (% kcal)	CARBOHYDRATE g (% kcal)	FAT g (% kcal)	Na (mEq)	K (mEq)	Ca (mg)	P (mg)	Fe (mg)	OSMOLALITY (mOsm/kg water)	SUGGESTED USES
Alimentum (Ross)	0.67 (20)	19 (11) Casein hydrolysate Cystine, Tyr, Trp Methionine	69 (41) Sucrose 67% Modified tapioca starch	38 (48) MCT oil (50%) Safflower oil (40%) Soy oil (10%)	13	20	709	507	12	370	Infants with food allergies, protein or fat malabsorption
Alsoy (Carnation)	0.67 (70)	19 (11) Soy Isolate Methionine	75 (44) Sucrose Maltodextrin	36 (45) Soy oil	10	20	709	412	12	200	Infants with allergy to cow's milk, lactose malabsorption, galactosemia
Enfamil [w/Fe] (Mead Johnson)	0.67 (20)	14 (9) Nonfat milk Demineralized whey	73 (43) Lactose	36 (48) Palm olein (45%) Soy oil (20%) Coconut oil (20%) HO Sun oil (15%)	8	19	530	360	5 [12.5]	300	Infants with normal GI tract
Enfamil AR (Mead Johnson)	0.67 (20)	16.7 (10) Nonfat milk Demineralized whey	73 (44) Lactose (57%) Rice starch (30%) Maltodextrins (13%)	34 (46) Palm olein (45%) Soy oil (20%) Coconut oil (20%) HO sun oil (15%)	11	18	520	353	12	230	When a thickened feeding is desired
Enfamil 24 [w/Fe] (Mead Johnson)	0.8 (20)	17 (9) Nonfat milk Whey	88 (43) Lactose	43 (48) Palm olein (45%) Soy oil (20%) HO Sun oil (15%)	10	22	630	430	6 [15]	360	Infants with normal GI tract requiring additional calories

Continued

From Cox J: Nutrition. In Siberry GK, Iannone R (eds): *The Harriet Lane handbook: a manual for pediatric house officers*, ed 15, St Louis, 2000, Mosby.

III

TABLE 3-34 Infant Formula Analysis (Per Liter)—cont'd

FORMULA	kcal/ml (kcal/oz)	PROTEIN g (% kcal)	CARBOHYDRATE g (% kcal)	FAT g (% kcal)	Na (mEq)	K (mEq)	Ca (mg)	P (mg)	Fe (mg)	OSMOLALITY (mOsm/kg water)	SUGGESTED USES
Enfamil Premature Formula 20 [w/Fe] (Mead Johnson)	0.67 (20)	20 (12) Demineralized whey Nonfat milk	75 (44) Corn syrup solids Lactose	35 (44) MCT oil (40%) Soy oil Coconut oil	11	18	1120	560	1.7 [12]	260	Preterm infants
Enfamil Premature Formula 24 [w/Fe] (Mead Johnson)	0.8 (24)	24 (12) Demineralized whey Nonfat milk	9 (44) Corn syrup solids Lactose	41 (44) MCT oil (40%) Soy oil Coconut oil	14	21	1340	670	2 [15]	310	Preterm infants
Enfamil 22 with iron (Mead Johnson)	0.73 (22)	20.6 (11) Nonfat milk Demineralized whey	79 (43) Corn syrup solids Lactose	39 (48) HO sun oil Soy oil MCT oil Coconut oil	11	20	890	490	13	—	Preterm infants after hospital discharge until goal catch-up growth
Evaporated milk formula*	0.69 (21)	28 (16) Cow's milk	75 (43) Lactose Corn syrup	33 (43) Butterfat	20	33	1130	870	2	—	Infants with normal GI tract; need vitamin C and iron supplement
Follow-up (Carnation)	0.67 (20)	18 (10) Nonfat milk	89 (53) Corn syrup (43%) Lactose (37%)	28 (37) Palm olein (47%) Soy oil (26%) Coconut oil (21%) HO saff oil (6%)	11	23	912	608	13	328	Infants 4-12 months with normal GI tract
Follow-up Soy (Carnation)	0.67 (20)	21 (12) Soy isolate Methionine	81 (48) Maltodextrin Sucrose	29 (40) Palm olein (47%) Soy oil (26%) Coconut oil (21%) HO saff oil (6%)	12	20	912	608	12	200	Infants 4-12 months with allergy to cow's milk, lactose malabsorption, galactosemia

Good Start (Carnation)	0.67 (20)	16 (10) Hydrolyzed whey	74 (44) Lactose Maltodextrins	3.5 (46) Palm olein (47%) Soy oil (26%) Coconut oil (21%) HO saff oil (6%)	7	17	432	243	10	265	Infants with normal GI tract
Isomil (Ross)	0.67 (20)	17 (10) Soy isolate Methionine	70 (41) Corn syrup Sucrose	37 (49) Soy oil Coconut oil	13	19	709	507	12	230	Infants with allergy to cow's milk, lactose malabsorption, galactosemia
Isomil DF (Ross)	0.67 (20)	18 (11) Soy isolate Methionine	68 (40) Corn syrup Sucrose Soy fiber	37 (49) Soy oil Coconut oil	13	19	709	507	12	240	Short-term management of diarrhea; contains fiber
Lactofree (Mead Johnson)	0.67 (20)	14 (9) Milk protein isolate	7 (43) Corn syrup solids	36 (48) Palm olein (45%) Soy oil (20%) Coconut oil (20%) HO Sun oil (15%)	9	19	550	370	12	200	Infants with lactose malabsorption
MJ3232A (Mead Johnson)	0.42 (12.6)	19 (17) Casein hydrolysate Cystine, Tyr, Trp	28 (25) Tapioca starch CHO selected by physician	28 (57) MCT oil (85%) Corn oil (15%)	13	19	630	420	13	250	Infants with severe CHO intolerance (CHO must be added)
Neocate (Scientific Hospital Supply)	0.69 (21)	20 (12) Free amino acids	78 (47) Corn syrup solids	32 (41) Safflower oil Coconut oil Soy oil	8	16	826	620	10	342	Infants with severe food allergies

Continued

From Cox J: Nutrition. In Siberry GK, Iannone R (eds): *The Harriet Lane handbook: a manual for pediatric house officers*, ed 15, St Louis, 2000, Mosby.
*Thirteen ounces evaporated whole milk, 119 ounces water, 12 tbsp corn syrup.

III

TABLE 3-34　Infant Formula Analysis (Per Liter)—cont'd

FORMULA	kcal/ml (kcal/oz)	PROTEIN g (% kcal)	CARBOHYDRATE g (% kcal)	FAT g (% kcal)	Na (mEq)	K (mEq)	Ca (mg)	P (mg)	Fe (mg)	OSMOLALITY (mOsm/kg water)	SUGGESTED USES
Nutramigen (Mead Johnson)	0.67 (20)	19 (11) Casein hydrolysate Cystine, Tyr, Trp	74 (44) Corn syrup solids Modified cornstarch	34 (45) Palm olein (45%) Soy oil (20%) Coconut oil (20%) HO Sun oil (15%)	14	19	640	430	13	320	Infants with food allergies
Portagen (Mead Johnson)	0.67 (20)	24 (14) Na caseinate	78 (46) Corn syrup solids Sucrose	32 (40) MCT oil (85%) Corn oil (15%)	16	22	640	470	13	230	Infants with fat malabsorption
Pregestimil (Mead Johnson)	0.67 (20)	19 (11) Casein hydrolysate Cystine, Tyr, Trp	69 (41) Corn syrup solids (60%) Modified cornstarch (20%) Dextrose (20%)	38 (48) MCT oil (55%) Corn oil (20%) Soy oil (12.5%) HO Saff oil (12.5%)	11	19	640	430	13	320	Infants with food allergies, protein or fat malabsorption
ProSobee (Mead Johnson)	0.67 (20)	20 (12) Soy isolate Methionine	73 (42) Corn syrup solids	37 (48) Palm olein (45%) Soy oil (20%) Coconut oil (20%) HO Sun oil (15%)	10	21	710	560	12	200	Infants with allergy to cow's milk, lactose malabsorption, galactosemia
RCF† (Ross) [w/Fe]	0.4 (12)	20 (20) Soy isolate	— Selected by physician	36 (80) Soy oil Coconut oil	13	19	709	507	12	—†	Infants with severe CHO intolerance (CHO must be added) Modified for ketogenic diet

Formula	kcal/mL (kcal/oz)	Protein g (% cal) source	CHO g (% cal) source	Fat g (% cal) source							Indications
Similac [w/Fe] (Ross)	0.67 (20)	14 (8) Nonfat milk Whey protein	73 (43) Lactose	36 (49) Soy oil Coconut oil HO saff oil	7	18	527	284	1.5 [12]	300	Infants with normal GI tract
Similac 24 [w/Fe] (Ross)	0.8 (24)	22 (11) Nonfat milk	85 (42) Lactose	43 (47) Soy oil Coconut oil	12	27	726	565	1.8 [15]	380	Infants with normal GI tract requiring additional calories
Similac Lactose Free (Ross)	0.67 (20)	14.5 (9) Milk isolate	72.3 (43) Corn syrup solids Sucrose	36.5 (49) Soy oil Coconut oil	9	18.5	568	378	12	230	Infants with lactose malabsorption
Similac Neosure (Ross)	0.75 (22)	19 (10) Nonfat milk Whey	77 (41) Corn syrup solids (50%) Lactose (50%)	41 (49) MCT oil Soy oil Coconut oil HO saff oil	11	27	784	463	13	250	Preterm infants, after hospital discharge, until goal catch-up growth
Similac PM 60/40 (Ross)	0.67 (20)	15 (9) Whey Na caseinate	69 (41) Lactose	38 (50) Soy oil Coconut oil Corn oil	7	15	378	189	1.5	280	Infants who require lowered calcium and phosphorus levels
Similac Special Care 20 [w/Fe] (Ross)	0.67 (20)	18 (11) Nonfat milk Whey	72 (42) Corn syrup solids Lactose	37 (49) MCT oil Soy oil Coconut oil	13	22	1216	676	2.5 (12)	235	Preterm infants
Similac Special Care 24 [w/Fe] (Ross)	0.8 (24)	22 (11) Nonfat milk Whey	86 (42) Corn syrup solids Lactose	44 (49) MCT oil Soy oil Coconut oil	15	27	1452	806	3 [15]	280	Preterm infants

From Cox J: Nutrition. In Siberry GK, Iannone R (eds): *The Harriet Lane handbook: a manual for pediatric house officers*, ed 15, St Louis, 2000, Mosby.
†Available as concentrated liquid. Nutrient values vary depending on amount of added carbohydrate (CHO) and water. A total of 12 fl oz concentrated liquid with 15 g CHO and 12 fl oz water yields 20 kcal/fl oz formula with 68 g CHO/L.

III

TABLE 3-35 Human Milk and Fortifiers Analysis (Per Liter)

FORMULA	kcal/ml (kcal/oz)	PROTEIN g (% kcal)	CARBOHYDRATE g (% kcal)	FAT g (% kcal)	Na (mEq)	K (mEq)	Ca (mg)	P (mg)	Fe (mg)	OSMOLALITY (mOsm/kg water)	SUGGESTED USES
Human milk (mature)	0.69 (20)	9 (5) Human milk protein	73 (42) Lactose	42 (54) Human milk fat	8	13	280	147	0.4	286	Infants
Preterm human milk*	0.67 (20)	14 (8) Human milk protein	66 (40) Lactose	39 (52) Human milk fat	11	15	248	128	1.2	290	Preterm infants
Enfamil Human Milk Fortifier (per packet) (Mead Johnson)	3.5 (—)	0.15 (20) Whey protein concentrate Na caseinate	0.68 (76) Corn syrup solids	0.02 (3.9) From caseinate Lactose	0.08	0.1	23	11	0	—	Fortifier for preterm human milk
Similac Natural Care Human Milk Fortifier (Ross)	0.8 (24)	22 (11) Nonfat milk Whey protein concentrate	86 (42) Corn syrup solids Lactose	44 (47) MCT oil Soy oil Coconut oil	15	26.6	1694	935	3	280	Fortifier for preterm human milk
Preterm Human Milk + Similac Natural Care 75:25 ratio	0.7 (21)	16 (9) Human milk protein Nonfat milk Whey protein concentrate	71 (40) Lactose Corn syrup solids	40 (51) Human milk fat MCT oil Soy oil Coconut oil	12	18	610	330	1.65	288	Preterm infants

Formula											
Preterm Human Milk + Similac Natural Care 50:50 ratio	0.74 (22)	18 (10) Human milk protein Nonfat milk protein Whey protein concentrate	71 (40) Lactose Corn syrup solids	41 (50) Human milk fat MCT oil Soy oil Coconut oil	13	21	971	531	2.1	285	Preterm infants
Preterm Human Milk + Similac Natural Care 25:75 ratio	0.77 (23)	19.9 (10) Nonfat milk Whey protein concentrate Human milk protein	81 (42) Lactose Corn syrup solids	43 (50) MCT oil Soy oil Coconut oil Human milk fat	14	24	1332	734	2.5	282	Preterm infants
Preterm Human Milk + Enfamil Human Milk Fortifier (1 pkt/50 ml)	0.73 (22)	17.3 (9) Human milk protein Whey protein concentrate Na caseinate	79 (43) Lactose Corn syrup solids	39 (48) Human milk fat	12	16	688	348	1.2	350	Preterm infants
Preterm Human Milk + Enfamil Human Milk Fortifier (1 pkt/25 ml)	0.78 (24)	20.5 (10) Human milk protein Whey protein concentrate Na caseinate	91 (46) Lactose Corn syrup solids	39 (44) Human milk fat	13	17	1166	561	1.2	410	Preterm infants

From Cox J: Nutrition. In Siberry GK, Iannone R (eds): *The Harriet Lane handbook: a manual for pediatric house officers*, ed 15, St Louis, 2000, Mosby.
*Composition of human milk varies with maternal diet, stage of lactation, within feedings, diurnally, and among mothers.

III

TABLE 3-36 Toddler and Young Child Formula Analysis (Per Liter)

FORMULA	kcal/ml (kcal/oz)	PROTEIN g (% kcal)	CARBOHYDRATE g (% kcal)	FAT g (% kcal)	Na (mEq)	K (mEq)	Ca (mg)	P (mg)	Fe (mg)	OSMOLALITY (mOsm/kg water)	SUGGESTED USES
Compleat Pediatric (Novartis)	1 (30)	38 (15) Meats Vegetables Na caseinate Ca caseinate	125 (50) Vegetables Fruit Hydrolyzed cornstarch	39 (35) HO sun oil Soy oil MCT oil	30	38	1000	1000	13	380	For those who desire a blenderized tube feeding
Cow's milk, whole	0.63 (19)	Cow's milk 34 (22)	Lactose 48 (31)	34 (49) Butterfat	22	40	1226	956	0.5	285	Children >1 year of age with normal GI tract
Elecare (Ross)	1 (30)	30 (15) Free L-amino acids	110 (44) Corn syrup solids	47.6 (42) HO saff oil MCT oil Soy oil	19.6	38.4	1082	808	17	596	Children with malabsorption, protein allergy
Kindercal (contains fiber) (Mead Johnson)	1.06 (32)	34 (13) Na caseinate	135 (50) Maltodextrins (83%) Sucrose (17%)	44 (37) Canola oil (50%) HO sun oil (15%) Corn oil (15%) MCT oil (20%)	16	34	850	850	11	310	Tube feeding and oral supplement for children with normal GI tract
L-Emental Pediatric (GalaGen/ Nutrition, Medical)	0.8 (24)	24 (12) Free L-amino acids	130 (63) Maltodextrins Modified starch	24 (25) Soy oil MCT oil (68%)	17	31	970	800	10	360	Children with malabsorption, protein allergy
Neonate One Plus (Scientific Hospital Supply)	1 (30)	25 (10) Free amino acids	146 (58) Maltodextrins Sucrose	35 (32) MCT oil (35%) Safflower oil Canola oil	9	24	620	620	8	835	Children with malabsorption, protein allergy

Formula	kcal/ml (kcal/oz)	Protein g (% kcal)	Carbohydrate g (% kcal)	Fat g (% kcal)	Na (mEq)	K (mEq)	Ca (mg)	P (mg)	Fe (mg)	Osmolality (mOsm/kg water)	Suggested uses
Next Step (Mead Johnson)	0.67 (20)	17 (10) Nonfat milk	74 (45) Lactose Corn syrup solids	34 (45) Palm olein (45%) Soy oil (20%) Coconut oil (20%) HO sun oil (15%)	12	22	800	560	12	270	Toddlers with normal GI tract
Next Step Soy (Mead Johnson)	0.67 (20)	22 (13) Soy protein	79 (47) Corn syrup solids Sucrose	29 (40) Palm olein (45%) Soy oil (20%) Coconut oil (20%) HO sun oil (15%)	13	26	767	600	12	260	Toddlers with cow's milk allergy, galactosemia
Nutren Junior (also with fiber) (Clintec)	1 (30)	30 (12) Casein Whey	128 (51) Maltodextrins Sucrose Soy polysaccharides	42 (37) Soy oil Canola oil MCT oil	20	34	1000	800	14	350	Tube feeding and oral supplement for children with normal GI tract
PediaSure (also with fiber) (Ross)	1 (30)	30 (12) Na caseinate Whey protein	110 (44) Hydrolyzed cornstarch (70%) Sucrose (30%) (Soy fiber)	50 (44) HO saff oil (50%) Soy oil (30%) MCT oil (20%)	16.5	33.5	970	800	14	310	Tube feeding and oral supplement for children with normal GI tract

From Cox J: Nutrition. In Siberry GK, Iannone R (eds): *The Harriet Lane handbook: a manual for pediatric house officers*, ed 15, St Louis, 2000, Mosby.

Continued

III

TABLE 3-36 Toddler and Young Child Formula Analysis (Per Liter)—cont'd

FORMULA	kcal/ml (kcal/oz)	PROTEIN g (% kcal)	CARBOHYDRATE g (% kcal)	FAT g (% kcal)	Na (mEq)	K (mEq)	Ca (mg)	P (mg)	Fe (mg)	OSMOLALITY (mOsm/kg water)	SUGGESTED USES
Peptamen Junior (Clintec)	1 (30)	30 (12) Hydrolyzed whey	138 (55) Maltodextrin Sucrose (flavored) Cornstarch	38.5 (33) MCT oil (60%) Soy oil Canola oil Lecithin	20	34	1000	800	14	260 (unflavored) 365 (flavored)	Children with malabsorption
ProPeptide for Kids (GalaGen/ Nutrition, Medical)	1 (30)	30 (12) Enzymatically hydrolyzed whey protein	137.5 (55) Maltodextrin Sucrose Cornstarch	38.5 (33) Medium-chain triglycerides (18.5%) Soy oil (22%) Canola oil (60%)	20	34	1000	800	14	360	Children with malabsorption
Resource Just for Kids (Novartis)	1 (30)	30 (12) Na caseinate Ca caseinate Whey protein concentrates	110 (44) Hydrolyzed cornstarch Sucrose	50 (44) HO Sun oil Soy oil MCT oil	17	33	1140	800	14	390	Tube feeding and oral supplement for children with normal GI tract
Vivonex Pediatric (Novartis)	0.8 (24)	24 (12) Free amino acids	130 (63) Maltodextrin Modified starch	24 (25) MCT oil (68%) Soy oil (32%)	17	31	970	800	10	360	Children with malabsorption, protein allergy

From Cox J: Nutrition. In Siberry GK, Iannone R (eds): *The Harriet Lane handbook: a manual for pediatric house officers*, ed 15, St Louis, 2000, Mosby.

TABLE 3-37   Older Child & Adult Formula Analysis (Per Liter)

FORMULA	kcal/ml (kcal/oz)	PROTEIN g (% kcal)	CARBOHYDRATE g (% kcal)	FAT g (% kcal)	Na (mEq)	K (mEq)	Ca (mg)	P (mg)	Fe (mg)	OSMOLALITY (mOsm/kg water)	SUGGESTED USES
Carnation Instant Breakfast w/whole milk (Clintec)	1.2 (36)	53 (18) Cow's milk	161 (54) Lactose Maltodextrin Sucrose	34 (26) Butterfat	42	67	1632	1400	17	590	High-calorie supplement for patients with normal GI tract
Criticare HN (Mead Johnson)	1.06 (32)	38 (14) Hydrolyzed casein Amino acids	220 (81.5) Maltodextrin Modified cornstarch	53 (4.5) Safflower oil	27	34	530	530	9.5	650	Patients with malabsorption
Deliver 2.0 (Mead Johnson)	2 (60)	75 (15) Ca caseinate Na caseinate	200 (40) Corn syrup	102 (45) Soy oil (70%) MCT oil (30%)	35	43	1000	1000	18	640	Oral supplement or tube feeding for patients with fluid restriction or increased calorie needs
Ensure (Ross)	1.06 (32)	37 (14) Na caseinate Ca caseinate Soy protein	145 (55) Corn syrup (70%) Sucrose (30%)	37 (32) Corn oil	36	40	530	530	9.6	470	Oral supplement or tube feeding for patients with normal GI tract
Ensure Plus (Ross)	1.5 (45)	55 (15) Na caseinate Ca caseinate Soy protein	200 (53) Corn syrup Sucrose	53 (32) Corn oil	46	50	705	705	13	690	Oral supplement or tube feeding for patients with higher calorie needs, normal GI tract
Ensure with Fiber (Ross)	1.1 (33)	40 (15) Na caseinate Ca caseinate Soy protein	162 (55) Hydrolyzed cornstarch (58%) Sucrose (32%) Soy polysaccharide (10%)	37 (31) Corn oil	37	43	719	719	13	480	Oral supplement or tube feeding with fiber, normal GI tract

Continued

From Cox J: Nutrition. In Siberry GK, Iannone R (eds): *The Harriet Lane handbook: a manual for pediatric house officers*, ed 15, St Louis, 2000, Mosby.

III

TABLE 3-37 Older Child & Adult Formula Analysis (Per Liter)—cont'd

FORMULA	kcal/ml (kcal/oz)	PROTEIN g (% kcal)	CARBOHYDRATE g (% kcal)	FAT g (% kcal)	Na (mEq)	K (mEq)	Ca (mg)	P (mg)	Fe (mg)	OSMOLALITY (mOsm/kg water)	SUGGESTED USES
Glucerna (Ross)	1 (30)	42 (17) Na caseinate Ca caseinate	94 (33) Glucose polymers (53%) Soy polysaccharide (25%) Fructose (21%)	56 (50) HO saff oil (85%) Soy oil (15%)	40	40	704	704	13	375	Patients with impaired glucose tolerance, also contains fiber
Isocal (Mead Johnson)	1.06 (32)	34 (13) Na caseinate Ca caseinate Soy protein	135 (50) Maltodextrin	44 (37) MCT oil (20%) Soy oil (80%)	23	34	630	530	10	270	Tube feeding for patients with normal GI tract
Jevity (Ross)	1.06 (32)	44 (17) Na caseinate Ca caseinate	152 (53) Hydrolyzed cornstarch Soy polysaccharide	36 (30) HO saff oil (50%) Canola oil (30%) MCT oil (20%)	40	40	909	758	14	300	Tube feeding with fiber, normal GI tract
L-Emental (GalaGen/ Nutrition, Medical)	1 (30)	38 (15) Free l-amino acids	205 (82) Maltodextrins	2.85 (2.5) Safflower oil	20	20	500	500	9	630	Patients with malabsorption, protein allergy
L-Emental Plus (Nutrition, Medical)	1 (30)	45 (18) Free l-amino acids	190 (76) Maltodextrins	6.7 (6) Soy oil	26	27	556	556	10	650	Patients with malabsorption, protein allergy
Lipisorb (Mead Johnson)	1.35 (40)	57 (17) Na caseinate Ca caseinate	161 (48) Maltodextrin Sucrose	57 (35) MCT oil (85%) Soy oil (15%)	59	43	850	850	15	630	Patients with fat malabsorption
Nepro (Ross)	2 (60)	70 (14) Ca caseinate Mg caseinate Na caseinate	215 (43) Hydrolyzed cornstarch (88%) Sucrose (12%)	96 (43) HO saff oil (90%) Soy oil (10%)	36	27	1373	686	19	635	Patients with renal failure undergoing dialysis

Formula	Cal/mL (serving)	Protein g (%) source	Carbohydrate g (%) source	Fat g (%) source							Comments
Nutren 2.0 (Clintec)	2 (60)	80 (16) K caseinate Ca caseinate	196 (39) Sucrose Corn syrup solids Maltodextrin	106 (45) MCT oil (75%) Canola oil Corn oil Soy oil Lecithin	57	49	1340	1340	24	720	Oral supplement or tube feedings for patients with fluid restriction or increased calorie needs
Nutrivent (Clintec)	1.5 (45)	68 (18) Ca caseinate K caseinate	100 (27) Maltodextrin Sucrose	95 (55) MCT oil (40%) Canola oil (43%) Corn oil (13%) Lecithin (4%)	50	42	1200	1200	18	330	Patients requiring higher percentage of calories from fat
Osmolite (Ross)	1.06 (32)	37 (14) Na caseinate Ca caseinate Soy protein	145 (55) Hydrolyzed cornstarch	38 (31) HO saff oil (50%) Canola oil (30%) MCT oil (20%)	28	26	530	530	9.5	300	Tube feeding for patients with normal GI tract
Peptamen (Clintec)	1 (30)	40 (16) Hydrolyzed whey	127 (51) Maltodextrin (88%) Hydrolyzed cornstarch (12%)	39 (33) MCT oil (67%) Sunflower oil (18%) Lecithin (6%) Milk fat (9%)	22	32	800	700	120	270	Patients with malabsorption
Promote (Ross)	1 (30)	63 (25) Na caseinate Ca caseinate Soy protein	130 (52) Hydrolyzed cornstarch (91%) Sucrose (9%)	26 (23) HO saff oil (50%) Canola oil (30%) MCT oil (20%)	40	51	960	960	14	330	Oral supplement or tube feeding for patients with increased protein needs

Continued

From Cox J: Nutrition. In Siberry GK, Iannone R (eds): *The Harriet Lane handbook: a manual for pediatric house officers*, ed 15, St Louis, 2000, Mosby.

III

TABLE 3-37 Older Child & Adult Formula Analysis (Per Liter)—cont'd

FORMULA	kcal/ml (kcal/oz)	PROTEIN g (% kcal)	CARBOHYDRATE g (% kcal)	FAT g (% kcal)	Na (mEq)	K (mEq)	Ca (mg)	P (mg)	Fe (mg)	OSMOLALITY (mOsm/kg water)	SUGGESTED USES
ProPeptide (unflavored) (GalaGen/Nutrition, Medical)	1 (30)	40 (16) Hydrolyzed whey	127 (51) Maltodextrins Starch	39 (33) Sunflower oil (30%) MCT oil (70%)	22	32	800	700	14	270	Patients with malabsorption
Pulmocare (Ross)	1.5 (45)	63 (17) Na caseinate Ca caseinate	106 (28) Hydrolyzed cornstarch (46%) Sucrose (54%)	92 (55) Corn oil	57	44	1056	1056	19	465	Patients requiring higher percentage of calories from fat
Respalor (Mead Johnson)	1.5 (45)	76 (20) Ca caseinate Na caseinate	148 (39) Corn syrup Sucrose	71 (41) Canola oil (70%) MCT oil (30%)	55	38	710	710	13	580	Patients requiring higher percentage of calories from fat
Scandishake w/whole milk (Scandipharm)	2.5 (75)	50 (8) Cow's milk	292 (47) Lactose Maltodextrin Soy oil	125 (45) Coconut oil Safflower oil Palm oil	240	103	391	478	trace	1094	High-calorie supplement and for fat malabsorption
Suplena (Ross)	2 (60)	30 (6) Na caseinate Ca caseinate	255 (51) Hydrolyzed cornstarch (90%) Sucrose (10%)	96 (43) HO saff oil (90%) Soy oil (10%)	34	29	1385	728	19	600	Patients with renal failure not undergoing dialysis
Boost High Protein (Mead Johnson)	1 (30)	61 (24) Na caseinate Ca caseinate Soy protein	140 (55) Corn syrup Sucrose	23 (21) Partially hydrogenated soy oil	40	54	1010	930	17	650	Oral supplement or tube feeding for patients with increased protein needs
Boost Plus (Mead Johnson)	1.5 (45)	61 (16) Na caseinate Ca caseinate	190 (50) Corn syrup solids Sucrose	57 (34) Corn oil	37	38	850	850	15	670	Oral supplement or tube feeding for patients with high calorie needs, normal GI tract

Product	Cal/mL (%)	Protein g (%) / Source	Carbohydrate g (%) / Source	Fat g (%) / Source						Osmolality	Indications
Boost with Fiber (Mead Johnson)	1.06 (30)	46 (17) Na caseinate Ca caseinate Soy protein	140 (53) Maltodextrin Sucrose	35 (30) Corn oil	31	36	850	710	13	480	Oral supplement or tube feeding with fiber, normal GI tract
Tolerex (Novartis)	1 (30)	21 (8) Free amino acids	230 (91) Maltodextrin	1.5 (1) Safflower oil	20	31	560	560	10	550	Patients with malabsorption or severe food allergy
Traumacal (Mead Johnson)	1.5 (45)	82 (22) Na caseinate Ca caseinate	142 (38) Corn syrup Sucrose	68 (40) Soy oil (70%) MCT oil (30%)	51	36	750	750	9	560	Patients with increased protein and calorie needs
Ultracal (Mead Johnson)	1.06 (30)	44 (17) Na caseinate Ca caseinate	123 (46) Maltodextrin Soy fiber Oat fiber	45 (37) MCT oil (40%) Canola oil (60%)	40	41	850	850	15	310	Oral supplement or tube feeding with fiber, normal GI tract
Vital HN (Ross)	1 (30)	42 (17) Hydrolyzed whey, meat, and soy (87%) Free amino acids (13%)	185 (74) Hydrolyzed cornstarch (83%) Sucrose (17%) Lactose (<0.5%)	11 (9) Safflower oil (55%) MCT oil (45%)	25	36	667	667	12	500	Patients with malabsorption
Vivonex Plus (Novartis)	1 (30)	45 (18) Free amino acids	190 (76) Maltodextrin	6.7 (6) Soybean oil	27	28	560	560	10	650	Patients with malabsorption or severe food allergy
Vivonex TEN (Novartis)	1 (30)	38 (15) Free amino acids	210 (82) Maltodextrin	2.8 (3) Safflower oil	20	20	500	500	9	630	Patients with malabsorption or severe food allergy

From Cox J: Nutrition. In Siberry GK, Iannone R (eds): *The Harriet Lane handbook: a manual for pediatric house officers*, ed 15, St Louis, 2000, Mosby.

III

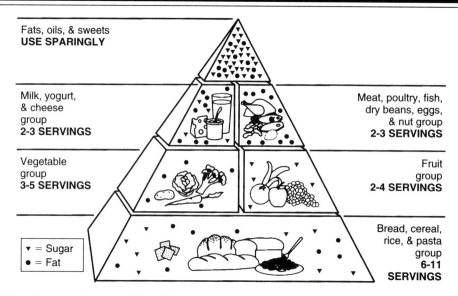

Fig. 3-53 **Food guide pyramid: guide to daily food choices.** (From US Department of Agriculture, US Department of Health and Human Services.)

TABLE 3-38 **Step 1 and Step 2 Diets**

NUTRIENT	STEP 1 DIET	STEP 2 DIET
Calories	Adequate to promote normal growth and development	Same
Total fat	≤30% of calories	Same
Saturated fat	<10% of calories	<7% of calories
Polyunsaturated fat	Up to 10% of calories	Same
Monounsaturated fat	Remaining fat calories	Same
Cholesterol	<300 mg/day	<200 mg/day
Carbohydrates	Approximately 55% of calories	Same
Protein	About 15%-20% of calories	Same

III

Section 8
EMERGENCY MEDICINE

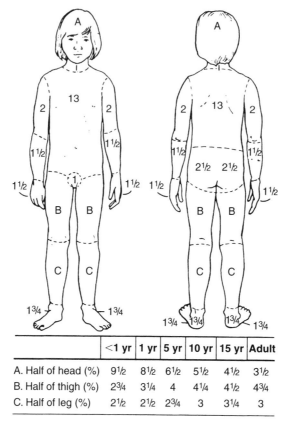

	<1 yr	1 yr	5 yr	10 yr	15 yr	Adult
A. Half of head (%)	9½	8½	6½	5½	4½	3½
B. Half of thigh (%)	2¾	3¼	4	4¼	4½	4¾
C. Half of leg (%)	2½	2½	2¾	3	3¼	3

Fig. 3-54   Burn assessment chart. (From Barkin RM, Rosen P: *Emergency pediatrics,* ed 5, St Louis, 1999, Mosby.)

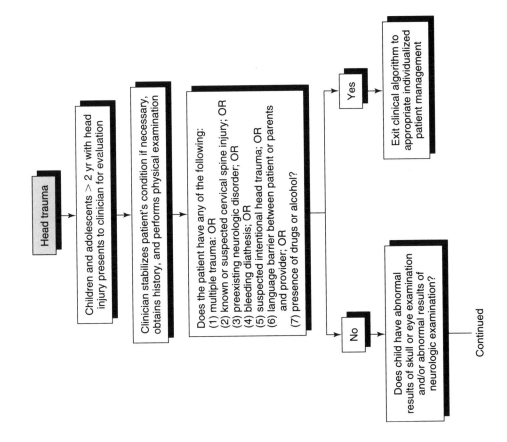

Head trauma

Children and adolescents > 2 yr with head injury presents to clinician for evaluation

Clinician stabilizes patient's condition if necessary, obtains history, and performs physical examination

Does the patient have any of the following:
(1) multiple trauma: OR
(2) known or suspected cervical spine injury; OR
(3) preexisting neurologic disorder; OR
(4) bleeding diathesis; OR
(5) suspected intentional head trauma; OR
(6) language barrier between patient or parents and provider; OR
(7) presence of drugs or alcohol?

Yes

Exit clinical algorithm to appropriate individualized patient management

No

Does child have abnormal results of skull or eye examination and/or abnormal results of neurologic examination?

Continued

III

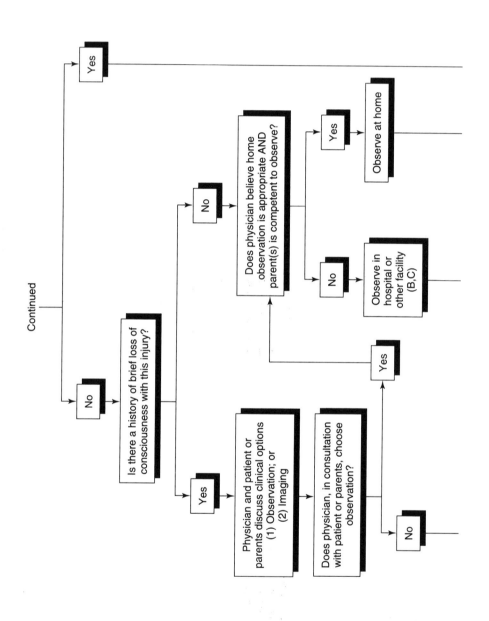

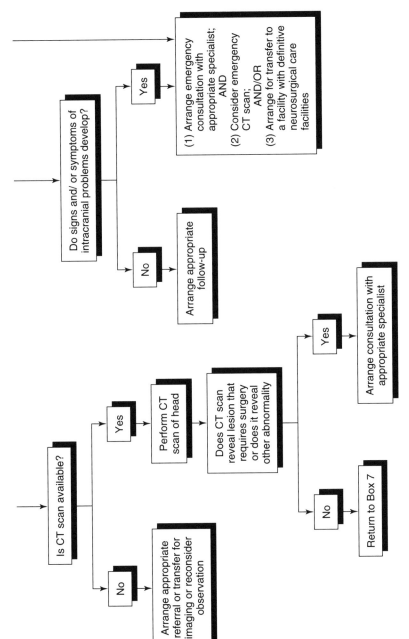

Fig. 3-55   Algorithm for the evaluation and triage of children and adolescents with minor head trauma. *CT,* Computed tomography. (From *Pediatrics* 104:1407, 1999.)

III

BOX 3-3 Children's Coma Scale (Children <4 Years of Age)

Eye Opening	Score
Spontaneous	4
Reaction to speech	3
Reaction to pain	2
No response	1

Best Motor Response

	Score
Spontaneous (obeys verbal command)	6
Localizes pain	5
Withdraws in response to pain	4
Abnormal flexion in response to pain	2
No response	1

Best Verbal Response

		Score
Smiles, oriented to sounds, follows objects		5
Crying consolable		4
Interacts inappropriate		4
Intermittantly consolable		3
Moaning/irritable		3
Inconsolable	Restless	2
No response	No response	1

GCS Total 3-15

BOX 3-4 Glascow Coma Scale (Age 4-Adult)

Eye Opening	Score
Open	
Spontaneously	4
To verbal command	3
To pain	2
No response	1

Best Motor Response

	Score
To Verbal Commands	
Obeys	6
To Painful Stimulus	
Localizes pain	5
Flexion-withdrawl	4
Flexion-abnormal	3
Extension	2
No response	1

Best Verbal Response

	Score
Oriented and converses	5
Disoriented and converses	4
Inappropriate words	3
Incomprehensible sounds	2
No response	1

GCS Total 3-15

Section 9
SPORTS MEDICINE

TABLE 3-39 Medical Conditions and Sports Participation

This table is designed to be understood by medical and nonmedical personnel. In the *Explanation* section below, "needs evaluation" means that a physician with appropriate knowledge and experience should assess the safety of a given sport for an athlete with the listed medical condition. Unless otherwise noted, this is because of the variability of the severity of the disease or of the risk of injury among the specific sports in Box 3-5, or both.

CONDITION	MAY PARTICIPATE?
Atlantoaxial instability (instability of the joint between cervical vertebrae 1 and 2)	Qualified yes
Explanation: Athlete needs evaluation to assess risk of spinal cord injury during sports participation.	
Bleeding disorder	Qualified yes
Explanation: Athlete needs evaluation.	
Cardiovascular diseases	
Carditis (inflammation of the heart)	No
Explanation: Carditis may result in sudden death with exertion.	
Hypertension (high blood pressure)	Qualified yes
Explanation: Those with significant essential (unexplained) hypertension should avoid weight and power lifting, body building, and strength training. Those with secondary hypertension (hypertension caused by a previously identified disease) or severe essential hypertension need evaluation.	
Congenital heart disease (structural heart defects present at birth)	Qualified yes
Explanation: Those with mild forms may participate fully; those with moderate or severe forms, or who have undergone surgery, need evaluation. The 26th Bethesda Conference defined mild, moderate, and severe disease for common cardiac lesions.	
Arrhythmia (irregular heart rhythm)	Qualified yes
Explanation: Those with symptoms (chest pain, syncope, dizziness, shortness of breath, or other symptoms of possible dysrhythmia) or evidence of mitral regurgitation (leaking) on physical examination need evaluation. All others may participate fully.	
Heart murmur	Qualified yes
Explanation: If the murmur is innocent (does not indicate heart disease), full participation is permitted. Otherwise, the athlete needs evaluation (see "Congenital Heart Disease" and "Mitral Valve Prolapse" above).	
Cerebral palsy	Qualified yes
Explanation: Athlete needs evaluation.	
Diabetes mellitus	Yes
Explanation: All sports can be played with proper attention to diet, blood glucose concentration, hydration, and insulin therapy. Blood glucose concentration should be monitored every 30 min during continuous exercise and 15 min after completion of exercise.	
Diarrhea	Qualified no
Explanation: Unless disease is mild, no participation is permitted, because diarrhea may increase the risk of dehydration and heat illness (see "Fever").	
Eating disorders Anorexia nervosa Bulimia nervosa	Qualified yes
Explanation: These patients need both medical and psychiatric assessment before participation.	

From American Academy of Pediatrics, Committee on Sports Medicine and Fitness: *Pediatrics* 107:1205, 2001.

Continued

TABLE 3-39   Medical Conditions and Sports Participation—cont'd

CONDITION	MAY PARTICIPATE?
Eyes	Qualified yes
Functionally one-eyed athlete	
Loss of an eye	
Detached retina	
Previous eye surgery or serious eye injury	
Explanation: A functionally one-eyed athlete has a best corrected visual acuity of <20/40 in the worse eye. These athletes would suffer significant disability if the better eye was seriously injured as would those with loss of an eye. Some athletes who have previously undergone eye surgery or had a serious eye injury may have an increased risk of injury because of weakened eye tissue. Availability of eye guards approved by the American Society for Testing Materials (ASTM) and other protective equipment may allow participation in most sports, but this must be judged on an individual basis.	
Fever	No
Explanation: Fever can increase cardiopulmonary effort, reduce maximum exercise capacity, make heat illness more likely, and increase orthostatic hypotension during exercise. Fever may rarely accompany myocarditis or other infections that may make exercise dangerous.	
Heat illness, history of	Qualified yes
Explanation: Because of the increased likelihood of recurrence, the athlete needs individual assessment to determine the presence of predisposing conditions and to arrange a prevention strategy.	
Hepatitis	Yes
Explanation: Because of the apparent minimal risk to others, all sports may be played that the athlete's state of health allows. In all athletes, skin lesions should be covered properly, and athletic personnel should use universal precautions when handling blood or body fluids with visible blood.	
HIV infection	Yes
Explanation: Because of the apparent minimal risk to others, all sports may be played that the state of health allows. In all athletes, skin lesions should be properly covered, and athletic personnel should use universal precautions when handling blood or body fluids with visible blood.	
Kidney: absence of one	Qualified yes
Explanation: Athlete needs individual assessment for contact/collision and limited contact sports.	
Liver: enlarged	Qualified yes
Explanation: If the liver is acutely enlarged, participation should be avoided because of risk of rupture. If the liver is chronically enlarged, individual assessment is needed before collision/contact or limited contact sports are played.	
Malignant neoplasm	Qualified yes
Explanation: Athlete needs individual assessment.	
Musculoskeletal disorders	Qualified yes
Explanation: Athlete needs individual assessment.	
Neurologic disorders	
History of serious head or spine trauma, severe or repeated concussions, or craniotomy.	Qualified yes
Explanation: Athlete needs individual assessment for collision/contact or limited contact sports, and also for noncontact sports if there are deficits in judgment or cognition. Recent research supports a conservative approach to management of concussion.	
Seizure disorder, well controlled	Yes
Explanation: Risk of convulsion during participation is minimal.	
Seizure disorder, poorly controlled	Qualified yes
Explanation: Athlete needs individual assessment for collision/contact or limited contact sports. Avoid the following noncontact sports: archery, riflery, swimming, weight or power lifting, strength training, or sports involving heights. In these sports, occurrences of a convulsion may be a risk to self or others.	

From American Academy of Pediatrics, Committee on Sports Medicine and Fitness: *Pediatrics* 107:1205, 2001.

TABLE 3-39 Medical Conditions and Sports Participation—cont'd

CONDITION	MAY PARTICIPATE?
Obesity	Qualified yes
Explanation: Because of the risk of heat illness, obese persons need careful acclimatization and hydration.	
Organ transplant recipient	Qualified yes
Explanation: Athlete needs individual assessment.	
Ovary: absence of one	Yes
Explanation: Risk of severe injury to the remaining ovary is minimal.	
Respiratory	
Pulmonary compromise including cystic fibrosis	Qualified yes
Explanation: Athlete needs individual assessment, but generally all sports may be played if oxygenation remains satisfactory during a graded exercise test. Patients with cystic fibrosis need acclimization and good hydration to reduce the risk of illness.	
Asthma	Yes
Explanation: With proper medication and education, only athletes with the most severe asthma will have to modify their participation.	
Acute upper respiratory infection	Qualified yes
Explanation: Upper respiratory obstruction may affect pulmonary function. Athlete needs individual assessment for all but mild disease (see ''Fever'' earlier).	
Sickle cell disease	Qualified yes
Explanation: Athlete needs individual assessment. In general, if status of the illness permits, all but high exertion, collision/contact sports may be played. Overheating, dehydration, and chilling must be avoided.	
Sickle cell trait	Yes
Explanation: It is unlikely that individuals with sickle cell trait (AS) have an increased risk of sudden death or other medical problems during athletic participation except under the most extreme conditions of heat, humidity, and possibly increased altitude. These individuals, like all athletes, should be carefully conditioned, aclimatized, and hydrated to reduce any possible risk.	
Skin: boils, herpes simplex, impetigo, scabies, molluscum contagiosum	Qualified yes
Explanation: While the patient is contagious, participation in gymnastics with mats, martial arts, wrestling, or other collision/contact or limited contact sports is not allowed.	
Spleen, enlarged	Qualified yes
Explanation: Patients with acutely enlarged spleens should avoid all sports because of risk of rupture. Those with chronically enlarged spleens need individual assessment before playing collision/contact or limited contact sports.	
Testicle: absent or undescended	Yes
Explanation: Certain sports may require a protective cup.	

III

BOX 3-5 Classification of Sports by Contact

Contact/Collision		Limited Contact		Noncontact	
Basketball	Lacrosse	Baseball	Racquetball	Archery	Orienteering
Boxing*	Martial arts	Bicycling	Skating	Badminton	Power lifting
Diving	Rodeo	Cheerleading	Ice	Body building	Race walking
Field hockey	Rugby	Canoeing/kayaking	Inline	Bowling	Riflery
Football	Ski jumping	(white water)	Roller	Canoeing/kayaking	Rope jumping
Tackle	Soccer	Fencing	Skiing	(flat water)	Running
Ice hockey†	Team handball	Field events	Cross-country	Crew/rowing	Sailing
	Water polo	High jump	Downhill	Curling	Scuba diving
	Wrestling	Pole vault	Water	Dancing	Swimming
		Floor hockey	Skateboarding	Field events	Table tennis
		Football	Snowboarding	Discus	Tennis
		Flag	Softball	Javelin	Track
		Gymnastics	Squash	Shot put	Weight lifting
		Handball	Ultimate Frisbee	Golf	
		Horseback	Volleyball		
		riding	Windsurfing/surfing		

From American Academy of Pediatrics, Committee on Sports Medicine and Fitness: *Pediatrics* 107:1205, 2001.
*Participation not recommended.
†The AAP recommends limiting the amount of body checking allowed for hockey players 15 years and younger to reduce injuries.

BOX 3-6 Summary of Recommendations for Management of Concussion in Sports

A *concussion* is defined as head-trauma—induced alteration in mental status that may or may not involve loss of consciousness. Concussions are graded in three categories. Definitions and treatment recommendations for each category are presented below.

Grade 1 Concussion

- **Definition:** Transient confusion, no loss of consciousness, and a duration of mental status abnormalities of <15 minutes.
- **Management:** The athlete should be removed from sports activity, examined immediately and at 5-minute intervals, and allowed to return that day to the sports activity only if postconcussive symptoms resolve within 15 minutes. Any athlete who incurs a second Grade 1 concussion on the same day should be removed from sports activity until asymptomatic for 1 week.

Grade 2 Concussion

- **Definition:** Transient confusion, no loss of consciousness, and a duration of mental status abnormalities of ≥15 minutes.
- **Management:** The athlete should be removed from sports activity and examined frequently to assess the evolution of symptoms, with more extensive diagnostic evaluation if the symptoms worsen or persist for >1 week. The athlete should return to sports activity only after asymptompatic for 1 full week. Any athlete who incurs a grade 2 concussion subsequent to a grade 1 concussion on the same day should be removed from sports activity until asymptomatic for 2 weeks.

Grade 3 Concussion

- **Definition:** Loss of consciousness, either brief (seconds) or prolonged (minutes or longer).
- **Management:** The athlete should be removed from sports activity for 1 full week without symptoms if the loss of consciousness is brief or 2 full weeks without symptoms if the loss of consciousness is prolonged. If still unconscious or if abnormal neurologic signs are present at the time of initial evaluation, the athlete should be transported by ambulance to the nearest hospital emergency department. An athlete who suffers a second grade 3 concussion should be removed from sports activity until asymptomatic for 1 month. Any athlete with an abnormality on computed tomography or magnetic resonance imaging brain scan consistent with brain swelling, contusion, or other intracranial pathology should be removed from sports activities for the season and discouraged from future return to participation in contact sports.

From Quality Standards Subcommittee, American Academy of Neurology. In summary of recommendations for management of concussion in sports, *MMWR Morb Mortal Wkly Rep* 46(10):226, 1997.

III

BOX 3-7 Knee Maneuvers

Knee Valgus Stress Test

To test medial collateral ligament

Patient: Supine, leg extended and supported by examiner

Examiner: Beside extremity tested, with one hand on distal lateral femur and other on medial tibia below the joint line

Technique: Apply medial pressure on femur while distracting tibia laterally. Note amount of opening of medial knee. It should be minimal. Compare with other leg.

Knee Varus Stress Test

To test lateral collateral ligament

Patient: Supine, leg extended and supported by examiner

Examiner: Beside extremity tested, with one hand on distal medial femur and other on the lateral tibia below the joint line

Technique: Apply lateral pressure on the femur while distracting the tibia medially. Note amount of opening of lateral knee. It should be minimal. Compare with other leg.

McMurray Sign

To test for tears in medial and lateral menisci

Patient: Supine and relaxed with knee completely bent

Examiner: Standing at the side of the injured limb

Technique: Grasp the heel and rotate the foot externally while abducting the leg and extending the knee. A click or pain is significant for lateral tear. Opposite maneuver can be positive for medial tear and is done by rotating the foot internally and abducting the leg while extending the knee.

Apprehension Test

To test for patella subluxation

Patient: Seated

Examiner: Hand on affected patella

Technique: Gently push the patella laterally. A start of apprehension is positive. If negative, examiner can extend the knee and then passively flex the knee while gently pushing the patella laterally.

Anterior Drawer Sign

To test the anterior cruciate

Patient: Supine, hip flexed 45 degrees, knee flexed 90 degrees

Examiner: Sitting on patient's ipsilateral foot

Technique: Place hands around the tibia just below the joint line. Apply anterior force and note the amount of anterior motion. Always compare with other knee.

Lachman Test

When the knee cannot be flexed

Patient: Supine, hip, and knee extended

Examiner: Standing beside patient

Technique: Grasp the femus with one hand and the tibia below the joint line. Apply a distracting force to the tibia and note the excursion.

Posterior Drawer Sign

To test the posterior cruciate

Patient: Supine, hip flexed 45 degrees, knee flexed 90 degrees

Examiner: Sitting on patient's ipsilateral foot

Technique: Same as anterior drawer sign, except apply posterior force on tibia.

From Driscoll CE et al: *The family practice desk reference*, ed 3, St Louis, 1996, Mosby.

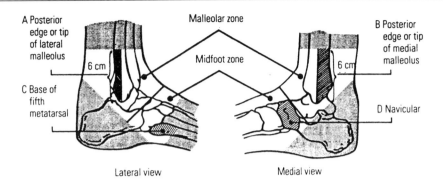

An ankle radiographic series is only required if there is any pain in the malleolar zone and any of these
    findings is present:
(1) bone tenderness at A
(2) bone tenderness at B
(3) inability to bear weight both immediately and in the ED

A foot radiographic series is only required if there is any pain in midfoot zone and any of these findings is
    present:
(1) bone tenderness at C
(2) bone tenderness at D
(3) inability to bear wieght both immediately and in the ED

Fig. 3-56   Ottawa ankle rules. (Courtesy Stiell IG, Greenberg GH, McKnight RD, Wells GA, Ottowa
Civic Hospital, Ottowa, Ontario, Canada.)

Section 10
NEUROLOGY

TABLE 3-40 **Office Hearing Tests**

TEST	METHOD	INTERPRETATION
Weber's test	512-Hz tuning fork placed on top of the head; patient is asked which ear tone is heard	*Normal:* sound heard in midline *Conductive loss:* sound heard on affected side *Neurosensory loss:* sound heard on unaffected side
Rinne's test	512-Hz tuning fork held against mastoid; when sound is no longer heard, duration of bone conduction is noted; fork transferred to ½ inch from ear; air conduction should be twice as long as bone and louder	*Air > bone:* normal (+) test *Bone > air:* conductive hearing loss (–) test
Whispered voice	Occlude opposite ear; whisper softly, from 2 feet away; do not use a question that is answered by "yes" or "no"	Usually indicates 20-dB hearing loss if not perceived
Watch tick	Hold watch 2 inches from ear	Indicates high-frequency loss if not perceived; if heard, 98% chance of hearing all lower frequencies normally
Schwabach's test	512-Hz tuning fork is pressed alternately to examiner's mastoid, then to patient's mastoid	When hearing is normal, both patient and examiner cease to hear the tuning fork at the same time; if patient hears the tuning fork longer than an examiner with normal hearing, this indicates middle ear (conductive) loss; if examiner with normal hearing hears the tuning fork longer, the patient has sensorineural loss

From Driscoll CE et al: *The family practice desk reference,* ed 3, St Louis, 1996, Mosby.

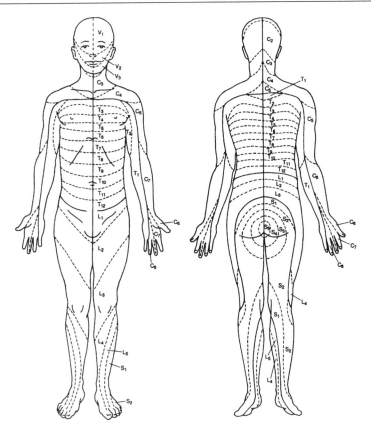

Fig. 3-57   Spinal dermatomes. (From Siberry GK, Iannone R [eds]: *The Harriet Lane handbook: a manual for pediatric house officers,* ed 15, St Louis, 2000, Mosby.)

III

TABLE 3-41 **Characteristics of Abnormal Movements**

MOVEMENT	SPEED	LOCATION	DIRECTION	STEREOTYPE	RHYTHMICITY	INTERVAL
Athetosis	Slow	Most prominent in distal limbs	Axial rotations (writhing) and hyperextension	Common; continuous movement in extremity	Not rhythmic	Continuous, amplitude increased by excitement
Ballismus	Rapid	Proximal, especially at shoulder; also at hip; sometimes trunk, face, and muscles of respiration	Hurling, flinging, throwing, kicking, circumducting	Constant location; movements vary	Not rhythmic	0.5-120 seconds
Chorea	Rapid	Generalized; may be unilateral	Primarily at right angles to axis; also facial grimacing; flexion and extension	None; movements generally dance from joint to joint; when proximal and severe may appear semipurposeful	Not rhythmic	0.5-5 seconds
Dystonia	Rapid, slow; very slow relaxation	Trunk, head, extremities	Any, often twisting	Common; because of location of movements, relative strength of contracting muscles	Irregular	Irregular
Myoclonus	Very rapid	Localized or generalized	Any	Stereotyped	Irregular	0.5-5 seconds
Tic	Rapid	Usually in area supplied by motor cranial nerve (face, shoulder, neck)	Rotational; away	Stereotyped	Irregular	1 second to minutes
Tremor	Variable	Usually localized, often in hand	Complex or simple	Extreme stereotype	Very rhythmic; may be irregular	0.1-1 second

From McMillan JA, Stockman JA III, Oski FA (eds): *The whole pediatrician catalog: a compendium of clues to the diagnosis and management*, Philadelphia, 1979, WB Saunders.

Section 11
CONTRACEPTION

 BASIC INFORMATION

■ DEFINITION
Contraception is the voluntary prevention of conception or impregnation.

■ SYNONYMS
- Birth control
- Oral contraceptive pills (OCPs): the pill
- Depo-Provera (depo)
- Intrauterine device (IUD)
- Norplant

■ ICD-9CM CODES
V25.09 Contraceptive advice or counseling NEC
V25.40 Contraceptive maintenance or examination
V25.01 Prescribing or use of oral contraceptive agent
V25.41 Contraceptive maintenance oral contraceptive
V25.02 Prescribing or use of specified agent NEC
V25.49 Contraceptive maintenance specified method NEC
V25.02 Fitting of diaphragm
V25.10 Insertion intrauterine contraceptive device
V25.42 Contraceptive maintenance intrauterine device
V25.50 Insertion subdermal implantable
V25.43 Contraceptive maintenance subdermal implantable
V25.42 Removal or reinsertion device (in situ)

■ EPIDEMIOLOGY
- Approximately 76% of adolescent women use contraception for their first episode of premarital sex.
  1. Condoms: 83%
  2. OCPs: 11%
  3. Withdrawal: 5%
- Current use for 15- to 19-year-old women is as follows:
  1. OCPs: 33%
  2. Condoms: 30%
  3. Depo: 8%
  4. Withdrawal: 3%
  5. Norplant: 2%
  6. Abstinence: 1%
- Adolescents are less likely to use contraception consistently or effectively.
- Barriers to contraception include inadequate knowledge, access issues (e.g., cost, transportation, confidentiality), and adolescent developmental issues (e.g., peers, denial of risk).

HORMONAL CONTRACEPTION
Hormonal contraception inhibits ovulation, thickens cervical mucus, causes premature luteolysis, and causes endometrial changes that hamper implantation. (See Table 3-43 for failure rates; also see end of section "OCP Information.")
- Oral contraceptive pills
  1. Combined (estrogen and progestin): monophasic, triphasic, 28- and 21-day packs
     a. OCPs containing 30 to 35 µg ethinyl estradiol commonly used
     b. If estrogen side effects problematic, 20 µg useful
     c. Newer progestins: norgestimate, desogestrel; have less androgen effects
     d. Desogestrel: question of link with venous thromboembolic events; not first-line choice
  2. Progestin only
     a. Less efficacious, more breakthrough bleeding
- Depo-Provera
  1. Medroxyprogesterone acetate
  2. 150 mg intramuscularly every 12 weeks
- Norplant
  1. Levonorgestrel in six silastic rods inserted subdermally in arm
  2. Effective for 5 years

■ COMMON CONCERNS
- Missed dose of OCP
  1. See Fig. 3-58.
- Breast cancer
  1. OCPs
     a. No significant increase: small apparent increased risk because of diagnostic bias/random chance
     b. No relationship to age, preparation, reproductive history, family history, age of menarche, duration of use
     c. Tumors in OCP users more likely localized to breast
  2. Depo
     a. Highest risk is in first 3 months of use and those younger than age 35.
     b. No increase is seen in ever users or with more than 5 years of use.
     c. Apparent increase may represent increased detection or increased growth of existing tumor.
- Cardiovascular/metabolic
  1. OCPs
     a. Smokers older than 35 are at highest risk for coronary heart disease and stroke.
     b. Less than 5% develop hypertension.
     c. Low-dose pills produce minimal changes in lipids and glucose tolerance.
     d. Improvement in bone density is seen.

III

TABLE 3-42 **Contraindications (World Health Organization) of Hormonal Contraception**

	OCP	DEPO	NORPLANT
Thromboembolic event	X	O	O
Cerebrovascular accident, coronary artery disease, ischemic heart disease	X	*	*
Diabetes with vascular disease	X	*	#
Breast cancer (current)	X	X	X
Pregnancy	X	X	X
Liver disease	X	*	*
Migraine with focal neurologic symptoms	X	#	#
Surgery with prolonged immobilization	X	O	O
Hypertension 160/100+ mm Hg or with vascular disease	X	1	1
Hypertension 140-179/90-109 mm Hg	2	#	O
Hypertension 180/110+ mm Hg	X	3	#
Unexplained vaginal bleeding	*	X	X
Gallbladder disease	*	O	O

X, Refrain from providing; ***, exercise caution; *#*, advantages generally outweigh risks; *O*, do not restrict; *1*, see next category; *2*, for OCPs blood pressure 140-159/100-109 mm Hg—advantages outweigh risks; *3*, for depo significant hypertension should be evaluated individually and one should exercise caution since the lack of estrogen combined with the fall in high-density lipoprotein (HDL) cholesterol levels may increase the risk of cardiovascular complications. See also text on pp. 877-879.

2. Depo
   a. Can cause decreased HDL; increased low-density hypoprotein (LDL)
   b. No significant cardiovascular changes, thromboembolic events
   c. Slightly exaggerated insulin response to glucose tolerance test
   d. Decrease in bone density
3. Norplant
   a. No significant changes in lipid levels are observed.
   b. Hypertension is not common.
   c. Some studies show improved bone density.
- Menstrual pattern
  1. OCPs
     a. Initial breakthrough bleeding usually resolves after a few packs, and OCPs can regulate menses.
     b. Patients taking low-dose pills (20 µg) and progestin-only pills are most likely to have breakthrough bleeding.
     c. Menses become shorter and lighter over time.
  2. Depo
     a. Approximately 70% of patients have irregular menses: amenorrhea or spotting.
     b. More than half have amenorrhea by end of year 1, 70% by year 2.

   c. Treat bleeding with nonsteroidal anti-inflammatory drugs (NSAIDs), Premarin, or OCP.
3. Norplant
   a. Approximately 70% of patients have irregular menses.
   b. More than one third of patients will have increased bleeding and spotting in year 1.
   c. Regular cycles after year 1 are seen in 50% to 60% of patients.
   d. Treat bleeding with NSAIDs, Premarin, or OCP.
- Infertility
  1. No hormonal methods cause infertility.
  2. Delay in return of regular ovulatory cycles is more common with Depo compared with OCPs or Norplant.
- Weight gain
  1. OCPs and Norplant may cause similar small increases in weight.
  2. Depo may cause significant weight gain as a result of increased appetite.
- Headaches
  1. OCPs
     a. Migraine with focal neurologic symptoms associated with possible increased risk of stroke are reported.

TABLE 3-43 Contraception–Failure Rates

	LOWEST EXPECTED (%)	USUAL (%)
OCPs		3-5%
Combined	0.1	
Progestin	0.5	
Depo-Provera	0.3	0.3
Norplant	0.05	0.05
Male condom	3	14
Female condom	5	21
IUD (copper)	0.6	0.8
IUD (progesterone)	1.5	2.0
Diaphragm	6	20
Cap		
Parous	26	40
Nulliparous	9	20
Sponge		
Parous	20	40
Nulliparous	9	20
Withdrawal	4	19
Rhythm		25
None	85	85

IUD, Intrauterine device.

  b. Estrogen withdrawal may be associated with migraine: Mircet is newer pill with fewer nonhormonal days (ethinyl estradiol in last week of 28-day cycle may be helpful).
  2. Depo and Norplant
    a. Advantages outweigh risks for migraine, even with focal neurologic symptoms.
    b. Norplant: If severe headache with blurred vision or papilledema occurs, discontinue use.
- Depression
  1. OCPs
    a. No evidence that there is significant increase
  2. Depo and Norplant
    a. Some depression with progestin-only contraceptives

  b. Depo more of a problem because cannot discontinue immediately
- Drug interactions
  1. OCPs and Norplant
    a. Hepatic enzyme–inducing drugs (i.e., antibiotics, antiepileptic medications) may decrease efficacy.
  2. Depo
    a. No significant interactions

■ METHOD-SPECIFIC BENEFITS
- OCPs may lead to improvement in benign breast disease, dysmenorrhea, dysfunctional bleeding, anemia, bone density, ovarian cycsts, pelvic inflammatory disease, acne, hirsutism, and uterine and ovarian cancer.
- Depo-Provera leads to improvement in dysmenorrhea, endometrial cancer, anemia, breast tenderness, pelvic inflammatory disease (PID), seizures, and sickle cell disease (decreases sickling, increases red blood cell survival)
  1. Easier compliance than OCPs
  2. Confidentiality because not hiding method and not visible
- Norplant possibly improves bone density and has the fewest issues with compliance.

EMERGENCY CONTRACEPTION
■ METHODS
- Emergency oral contraceptive pills (ECP)
  1. Combined OCPs such as Preven
  2. Progestin only (levonorgestrel, Plan B), less nausea; may be advantageous
  3. Multiple doses of standard OCPs (see Table 3-44)
- Copper IUD

■ MECHANISM OF ACTION
- ECPs
  1. Inhibit or delay ovulation
  2. Cause changes in endometrium: prevent implantation
  3. Cause luteolysis
  4. Prevent fertilization
  5. Do not disrupt existing pregnancy
- Copper IUDs
  1. Prevent fertilization
  2. Interfere with implantation

■ EFFICACY
- Reduces risk of pregnancy as follows:
  1. At least 75%: combined OCP
  2. Approximately 89%: Plan B
  3. Approximately 99%: copper IUD

III

■ **PRESCRIBING INFORMATION**
- Take pills within 72 hours of unprotected sex.
  1. Preven: 2 pills every 12 hours for total of 4 pills
  2. Plan B: 1 pill every 12 hours for total of 2 pills
     a. Plan B has significantly less nausea and vomiting than Preven
  3. See Table 3-44 for emergency contraception with commonly used OCPs.
- Take antiemetic 30 to 60 minutes before ECP.
- Insert copper IUD within 5 to 7 days of unprotected intercourse.
- Emergency Contraceptive Hotline: 800-NOT-2-LATE.
- Consider prophylactic prescription of ECP.

NONHORMONAL CONTRACEPTION
■ **METHODS**
- Condoms
  1. Male: latex, polyurethane, natural skin
  2. Female: polyurethane
- Spermicides
  1. Nonoxynol-9
  2. Suppository, film, foam, jelly
- Diaphragm
  1. Dome-shaped latex cup used with spermicide
  2. Fit by clinician, sizes 50 to 95 mm in diameter
  3. Arching, coil, and flat spring versions
  4. Effective for 6 hours after insertion
- Cervical cap
  1. Dome-shaped latex cap used with spermicide
  2. Fit by trained clinician, four sizes available
     a. About 6% to 10% of women cannot be fit.
  3. Effective for 48 hours without additional spermicide
- IUD
  1. Copper: copper T, effective for 10 years
  2. Progesterone: Progestasert effective for 1 year
     a. This IUD contains progesterone in the vertical stem.
- Sponge
  1. Polyurethane sponge containing nonoxynol-9
  2. Effective for 24 hours after insertion
  3. To be reintroduced into the market in near future

■ **MECHANISM OF ACTION**
- Barrier: condom, diaphragm, cap
- Spermicidal: spermicide, IUD, diaphragm, sponge, cap
- Thicken cervical mucus: progesterone IUD
- Inhibit fertilization: IUD

■ **METHOD SPECIFIC ISSUES**
- Male condom
  1. Need to discuss and demonstrate proper use
  2. When used with spermicide, 98% to 99% effective against pregnancy
  3. Polyurethane available if person is allergic to latex
  4. Cannot use with oil-based lubricants, except polyurethane brand
     a. Spermicidal condoms may increase risk of human immunodeficiency (HIV) transmission if inflammation occurs in individual sensitive to spermicide
- Female condom
  1. Need to explain and demonstrate proper use
  2. Correct use more difficult than male condom
  3. Can be noisy; may need extra lubricant
  4. Need to be comfortable touching genitalia to insert
  5. Can be inserted before sex
  6. Can use with oil-based lubricants
- Spermicide
  1. Foam or jelly immediately active
  2. Film or suppository active in 10 to 15 minutes
  3. Individuals sensitive or allergic: may have increased HIV transmission risk
- Diaphragm
  1. Refitting required postpartum or with 10-pound weight change
  2. Cannot use with oil-based lubricant
  3. Must use with spermicide for optimal efficacy; add additional spermicide for each sexual act
  4. Can be inserted up to 6 hours before sex
  5. Must be left in place 6 hours after sex
  6. Should be removed within 24 hours because of toxic shock risk
  7. Increased risk of urinary tract infection (UTI), bacterial vaginosis, yeast infection, toxic shock
- Cap
  1. More difficult to insert than diaphragm
  2. Must use with spermicide for optimal efficacy
  3. Cannot use with oil-based lubricants
  4. Can be inserted before sex: need at least 30 minutes between insertion and sexual intercourse
  5. Must be left in place 6 hours after sex
  6. Should be removed within 48 hours because of toxic shock risk
- Sponge
  1. Must be left in place 6 hours after intercourse
  2. Risk of toxic shock if left in more than 24 to 30 hours
  3. Can be difficult to remove
  4. Can cause vaginal dryness
  5. Increased risk of UTI, yeast, bacterial vaginosis
- IUD
  1. Popularity returning
  2. Easy compliance

3. Risks: perforation, pain and bleeding, expulsion
   a. More expulsions: nulliparous, younger, during menses, first 3 months of use
4. Risk of PID greatest at time of insertion and in a few weeks after insertion
5. Spontaneous abortion possible if left in past first trimester
6. Absolute contraindications: malignant disease of the uterus or cervix, vaginal bleeding of unclear etiology, pregnancy, active PID
7. Relative contraindications: multiple sexual partners, sexually transmitted disease exposure
8. Most appropriate: if parous, mutually monogamous relationship

REFERENCES

1. Grimes DA (ed): Issues of *The Contraception Report,* Totowa, NJ, Emron. Fax: 201-720-6080. Presented as a monograph, several issues per year presenting continuing research into present and future contraceptive methods.
2. Grimes DA et al: *Modern contraception,* Totowa, NJ, 1997, Emron.
3. Hatcher RA et al: *Contraceptive technology,* ed 17, New York, 1998, Ardent Media, Inc.

Author: **Paula K. Braverman, M.D.**

■ ORAL CONTRACEPTIVE PILL (OCP) INFORMATION*

1. **OCP contraindications** (for all OCPs containing estrogen)
   a. Refrain from providing (WHO category 4): History of thrombophlebitis/thromboembolic disease, stroke, ischemic structural heart disease, structural heart disease with complications, breast/liver cancer, estrogen-dependent neoplasia, acute liver disease, benign hepatic adenoma, diabetes with complications, headaches with focal neurologic symptoms, major surgery with prolonged immobilization or any surgery on the legs, hypertension with pressures 160+/100+ mm Hg.
   b. Exercise caution (WHO category 3): Undiagnosed abnormal vaginal/uterine bleeding, use of drugs that affect liver enzymes, gallbladder disease.
   c. Advantages generally outweigh disadvantages (WHO category 2): Headaches without focal neurologic symptoms, diabetes without complications, major surgery without prolonged immobilization, sickle cell disease, moderate hypertension (140-159/100-109 mm Hg), undiagnosed breast mass.
2. **Instructions for use**
   a. Sunday start most common method.

*From Straub DM: Adolescent medicine. In Siberry GK, Iannone R (eds): *The Harriet Lane handbook: a manual for pediatric house officers,* ed 15, St Louis, 2000, Mosby.

b. Start with low-dose estrogen pill (=30-35 µg).
c. 21 days hormonal pills, 7 days inactive pills.
d. Advise patient about need for back-up methods during first month of use and need for STD prevention.
e. Pelvic examination recommended at baseline or during first 3-6 months of use, then annually to test for STDs and perform Pap smears.
f. 2-3 visits a year to monitor for compliance, BP, side effects.

3. **Side effects (ACHES)**
   a. **A**bdominal pain (pelvic vein/mesenteric vein thrombosis, pancreatitis).
   b. **C**hest pain (pulmonary embolism, myocardial infarction).
   c. **H**eadaches (thrombotic/hemorrhagic stroke, retinal vein thrombosis).
   d. **E**ye symptoms (thrombotic/hemorrhagic stroke, retinal vein thrombosis).
   e. **S**evere leg pain (thrombophlebitis of the lower extremity, venous thrombosis).

■ ADVICE FOR PATIENTS WHO HAVE MISSED ORAL CONTRACEPTIVE PILLS (Fig. 3-58)

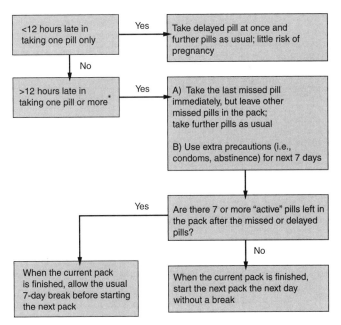

Fig. 3-58   Advice for patients who have missed oral contraceptive pills. Based on the "7-day rule" that seven consecutive pills are enough to "put the ovaries to sleep," so a pill-free interval of greater than 7 days risks ovulation. This algorithm is based on exogenous hormone for 21 days of the 28-day cycle; in packs with 28 days of pills, the "7-day break" represents the hormone-free pills. *If two or more pills are missed, if they were all from the first seven in the pack, and if unprotected intercourse occurred since the end of the last pack, emergency contraception is indicated in addition to (A) and (B) (see Table 3-44). (From Guillebaud J: *Fertil Contol Rev* 4:18, 1995.)

■ **EMERGENCY CONTRACEPTION USING OCPs**
(Table 3-44)
1. Instructions for use
   a. To reduce the chance of nausea, recommend an antiemetic dose 30 to 60 minutes before the first dose of emergency contraception.
   b. The first dose should be taken as soon as possible after unprotected sex but must be within the first 72 hours.
   c. The second dose should be taken 12 hours after the first dose; do not take any extra pills.
   d. Use only one type of pill.
   e. Recommend the use of condoms, spermicides, or a diaphragm during sex after taking emergency contraception until the next menstrual period; ensure proper regular birth control for the future.
   f. Perform pregnancy test if there is no menstrual period within 3 weeks of ECP treatment.

TABLE 3-44 Emergency Contraception Using Standard OCPs

TRADE NAME	FORMULATION	PILLS PER DOSE
Ovral	0.05 mg ethinyl estradiol, 0.50 mg norgestrel	2 white pills
Lo-Ovral	0.03 mg ethinyl estradiol, 0.30 mg norgestrel	4 white pills
Nordette	0.03 mg ethinyl estradiol, 0.15 mg levonorgestrel	4 light-orange pills
Levlen	0.03 mg ethinyl estradiol, 0.15 mg levonorgestrel	4 light-orange pills
Triphasil	0.03 mg ethinyl estradiol, 0.125 mg levonorgestrel	4 yellow pills
Trilevlen	0.03 mg ethinyl estradiol, 0.125 mg levonorgestrel	4 yellow pills
Alesse	0.02 mg ethinyl estradiol, 0.10 mg levonorgestrel	5 pink pills

Data from Program for Applied Technologies (PATH), *Emergency contraception: resource for providers*, Seattle, 1997, PATH.

Section 12
INTERPRETATION
OF SELECTED
LABORATORY VALUES

TABLE 3-45   Neonatal Hemoglobin (Hb) Electrophoresis Patterns*

FA	Fetal Hb and adult normal Hb; the normal newborn pattern.
FAV	Indicates the presence of both HbF and HbA. However, an anomalous band (V) is present, which does not appear to be any of the common Hb variants.
FAS	Indicates fetal Hb, adult normal HbA and HbS, consistent with benign sickle cell trait.
FS	Fetal and sickle HbS without detectable adult normal HbA. Consistent with homozygous sickle Hb genotype (S/S) or sickle β-thalassemia, with manifestations of sickle cell anemia during childhood.
FC†	Designates the presence of HbC without adult normal HbA. Consistent with clinically significant homozygous HbC genotype (C/C), resulting in a mild hematologic disorder presenting during childhood.
FSC	HbS and HbC present. This heterozygous condition could lead to the manifestations of sickle cell disease during childhood.
FAC	HbC and adult normal HbA present, consistent with benign HbC trait.
FSAA$_2$	Heterozygous HbS/β-thalassemia, a clinically significant sickling disorder.
FAA$_2$	Heterozygous HbA/β-thalassemia, a clinically benign hematologic condition.
F†	Fetal HbF is present without adult normal HbA. Although this may indicate a delayed appearance of HbA, it is also consistent with homozygous β-thalassemia major, or homozygous hereditary persistence of fetal HbF.
FV†	Fetal HbF and an anomalous Hb variant (V) are present.
AF	May indicate prior blood transfusion. Submit another filter paper blood specimen when the infant is 4 mo of age, at which time the transfused blood cells should have been cleared.

From Ebel BE, Raffini L: Hematology. In Siberry GK, Iannone R (eds): *The Harriet Lane handbook: a manual for pediatric house officers*, ed 15, St Louis, 2000, Mosby.
*Hemoglobin variants are reported in order of decreasing abundance; for example, *FA* indicates more fetal than adult hemoglobin.
†Repeat blood specimen should be submitted to confirm the original interpretation.

III

TABLE 3-46 Classification of Anemia

RETICULOCYTE COUNT	MICROCYTIC ANEMIA	NORMOCYTIC ANEMIA	MACROCYTIC ANEMIA
Low	Iron deficiency	Chronic disease	Folate deficiency
	Lead poisoning	Red blood cell aplasia (TEC, infection, drug induced)	Vitamin B_{12} deficiency
	Chronic disease		Aplastic anemia
		Malignancy	
	Aluminum toxicity		Congenital bone marrow dysfunction (Diamond-Blackfan or Fanconi syndromes)
		Juvenile rheumatoid arthritis	
	Copper deficiency		
		Endocrinopathies	Drug induced
	Protein malnutrition		
		Renal failure	Trisomy 21
			Hypothyroidism
Normal	Thalassemia trait	Acute bleeding	—
	Sideroblastic anemia	Hypersplenism	
		Dyserythropoietic anemia II	
High	Thalassemia syndromes	Antibody-mediated hemolysis	Dyserythropoietic anemia I, III
	Hemoglobin C disorders	Hypersplenism	Active hemolysis
		Microangiopathy (HUS, TTP, DIC, Kasabach-Merritt)	
		Membranopathies (spherocytosis, elliptocytosis)	
		Enzyme disorders (G6PD, pyruvate kinase)	
		Hemoglobinopathies	

From Oski FA: Personal communication. In Ebel BE, Raffini L: Hematology. In Siberry GK, Iannone R (eds): *The Harriet Lane handbook: a manual for pediatric house officers,* ed 15, St Louis, 2000, Mosby.

DIC, Disseminated intravascular coagulation; *G6PD,* glucose-6-phosphate dehydrogenase; *HUS,* hemolytic uremic syndrome; *TEC,* transient erythroblastopenia of childhood; *TTP,* thrombotic thrombocytopenic purpura.

TABLE 3-47 **Common Causes of Microcytic Anemia**

	IRON DEFICIENCY	β-THALASSEMIA TRAIT	CHRONIC INFLAMMATION
Reticulocyte count	Low	Normal to ↑	Normal
RDW	↑	↓	Normal
Ferritin	↓	Normal to ↑	Normal to ↑
FEP	↑	Normal	↑
Iron	↓	Normal	↓
TIBC	↑	Normal	↓
Electrophoresis	Normal	↑ HbA$_2$	Normal
ESR	Normal	Normal	↑
Smear	Hypochromic, target cells, microcytic, fine basophilic stippling	Normochromic, microcytic, coarse basophilic stippling	Variable

From Ebel BE, Raffini L: Hematology. In Siberry GK, Iannone R (eds): *The Harriet Lane handbook: a manual for pediatric house officers,* ed 15, St Louis, 2000, Mosby.
ESR, Erythrocyte sedimentation rate; *FEP,* free erythrocyte protoporphrin; *Hb,* hemoglobin; *RDW,* red cell distribution width; *TIBC,* total iron-binding capacity.

III

TABLE 3-48 **Evaluation of Liver Function Tests**

ENZYME	SOURCE	INCREASED	DECREASED	COMMENTS
AST/ALT	Liver Heart Skeletal muscle Pancreas Red blood cells Kidney	Hepatocellular injury Rhabdomyolosis Muscular dystrophy Hemolysis Liver cancer	Vitamin B$_6$ deficiency Uremia	ALT more specific than AST for liver AST > ALT in hemolysis AST/ALT >2 in 90% of alcohol disorders in adults
Alkaline phosphatase	Liver Osteoblasts Small intestine Kidney Placenta	Hepatocellular injury Bone growth, disease, trauma Pregnancy Familial	Low phosphate Wilson's disease Zinc deficiency Hypothyroidism Pernicious anemia	Highest in cholestatic conditions Must be differentiated from bone source
GGT	Bile ducts Renal tubules Pancreas Small intestine Brain	Cholestasis Newborn period Induced by drugs	Estrogen therapy Artificially low in hyperbilirubinemia	Not found in bone Increased in 90% primary liver disease Biliary obstruction Intrahepatic cholestasis Induced by alcohol Specific for hepatobiliary disease in nonpregnant patient
5'-NT	Liver cell membrane Intestine Brain Heart Pancreas	Cholestasis		Specific for hepatobiliary disease in nonpregnant patient
NH$_3$	Bowel Bacteria Protein metabolism	Hepatic disease secondary to urea cycle dysfunction Hemodialysis Valproic acid treatment Urea cycle enzyme deficiency Organic acidemia and carnitine deficiency		Converted to urea in liver

From Gleason BK: Gastroenterology. In Siberry GK, Iannone R (eds): *The Harriet Lane handbook: a manual for pediatric house officers*, ed 15, St Louis, 2000, Mosby.
Alk phos, Alkaline phosphatase; *AST/ALT*, aspartate aminotransferase/alanine aminotransferase; *GGT*, γ-glutamyl transpeptidase; *5'-NT*, 5'-nucleotidase.

Section 13
SELECTED TESTS

■ FETAL HEMOGLOBIN (APT TEST)*

1. **Purpose:** To differentiate fetal blood from swallowed maternal blood.
2. **Method:** Mix specimen with an equal quantity of tap water and centrifuge or filter. Add 1 part of 0.25 mMol/L (1%) NaOH to 5 parts of supernatant.
   Note: Specimen must be bloody, and supernatant must be pink for proper interpretation.
3. **Interpretation:** A pink color persisting over 2 minutes indicates fetal hemoglobin. Transition from pink to yellow within 2 minutes indicates adult hemoglobin.

*From Gleason BK: Gastroenterology. In Siberry GK, Iannone R (eds): *The Harriet Lane handbook: a manual for pediatric house officers,* ed 15, St Louis, 2000, Mosby.

III

■ BEDSIDE COLD AGGLUTININ TEST

- One milliliter of the patient's blood is drawn into a tube containing anticoagulant (the tube used for prothrombin determinations is best).
- Before cooling, examination of the tube shows a smooth coating of the tube by red cells.
- The blood is cooled to 4° C by placing it in a standard refrigerator.
- After 3 to 4 minutes, the tube is examined for evidence of macroscopic agglutination as the tube is rolled.
- The tube is then rewarmed to 37° C in an incubator, or by exposure to body heat, and the agglutination disappears.
- A positive result correlates with a laboratory titer of 1:64 or greater.

■ OSMOTIC FRAGILITY
Methodology
The osmotic fragility test assesses the presence or absence of spherocytes and roughly gauges their quantity in the red cell population. Increasing proportions of red blood cells lyse upon exposure to increasingly hypoosmotic saline solutions.

The test does not distinguish between spherocytes in hereditary spherocytosis and in acquired autoimmune hemolytic anemia; the test only indicates that a proportion of the red cells have decreased surface:volume ratios and are more susceptible to lysis in hypoosmotic solutions. Cells with increased surface:volume ratios, such as occur in thalassemias and iron deficiency, may also show decreased osmotic fragility.

Clinical Significance
Erythrocyte osmotic fragility is most often requested in the workup of possible cases of hereditary spherocytosis.

REFERENCES
1. Elghetany MT, Davey FR: Erythrocytic disorders. In Henry JB (ed): *Clinical diagnosis and management by laboratory methods,* ed 19, Philadelphia, 1996, WB Saunders.
2. Kjeldsberg C et al: *Practical diagnosis of hematologic disorders,* ed 3, Chicago, 2000, ASCP Press.

III

■ **SCHILLING TEST**

Why the Schilling Test Is Performed*

The Schilling test is performed to evaluate vitamin B_{12} absorption. Ingested vitamin B_{12} combines with intrinsic factor (produced in the stomach) and is absorbed in the distal ileum.

How the Schilling Test Is Performed

1. The patient may fast (except for water) for 8 hours before starting the test, then he or she may eat normally.
2. An intramuscular injection of nonradioactive vitamin B_{12} is given to bind available vitamin B_{12} receptor sites. This facilitates rapid excretion of radioactive vitamin B_{12}, if it is absorbed, because there are no places in the body for it to adhere.
3. Urinary B_{12} levels are measured after oral ingestion of a small amount of radioactive vitamin B_{12}.
    a. Either the one-stage Schilling test (without intrinsic factor) or the two-stage Schilling test (with intrinsic factor) may be used.
    b. A 24-hour urine sample is needed.

Normal Values

Excretion of 8% to 40% of the radioactive vitamin B_{12} within 24 hours is normal.

---

*From *Mosby's medical encyclopedia,* St Louis, 1998, Mosby.

Interfering Factors

• Renal insufficiency (inadequate kidney function)
• Hypothyroidism
• Laxatives (may decrease the rate of absorption)

What Abnormal Results Mean

Pernicious anemia results when absorption of vitamin B_{12} is inadequate. This may be caused by malabsorption, intestinal inflammation, a deficiency of vitamin B_{12} in the diet, or a deficiency of intrinsic factor.

Abnormal one- and two-stage Schilling tests may indicate the following:

• Biliary disease
• Celiac disease (sprue)
• Hypothyroidism
• Liver disease

Lower-than-normal amounts of vitamin B_{12} absorption may indicate the following:

• Biliary disease, resulting in malabsorption (inadequate absorption of nutrients from the intestinal tract)
• Intestinal malabsorption (e.g., related to sprue or celiac disease)
• Liver disease (causing malabsorption)
• Pernicious anemia

Additional conditions under which the test may be performed include the following:

• Anemia of B_{12} deficiency
• Blind loop syndrome
• Megaloblastic anemia

Section 14
TOPICAL STEROIDS

TABLE 3-49 **Topical Steroid Potency Ranking**

These commonly used topical steroids are listed by potency group. With Group I as the superpotent category, in descendind order, Group VII is the least potent. There is no significant difference between agents *within* Groups II through VII (compounds are simply listed alphabetically). Within Group I, however, Temovate and Ultravate are more potent than the others.

GROUP	BRAND NAME	GENERIC NAME	GENERIC EQUIVALENT ?	SIZES (g; unless noted)
I	Temovate cream 0.05%	Clobetasol proprionate	Yes	15, 30, 45, 60
	Temovate ointment 0.05%			15, 30, 45, 60
	Ultravate cream 0.05%	Halobetasol proprionate	No	15, 50
	Ultravate ointment 0.05%			15, 50
	Diprolene ointment 0.05%	Betamethasone dipropionate	Yes	15, 45
	Psorcon ointment 0.05%	Diflorasone diacetate	Yes	15, 30, 60
II	Cyclocort ointment 0.1%	Amicinonide	No	15, 30, 60
	Diprolene AF cream	Betamethasone dipropionate	Yes	15, 50
	Elocon ointment 0.1%	Mometasone furoate	No	15, 45
III	Aristocort A ointment 0.1%	Triamcinolone acetonide	Yes	15, 60
	Cutivate ointment 0.005%	Fluticasone propionate	No	15, 30, 60
	Cyclocort cream 0.1%	Amicinonide	No	15, 30, 60
	Cyclocort lotion 0.1%			20, 60 ml
IV	Elocon cream 0.1%	Mometasone furoate	No	15, 45
	Elocon lotion 0.1%			30, 60 ml
	Synalar ointment 0.025%	Flucinolone acetonide	Yes	15, 60
	Westcort ointment 0.2%	Hydrocortisone valerate	Yes	15, 45, 60, 120
V	Cordran cream 0.05%	Flurandrenolide	No	15, 30, 60
	Cutivate cream 0.05%	Fluticasone propionate	No	15, 30, 60
	Locoid Lipocream 0.1%	Hydrocortisone butyrate	No	15, 45
	Locoid cream 0.1%	Hydrocortisone butyrate	No	15, 45
	Locoid ointment 0.1%			15, 45
	Locoid solution 0.1%			20, 60 ml
	Synalar cream 0.025%	Flucinolone acetonide	Yes	15, 60
	Westcort cream 0.2%	Hydrocortisone valerate	Yes	15, 45, 60
VI	Aclovate cream 0.05%	Aclometasone dipropionate	No	15, 45, 60
	Aclovate ointment 0.05%			15, 45, 60
	Synalar cream 0.01%	Flucinolone acetonide	Yes	15, 60
	Synalar solution 0.01%			20, 60 ml
	Desowen cream 0.05%	Desonide	Yes	15, 60
	Desowen lotion 0.05%		No	59, 118 ml
VII	Pramosone cream 1.0%	Hydrocortisone acetate and	No	30, 60
	Pramosone cream 2.5%	Pramoxine HCl 1%		30, 60
	Pramosone lotion 1.0%			2, 4, 8 oz
	Pramosone lotion 2.5%			2, 4 oz
	Pramosone ointment 1.0%			30
	Pramosone ointment 2.5%			30
	Hytone cream 2.5%	Hydrocortisone	Yes	30, 60
	Hytone lotion 2.5%			60 ml
	Hytone ointment 2.5%			30

. . . and others containing dexamethasone, flumetholone, prednisolone, methylprednisolone

Courtesy Ferndale Laboratories, Ferndale, Michigan, February 2001.

III

INDEX

Page numbers followed by f indicate figures; t, tables.